CARE OF THE HIGH-RISK NEONATE

CARE OF THE HIGH-RISK NEONATE

Fifth Edition

Marshall H. Klaus, MD
Adjunct Professor of Pediatrics
University of California, San Francisco
San Francisco, California

Avroy A. Fanaroff, MB (Rand), FRCPE
Eliza Henry Barnes Chair in Neonatology
Professor of Pediatrics and Neonatology in
    Reproductive Biology
Case Western Reserve University School of Medicine
Co-Director, Division of Neonatology
Rainbow Babies and Children's Hospital of University
    Hospitals of Cleveland
Cleveland, Ohio

SAUNDERS
An Imprint of Elsevier

SAUNDERS
An Imprint of Elsevier
The Curtis Center
Independence Square West
Philadelphia, PA 19106

Library of Congress Cataloging-in-Publication Data

Care of the high-risk neonate / Marshall H. Klaus, Avroy A. Fanaroff—5th ed.

p.   cm.

ISBN 0–7216–7729–0

I. Neonatal intensive care.   I. Fanaroff, Avroy A.   II. Title.

RJ253.5. K55 2001   618.92′01—dc21   00-058343

Acquisitions Editor: Dolores Meloni
Project Manager: Agnes Hunt Byrne
Production Manager: Norman Stellander
Illustration Specialist: John Needles

CARE OF THE HIGH-RISK NEONATE   ISBN 0–7216–7729–0

Last digit is the print number: 9   8   7   6   5   4   3

This book is dedicated to all students of perinatology, our patients and their parents, and to Phyllis, Susan, Alisa, and Sarah Klaus; David, Laura, Michael and Abigail Klaus; Laura, David, Emily, Sharon, and Benjamin Abada; Roslyn, Jonathan, and Amanda Fanaroff; Jodi, Peter, Austin, and Morgan Tucker.

CONTRIBUTORS

Ellis D. Avner, MD
Professor of Pediatrics, Case Western Reserve
University School of Medicine; Pediatrician-in-
Chief, Rainbow Babies and Children's Hospital of
University Hospitals of Cleveland, Cleveland, Ohio
The Kidney

Jill E. Baley, MD
Associate Professor of Pediatrics, Case Western
Reserve University School of Medicine; Medical
Director, NICU Step-Down Unit, Rainbow Babies
and Children's Hospital of University Hospitals of
Cleveland, Cleveland, Ohio
Neonatal Infections

Eduardo Bancalari, MD
Professor of Pediatrics, Director, Division of
Neonatology, University of Miami School of
Medicine, Miami, Florida
Respiratory Problems

Michael M. Brook, MD
Associate Professor of Clinical Pediatrics,
University of California, San Francisco, School of
Medicine, San Francisco, California
The Heart

Waldemar A. Carlo, MD
Dixson Professor of Pediatrics, University of
Alabama at Birmingham; Director, Division of
Neonatology; Director of Newborn Nurseries,
University Hospital, The Children's Hospital of
Alabama, Birmingham, Alabama
Assisted Ventilation

D. Wade Clapp, MD
Associate Professor of Pediatrics and Microbiology
and Immunology, Indiana University School of
Medicine, Indianapolis, Indiana
Hematologic Problems

Ira D. Davis, MD, MS
Associate Professor, Case Western Reserve
University School of Medicine; Director of
Pediatric Nephrology, Rainbow Babies and
Children's Hospital of University Hospitals of
Cleveland, Cleveland, Ohio
The Kidney

Arthur E. D'Harlingue, MD
Division of Neonatology, Children's Hospital,
Oakland, California
*Recognition, Stabilization, and Transport of the
High-Risk Newborn*

David J. Durand, MD
Division of Neonatology, Children's Hospital,
Oakland, California
*Recognition, Stabilization, and Transport of the
High-Risk Newborn*

Avroy A. Fanaroff, MB (Rand), FRCPE
Eliza Henry Barnes Chair in Neonatology; Professor
of Pediatrics, Case Western Reserve University
School of Medicine; Co-Director, Division of
Neonatology, Rainbow Babies and Children's
Hospital of University Hospitals of Cleveland,
Cleveland, Ohio
*Antenatal and Intrapartum Care of the High-Risk
Infant; The Physical Environment; Nutrition and
Selected Disorders of the Gastrointestinal Tract:
Part Two, Selected Disorders of the Gastrointestinal
Tract and Part Three, Necrotizing Enterocolitis*

Johanna Goldfarb, MD
Staff, Cleveland Clinic Foundation; Chief, Section
of Pediatric Infectious Diseases, Cleveland Clinic
Foundation, Cleveland, Ohio
Neonatal Infections

Maureen Hack, MB, ChB
Professor of Pediatrics and Reproductive Biology,
Case Western Reserve University School of
Medicine; Division of Neonatology, Rainbow
Babies and Children's Hospital of University
Hospitals of Cleveland, Cleveland, Ohio
The Outcome of Neonatal Intensive Care

Michael A. Heymann, MD
Professor of Pediatrics Emeritus, Cardiovascular
Research Institute Investigator Emeritus, University
of California, San Francisco, School of Medicine,
San Francisco, California
The Heart

Leta Houston Hickey, RN, MSN, cNNP
Nurse Practitioner, Division of Neonatology,
Rainbow Babies and Children's Hospital of
University Hospitals of Cleveland, Cleveland, Ohio
Drug Compatibility

Satish C. Kalhan, MBBS, FRCP
Professor, Departments of Pediatrics and
Reproductive Biology; Director, Robert Schwartz
MD Center for Metabolism and Nutrition, Case
Western Reserve University School of Medicine;
Attending Neonatologist, MetroHealth Medical
Center, Cleveland, Ohio
*Nutrition and Selected Disorders of the
Gastrointestinal Tract: Part One, Nutrition for the
High-Risk Infant*

William Keenan, MD
Professor of Pediatrics and Obstetrics and
Gynecology, Saint Louis University School of
Medicine; Director, Neonatal-Perinatal Medicine,
Cardinal Glennon Children's Hospital, St. Louis,
Missouri
Resuscitation of the Newborn Infant

John H. Kennell, MD
Professor of Pediatrics, Case Western Reserve
University School of Medicine; Pediatrician,
Division of Behavioral Pediatrics, Rainbow Babies
and Children's Hospital of University Hospitals of
Cleveland, Cleveland, Ohio
Care of the Parents

**Robert Kiwi, MD, MB, ChB, FRCOG,
FACOG**
Associate Professor of Reproductive Biology, Case
Western Reserve University School of Medicine,
Cleveland, Ohio
*Antenatal and Intrapartum Care of the High-Risk
Infant*

Marshall H. Klaus, MD
Adjunct Professor of Pediatrics, University of
California, San Francisco, California
The Physical Environment; Care of the Parents

Robert M. Kliegman, MD
Professor and Chair, Department of Pediatrics,
Medical College of Wisconsin; Pediatrician-in-
Chief, Pamela and Leslie Muma Chair in
Pediatrics, Children's Hospital of Wisconsin,
Milwaukee, Wisconsin
*Nutrition and Selected Disorders of the
Gastrointestinal Tract: Part Three, Necrotizing
Enterocolitis; Problems in Metabolic Adaptation:
Glucose, Calcium, and Magnesium*

Linda Lefrak, RN, MS
Neonatal Clinical Nurse Specialist, Children's
Hospital, Oakland, California
*Nursing Practice in the Neonatal Intensive Care
Unit*

Carolyn Houska Lund, RN, MS, FAAN
Adjunct Professor, School of Nursing, University of
California, San Francisco; Neonatal Clinical Nurse
Specialist, ECMO Coordinator, Intensive Care
Nursery, Children's Hospital, Oakland, California
*Nursing Practice in the Neonatal Intensive Care
Unit*

M. Jeffrey Maisels, MB, BCh
Clinical Professor of Pediatrics, Wayne State
University School of Medicine, Detroit; Clinical
Professor of Pediatrics and Communicable
Diseases, University of Michigan Medical School,
Ann Arbor; Chairman, Department of Pediatrics,
William Beaumont Hospital, Royal Oak, Michigan
Neonatal Hyperbilirubinemia

Richard J. Martin, MB, FRACP
Professor of Pediatrics, Case Western Reserve
University School of Medicine; Director, Division
of Neonatology, Rainbow Babies and Children's
Hospital of University Hospitals of Cleveland,
Cleveland, Ohio
Respiratory Problems

Lawrence J. Nelson, PhD, JD
Lecturer, Santa Clara University; Faculty Scholar,
Markkula Center for Applied Ethics, Santa Clara
University, Santa Clara, California
Ethical Issues in the Perinatal Period

Susan Niermeyer, MD
Associate Professor of Pediatrics, University of
Colorado School of Medicine; Director of Neonatal
Education, The Children's Hospital, Denver,
Colorado
Resuscitation of the Newborn Infant

Roderic H. Phibbs, MD
Professor of Pediatrics, University of California,
San Francisco, School of Medicine, San Francisco,
California
Hematologic Problems

William B. Pittard, III, MD, MPH
Vice Chairman, Department of Pediatrics; Professor
of Pediatrics, Division of Pediatrics and
Epidemiology and Health Systems Research,
Medical University of South Carolina, Charleston,
South Carolina
*Classification and Physical Examination of the
Newborn Infant*

Pamela T. Price, PhD, RD, CNSD
Postdoctoral Research Fellow, USDA/ARS
Children's Nutrition Research Center, Department
of Pediatrics, Baylor College of Medicine, Houston,
Texas
*Nutrition and Selected Disorders of the
Gastrointestinal Tract: Part One, Nutrition for the
High-Risk Infant*

Michael D. Reed, PharmD, FCCP, FCP
Professor of Pediatrics, Department of Pediatrics,
Case Western Reserve University School of
Medicine; Director, Pediatric Clinical
Pharmacology and Toxicology, Division of
Pediatric Pharmacology and Critical Care, Rainbow
Babies and Children's Hospital of University
Hospitals of Cleveland, Cleveland, Ohio
Drug Dosing Table

Ricardo J. Rodriguez, MD
Assistant Professor of Pediatrics, Case Western
Reserve University School of Medicine; University
Hospitals of Cleveland, Cleveland, Ohio
*Drugs Used for Emergency and Cardiac Indications
in Newborns; Drug Dosing Table; Umbilical Vessel
Catheterization*

Mark S. Scher, MD
Professor of Pediatrics and Neurology, Case
Western Reserve University School of Medicine;
Director, Pediatric Neurology, Director, Fetal and
Neonatal Neurology, Rainbow Babies and
Children's Hospital of University Hospitals of
Cleveland, Cleveland, Ohio
Brain Disorders of the Fetus and Neonate

Dinesh M. Shah, MD
Associate Professor of Reproductive Biology, Case
Western Reserve University School of Medicine;
Director, Maternal-Fetal Medicine, University
MacDonald Women's Hospital, Cleveland, Ohio
*Antenatal and Intrapartum Care of the High-Risk
Infant*

Kevin M. Shannon, MD
Professor of Pediatrics, University of California,
San Francisco, School of Medicine, San Francisco,
California
Hematologic Problems

Ilene R. S. Sosenko, MD
Professor of Pediatrics, Division of Neonatology,
University of Miami School of Medicine, Miami,
Florida
Respiratory Problems

W. Michael Southgate, MD
Associate Professor of Pediatrics, Medical
University of South Carolina; Medical Director,
Neonatal Intensive Care Unit, Children's Hospital
of the Medical University of South Carolina,
Charleston, South Carolina
*Classification and Physical Examination of the
Newborn Infant*

David F. Teitel, MD
Professor of Pediatrics, University of California,
San Francisco, School of Medicine, San Francisco,
California
The Heart

Andrew P. Ten Eick, PharmD
Clinical Assistant Professor, College of Pharmacy,
University of Oklahoma; Children's Hospital of
Oklahoma, Oklahoma City, Oklahoma
Drug Dosing Table

Beth A. Vogt, MD
Assistant Professor of Pediatrics, Case Western
Reserve University School of Medicine; Director of
Dialysis Services, Rainbow Babies and Children's
Hospital of University Hospitals of Cleveland,
Cleveland, Ohio
The Kidney

Deanne Wilson-Costello, MD
Assistant Professor of Pediatrics, Case Western
Reserve University School of Medicine; University
Hospitals of Cleveland, Cleveland, Ohio
*Nutrition and Selected Disorders of the
Gastrointestinal Tract: Part Three, Necrotizing
Enterocolitis*

COMMENTERS

Cynthia F. Bearer, MD, PhD
Assistant Professor of Pediatrics and
Neurosciences, Division of Neonatology, Case
Western Reserve University School of Medicine;
Co-Director, Neonatology Training Program,
Rainbow Babies and Children's Hospital of
University Hospitals of Cleveland, Cleveland, Ohio

Denise Campbell, PhD
Assistant Professor of Medicine, Department of
Community Health, University of Calgary, Calgary,
Alberta, Canada

Waldemar A. Carlo, MD
Dixson Professor of Pediatrics, University of
Alabama at Birmingham; Director, Division of
Neonatology; Director of Newborn Nurseries,
University Hospital, The Children's Hospital of
Alabama, Birmingham, Alabama

Maureen Hack, MB, ChB
Professor of Pediatrics and Reproductive Biology,
Division of Neonatology, Case Western Reserve
University School of Medicine; Director, High-Risk
Follow-up, Rainbow Babies and Children's
Hospital of University Hospitals of Cleveland,
Cleveland, Ohio

John Kattwinkel, MD
Professor of Pediatrics, University of Virginia
School of Medicine; Chief of Neonatology,
University of Virginia Health Sciences Center,
Charlottesville, Virginia

Albert Okken, MD
Professor of Pediatrics, Wilhemina Children's
Hospital, University Medical Center, Utrecht, The
Netherlands

Edward J. Quilligan, MD
Professor of Obstetrics and Gynecology (Emeritus),
University of California, Irvine, College of
Medicine, Irvine, California

Mildred T. Stahlman, MD
Professor of Pediatrics (Emeritus), Vanderbilt
University School of Medicine, Nashville,
Tennessee

Norman S. Talner, MD
Professor of Pediatrics, Political Professor of
Pediatrics (Cardiology), Duke University School of
Medicine, Duke University Medical Center,
Durham, North Carolina

Reginald Tsang, MB, BS
Professor of Pediatrics and Obstetrics and
Gynecology, University of Cincinnati College of
Medicine and Children's Research Foundation,
Cincinnati, Ohio

Roberta G. Williams, MD
Professor and Chair, Department of Pediatrics,
Keck School of Medicine, University of Southern
California, Los Angeles; Vice President of
Pediatrics and Academic Affairs, The Children's
Hospital, Los Angeles, California

◆ PREFACE

Remarkably it has been 27 years since the first edition of *Care of the High-Risk Neonate* was published. Great strides have been taken in the care of high-risk infants, and the outcome for the most complex neonatal disorders is more favorable. Survival rates for even the most immature infants have improved enormously; however, the severe morbidity and long-term neurodevelopmental handicaps among this population remain a major concern. The foundations for the practice of evidence-based neonatology have been laid by a large number of multicenter, randomized trials. Meta-analyses and summation of these trials in the Cochrane Database and other contemporaneous publications assist the practitioners in formulating their care pathways and help ensure the best possible outcomes.

To incorporate the major advances that have occurred since the fourth edition as well as to view the field of neonatal-perinatal medicine in a critical fashion, all the chapters of this fifth edition have undergone significant revision. We are pleased to once again welcome several new contributors. One third of the chapters have been rewritten by new contributors who have diligently adhered to the basic format but presented a host of new ideas, fresh approaches, and differing views.

New information is presented in the form of text, critical comments, case problems, or simple questions. Overall, our objective has remained the same: to stimulate the readers and to provide a sound physiologic and experimental basis for perinatal care.

We have been most gratified to learn that this book continues to serve as a guide and companion for neonatal health care providers in many parts of the world. Our task of completing this fifth edition has been most pleasurable because of the expert editorial assistance provided by Bonnie Siner and Dolores Meloni at W.B. Saunders. We are deeply indebted to them as well as to the many contributors and commenters.

MARSHALL H. KLAUS
AVROY A. FANAROFF

CONTENTS

Antenatal and Intrapartum Care of the High-Risk Infant

Avroy A. Fanaroff
Robert Kiwi
Dinesh M. Shah

> Everything ought to be done to ensure that an infant be born at term, well developed, and in a healthy condition. But in spite of every care, infants are born prematurely.
>
> *Pierre Budin,* The Nursling

Parallel to the significant improvements in care of the premature and sick neonate, extensive technology concerned with the evaluation and supervision of the high-risk fetus has developed.[35, 150, 153, 180] Initially stimulated in the 1960s by the pioneering work with amniotic fluid analysis in Rh-isoimmunized pregnancy, this technology has evolved and expanded at a rapid rate. Hormonal assessments of fetoplacental function; fetal scalp blood determinations of fetal homeostasis, electronic monitoring of the fetal heart rate (FHR) during and before labor; biochemical estimations of fetal pulmonary maturity; ultrasonic measurements of fetal head size, fetal growth, and fetal activity; and detailed ultrasonic evaluation of fetal anatomy have all become commonplace procedures.[6, 8, 57]

The inner sanctum of the fetus has been penetrated and it has become commonplace to detect many genetic and antenatal abnormalities before delivery. Visualization of the fetus by fetoscopy and ultrasonic recording of fetal respiration, tone, and state, together with monitoring of fetal behavioral responses are an integral part of antepartum care. Detailed studies of fetal cardiac and renal anatomy and function present valuable information to the perinatal team.[52, 53] The capabilities of accurate diagnosis and treatment of fetal disorders have expanded rapidly so that fetal blood sampling, major surgical interventions such as repair of a diaphragmatic hernia, and excision of CCAM (congenital cystic adenomatoid malformation) or even correction of neural tube defects may be accomplished without interrupting the pregnancy.[55, 69, 71] Furthermore,

intravascular transfusions for Rh isoimmune fetal anemia or other causes of reversible fetal anemia as well as medical treatment of fetal arrhythmias are possible.

EDITORIAL COMMENT: Minimally invasive fetal surgery appears to constitute a feasible approach to nonlethal fetal malformations that result in progressive and disabling organ damage. The concept that performing in utero surgery could protect the exposed but initially well-developed and uninjured spinal cord, prevent secondary neural injury, and preserve neural function in the human fetus with myelomeningocele has become a reality.

◆ ———

Meuli M, Meuli-Simmen C, Hutchins GM, et al: The spinal cord lesion in human fetuses with myelomeningocele: implications for fetal surgery. J Pediatr Surg 32:448–452, 1997.
Tulipan N, Hernanz-Schulman M, Bruner JP: Reduced hindbrain herniation after intrauterine myelomeningocele repair: A report of four cases. Pediatr Neurosurg 29:274–278, 1998.

These and other sophisticated approaches have rapidly become routine components of clinical care. However, many of these procedures are expensive and need quality laboratory support, and their results are not always easy to interpret. Advanced training and accreditation for obstetric perinatologists have followed the introduction of new technology, but in this, as in other allied areas, the supply of personnel remains limited. Furthermore, epidemiologic studies have indicated that only a small percentage of all pregnant women manifest risk features that necessitate these intensive interventions. Practicalities demand that they be applied in an appropriately effective fashion because underutilized personnel and facilities will not be tolerated by a society increasingly concerned with maximizing cost-benefit ratios and reducing costs.

COMMENT: Nor should overutilization be tolerated. Although perinatal technologies and services are available, their use must be based on a reasonable amount of information about risks, benefits, and alternatives. Health care providers must be vigilant to avoid indiscriminate use of tests and facilities since they may result in more harm than benefits.

Denise Campbell

Nevertheless, in many centers of excellence, the appropriate utilization of the available technology appears to have contributed to marked reductions of perinatal mortality even among groups of very high-risk patients.[135, 191] It is hoped that wider and more uniform application of these newer concepts of care after controlled studies evaluating their benefits may, in part, offer a solution to the longstanding problem of unacceptably high perinatal mortality and morbidity in the United States. Overall, perinatal mortality rates have decreased dramatically, such that most centers are reporting a rate of 9 in 1000 live births in the surfactant era.[167, 191] Nonetheless, urgent need to tackle the problem of prematurity to reduce these rates further persists. The recent declines in mortality rates have been attributed to improved neonatal care, with no evidence to date of any impact on the prematurity rate. Neonataologists and perinatologists cannot claim all the credit for reductions in neonatal mortality. Changes in the birth weight and gestational age makeup of the newborn population accounted for 34% of the reduction in neonatal mortality rates in North Carolina from 1968 to 1977. Doing away with poverty would have an even greater effect in reducing the prematurity rate and the number of neonatal deaths.

Because many of the determinants of neonatal outcome relate directly to intrauterine and intrapartal events, continued improvement in perinatal care is contingent on a team approach to high-risk pregnancies. Obstetricians, midwives, nurses, pediatricians, and family physicians collaboratively must develop comprehensive protocols of management that will ensure the best results for the maximum number of mothers and infants.

Maximizing the benefits of the available

technology requires regionalization—specifically, the development of a network of providers of perinatal care within a defined geographic area to implement the following objectives: (1) the identification of high-risk pregnancies early in the perinatal period, (2) the further identification of high-risk factors within the intrapartum period, (3) the development of interhospital agreements on criteria for transfer of mothers and infants within the network, (4) the development of support systems of consultation, laboratory services, education, and transportation within a region, and (5) the development of a record-keeping system that will allow adequate monitoring of the performance of the entire program.[100, 156]

EDITORIAL COMMENT: Paneth et al[139] noted that the mortality rate for full-term, appropriate size for gestational age infants in New York was not influenced by hospital of birth. However, the risk for death increased 24% if preterm infants were delivered at level I or II centers as compared with level III units. These small infants constituted only 12% of the births but accounted for 70% of the deaths. Extrapolation of these data to the rest of the United States makes a compelling case for delivery of preterm infants at tertiary centers.

Phibbs et al[145] examined the effects of neonatal intensive care unit (NICU) patient volume and the level of NICU care available at the hospital of birth on neonatal mortality for all nonfederal hospitals in California with maternity services. Hospitals were classified by the level of NICU care available (no NICU: level I; intermediate NICU: level II; expanded intermediate NICU: level II+: tertiary NICU: level III) and by the average patient census in the NICU. They observed that patient volume and level of NICU care at the hospital of birth both had significant effects on mortality. Compared with hospitals without an NICU, infants born in a hospital with a level III NICU with an average NICU census of at least 15 patients per day had the lowest risk-adjusted neonatal mortality rate. Furthermore, despite the differences in outcomes, costs for the birth of infants born at hospitals with large level III NICUs were not more than those for infants born at other hospitals with NICUs. The original principles of regionalization hold true despite efforts of managed care organizations to disrupt the process.

◆ IDENTIFYING THE PATIENT AT RISK

Early identification of the high-risk population associated with the largest proportion of untoward perinatal outcomes has become a priority for the obstetric care delivery system. Many of the principal determinants of perinatal morbidity and mortality have been delineated. Included among these are maternal age, race, socioeconomic status, nutrition, past obstetric history, associated medical illness, and current pregnancy problems.

Careful analysis indicates that these determinants of morbidity and mortality are composed of historical factors existing before pregnancy as well as factors and events associated directly with pregnancy. Together these have provided the basis for the development of several assessment techniques capable of distinguishing most of the high-risk patients from the low-risk patients before delivery.

In 1969, Nesbitt and Aubry[133] indicated that 29% of pregnant women could objectively be identified as being at increased risk. The outcome of pregnancy among these women was judged unsatisfactory by the occurrence of premature birth, low-birthweight, perinatal mortality, neonatal depression, and respiratory distress syndrome at a rate twice that of the normal population. In Canada, similar results were obtained on more diverse groups of pregnant women by Goodwin et al.[60] Hobel et al[74] described a risk assessment system that included intrapartum as well as prenatal risk factors and identified four subgroups of patients with ascending rates of perinatal mortality and neonatal morbidity. In a prospective study of a low socioeconomic population, 18% of pregnant women were categorized as being at high risk both prenatally and intrapartally, and it was from this group that the poorest outcomes were obtained.

In many communities, perinatal teams use uniform record keeping and risk identification across broad populations of pregnant women. In this manner it is hoped to better define high-risk indicators among diverse socioeconomic groups.

Prematurity remains the most significant perinatal problem, accounting for 75% of all perinatal deaths. In the United States, the prematurity rate (~10%) has remained remarkably constant. In San Francisco, Creasy et al,[34] in an effort to identify and intervene in those cases in which patients are at greatest risk of delivering prematurely, developed an evaluation (scoring) system that takes into account (1) the patient's socioeconomic status, (2) her past history, (3) her daily habits, and (4) current pregnancy events. The patients were evaluated at their first office visit and again between 25 and 28 weeks' gestation. Those with a score of 10 were classified as being at high risk for preterm delivery (Table 1–1).

Of high-risk patients, 30% delivered prematurely, in contrast to only 2.5% among the low-risk group. In the second phase of the study, those identified as high risk were observed closely and instructed to report immediately any signs or symptoms compatible with early onset of labor. Furthermore, the perinatal staff received in-service education emphasizing (1) the need to respond promptly to any subtle signs of preterm labor, (2) the need to admit and observe closely with electronic monitoring those patients with mild signs of early preterm labor or cervical dilation, (3) the need to attempt tocolysis aggressively when premature labor was present, and (4) an awareness of the contraindications and side effects of tocolysis. Institution of these protocols resulted in a decrease in the prematurity rate from 6.75% to 2.4%. Bouyer et al,[17] using a program comprising (1) risk identification via a scoring system, (2) education of women at risk with emphasis on lifestyle and evaluation of uterine contraction and fetal movement, and (3) obligatory rest and a diminished workload for women identified at risk, were able to significantly reduce the prematurity rate in a region of France from 6% to 4% with a marked reduction in deliveries at less than 32 weeks' gestation.

Strategies to improve the outcome of premature babies have focused on antenatal prevention of conditions associated with low-birth-weight, together with intensive education, extensive intrapartum evaluation, and monitoring with sophisticated and aggressive care of the low-birth-weight fetus and infant. Simple measures in antenatal care such as elimination of cigarette smoking, improved nutrition, eradication of genitourinary tract infection, and increased awareness of the hazards of preterm birth have contributed to lower rates of prematurity.

EDITORIAL COMMENT: The goal of tocolytic therapy is to reduce neonatal morbidity and mortality by delaying delivery until 34 weeks of gestation, or at least for 48 hours, to allow time for the therapeutic effects of corticosteroids. Nitroglycerin, a nitric oxide donor, successfully

Table 1–1. Scoring System for Risk of Preterm Delivery

Points*	Socioeconomic Status	Past History	Daily Habits	Current Pregnancy
1	Two children at home Low socioeconomic status	One abortion <1 y since last birth	Works outside home	Unusual fatigue
2	<20 y >40 y Single parent	Two abortions	>10 cigarettes/d	<13 lb gain by 32 wk Albuminuria Hypertension Bacteriuria
3	Very low socioeconomic status <150 cm <45 kg	Three abortions	Heavy work Long, tiring trip	Breech at 32 wk Weight loss of 2 kg Head engaged Febrile illness
4	<18 y	Pyelonephritis		Metrorrhagia after 12 wk of gestation Effacement Dilation Uterine irritability
5		Uterine anomaly Second-trimester abortion Diethylstilbestrol exposure		Placenta previa Hydramnios
10		Premature delivery Repeated second trimester abortion		Twins Abdominal surgery

*Score is computed by addition of number of points given any item. 0–5 = low risk; 6–9 = medium risk; ≥10 = high risk.
Adapted from Creasy R, Gummer B, Liggins G: System for predicting spontaneous preterm birth. Obstet Gynecol 55:692, 1980. Reprinted with permission of the American College of Obstetricians and Gynecologists.

inhibits uterine contractions in sheep and monkeys and is one of the newer agents undergoing evaluation in humans.

These regionally successful programs have not easily been replicated when these principles were applied to a broader population base and consequently have not translated into a successful national strategy. In particular, the scoring systems as outlined herein have not been discriminating enough to identify patients at risk in order to implement an appropriate intervention program.

EDITORIAL COMMENT: The potential benefits and cost savings of reducing the number of premature deliveries assume astronomic proportions. Because there is no single "magic bullet," it is imperative to apply the knowledge gained from large controlled trials and the principles founded on the molecular mechanisms of human parturition. These include avoidance of multifetal pregnancies resulting from iatrogenic excesses of assisted reproduction and appropriate identification and treatment of sexually transmitted and genitourinary infections including bacterial vaginosis and group B streptococcal bacteriuria.[57] By applying such aggregate knowledge to women at risk for preterm birth MacGregor significantly reduced the rate

of prematurity by half with estimated yearly savings of $2.5 million.[106]

The search for other indicators of premature labor or premature rupture of membranes continues with renewed vigor.

◆ EVALUATION OF FETUS AND SUPERVISION OF CARE

Improved physiologic understanding and multiple technologic advancements now provide the obstetrician with tools for objective evaluation of the fetus. In particular, specific information can be sought and obtained relative to fetal anatomy, growth, well-being, and functional maturity, and these data are used to provide a rational approach to clinical management of the high-risk infant before birth. For detailed reviews of the many new physical, hormonal, and biochemical approaches to prenatal and fetal assessments, refer to more comprehensive obstetric texts.[25, 35, 71] This section summarizes the clinical applications of the most widely used techniques as background for a discussion of practical clinical problems.

Monitoring Fetal Growth

It is important to emphasize that no test or laboratory procedure can supplant the data obtained from a careful history and physical examination. Ultimately, the results of all of the newer techniques have to be interpreted in light of the true or presumed gestational age of the fetus. It is, therefore, essential that the initial pregnancy visit be concerned with a thorough documentation of information relative to the regularity of the patient's menstrual cycles, use of oral contraceptive agents, date of last menstrual period, pregnancy test results, and the like. The initial and subsequent physical examinations are then approached with these facts in mind to ascertain whether the uterine size and growth are consistent with the supposed length of gestation. Similarly, the milestones of quickening (16 to 18 weeks) and fetal heart tone auscultation by Doppler ultrasound (12 to 14 weeks) and fetoscope (18 to 22 weeks) are important and need to be systematically recorded. Although most of this information is gathered early in pregnancy, it may not be used until later in gestation when decisions regarding the appropriateness of fetal size and the timing of delivery are contemplated.

Irregular menstrual cycles, use of oral contraceptives around the conception cycle (resulting in delayed ovulation), and discrepancies in either direction of size versus dates or expected gestational age indicate the need for an ultrasound evaluation to determine the fetal gestational age on the basis of biometric parameters. Ultrasound is a technique by which short pulses (2 μs) of high-frequency (approximately 2.5 MHz), low-intensity sound waves are transmitted from a piezoelectric crystal (transducer) through the maternal abdomen to the uterus and the fetus. The echo signals reflected back from tissue interfaces provide a two-dimensional picture of the uterine wall, placenta, amniotic fluid, and fetus. Diagnoses of multiple gestation, fetal structural abnormalities, abnormally implanted placentae, and uterine or placental pathologic conditions can be made by this technique. Serial measurements of the fetus can provide a reliable indicator of fetal growth. Furthermore, ultrasound is extensively used to assess fetal well-being and to study fetal physiology. Some indications for ultrasound are contained in Table 1–2. In many instances,

Table 1–2. Uses of Ultrasound

Confirmation of pregnancy
Determination of
Gestational age
Fetal number and presentation
Placental location (vaginal bleeding)
Fetal anatomy (previous malformations)
Assessment of
Size/date discrepancy
Fetal well-being (biophysical profile—fetal tone, movements, and respiration)
Volume of amniotic fluid (suspected oligohydramnios or polyhydramnios)
Fetal arrhythmias
Fetal anatomy (abnormal alpha-fetoprotein)
Assist with procedures
Amniocentesis
Intrauterine transfusion

ultrasound is performed to comply with the mother's request only.

In the first trimester, the gestational age of the fetus is assessed by a crown-to-rump measurement. After the 13th week of gestation, measurement of the fetal biparietal diameter (BPD) or cephalometry is the most commonly used technique (Fig. 1–1). Before 20 weeks' gestation, this measurement provides a good estimation of gestational age within a range of plus or minus 10 days. After 20 weeks' gestation, the predictability of the measurement is less reliable, so an initial examination should be obtained before this state whenever possible. Such early examination also assists in interpretation of triple screen results as well in detection of major malformations. Follow-up examinations can then be done to ascertain whether fetal growth in utero is proceeding at a normal rate.

COMMENT: Low birth weight, defined as weight of less than 5 pounds, which results from either preterm delivery or intrauterine growth failure, is a universally recognized marker for poor perinatal outcome. The finding by Smith et al[163] that suboptimal growth during the first trimester predicts extreme premature birth and low birth weight at term gestation is not surprising.

Smith reported that, although significantly more infants who had subnormal first trimester growth were of low birth weight, the rate of perinatal death did not differ between those who were smaller than expected during the first trimester compared with those who were normal or larger than expected. Modern perinatal care has practically eliminated deaths of babies at term gestation except in cases of major con-

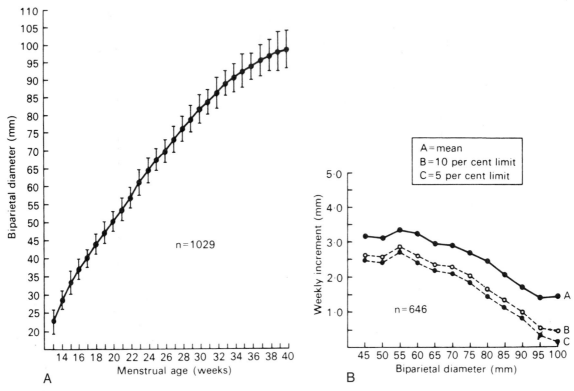

Figure 1–1. *A,* Mean fetal biparietal diameter (mm) ± 2 SD for each week of pregnancy from 13 weeks to term. *B,* Mean growth rate of fetal biparietal diameter with lower tolerance limits related to size of biparietal diameter. (From Campbell S: Fetal growth. In Beard R, Nathanielez P (eds): Fetal Physiology and Medicine: The Basis of Perinatology. Philadelphia: WB Saunders, 1976.)

genital malformations and rare cases of infection and asphyxia. Some maintain that the majority of term low-birth-weight children represent the normal distribution of growth rather than pathology.[27] On follow-up, these children have fairly good outcomes, with the exception of those born following asphyxia or with subnormal head growth and major congenital malformations.[86]

Maureen Hack

When fetal growth is retarded, however, brain sparing may result in an abnormal ratio of growth between the head and the rest of the body. Because the BPD may then remain within normal limits, other measurements are needed to detect the true retardation of growth. Campbell[20] has found that measurement of the ratio between the circumferences of head and abdomen is particularly valuable under these circumstances. During the second trimester of pregnancy, the normal ratio is greater than 1 in favor of the head, but after 36 weeks' gestation, there is a reversal and the abdominal circumference (AC) predominates. In many cases of

growth retardation, this reversal is not seen (Fig. 1–2).

Femur length (FL), which may be less affected by alterations in growth than the head or abdomen, is used to aid in determining gestational age and to identify the fetus with abnormal growth. Serial assessment of growth and deviations from normal, including both macrosomia and growth retardation, helps to identify the fetus at risk during the perinatal period (see Chapter 4). Nonetheless, only approximately 50% of growth-retarded fetuses are identified before delivery. Calculation of estimated fetal weight (EFW) based on various fetal biometric parameters (BPD, head circumference [HC], AC, and FL) plotted against gestational age using various sonographic nomograms is an extremely useful method for serial assessment of fetal growth. Sophisticated computer software to serially plot EFW and provide percentile ranking of a given fetus are in common use at major perinatal centers.

EDITORIAL COMMENT: Guidetti et al[65] evaluated the efficacy of different methods of EFW

Figure 1–2. Head-to-abdomen (H/A) circumference ratio in small-for-dates (SFD) fetuses (i.e., below 5th percentile weight for gestation) and three fetuses with cephalic abnormalities; these are plotted on normal H/A ratio graph showing mean, 95th, and 5th percentile confidence limits. Of the 25 small-for-dates fetuses, 22 had ratios above 95th percentile limit, and two fetuses who died (+) had high ratios. Hydrocephalus *(H)* is associated with very high and microcephaly *(M)* with very low H/A ratios. (From Campbell S: Fetal growth. In Beard R, Nathanielez P (eds): Fetal Physiology and Medicine: The Basis of Perinatology. Philadelphia: WB Saunders, 1976.)

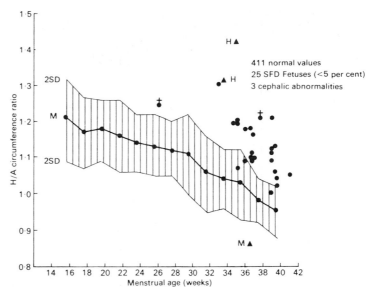

using sonographic measurements of the abdominal circumference, BPD, and FL, either alone or in combination in fetuses with suspected growth retardation. They reported that 75% of the EFWs using all three parameters, performed within 7 days of delivery, were within 110% of the actual birth weight. Estimates of fetal weight incorporating FL correlated best with actual birth weight.

In prospective studies using antenatal ultrasound,[6, 14, 157] no differences were noted in neonatal outcome from pregnancies in which ultrasound was not used. Nonetheless, early ultrasound has resulted in more confident establishment of dates, earlier detection of multiple gestation, and earlier diagnosis and more active intervention for infants with intrauterine growth retardation. Furthermore, no adverse, short-term effects from ultrasound have been noted. More women who had been screened with ultrasound required antenatal hospitalization.

A clear role for antenatal ultrasound has been established, and it is valuable in dating pregnancies, diagnosing multiple pregnancies, monitoring intrauterine growth, and detecting congenital malformation, (Fig. 1–3), as well as locating the placental site. Ultrasound is valuable when performing amniocentesis or attempting other invasive procedures such as intrauterine transfusions. Ultrasound may be used during labor to resolve problems related to vaginal bleeding, size or date discrepancies, suspected abnormal presentation, loss of fetal heart

tones, delivery of a twin, attempted version of a breech presentation, and diagnosis of fetal anomalies.[157]

Assessing Fetal Condition Antepartum (Table 1–3)

The most widely used tests to evaluate the function and reserve of the fetoplacental unit and the well-being of the fetus before labor are stress and nonstress monitoring of the fetal heart rate (FHR), monitoring of fetal state and activity, and amnioscopy. Studies of fetal movements and respirations incorporated as part of the multivariable assessment (see discussion of fetal biophysical profile) continue to be used clinically.[99]

Antepartum Fetal Heart Rate Monitoring

Antepartum electronic monitoring of the FHR has provided a useful approach to fetal evaluation. The oxytocin challenge test described by Ray et al[148] records the responsiveness of the FHR to the stress of induced uterine contractions and thus attempts to assess the functional reserve of the placenta. A negative test (no FHR decelerations in response to adequate uterine contractions) gives reassurance that the fetus is not in immediate jeopardy.[189] Similar information may be obtained by evaluating the response of the FHR to spontaneous uterine contrac-

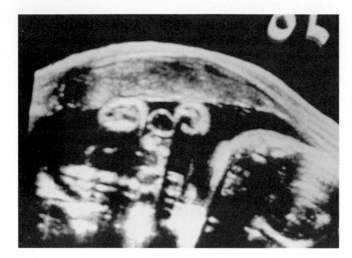

Figure 1–3. Gastroschisis with polyhydramnios.

tions and perhaps also from the resting heart rate patterns without contractions.[152, 158] Baseline variability of the FHR and accelerations of the rate with fetal motion have been reported as good indicators of the response to subsequent stress testing and of fetal well-being[152] (Table 1–4).

The contraction stress test evaluates uteroplacental function and was traditionally performed by initiating uterine contractions with oxytocin (Pitocin). Because continuous supervision and an electronic pump is required for regulated oxytocin infusion, and because of the invasiveness of intravenous infusion, attempts have been made to induce uterine contractions with nipple stimulation either by automanipulation or with warm compresses. Nipple stimulation has a variable success rate and, because of inability to regulate the contractions as well as concerns raised by the observation of uterine hyperstimulation accompanied by FHR decelerations, it has not gained wide acceptance. Nonetheless, breast stimulation provides an alternative, cheap technique for initiating uterine contractions and evaluating placental reserve.[89]

An antepartum demise of 1 to 4 in 1000 may be anticipated despite a reactive nonstress test (NST). The frequency of doing an NST is also important. In certain high-risk pregnancies in which the fetal status may change in less than a week (e.g., insulin-dependent diabetes mellitus in pregnancy), an NST performed twice a week at equidistant intervals results in lower perinatal mortality rate (less than 1 in 1000). On the other hand, in up to 90% of patients, a nonreactive NST indicates a fetal sleep state and is not associated with fetal jeopardy.[172] Vibroacoustic stimulation, using devices emitting sound levels of approximately 80 dB at a frequency of 80 Hz, results in FHR acceleration and reduces the rate of falsely worrisome NSTs. Thus, the specificity of the NST may be improved by adding sound stimulation.

The modified NST comprises vibroacoustic stimulation, initiated if no acceleration is noted within 5 minutes during the standard NST. Because reactivity is defined by two

Table 1–3. Assessment of the Fetus

Throughout Pregnancy

Gestational age: history, uterine growth, quickening, first heart sounds, ultrasound
Fetal growth
Serology, maternal antibodies
Amniotic fluid volume
Ultrasound: fetal number, growth, anomalies, fetal well-being
Risk assessment

First and Second Trimesters

Alpha-fetoprotein
Chorionic villus sampling
Amniocentesis
Cordocentesis

Third Trimester

Nonstress, stress tests
Formal fetal movement counting
Fetal biophysical profile
Amniotic fluid phospholipids and bilirubin

Perinatal Period

Continuous fetal heart rate monitoring
Fetal scalp pH
Cord blood gases

Table 1–4. Criteria for Interpreting Nonstress Test (NST) and Acoustic Stimulation Test (AST)

Reactivity Terms	Criteria
Reactive NST	Two fetal heart rate (FHR) accelerations of at least 15 bpm, lasting a total of 15 s, in 10-min period
Nonreactive NST	No 10-min window containing two acceptable (as defined by reactive NST) accelerations for maximum of 40 min
Reactive AST	Two FHR accelerations of at least 15 bpm, lasting a total of 15 s, within 5 min after application of acoustic stimulus or one acceleration of at least 15 bpm above baseline lasting 120 s.
Nonreactive AST	After three applications of acoustic stimulation at 5-min intervals, no acceptable accelerations (as defined by reactive AST) for 5-min after third stimulus

accelerations within 10 minutes, the sound is repeated if 9 minutes have elapsed since the first acceleration.

EDITORIAL COMMENT: While the effectiveness of *vibroacoustic stimulation* in assessing the health of the fetus continues to be studied, its safety for the fetus has come under scrutiny. Detailed evaluation of 10 healthy women with normal pregnancies of 37 to 40 weeks' gestation noted that stimulation with an electronic artificial larynx (EAL) *induced excessive fetal movements sometimes lasting as long as an hour, a prolonged tachycardia, nonphysiologic state changes, and a disorganization and change in the distribution of fetal behavioral states.*[182] Using simultaneous ultrasound during stimulation, Smith et al surprisingly *noted that 20 of 21 fetuses urinated at its onset.* Although during labor 47% of fetuses do not respond to EAL despite normal blood gases, during antenatal testing the absence of a response could simply mean the fetus is sleeping. Is this device harmful when it causes most fetuses to urinate and some fetuses to move for longer than an hour?

Clark[28] reported that, when using the modified NST, the testing time averaged 10 minutes, 2% of the tests were nonreactive, intervention was indicated in 3%, and mortality rate was low (0.01%).

Quicker and as effective as the contraction stress test or the biophysical profile, the modified NST has become the testing scheme of choice.

Monitoring Fetal Activity

Fetal movement has gained increased attention as an expression of fetal well-being in utero. It has been monitored simply by maternal recording of perceived activity or us-

ing pressure-sensitive electromechanical devices and real-time ultrasound. Fetal inactivity is generally defined as less than three movements per hour. Whereas evidence of an active or vigorous fetus is reassuring, an inactive fetus is not necessarily an ominous finding and may merely reflect fetal state (fetal activity is reduced during quiet sleep, by certain drugs including alcohol and barbiturates, and by cigarette smoking). Nonetheless, fetal inactivity requires prompt reassessment including real-time ultrasound or electronic FHR monitoring.

Formal Fetal Movement Counting[61, 123]

With a goal of decreasing the stillbirth rate near term, there has been an increased tendency to use fetal movements as an indicator of fetal well-being. The test is simple and can be administered frequently by a compliant and perceptive mother, preferably every night when the fetus is more active. The mother documents how long it takes to feel 10 kicks and maintains accurate "kick sheets" for review by the medical staff. Fifty percent of women feel 10 kicks in less than 20 minutes, and if the woman does not feel 10 kicks in 2 hours, she is instructed to come to the hospital for an NST. The use of kick counts has been associated with a 50% increase in the number of NSTs and an increased rate of obstetric intervention for fetal compromise. Moore and Piacquadio,[123] with the aid of historical control subjects, noted that the test reduced fetal mortality rate, but a larger prospective controlled trial from Europe failed to demonstrate that routine formal fetal movement counting achieved such an effect. The test is certainly worth instituting for selected high-risk patients as they approach term. It has the advantages of being inexpensive and of providing continual reassurance to anxious mothers between fetal evaluation visits, especially in high-risk conditions wherein the fetal status may change in a short time (e.g., insulin-dependent diabetes mellitus [IDDM]).

Fetal Biophysical Profile

Antepartum stillbirths account for 66% of all perinatal deaths and are the result predominantly of chronic asphyxia and congenital malformations. There is an urgent need to detect developing fetal asphyxia accurately in order to intervene and reduce fetal wastage appropriately. A composite of fetal functions, the biophysical profile, has emerged to address this issue.

EDITORIAL COMMENT: Fretts and associates[48] reported on the changing patterns of fetal death over 3 decades. The fetal death rate (per 1000 births) diminished from 11.5 in the 1960s to 5.1 in the 1980s. Significant changes over this time period include virtual elimination of fetal deaths caused by intrapartum asphyxia and Rh isoimmunization and significant decreases in unexplained fetal deaths and those caused by fetal growth retardation. The continued toll is due to intrauterine infections, lethal malformations, growth retardation, and abruptio placentae, which remains the largest identifiable cause of fetal death.

Six variables—the NST, fetal movements, fetal breathing movements, fetal tone, amniotic fluid volume, and placental grading—constitute the fetal biophysical profile (Table 1–5). A modified biophysical profile refers to sonographic components of the composite test (i.e., excludes NST) and is commonly used as a follow-up test for a nonreactive NST. There has been much debate regarding the pros and cons of each component of this evaluation. However, in a prospective evaluation, normal tests were highly predictive of a good neonatal outcome. In contrast, each abnormal variable was associated with a high false-positive rate. Vintzileos et al[181] noted that the absence of fetal movements was the best predictor of abnormal FHR patterns in labor (80%), the nonreactive NST best predicted meconium-stained amniotic fluid (33%), and decreased tone was the best predictor of perinatal death. The biophysical profile was far superior to the contraction stress test in predicting the hypoxic fetus (71% versus 16%). Because

Table 1–5. Technique of Biophysical Profile Scoring

Biophysical Variable	Normal (score = 2)	Abnormal (score = 0)
Fetal breathing movements	At least 1 episode of at least 30-s duration in 30-min observation	Absent or no episode of ≥30 s in 30 min
Gross body movement	At least three discrete body/limb movements in 30 min (episodes of active continuous movement considered as single movement)	Two or fewer episodes of body/limb movements in 30 min
Fetal tone	At least one episode of active extension with return to flexion of fetal limb(s) or trunk; opening and closing of hand considered normal tone	Either slow extension with return to partial flexion or movement of limb in full extension or absent fetal movement
Reactive fetal heart rate	At least two episodes of acceleration of ≥15 bpm and a least 15-s duration associated with fetal movement in 30 min	Less than two accelerations or accelerations <15 bpm in 30 min
Qualitative amniotic fluid volume	At least one pocket of amniotic fluid that measures at least 1 cm in two perpendicular planes	Either no amniotic fluid pockets or a pocket <1 cm in two perpendicular planes

From Manning F, Morrison I, Lange I, et al: Antepartum determination of fetal health: Composite biophysical profile scoring. Clin Perinatol 9:285, 1982.

the biophysical profile incorporates ultrasonic evaluation of the fetus and may result in the detection of anatomic abnormalities, some investigators have proposed that it should be used as the primary method of fetal surveillance.

Experience with composite biophysical profile scoring has been encouraging, with a reduction in perinatal mortality rate and increased detection of fetal anomalies. A high sensitivity (few fetal asphyxial deaths) and high specificity (minimal inappropriate intervention) are noted from these reports. This contrasts sharply with the high incidence of false-positive tests observed with single assessments such as fetal movements or fetal breathing. A normal fetal biophysical profile appears to indicate intact central nervous system (CNS) mechanisms, whereas factors depressing the fetal CNS reduce or abolish fetal activities. Thus, hypoxemia decreases fetal breathing and, with acidemia, reduces body movements. CNS stimulants increase fetal activities. The biophysical profile offers a broader approach to fetal well-being. Perinatologists have become attuned to doing multiple tests in evaluating fetal well-being, resulting in wider acceptance of the biophysical profile.

Alpha-Fetoprotein

Alpha-fetoprotein (AFP) is a fetal serum protein genetically and biochemically related to albumin. It has become a valuable marker not only in the prenatal detection of open neural tube defects but also in identifying fetuses likely to have chromosomal abnormalities.[116]

Maternal serum AFP measurement has proven to be the most effective prenatal screening program yet devised. The fetal liver is the primary site of synthesis of AFP and by 15 to 20 weeks of pregnancy, AFP is a major component of fetal serum. The AFP in amniotic fluid at 15 to 20 weeks is mainly derived from fetal urination with a small contribution through the fetal skin. Any pregnancy complication or birth defect that causes fetal serum to leak or exude into the amniotic fluid elevates amniotic fluid AFP and subsequently maternal serum AFP levels. Examples include anencephaly, open spina bifida, epidermolysis bullosa, gastroschisis, omphalocele, and amniotic bands. Furthermore, abnormalities in the volume of amniotic fluid may be reflected by abnormal AFP values. Additionally, a fetomaternal bleed may also result in elevated maternal AFP levels without increasing amniotic fluid levels.

Studies in the United Kingdom documented the correlation of an elevated amniotic fluid AFP level between 16 and 18 weeks' gestation with open neural tube defects. Subsequent testing demonstrated elevated maternal serum AFP levels as well for those fetuses with open defects, and this knowledge has been translated into worldwide screening programs that use maternal serum. These programs have been very successful, particularly when it is noted that neural tube defects predominantly occur (95%) in families with no prior history of such defects. The analysis of amniotic fluid has proved to be a reliable, accurate diagnostic test for open neural tube defects, with a 98% to 99% correlation between amniotic fluid AFP values (plus 3 or more standard deviations from the mean) and affected fetuses.

In addition to open neural tube defects, fetal demise and other fetal anomalies also have an elevated amniotic fluid AFP level; these include abdominal wall defects (gastroschisis and omphalocele), upper gastrointestinal obstruction, congenital nephrosis, and Turner syndrome.

A new correlation between low maternal serum AFP levels and fetal anomaly has also been recognized. First reported by Merkatz et al,[116] this phenomenon has been confirmed in a number of studies. Pregnancies involving fetuses with chromosomal aneuploidy, particularly trisomy 21 but also trisomy 18, have serum and amniotic fluid AFP levels significantly below the normal median. Application of this method can be of great value in identifying pregnancies at risk, particularly for mothers younger than 35 years of age.

Human chorionic gonadotropin (hCG) is elevated in women carrying aneuploid fetuses, unconjugated estriol is lower in women carrying fetuses with trisomy 21, and maternal serum AFP may be reduced with chromosomal abnormalities. The triple screen in which determinations of AFP are considered in conjunction with hCG and estriol have improved the reliability with which spina bifida and trisomy 21 are identified.[118, 127, 184, 185]

Although it will probably never be possible to eradicate neural tube defects, progress has been made in diminishing their incidence, identifying and characterizing the defects, counseling families who choose to continue a pregnancy, and decreasing morbidity by optimizing management at the time of delivery. Incidentally, the prevalence of neural tube defects is naturally declining in the United States in all regions as monitored by the Centers for Disease Control and Prevention. The triumph for perinatal medicine has all been the result of beautifully integrated epidemiologic studies, prospective screening trials, rapid improvement in ultrasound imaging, implementation of rapidly evolving techniques of prenatal diagnosis, and better preoperative and postoperative care of mother and baby.

Trisomy 21 Screening

Screening of maternal serum to identify fetuses with Down syndrome is routinely offered during the second trimester of pregnancy. Prenatal screening by means of serum assays or ultrasonographic measurements, either alone or in combination, may also be possible in the first trimester. Neilson[131] notes that trisomic fetuses with pronounced nuchal translucency are more likely to die in utero.

Maternal age and abnormalities of serum pregnancy-associated plasma protein A and free β-hCG detects about 60% of affected fetuses by 10 to 14 weeks' gestation. The combination of maternal age and quadruple screening test, including Inhibin A, alpha-fetoprotein, hCG, and unconjugated estriol, can detect approximately 75% of affected fetuses by 15 to 22 weeks' gestation. Haddow's series included a total of 48 pregnancies affected by Down syndrome and 3169 unaffected pregnancies studied before 14 weeks of gestation. The rates of detection of Down syndrome for the five serum markers were as follows: 17% for alpha-fetoprotein, 4% for unconjugated estriol, 29% for hCG, 25% for the free beta subunit of hCG, and 42% for pregnancy-associated protein A, with false-positive rates of 5%. They concluded that screening for Down syndrome in the first trimester is feasible, with use of measurements of pregnancy-associated protein A and either hCG or its free beta subunit in maternal serum. Nuchal translucency is increased at 10 to 13 weeks in trisomy 21 fetuses, but its role alone or in combination

with the aforementioned serum markers is still being evaluated. The skin edema in fetal trisomies is characterized by specific alterations of the extracellular matrix attributable to altered gene dosage.[183]

The accuracy of nuchal translucency measurement varies between examiners and between patients, likely in relation to examiner skill and image resolution. The size of translucency varies slightly with gestational age and crown-rump length and is independent of maternal age. Most authors have used a nuchal thickness of at least 2.5 mm or 3 mm to define abnormal, although some have suggested that the normal variation with gestation requires that different thresholds be used at different gestational ages. The presence of a thickened nuchal translucency is associated with chromosomal abnormality and perhaps with structural abnormality even when the karyotype is normal. D'Ottavio[41] found that increased nuchal translucency thickness (≥ 4 mm) at the 13- to 15-week scan was the most effective marker for chromosomal defects.

Because of the reported variations in the populations studied, the methods used, and the results of screening, it is inappropriate at this time to assign a numeric risk to any individual patient with this finding. Pandya,[138] in what was considered to be a "nonrepresentative population,"[151] reported that at 10 to 14 weeks' gestation the sensitivity of fetal neck translucency was 77% and the specificity 95%.[138] Haddow noted that measurements of nuchal translucency varied considerably between centers and could not be reliably incorporated into their calculations. Pajkrt[137] examined the effectiveness of nuchal translucency measurement in the detection of trisomy 21 in a low-risk population. A nuchal translucency of 3 mm or more identified 67% of the fetuses with trisomy 21, for an invasive testing rate of 2.2%. Screening by maternal age would have diagnosed six of nine fetuses (67%) with trisomy 21 for an invasive testing rate of 24%. After doing various risk assessments, the researchers concluded that nuchal translucency measurement is an effective screening method for trisomy 21 in an unselected obstetric population. In Greece, Theodoropoulos[173] reported that the combination of fetal nuchal translucency and maternal age were an effective means of screening for chromosomal abnormalities. An adjusted risk of 1 in 300 or more identified 10 of 11 fetuses with trisomy 21 and all 11 fetuses with other chromosomal defects.

Prenatal diagnosis of trisomy 21 currently relies on assessment of risk followed by invasive testing in the 5% of pregnancies at the highest estimated risk. Factoring in maternal age and combining first trimester ultrasonography with early serum screening may ultimately prove to be the most efficient means of screening for chromosomal anomaly, but although Snijders'[164] series included these criteria and detected almost 80% of affected pregnancies, it still required about 30 invasive tests to confirm the identification of one affected fetus.

EDITORIAL COMMENT: Prenatal screening for trisomy 21 incorporates estimation of risk on the basis of maternal age, serum concentration of various analytes, and ultrasound measurements. Because only 20% of infants with trisomy 21 are born to women 35 years or older, maternal age by itself has too low a sensitivity. During the first trimester, screening for Down syndrome uses ultrasound measurement of nuchal translucency (at 10 to 14 weeks' gestation) and measurements of the free beta subunit of hCG. This increases the sensitivity of first trimester screening to 80%. Second trimester screening has been improved by the addition of serum inhibin measurements to the triple screen, which included maternal serum alpha-

fetoprotein concentration (low), serum hCG (elevated), and unconjugated estriol (low). Wald et al[187] proposed a new screening algorithm in which measurements obtained during both trimesters are integrated to provide a single estimate of a woman's risk of having a pregnancy affected by Down syndrome. They used data from published studies of various screening methods employed during the first and second trimesters. When they used a risk of 1 in 120 or greater as the cutoff to define a positive result on the integrated screening test, the rate of detection of Down syndrome was 85%, with a false-positive rate of 0.9%. To achieve the same rate of detection, current screening tests would have higher false-positive rates (5% to 22%) (Fig. 1–4). If the integrated test were to replace the triple test (measurements of serum alpha-fetoprotein, unconjugated estriol, and hCG), currently used with a 5% false-positive rate, for screening during the second trimester, the detection rate would be higher (85% vs. 69%), with a reduction of four fifths in the number of invasive diagnostic procedures and consequent losses of normal fetuses. Although the integrated test detects more cases of Down syndrome with a much lower false-positive rate than the best currently available test, it may not gain wide acceptance because patients detected as high risk in the first trimester are more likely to choose chorionic villus sampling (CVS) than wait for the repeat screening during the second trimester.

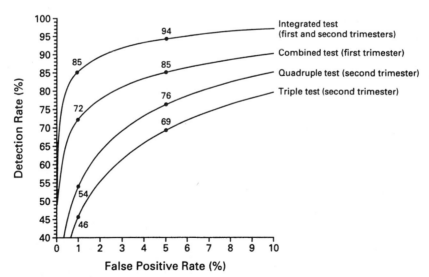

Figure 1–4. Rates of detection of Down syndrome and false positive rates for various screening tests. The triple test includes measurements of serum alpha-fetoprotein, unconjugated estriol, and human chorionic gonadotropin in the second trimester. The quadruple test includes measurements of serum alpha-fetoprotein, unconjugated estriol, human chorionic gonadotropin, and inhibin A in the second trimester. The combined test includes measurements of serum pregnancy-associated plasma protein A, free beta subunit of human chorionic gonadotropin, and nuchal translucency in the first trimester. The integrated test includes measurements of serum pregnancy-associated plasma protein A and nuchal translucency in the first trimester and measurements of serum alpha-fetoprotein, unconjugated estriol, human chorionic gonadotropin, and inhibin A in the second trimester.

Chorionic Villus Sampling[76, 150]

CVS is a method of prenatal diagnosis of genetic abnormalities that can be used during the first trimester of pregnancy. The major indications for chorionic villus sampling are to detect disorders related to maternal age and those that are sex linked, and to detect single gene disorders and hemoglobinopathies. Rhoads[150] reported that successful cytogenetic diagnoses were accomplished from 98% of 2235 attempts at CVS and from 99.4% of 651 amniocenteses. The total loss of desired pregnancies was 7% in the CVS group and 6% in the amniocentesis group. Thus, CVS permits early and accurate diagnosis but is not without hazard and should be used selectively.[150]

Although a screening test to identify a "high-risk" population would greatly improve the ability to diagnose congenital and acquired disease, the formulation of a noninvasive prenatal test that would provide all the diagnostic information currently available by amniocentesis and CVS without the risk of an invasive procedure remains a sentinel risk.

EDITORIAL COMMENT: A randomized trial (Medical Research Council) involving 3248 patients from 31 centers demonstrated that the policy of CVS in the first trimester reduced the chances of a successful pregnancy outcome by 4.6% (95% confidence intervals [CI] 1.6–7.5) when compared with second trimester amniocentesis. This was attributed to an increase in both spontaneous fetal deaths before 20 weeks and terminations of pregnancy for chromosomal anomalies. The observation of severe limb abnormalities following early (8 to 9 weeks) CVS raises further concerns.[76] The ideal time for performing CVS is between 10 and 12 weeks' gestation. Also, the consensus opinion, borne out by meta-analysis of the available data, is that CVS does not increase the risk for limb abnormalities. In the quest for earlier diagnosis, embryoscopy, a new invasive technique for direct visualization of the first trimester conceptus, has been used before elective termination. Incredibly clear pictures of the developing embryo are obtained, but it remains to be proven that the technique is safe and superior to transvaginal ultrasonography.

Assessing Fetal Maturity

The introduction of amniocentesis for study of amniotic fluid and Rh-immunized women paved the way for development of the battery of tests currently available to assess fetal maturity. The initial methods developed were based on amniotic fluid levels of creatinine, bilirubin, and fetal fat cells, and these provided a good correlation with fetal size and gestational age. They were, however, inadequate predictors of fetal pulmonary maturity.[115]

Amniocentesis to assess fetal pulmonary maturity is the currently accepted technique. Lecithin and sphingomyelin are present in amniotic fluid, and their relative ratios can be used for assessment of pulmonary maturity.[54] The risk of respiratory distress syndrome (RDS) is least when the ratio of lecithin to sphingomyelin (L:S) is greater than 2. However, this does not preclude the development of RDS in certain circumstances (i.e., IDDM or erythroblastosis). The presence of phosphatidylglycerol is a good indication of lessened risk of RDS with fewer false-negative results.

Because RDS is a frequent consequence of premature birth and a major component of neonatal morbidity and mortality in many high-risk situations, it was critical that an antenatal assessment of pulmonary status be developed. After it was found that the pulmonary surface-active materials needed for lung stabilization could be detected in the amniotic fluid and that their concentrations increased with gestational age, it followed that amniotic fluid analysis might yield insight into pulmonary maturation. Gluck and Kulovich[54] first measured the amniotic fluid L:S ratio in the third trimester of pregnancy and demonstrated its clinical application for the prediction of RDS (Fig. 1–5).

EDITORIAL COMMENT: RDS is the most common complication in preterm infants and is a significant, but diminishing, cause of death and severe morbidity. Thirty years of research has documented the beneficial effect of antenatal corticosteroids on fetal lung maturation. As a result, antenatal corticosteroids in combination with postnatal surfactant remains the mainstay of prevention and therapy for RDS in preterm infants. In 1994, a National Institutes of Health (NIH) consensus panel, on the basis of available evidence, recommended the use of corticosteroid therapy for delivery anticipated before 34 weeks of gestation when the fetal membranes are intact and before 32 weeks of gestation when the membranes are ruptured.[130] The beneficial effects of corticosteroid administration appear to be the greatest if more than 24 hours and less than 7 days have elapsed between

Figure 1–5. Abnormal elevations of lecithin/sphingomyelin (L:S) ratio as compared with curve of progress of L:S ratio of normal pregnancy. A = Chronic stress, retroplacental bleeding; B = acute stress, membranes ruptured 72 to 96 hours; C = acute stress, placental infarction; and D = chronic stress, postmaturity. (From Gluck L, Kulovich M: Lecithin-sphingomyelin ratios in amniotic fluid in normal and abnormal pregnancy. Am J Obstet Gynecol 115:539, 1973.)

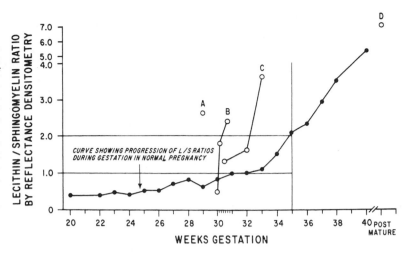

initial administration of therapy and actual delivery. However, even partial courses appear to have been beneficial. At the time of the consensus conference, corticosteroids were used in less than 20% of eligible patients, but since the conference, that number has increased to nearly 80%. Antenatal corticosteroids have decreased the incidence and severity of respiratory distress, lowered the mortality rate, and significantly reduced the incidence of major intraventricular hemorrhage. Antenatal exposure to betamethasone, but not dexamethasone, is associated with a decreased risk of cystic periventricular leukomalacia among very premature infants.[10] An important secondary benefit of corticosteroid administration is the reduction in the cost and duration of neonatal hospitalization. The optimal number of courses of antenatal corticosteroids for lung maturation remains unclear. On the basis of a retrospective analysis of multiple courses of antenatal corticosteroids, Banks[8] reported that they did not improve outcome and were associated with increased mortality rate, decreased fetal growth, and prolonged adrenal suppression.

Because thyrotropin-releasing hormone (TRH) also accelerated pulmonary maturation, and there are still many infants with chronic lung disease, TRH was added to antenatal corticosteroids. A number of large multicenter trials universally reported that the combination regimen did not reduce the frequency of RDS or improve the outcome of preterm neonates compared with the use of corticosteroids alone.[7, 31, 37]

There are several advocates of the direct quantitative measurement of lecithin rather than the more qualitative L:S ratio. The introduction of the foam stability test by Clements and coworkers[29] provided a rapid, simple, inexpensive test for surfactant. As with the L:S ratio itself, this test provides two

limits of reliable prognostic usefulness and an intermediate zone with more equivocal results. False-positive and false-negative results have been reported with both methods.[174] Investigators have noted that confirmation of the presence of phosphatidyl glycerol, a component of the more mature surfactant complex, reduces the incidence of false-positive tests. Nonetheless, in uncomplicated, unstressed situations such as elective repeat cesarean section, any of these techniques are useful, and their use should be encouraged, taking into consideration the risk of amniocentesis.

Phosphatidylglycerol can be measured by rapid tests and is not influenced by blood or vaginal secretion, and is therefore a good indication (in the presence of a positive test) of pulmonary maturity when sampled from a vaginal pool of fluid. Other tests have been used to reduce testing time and to increase the ease of interpretation. These include the foam stability (shake) test[29,] the Lamadex-FSI test[159,] and the amniotic fluid absorbance test at 650 nm.[176] Lamellar body counts—size similar to platelets—is a standard hematology counter that can be used; values of 30,000 to 50,000/μL indicate maturity.[4] The use of amniotic fluid testing for elective delivery at term has been replaced by accurate dating using ultrasound,[1] either crown-rump length at 6 to 11 weeks and an ultrasound at 12 to 20 weeks combined with additional evidence of gestational length at 30 weeks fetal heart tones (FHT) by Doppler or 36 weeks since a positive pregnancy test.[1] If any of these confirm a gestational age of 39 weeks, amniocentesis can be waived for delivery.

However, in many high-risk conditions, the developmental biochemical maturation of the fetal lung may be altered, at least as measured by the L:S ratio.[54] Acceleration of mature L:S ratios has been reported in maternal hypertensive states, sickle cell disease, and narcotics addiction, as well as with intrauterine growth retardation (IUGR) and prolonged premature rupture of membranes.[54] Considerable investigative interest currently centers around the regulatory mechanism leading to such accelerated pulmonary maturation. Experiments in pregnant rabbits and sheep have demonstrated that glucocorticoids can stimulate the appearance of surface-active material in the alveoli of the lungs of the fetuses of these species, presumably by enzyme induction.[122] Chronic intrauterine stress may initiate earlier lung maturation to permit a premature extrauterine adaptation, but the need persists for careful controlled studies to document this phenomenon in independent high-risk circumstances. In contrast, a delay in the appearance of lung maturation is seen in the infants of some diabetic mothers, particularly where there is macrosomia, presumably as the result of poor regulation of maternal blood sugar. The interface between receptors for insulin and cortisone has been implicated in this regard. In diabetic pregnancies, the presence of phosphatidylglycerol (PG) is generally considered necessary, in addition to a mature L:S ratio, in order to establish pulmonary maturity.

Furthermore, studies of patients in whom respiratory distress syndrome occurred in the presence of mature foam stability tests call attention to the separate roles of (1) surfactant deficiency, (2) fetal immaturity, and (3) intrapartum asphyxia in the pathogenesis of this disorder.[174]

Doppler Velocimetry[103, 165]

Doppler velocimetry has been used to assess the fetoplacental circulation since 1978 but still has a limited role in fetal evaluation.[103] Because the placental bed is characterized by low resistance and high flow, the umbilical artery maintains flow throughout diastole. Diastolic flow steadily increases from 16 weeks' gestation to term. A decrease in diastolic flow, indicated by an elevated systolic-to-diastolic ratio, reflects an increase in downstream placental resistance. A normal waveform is considered reassuring and presumes normal fetal oxygenation. Elevated systolic-to-diastolic ratios are best interpreted in conjunction with NSTs and the fetal biophysical profile. Absent or reversed diastolic flow (defined as the absence or reversal of end-diastolic frequencies before the next systolic upstroke) in the umbilical artery is regarded as an ominous finding. It has been associated with maternal disease (hypertension or diabetes), uteroplacental insufficiency, and fetal and neonatal problems such as growth retardation, major malformations, or necrotizing enterocolitis. To manage such cases, it is important to know the fetal karyotype, fetal anatomy, and other assessments of fetal well-being. In the absence of fetal karyotype or other structural abnormalities, it is extraordinarily unlikely to find absent end diastolic flow without associated obvious FHR abnormalities, at least persistent absence of decelerations and absent long-term variability.

Percutaneous Fetal Umbilical Blood Sampling (Cordocentesis)[69, 73, 153]

Percutaneous fetal umbilical blood sampling (PUBS), or cordocentesis, provides direct access to the fetal circulation for both diagnostic and therapeutic purposes. The procedure is carried out under high-resolution ultrasound guidance and has had a major impact on the evaluation and treatment of the residual patients with Rh isoimmunization and other causes of severe fetal anemia (e.g., parvovirus-induced hydrops fetalis or induced hemolytic anemia) in pregnancy. Other indications for PUBS include rapid karyotyping in the evaluation of fetal malformations detected later in pregnancy, evaluation of fetal acid-base status, and evaluation of fetal metabolic, endocrine (e.g., thyroid function), and infectious diseases—notably toxoplasmosis and other hematologic disorders including hemoglobinopathies, thrombocytopenia, and twin-to-twin transfusions. The technique may also be used for directly transfusing or administering medications to the fetus.

Fetal Treatment

A combination of medical and surgical therapies is available for the prevention and treatment of fetal disorders. As noted in Table 1–6, these range from simple dietary supplements (which prevent birth defects) to complex surgical procedures, usually mandated by severe fetal compromise with hydrops fetalis or gross disturbances in the volume of amniotic fluid. The development of invasive fetal therapy can be attributed to advances in prenatal ultrasonography. Ultrasonography has been critical in following the natural history of many of the birth defects and disorders. It has also permitted early identification of the structural anomalies and served as a guide for the minimally invasive prenatal therapy as well as intraoperative monitoring during open fetal surgery.

Direct or indirect treatment of the fetus continues to evolve slowly. These treatments include short-term oxygen therapy for IUGR, blood transfusions for fetal anemia, antibiotics (e.g., spiramycin and sulfonamides) for toxoplasmosis, steroid replacement for congenital adrenal hyperplasia, stem cell therapy for immune deficiency disorders, therapy for fetal arrhythmias, and thyroxine instillation for severe hypothyroidism.

Pioneering studies by Harrison and colleagues[69] have paved the way for surgical exploration of the fetus. They have successfully repaired congenital diaphragmatic hernias and excised cystadenomatous malformations of the lung. Rarely, infants with hydrocephalus or hydronephrosis are candidates for in utero interventions, but infants with neural tube defects may benefit from intrauterine surgery.

Monitoring the Fetus During Labor[87]

Selected high-risk pregnancies should be closely monitored during labor. Of 83 term intrapartum fetal deaths reported, 47 occurred in mothers who had at least one of the criteria for high risk based on the individual pregnancy history alone. Careful monitoring with appropriate operative intervention might salvage a significant number of these infants.

Counting the FHR between contractions using a stethoscope is an inadequate method of determining early evidence of fetal distress, because significant rate changes occur early during a contraction and persist for a short time after the contraction ends. This is a period when fetal heart tones are least audible with a stethoscope. Furthermore, it is difficult to objectively evaluate audible data in the same manner as a recorded continuous FHR, and auscultation data cannot be subjected to peer evaluation. By continuously monitoring intrauterine pressure and FHR using continuous ultrasound (Doptone) or, when the fetal scalp is accessible, a scalp electrode attached to a recording monitor, significant abnormalities can be detected at a time when operative intervention has a greater chance of promoting delivery of a live, neurologically intact newborn infant.

Table 1–6. An Overview of Fetal Therapy

Prevention of Birth Defects

Folic acid
Periconceptual glucose control in diabetes

Hormonal Therapy

Thyroid hormone
Antenatal corticosteroids for acceleration of
  pulmonary maturation
Corticosteroids for congenital adrenal hyperplasia

Prevention and Treatment of Anemia/Jaundice

Anti-D globulin (Rhogam) at 28 weeks to prevent
  erythroblastosis
Direct transfusions for severe anemia/hydrops

Treatment and Prevention of Infection

Spiramycin for toxoplasmosis
Zidovudine or other agents for human
  immunodeficiency virus
Antibiotics for premature rupture of membranes
Intrapartum penicillin for group B streptococcal
  disease

Treatment of Cardiac Arrhythmias

Agents administered to mother, injected into
  amniotic fluid or directly into the fetus

Fetal Surgery: Highly Selected Cases

Usually with hydrops fetalis or gross alterations in
  amniotic fluid volume
Congenital diaphragmatic hernia
Congenital cystic adenomatoid malformation
Fetal hydrothorax
Sacrococcygeal teratoma
Obstructive uropathy
Fetal airway obstruction due to giant neck masses
Neural tube defects

EDITORIAL COMMENT: Nelson and others found that there was an increased risk of cerebral palsy associated with multiple late decelerations and decreased variability of the FHR, but the false-positive rate was extremely high. No association existed between the highest or low-

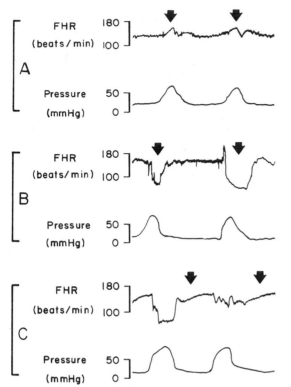

Figure 1–6. Changes in FHR during uterine contractions as reflection of fetal distress. Arrows indicated transient tachycardia *(A)*, variable deceleration *(B)*, and variable deceleration with slow recovery after uterine relaxation *(C)*. Pressure is uterine pressure. (See text for explanation.)

Table 1–7. Fetal Heart Rate Patterns and Underlying Mechanisms

Reflecting Fetal Reserve	
Normal baseline heart rate and FHR	Intact autonomic cardiovascular reflexes
Tachycardia (>160 bpm)	Prematurity, maternal fever, acidosis
Diminished variability (<6 bpm variation)	"Sleep cycle," drug effects, acidosis, congenital anomaly
Bradycardia (<120 bpm)	Normal variant, congenital heart block, cardiac anomaly, maternal hypothermia
Sinusoidal pattern	Anemia, hypoxia, drug effect
Reflecting Acute Environmental Change	
Early deceleration	Head compression
Variable deceleration	Cord compression, acute hemorrhage
Late deceleration	Contraction-induced hypoxia
Acceleration	Intact autonomic response to intrinsic or extrinsic stimuli

Modified from Clark SL, Miller FC: Scalp blood sampling—F.H.R. patterns tell you when to do it. Contemp Obstet Gynecol 21:47, 1984.

est FHR recorded for each child and cerebral palsy.

♦ ——————

Nelson KB, Dambrosia JM, Ting TY, Grether JK: Uncertain value of electronic fetal monitoring in predicting cerebral palsy. N Engl J Med 334:613–618, 1996.

Transient tachycardia with heart rates of more than 160 beats per minute (Fig. 1–6*A*) may be an isolated finding. It frequently precedes a variable deceleration pattern as a brief episode (see Fig. 1–6*B* and *C*), which may reflect umbilical cord venous compression. A late deceleration pattern (Fig. 1–7)

is commonly associated with uteroplacental insufficiency. Either of these patterns may be compatible with fetal distress (Table 1–7).

Sampling blood from the fetal scalp during labor is another method used for monitoring the fetuses in selected high-risk pregnancies usually when fetal distress is suspected based on the FHR pattern. The procedure can be done when membranes are ruptured, the cervix is dilated 3 to 4 cm, and the fetal vertex is well applied to the cervix. A fetal scalp puncture (only a few millimeters deep) is made under direct visualization, and a sample is collected in a heparinized capillary tube. The values for acid-base parameters on fetal scalp blood correspond to those obtained from the umbilical cord at cesarean section. The most reliable parameter reflecting the presence of fetal

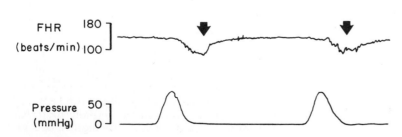

Figure 1–7. Changes in FHR during uterine relaxation as reflection of fetal distress. Arrows indicate late deceleration pattern with slow recovery after uterine relaxation. Pressure is uterine pressure. (See text for explanation.)

hypoxia and acidosis has been pH.[12] There is a high correlation with fetal distress when the fetal scalp pH is less than 7.15 in the presence of normal maternal blood pH. However, a significant number of infants with low pH are born vigorous and with essentially normal acid-base status.[94]

At present, continuous FHR monitoring is the preferred method of identifying fetal distress. Fetal scalp pH is measured when the FHR record is difficult to interpret or in the presence of decelerations. Complications of fetal scalp blood sampling and fetal scalp electrode monitoring include significant fetal blood loss and infections in the newborn, but occur rarely. An alternative to fetal scalp pH determination is digital stimulation of the fetal scalp in the absence of uterine contractions and when the FHR is at the baseline. A positive test (i.e., an acceleration [15 bpm for 15 seconds] response to such stimulation) is considered fairly reliable evidence of the absence of fetal acidosis, and clinical investigation supports its use. Fetal scalp stimulation is generally used to obtain reassurance about the fetal status when obtaining fetal scalp pH is not feasible because of inadequate cervical dilatation and when the FHR pattern is not obviously ominous.

Principles Related to FHR Monitoring[25, 35] (see Table 1–7)

The normal antepartum FHR record is characterized by a normal baseline, normal long-term variability, and the presence of accelerations (2/20 min; >15 to 20 bpm) and the absence of decelerations with contractions.

- Continuous electronic monitoring of FHR complemented by fetal scalp blood pH best evaluates intrapartum fetal well-being.
- Whereas a normal FHR pattern accurately predicts a nondepressed infant (Apgar >7), even with apparently ominous FHR abnormalities, only 50% of the neonates are depressed. Unnecessary interventions (e.g., cesarean section based on FHR abnormalities alone during labor) can be diminished by assessing fetal scalp blood pH or by additional monitoring of fetal echocardiogram (ECG).
- In the presence of normal FHR variability, infants with late decelerations are unlikely to be acidotic. However, if there are late decelerations accompanied by diminished baseline variability together with baseline tachycardia, there is a 60% chance that the fetus is acidotic.
- Neither baseline bradycardia (FHR <120 bpm) nor tachycardia (FHR >160 bpm) alone is predictive of acidosis.
- Baseline tachycardia may be due to early asphyxia but is more frequently the result of maternal fever, fetal infection, maternal drugs, or prematurity.
- Persistent fetal bradycardia with good beat-to-beat variability is generally not associated with acidosis. It is more likely to be the result of drugs (medications) or fetal cardiac anomalies.
- Variability is a measure of fetal reserve. Both long- and short-term variability should be evaluated. Decreased variability is suggestive of fetal acidosis. Normal baseline variability and accelerations occurring spontaneously or after stimulation indicate intact fetal reserves.
- The occurrence of decelerations except for sporadic mild variable decelerations before labor signifies antepartum hypoxia. The hypoxia may be mild and may not necessarily compromise the fetus. Persistent or repetitive late and marked atypical variable decelerations before labor are always ominous and require expeditious intervention. Ominous features of variable decelerations include a slow return to a baseline, an increasing baseline, and a transient smooth increase in baseline following a variable deceleration.
- Absent or decreased FHR variability, with fetal tachycardia and late decelerations, has a high association with acidosis.
- Flat tracing (i.e., absence of both long-term and short-term variability with a "straight line" record) may be an ominous finding and requires urgent evaluation (e.g., biophysical profile [BPP]) and consideration of intervention.
- If more than one third of contractions are associated with late decelerations or if more than 20 late decelerations are noted during labor, the baby is likely to be physiologically depressed. The depth of the deceleration does not cor-

relate with the likelihood of acidosis and, in fact, some shallow decelerations may indicate the inability of the depressed (resulting from hypoxemia) fetal parasympathetic system to decrease FHR and is more likely associated with acidosis.

- Variable decelerations of less than 15 bpm are considered mild, 15 to 60 bpm moderate, and 60 bpm severe. Neither the degree of decrease of FHR frequency during variable decelerations nor their number appeared to be significant factors in neonatal depression. The duration of the deceleration is most important. Prolonged decelerations of 2 minutes or more are associated with significant fetal asphyxia. They may be induced by uterine hypertonus, local anesthesia, vaginal examination, or an active second stage of labor with the mother bearing down. Because the etiology may be nonrecurrent, a single prolonged deceleration—which is followed by a return to baseline with good beat-to-beat variability—is not ominous. If there is a recurrence, delivery must be expedited.
- If there is an increase in FHR at the time of obtaining a blood gas sample, the pH is usually normal. This is also true of acceleration response after digital stimulation of the fetal scalp.
- In the fetus with decreased beat-to-beat variability, acoustic or scalp stimulation may induce FHR acceleration, indicating fetal well-being.
- Criteria for fetal distress include the following: (1) persistent late decelerations, regardless of depth, (2) persistent severe variable decelerations, notably those with slower return to baseline, (3) prolonged decelerations, and (4) sinusoidal pattern.

Treatment of Fetal Distress In Utero

Administration of a high concentration of oxygen to the mother of a distressed fetus is one of the few methods of treating acute fetal asphyxia.

COMMENT: Although the rise in fetal Po_2 associated with maternal oxygen inhalation is small, this may be reflected in a significant increase in fetal oxygen saturation because of the shift to the left and steep slope of the oxygen hemoglobin dissociation curve for fetal hemoglobin, especially at low Po_2s.

Mildred T. Stahlman

Repositioning the mother in labor occasionally may relieve acute fetal asphyxia caused by mechanical compression of the umbilical cord. Maternal hypotension caused by compression of the inferior vena cava may produce fetal asphyxia by decreasing uterine blood flow and oxygenation. This may be relieved by rotating the mother from a supine to a lateral position. If FHR indicates fetal compromise and it is confirmed by fetal scalp pH or lack of scalp stimulation response, a prompt delivery may be indicated. The method of delivery, operative vaginal or cesarean section, will depend on cervical dilatation, station, and position of the fetal head.

COMMENT: Prolonged preparation of the mother on the delivery or operating table in a supine position (for instance, during the preparation for cesarean delivery) may bring about these adverse effects at a time when monitoring is frequently discontinued.

Mildred T. Stahlman

Adequate preparation is desirable for prompt effective resuscitation of the newborn. The pediatrician should be alerted when a decision is being made to intervene operatively for a fetus in distress (Table 1–8) (also see Chapter 2, Resuscitation of the Newborn Infant). Fetal distress may or may not be associated with asphyxia. Asphyxia is generally described as the presence of hypoxemia and acidosis, and its diagnosis requires evidence of multiple end-organ damage, such as brain (encephalopathy) or kidney (renal failure) damage.

◆ SELECTED MATERNAL DISORDERS AND THEIR EFFECTS ON THE FETUS

Pregnancy-Induced Hypertension[39]

Hypertensive disorders with a host of different etiologies affect 7% to 10% of pregnant women. The term *preeclampsia* is used to denote the syndrome that occurs predominantly in 5% to 7% of primigravid pregnancies. Preeclampsia is a complex clinical syndrome with hypertension representing only

Table 1–8. Planning Care of High-Risk Infant

Fetal Disorders (suspected or confirmed)

Size for date discrepancy
Abnormal karyotype
Polyhydramnios or oligohydramnios
Hydrops fetalis
Fetal anomalies
Abnormal alpha-fetoprotein determination
Abnormal stress or nonstress contraction test
Reduced biophysical profile score
Reduced fetal movement
Immature L:S ratio
Cardiac dysrhythmias

Maternal Problems

Pregnancy-associated hypertension
Diabetes
Previous stillbirth or neonatal death
Maternal age <18 y or >34 y
Anemia or abnormal hemoglobin
Rh sensitization
Maternal infection
Prematurity or postmaturity
Malnutrition or poor weight gain
Premature rupture of membranes
Antepartum hemorrhage
Collagen vascular disorders
Drug therapy
Maternal drug or alcohol abuse
Multiple gestation

***Intrapartum Factors Associated With Maternal/
Fetal Compromise***

Extreme prematurity or postmaturity
Placenta previa or abruptio placentae
Abnormal presentation
Prolapsed cord
Prolonged rupture of membranes >24 h
Maternal fever or chorioamnionitis
Abnormal labor pattern
Prolonged labor >24 h
Prolonged second stage of labor (>2 h)
Persistent fetal tachycardia
Persistent abnormal fetal heart rate (FHR) pattern
Loss of beat-to-beat variability in FHR
Meconium-stained amniotic fluid
Fetal acidosis
General anesthesia
Narcotic administered to mother within 4 h of delivery
Cesarean delivery
Difficult delivery

one manifestation. The syndrome is characterized by the sequential development of facial and hand edema, hypertension, and proteinuria after the 20th week of gestation. If seizures supervene, then the condition is known as eclampsia. The etiology is still unknown, although the pathogenesis is becoming more clearly delineated. Events implicated in the development of preeclampsia include incomplete trophoblastic invasion of the maternal spiral arteries, poor trophoblastic perfusion, activation of renin–angiotensin system, endothelial cell injury with activation of coagulation, and altered endothelial permeability. The goal is to detect the onset of preeclampsia early and to intervene so that severe complications for the mother and fetus are prevented.

According to the World Health Organization (WHO) preeclampsia is defined by blood pressure greater than 140/90 mm Hg and proteinuria greater than 300 mg/L in 24 hours. The presence of proteinuria greater than 5 g/L, a persistent diastolic pressure greater than 110 mm Hg, platelet count of less than 100,000/mm^3 (low platelets), elevated liver enzymes (EL) or jaundice, hemolysis (HE), oliguria of less than 400 mL/24 h, and symptoms including epigastric pain, visual disturbance, or severe headache identify the sickest women, those with the so-called HELLP syndrome.

Close supervision of all hypertensive pregnant women with frequent evaluation of fetal growth and well-being is indicated. Current data suggest that aspirin may not prevent preeclampsia and calcium may not prevent hypertensive disorders except in a nutritionally deprived population.

EDITORIAL COMMENT: Preeclampsia, defined as hypertension and proteinuria, or nondependent edema after 20 weeks' gestation, is a common pregnancy disorder. Early clinical trials and a meta-analysis suggested that low-dose aspirin prevented preeclampsia without harming the mother or fetus. Caritis et al randomly treated a high-risk group of women (pregestational, insulin-dependent diabetes, chronic hypertension, multiple gestations, or previous preeclampsia) with 60 mg of aspirin a day or placebo between the 13th and 26th week of pregnancy. They were unable to reduce the incidence of preeclampsia, but did find a trend toward a reduction in preterm deliveries and perinatal deaths among the aspirin-treated group. The role of aspirin has, thus, not yet been fully resolved.

◆

Imperiale TF, Petrulis AS: A meta-analysis of low dose aspirin to prevent pregnancy-induced hypertensive disease. JAMA 266:260–264, 1991.
Caritis S, Sibai B, Hauth J, et al: Low dose aspirin to prevent preeclampsia in women at high risk. N Engl J Med 338:701–705, 1998.

Diabetic Pregnancy[188]

Major advances in the knowledge of carbohydrate metabolism provide the opportunity for improved screening and identification of the gestational diabetic woman. Physiologic studies currently offer a better rationale for management of both the chemical and the overt diabetic pregnant woman and her fetus. Furthermore, the increased risks for stillbirth, prematurity, and neonatal morbidity associated with diabetes pose a direct challenge to the efficacy of both antenatal surveillance and neonatal intensive care.

Despite insulin therapy, the perinatal mortality rate among offspring of diabetic mothers continues to be extraordinarily high. The infant survival rate at the Joslin Clinic from 1922 to 1938 was only 54%. From 1938 to 1958, the survival rate improved to 86%, and from 1958 to 1974, a 90% survival was achieved. Thus, the combined toll from stillbirth and neonatal death may persist at five times the rate of nondiabetic women, even at major medical centers. Where care is less intensive, perinatal mortality rate for diabetics of 20% to 30% still exists.

Based on the increased risk of stillbirth during the last month of pregnancy, preterm delivery at 36 to 37 weeks' gestation was the generally accepted recommendation for many years.[51] Möller[119] was one of the first to strive for an avoidance of premature deliveries. In 1970, she reported from Sweden a series of diabetic women carried closer to term when blood sugar regulation comparable to the nondiabetic pregnancy had been achieved and when evidence of fetal jeopardy or pregnancy complications such as toxemia did not appear. The perinatal mortality rate in her series of 47 patients was 2.1% as compared with a 21% mortality rate in a prior series from the same obstetric unit.

Similar favorable results have been reported from other institutions both in Europe and in the United States.[66, 142, 154] Gyves et al[66] described a reduction in perinatal mortality rate from 13.5% to 4.1% in a group of 96 diabetic patients in whom the modern technology was applied and preterm delivery was not routinely employed. These statistics continue to improve.

For many years, good control of maternal blood sugar concentration has been considered important for the well-being of the fetus of the diabetic mother. However, wide differences of opinion exist as to what constitutes good control. The fasting plasma glucose concentration in pregnancy, in both normal and diabetic mothers, has been shown to be lower than in women in the nongravid state. The continuous siphoning of glucose by the fetus profoundly affects maternal carbohydrate metabolism and, as a result, fasting glucose levels are 15 to 20 mg/dL lower during pregnancy than postpartum. Furthermore, physiologic studies describing diurnal profiles for blood glucose concentrations in normal pregnancies have shown a remarkable constancy of these concentrations throughout the day. The fetus is thus, under normal circumstances, provided with a constant glucose environment.

These physiologic principles have provided a rational basis for the care of pregnant diabetic women, and the importance of rigid blood glucose control has been illustrated by several clinical studies. The marked improvement in perinatal mortality rates and morbidity obtained by Möller[119] and Gyves et al[66] was with a mean preprandial blood glucose concentration kept close to 100 mg/dL, particularly during the third trimester. The latter series also described a significant reduction in macrosomia among the infants of such well-controlled diabetic mothers. Karlsson and Kjellmer[80] reported that their perinatal mortality rate could be directly correlated with maternal mean blood glucose concentrations. When mean concentrations were greater than 150 mg/dL, the mortality rate was 23.6%. At concentrations between 100 and 150 mg/dL, the rate declined to 15.3%, and at less than 100 mg/dL a 3.8% mortality was achieved. The King's College group in London reported on deliveries of 100 diabetic pregnant women in whom the mean preprandial blood glucose concentrations were maintained at approximately 100 mg/dL. There was no perinatal loss in this series.

Because improvements in obstetric and neonatal management have evolved over the same time span as these studies of intensive blood sugar control, it is difficult to attribute marked improvements in outcome to only one variable. Nevertheless, it seems prudent that the therapeutic objective in pregnant diabetic patients be an effort at normalization of plasma glucose throughout the day. This approach should apply to the woman with gestational diabetes as well as to the woman who was diabetic before pregnancy.

Principles of Management of Diabetes in Pregnancy

1. Metabolic derangements are the major abnormality affecting individuals with diabetes mellitus.

2. Pregnant women with diabetes should be managed by suitably trained individuals and teams who comprehensively monitor mother and fetus throughout pregnancy (Table 1–9).
3. Optimal care of women with diabetes must begin before conception because it has been demonstrated that careful preconception control of diabetes reduces the incidence of major anomalies.
4. All pregnancies should be screened so that women with gestational diabetes can be identified and appropriately managed.

Management of Diabetic Women Before Conception

The rationale of the preconception program for diabetic women is to optimize the pregnancy outcome for the woman and her off-

Table 1–9. Clinical Status of Diabetes: Timing of Assessments

Assessment	Non–Insulin-Dependent	Insulin-Dependent, No Vasculopathy	Insulin-Dependent, With Vasculopathy
Maternal			
History/physical examination	Preconceptual/initial visit	Preconceptual/initial visit	Preconceptual/initial visit
Ophthalmologic evaluation*			
No known abnormality	Preconceptual/initial visit	Preconceptual/early first trimester	Preconceptual/early first trimester
Known abnormality	Each trimester	Each trimester	Each trimester as indicated
Electrocardiogram†	NI	Preconceptual/initial visit‡	Preconceptual/initial visit†
Prenatal screen panel and bacteriuria screen	Preconceptual/initial visit	Preconceptual/initial visit	Preconceptual/initial visit
Glycosylated proteins‡	NI	Initial visit/delivery‡	Initial visit/delivery‡
Thyroid panel screen	NI	Preconceptual/initial visit (repeat monthly until normal)	Preconceptual/initial visit (repeat monthly until normal)
Creatinine clearance	NI	Preconceptual/initial visit (if abnormal, each trimester)	Preconceptual/initial visit (if abnormal, each trimester)
Urine protein			
Dipstick	Serially	Serially	Serially
24 h	NI	≥1 + by dipstick	≥1 + by dipstick
Lipid profile	NI	Preconceptual/initial visit	Preconceptual/initial visit
Fetal (weeks' gestation)			
Alpha-fetoprotein (maternal serum)	16–18	16–18	16–18
Ultrasonography			
Dating/anomaly screen	18–22	18–23	18–22
Echocardiography	NI	20–24	20–24
Fetal growth/development	37–39§	30–32; 37–39	30–32; 37–39
Fetal movement§	36 to intervention§	34 to intervention§	30 to intervention§
CST/NST (biophysical profile: backup)§	NI	32–34 to intervention§	32–34 to intervention§
Lung maturity documentation	If intervention <38 wk	If intervention <39 wk	If intervention <39 wk

NI, Not routinely indicated.
*Implies pupillary dilation.
†Advised with diabetes >10 y duration or known cardiovascular disease or abnormal lipid profile.
‡More frequently if used as compliance evaluator.
§Earlier or more frequent assessment dependent on clinical status (e.g., evidence of intrauterine growth retardation or multiple gestation).
From *Guidelines for Care: California Diabetes and Pregnancy Program.* Maternal and Child Health Branch, Department of Health Services, 1986.

spring. Optimal care of gravidas with pre-pregnancy diabetes must begin before conception. A well-disciplined, well-coordinated, and well-organized multidisciplinary team and a compliant patient are the prime ingredients for a successful pregnancy outcome. The team comprises internists, perinatologists, and selected other medical subspecialists; a nutritionist, a social worker, and other perinatal nurse specialists who coordinate the dietary needs; and specialists in ongoing education, exercise, and blood glucose regulation. The goal is to achieve a mean fasting glucose of less than 100 mg/dL and a 2-hour postprandial level around 120 mg/dL. Glycosylated hemoglobin should be maintained within the normal range. The objective is to achieve glycemic control before conception and throughout embryogenesis and then continue throughout gestation. In this way, major abnormalities may be averted. In addition, prophylactic folate supplementation is advocated during the periconceptual period to reduce the risk of neural tube defects. Strict glucose control may also diminish other perinatal complications including intrauterine demise, macrosomia, and neonatal disorders such as hypoglycemia and polycythemia. Ongoing surveillance, continued education, and careful monitoring throughout the pregnancy are necessary to achieve optimal maternal and perinatal outcome.

Outpatient management of the diabetic pregnancy has replaced the obligatory period of hospitalization. However, in the face of deteriorating glycemic control, maternal complications including hypertensive disorders, infection, preterm labor, or evidence of fetal compromise, hospitalization is mandated.

A comprehensive program devised by the California Maternal and Child Health Division is outlined in Table 1–9.

A critical determinant of the outcome of diabetic pregnancy is the timing of delivery. The risk of intrauterine death increases as term approaches. On the other hand, the infant delivered preterm is exposed to the risks of prematurity, particularly that of respiratory distress, which may result in neonatal loss. The risk of RDS is higher in diabetic pregnancies compared with nondiabetic pregnancies. Over the past 25 years, the feasibility of extending the gestational period and of individualizing delivery timing for the diabetic mother has been en-hanced by the availability of objective tests for fetal surveillance.

Because the major consequence of premature birth is respiratory distress, fetal pulmonary functional maturity is the most critical objective of current care. Biochemical estimations of this maturity can be obtained from the amniotic fluid with either the L:S ratio[54] or the foam stability test.[29] These determinations provide an important dimension in the management of the pregnant diabetic woman, particularly when maternal blood sugar control has been good and a normal physiologic milieu has been approximated.

Congenital malformations have assumed a major role in diabetic pregnancies. Simpson et al,[161] in a prospective study, documented a 6.6% incidence of major anomalies among offspring of diabetic mothers as compared with a 2.4% incidence in control mothers. (Other centers report even higher rates.) Because the anomaly rate in those patients whose diabetes was aggressively managed was similar to that observed by others in patients whose diabetes was less vigorously managed, the researchers hypothesized that abnormal development had occurred before the patients entered the study. There is a major emphasis on carefully managing diabetes before conception and even in the first trimester to reduce the high anomaly rate associated with diabetic pregnancies.

Patients with high hemoglobin (Hb) A_{1C} (variably defined as greater than 7.99 or greater than 9.0) have extremely high (22.5% to 40%) risk of congenital malformation compared with women whose HbA_{1C} is less than that level (5%). This is supported by data generated by Ylinen et al,[194] who measured maternal HbA_{1C} as an indication of maternal hyperglycemia during pregnancy to determine its relationship to fetal malformations. Maternal HbA_{1C} was measured at least once before the end of the 15th week of gestation in 139 insulin-dependent patients who delivered after 24 weeks' gestation. The mean initial HbA_{1C} was 9.5% of the total hemoglobin concentration in the 17 pregnancies complicated by malformations, which was significantly higher than in pregnancies without malformations (8.0%). Fetal anomalies occurred in 6 of 17 cases (35%) with values initially of 8% to 9.9%, and only 3 of 63 (5%) anomalies occurred in babies of patients who had an initial level less than 8%. These data support the notion that there is an increased risk of malformation associated with poor glucose control. Unplanned pregnancies should be avoided in diabetic women, and determination of HbA_{1C} before conception may assist in planning the optimal time for conception.

EDITORIAL COMMENT: Many studies confirm the extensive work of Fuhrman and coworkers[48a] that strict diabetic control before conception significantly reduces the incidence of congenital malformations. To have a meaningful effect, this information must be widely disseminated. It is unfortunate that these results have not been achieved because appropriate preconceptional control was not attempted. The reasons for this remain undefined, but are probably shared, for example, (1) unplanned nature of pregnancies (i.e., lack of planned, or recommendation for, contraception by internist), (2) noncompliance by the patient, and (3) lack of effort by health care provider (generally internist) to attempt to achieve good control because of lack of consideration of the possibility of pregnancy.

The application of current technology thus provides the clinical team with the means of minimizing both fetal death in utero and preventable neonatal morbidity and mortality from the hazards of prematurity. Together with intensive control of maternal blood glucose, the technology of fetal surveillance offers the possibility of normalizing perinatal outcomes in large numbers of diabetic pregnancies.

Obstetric Management of the Low-Birth-Weight Infant

Low birth weight is the key determinant of perinatal outcome.[46, 167] Major obstetric complications resulting in delivery of very low-birth-weight infants include premature rupture of membranes (PROM) (75%), premature labor (45%), multiple gestation (16%), amnionitis (14%), and premature separation of the placenta (7%). The rationale for a group of specific obstetric interventions directed at optimizing the outcome of low-birth-weight infants currently exists and is illustrated in the following section. The following basic principles apply:

1. Prevent prematurity through maximal antenatal care, avoidance of unnecessary

iatrogenic interventions, and conservative management of pregnancy problems whenever feasible. Specifically, screening and treatment of bacterial vaginosis is generally applied to patients deemed at high risk for preterm labor and PROM. These generally include patients with a history of such complications in previous pregnancies and those from low socioeconomic strata and with multiple sexual partners.
2. Inhibit premature labor pharmacologically when favorable conditions permit.
3. Avoid asphyxia and expedite delivery when the intrauterine environment becomes too unfavorable for allowing further fetal maturation.
4. Avoid excessive medications or the inappropriate use of anesthetic agents that may depress the low-birth-weight infant.
5. Maintain a controlled delivery of the low-birth-weight infant—this is critical in avoiding birth trauma and injury. Cesarean delivery is favored over arduous inductions of labor or extensive vaginal manipulations. A more liberal consideration of cesarean sections for fetal indication in the low-birth-weight and very low-birth-weight group, and the willingness of the obstetrician to perform cesarean sections at a gestation age of 23 to 26 weeks is likely to result in an increase, both in intact survival and in survival with serious morbidity. This approach also was associated with a reduced neonatal mortality rate.[16]
6. Anticipate problems and communicate management plans to neonatal and nursing colleagues. The team approach furthers a continuity of care between the delivery room and the nursery.
7. Promote healthy maternal-infant attachments by avoiding separations, maintaining an air of optimism, and maintaining a positive, supportive approach to the emotional needs of both parents.

Pharmacologic Inhibition of Premature Labor

For properly selected patients, the option to inhibit uterine contractions must be available when premature onset of labor cannot be prevented. When such treatment is contraindicated or unsuccessful, optimal obstetric management and expert neonatal care need to be ready to maximize the outcome for the very small premature infant. After exclusion of cases in which arrest of labor is either contraindicated or likely to fail because of advanced state of labor, a group of patients remains for whom a program of pharmacologic control of labor can materially improve the perinatal outcome (approximately 25% of patients delivering premature infants).[81]

Pharmacologic inhibition of threatened premature labor is generally contraindicated under the following conditions: (1) severe pregnancy-induced hypertension, (2) active vaginal bleeding, (3) advanced dilation of the cervix (>4 to 5 cm), (4) chorioamnionitis, (5) coexisting medical problems such as hyperthyroidism or cardiovascular disease, (6) evidence of severe IUGR or chronic fetal distress, and (7) the presence of a fetal anomaly incompatible with life, or fetal demise.

Time-honored approaches to therapy have included the use of bed rest, intravenous (IV) fluids, tranquilizers, sedatives, and narcotics. Because it remains difficult to distinguish those patients in true early labor from those in false labor, each of these approaches has, at times, been credited with some degree of success by obstetricians. However, it is agreed that their actual therapeutic influence on inhibiting the myometrium is minimal; the groups of drugs used have the potential for depressing the very small premature infant and should be discontinued completely when delivery appears inevitable. Castrén et al[24] have emphasized the therapeutic value derived from placebos when the mother is assigned to bed rest and is reassured that she is being treated.

It is in light of such background that the evaluation and introduction of pharmacologic agents for the control of premature labor have posed particular difficulties. Patient selection, criteria for premature labor, and suitable control subjects are the areas of greatest controversy.

The commonly used method for clinical suppression of premature labor has been treatment with β-adrenergic stimulators, an approach in use since the early 1960s. Stimulation of myometrial β-receptors inhibits activity as it does in smooth muscles. The myocardium responds with increased activity when its β-receptors are stimulated.

Ritodrine hydrochloride was the first of the agents to undergo rigorous clinical investigation in the United States. Whereas ritodrine was specifically synthesized for its predominant β_2 effect, by which uterine relaxation is achieved, there is invariably a degree of β_1 stimulation, resulting in tachycardia, widened pulse pressure, tremor, and restlessness. Additionally, ritodrine causes fluid retention, a short-lived elevation in blood glucose, and a decrease in hematocrit and potassium.

In a multicenter series of randomized, prospective, double-blind studies, ritodrine was compared with either ethanol or placebo in the treatment of idiopathic preterm labor. When compared with control subjects, offspring of ritodrine-treated mothers experienced a significantly reduced incidence of neonatal death and RDS; also, a significantly higher proportion of these infants achieved a gestation of greater than 36 weeks or a birth weight or more than 2500 g, or both. There was thus a significant prolongation of pregnancy in the ritodrine-treated patients.[9, 21] In patients who do not tolerate tachycardia or tremor associated with ritodrine or in those with diabetes or hyperthyroidism, magnesium sulfate or indomethacin may be used for tocolysis.

Indomethacin, magnesium sulfate, and calcium channel blockers (nifedipine) all have their clinical proponents. Magnesium sulfate, because of its minimal side effects, and terbutaline, a β-mimetic with clinical pharmacology features similar to ritodrine, have also been used as tocolytics. Several major centers also use indomethacin because of its minimal maternal cardiac effects. Its use should be avoided past 32 weeks' gestation because of the serious risk of closure of the fetal ductus arteriosus.

EDITORIAL COMMENT: After women have received indomethacin, the preterm infant is more likely to be unresponsive to indomethacin therapy for a clinically significant patent ductus arteriosus.

Nonetheless, assessment of the efficacy of various treatment modalities of preterm labor has been difficult. Because the exact mechanisms that trigger the onset of either term or preterm labor remain incompletely understood, efficacy can only be assessed in terms of subsequent clinical events rather than precise or discriminating biochemical or physiologic parameters. Furthermore, there is a significant margin of error attendant to an accurate diagnosis of preterm labor made early enough for the interventions to work effectively. Criteria establishing premature labor vary among physicians and institutions. Those centers with a positive attitude to arresting premature labor pharmacologically tend to intervene earlier, with a greater chance for success, but there is also the likelihood of overtreating patients in false labor. On the other hand, those less enamored of the available agents who await clear evidence of progressive labor may be risking delays in instituting treatment. By the time unquestionable changes in cervical effacement and dilation can be documented, it may be too late for effective inhibition of uterine activity.

Table 1–10 summarizes the analysis of a number of controlled studies with tocolytics.

In summary, β-mimetics, ritodrine and terbutaline, magnesium sulfate and inhibitors of prostaglandin synthesis, primarily Indocin, have emerged as the group of agents likely to inhibit preterm labor. These groups of agents have been effective in postponing delivery; however, neither the prematurity rate nor infant morbidity has been successfully reduced. These agents do buy time for the perinatal team to establish a care plan for the mother and infant. This includes arranging for delivery in an appropriate level of care and administration of steroids to accelerate pulmonary maturation. The task for the perinatologist is to distinguish those women truly in need of tocolysis as well as to identify the ideal tocolytic agent.[25, 81, 92]

EDITORIAL COMMENT: Preterm birth complicates just more than 10% of all pregnancies. Prematurity accounts for the bulk of the neonatal deaths and a significant proportion of the neurologic disability including cerebral palsy. The standout risk factors for premature delivery include a history of preterm birth, fetal fibro-nectin, bacterial vaginosis, short cervical length, and abnormal body mass index. The history of a previous preterm birth and determining body mass index may be the initial red flags that identify women at risk who will then be more closely supervised and monitored for the rest of the pregnancy. There may be remedies for bacterial vaginosis, which accounted for 40% of the attributable risk for spontaneous preterm birth at less than 32 weeks. Clinicians have a better handle on what to do with pregnancies in which fetal fibronectin is detected. No doubt many obstetricians need to learn that the predicted recurrence risk is increased by two- to four-fold in women with a positive, compared with a negative, fetal fibronectin, and the risk of premature delivery increases as cervical length shortens in both fetal fibronectin-positive and fetal fibronectin-negative women. These data may be useful in caring for women with a history of preterm birth and in designing studies to prevent recurrent premature delivery.[59]

However according to the sage words of Goldenberg and Rouse, "Most interventions designed to prevent preterm birth do not work, and the few that do, including treatment of urinary tract infection, cerclage, and treatment of bacterial vaginosis in high-risk women are not universally effective and are applicable to only a small percentage of women at risk for preterm birth. A more rational approach to intervention will require a better understanding of the mechanisms leading to preterm birth. In the meantime substantial reductions in preterm delivery are unlikely to be achieved."[59] Prevention of prematurity is not imminent but the seeds for success have been sown.

Fetal fibronectin (FFN) is a complex glycoprotein, confined to the decidual area of the uterus, and can be detected by a monoclonal antibody immunoassay.

FFN is present in cervicovaginal secretions during the first 24 weeks of pregnancy and diminishes thereafter. The presence of FFN after 24 weeks is consistent with preterm delivery in symptomatic women. Use of FFN assays is valuable in assessing the risk of delivery in symptomatic women. A negative FFN is associated with delivery in 1 in 125 women in 14 days

Table 1–10. Meta-analysis—Tocolytics

Efficacy Criterion	Tocolysis (%)	Control (%)	OR	95% CI
Preterm birth	47	47.5	0.95	0.77–1.17
Perinatal death	2.5	1.3	1.73	0.80–3.22
Neonatal RDS	9.4	9	1.06	0.72–1.55
Intraventricular hemorrhage	3.8	2.8	1.36	0.70–2.64
NEC	1.9	0.8	1.9	0.64–5.61
NICU admission	23.5	23.6	1.03	0.75–1.42

CI, confidence interval; NEC, necrotizing enterocolitis; NICU, neonatal intensive care unit; OR, odds ratio; RDS, respiratory distress syndrome.
Adapted from Sanchez-Ramos L, Kaunitz AM, Gaudier FL, et al: Efficacy of maintenance therapy after tocolysis: A meta-analysis. Am J Obstet Gynecol 181:484, 1999.

or less; a positive FFN, on the other hand, is associated with deliveries in 1 in 6 women in 14 days or less.[141] Lockwood et al[92] reported that FFN in cervical or vaginal secretions had a positive predictive value of 83% for preterm delivery with a sensitivity of 82%.

One of 12 high-risk, asymptomatic women with a negative FFN will deliver at less than 37 weeks, whereas, with a positive FFN, 50% of women deliver at less than 37 weeks.[109]

Salivary estriol (SE) reflects unbound, unconjugated, biologically active estriol in maternal serum. There is an abrupt increase in estriol at the onset of labor. McGregor et al evaluated an enzyme-linked immunosorbent assay for salivary estriol in 241 singleton pregnancies.[105] They found a slow increase in estriol levels 3 weeks before delivery. Women who delivered preterm had higher levels earlier in pregnancy.

A sample SE level greater than or equal to 2.3 ng/mL had a 71% sensitivity and 77% specificity, and a false-positive rate of 23%—reflecting a more accurate prediction for preterm labor, 71% vs. 37%, and preterm birth, 51% vs. 34%.

A follow-up study confirmed the findings: an SE of 7.1 mL amongst high-risk patients proved a positive predictive value of 26% and a negative predictive value of 94%.

Multiple endocrine markers, including inhibin, relaxin, and corticotropin-releasing hormone (CRH), are being evaluated for use as a screening tool for preterm labor. The use of multiple tests, including monitored data, cervical length, cervicovaginal FFN, and a panel of endocrine and inflammatory markers may ultimately lead to the definitive diagnosis of preterm labor in women at risk.

To reduce the prematurity rate and its related morbidity and mortality, it is necessary to understand the etiology of preterm labor and PROM, and then address the etiologic causes. The role of subclinical intra-amniotic infections, as evidenced by the presence of inflammatory proteins like proinflammatory cytokines, is being recognized as markers associated with serious perinatal morbidities, including cerebral palsy[195] and periventricular leukomalacia.

Leitich et al concluded from their meta-analysis of 27 studies "that among patients with symptoms of preterm labor, cervico-vaginal fetal fibronectin appears to be among the most effective predictors of preterm labor."

◆

Leitich H, Egarter C, Kaider A, et al: Cervical fetal fibronectin as a marker for preterm delivery: A meta-analysis. Am J Obstet Gynecol 180:1169–1176, 1999.

◆ INTRAUTERINE GROWTH RETARDATION

IUGR is associated with significantly increased rates of both perinatal mortality and

long-term morbidity.[42, 64] Before the widespread use of ultrasound, most studies revealed that only a small percentage of IUGR infants were actually identified before birth. Improved perinatal outcome depends on early identification, which requires an awareness of developing signs of uterine growth lag. Confirmation of diagnosis, based on continued lack of clinical growth or serial ultrasonography, still requires a delay, often of several weeks, following initial suspicions. On the other hand, even when an awareness of the problem exists and a high index of suspicion is maintained, a significant number of false-positive diagnoses will result, especially when there is coincident ambiguity in pregnancy dating. Beard and Roberts[13] reported that in 35% of their suspected cases the infants turned out not to be growth retarded. In our own studies, 50% of patients with suspected IUGR of the fetus eventually delivered an infant whose weight was appropriate for gestational age, although conservative management and prolonged bed rest may well have been ameliorating in some instance.

EDITORIAL COMMENT: The most important reason for the inability to diagnose deficiency of fetal growth antenatally may be the current sonographic parameters used for diagnosis and the approach to defining growth restriction. It is well recognized that as many as two thirds of the fetuses less than the 10th percentile may actually be constitutionally small. However, because 33% are truly growth retarded with attendant morbidities, perinatologists still continue to use estimates less than the 10th percentile as the criterion for planned delivery. This approach does not address fetuses that are within the normal range of the 10th to 90th percentile, but may actually be growth retarded. An approach to serially plot fetal growth and detect deviations from normal toward growth retardation may be better to detect all truly growth-retarded fetuses. However, the threshold for such deviation from normal and the degree of growth deviation that correlate with perinatal morbidities remain to be defined.

Once the identification of possible growth retardation has been made, a close follow-up is recommended and a severe case may require hospitalization. Bed rest, nutritional support, and, when appropriate, control of maternal blood pressure constitute the therapeutic approach for both mother and baby. Placental perfusion, however, must not be compromised by overly aggressive treatment of maternal hypertension. This caution is a legacy of studies regarding a shift in the autoregulatory zone of cerebral flow in hypertensive, older males. There is no clinical evidence that appropriate treatment of hypertension and normalization of blood pressure in pregnancy is associated with any adverse consequences.

Fetal growth and well-being are evaluated by regular clinical measurements of fundal height and ultrasonographic measurements of fetal growth. Additional tests of fetal well-being include biophysical profiles, NST, and Doppler velocimetry of umbilical arteries. The decision regarding appropriate timing of delivery rests on whether the fetus will continue to benefit from its environment in utero or whether it will profit more from premature delivery. Aggressive intervention increases the risk of fetal immaturity, particularly when the diagnosis of IUGR has not been fully substantiated. Expectant management, on the other hand, may result in intrauterine death or irreversible damage to a surviving neonate.

To date, none of the current laboratory estimations of fetal well-being have been able to provide supportive data adequate to formulate a clear decision.[99] As a result, one commonly advocated approach is to deliver the growth-retarded baby following earliest evidence of pulmonary maturity by amniotic fluid analysis or reasonable estimation of pulmonary maturity based on accurate gestational age data. However, amniocentesis in cases of IUGR, particularly those identified before 35 weeks, is often complicated by the presence of oligohydramnios and by difficulty in obtaining the amniotic fluid specimen. Traumatic taps may force unplanned interventions and, at times, may further compromise fetal homeostasis. These patients require management and amniocentesis in specialized centers.

In our hands, the use of antepartum cardiotachography without oxytocin (i.e., NST twice a week or more frequently in hospitalized patients) or daily NST supported by biophysical profile (BPP) has proved to be an aid in individualizing the timing of delivery in such situations involving suspected IUGR. Delivery is expedited at any time beyond 28 weeks' gestation if FHR abnormalities suggestive of fetal compromise are observed in response to spontaneous uterine contractions. Otherwise, expectant management is advocated, and prolongation of the time in utero is sought. The ominous significance of a positive contraction stress test (CST) was described initially by Fairbrother et al,[44] who observed the presence of late deceleration FHR patterns in response to Braxton Hicks contractions in four infants who were severely growth retarded and born before 35 weeks' gestation. Two infants were delivered by immediate cesarean section and did well, whereas the other two were not delivered immediately and died within days of the observation. There has been extensive experience confirming the ominous significance of a positive NST.

◆ EXPECTANT MANAGEMENT FOR PREMATURE RUPTURE OF FETAL MEMBRANES

Depending on the definition used, the reported incidence for pregnancies complicated by PROM generally varies from 7% to 20%. The incidence among women delivering preterm ranges between 40% and 60%. Furthermore, perinatal mortality rate among premature infants is markedly increased when there has been coexisting PROM. In a 1-year retrospective study from the University of California, Los Angeles, 16% of all perinatal deaths were associated with PROM. The vast majority of these deaths were among low-birth-weight infants.

The obstetric management of this major complication remains controversial.[50, 140] There has been strong advocation of an aggressive or dynamic management that favors early delivery of the fetus by induction of labor or cesarean section. Equally strong is advocation, particularly when the fetus is premature, of an approach predicated on a hands-off policy of expectant management.[132] This latter approach has as its objective the continued growth of the fetus unless labor, infection, or fetal maturation dictates otherwise.

EDITORIAL COMMENT: There is considerable divergence of opinion among perinatologists as to what constitutes expectant management. Whereas all agree that ultrasonographic evaluation is an integral component of evaluation, all other issues relating to diagnostic follow-up and treatment are heatedly debated.

When membranes rupture at term, 70% of women begin to labor within 24 hours and 95% within 72 hours. The latency increases with preterm PROM so that at 20 to 26 weeks' gestation the mean latency period is 12 days and at 32 to 34 weeks' gestation it is only 4 days. PROM, defined as rupture of the fetal membranes prior to labor, is the leading cause of preterm delivery, hence a major contributor to perinatal morbidity and mortality. There are many causes of PROM. At the molecular level, diminished collagen synthesis, altered collagen structure, and accelerated collagen degradation have all been implicated, with infection always lurking in the background. The consequences for the fetus are varied and range from sepsis and minor deformations to pulmonary hypoplasia and periventricular leukomalacia. In studying the natural history of PROM (between 20 and 36 weeks), Nelson reported that the maternal infection rate was 22% and the perinatal death rate 8%. Vaginal bleeding, smoking, and a history of PROM are prominent risk factors, and there is a strong association with group B *Streptococci,* bacterial vaginosis, *Trichomonas, Chlamydia,* and gonorrhea. There is an expanding body of evidence that antibiotic therapy increases the latency to delivery, reduces chorioamnionitis, endometritis, neonatal sepsis, and RDS.[43, 93, 110, 111, 132]

At term, approximately 80% to 90% of women who experience ruptured membranes progress to spontaneous labor within 24 hours, so any controversy regarding management at term pertains principally to a small minority of patients. However, when preterm pregnancies are considered, only 35% to 50% of women will be in labor within 24 hours, and the probability of an infant not being delivered within 72 hours after PROM is reported to be about 30%. In general, the earlier in gestation that rupture occurs, the greater the likelihood of delay in onset of labor. Some patients experience delays of 14 days of more, and such an extension of gestation for the small premature infant can be of critical benefit.

The interval between occurrence of membrane rupture and onset of regular uterine contractions resulting in progressive cervical dilation is defined as the latent period. The longer the latent period, the greater the risk of the eventual development of amnionitis. However, the lower the gestational age, the longer the latent period. Association of a longer latency period with infection and chorioamnionitis is simply reflective of the association of infection at a low gestational age, and thereby the role of infection as an etiologic factor in causing the PROM and premature delivery. Therefore, the expectant management of PROM in the preterm gesta-

tion represents a balancing of the risks of low-birth-weight delivery versus the risk of infection. The likelihood of infection, in turn, is directly related to the number and frequency of vaginal examinations, especially in the intrapartum period. It can be argued that such examinations serve little useful purpose and that in most instances they can be avoided entirely to minimize infection. Because the most frequent cause of perinatal death in the low-birth-weight group with PROM is prematurity itself, at our institution expectant management is advocated.

EDITORIAL COMMENT: The most serious consequence of PROM is preterm delivery, with the ultimate chance of survival dependent on gestational age at delivery. Clinically manifest infection is the next major hazard, compounded by the immature host defense systems together with the fact that the bacteriostatic properties of amniotic fluid increase with advancing gestational age. Pulmonary hypoplasia and the deformation syndrome associated with oligohydramnios represent another potentially lethal peril for the fetus. Rotschild[155] reported that the risk of pulmonary hypoplasia is significant only if rupture occurred before 26 weeks' gestation. Pulmonary hypoplasia may be suspected if the chest circumference or lung length as determined ultrasonographically falls below the fifth percentile.

Delivery of a small premature infant and PROM is generally avoided until labor ensues or infection supervenes. In those instances when early clinical manifestations of amnionitis, such as low-grade fever, leukocytosis, or uterine tenderness, appear, the strategy is reversed, and delivery is expedited within a few hours.

COMMENT: If one is going to manage PROM conservatively, it is important to look for signs of infection. In addition to monitoring for fetal tachycardia, maternal temperature should be obtained frequently because these are the first indicators of intra-amniotic infection. Examination of the amniotic fluid for bacteria is helpful, but the presence of white blood cells in the amniotic fluid does not correlate well with subsequent maternal infection. If signs of infection develop, antibiotics should be given and the fetus delivered.

Edward Quilligan

Our experience at MacDonald Women's Hospital has been consistent with that of the Denver group, whose data first demonstrated that neonatal sepsis developed in less than 2% of infants of mothers with PROM who are conservatively managed and that the perinatal mortality rate for low-birth-weight infants is not increased by this conservative approach. Furthermore, in contrast to other reports, our experience indicates that such management can be appropriate for patients from poor socioeconomic environments as well as for patients from other socioeconomic environments.

Garite et al[50] observed 251 patients with PROM prospectively to evaluate the maternal and neonatal effects of chorioamnionitis. The period of gestation ranged from 28 to 34 weeks at time of rupture. Intrauterine infection occurred in 19% before delivery. Fetal tachycardia, maternal leukocytosis, and uterine contractions were not predictive of intrauterine infection in afebrile patients; however, amniocentesis positive for bacteria either with Gram stain or with subsequent positive culture correlated with antenatal maternal fever. Postpartum endometritis was the only major maternal complication associated with chorioamnionitis. Neonatal outcome—as evidenced by an increased perinatal mortality rate and a higher incidence of neonatal infection and RDS—was adversely affected in the presence of maternal fever before the onset of labor, a prognostically ominous sign for the fetus.

Patients with PROM are admitted to the hospital and placed at bed rest. Careful abdominal examination is performed to evaluate the fetal size, presentation, and estimated station. In many instances, the diagnosis of PROM can be confirmed by history and perineal inspection without requiring vaginal examination. The continued leakage of amniotic fluid from the vagina is often obvious, and Nitrazine testing or the collection of fluid for ferning can be performed at the introitus. The vagina is examined by sterile speculum under aseptic conditions only when the diagnosis remains questionable and visualization of the cervix or posterior vaginal pool is necessary for confirmation. Digital examinations are avoided in that they may add significantly to the risk of infection and usually add little to either diagnosis or management. Particularly when on Leopold's maneuvers the presenting part has been found to be high and floating free from the pelvis, it should not come as a surprise that the examining fingers find only a "long and closed" cervix.

Furthermore, visual inspection of the cervix during speculum examination is generally adequate for clinical management of these patients.

A period of electronic monitoring of the FHR and uterine activity is routinely initiated by external cardiotachography. The absence of progressive labor with or without occasional mild contractions is documented. Fetal tachycardia may be an early indicator of incipient amnionitis, and its finding should be considered significant. Usually mild variable decelerations with uterine contractions reflect mild occult cord compression resulting from oligohydramnios and is usually of no serious consequence because cord prolapse is not a common complication of PROM. In early gestations complicated by PROM, the incidence has been reported to be as low as 0.7% to 3.0%, which is only slightly higher than in the general population. Moderate or severe variable decelerations necessitate an evaluation for cord prolapse.

Other therapies that continue to be evaluated include the prophylactic use of antibiotics with or without tocolytics, the use of corticosteroids to induce pulmonary maturity, and induction of labor if pulmonary maturity has been established. Prophylactic antibiotics do not appear to reduce either amnionitis or neonatal infection, and data are omitted on the effectiveness of tocolytics coincident with the rupture of membranes and before the onset of labor. Prophylactic antibiotics (PCN/Sulbactam) may improve neonatal morbidity and mortality risks. In addition, antibiotics may prolong the latent phase and, therefore, further reduce the prematurity risk. In a study by Lovett et al[93] (double blind, randomized, controlled) of 112 women, the total frequency of neonatal mortality, sepsis, and RDS was subsequently lowered and birth weight increased with antibiotics and steroids as compared with steroids alone. Indiscriminate use of antibiotics have potential risk of neonatal sepsis by resistant organisms.

It is the complications of prematurity per se, notably RDS, that are the principal threats to the very low-birth-weight infant with associated PROM. Reports are contradictory as to whether PROM decreases the chance of RDS. Yoon and Harper[195] first suggested that rupture of membranes more than 24 hours before delivery protected against the development of RDS. Other investigators reporting similar findings suggested acceleration of fetal lung maturation by endogenous corticosteroids.[111] Another study focusing retrospectively on the incidence of RDS with PROM found no such protective influence.

◆ PRETERM CORTICOSTEROID THERAPY FOR FETAL MATURATION

The role of exogenous corticosteroids in preventing RDS has been the focus of much attention. Crowley has reviewed all the controlled trials and concluded that the administration of betamethasone, dexamethasone, or hydrocortisone is associated with a 40% to 60% reduction in the risks of neonatal respiratory distress.[130] Therefore, we recommend the use of corticosteroids to enhance pulmonary maturation in all pregnancies between 24 and 34 weeks' gestation, even those complicated by PROM.

Glucocorticoids play a major role in development of the fetal lung and are stimulators of surfactant synthesis. Liggins[91] was the first to demonstrate a more favorable outcome in a betamethasone-treated group as compared with a control group. There were reduced incidences of RDS, pneumonia, intraventricular hemorrhage, and perinatal mortality recorded in the betamethasone-treated group. Infants born less than 1 day or more than 7 days after steroid therapy and those greater than 34 weeks' gestation demonstrated no benefit from treatment. More recent studies demonstrate the maximum benefits after 24 hours, but all parties appear to benefit, regardless of sex or gestational age. The reduction in the risk of RDS is accompanied by reductions in periventricular hemorrhage and mortality rate.

EDITORIAL COMMENT: These benefits are achieved without any detectable increase in the risk of maternal, fetal, or neonatal infection, even in the presence of prolonged rupture of membranes.[36, 130] Corticosteroids are given to almost 80% of women who deliver infants with birth weights less than 1500 g.[167] Recent data suggest adverse effects on the mother and neonate from recurrent weekly administration of steroids in undelivered patients.[8] In view of the fact that benefits are obtained up to 2 weeks after a single dose is administered, we now wonder if it is adequate to repeat steroid administration every 2 weeks if the threat of preterm delivery is significant, which would apply to all cases with PROM and patients requiring continued hospitalization for premature labor with intact membranes.

Banks and others performed a post hoc nonrandomized analysis on 710 neonates of 25–32 weeks' gestation who were born to mothers enrolled in the North American Thyrotropin-Releasing Hormone Trial and who received 1, 2, or ≥3 courses of antenatal corticosteroids. There was no detectable clinical difference in incidence of respiratory distress syndrome, chronic lung disease, and intraventricular hemorrhage related to courses of antenatal corticosteroids, and outcome was similar for infants delivered at 7–13 days compared with those delivered at 1–6 days after receiving antenatal corticosteroids. Compared with those who received a single course, neonates who received 2 courses had lower birth weights (-39 g, $P = .02$), and those receiving ≥3 courses had increased risk of death (adjusted odds ratio, 2.8; 95% CI, 1.3–5.9; $P = .01$) and lower levels of plasma cortisol at age 2 hours. A recently concluded NICHD sponsored consensus conference concluded that "data from currently available studies assessing benefits and risks are inadequate to argue for or against the use of repeat or rescue courses of antenatal corticosteroids for fetal maturation." Randomized clinical trials to address the efficacy and safety are under way.

◆ ─────

Banks BA, Cnaan A, Morgan MA, et al: Multiple courses of antenatal corticosteroids and outcome of premature neonates. North American Thyrotropin-Releasing Hormone Study Group. Am J Obstet Gynecol 181:709–717, 1999.

Antenatal Corticosteroids Revisited: Repeat Courses, August 17–18. 2000 NIH Consensus Statement 17(2):1–10. http://odp.od.nih.gov/consensus

◆ AMNIOINFUSION[75, 128, 169]

Severe variable or umbilical cord compression decelerations are defined as decelerations that last for greater than 60 seconds in which the deceleration nadir is less than 60 bpm. The nadir heart rate of less than 60 bpm approximates the atrioventricular nodal rate and thereby implies maximal vagal stimulation. Severe cord compression leads to metabolic acidosis. Severe variable decelerations are encountered with PROM, severe oligohydramnios, nuchal cord, true knot in the cord, and cord prolapse. Standard therapy for severe variable decelerations includes changing the maternal position, discontinuation of oxytocics, ruling out cord prolapse, and administration of 100% oxygen to the mother by face mask. Amnioinfusion represents an alternative approach to the treatment of oligohydramnios, FHR abnormalities, and meconium-stained fluid in labor. Amnioinfusion is considered when variable decelerations do not respond to standard therapy. Preliminary controlled trials indicate that the restoration of amniotic fluid volume by means of saline infusion relieves cord compression and reduces the incidence of variable decelerations.

EDITORIAL COMMENT: The Oxford Database of Perinatal Trials[75] notes seven randomized trials that showed similar results, with improvement in proxy measures of infant well-being but no clear-cut effects on more substantive outcomes. Further trials with large enough numbers are still required to evaluate whether the procedure has an effect on clinical outcome.

◆ LIMITS OF VIABILITY

There remains considerable controversy as to what constitutes the definition of the limits of viability. This is a "moving target" and the controversy will not be resolved soon. It is important to recognize that the available survival and outcome data apply to groups in general, and the risks may be greater or less for the individual under consideration. Decisions regarding active resuscitation and viability should take into consideration all the available factors, including projected birth weight, gestational age, gender, and maternal history. On many occasions the perinatal team is confronted by the imminent delivery of a patient with uncertain dates following a pregnancy with no prenatal care. Estimated birth weight and gender may be available if there is time for an ultrasound examination. Gestational age may be difficult to determine. It is apparent that the outlook is vastly different at 24$\frac{1}{7}$ weeks for a male infant who weighs 550 g than for a female infant who will weigh 900 g at 24$\frac{6}{7}$ weeks. Both are 24 weeks' gestation. The outcome data for infants according to birth weight, gestational age, and gender are presented in Figure 1–8.

There are no well-defined guidelines regarding the obstetric management of extremely low-birth-weight infants. The Fetus and Newborn Committee, Canadian Pediatric Society, Maternal-Fetal Medicine Committee, and Society of Obstetricians and Gynecologists of Canada[47] have been directive with regard to management of women with the threatened birth of an infant of extremely low gestational age. Fetuses with gestational age of less than 22 weeks are not viable and those with an age of 22 weeks are rarely viable. Their mothers are not, therefore, candidates for cesarean section, and the newborns would be provided with compassionate care, rather than active treatment. The outcomes for infants with a gestational age of 23 and 24 weeks vary greatly. Careful consideration should be given to the limited benefits for the infants versus the potential harm for the mothers of cesarean section together with the plans for resuscitation. At age 25 to 26 weeks' gestation, most

Figure 1–8. Estimated mortality by birth weight, gestational age, and gender. (Data from Stevenson DK, Wright LL, Lemons JA, et al: Very low birth weight outcomes of the National Institute of Child Health and Human Development Neonatal Research Network. January 1993 through December 1994, Am J Obstet Gynecol 179:1632, 1998.)

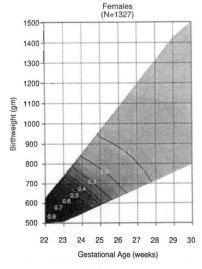

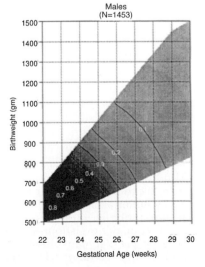

of the infants are expected to survive without severe disability. At these gestational ages, cesarean section when indicated and full neonatal resuscitation and treatment are recommended.

◆ CESAREAN SECTION FOR PREMATURE DELIVERY

Premature deliveries of very low-birth-weight infants are associated with a greatly increased incidence of breech presentations.[18] When compared with cephalic presentations, breech births, with or without associated prematurity, demonstrate increased incidence of perinatal mortality and morbidity stemming from associated birth trauma, growth retardation, prolapse of the umbilical cord, placental accidents, fetal anomalies, and multiple gestation. Whereas the overall incidence of breech presentation is only 3% to 4% of deliveries, for infants weighing less than 1500 g at birth, the incidence may be 30% or greater. An analysis of more than 30,000 deliveries at MacDonald Women's Hospital revealed that more than one fourth of all breech births occurred at or before 34 weeks' gestation.

How should the preterm breech delivery be managed? Most centers increasingly tend to use cesarean section as the mode of delivery for all but the most uncomplicated of breech presentations.[147] Because vaginal delivery of a fetus in breech presentation entails delivery of successively larger fetal parts, most complications have to be anticipated in advance. With a premature fetus, the size of the head is even greater in relation to that of the buttocks than with a term fetus, and the chance for entrapment is markedly increased. Trauma to the fetus, cord complications, or a period of hypoxia may prove particularly disastrous for a tiny infant, for whom there is a much narrower margin for error. Cesarean section as a preferable method of delivery appears at least as rational for this group as for any other category of breech deliveries.

EDITORIAL COMMENT: Breech presentation occurs in 3% to 5% of deliveries and can be managed by either a trial of vaginal breech delivery, external cephalic version (ECV), or cesarean section. A postal questionnaire was completed by 82% of Scottish consultant obstetricians and revealed wide variations in practice. One fifth of respondents apparently resorted to elective cesarean, many performed ECV before 37 weeks, even though spontaneous version might occur, and approximately 20% never performed an ECV.[193] Coco and Silverman imply that external version has made a resurgence in the past 15 years because of a strong safety record and a success rate of about 65%. They conclude that the use of external cephalic version can produce considerable cost savings in the management of the breech fetus at term. "It is a skill easily acquired by family physicians and should be a routine part of obstetric practice."[30] This does not appear to be a consensus opinion. From Norway, Albrechtsen and colleagues reported that breech and cesarean delivery lowered the subsequent pregnancy rate, probably because of the woman's decision not to reproduce. Thus, preconceptional counseling with information, support, and reassurance regarding future pregnancies and deliveries might reduce the discouraging effect. They commented on the high odds ratio of recurrence of breech, which suggests effects of recurring specific causal factors of either genetic or more permanent environmental origin.[3] Daniel and coworkers studied the umbilical cord blood acid-base values of 30 uncomplicated, vaginal breech delivery term neonates and compared them with double the number of control subjects. The values from the breech deliveries differ significantly from those of uncomplicated, cephalic-vaginal delivery neonates. The umbilical cord artery blood pH and pO_2 were significantly lower and the pCO_2 was significantly higher. These differences may represent a greater degree of acute cord compression that reflects the different mechanisms of labor in vaginal breech delivery.[38] Guidelines are required to ensure safe, consistent practice and avoid unnecessary cesarean sections for the term breech.[78]

ECV before term has been advocated at some centers, but the procedure has failed to reduce the incidence of breech birth, cesarean delivery rates, or perinatal outcome. On the other hand, the procedure has been successful at term.

An increase in perinatal mortality rate in breech delivery has been shown to correlate with birth weights in amounts decreasing from 2500 g. One study contrasted a perinatal mortality rate of 51 per 1000 in breech deliveries of term fetuses for primigravidas with a mortality rate of 310 per 1000 in breech deliveries of premature fetuses weighing between 1000 and 2499 g. Goldenberg and Nelson[58] found that during labor the premature fetus in breech presentation was 16 times more likely to die than the premature fetus in vertex presentation. Although the corrected perinatal mortality rate for breech deliveries in their study was greater than that for vertex deliveries in every weight category, the difference was greatest and statistically significant between 750 and 1500 g.

A study at MacDonald Women's Hospital demonstrated that, at each stage of gestation, the incidence of intrapartum stillbirths, neonatal deaths, and low Apgar scores increased for breech as compared with nonbreech deliveries.[18] Furthermore, from as early as 32 weeks' gestation onward, vaginal delivery could be shown to result in higher rates of perinatal loss and lower Apgar scores than did cesarean delivery. In fact, it was in the gestational period of 32 to 35 weeks that the most measurable advantage could be ascribed to cesarean delivery of the fetus in breech presentation rather than to vaginal delivery. The period covered by this study preceded many of the recent advances in neonatal care that have resulted in improved survival expectations for the tiny infant weighing 1000 to 1500 g. Few cesarean deliveries were performed before 32 weeks, and, as a consequence, there were no data available to evaluate the potential benefits of cesarean delivery for breech presentations in the gestational period of 28 to 31 weeks. Currently, more than 50% of all low-birth-weight infants are delivered by cesarean section, including the vast majority with abnormal position.

Many obstetric perinatologists, therefore, accept that modern management of premature, low-birth-weight fetuses in breech presentation includes the widespread use of cesarean delivery. Depending on the supporting neonatal services available within an institution, opinions may vary as to how early in gestation such an approach should be adopted.

More recently, with an improved outcome for smaller, less mature infants, these criteria have been expanded. The lower limits of expected weight and gestational age remain fuzzy. With the limits of viability creeping lower and a 50% survival rate anticipated as early as 24 weeks' gestation, more cesarean deliveries are performed for smaller, less mature infants than ever before. It must be acknowledged, however, that several problems with the premature fetus in breech presentation remain unsolved and merit discussion.

Cesarean delivery cannot be used for all circumstances. Many breech deliveries of very small, potentially viable infants occur after rapid, unanticipated labors in which there may be little opportunity to prepare for cesarean delivery. Furthermore, having to set a lower limit for fetal weight and gestational age, particularly in view of the known maternal risks of cesarean delivery, means that errors in judgment will occur. Infants who are larger than anticipated may be delivered vaginally when there is a desire to avoid unnecessary procedures on women who might deliver previable infants. Ultrasound cephalometry may be helpful in this regard but only when there is adequate time and accessibility to the labor suite for an accurate examination. Sonographic equipment should be readily available in the labor and delivery suites for the purpose of obtaining fetal biometry to apply to such clinical decision making. These clinical decisions should also take into account maternal considerations and it must be understood that these are subject to error.

A second problem with the more liberal use of cesarean deliveries for the premature fetus in breech presentation stems from the high incidence of associated congenital anomalies. Most series on premature breeches provide corrected perinatal mortality rates, eliminating both the high incidence of stillbirths before labor and the serious anomalies. Congenital abnormalities are more frequent in infants of breech deliveries as compared with infants of nonbreech deliveries at all durations of gestation. The MacDonald Women's Hospital data demonstrated that the percentage of congenital anomalies in infants of breech deliveries peaks at about 35 weeks and that in the period between 30 and 35 weeks the anomaly rate for infants delivered in breech presentation is 10% to 15%. This increased incidence of fetal anomalies further emphasizes the need for ultrasound equipment in the labor and delivery suite.

Chervenak et al raised the question of whether routine cesarean delivery is necessary for vertex-breech or vertex-transverse twin gestations. Analysis of a 5-year experience at Yale University documented first the high proportion (97%) of twins confirmed before labor. Seventy-eight percent of the vertex-breech and 53% of vertex-transverse twins were delivered vaginally by breech extraction for a total of 76 second twins. Infants with birth weights less than 1500 g had low 5-minute Apgar scores (67%) and accounted for the six neonatal deaths. These data support the concept of cesarean delivery for infants weighing less than 1500 g with abnormal presentations.

Extending the indications for cesarean delivery to include those described specifically for the very low-birth-weight infant creates a new set of experiences for the contemporary obstetrician. The traditional transverse lower uterine segment incision, which has proved so successful for delivery of most term infants, may not always be ideal for cesarean delivery done for extremely premature infants. This is particularly true with very small breech or twin premature fetuses.

EDITORIAL COMMENT: Malloy analyzed the mode of delivery for infants with birth weight less than 1500 g across centers in the NICHD Neonatal Research Network. He reported that 50% of infants between 750 and 1500 g were delivered by cesarean but only 33% between 501 and 749 g. When controlling for maternal and fetal factors, he failed to demonstrate a protective effect of cesarean delivery for early neonatal death or intraventricular hemorrhage.

In 1995 and 1996 the cesarean section rate in the network for infants between 501 and 1500 gm was 53% and for those between 501 and 749 gm was 44%.

The overall rate of cesarean delivery continues to spiral in the United States, another problem that urgently needs to be addressed. The Dutch have demonstrated that high-quality care can be provided by midwives. Regional data reveal a perinatal mortality rate of 2.3 in 1000 among their low-risk patients not requiring referral to an obstetrician. Furthermore, the cesarean birth rate is extraordinarily low, and neonatal seizures, an indicator of the quality of perinatal care, are noted in less than 1 in 1000 deliveries.

Other authors have reported that a companion, or doula, assisting the women during the entire labor can also reduce the need for operative intervention by 50%. Myers was able to effectively reduce the number of cesarean births by requiring a second opinion before operative delivery, establishing objective criteria for the commonest indications, and reviewing all cesarean sections and physicians' rates of doing them.[98, 126, 178]

◆

Lemons JA, Wright L, Stevenson DK, et al: Very-low-birth-weight (VLBW) outcomes of the NICHD Neonatal Research Network, January 1995 through December 1996. Pediatrics, in press.

◆ QUESTIONS

◆ *How safe are diagnostic x-ray films for the fetus and newborn?*

Much of the current knowledge of the changes caused by x-ray radiation comes from the more immediately apparent results of large doses such as those from radiation therapy, radiation accidents, and atomic bomb explosions. To estimate the longer term effects of the much lower doses derived from diagnostic radiation, one can make theoretic extrapolations from the effects of large doses or use epidemiologic methods.

The latter approach was applied to offspring of mothers who had received diagnostic x-ray films for purposes of pelvic measurement during the latter part of pregnancy. Radiation is known to possibly damage the embryo even before its implantation in the uterus. Also, during embryogenesis in early pregnancy, relatively high levels of radiation have been shown to cause anomalies in experimental animals.

◆ *What constitutes a dangerous radiation exposure for the fetus?*

Kneale and Stewart[168] noted an increased incidence of the childhood cancer after in utero doses of about 2 rads. The consensus appears to be that there is an overall increase in risk, between 40% and 50% after prenatal irradiation of approximately 1 to 4 rads. Moore reported that approximately 15% of pregnant women undergo x-ray examination during pregnancy.

◆ *Is it possible to induce leukemia by diagnostic x-ray films? Are premature infants at greater risk?*

In this regard, evidence exists that mothers of leukemic children had been radiographed more frequently during the relevant pregnancy than those of normal children. The studies that showed this increased risk for leukemia, which may be as much as twofold, have been challenged by some because of unavoidable statistical bias. A case-controlled study of twins by Harvey and associates[72] found that twins in whom leukemia or other childhood cancer developed were twice as likely to have been exposed to x-rays in utero as twins who were free of disease.

In a chronologic sense the premature infant can be considered to be a fetus and some organ systems may be immature. It is doubtful, however, that the risk of induction of malignancies per unit of absorbed dose differs significantly in the fetus from that of adults who have also had whole body exposures. Moreover, most of the radiographic exposures of newborn infants concentrate on specific regions of the body, most often the chest, rather than the entire body. Consequently, fewer of the critical blood-forming areas of the newborn are exposed than would be the case during intrauterine life. Incidentally, the characteristics of scattered radiation are such that exposure of a carefully composed radiograph will result in negligible radiation of a neighboring patient.

Although it can be stated that there is an increased risk of inducing malignancy by radiation, even at very low levels, this risk is small when compared with the probability of cancer occurring naturally. The risk becomes more acceptable when it is appreciated in terms of the increased risk of morbidity or mortality that would result from not obtaining diagnostic x-ray studies from critically ill infants. Theoretically, during a lifetime, nearly 2000 chest radiographs would be necessary to cause any appreciable increase in probability of occurrence of a fatal malignancy over the natural incidence.

It has been only in relatively recent years that large numbers of premature babies have survived. The more immediate effects of the various medical advances necessary for this increased survival are currently becoming known. However, the latency period between delivery and effect of low-dose diagnostic radiation is measured in years and decades. Although one can be optimistic, the eventual outcome is unknown. In the meantime, it is up to the many concerned neonatologists, radiologists, and technicians to improve radiographic techniques, to substitute less invasive methods whenever possible, and to exercise care and judgment in the use of diagnostic radiation for this fragile portion of the human population.

EDITORIAL COMMENT: Wilson-Costello et al examined the radiation doses from radiographs of infants of less than 750 g birth weight. The infants had a mean of 31 radiographs performed. Nonetheless, she concluded that the radiation doses were small in comparison with the range of doses that form the basis of risk estimates for cancer. Infants with chronic lung disease and necrotizing enterocolitis were exposed to the largest doses and the surface organs (skin, breast, and thyroid) received the largest radiation doses. We should protect the gonads whenever possible at the time of the radiograph.

◆

Wilson-Costello D, Rao PS, Morrison S, Hack M: Radiation exposure from diagnostic radiographs in extremely low birth weight infants. Pediatrics 97:369–374, 1996.

◆ When should a fetus be delivered if the NST is nonreactive?

In interpreting any assessment of fetal well-being, the whole pregnancy profile should always be reviewed before any judgments concerning intervention are made. Following are indications for delivery with a nonreactive NST:

- ◆ Persistently nonreactive NST followed by a biophysical profile of less than 4 or a positive contraction stress test (CST).
- ◆ Oligohydramnios in term or post-term fetus. (The definition of oligohydramnios is based on the ultrasound and includes the semiquantitative assessment wherein a four-quadrant sum of less than 5 cm is considered abnormal.)
- ◆ Variable decelerations in the presence of oligohydramnios. (In general, if there are variable decelerations during the NST in a term infant, a CST is done. If the CST accentuates variables, then deliver; if it does not, manage expectantly.)
- ◆ Any significant decelerations in a fetus past 42 weeks' gestation.

◆ Which tocolytic agents should be used for the pregnant woman with insulin-dependent diabetes?

Maternal side effects are inevitable with β-mimetic drug treatment and are accentuated in the woman with diabetes. If tocolysis is indicated in a diabetic pregnancy, IV magnesium sulfate has been recommended. Parenteral β-agonists may produce hyperglycemia, lactic acidosis, hypokalemia, and diabetic ketoacidosis. Furthermore, their chronotropic effects on the maternal myocardium preclude their use in pregnant women with insulin-dependent diabetes and vascular disease.

◆ How frequently are diagnostic ultrasound, x-ray examinations, and electronic fetal monitors used?

Currently, almost 80% of pregnancies receive an ultrasound during pregnancy and

58% of women have two or more ultrasound examinations. The most common indication is to establish dates and gestational age. Of pregnant women surveyed, 15% underwent x-ray examination and 75% were monitored electronically during labor (55% with external monitors, 20% with internal monitors).[121]

EDITORIAL COMMENT: In the United States, almost every pregnant woman has at least one ultrasound at around 18 to 20 weeks. An anatomic survey is done at this time.

◆ TRUE OR FALSE

◆ Ultrasonography may produce major anatomic malformations in the fetus.

Diagnostic ultrasonography is performed millions of times annually in the United States for fetal visualization and gestational aging. The Food and Drug Administration issued a report (8.2:8190) expressing concerns about ultrasonography. Very high-intensity sound produces biologic effects.[5] Mouse tissue exposed to pulsed ultrasound, similar to the intensity used in most commercial ultrasound instruments, reveals tissue changes. Whether these results apply to human tissue cells is unknown. Although acute dramatic effects are unlikely, less obvious long-term or cumulative effects remain unexplored. Furthermore, even assuming there is a small biologic risk from ultrasound, the benefits far outweigh any such risk. The statement is false, but there is never room for complacency.

◆ Diminished amniotic fluid has a serious implication for the fetus.

Reduced amniotic fluid is defined by ultrasound when no vertical pool measures 30 mm.[37] The best definition of oligohydramnios is based on the four-quadrant amniotic fluid index, a semiquantitative form of amniotic fluid volume assessment. A four-quadrant sum of 5 cm or greater is considered normal. The association between oligohydramnios and renal anomalies has long been recognized. Mercer et al[112] reviewed ultrasound for detection of diminished amniotic fluid and eliminated those cases secondary to rupture of membranes. A 7% malformation rate was noted, and if diminished amniotic fluid was present before 27 weeks, outcome was poorer. Crowley et al[36] noted

more meconium staining, fetal distress, and growth retardation in pregnancies with decreased amniotic fluid. The statement is true.

◆ Amniocentesis should be a routine part of the management of patients with PROM.

Some investigators would support this notion because knowledge of the L:S ratio, Gram stains, and quantitative colony counts would dictate further management policies. Thus, if the L:S ratio is mature or the Gram stain shows evidence of bacteria, regardless of gestational age, delivery is expedited. Not everyone would agree that amniocentesis should be routine even with ultrasound guidance. The statement is false.

◆ Amniocentesis and determination of alpha-fetoprotein should be performed in pregnancies subsequent to one that produced an infant with a neural tube defect.

Open neural tube defects have an increased recurrence rate of 1 in 20 with a previously affected child, and this risk is even greater when two previous children have been affected. Routine antenatal screening of amniotic fluid alpha-fetoprotein concentration together with careful ultrasonographic study of the fetus is thus recommended in such pregnancies.[115] The statement is true.

◆ Women with gestational diabetes may contribute significantly more to perinatal mortality than do women with insulin-dependent diabetes.

Because the incidence of gestational diabetes far exceeds that of the overt form, its potential impact on perinatal outcome for a defined population may be more significant. It has been estimated that many pregnancies in the United States have resulted in perinatal death from undiagnosed or untreated gestational diabetes. Therefore, the importance of screening for abnormal glucose tolerance during pregnancy must be reemphasized.[154] In identification of the woman with gestational diabetes, suggestive clinical features include a family history of diabetes, a prior delivery of a baby weighing more than 4000 g, maternal obesity, a prior unexplained stillbirth, neonatal death, or major fetal anomaly. Glucose in a second fasting urine specimen and clinical hydramnios are additional factors that raise the index of suspicion during pregnancy. The statement is true.

REFERENCES

1. ACOG Educational Bulletin 230, November 1996.
2. Albrechtsen S, Rasmussen S, Dalaker K, Irgens LM: Reproductive career after breech presentation: Subsequent pregnancy rates, interpregnancy interval, and recurrence. Obstet Gynecol 92:345–350, 1998.
3. Alexander GR, Himes JH, Kaufman RB, et al: A United States national reference for fetal growth. Obstet Gynecol 87:163, 1996.
4. Ashwood ER, Palmer SE, Taylor JS, Pingree SS: Lamellar body counts for rapid total lung maturity testing. Obstet Gynecol 81:619–624, 1993.
5. Baker ML, Dalrymple GV: Biological effects of diagnostic ultrasound: A review. Radiology 126:479, 1978.
6. Bakketeig LS, Jacobsen G, Brodtkorb CJ, et al: Randomized controlled trial of ultrasonographic screening in pregnancy. Lancet 2:207, 1984.
7. Ballard RA, et al: Antenatal thyrotropin-releasing hormone to prevent lung disease in preterm infants. North American Thyrotropin-Releasing Hormone Study Group. N Engl J Med 338:493, 1998.
8. Banks BA, Cnaan A, Morgman MA, et al: Multiple courses of antenatal corticosteroids and outcome of premature neonates. North American Thyrotropin-Releasing Hormone Study Group. Am J Obstet Gynecol 181:709, 1999.
9. Barden TP, Peter JB, Merkatz IR: Ritodrine hydrochloride: A betamimetic agent for use in preterm labor. I. Pharmacology, clinical history, administration, side effects and safety. Obstet Gynecol 56:1, 1980.
10. Baud O, Foix-L'Helias L, Kaminski M, et al: Antenatal glucocorticoid treatment and cystic periventricular leukomalacia in very premature infants. N Engl J Med 341:1190, 1999.
11. Bauer C, Stern L, Colle E: Prolonged rupture of membranes associated with a decreased incidence of respiratory distress syndrome. Pediatrics 53:7, 1974.
12. Beard R, Morris E, Clayton S: pH of foetal capillary blood as an indicator of the condition of the foetus. J Obstet Gynaecol Br Cwlth 74:812, 1967.
13. Beard R, Roberts G: A prospective approach to the diagnosis of intrauterine growth retardation. Proc R Soc Med 63:501, 1970.
14. Bennett MJ, Little G, Dewhurst Sir J, et al: Predictive value of ultrasound measurement in early pregnancy: A randomized controlled trial. Br J Obstet Gynaecol 89:338, 1982.
15. Bishop E, Wouterez T: Isoxsuprine, a myometrial relaxant. Obstet Gynecol 17:442, 1961.
16. Bottoms SF, the National Institute of Child Health and Human Development Network of Maternal-Fetal Medicine Units: Obstetric determinants of neonatal survival: Influence of willingness to perform cesarean delivery on survival of extremely low-birth-weight infants. Am J Obstet Gynecol 176:960, 1997.
17. Bouyer J, Papiernik E, Dreyfus J: Prevention of preterm birth and perinatal risk reduction. Isr J Med Sci 22:313, 1986.
18. Brenner W, Bruce R, Hendricks C: The characteristics and perils of breech presentation. Am J Obstet Gynecol 118:700, 1974.
19. Bross I, Natarajan N: Genetic damage from diagnostic radiation. JAMA 237:2399, 1977.
20. Campbell S, Warsof SL, Little D, Cooper DJ: Routine ultrasound screening for the prediction of gestational age. Obstet Gynecol 65:613, 1985.
21. Caritis SN, Edelstone DI, Mueller-Heubach EA: Pharmacologic inhibition of preterm labor. Am J Obstet Gynecol 133:557, 1979.
22. Carrera JM, Torrents M, Mortera C, Cusi V, Muñoz A: Routine prenatal ultrasound screening for fetal abnormalities: 22 years' experience. Ultrasound Obstet Gynecol 5:174, 1995.
23. Casals E, Fortuny A, Grudzinskas JG, et al: First-trimester biochemical screening for Down syndrome with the use of pAPP-A, AFP, and β-hCG. Prenat Diagn 6:405, 1996.
24. Castrén O, Gummerus M, Saarikoski S: Treatment of imminent premature labor. Acta Obstet Gynecol Scand 54:95, 1975.
25. Chalmers I, Enkin M, Keirse MJN, eds: Effective Care in Pregnancy and Childbirth. Oxford, England: Oxford University Press, 1989.
26. Chapman SJ, et al: Benefits of maternal corticosteroid therapy in infants weighing ≤1000 grams at birth after preterm rupture of amnion. Am J Obstet Gynecol 180:677, 1999.
27. Chard T, Yoon A, Macintosh M: The myth of fetal growth retardation at term. Br J Obstet Gynaecol 100:1076, 1993.
28. Clark SL, Sabey P, Jolley K: Non-stress testing with acoustic stimulation and amniotic fluid volume assessment: 5973 tests without unexpected fetal death. Am J Obstet Gynecol 160:694, 1989.
29. Clements J, Platzker A, Tierney D, et al: Assessment of the risk of the respiratory distress syndrome by a rapid test for surfactant in amniotic fluid. N Engl J Med 286:1077, 1972.
30. Coco AS, Silverman SD: External cephalic version. Am Fam Physician 58:731, 742, 1998.
31. Collaborative Santiago Surfactant Group: Collaborative trial of prenatal thyrotropin-releasing hormone and corticosteroids for prevention of respiratory distress syndrome. Am J Obstet Gynecol 178: 33, 1998.
32. Cooper RL, Goldenberg RL, Das A, et al: The preterm prediction study: Maternal stress is associated with spontaneous preterm birth at less than thirty-five weeks' gestation. Am J Obstet Gynecol 175:1286, 1996.
33. Corwin MJ, Mou SM, Sunderji SG, et al: Multicenter randomized clinical trial of home uterine activity monitoring: Pregnancy outcomes for all women randomized. Am J Obstet Gynecol 175:1281, 1996.
34. Creasy R, Gummer B, Liggins G: System for predicting spontaneous preterm birth. Obstet Gynecol 55:692, 1980.
35. Creasy RK, Resnik R, eds: Maternal-Fetal Medicine: Principles and Practice. 3rd ed. Philadelphia: WB Saunders, 1998.
36. Crowley P, O'Herlihy C, Boylan P, et al: The value of ultrasound measurement of amniotic fluid volume in the management of prolonged pregnancies. Br J Obstet Gynaecol 91:444, 1984.
37. Crowther CA, Hill JE, Haslam RR, Robinson JS: Australian Collaborative Trial of Antenatal Thyrotropin-Releasing Hormone: Adverse effects at 12 month follow-up. ACTOBAT Study Group. Pediatrics 99:311, 1997.

38. Daniel Y, Fait G, Lessing JB, et al: Umbilical cord blood acid-base values in uncomplicated term vaginal breech deliveries. Acta Obstet Gynecol Scand 77:182, 1998.

39. Davey DA, MacGillivray I: The classification and definition of the hypertensive disorders of pregnancy. Am J Obstet Gynecol 158:892, 1988.

40. David RJ, Siegel E: Decline in neonatal mortality, 1968 to 1977: Better babies or better care? Pediatrics 71:531, 1983.

41. D'Ottavio G, Meir YJ, Rustico MA, et al: Screening for fetal anomalies by ultrasound at 14 and 21 weeks. Ultrasound Obstet Gynecol 110:375, 1997.

42. Drillien C: The small-for-dates infant: Etiology and prognosis. Pediatr Clin North Am 17:9, 1970.

43. Egarter C, Leitich H, Karas H, et al: Antibiotic treatment in preterm premature rupture of membranes and neonatal morbidity: A meta-analysis. Am J Obstet Gynecol 174:589, 1996.

44. Fairbrother P, VanCoeverden De Groot H, Coetzee E, et al: The significance of prelabour type II deceleration of fetal heart rate in relation to Braxton-Hicks contractions. S Afr Med J 48:2391, 1974.

45. Fanaroff AA, Martin RM, Miller MJ: Identification and management of high-risk problems in the neonate. In Creasy RK, Resnik R, eds: Maternal-Fetal Medicine. 5th ed. Orlando: WB Saunders, 1998.

46. Fanaroff A, Merkatz I: Modern obstetrical management of the low birth weight infant. Clin Perinatol 4:215, 1977.

47. Fetus and Newborn Committee, Canadian Pediatric Society: Management of the woman with threatened birth of an infant of extremely low gestational age. Can Med Assoc J 151:547, 1994.

48. Fretts RC, Boyd ME, Usher RH, Usher HA: The changing pattern of fetal death, 1961–1988. Obstet Gynecol 79:35, 1992.

48a. Fuhrman K, Reiber H, Semmler K, et al: Prevention of congenital malformations in infants of insulin-dependent diabetic mothers. Diabetes Care 6:219, 1983.

49. Gagnon RJ, Patrick J, Foreman J, et al: Stimulation of human fetuses with sound and vibration. Am J Obstet Gynecol 155:848, 1986.

50. Garite TJ, Freeman RK, Linzey EM, et al: Prospective randomized study of corticosteroids in the management of premature rupture of the membranes and premature gestation. Am J Obstet Gynecol 141:508, 1981.

51. Gellis S, Hsia D: The infant of the diabetic mother. Am J Dis Child 97:1, 1959.

52. Gluck L: Modern Perinatal Medicine. Chicago: Year Book Medical, 1974.

53. Gluck L, Kulovich MV, Borer RC Jr, et al: Diagnosis of respiratory distress by amniocentesis. Am J Obstet Gynecol 109:440, 1971.

54. Gluck L, Kulovich M: Lecithin-sphingomyelin ratios in amniotic fluid in normal and abnormal pregnancy. Am J Obstet Gynecol 115:539, 1973.

55. Golbus MS, Loughman WD, Epstein CJ, et al: Prenatal genetic diagnosis in 3,000 amniocenteses. N Engl J Med 300:157, 1979.

56. Goldenberg RL for the NICHD Maternal Fetal Medicine Units Network: The preterm prediction study: Fetal fibronectin testing and spontaneous preterm birth. Obstet Gynecol 87:643, 1996.

57. Goldenberg RL, Iams JD, Mercer BM, et al for the Maternal-Fetal Medicine Units Network of the National Institute of Child Health and Human Development, Bethesda, MD: The preterm prediction study: The value of new vs standard risk factors in predicting early and all spontaneous preterm births. Am J Public Health 88:233, 1998.

58. Goldenberg R, Nelson K: The premature breech. Am J Obstet Gynecol 127:240, 1977.

59. Goldenberg RL, Rouse DJ: Prevention of premature birth. N Engl J Med 339:313, 1998.

60. Goodwin J, Dunne J, Thomas B: Antepartum identification of the fetus at risk. Can Med Assoc J 101:458, 1969.

61. Grant A, Elbourne D, Valentin L, Alexander S: Routine formal fetal movement counting and risk of antepartum late death in normally formed singletons. Lancet 2:345, 1989.

62. Grant A, Penn ZJ, Steer PJ: Elective or selective caesarean delivery of the small baby? A systematic review of the controlled trials. Br J Obstet Gynaecol 103:1197, 1996.

63. Gregg E: Radiation risks with diagnostic x-rays. Radiology 123:447, 1977.

64. Gruenwald P: Infants of low birth weight among 5,000 deliveries. Pediatrics 34:157, 1964.

65. Guidetti DA, Divon MY, Braverman JJ, et al: Sonographic estimates of fetal weight in the intrauterine growth retardation population. Am J Perinatol 7:5, 1990.

66. Gyves M, Rodman H, Little A, et al: A modern approach to management of pregnant diabetics: A two-year analysis of perinatal outcomes. Am J Obstet Gynecol 128:606, 1977.

67. Hack M, Fanaroff A, Klaus M, et al: Neonatal respiratory distress following elective delivery—A preventable disease? Am J Obstet Gynecol 126:43, 1976.

68. Haddow JE, Palomaki GE, Knight GJ, et al: Screening of maternal serum for fetal Down's syndrome in the first trimester. N Engl J Med 338:955, 1998.

69. Harrison MR, Adzick NS, Longaker MT, et al: Successful repair in utero of a fetal diaphragmatic hernia after removal of herniated viscera from the left thorax. N Engl J Med 322:1582, 1990.

70. Harrison MR, Filly RA, Golbus MS, et al: Fetal treatment. N Engl J Med 307:1651, 1982.

71. Harrison MR, Golbus MS, Filly RA: The Unborn Patient: Prenatal Diagnosis and Treatment. New York: Grune & Stratton, 1984.

72. Harvey EB, Boice JD, Honeyman J, et al: Prenatal x-ray exposure and childhood cancer in twins. N Engl J Med 312:541, 1985.

73. Hobbins J, Grannum P, Romero R, et al: Percutaneous umbilical blood sampling. Am J Obstet Gynecol 152:1, 1985.

74. Hobel C: Recognition of the high-risk pregnant woman. In Spellacy W, ed: Management of the High-Risk Pregnancy. Baltimore: University Park Press, 1975, p 1.

75. Hofmeyer GJ: Overviews of amnioinfusion. In Chalmers I, Enkin M, Keirse MJN, eds: Effective Care in Pregnancy and Childbirth. Oxford, England: Oxford University Press, 1989.

76. Hsick FJ, Chen D, Tsing LH: Limb-reduction defects and chorion villus sampling. Lancet 337:1091, 1991.

77. Iams JD, et al: The preterm prediction study: Recurrence risk of spontaneous preterm birth. National Institute of Child Health and Human Development Maternal-Fetal Medicine Units Network. Am J Obstet Gynecol 178:1035, 1998.

78. Irion O, Almagbaly PH, Morabia A: Planned vaginal delivery versus elective caesarean section: A study of 705 singleton term breech presentations. Br J Obstet Gynaecol 105:710, 1998.
79. Jackson M, Rose NC: Diagnosis and management of fetal nuchal translucency. Semin Roentgenol 33:333, 1998.
80. Karlsson K, Kjellmer I: The outcome of diabetic pregnancies in relation to the mother's blood sugar level. Am J Obstet Gynecol 112:213, 1972.
81. Keirse MJNC, Grant A, King JF: Preterm labour. In Chalmers I, Enkin M, Keirse MJN, eds: Effective Care in Pregnancy and Childbirth. Oxford, England: Oxford University Press, 1989.
82. Keith RDF, Beckley S, Garibaldi JM, et al: A multicentre comparative study of 17 experts and an intelligent computer system for managing labour using the cardiotocogram. Br J Obstet Gynaecol 102:688, 1995.
83. Kimberlin DF, et al: Indicated versus spontaneous preterm delivery: An evaluation of neonatal morbidity among infants weighing ≤1000 grams at birth. Am J Obstet Gynecol 180:683, 1999.
84. Kimberlin DF, et al: The effect of maternal magnesium sulfate treatment on neonatal morbidity in ≤1000 gram infants. Am J Perinatol 15:635, 1998.
85. Kitzmiller JL, Gavin LA, Gin GD, et al: Preconception care of diabetes: Glycemic control prevents congenital anomalies. JAMA 265:731, 1991.
86. Kramer MS, Oliver M, McLean FH, et al: Impact of intrauterine growth retardation and body proportionality on fetal and neonatal outcome. Pediatrics 86:707, 1990.
87. Krebs HB, Petres RE, Dunn IJ, et al: Intrapartum fetal heart rate monitoring. I. Classification and prognosis of fetal heart rate patterns. Am J Obstet Gynecol 133:762, 1979.
88. Lauersen N, Merkatz I, Tejani N, et al: Inhibition of premature labor: A multicenter comparison of ritodrine and ethanol. Am J Obstet Gynecol 127:837, 1977.
89. Lenke RR: Use of nipple stimulation to obtain contraction stress test. Obstet Gynecol 63:345, 1984.
90. Liebeskind D, Bases R, Elequin F, et al: Diagnostic ultrasound: Effects on the DNA and growth patterns of animal cells. Radiology 131:177, 1979.
91. Liggins G: Prenatal glucocorticoid treatment: Prevention of respiratory distress syndrome. In Moore T: Report of the 70th Ross Conference on Pediatric Research. Columbus, OH: Ross Laboratories, 1976, p 97.
92. Lockwood CJ, Senyei AE, Dische MR, et al: Fetal fibronectin in cervical and vaginal secretions as a predictor of preterm delivery. N Engl J Med 325:669, 1991.
93. Lovett SM, Weiss JD, Diogo MJ, et al: A prospective, double-blind, randomized, controlled clinical trial of ampicillin-sulbactam for preterm premature rupture of membranes in women receiving antenatal corticosteroid therapy. Am J Obstet Gynecol 176:1030, 1997.
94. Low JA, Cox MJ, Karchmar EJ, et al: The prediction of intrapartum fetal metabolic acidosis by fetal heart rate monitoring. Am J Obstet Gynecol 135:299, 1981.
95. MRC Working Party on the Evaluation of Chorionic Villus Sampling: Medical Research Council European Trial of Chorion Villus Sampling. Lancet 337:1491, 1991.
96. Main DM, Richardson D, Gabbe SG, et al: Prospective evaluation of a risk scoring system for predicting preterm delivery in black inner city women. Obstet Gynecol 79:61, 1987; Perinatal Trials, 1990.
97. Malak TM, Sizmur F, Bell SC, et al: Fetal fibronectin in cervicovaginal secretions as a predictor of preterm birth. Br J Obstet Gynaecol 104:648, 1996.
98. Malloy MH, Onstad L, Wright E: Cesarean sections and birth outcome for very low birthweight infants. Obstet Gynecol 77:498, 1991.
99. Manning FA, et al: Fetal assessment based on fetal biophysical profile scoring: Experience in 19,221 referred high-risk pregnancies. II. Am J Obstet Gynecol 157:880, 1987.
100. March of Dimes Birth Defects Foundation, Committee on Perinatal Care: Toward improving the outcome of pregnancy: The 90s and beyond. New York: March of Dimes Birth Defects Foundation, 1993.
101. Margulis A: The lessons of radiobiology for diagnostic radiology. Am J Roentgenol 117:741, 1973.
102. Mazzi E, Herrera A, Herbert L: Neonatal intensive care and radiation. Johns Hopkins Med J 142:15, 1978.
103. McCallum WD, Williams CS, Napel S, et al: Fetal blood velocity waveform. Am J Obstet Gynecol 127:491, 1978.
104. McCormick M: Trends in rates of low birthweight in the United States. In Berendes HW, Kessel S, Yaffe S, eds: Advances in the Prevention of Low Birthweight. Washington, DC: National Center for Education in Maternal and Child Health, 1991.
105. McGregor JA: Salivary estriol as risk assessment for preterm labor: A prospective trial. Am J Obstet Gynecol 173:1337, 1995.
106. McGregor JA, French H, Parker R, et al: Prevention of premature birth by screening and treatment for common genital tract infections: Results of a prospective controlled evaluation. Am J Obstet Gynecol 173:157, 1995.
107. McKenna DS, et al: Effect of digital cervical examination on the expression of fetal fibronectin. J Reprod Med 44:796, 1999.
108. Meade TW, Ammala P, Aynsley-Green A, et al: Medical Research Council European Trial of Chorion Villus Sampling. Lancet 337:1491, 1991.
109. Meis PJ, et al: The preterm prediction study: Risk factors for indicated preterm births. Maternal-Fetal Medicine Units Network of the National Institute of Child Health and Human Development. Am J Obstet Gynecol 178:562, 1998.
110. Mercer BM: Management of preterm premature rupture of the membranes. Clin Obstet 41:870, 1998.
111. Mercer BM, Miodovnik M, Thurnau GR, et al: Antibiotic therapy for reduction of infant morbidity after preterm premature rupture of the membranes. A randomized controlled trial. National Institute of Child Health and Human Development Maternal-Fetal Medicine Units Network. JAMA 278:989, 1997.
112. Mercer LJ, Brown LG, Petres RE, et al: A survey of pregnancies complicated by decreased amniotic fluid. Am J Obstet Gynecol 149:355, 1984.
113. Merkatz IR, Fanaroff A: The regional perinatal network. In Sweeney W, Caplan R, eds: Advances in Obstetrics and Gynecology. Vol II. Baltimore: Williams & Wilkins, 1978, p 1.

114. Merkatz IR, Johnson K: Regionalization of perinatal care for the United States. Clin Perinatol 3:271, 1976.

115. Merkatz IR, Aladjem S, Little B: The value of biochemical estimations on amniotic fluid in management of the high-risk pregnancy. Clin Perinatol 1:301, 1974.

116. Merkatz IR, Nitowsky HM, Macri JM, et al: An association between low maternal serum alpha-fetoprotein and fetal chromosome abnormalities. Am J Obstet Gynecol 148:886, 1984.

117. Milunsky A: Symposium on the management of the high-risk pregnancy. Clin Perinatol 1:2, 1974.

118. Milunsky A, et al: Predictive values, relative risks, and overall benefits of high and low maternal alpha fetoprotein screening in singleton pregnancies: New epidemiologic data. Am J Obstet Gynecol 161:291, 1989.

119. Möller E: Studies in Diabetic Pregnancy. Lund: Student Literature, 1970.

120. Monson RR, MacMahon B: Prenatal x-ray exposure and cancer in children. In Boice JD, Faumeni JF, eds: Radiation Carcinogenesis: Epidemiology and Biologic Significance. New York: Raven Press, 1984, p 97.

121. Moore RM, Jeng LL, Kaczmarek RG, Placek PJ: Use of diagnostic ultrasound, x-ray examinations, and electronic fetal monitoring in perinatal medicine. J Perinatol 10:361, 1990.

122. Moore T: Lung maturation and the prevention of hyaline membrane disease. In Report of 70th Ross Conference on Pediatric Research. Columbus, OH: Ross Laboratories, 1976.

123. Moore TR, Piacquadio K: A prospective assessment on fetal movement screening to reduce fetal mortality. Am J Obstet Gynecol 160:1075, 1989.

124. Morrison JJ, Rennie JM, Milton PJ: Neonatal respiratory morbidity and mode of delivery at term: Influence of timing of elective caesarean section. Br J Obstet Gynaecol 102:101, 1995.

125. Mueller-Heuback E, Reddick D, Barnett B, Bente R: Preterm birth prevention: Evaluation of a prospective controlled randomized trial. Am J Obstet Gynecol 160:1172, 1989.

126. Myers SA, Gleicher N: A successful program to lower cesarean section rates. N Engl J Med 319:1511, 1988.

127. Nadel AS, Green JK, Holmes LB, et al: Absence of need for amniocentesis in patients with elevated levels of maternal serum alpha-fetoprotein and normal ultrasonographic examinations. N Engl J Med 323:557, 1990.

128. Nageotte MP, Freeman RK, Garite TJ, Dorchester W: Prophylactic intrapartum amnioinfusion in patients with preterm rupture of membranes. Am J Obstet Gynecol 153:557, 1985.

129. Nageotte MP, Towers CV, Asrat T, et al: The value of a negative antepartum test: Contraction stress test and modified biophysical profile. Obstet Gynecol 84:231, 1994.

130. National Institutes of Health Consensus Development Panel on the Effect of Corticosteroids for Fetal Maturation on Perinatal Outcomes: Effect of corticosteroids for fetal maturation on perinatal outcomes. JAMA 273:413, 1995.

131. Neilson JP: Assessment of fetal nuchal translucency test for Down's syndrome. Lancet 350:754, 1997.

132. Nelson LH, Anderson RL, O'Shea TM, Swain M: Expectant management of preterm premature rupture of membranes. Am J Obstet Gynecol 171:350, 1994.

133. Nesbitt R Jr, Aubrey R: High-risk obstetrics. II. Value of semi-objective grading system in identifying the vulnerable group. Am J Obstet Gynecol 103:972, 1969.

134. Newham JP, Godfrey M, Walters BJN, et al: Low dose aspirin for the treatment of fetal growth restriction: A randomized controlled trial. Aust N Z J Obstet Gynaecol 35:370, 1995.

135. O'Driscoll K, Foley M: Correlation of decrease in perinatal mortality and increase in cesarean section rates. Obstet Gynecol 61:1, 1983.

136. Ohel G, Horowitz E, Lander N, et al: Neonatal auditory acuity following in utero vibratory acoustic stimulation. Am J Gynecol 157:440, 1987.

137. Pajkrt E, van Lith JM, Mol BW, et al: Screening for Down's syndrome by fetal nuchal translucency measurement in a general obstetric population. Ultrasound Obstet Gynecol 12:163, 1998.

138. Pandya PP, Snijders RJM, Johnson SP, et al: Screening for fetal trisomies by maternal age and fetal nuchal translucency thickness at 10–14 weeks' gestation. Br J Obstet Gynaecol 102:957, 1995.

139. Paneth N, Keily JL, Wallenstein S, Susser M: The choice of place of delivery: Effect of hospital level on mortality in all singleton births in New York City. Am J Dis Child 141:60, 1987.

140. Parry S, Strauss JF III: Premature rupture of the fetal membranes. N Engl J Med 338:663, 1998.

141. Peaceman AM, Andrews WW, Thorp JM, et al: Fetal fibronectin as a predictor of preterm birth in patients with symptoms: A multicenter trial. Am J Obstet Gynecol 177:13, 1997.

142. Pederson J: The Pregnant Diabetic and Her Newborn: Problems and Management. Baltimore: Williams & Wilkins, 1967.

143. Petrie R, ed: Fetal monitoring. Clin Perinatol 9:231, 1982.

144. Phelan JP, Smith CV, Broussard P, et al: Amniotic fluid volume assessment using the four-quadrant technique in the pregnancy between 36 and 42 weeks gestation. J Reprod Med 32:540, 1987.

145. Phibbs CS, Bronstein JM, Buxton E, Phibbs RH: The effects of patient volume and level of care at the hospital of birth on neonatal mortality. JAMA 276:1054, 1996.

146. Pochin E: Radiology now: Malignancies following low radiation exposures in man. Br J Radiol 49:577, 1976.

147. Pritchard J, MacDonald P: Williams' Obstetrics. 15th ed. New York: Appleton-Century-Crofts, 1976.

148. Ray M, Freeman R, Pine S, et al: Clinical experience with the oxytocin challenge test. Am J Obstet Gynecol 114:1, 1972.

149. Reed NN, Mohajer MP, Sahota DS, et al: The potential impact of PR interval analysis of the fetal electrocardiogram [FECG] on intrapartum fetal monitoring. Eur J Obstet Gynecol Reprod Biol 68:87, 1996.

150. Rhoads GG, Jackson LG, Schlesselman SE, et al: The safety and efficacy of chorionic villus sampling for early prenatal diagnosis of cytogenetic abnormalities. N Engl J Med 320:609, 1989.

151. Richards DS, Cefalo RC, Thorpe JM, et al: Determinants of fetal heart rate response to vibroacous-

tic stimulation in labor. Obstet Gynecol 71:535, 1988.

152. Rochard F, Schifrin B, Goupil F, et al: Non-stressed fetal heart rate monitoring in the antepartum period. Am J Obstet Gynecol 126:699, 1976.

153. Rodeck CH: Fetoscopy and the prenatal diagnosis of inherited conditions. J Genet Hum 28:41, 1980.

154. Rodman H, Gyves M, Fanaroff A, et al: The diabetic pregnancy as a model for modern perinatal care. In New M, Fiser R Jr, eds: Diabetes and Other Endocrine Disorders During Pregnancy and in the Newborn: Progress in Clinical and Biological Research. Vol 10. New York: Alan R Liss, 1976.

155. Rotschild A, Ling EW, Puterman ML, Farquharson D: Neonatal outcome after premature rupture of the membranes. Am J Obstet Gynecol 162:46, 1990.

156. Ryan G: Toward improving the outcome of pregnancy: Recommendations for the regional development of perinatal health services. Obstet Gynecol 46:375, 1975.

157. Saari-Kemppainen A, Karjalainen O, Ylosalo P, Heinonen OP: Ultrasound screening and perinatal mortality: Controlled trial of systematic one-stage screening in pregnancy. (The Helsinki Ultrasound Trial). Lancet 336:387, 1990.

158. Schifrin B, Lapidus M, Doctor G, et al: Contraction stress test for antepartum fetal evaluation. Obstet Gynecol 45:433, 1975.

159. Sher G, Statland BE, Freer DE, Kraybill EN: Assessing fetal lung maturation by the foam stability index test. Obstet Gynecol 52:673, 1978.

160. Shy K, Luthy DA, Bennett FC, et al: Effects of fetal heart rate monitoring as compared with periodic auscultation, on the neurologic development of premature infants. N Engl J Med 322:588, 1990.

161. Simpson JL, Elias S, Martin AO, et al: Diabetes in pregnancy. Northwestern University series (1977–1981). I. Prospective study of anomalies in offspring of mothers with diabetes mellitus. Am J Obstet Gynecol 146:263, 1983.

162. Smith CV, Phelan JP, Platt LD, et al: Fetal acoustic stimulation testing. II. A randomized clinical trial with the non-stress test. Am J Obstet Gynecol 155:131, 1986.

163. Smith GCS, Smith MFS, McNay MMB, Fleming JEE: First-trimester growth and the risk of low birth weight. N Engl J Med 339:1817, 1998.

164. Snijders RJM, Noble P, Sebire N, et al for the Fetal Medicine Foundation First Trimester Screening Group: UK multicenter project on assessment of risk of trisomy 21 by maternal age and fetal nuchal translucency thickness at 10–14 weeks of gestation. Lancet 352:343, 1998.

165. Soothill PW, Bilardo CM, Nicolaides KH, et al: Relation of fetal hypoxia in growth retardation to mean blood velocity in the fetal aorta. Lancet 2:1118, 1986.

166. Steel JM, Johnstone FD, Hepburn DA, et al: Can pre-pregnancy care of diabetic women reduce the risks of abnormal babies? BMJ 301:1070, 1990.

167. Stevenson DK, Wright LL, Lemons JA, et al: Very low birth weight outcomes of the National Institute of Child Health and Human Development Neonatal Research Network, January 1993 through December 1994. Am J Obstet Gynecol 179:1632, 1998.

168. Stewart AM, Kneale GW: Radiation dose effects in relation to obstetric x-rays and childhood cancers. Lancet 1:1185, 1970.

169. Strong TH Jr, Hetzler LG, Sarno AP, Paul RH: Prophylactic intrapartum amnioinfusion: A randomized clinical trial. Am J Obstet Gynecol 162:1370, 1990.

170. Taylor K: Current status of toxicity investigation. J Clin Ultrasound 2:149, 1974.

171. Tegnander E, Eik-Nes SH, Johansen OJ, Linker DT: Prenatal detection of heart defects at the routine fetal examination at 18 weeks in a non-selected population. Ultrasound Obstet Gynecol 5:372, 1995.

172. Thacker SB, Berkelman RL: Assessing the diagnostic accuracy and efficacy of selected antepartum fetal surveillance techniques. Obstet Gynecol Surv 41:121, 1986.

173. Theodoropoulos P, Lolis D, Papageorgiou C, et al: Evaluation of first-trimester screening by fetal nuchal translucency and maternal age. Prenat Diagn 18:133, 1998.

174. Thibeault D, Hobel C: The interrelationship of the foam stability test, immaturity, and intrapartum complications in the respiratory distress syndrome. Am J Obstet Gynecol 118:56, 1974.

175. Todros T, Preve CU, Plazzotta C, et al: Fetal heart rate tracings: Observers versus computer assessment. Eur J Obstet Gynecol Reprod Biol 68:83, 1996.

176. Tsai MY, Josephson MW, Knox GE: Absorbance of amniotic fluid at 650 nm as a fetal lung maturity test: a comparison with the lecithin/sphingomyelin ratio and tests for disaturated phosphatidylcholine and phosphatidylglycerol. Am J Obstet Gynecol 146:963, 1983.

177. Turnbull AC: The lecithin/sphingomyelin ratio in decline. Br J Obstet Gynaecol 90:993, 1983.

178. Van Alten D, Eskes M, Treffers PE: Midwifery in the Netherlands: The Wormeveer study; selection, mode of delivery, perinatal mortality and infant morbidity. Br J Obstet Gynaecol 96:656, 1989.

179. van Wijngaarden WJ, Sahota DS, James DK, et al: Improved intrapartum surveillance with PR interval analysis of the fetal electrocardiogram: A randomized trial showing a reduction in fetal blood sampling. Am J Obstet Gynecol 174:1295, 1996.

180. Vintzileos AM: The relationships among the fetal biophysical profile, umbilical cord pH, and Apgar scores. Am J Obstet Gynecol 157:627, 1987.

181. Vintzileos AM, et al: The use and misuse of fetal biophysical profile. Am J Obstet Gynecol 156:527, 1987.

182. Visser GH, Mulder HH, Wit HP: Vibro-acoustic stimulation of the human fetus: Effect on behavioral state organization. Early Human Dev 19:285, 1989.

183. von Kaisenberg CS, Krenn V, Ludwig M, et al: Morphological classification of nuchal skin in human fetuses with trisomy 21, 18, and 13 at 12–18 weeks and in a trisomy 16 mouse. Anat Embryol [Berl] 197:105, 1998.

184. Wald NJ, et al: Maternal serum unconjugated oestriol as an antenatal screening test for Down's syndrome. Br J Obstet Gynaecol 95:334, 1988.

185. Wald NJ, et al: Maternal serum screening for Down's syndrome in early pregnancy. BMJ 297:883, 1988.

186. Wald NJ, Densem JW, George L, et al: Prenatal screening for Down's syndrome using inhibin-A as a serum marker. Prenat Diagn 16:143, 1996.

187. Wald NJ, Watt HC, Hackshaw AK: Integrated screening for Down's syndrome on the basis of tests performed during the first and second trimesters. N Engl J Med 341:461, 1999.

188. Warshaw JB, Hobbins JC, eds: Principles and Practice of Perinatal Medicine: Maternal, Fetal, and Newborn Care. Menlo Park, CA: Addison-Wesley, 1983.

189. Weingold A, DeJesus T, O'Keife J: Oxytocin challenge test. Am J Obstet Gynecol 123:466, 1975.

190. White P: Diabetes mellitus in pregnancy. Clin Perinatol 1:331, 1974.

191. Williams RL, Chen PM: Identifying the sources of the recent decline in perinatal mortality rates in California. N Engl J Med 306:4, 1982.

192. Wilson-Costello D, Rao PS, Morrison S, Hack M: Radiation exposure from diagnostic radiographs in extremely low birth weight infants. Pediatrics 97:369, 1996.

193. Yahya SZ, Williams J, Mathers A, et al: Variations in the management of singleton breech presentation throughout Scotland. Scott Med J 43:144, 1998.

194. Ylinen K, Aula P, Stenman UH, et al: Risk of minor and major fetal malformations in diabetics with high hemoglobin A1c values in early pregnancy. BMJ 289:345, 1984.

195. Yoon BH, Romero R, Kim CJ, et al: High expression of tumor necrosis factor-alpha and interleukin-6 in periventricular leukomalacia. Am J Obstet Gynecol 177:406, 1997.

Resuscitation of the Newborn Infant

Susan Niermeyer
William Keenan

The clinical experiences described in the 14th to 18th centuries helped establish much of the basis for modern neonatal resuscitation. In 1754, Benjamin Pugh urged the use of endotracheal intubation for asphyxiated newborns using his tube design of coiled wire and soft leather.[25] The publications of the Royal Humane Society between 1774 and 1776 commended the use of mouth-to-mouth resuscitation in stillborn infants. The Society promoted the resuscitation of newborn children by giving awards of merit in 1802, 1816, and 1857 to three midwives for their prominent role in successful resuscitation of large numbers of newly born children.[15] However, the methods employed in neonatal resuscitation continued to be a source of controversy. Even the European giant of pediatrics, August Ritter von Reuss, in his 1920 text *The Diseases of the Newborn,* recommended smacking the buttocks, alternating warm or hot baths, and giving mustard baths. He mentions the desirability of endotracheal tube ventilation but also cites Schultz's method as being most commonly used by obstetricians. This method is described as grasping the prone infant by both shoulders and swinging the child's body, forcing the lower part of the body on the chest and abdomen. This maneuver is repeated six to eight times between immersions in a water bath.[19] By 1933, Griffith's and Mitchell's pediatric text cautions against using any of the older methods, urges prompt establishment of a clear airway and the potential use of mouth-to-mouth ventilation, and describes placement of an endotracheal tube with mouth-to-tube ventilation.[8] In the 1950s, doctors Virginia Apgar and Stanley James provided a major stimulus to successful neonatal resuscitation through their systematic methods of evaluation of the newly born infants and early resuscitation steps.[4] In 1987, the

American Heart Association and the American Academy of Pediatrics began to provide a structured training program with accompanying text designed to incorporate new information and experience.[5]

Three to seven percent of newly born infants require some form of resuscitative intervention.[20] All infants require the basic steps in neonatal resuscitation, that is, prevention of heat loss (dry and provide warmth), clearing the airway (position and suction), support of breathing (stimulate), and evaluation of circulation (assess heart rate and color). Figure 2–1 illustrates the relationship between the steps in neonatal resuscitation. Diminishing numbers of ba-

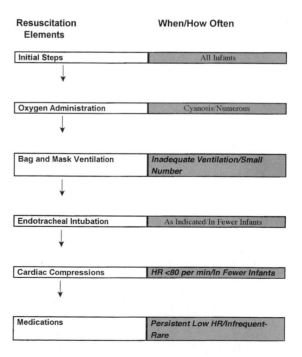

Figure 2–1. Abbreviated algorithm for neonatal resuscitation.

bies need supplemental oxygen, positive-pressure ventilation or intubation, chest compressions, or medications. Perlman recorded that, of 30,839 consecutively born infants, 39 (0.12%) required chest compressions or epinephrine. Inadequate ventilatory assistance was thought to account for the need for further resuscitation in 29 of the 39 infants.[18]

Among experts there is a wide variety in preferences for certain equipment, such as positive-pressure resuscitation bags and endotracheal tubes, and in ventilation styles. The unifying theme for these same experts, which may clarify the task for the beginning resuscitator, is the priority for establishing an airway and furnishing adequate ventilation for the resuscitation of the severely depressed newly born infant. A second important concept held by experts involves self-efficacy. Self-efficacy is confidence born of knowledge, practice, and a sense of responsibility that leads to successful performance. Understanding the elements of neonatal resuscitation and structured practice of the skills required will lead to successful resuscitation.[16]

◆ SUCCESSFUL APPROACH TO NEONATAL RESUSCITATION

Anticipation

The need for resuscitation can occur at any delivery. At every delivery there should be at least one person skilled in neonatal resuscitation whose sole responsibility is care of the newly born infant. Fully functional equipment necessary for a complete resuscitation should be in the delivery room for every birth. However, careful identification of risk factors can predict the need for extensive intervention in more than half of infants who require such resuscitation. Anticipation allows recruitment of additional personnel to assist with resuscitation and specific preparation of equipment and supplies.

Certain antepartum and intrapartum risk factors are associated with the need for neonatal resuscitation. These are summarized in Table 2–1. These risk factors can be predictive of respiratory depression or respiratory distress, intravascular volume loss, infection, asphyxia, or fetal malformations. The implications of each circumstance

Table 2–1. Examples of Risk Factors Associated with the Need for Resuscitation in the Newly Born Infant

Maternal

Premature/prolonged rupture of membranes
Bleeding in second or third trimester
Severe pregnancy-induced hypertension
Chronic hypertension
Substance abuse
Pharmacologic therapy (e.g., lithium, magnesium)
Diabetes mellitus
Chronic illness (e.g., anemia, significant heart disease)
Maternal infection
Heavy sedation
Previous fetal or neonatal death
No prenatal care

Fetal

Multiple gestation
Preterm gestation (especially <35 wk)
Post-term gestation (≥42 wk)
Size-date discrepancy
Intrauterine growth restriction
Rhesus isoimmunization/hydrops fetalis
Polyhydramnios and oligohydramnios
Reduced fetal movement before onset of labor
Congenital abnormalities
Intrauterine infection

Intrapartum

Fetal distress
Abnormal presentation
Prolapsed cord
Prolonged rupture of the membranes
Prolonged labor (or prolonged second stage of labor)
Precipitous labor
Antepartum hemorrhage (abruptio placenta, placenta previa)
Thick meconium staining of amniotic fluid
Nonreassuring fetal heart rate patterns
Narcotic administration to mother within 4 hours of delivery
Forceps delivery
Vacuum-assisted delivery
Cesarean section delivery

should be considered in assembling appropriately skilled personnel, designating roles in the resuscitation, selecting appropriately sized equipment, and organizing supplies to be immediately usable.

Personnel

At every delivery there should be one person who is solely responsible for the baby and who is capable of initiating resuscitation, including bag-and-mask ventilation. That person may have the skills required to perform a complete resuscitation, including endotracheal intubation, chest compressions, and medication administration. If not, a second person with complementary skills should be readily available to the delivery room.

If the baby is anticipated to be at high risk for neonatal resuscitation, at least two people should be present to manage the baby. One must have the skills to perform a complete resuscitation and usually provides airway management and ventilation. The second provides stimulation, monitors heart rate, and provides chest compressions, if necessary. Other individuals can serve as valuable assistants, for example, by preparing medication doses and recording interventions and times. Whenever possible, the resuscitation team should designate a leader and each team member should have an identified role before commencing the resuscitation. In the case of multiple births, each baby should have a separate resuscitation team.

Equipment

To avoid delay in resuscitation, the equipment and supplies to perform a complete resuscitation must be available at every delivery. This can be accomplished in a variety of ways. All delivery settings should have equipment for oxygen administration, bag-and-mask ventilation, and endotracheal intubation. Cesarean section delivery rooms, where many high-risk deliveries occur, may be stocked permanently with supplies for vascular access, volume expanders, and medications, as well as respiratory equipment. Low-risk labor-delivery-recovery rooms may be served by emergency carts or trays, which bring the supplies for advanced resuscitation to the delivery room at the time of birth. The responsibility for restocking of supplies and routine maintenance of equipment must be clearly designated. Equipment that is missing or non-operational (e.g., resuscitation bag or laryngoscope bulb) can compromise a resuscitation. A list of equipment for neonatal resuscitation is provided in Table 2–2.

An appropriate thermal environment should be available. When the need for resuscitation is anticipated, correct size respiratory equipment should be unpacked, prepared, and tested. If three or more persons make up the resuscitation team, volume expanders and drugs may be prepared as required. In other high-risk circumstances, volume expanders and medications may need to be prepared and labeled in advance.

Recognition

Successful performance of neonatal resuscitation relies on three key steps: evaluating the infant, deciding on the correct action to take, and taking that action. Once the action is taken, the cycle is repeated—evaluation, decision, action—based on the effect of the previous action and the resultant new findings (Fig. 2–2). For example, an infant just born is evaluated for breathing; he is found to be apneic. The decision is made to provide brief tactile stimulation. The infant's back is rubbed briefly while drying of the skin is completed. The infant is then reevaluated and found to be still apneic. At this point, the decision is made to provide positive-pressure ventilation. Bag-and-mask ventilation is initiated. The effect of the intervention is evaluated and the cycle of evaluation, decisions, and action begins again.

Three basic signs form the basis for evaluation: respirations, heart rate, and color. These are physical signs that serve as the indicators for the ABCs of resuscitation: airway, breathing, circulation. Respirations give information on airway and breathing, heart rate is a primary measure of circulation, and color is a measure of all three ABCs. Each member of the team must know the three key points for evaluation and employ the evaluation, decision, action cycle to work through a resuscitation algorithm. With a standardized approach to neonatal resuscitation, all team members work through the same decision tree and thus are coordinated in their responses. The evaluation, decision, action cycle is completed quickly in an actual resuscitation, and several actions may be in progress simultaneously.[13]

The Apgar score, developed by Dr. Virginia Apgar in 1952, provides an objective and sensitive measure of an infant's condition in the first minutes after birth.[1] While the Apgar score includes the three basic signs that are the basis for neonatal resuscitation (respirations, heart rate, color), it adds two neurologic elements (reflex irritability and tone). The score is assessed at 1 and 5 minutes after birth and every 5 minutes thereafter until the score is greater than or equal to 7. The Apgar score is not useful as an indicator of the need for resuscitation,

Table 2–2. Recommended Equipment and Drugs for Resuscitation of the Newly Born Infant

Equipment

Firm, padded resuscitation surface
Overhead warmer or other heat source
Light source
Clock
Warmed linens (infant hat optional)
Stethoscope
Suction catheter (6, 8, 10, 12, or 14 French)
Meconium suction device (to apply suction directly to endotracheal tube)
Feeding tube (8 French) and 20-mL syringe for gastric decompression
Oxygen supply (flow rate of up to 10 L/min) with flow meter and tubing
Portable oxygen cylinders
Face masks (various sizes)
Oropharyngeal airways (sizes 0 and 00)
Resuscitation system for positive pressure ventilation (any one)
   Face mask with T-piece
   Face mask with self-inflating bag and oxygen reservoir
   Face mask with flow-inflating bag, valve, and manometer
Laryngoscopes with straight blade, spare bulbs, and batteries
Endotracheal tubes (sizes 2.5, 3, 3.5, and 4 mm internal diameter)
Stylet
Supplies for fixation of endotracheal tubes and intravenous (IV) lines (e.g., scissors, tape, alcohol sponges)
Feeding tube or umbilical catheter (5 French) shortened for surfactant administration
Umbilical vein catheterization tray
Syringes with needles (assorted sizes)
IV cannulas (assorted sizes)
Electrocardiograph with cardiotachometer (optional)
Pulse oximeter (optional)
Exhaled CO_2 detector (optional confirmation for intubation)

Drugs

Epinephrine 1:10,000 concentration (0.1 mg/mL)
Volume expanders: normal saline, Ringer's lactate, blood
Naloxone hydrochloride: 1.0 mg/mL or 0.4 mg/mL solution
Sodium bicarbonate: 0.5 mEq/mL solution (4.2% concentration)
Dextrose: 5% and 10% solutions

---

because resuscitative efforts are most often initiated before 1 minute after birth. Apgar scores documenting infant status relative to resuscitative measures, especially when accompanied by a narrative of interventions and their timing, may be quite useful.

Techniques in Resuscitation

Using the ABCs as the overall framework for neonatal resuscitation, the components of the procedure can be identified as follows:

A—Establish an *A*irway
   Positioning
   Suctioning
   Endotracheal intubation (if necessary)
B—Initiate *B*reathing
   Tactile stimulation (drying, rubbing)
   Positive-pressure ventilation
C—Maintain *C*irculation

   Chest compressions
   Medications and volume expansion

All of the above steps are performed in an environment that maintains the infant's body temperature (The **ABCs**—*T*emperature, *A*irway, *B*reathing, *C*irculation).

Initial Steps

The initial steps of neonatal resuscitation should be performed at every delivery. Routine care includes prevention of heat loss by drying the infant, removing the wet linen, and providing a heat source and clearing the airway by positioning the neck slightly extended and, if required, suctioning secretions from the mouth and the nose. The initial steps may also include supporting respirations by tactile stimulation and oxygen administration as necessary.

   Minimizing heat loss of the newly born

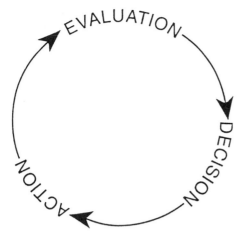

Figure 2–2. Action/evaluation/decision cycle. (Used with permission of the American Academy of Pediatrics. From Bloom RS, Cropley C, and the AHA/AAP Neonatal Resuscitation Program Steering Committee: Textbook of Neonatal Resuscitation. Elk Grove Village, IL: American Academy of Pediatrics: American Heart Association, 1994.)

infant avoids the metabolic problems associated with cold stress. An infant who requires resuscitation may be even more vulnerable to cold stress, making it important not to neglect this important step. When the temperature of the delivery setting is regulated to be comfortable for clothed adults, a source of radiant heat for the newly born infant can be quite helpful. Preheating an overhead warmer creates a warm surface on which to place the infant. Drying the scalp and face addresses a large proportion of the infant's surface area and facilitates subsequent steps in airway management. Drying of the body can be continued by a second delivery attendant while the head is positioned and the airway cleared. Wet linen should be removed from contact with the infant.

Opening the airway of the depressed newly born involves positioning the infant correctly and clearing the mouth and nose of secretions. Positioning of the head, with the neck slightly extended, serves to align the posterior pharynx, larynx, and trachea, thus facilitating easy air entry (Fig. 2–3). Both hyperextension and flexion of the neck can obstruct the airway. A rolled blanket or towel under the shoulders (generally less than 1 inch thick) can help maintain correct head position. Suctioning the mouth clears the largest volume of secretions from the airway first. This can generally be accomplished with a bulb syringe. Turning the in-

fant's head to the side allows secretions to pool in the cheek. Suctioning of the nares often results in a sneeze, cough, or cry. A suction catheter attached to mechanical suction (-80 to 100 cm H_2O) may be used to clear the airway. Vigorous or deep suction may produce vagal bradycardia and should be avoided.

Both drying and suctioning are forms of tactile stimulation, and, for many infants, these interventions are sufficient to initiate and support respirations. However, if the infant is not breathing or has inadequate respiratory effort, brief tactile stimulation may be given either by rubbing the back or slapping/flicking the soles of the feet. If the infant does not respond within a few seconds, positive-pressure ventilation should be initiated promptly. Gentle rubbing of the trunk or extremities may help support the rate and depth of respirations once breathing has been established.

Evaluation of the infant is ongoing during all of the aforementioned steps. The first question to be answered is *"Is the baby breathing?"* If the baby is apneic, gasping, or otherwise has ineffective respirations, the operator should supply positive-pressure ventilation. After the adequacy of ventilation is established, the second question is *"What is the infant's heart rate?"* If the heart rate is less than 100 beats per minute, positive-pressure ventilation should be continued or instituted. If the heart rate is less than 60 beats per minute, positive pressure should be continued or instituted and direct support of the cardiac output (chest com-

Correct

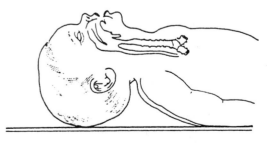

Neck slightly extended

Figure 2–3. Correct position for opening the airway. (Used with permission of the American Academy of Pediatrics. From Bloom RS, Cropley C, and the AHA/AAP Neonatal Resuscitation Program Steering Committee: Textbook of Neonatal Resuscitation. Elk Grove Village, IL: American Academy of Pediatrics: American Heart Association, 1994.)

pressions) should be supplied while positive-pressure ventilation is continued. If ventilation is adequate and the heart rate is greater than 100 beats per minute, the third question is *"Is the baby pink?"* If the breathing child has central cyanosis, then free-flow 100% oxygen should be administered at a flow rate of 5 L/min. This can be accomplished in many ways, including holding an oxygen mask or flow-inflating bag-and-mask gently on the face. Alternatively, oxygen may be delivered directly from the supply tubing with the hand cupped around the tubing to concentrate the flow around the nose and mouth. Oxygen should be administered until the infant's color is pink. Oxygen should be gradually, not abruptly, withdrawn while the infant's color is observed. If cyanosis recurs as oxygen is withdrawn, the oxygen should be increased to maintain a pink color until the infant can be monitored in a stabilization area. Cyanosis of the extremities, or acrocyanosis, is a common response to cooling stimuli and is neither a reflection of hypoxemia nor an indication for supplemental oxygen treatment.

Initial Steps of Resuscitation with Meconium-Stained Amniotic Fluid

If meconium is present in the amniotic fluid, the initial steps must be modified in some cases to assure a clear airway. When meconium has been noted, the person delivering the infant should suction the mouth and nasohypopharynx upon delivery of the head and before delivery of the shoulders and body.[4, 26] Once delivered, the infant should be immediately placed on a preheated radiant warmer, but before drying and stimulation is initiated, the infant should be rapidly assessed and classified as "vigorous" or "depressed" to determine whether tracheal suctioning is indicated. A vigorous infant cries spontaneously, has good muscle tone, and a heart rate greater than 100 beats/min. Tracheal suctioning may not be necessary. If the infant is vigorous, the initial steps of resuscitation can be continued as usual, with drying, positioning, and suctioning of the mouth and nares with a bulb syringe or 10- or 12-French suction catheter. If the baby is depressed, tracheal intubation for suctioning should be performed.

To perform tracheal suctioning, a laryngoscope is inserted and the mouth and posterior pharynx suctioned with a 12- or 14-

Table 2–3. Guidelines—Endotracheal Tube Size and Placement Depth

Weight (g)	Gestational Age (wk)	Endotracheal Tube Size (mm)
1000	<28	2.5
1000–2000	28–34	3.0
2000–3000	34–38	3.5
>3000	>38	3.5–4.0

Depth of placement (tip to lip); weight in kg plus 6 cm (e.g., 1000 g infant, 1 + 6 = 7 cm).

French suction catheter under direct vision to provide an unobstructed view of the glottis. The appropriate size endotracheal tube (Table 2–3) is inserted into the trachea and attached to a meconium aspirator device, which is, in turn, attached to a suction source (Fig. 2–4). Suction is applied as the tube is slowly withdrawn. If meconium is obtained, the procedure should be repeated once or twice, as necessary, until little meconium is removed or until substantial bradycardia indicates that further resuscitation should be initiated.

If the infant remains depressed after tracheal suctioning for meconium, positive-pressure ventilation should be provided, either by bag-and-mask or by endotracheal tube. This decision depends largely on the infant's degree of depression and the anticipated severity of respiratory illness. If the heart rate is very low (less than 60 beats/

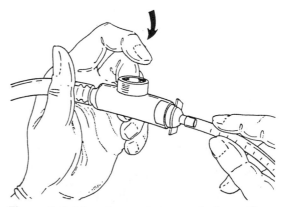

Figure 2–4. Meconium aspirator attached to wall suction. (Used with permission of the American Academy of Pediatrics. From Bloom RS, Cropley C, and the AHA/AAP Neonatal Resuscitation Program Steering Committee: Textbook of Neonatal Resuscitation. Elk Grove Village, IL: American Academy of Pediatrics: American Heart Association, 1994.)

min) and copious meconium was obtained with suctioning, or other antenatal indicators suggest significant ongoing depression, reintubation with a clean endotracheal tube should be considered for ventilation. Such rapid decision making requires teamwork between at least two individuals who are simultaneously evaluating the infant, communicating their findings, and performing resuscitative actions.

Advanced Support of Airway and Breathing: Bag-and-Mask Ventilation and Endotracheal Intubation

Adequate ventilation is the cornerstone of successful neonatal resuscitation. Active support of ventilation requires availability of properly functioning equipment, skill and confidence in performance of the techniques of bag-and-mask ventilation and endotracheal intubation, and effective use of the evaluation, decision, action cycle by members of the resuscitation team.

The indications for positive-pressure ventilation include (1) apnea unresponsive to brief stimulation, (2) gasping respirations, or (3) heart rate less than 100 beats/min. Continued central cyanosis despite adequate spontaneous ventilation may also be an indication for positive-pressure ventilatory support. Bag-and-mask ventilation can be performed with either a self-inflating bag (volume 240 to 750 mL) equipped with an oxygen reservoir and pressure-release valve or a flow-inflating bag (anesthesia bag) of volume 500 to 750 mL equipped with a pressure gauge and flow-control valve (Fig. 2–5). Each type of bag has advantages and disadvantages. Self-inflating bags deliver a tidal volume more reliably in the hands of persons who resuscitate babies infrequently[12]; however, some self-inflating bags cannot be used to deliver free-flow oxygen and a special adapter must be inserted to deliver continuous positive airway pressure (CPAP) or positive end-expiratory pressure (PEEP). High peak inspiratory pressures are achieved by overriding the pressure-release (pop-off) valve. Flow-inflating bags require a complete seal between mask and face to deliver a tidal volume. However, they can be used to deliver free-flow oxygen, CPAP or PEEP, and high peak inspiratory pressures. Inadvertent exposure of the infant to high airway pressures can be a risk with this type of bag.

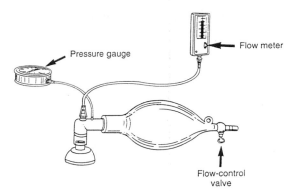

Figure 2–5. Resuscitation bag connects to flow meter and pressure gauge. (Used with permission of the American Academy of Pediatrics. From Bloom RS, Cropley C, and the AHA/AAP Neonatal Resuscitation Program Steering Committee: Textbook of Neonatal Resuscitation. Elk Grove Village, IL: American Academy of Pediatrics: American Heart Association, 1994.)

The choice of mask is important to ensure a complete seal between the mask and the face without injuring the eyes or other facial structures. Masks are commonly available in sizes for term and preterm infants; they may be obtained in sizes that fit infants 1000 g and smaller as well. Flexible masks with a cushioned rim provide the best seal with the least risk of trauma.

Selected equipment should be tested in advance of performing an actual resuscitation. The bag-and-mask is assembled and connected to a compressed gas source that delivers 100% oxygen. The flow should be adjusted between 5 and 10 L/min. While the mask is occluded against the palm of the hand, the bag should be squeezed to ensure the development of adequate pressures. If using a flow-inflating bag, the flow meter and flow-control valve should be adjusted to produce reinflation of the bag and the desired end-expiratory pressure.

To perform bag-and-mask ventilation, the infant should be positioned with the neck slightly extended. The mask should cover the nose and mouth, but not the eyes; it should be held against the face with the thumb and index finger while the third, fourth, and fifth fingers rest along the jaw. Universal recommendations for initial inflation pressures and inspiratory times are not available, but some experts have suggested the use of very long inflation times (2 to 3 seconds) for initial inflation breaths.[24] Adequate ventilation should produce easy chest wall movement at a rate of 40 to 60 breaths/min. Peak inspiratory pressures depend on the extent of lung disease and preceding inflation or lack thereof. Pressures in the range of 15 to 40 cm H_2O may be adequate to achieve lung inflation. If chest expansion is inadequate, the following steps should be taken: (1) reapply the mask, (2) reposition the head, (3) remove secretions from the mouth, (4) open the infant's mouth slightly, (5) ventilate with higher pressures. If bag-and-mask ventilation is continued for more than 2 minutes, an orogastric catheter should be inserted with little interruption of positive-pressure ventilation. The depth of catheter insertion should be estimated by the technique illustrated in Figure 2–6. The distance from the bridge of the nose to the earlobe and then to the xiphoid should be measured from the tip of the catheter. The catheter should be inserted through the mouth and its position confirmed by aspiration of gastric contents. The catheter should be left open and taped against the infant's cheek.

The ongoing effectiveness of bag-and-mask ventilation should be assessed by observation of chest wall movement, auscultation of breath sounds, monitoring of heart rate, and observation of skin color. Both underinflation and overinflation of the lungs can be hazardous. Because inflation pressures cannot be estimated clinically, use of a pressure manometer is recommended in the delivery room. In addition to trauma to the eyes or face, the complications of bag-and-mask ventilation include pulmonary air leak, intestinal distention elevating the dia-

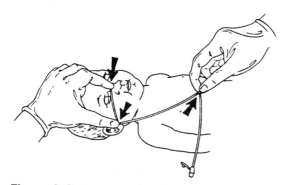

Figure 2–6. Estimating length of orogastric catheter for placement in stomach. (Used with permission of the American Academy of Pediatrics. From Bloom RS, Cropley C, and the AHA/AAP Neonatal Resuscitation Program Steering Committee: Textbook of Neonatal Resuscitation. Elk Grove Village, IL: American Academy of Pediatrics: American Heart Association, 1994.)

phragm, and compression of the lung in the case of diaphragmatic hernia.

When bag-and-mask ventilation is ineffective, despite attempts to optimize pressures and inflation times, endotracheal intubation is indicated. Other indications for intubation include the anticipated need for prolonged positive-pressure ventilation, surfactant administration, the need for tracheal suctioning (to remove meconium), and suspected diaphragmatic hernia. The need for chest compressions is a relative indication for placement of an endotracheal tube. The equipment for intubation is listed in Table 2–2. The estimated weight of the infant should guide selection of the correct size laryngoscope blade and endotracheal tube. Generally, a number 1 Miller laryngoscope blade is appropriate for term infants and a size 0 is appropriate for preterm infants. The appropriate sizes of tubes for infants of a given gestation and weight are listed in Table 2–3.

The procedure of intubation can be viewed as a series of steps. Preceding and between attempts at endotracheal tube placement, ventilation is supported with a bag-and-mask as the child's condition indicates. Successful performance of intubation depends both on skill and self-efficacy. The most crucial steps are visualization of landmarks and inserting the tube through the vocal cords.

The resuscitation team prepares the needed equipment and supplies, that is, laryngoscope, tape, suction, oxygen source, bag, mask, and endotracheal tube of the correct size. A variety of sizes should be available, because estimated weights may be inaccurate or malformations may necessitate a different size tube. The endotracheal tube can be shortened to 13 cm before intubation to eliminate dead space and may facilitate easy handling. A flexible stylet may be inserted, but the tip should not extend beyond the end of the endotracheal tube. The following steps are taken to accomplish endotracheal intubation:

1. Position the infant with the neck slightly extended.
2. Provide free-flow oxygen during the procedure.
3. Hold the laryngoscope with the left hand, open the mouth with the right index finger and insert the blade under the tongue.

4. Lift the laryngoscope blade upward and forward so that the blade is nearly parallel to the infant's body.
5. Visualize the landmarks of the epiglottis, vocal cords, and glottis (Fig. 2–7). If the esophagus is seen, withdraw the laryngoscope until the epiglottis drops into view. If the tongue is seen, advance the laryngoscope until it enters the vallecula or passes under the epiglottis.
6. Provide gentle external pressure over the cricoid cartilage of the trachea. This can be accomplished with the little finger of the hand holding the laryngoscope or an assistant can provide pressure.
7. Insert the slightly curved endotracheal tube with a motion through a C-shaped arc. Enter the mouth at the right corner and maintain visualization of the glottis to confirm that the tip of the tube passes through the vocal cords. Position the vocal cord guideline at the level of the vocal cords.
8. Limit each intubation attempt to 20 seconds. If an attempt is unsuccessful, provide bag-and-mask ventilation between attempts.
9. Confirm endotracheal tube position by auscultation (equal breath sounds in both axillae and absent breath sounds over the stomach) and chest wall movement.
10. Adjust the depth of intubation (if necessary), note the centimeter mark at the lip (see Table 2–3), and secure the endotracheal tube with tape.
11. Obtain chest x-ray film.
12. Shorten the endotracheal tube 4 cm beyond the lips (if necessary).

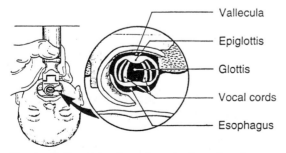

Figure 2–7. View of vocal cords through a laryngoscope. (Used with permission of the American Academy of Pediatrics. From Bloom RS, Cropley C, and the AHA/AAP Neonatal Resuscitation Program Steering Committee: Textbook of Neonatal Resuscitation. Elk Grove Village, IL: American Academy of Pediatrics: American Heart Association, 1994.)

Complications of intubation relate principally to hypoxia and trauma. Prolonged intubation attempts, tube malposition, apnea and bradycardia caused by laryngeal stimulation, and lack of free-flow oxygen may all aggravate preexisting hypoxemia. Lacerations, edema, or even airway perforation are examples of possible airway trauma. Confirmation of endotracheal tube placement by use of carbon dioxide detectors is commonly used in pediatric anesthesia and critical care. Few data regarding low-birth-weight infants are available but such adjunctive devices can prove valuable to confirm tracheal positioning of the tube before an x-ray film is available.[3]

Advanced Support of Circulation: Chest Compressions and Medications

Even though bradycardia usually resolves with adequate ventilation, persistent bradycardia is the indication for chest compressions to support cardiac output. The specific indication for chest compressions is a heart rate less than 60 beats/min despite 30 seconds of effective positive-pressure ventilation with 100% oxygen.[10, 14, 17] The infant should remain in the optimal position for ventilation, that is, supine with the neck slightly extended. Compressions may be performed using either the two-thumb method (encircling technique) or the two-finger method (Fig. 2–8). The two-thumb method is preferred because data suggest it may provide better coronary perfusion pressure; however, access to the umbilical cord for medication administration may be more easily obtained during two-finger compressions. Compressions should be performed over the lower third of the sternum, just below an imaginary line connecting the nipples. Compressions should be given 90 times/min and 30 ventilations should be interposed in a 3:1 compression-to-ventilation ratio (120 events/min). Compressions should be given to a depth of approximately one-third the anteroposterior diameter of the chest. Back support should be provided by the tips of the encircling fingers in the two-thumb method or by the second hand being placed under the back in the two-finger method. Compressions coordinated with ventilation (e.g., compress, compress, compress, breath, compress, compress, compress, breath) should be continued until the heart rate is greater than 60 beats/min.

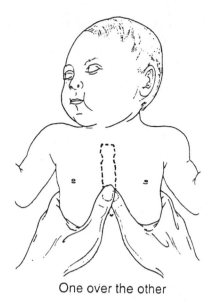

One over the other

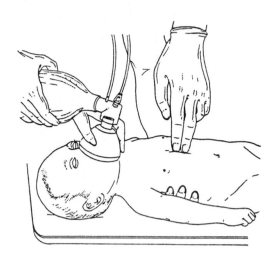

Figure 2–8. Cardiac compression techniques: thumb method and two-finger method. (Used with permission of the American Academy of Pediatrics. From Bloom RS, Cropley C, and the AHA/AAP Neonatal Resuscitation Program Steering Committee: Textbook of Neonatal Resuscitation. Elk Grove Village, IL: American Academy of Pediatrics: American Heart Association, 1994.)

Complications of chest compressions can include rib fractures, laceration of the liver, and pneumothorax. To minimize complications, compressions should be performed in the correct position, contact should be maintained with the chest during the release portion of the cycle, and just enough force to compress the chest one-third of its antero-posterior dimension and to generate a palpable pulse should be used.

When there is poor response to positive-pressure ventilation and chest compressions, the evaluation, decision, action cycle is repeated several times to continue along the neonatal resuscitation algorithm, while simultaneously reevaluating for technical or clinical problems that might interfere with ventilation or return of spontaneous circulation.

If the infant fails to respond to adequate ventilation and chest compressions, the next step in resuscitation is the administration of medications. At that point, intubation can be carried out (if not already performed) because the endotracheal route is the most rapid method to give epinephrine. Intubation provides a more secure airway and may facilitate the effectiveness of chest compressions.

The principal medications used in neonatal resuscitation are epinephrine, volume expanders, and sodium bicarbonate. Naloxone hydrochloride, a narcotic antagonist, is used for the specific indication of postnarcotic respiratory depression. Other drugs, such as calcium and atropine, may have a role in certain resuscitation circumstances outside the delivery room, but they are not helpful and may be harmful in resuscitation of the newly born infant. Epinephrine is indicated if the heart rate remains less than 60 beats/min after a minimum of 30 seconds of adequate positive-pressure ventilation and coordinated chest compressions. Epinephrine may be given via the endotracheal tube or intravenously. Even though endotracheal administration is rapid, absorption of the drug can be erratic and plasma concentrations variable. The intravenous route has the advantage of more dependable drug delivery and is necessary for administration of volume expanders and sodium bicarbonate.

The umbilical vein provides ready intravenous access in the newly born infant (see Table 2–2). Placement of a low-lying umbilical venous line can be accomplished quickly with the following steps:

1. Place a loose tie of umbilical tape around the base of the cord.
2. Prepare a 3.5- or 5-French umbilical catheter with normal saline flush, a three-way stopcock, and syringe.
3. Cut the cord with a sterile scalpel about 1 to 2 cm from the base and identify the large, thin-walled umbilical vein.

4. Insert the umbilical catheter into the vein just until free flow of blood is obtained when the catheter is aspirated. (This should be only a few centimeters into the vein.)
5. Clear any air bubbles from the catheter and stopcock; turn the stopcock off to the infant to disconnect and connect the medication syringe; follow medication with normal saline flush.

When resuscitation is complete, the low-lying umbilical line should be further secured or removed and the umbilical tape secured around the umbilical stump. Moving the infant with an unsecured low-lying umbilical line incurs a risk of bleeding.

Epinephrine should be given rapidly in a dose of 0.1 to 0.3 mL/kg of 1:10,000 solution. If there is not a prompt increase in heart rate to greater than 60 beats/min, the dose may be repeated every 3 to 5 minutes, possibly using the upper end of the dosing range. There is no evidence that high-dose epinephrine (10 times the usual dose) is useful in neonatal resuscitation, and it may be harmful, producing myocardial damage or intracranial hemorrhage.

Expansion of the circulating plasma volume may be required to maintain cardiac output, blood pressure, and peripheral perfusion. Volume expansion should be considered when there is evidence of acute blood loss (e.g., placental abruption, fetal-maternal hemorrhage, umbilical cord tear, acute neonatal hemorrhage), and possibly poor response to resuscitation (e.g., pallor, poor capillary refill, bradycardia unresponsive to positive-pressure ventilation and chest compressions). The choice of fluid for volume expansion is dictated by availability and the specific needs of the infant. Normal saline and lactated Ringer's solution are readily available. Whole blood or packed red blood cells may be indicated in cases of acute blood loss; however, this need must be anticipated in order to have blood available in the delivery room. Use of 5% albumin solution should be restricted to special circumstances because of expense, limited availability, risk of infectious disease, and unresolved questions regarding increased mortality risk associated with its use.[9]

Although acidosis often persists after a prolonged resuscitation, adequate circulation and ventilation usually lead to spontaneous correction of acidosis. Administration of sodium bicarbonate in resuscitation of the newly born infant remains controversial. Some authorities advise bicarbonate administration if all other steps in neonatal resuscitation have brought no improvement. Others do not give bicarbonate until a blood gas determination has documented the presence of significant metabolic acidosis and adequate ventilation. If given, sodium bicarbonate can be administered slowly by umbilical vein in a dose of 2 mEq/kg of 4.2% solution.

Intraosseous infusion has been reported in neonates.[6] Although drug absorption has been documented to be excellent from this space in older infants and children, equivalent data are not available for newly born infants at a variety of gestational ages. Furthermore, the technical difficulties of intraosseous infusion may be greater in very small infants, increasing the risks of trauma or extravasation. Umbilical vein catheterization remains the preferred route of administration for resuscitation drugs, but in the rare circumstance in which umbilical or other venous access cannot be obtained, or in the older neonate, intraosseous infusion might be considered.

If all the steps in neonatal resuscitation have been carried out, but the heart rate remains less than 60 beats/min, efforts should be redoubled to check several points:

1. Is the airway unobstructed by secretions and the endotracheal tube correctly positioned?
2. Is 100% oxygen being delivered?
3. Is chest wall movement adequate and are breath sounds equal bilaterally?
4. Are chest compressions being given to a depth adequate to produce a palpable pulse and are they being coordinated with ventilations?
5. Has epinephrine been delivered into the circulation?

Other complications and conditions that can interfere with response to resuscitation should again be considered; for example, pneumothorax, diaphragmatic hernia, hypovolemia, and congenital heart block. If the heart rate remains slow, but is present, continued resuscitation may still be successful. If the heart rate is absent, it becomes necessary to consider discontinuation of resuscitative efforts.

◆ NARCOTICS AND DEPRESSED RESPIRATION

If the mother has received narcotic analgesia and the infant's ventilatory effort is decreased, consideration should be given to the administration of a narcotic antagonist. Naloxone hydrochloride 0.1 mg/kg/dose given intravenously, intramuscularly, subcutaneously, or via endotracheal tube is recommended. Narcotic antagonists are not a substitute for the effective support of ventilation as described earlier.

◆ SUBSTANCE ABUSE

The need for resuscitation is likely to be increased in children born of women taking illegal drugs. Short gestation, intrauterine growth retardation, and maternal illness are all associated with the increased need for resuscitation.

Avoidance of narcotic antagonist use when the infant has been chronically exposed to morphine-class drugs is important. Administration of narcotic antagonists to infants of heroin-addicted mothers has been reported to precipitate severe and immediate withdrawal symptoms.

◆ VERY LOW-BIRTH-WEIGHT INFANTS AND RESUSCITATION

Delivery room resuscitation including positive-pressure ventilation is frequently required in the care of low-birth-weight infants. Steps to prepare for a likely demanding resuscitation are outlined earlier. Particular attention to the minimization of thermal stress is required. Surfactant deficiency is common and provision should be made for the early administration of exogenous surfactant. A myriad of possible clinical problems such as hypotension, hypoglycemia, and respiratory insufficiency may require attention immediately following resuscitation.

Experience in the Vermont-Oxford Network neonatal centers between 1994 and 1996 suggests that aggressive delivery room resuscitation of the very low-birth-weight infant can be efficacious. For infants with birth weights less than 1000 g, chest compressions or the administration of epinephrine was associated with a survival rate of 53.8% versus 74.9% in infants who did not receive these interventions.[7]

◆ CONGENITAL DIAPHRAGMATIC HERNIA

A variety of problems that occur with congenital diaphragmatic hernia might alter the approach to required resuscitation. Assiduous resuscitation is often required, although occasional infants are asymptomatic and do not require resuscitation in the newborn period. If the diagnosis of congenital diaphragmatic hernia is being considered, bag-and-mask ventilation should be avoided in favor of ventilation via an endotracheal tube. High ventilating pressures via bag-and-mask force some gas down the esophagus and can distend intrathoracic intestine, further compromising ventilation and circulation. Decompression of the stomach with a large-bore nasogastric or orogastric tube should be instituted as soon as possible. Pulmonary hypoplasia is a frequent feature of congenital diaphragmatic hernia. Adequate ventilatory support, while minimizing the risk of a tension pneumothorax, is often difficult. Sedation or paralysis sometimes is helpful in these difficult situations. Tension pneumothoraces frequently occur and can be life-threatening. Support of the cardiac output with catecholamines and measures to achieve pulmonary vasodilatation are often required. Support with extracorporeal membrane oxygenation as either a time-limited rescue or as a perioperative technique has been used in many centers.

◆ AIR LEAKS

The occurrence of a tension pneumothorax can compromise both ventilation and cardiac output. Vigorous ventilatory and circulatory support should be instituted and continued as indicated while timely evacuation of the pneumothorax is carried out.

◆ HYDROPS

The prognosis and signs of generalized fetal edema relate to a diverse set of possible etiologies. Preparation for a challenging resuscitation and possible specific treatments remain a key to success. Some additional concepts might be considered. Many of these infants may require demanding attention to the establishment of an airway and adequate respiratory support. The need for resuscitation is frequent. Surfactant deficiency, which is common in hydrops, can be immediately treated with exogenous surfactant delivered via an endotracheal tube. Severe anemia can be treated with simple or modified exchange transfusion with packed red blood cells. Supraventricular tachycardia can be treated with measures such as adenosine, digoxin, or countershock, as indicated.

◆ AIRWAY OBSTRUCTION

Airway obstruction is a frightening prospect in the newborn requiring resuscitation. Bag-and-mask ventilation can be quite effective even when an endotracheal tube cannot be placed. Occasionally, placement of an endotracheal tube over a flexible bronchoscope that has passed beyond the vocal cords can be used. The laryngeal mask airway may provide an effective airway adjunct when used by trained persons. Immediate tracheostomy has been considered by a number of experts but remains a last resort. Once resuscitation has been carried out and ventilation is supported, more specific treatment for the obstructing condition can be planned.

◆ DECISIONS TO RESUSCITATE

Resuscitation decisions regarding the severely depressed newly born infant are challenging. The survival and the quality of survival in infants born with Apgar scores of zero are shown in Table 2–4. Many of the surviving children probably were affected

Table 2–4. Outcome in Resuscitated Newly Born Infants with Initial Apgar Score of Zero

	Total	Survived	Normal
Scott[21]	15	7	6/7
Steiner[22]	14	6	4/6
Thompson[23]	4	2	2/2
Jain[11]	93	33	14/23
Casulaz[5]	48	26	15/26
TOTAL	174	74 (42%)	41/64* (64%)

*Follow-up in 64 of 74 (86%)

by acute perinatal problems shortly before birth. Review of the same studies suggests that nonresponsiveness after 10 to 15 minutes of resuscitation is associated with very low survival rates and that the possibility of intact survival is essentially nil.

CASE PROBLEMS

Case One

Term—rapid delivery. *A 28-year-old woman whose fourth pregnancy is at term (39 5/7 weeks) arrives at the labor and delivery department with contractions every 3 minutes. Membranes ruptured approximately 1 hour before arrival at the hospital; the fluid was clear. Over the next 4 hours, cervical dilation increases to 6 cm; thereafter, cervical dilation rapidly progresses to complete and spontaneous vaginal vertex delivery after a 10-minute second stage. A female infant emerges limp and apneic.*

◆ *What are the initial steps in resuscitation of this infant?*

The infant should be dried, while simultaneously her head is positioned and her airway cleared. Wet linen should be removed from contact with the infant, and respirations assessed. If the baby is not breathing after the stimulation of drying and suctioning, specific stimulation such as rubbing the back or slapping the soles of the feet may be given for a few seconds while free-flow oxygen is administered in case the infant initiates spontaneous breathing.

◆ *The infant remains apneic. What is the next step in resuscitation?*

If tactile stimulation fails to trigger spontaneous respirations, positive-pressure ventilation is necessary. In this infant who has not taken a spontaneous breath since delivery, it is important to deliver "opening breaths" with adequate inspiratory time and pressure to begin to establish the residual volume of the lung. One way to accomplish this is to use an inspiratory time of 1 to 2 seconds and pressure in the range of 20 to 40 mm Hg. Subsequent breaths should be delivered at a rate of 40 to 60 breaths/min with peak inspiratory pressure that produces an easy rise of the chest wall.

◆ *The chest wall does not rise with positive-pressure ventilation. What steps should be taken?*

The most common reasons for inadequate chest wall expansion with bag-and-mask ventilation are an inadequate seal between the mask and the face and incorrect head position. Check the seal between the mask and face, then make sure that the head is not flexed or hyperextended. If these interventions fail to improve the ventilation, again clear the mouth of secretions and open the mouth when reapplying the mask. Finally, if good chest wall movement still has not been achieved, increase the peak inspiratory pressure. At this point, it is important to check the heart rate. If adequate ventilation has been established, the heart rate should be greater than 60 beats/min and, usually, will increase rapidly as a result of adequate lung expansion. If ventilation remains inadequate, the heart rate may remain low. In this case, further efforts must be made to improve lung expansion, either by continued bag-and-mask ventilation or by intubation.

◆ *The heart rate is 80 and easy chest wall movement is noted. What action is indicated?*
Bag-and-mask ventilation should be continued until spontaneous respirations return. The type and timing of the intervention should be documented.

The infant's heart rate quickly increases to 130 by 1 minute after delivery and her color becomes centrally pink. She cries spontaneously by 2 minutes and establishes regular respirations immediately after that. Positive-pressure ventilation is stopped, but free-flow oxygen held close to the face is continued. The infant is provided tactile stimulation to encourage deep spontaneous respirations. The oxygen is gradually withdrawn and the infant remains pink. The Apgar score is 5 at 1 minute (0 respirations, 2 heart rate, 1 color, 1 tone, 1 reflex irritability) with positive-pressure ventilation and 9 at 5 minutes (2 respirations, 2 heart rate, 1 color, 2 tone, 2 reflex irritability) without supplemental oxygen.

◆ *How should this infant be cared for during transition?*
The infant requires continued close observation during transition because the need for initial resuscitation may signal further difficulty. However, the rapid response to adequate ventilation and absence of need for supplemental oxygen permit consideration that the infant can remain with her mother for bedside transition. Respiratory rate, color, heart rate, and signs of respiratory distress must be monitored frequently in the first hour. Thermal stability can be assured by swaddling or providing skin-to-skin contact on the mother's chest, with covering blankets.

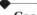

Case Two
Post-term with meconium and apnea. *A 20-year-old woman is admitted for induction of labor at 41 4/7 weeks' gestation of her first pregnancy. Membranes are ruptured artificially and the fluid is noted to be meconium-stained. Labor progresses with reassuring fetal heart rate monitoring until the second stage, when moderate variable decelerations are noted with pushing. The infant is delivered vaginally, but requires reduction of the cord around the neck x 2 prior to delivery of the body. The infant's face is noted to be bruised with petechiae and the infant does not cry spontaneously at delivery.*

◆ *What is the first step in this infant's resuscitation?*
When meconium is present in the amniotic fluid and the infant is depressed at the time of birth, tracheal suctioning to clear the airway of meconium is indicated before proceeding with other basic resuscitation steps. Thus, the infant must be rapidly assessed to classify him as "vigorous" or "depressed." An infant with no respirations or gasping respirations, heart rate less than 100 beats/min, or decreased muscle tone is considered depressed. He is given quickly to the resuscitation team and a person skilled in endotracheal intubation proceeds immediately with endotracheal intubation for suctioning.

The posterior pharynx is cleared of secretions and meconium with a suction catheter to provide a clear view of the vocal cords. The infant is intubated with a 3.5 endotracheal tube, which is connected to wall suction via an adapter, and suction (−80 to −100 cm H2O) is applied as the endotracheal tube is withdrawn. No meconium is obtained from the trachea. The infant remains apneic.

◆ *What is the next step in this infant's resuscitation?*
The infant has not yet been provided all the initial steps of basic resuscitation. He should be dried rapidly and the wet linen removed from contact. The head should be repositioned to open the airway and the baby could be provided brief tactile stimulation by rubbing the back or flicking the soles of the feet while free-flow oxygen is provided.

The infant cries and spontaneous respirations are maintained with continued drying and tactile stimulation. Heart rate at 1 minute after birth is 120, but the infant remains centrally and peripherally cyanotic. His 1-minute Apgar score is

7 (2 respirations, 2 heart rate, 0 color, 1 tone, 2 reflex irritability). He slowly becomes pink over his trunk, chest, and mucous membranes, and free-flow oxygen is gradually withdrawn, with maintenance of good color. The 5-minute Apgar score is 8 (2 respirations, 2 heart rate, 1 color, 1 tone, 2 reflex irritability).

◆ *What risk factors should be considered in the postresuscitation care of this infant?*

Even though no meconium was recovered from below the vocal cords, this infant remains at risk for respiratory problems related to parenchymal lung disease or complications of intubation. Transient tachypnea of the newborn or meconium aspiration syndrome might develop. Intubation carries with it risks of airway trauma, resulting in vocal cord injury and stridor, lacerations, or edema of pharyngeal/laryngeal structures. By virtue of gestational age greater than 40 weeks and need for resuscitation, the infant may be at higher risk for hypoglycemia during the transition period.

◆

Case Three

Moderately preterm with volume loss. *A 19-year-old woman in her first pregnancy experiences the spontaneous onset of labor at 36 weeks by uncertain dates and late fetal ultrasound. She arrives at the hospital just before spontaneous rupture of membranes, which yields clear fluid. The fetus is vertex, occiput posterior. Late decelerations with pushing prompt application of a vacuum device to complete delivery. After 14 minutes, the infant is delivered, but emerges apneic, pale, and cyanotic.*

◆ *What is the first step in resuscitation?*

The initial steps of resuscitation should be completed quickly in this infant who will likely need advanced intervention. The baby should be placed on a preheated radiant warmer and dried, while the head is positioned and the airway suctioned. Wet linen should be removed from contact with the infant and tactile stimulation may be given, but positive-pressure ventilation with bag-and-mask should be initiated rapidly.

The infant has easy chest wall movement with bag-and-mask ventilation. The heart rate after approximately 30 seconds is 160 beats/min. He has no respiratory effort and is pale and bruised.

◆ *What are the possible causes of his continued distress?*

With adequate chest wall movement, adequate ventilation seems likely; however, auscultation of the chest is important to assure good air exchange and help assess the need for intubation to continue ventilation. Low circulating blood volume can produce tachycardia; at delivery, this often relates to blood loss or failure of the infant to receive an adequate placental transfusion. Rapid cord clamping, cord entanglement, obstruction, or avulsion can result in failure of the placental transfusion. Laceration of the placenta, placenta previa, or severe abruption can also reduce the blood volume available to the baby. Hypovolemia may also result from bleeding into a closed space, such as the abdomen or the scalp. Plasma volume loss may be encountered in sepsis with capillary leak or in fetal hydrops. Primary problems of cardiac contractility may result from asphyxial injury to the myocardium, sepsis, or certain forms of congenital heart disease, such as congenital heart block or critical aortic stenosis with left ventricular damage in utero.

On a rapid physical assessment, there continues to be good air entry with bag-and-mask ventilation using modest peak airway pressure. There is no cardiac murmur or gallop rhythm. Although there is no evidence of hydrops, the scalp is very boggy and bruised and the infant is strikingly pale.

◆ *What intervention is most likely to address the cause of the persistent distress?*

With the physical findings of pallor and boggy scalp, hypovolemia caused by blood loss into an enclosed space seems the most likely explanation for the poor response to initial resuscitation. Acute volume expansion with 10 mL/kg of isotonic crystalloid fluid is the indicated intervention. The preferred route for volume administration during delivery room resuscitation is the umbilical vein. To minimize time needed for placement and potential complications, the catheter is inserted just below the skin surface, until a blood return is obtained. Crystalloid, such as normal saline or lactated Ringer's solution, is preferred for initial volume expansion because of its immediate availability, lower cost, lower infectious risk, and equivalent benefit to protein-containing solutions.

An amount of 10 mL/kg of normal saline is given over 5 minutes. Perfusion is slightly better and the infant has several gasping respirations, then begins a more regular respiratory pattern. A second dose of normal saline is administered, with decrease in the heart rate to 140 beats/minute.

◆ *What conditions should be considered in the differential diagnosis of hypovolemia in this infant?*

The most likely causes of hypovolemia include subgaleal hemorrhage or other bleeding into structures of the scalp and cranium. Bleeding may occur at various levels around and within the skull. Capillary bleeding and edema in the scalp itself make up a caput; shear stress on the bridging veins that cross the tissue plane below the skin and muscles of the scalp can result in subgaleal hemorrhage. Bounded by the aponeuroses of the scalp muscles as they insert at the nape of the neck, over the ear, and along the supraorbital ridge, this potential space can contain a large portion of the blood volume of a newly born infant. Blood collections under the periosteum of the skull bones are termed cephalohematomas. Bleeding may also occur within the skull in the form of subdural, intraventricular, or parenchymal hemorrhage. Other causes of volume loss, such as vasa previa, deserve investigation as well. Consideration should be given to any evidence for interruption of the usual placental transfusion, such as tight nuchal cord, knot or clot in the cord, or avulsion of the cord. Fetal-to-maternal hemorrhage can also result in hypovolemia. Acute or chronic hemolysis and fetal anemia may also be associated with hypovolemia.

◆ *What monitoring and laboratory studies should be carried out?*

Initial monitoring should include cardiorespiratory monitoring, pulse oximetry, and blood pressure, as well as measurement of occipitofrontal head circumference (OFC). Immediate laboratory studies include complete blood count, reticulocyte count, blood type, and Coombs with cross-match for packed red blood cells. Kleihauer-Betke stain should be considered to investigate fetal-to-maternal hemorrhage and the placenta should be examined. Cord blood gases may be useful in timing the onset of distress, and arterial blood gases should be considered if the infant is hypotensive or requires supplemental oxygen.

◆ *What further resuscitation/stabilization measures might be anticipated?*

If the cause of hypovolemia is self-limited (e.g., low-volume placental transfusion), the infant may remain stable without additional resuscitative measures. Need for additional expansion of the blood volume should be considered. If the volume loss is progressive, as often occurs with subgaleal hemorrhage, the infant may rapidly become unstable. Continuous monitoring of blood pressure (arterial catheter), heart rate, oxygenation/circulation, and urine output, as well as serial monitoring of hematocrit, coagulation studies, and OFC are necessary to detect changes as rapidly as possible. Central venous access is useful both for central venous pressure monitoring and rapid volume replacement. Volume replacement might include red cells and fresh frozen plasma in addition to crystalloid and colloid solutions.

◆

Case Four

Term with severe asphyxia. *A 32-year-old gravida 3, para 2 woman is seen in the labor and delivery department for evaluation of decreased fetal movement in the preceding 24 hours. External fetal heart rate monitoring reveals a fetal heart rate of 100 beats/min with absent variability and occasional decelerations to 60 beats/min in the absence of contractions. An emergency cesarean section is performed under general anesthesia. Upon incision of the uterus, the amniotic fluid is found to be stained with thick meconium. The infant emerges limp, pale, cyanotic, and takes one gasping breath on the way to the open warmer.*

◆ *What is the first step in resuscitation?*

This infant is clearly depressed and needs positive-pressure ventilation and potentially has meconium in the trachea. The first step is to intubate for tracheal suctioning. Establishment of a clear airway and ventilation is the pressing task.

The infant is intubated with a 3.5 endotracheal tube, with return of a significant amount of thick meconium from below the cords. The heart rate is 20 beats/min.

◆ *What is the next step in resuscitation?*

Although the airway may not have been thoroughly cleared of meconium, the need for further efforts to clear the airway is outweighed by the need for ventilatory support in the asphyxiated infant. Endotracheal intubation will ensure a secure airway during chest compressions, provide a route for epinephrine administration, and permit intermittent airway suctioning as required. As soon as ventilation is confirmed by chest wall rise and auscultation, coordinated chest compressions should be provided, with 90 compressions and 30 interposed breaths each minute. Preparations should be initiated for administration of medications and placement of an umbilical venous catheter.

After 30 seconds of ventilation per endotracheal tube and chest compressions, the heart rate continues to be 20 beats/min. Epinephrine is administered per endotracheal tube at a dose of 0.2 mL/kg of 1:10,000 solution. The heart rate remains 20 beats/min.

◆ *What circumstances could account for persistent bradycardia and cyanosis in this infant?*

In addition to endotracheal tube malposition, causes for persistent bradycardia and cyanosis in this infant can be classified as pulmonary parenchymal disease, obstructive airway problems, pulmonary vascular disease, cardiac injury, or structural malformations. In utero aspiration of meconium is likely, given the history of 24 hours of decreased fetal movement and a gasping respiration at birth. Meconium may already be present at the level of the alveoli and the pneumonitis associated with meconium aspiration may be developing. In addition, asphyxia can lead to pulmonary capillary leak, and meconium is known to inactivate surfactant in vitro; both circumstances contribute to a picture of poorly compliant lungs with impaired gas exchange. Pneumonia or sepsis must be considered as underlying causes that may have triggered the fetal distress. Meconium may also cause airway obstruction, especially when thick and particulate, as in this case. Partial obstruction on inspiration may become a complete obstruction in the exhalation phase, resulting in a pneumothorax. Especially with chronic fetal distress, changes may occur in the fetal pulmonary vasculature before delivery, manifesting as persistent pulmonary hypertension, changes which may be exacerbated by the hypoxia and acidosis of asphyxia. Asphyxial injury to the myocardium can also be a contributor in this case. Measurement of cord blood gases can give some indication of the degree of biochemical abnormality experienced by the fetus. Finally, structural malformations, such as congenital heart disease or congenital diaphragmatic hernia, cannot be excluded, even though more immediate possibilities exist.

◆ *What actions should be taken in light of the infant's poor response to resuscitation?*

Correct positioning of the endotracheal tube should be confirmed and adequacy of venti-

lation reassessed, especially with respect to differential caliber of breath sounds between right and left sides. Airway suctioning via the endotracheal tube may remove further obstructing meconium. While chest compressions are continued, a second dose of 1:10,000 epinephrine 0.1 to 0.3 mL/kg should be given via the endotracheal tube and an umbilical venous line inserted just until blood return is obtained. Epinephrine may then be given directly into the central circulation at a dose of 0.1 to 0.3 mL/kg of 1:10,000 solution.

After two intravenous doses of epinephrine, the heart rate increases to 110 beats/min. The infant resumes gasping respirations at approximately 20 minutes after delivery. Assisted ventilation is continued. Cord gases show a venous pH of 6.81, pCO_2 110, pO_2 14, base excess − 20; arterial pH 6.75, pCO_2 112, pO_2 12, base excess − 22.

◆ *What steps should be taken immediately for further stabilization?*

In addition to cardiorespiratory monitoring, preductal and postductal pulse oximetry, and blood pressure, an immediate heel-stick glucose should be checked. If glucose is low, a bolus of $D_{10}W$ in a volume of 2 mL/kg followed by a constant infusion may be given by the low-lying umbilical venous line. Immediate steps should be taken to place central arterial and venous lines and obtain blood for arterial blood gases, blood culture, and complete blood count. Chest and abdominal x-ray studies should be obtained to confirm correct line position and assess pulmonary parenchymal disease. Bicarbonate therapy in response to cord gases may not be beneficial; evidence of clearing metabolic acidosis on the initial arterial blood gas study from the infant after delivery would support continued expectant management, with attention to blood pressure, oxygenation, and ventilation as the mainstays of therapy. Early echocardiography to define contractility and volume status as well as pulmonary artery pressures may help guide initial management—that is, choice of ventilation modality and usefulness of pulmonary vasodilator therapy.

◆ *What information is important to communicate to the parents of this infant following resuscitation?*

The parents should be reassured that they responded appropriately to the warning sign of decreased fetal movement. They should be informed of the evidence of fetal compromise and the possible consequences, including heart, kidney, and brain injury. The natural course of meconium aspiration, its complications, and methods of treatment should be outlined.

◆─────────────────────────────

Case Five

Extremely low-birth-weight with pneumonia/ sepsis. *A 36-year-old woman is seen by her perinatologist at 26 2/7 weeks' gestation of her first pregnancy. She has experienced a gush of clear fluid. The pregnancy was conceived by in vitro fertilization. Rupture of membranes is confirmed. Uterine irritability quiets with fluid administration and bedrest, and fetal heart rate monitoring is reassuring; the fetus is in vertex presentation. Two doses of betamethasone are administered and the mother is kept at strict bedrest in the hospital. She is given prophylactic ampicillin. Five days later, she complains of low back pain and is found to be 4 cm dilated with an active contraction pattern. Her temperature increases to 103.5°F and the fetal heart rate is between 180 and 190. Urgent cesarean section is performed. The baby emerges limp and apneic.*

◆ **What should be prepared for the resuscitation of this infant?**
Antenatal ultrasound should provide an estimated fetal weight (EFW). In this case, the EFW is 730 g and appropriate preparations can be made for thermoregulation and airway management. The overhead warmer should be preheated and stocked with warm linen, if available. Supplemental heat may also be provided with a chemically activated heat pad under the blankets. A 2.5 mm endotracheal tube and 0 laryngoscope blade should be prepared and checked. The suction and flow-inflating bag should be checked and a "micropremie" mask obtained for bag-and-mask ventilation. A stethoscope of appropriate size should be available at the warmer. In addition, supplies for placement of umbilical venous catheter, volume expansion, and medication administration should be readily available. A transport isolette and portable oxygen should be readied if the intensive care nursery is not immediately adjacent to the operating room.

At least two persons should be assigned exclusively to care for the infant; one should be skilled in endotracheal intubation. A third person should be available for more extensive resuscitation, such as medication administration.

◆ **What is the first step in the resuscitation of this infant?**
The infant should receive the basic steps of neonatal resuscitation, including drying, positioning, suctioning of the airway—all performed quickly under the preheated radiant warmer. In the case of an extremely low-birth-weight infant who is apneic at birth, the person responsible for airway management may choose to intubate immediately after clearing the airway to visualize the cords adequately. Bag-and-mask ventilation can be accomplished effectively, even in small infants; however, exogenous surfactant administration may be another indication for intubation.

The infant is successfully intubated and ventilation is initiated with two opening breaths, using peak inspiratory pressure of 30 and inspiratory times of 1 second. Ventilation is then continued with pressures of approximately 22/4 and rate of 60; the chest wall does not rise and the heart rate at 30 seconds after intubation is 40 beats/ minute.

◆ **What circumstances could account for persistent bradycardia and cyanosis in this infant?**
Endotracheal tube malposition is problematic in extremely low-birth-weight infants. Esophageal intubation, deep right mainstem intubation, or dislodgment of tracheal intubation into the posterior pharynx or esophagus all occur frequently. After confirming correct tube placement in this infant, parenchymal lung disease or airway obstruction/ pneumothorax are the most likely causes of poor chest wall movement and persistent bradycardia and cyanosis.

Chest compressions are begun, interposed with ventilation at a rate of 90 compressions and 30 breaths per minute. The endotracheal tube is suctioned for a moderate amount of clear fluid and ventilation is continued with pressures up to 30 cm H_2O. A dose of epinephrine 1:10,000 solution 0.3 mL/kg is given via the endotracheal tube. The heart rate remains 40 beats/min and the infant is noted to have very constricted peripheral circulation.

◆ **What actions should be taken in light of the infant's poor response to resuscitation?**
Adequacy of ventilation should be reassessed. Although a peak inspiratory pressure of 30 cm H_2O is high in an infant weighing 730 g, it may be insufficient to establish lung inflation in the face of surfactant deficiency and pneumonia. Pressures should be increased until easy chest wall movement is noted and air exchange is audible bilaterally. Careful auscultation should

be performed periodically to assure that pneumothorax is not the cause of poor oxygenation/ventilation. A central venous catheter should be placed for intravenous administration of epinephrine. Volume expansion with 10 mL/kg of normal saline might be considered, because sepsis can be accompanied by capillary leak and hypovolemia, as well as depression of myocardial contractility.

Adequate air exchange is finally achieved with peak inspiratory pressures of 45 cm H_2O. Heart rate rises to 140 beats/min simultaneous with completion of the volume bolus, following an intravenous dose of epinephrine 1:10,000 solution 0.3 mL/kg. After several breaths, pressures are decreased to 40 and then 35 cm H_2O with maintenance of heart rate and improving, pink color. The infant is transported to the neonatal intensive care unit and supported with mechanical ventilation.

◆ *What steps should be taken immediately for further stabilization?*

In addition to cardiorespiratory monitoring, pulse oximetry, and blood pressure, an immediate heel-stick glucose should be checked. If glucose is low, a bolus of $D_{10}W$ in a volume of 2 mL/kg may be given followed by a constant infusion. Immediate steps should be taken to place central arterial and venous lines and obtain blood for arterial blood gases, blood culture, and complete blood count. Antibiotic therapy should be initiated. Chest and abdominal x-ray studies should be obtained to confirm correct line position and assess pulmonary parenchymal disease. Exogenous surfactant should be administered if not already given.

◆ *What information should be provided to the parents of this infant after resuscitation?*

Information on survival at 27 weeks' gestation and 730 g should be presented—specific survival figures for the delivering institution should be used, if available. Parents should be cautioned that survival probabilities are often lower when prematurity is complicated by superimposed infection. The importance of the child's response to initial therapy should be discussed. Discussion of perinatal depression should include the importance of long-term follow-up, as for any premature infant of this age and weight.

REFERENCES

1. Apgar V: A proposal for a new method of evaluation of the newborn infant. Curr Res Anesth Analg 13:260–267, 1953.
2. Apgar V, James LS: Futher observations on the newborn scoring system. Am J Dis Child 104:419, 1962.
3. Aziz HF, Martin JB, Moore JJ: The pediatric disposable end-tidal carbon dioxide detector role in endotracheal intubation in newborns. J Perinatol 19:110–113, 1999.
4. Carson BS, Losey RW, Bowes WA, et al: Combined obstetric and pediatric approach to prevent meconium aspiration syndrome. Am J Obstet Gynecol 126:712, 1976.
5. Casulaz D, Marlow N, Speidel B: Outcome of resuscitation following unexpected apparent stillbirth. Arch Dis Child B Fetal Neonatal Ed 78:F112–F115, 1998.
6. Ellemunter H, Simma B, Trawoger R, Maurer H: Intraosseous lines in preterm and full term neonates. Arch Dis Child Fetal Neonatal Ed 80:F74–F75, 1999.
7. Finer NN, Horbor JD, Carpenter JH (for the Vermont Oxford Network): Cardiopulmonary resuscitation in the very low birth weight infant: The Vermont Oxford Network Experience. Pediatrics 104:428–431, 1999.
8. Griffith JPC, Mitchell AG: The diseases of infants and children. 1933, pp 227–233.
9. Human albumin administration in critically ill patients: Systemic review of randomised controlled trials. Cochrane Injuries Group Albumin Reviewers. BMJ 317:235–240, 1998.
10. International Guidelines 2000 for Cardiopulmonary Resuscitation and Emergency Cardiac Care. Part II: Neonatal Resuscitation. Circulation 102(Suppl I): I-343, 2000.
11. Jain L, Ferre C, Vidyasagar D, et al: Cardiopulmonary resuscitation of apparently stillborn infants: Survival and long-term outcome. J Pediatr 118:778–782, 1991.
12. Kanter RK: Evaluation of mask-bag ventilation in resuscitation of infants. Am J Dis Child 141:761–763, 1987.
13. Kattwinkel J (ed): Textbook of Neonatal Resuscitation, 4th ed. Elk Grove Village, IL and Dallas, TX: American Academy of Pediatrics and American Heart Association, 2000.
14. Kattwinkel J, Niermeyer S, Nadkarni V, et al: An advisory statement from the pediatric working group of the International Liaison Committee on Resuscitation. Circulation 99:1927–1938, 1999.
15. Keith A: The mechanism underlying the various methods of artificial respiration. Lancet 1:825–828, 1909.
16. Mailbach EW, Schieber RA, Carroll MFB: Self-efficacy in pediatric resuscitation: Implications for education and performance. Pediatrics 97:94–99, 1996.
17. Niermeyer S, et al: International Guidelines for Neonatal Resuscitation: An Excerpt from the Guidelines 2000 for Cardiopulmonary Resuscitation and Emergency Cardiovascular Care: International Consensus on Science Pediatrics 106(3): 2000. http://www.pediatrics.org/cgi/content/fun/106/3/e29.
18. Perlman JM, Risser R: Cardiopulmonary resuscitation in the delivery room. Arch Pediatr Adolesc Med 149:20–25, 1995.
19. Ritter von Reuss A: The diseases of the newborn. London: John Bale, 1920, pp 276–290.
20. Saugstad OD: Practical aspects of resuscitating as-

phyxiated newborn infants. Eur J Pediatr 157:S11–S15, 1998.

21. Scott H: Outcome of very severe birth asphyxia. Arch Dis Child 51:712–716, 1976.

22. Steiner H, Naligan G: Perinatal cardiac arrest: Quality of the survivors. Arch Dis Child 50:696–702, 1975.

23. Thompson A, Searle M, Russell G: Quality of life after severe birth asphyxia. Arch Dis Child 52:620–626, 1977.

24. Vyas H, Milner AD, Hopkin IE, Boon AW: Physiologic responses to prolonged slow-rise inflation in the resuscitation of the asphyxiated newborn infant. J Pediatr 99:635–639, 1981.

25. White GMJ: Evolution of endotracheal and endobronchial intubation. Br J Anaesth 32:235–246, 1960.

26. Wiswell TE, Fuloria M: Management of meconium-stained amniotic fluid. Clin Perinatol 26:659, 1999.

Recognition, Stabilization, and Transport of the High-Risk Newborn

Arthur E. D'Harlingue
David J. Durand

At delivery, the newborn infant must make a complicated transition from intrauterine to extrauterine life. Although most newborns make this adaptation without difficulty, the first few hours of life can be a precarious time for the high-risk infant. Health care professionals who provide care to newborns must anticipate the problems of the high-risk infant before presentation. Early recognition of high-risk factors in the maternal history and of significant findings in the newborn allows for timely and appropriate monitoring and treatment. The goal of this approach of active anticipation and intervention is to prevent the development or progression of more serious illness and to minimize the risk of both morbidity and mortality in the high-risk newborn. A newborn infant should receive a level of care specific to his or her unique needs. If an infant is critically ill, it is essential to intervene rapidly and effectively in order to stabilize the infant. In contrast, some infants with perinatal risk factors may do quite well postnatally. After an initial assessment and careful observation, such an infant might be advanced to well newborn care. This chapter outlines an approach to the preparation for and management of the high-risk infant in the first hours of life, including initial stabilization and transport.

◆ MATERNAL HISTORY

During fetal growth the infant is somewhat protected in the intrauterine environment. However, in the course of a pregnancy the health of the mother impacts upon the well-being of the fetus.[34, 35] Both acute and chronic maternal illnesses can adversely affect embryogenesis and fetal growth and maturation. Maternal nutrition, medica-

tions, smoking, and drug use all affect the growth and development of the fetus. Such prenatal maternal factors may continue to have effects on the postnatal course of the newborn. Intrapartum factors including obstetric complications, maternal therapy, and mode of delivery may also impact on the condition of the newborn infant.

It is essential to obtain a complete maternal history in order to anticipate and prepare for a high-risk newborn. The physician should obtain this information before the delivery of the infant whenever possible. The maternal record should be reviewed including the current hospital chart and the prepartum record. Particular attention should be paid to the results of maternal prenatal laboratory studies, peripartum cultures, underlying maternal illnesses, and peripartum complications (Table 3–1). Maternal illnesses and medical problems have an important impact on the well-being of the fetus and the newborn (Table 3–2). Discussion with the obstetrician and nursing staff are essential to clarify the current status of both the mother and infant. When high-risk factors are identified, the physician and nursery staff are then prepared to deal with the anticipated problems of the newborn during delivery and subsequent hospital course.

Maternal Diseases

Maternal diabetes mellitus affects the fetus from prior to conception and throughout the entire pregnancy. Uncontrolled diabetes during the periconceptional period and during early embryogenesis increases the risk for fetal malformations including congenital heart disease, limb abnormalities, and central nervous system anomalies.[20] Small left

Table 3–1. Review of Obstetric and Perinatal History

Routine prenatal care
  Last menstrual period
  Estimated date of conception (by dates and
    ultrasound)
  Onset of prenatal care
Previous pregnancies
  Number
  Outcome of each
  Previous prenatal, intrapartum, neonatal
    complications
Maternal laboratory studies
  Blood type and Rh
  Antibody screen
  Rapid plasma reagin
  Hepatitis B surface antigen
  Rubella immunity
  Human immunodeficiency virus antibody
  Alpha-fetoprotein
  Results of cultures or antibody titers
Maternal illnesses and infections
  Diabetes
  Hypertension
  Thyroid disease
  Seizure disorder
  Sexually transmitted diseases (gonorrhea,
    syphilis, chlamydia, herpes)
Pregnancy-related conditions
  Pregnancy-induced hypertension
  Chorioamnionitis
  Premature labor (use of tocolytics)
Maternal medications and drug use
  Steroids
  Tocolytics
  Antibiotics
  Sedatives
  Analgesics
  Anesthetics
  Tobacco
  Alcohol
  Marijuana
  Cocaine
  Amphetamines
  Heroin or methadone
  Phencyclidine (PCP)
	Fetal laboratory studies
	  Amniotic fluid lung maturity studies
	  Fetal chromosome results
	  Amniotic fluid delta 450 to assess fetal bilirubin
	  Cordocentesis labs (complete blood count, platelet
	    count)
	  Scalp pH
	Fetal status
	  Singleton, twins, and so on
	  Ultrasound findings (weight, gestational age,
	    anomalies, intrauterine growth retardation)
	  Amniotic fluid (polyhydramnios, oligohydramnios,
	    meconium staining)
	  Time of rupture of membranes
	  Cord injuries or prolapse
	  Results of fetal heart rate monitoring
	  Maternal bleeding; placenta previa, abruptio
	    placentae
	Delivery
	  Method of delivery: vaginal or cesarean section
	    (indication)
	  Instrumentation at delivery: forceps, vacuum
	  Presentation and position
	  Prolonged second stage
	  Shoulder dystocia
	  Cord complications: nuchal cord, true knot,
	    laceration, avulsion
	Social factors
	  Maternal support system
	  History of family violence, neglect, or abuse
	  Previous childen in foster care
	  Stable living situation, homelessness
	  History of depression, psychosis	

colon syndrome, femoral hypoplasia–unusual facies syndrome, and caudal regression syndrome are particularly associated with maternal diabetes. Poor diabetic control with resulting chronic hyperglycemia during the third trimester leads to fetal macrosomia, which increases the risk for birth trauma and the need for cesarean delivery. Fetal lung maturation is also impaired by maternal diabetes, increasing the risk for respiratory distress syndrome even in near-term infants. The infant of the diabetic mother is at risk for hypoglycemia, hypocalcemia, hypomagnesemia, polycythemia, and hyperbilirubinemia.

Maternal thyroid disease can have a wide variety of effects on the newborn, depending on the combined effects of maternal transplacental antithyroid antibodies and thyroid medications. The neonate born to a mother with Graves disease can be hypothyroid, euthyroid, or hyperthyroid at birth. When the mother's Graves disease is well controlled with medications (e.g., propylthiouracil) during the pregnancy, then the infant is usually euthyroid at birth. However, as the effects of maternal antithyroid medication wear off, persistent maternal antithyroid antibodies may stimulate the neonatal thyroid gland and cause thyrotoxicosis.

Maternal preeclampsia has a number of adverse effects on the fetus and the new-

Table 3–2. Maternal Medical Conditions and the Newborn

Maternal Condition	Potential Effects upon the Fetus or Newborn
Endocrine, Metabolic	
Diabetes mellitus	Hypoglycemia, macrosomia, hyperbilirubinemia, polycythemia, increased risk for birth defects, birth trauma, small left colon syndrome, cardiomyopathy, and respiratory distress syndrome
Hypoparathyroidism	Fetal hypocalcemia, neonatal hyperparathyroidism
Hyperparathyroidism	Neonatal hypocalcemia and hypoparathyroidism
Graves disease	Fetal and neonatal hyperthyroidism, intrauterine growth retardation, prematurity
Obesity	Macrosomia, birth trauma
Phenylketonuria (untreated pregnancies)	Mental retardation, microcephaly, congenital heart disease
Cardiopulmonary	
Asthma	Increased rates of prematurity, toxemia, and perinatal loss
Congenital heart disease	Effects of cardiovascular drugs
Pregnancy-induced hypertension	Premature delivery caused by uncontrolled hypertension or eclampsia
	Uteroplacental insufficiency, abruptio placentae, fetal loss, growth retardation, thrombocytopenia, neutropenia
Hematologic	
Severe anemia (hemoglobin <6 mg/dL)	Impaired oxygen delivery, fetal loss
Iron deficiency anemia	Reduced iron stores, lower mental and developmental scores in follow-up
Idiopathic thrombocytopenic purpura	Thrombocytopenia, central nervous system (CNS) hemorrhage
Fetal platelet antigen sensitization	Thrombocytopenia, CNS hemorrhage
Rh or ABO sensitization	Jaundice, anemia, hydrops fetalis
Sickle cell anemia	Increased prematurity and intrauterine growth retardation
Infectious	
Chorioamnionitis	Increased risk for neonatal sepsis, prematurity
Gonorrhea	Ophthalmia neonatorum
Hepatitis A	Perinatal transmission
Hepatitis B	Perinatal transmission, chronic hepatitis, hepatic carcinoma
Herpes simplex	Encephalitis, disseminated herpes (risk of neonatal disease is much higher with primary than recurrent maternal infection)
Human immunodeficiency virus	Twenty-five percent risk of infectious transmission, lower with zidovudine use
Syphilis	Congenital syphilis, growth retardation
Tuberculosis	Perinatal and postnatal transmission
Inflammatory, Immunologic	
Systemic lupus erythematosus	Fetal death, spontaneous abortions, heart block, neonatal lupus, thrombocytopenia, neutropenia, hemolytic anemia
Inflammatory bowel disease	Increase in prematurity, fetal loss, and growth retardation
Renal, Urologic	
Urinary tract infection	Prematurity, intrauterine growth retardation
Chronic renal failure	Prematurity, intrauterine growth retardation
Transplant recipients	Prematurity, intrauterine growth retardation, possible effects of maternal immunosuppressive therapy and mineral disorders

born. When preeclampsia occurs early in the pregnancy, it may have severe effects on fetal growth. Fetal distress caused by preeclampsia may necessitate premature delivery of the infant before maturation of the lungs. Preeclampsia also causes neonatal neutropenia and thrombocytopenia.

Particular attention must be paid to infectious illnesses during the pregnancy and in the perinatal period. The results of the prenatal Venereal Disease Research Laboratory (VDRL) tests, as well as any maternal treatment for syphilis, should be recorded in the neonatal record. In communities with a high prevalence of syphilis or in high-risk patients, repeat testing (despite negative prenatal results) of the mother for syphilis at the time of delivery should be considered. All women should be tested for hepatitis B surface antigen during pregnancy, and all neonates born to positive mothers should receive both hepatitis B immunoglobulin and hepatitis B vaccine. Maternal testing for antibody to the human immunodeficiency virus (HIV) should be encouraged, particularly in high-risk populations. The HIV-positive mother should be given zidovudine prenatally and through the intrapartum course. When such maternal therapy is combined with neonatal treatment for 6 weeks with zidovudine, the incidence of vertical transmission of HIV was reduced from 25% to 8%.[15] Even if maternal treatment with zidovudine is limited to the peripartum period, or the infant is started on treatment within 48 hours of birth, the risk of transmission of HIV to the newborn can be reduced.[37] Any infant born to a mother with a positive HIV antibody or other evidence of HIV infection should be referred for appropriate evaluation and possible treatment.

Active maternal genital infection with herpes simplex virus (HSV) with ruptured membranes or vaginal delivery puts the infant at risk for neonatal herpes disease. The risk for vertical transmission of HSV is particularly high when the mother has active primary infection at the time of delivery or the infant is born prematurely. In contrast, with recurrent maternal herpes, the risk for vertical transmission of HSV is well below 5%.[27]

Maternal chorioamnionitis increases the risk for bacterial sepsis in the newborn, particularly in the premature infant. The results of amniotic fluid cultures may be helpful in anticipating possible pathogens in the new-born. It is strongly encouraged to follow the recommendations of the Centers for Disease Control and the American Academy of Pediatrics regarding the use of intrapartum prophylactic antibiotics for mothers at risk to transmit group B streptococcus to their infants.[5, 13]

Maternal Medications

Medications given to the mother may have adverse effects on the fetus (Table 3–3).[12, 28] One area of great concern has been the risk for fetal malformations caused by use of maternal drugs. Because organogenesis occurs primarily in the first 12 weeks of gestation, the fetus can easily be exposed to a variety of potentially teratogenic toxins and drugs before a woman knows she is pregnant or before the first prenatal visit. Appropriate counseling about the dangers of maternal drugs on the fetus is further complicated by the lack of prenatal care in some high-risk populations. Hence, the issue of medications and drugs during pregnancy is truly a public health issue. Women of childbearing age need to be educated about the potential risk associated with use of medications (both prescribed and over the counter) and illicit drugs before conception and embryogenesis. Besides their teratogenic potential, maternal medications can have a variety of other effects on the fetus and newborn. Fetal growth can be impaired by antineoplastic agents, heroin, cocaine, irradiation, and some anticonvulsants. Drugs used for tocolysis of labor can cause symptoms in the neonate. β-Sympathomimetics are associated with neonatal hypoglycemia resulting from the mobilization of glycogen from the fetal liver. Magnesium sulfate, which is used for treatment of preterm labor and preeclampsia, depresses respiratory effort and can lead to respiratory failure in the newborn. In contrast, prenatal steroids for fetal lung maturation are generally safe and without adverse effects on the newborn.

Illicit and recreational drug use among pregnant women remains a major problem that affects both the fetus and the newborn. Maternal heroin and methadone use cause neonatal abstinence syndrome, which is characterized by irritability, hypertonia, jitteriness, seizures, sneezing, tachycardia, diarrhea, and difficulties with feedings.[3] These withdrawal effects can be prolonged, partic-

Table 3–3. Maternal Medications and Toxins: Possible Effects on the Fetus and Newborn

Medication	Effect on Fetus and Newborn
Analgesics and Anti-inflammatories	
Acetaminophen	Generally safe except with maternal overdose
Aspirin	Hemorrhage, premature closure of ductus arteriosus, pulmonary artery hypertension (effects not seen at ≤100 mg/day)
Opiates	Neonatal abstincence syndrome with chronic use
Ibuprofen	Reduced amniotic fluid volume when used in tocolysis; risk for premature ductus arteriosus closure and pulmonary hypertension
Indomethacin	Closure of fetal ductus arteriosus and pulmonary artery hypertension
Meperidine	Respiratory depression peaks 2 to 3 hours after maternal dose
Propoxyphene	Drug withdrawal reported
Anesthetics	
General anesthesia	Respiratory depression of infant at delivery with prolonged anesthesia just before delivery
Lidocaine	High serum levels cause central nervous system (CNS) depression; accidental direct injection into the fetal head causes seizures
Antibiotics	
Aminoglycosides	Ototoxicity reported after use of kanamycin and streptomycin
Cephalosporins	Some drugs in this group displace bilirubin from albumin
Isoniazid	Risk for folate deficiency
Metronidazole	Potential teratogen and carcinogen, but not proven in humans
Penicillins	Generally no adverse effect
Tetracyclines	Yellow-brown staining of infant's teeth (when given at ≥5 months' gestation); stillbirth and prematurity due to maternal hepatotoxicity
Sulfonamides	Some drugs in this group displace bilirubin from albumin; can cause kernicterus
Trimethoprim	Folate antagonism
Vancomycin	Potential for ototoxicity
Anticonvulsants	
Carbamazepine	Neural tube defects; midfacial hypoplasia
Phenobarbital	Withdrawal symptoms, hemorrhagic disease; midfacial hypoplasia
Phenytoin	Hemorrhagic disease; fetal hydantoin syndrome: growth and mental deficiency, midfacial hypoplasia, hypoplasia of distal phalanges
Trimethadione	Fetal trimethadione syndrome: growth and mental deficiency, abnormal facies (including synophrys with upslanting eyebrows), cleft lip and palate, cardiac and genital anomalies
Valproic acid	Neural tube defects, midfacial hypoplasia
Anticoagulants	
Warfarin (Coumadin)	Warfarin embryopathy: stippled epiphyses, growth and mental deficiencies, seizures, hypoplastic nose, eye defects, CNS anomalies including Dandy-Walker syndrome
Heparin	No direct adverse effects upon the fetus
Antineoplastics	
Aminopterin	Cleft palate, hydrocephalus, meningomyelocele, growth retardation
Cyclophosphamide	Growth retardation, cardiovascular and digital anomalies
Methotrexate	Absent digits, CNS malformation
Antithyroid Drugs	
Iodide-containing drugs	Hypothyroidism
Methimazole	Hypothyroidism, cutis aplasia
Potassium iodide	Hypothyroidism and goiter, especially with chronic use
Propylthiouracil	Hypothyroidism
[131]I	Hypothyroidism, partial to complete ablation of thyroid gland

Table continued on following page

Table 3–3. Maternal Medications and Toxins: Possible Effects on the Fetus and Newborn *Continued*

Medication	Effect on Fetus and Newborn
Antivirals	
Acyclovir	No adverse effects reported; use reserved for life-threatening maternal illness
Ribavirin	Teratogenic and embryolethal in animals
Zidovudine	Potential for fetal bone marrow suppression; combined maternal and neonatal treatment reduces perinatal transmission of human immunodeficiency virus
Cardiovascular Drugs and Antihypertensives	
Angiotensin-converting enzyme inhibitors	Fetal hypocalvaria, oligohydramnios and fetal compression, oliguria, renal failure
β-Blockers (propranolol)	Neonatal bradycardia, hypoglycemia
Calcium channel blockers	If maternal hypotension occurs, this could affect placental blood flow
Diazoxide	Hyperglycemia; decreased placental perfusion with maternal hypotension
Digoxin	Fetal toxicity with maternal overdose
Hydralazine	If maternal hypotension occurs, this could affect placental blood flow
Methyldopa	Mild, clinically insignificant decrease in neonatal blood pressure
Diuretics	
Furosemide	Increases fetal urinary sodium and potassium levels
Thiazides	Thrombocytopenia, hypoglycemia, hyponatremia, hypokalemia
Hormones and Related Drugs	
Androgenics (danazol)	Masculinization of female fetuses
Corticosteroids	Cleft palate in animals but not humans
Diethylstilbestrol (DES)	DES daughters: vaginal adenosis, genital tract anomalies, increased incidence of clear cell adenocarcinoma, increased rate of premature delivery in future pregnancy DES sons: possible increase in genitourinary anomalies
Estrogens, progestins	Risk for virilization of female fetuses reported with progestins; small, if any, risk for other anomalies
Insulin	No apparent direct adverse effects, uncertain risk of maternal hypoglycemia
Tamoxifen	Animal studies suggest potential for DES-like effect
Sedatives, Tranquilizers, and Psychiatric Drugs	
Barbiturates	Risk for hemorrhage and drug withdrawal
Benzodiazepines	Drug withdrawal; cleft lip/palate in animals but not humans
Fluoxetine	No obvious effect on neurodevelopment
Lithium	Ebstein anomaly, diabetes insipidus, thyroid depression, cardiovascular dysfunction
Thalidomide	Limb deficiency, cardiac defects, ear malformations
Tricyclic antidepressants	No obvious effect on neurodevelopment; nortriptyline: neonatal urinary retention; imipramine: neonatal withdrawal
Social and Illicit Drugs	
Alcohol	Fetal alcohol syndrome (see text)
Amphetamines	Withdrawal, prematurity, decreased birth weight and head circumference, cerebral injury
Cocaine	Decreased birth weight, microcephaly, prematurity, abruptio placentae, decreased placental blood flow, stillbirth, cerebral hemorrhage; possible teratogen: genitourinary, cardiac, facial, limb
Heroin	Increased incidence of low birth weight and small for gestational age, drug withdrawal, postnatal growth and behavioral disturbances; decreased incidence of respiratory distress syndrome
Marijuana	Elevated blood carboxyhemoglobin; possible cause of shorter gestation, dysfunctional labor, intrauterine growth retardation, and anomalies
Methadone	Increased birth weight as compared to heroin, drug withdrawal (worse than with heroin alone)

Table 3–3. Maternal Medications and Toxins: Possible Effects on the Fetus and Newborn *Continued*

Medication	Effect on Fetus and Newborn
Phencyclidine (PCP)	Irritability, jitteriness, hypertonia, poor feeding
Tobacco smoking	Elevated blood carboxyhemoglobin; decreases birth weight by 175 to 250 g, increased prematurity rate, increased premature rupture of membranes, placental abruption and previa, increased fetal death, cleft lip
Tocolytics	
Magnesium sulfate	Respiratory depression, hypotonia, bone demineralization with prolonged (weeks) use for tocolysis
Ritodrine	Neonatal hypoglycemia
Terbutaline	Neonatal hypoglycemia
Vitamins and Related Drugs	
A (preformed, not carotene)	Excessive doses ($\geq$50,000 IU/day) may be teratogenic
Acitretin	Activated form of etretinate (see below)
D	Megadoses may cause hypercalcemia, craniosynostosis
Etretinate	Limb deficiency, neural tube defect; ear, cardiac, and CNS anomalies
Folate deficiency	Neural tube defects
Isotretinoin (13-cis-retinoic acid)	Ear, cardiac, CNS, and thymic anomalies
Menadione (vitamin K_3)	Hyperbilirubinemia and kernicterus
Phytonadione (vitamin K_1)	No adverse effect
Miscellaneous	
Anticholingergics	Neonatal meconium ileus
Antiemetic	Doxylamine succinate and/or dicyclomine HCl with pyridoxine reported to be teratogens, but bulk of evidence is clearly negative
Aspartame	Contains phenylalanine; potential risk to fetus of a mother with phenylketonuria
Chorionic villus sampling (CVS)	Limb deficiency with early CVS
Irradiation	Adverse effects primarily associated with therapeutic, not diagnostic doses, and is dose dependent: fetal death, microcephaly, growth retardation
Lead	Decreased IQ (dose related)
Methylene blue	Hemolytic anemia, hyperbilirubinemia, methemoglobinemia; intra-amniotic injection in early pregnancy associated with intestinal atresia
Methylmercury	CNS injury, neurodevelopmental abnormalities, microcephaly
Misoprostol	Moebius sequence
Oral hypoglycemics	Neonatal hypoglycemia
Polychlorinated biphenyls	Cola skin coloration, minor skeletal anomalies, neurodevelopmental deficits

ularly with methadone exposure. Intrauterine narcotic exposure is also associated with intrauterine growth retardation, poor postnatal growth, and abnormal neurodevelopmental outcome. Maternal cocaine exposure has also been reported to be associated with neurobehavioral disturbances in the newborn, although true withdrawal symptoms are less pronounced than with heroin or methadone.[19] In utero cocaine exposure affects fetal growth, and such infants tend to have a lower birth weight and smaller head circumference. Cocaine use in pregnancy is associated with neonatal cerebral hemorrhage, premature delivery, abruptio placentae, and stillbirth. There is conflicting data about the role of prenatal cocaine exposure and the risk for congenital malformations (including intestinal atresia, urogenital anomalies, and limb reduction anomalies), and necrotizing enterocolitis.[24] Prenatal opiate and cocaine exposure is associated with an increased incidence of sudden infant death syndrome.[16] Persistent illicit drug activity in the mother or other family members can continue to affect the care of the high-risk infant throughout the hospitalization and at the time of discharge, especially if the infant requires any type of special treatment at home. The management of the dysfunctional drug-exposed family can be as difficult as the care of the sick newborn.

Prenatal alcohol use has serious adverse effects on the fetus that can present as problems in the neonatal period and beyond. The greatest risk to the fetus seems to be associated with heavy chronic drinking during the pregnancy (four to six drinks per day). However, with even more modest alcohol consumption (e.g., two drinks per day), effects have been noted in some studies. The most extreme result of maternal alcohol use is fetal alcohol syndrome.[7] Signs of this syndrome at birth may include intrauterine growth retardation, central nervous system problems (microcephaly, irritability, tremulousness), facial dysmorphic features, congenital heart disease, and ear, eye, and limb (joint contractures, nail hypoplasia) anomalies. The facial dysmorphic features include short palpebral fissures, thin upper lip, smooth philtrum, maxillary hypoplasia, and a short nose. Later in life, these infants may have continued poor growth, neurobehavioral problems, and low IQ scores. Many infants exposed to alcohol in utero do not have sufficient physical features or anomalies required to make the diagnosis of fetal alcohol syndrome. However, these same infants may still demonstrate neurobehavioral and motor problems, which have been referred to as fetal alcohol effects.[7]

Maternal smoking increases blood levels of carboxyhemoglobin and impairs oxygen delivery to the fetus. Smoking is associated with a decrease in birth weight of 175 to 250 g. Several studies have suggested that nonsmoking mothers who are exposed to environmental tobacco smoke are more likely to have low birth weight infants than mothers with minimal tobacco exposure. Maternal smoking has also been implicated in placental abruption, preterm delivery, and postnatal respiratory illnesses. Whether prenatal exposure to tobacco causes an increased incidence of congenital malformations is unclear. However, a recent meta-analysis of previous studies found a small but significant effect of maternal smoking during the first trimester upon the incidence of cleft lip and palate.[40]

◆ PREPARATIONS FOR DELIVERY

After the maternal record has been reviewed, the physician should meet with the parents, before the delivery of the infant. Important information regarding the prena-

tal course is not always reflected in the hospital obstetric record, particularly if prenatal care was lacking or fragmented, and this information may be available from the mother. If the delivery of a premature infant is expected, it is appropriate to explain the role of the pediatrician or neonatologist in the delivery room, as well as resuscitation and subsequent management procedures (Table 3–4). Aspects of the anticipated hospital course for a sick premature infant should be discussed. Preparing parents for the prolonged hospitalization of a premature infant begins to build the foundations of trust and communication that will be needed between the family and the medical team. If time is limited because of the imminent delivery of the infant, the physician should at least introduce himself or herself to the parents and briefly explain the anticipated resuscitation procedures.

Depending on the type and severity of anticipated problems, specific equipment or extra personnel may be needed in the delivery room. For example, if an infant is known to have hydrops with pleural effusions and ascites, then the resuscitation team should have equipment fully prepared before the delivery for needle thoracentesis, chest tube drainage, intubation, ventilation, and umbilical catheterization. For such a high-risk delivery, the presence of two physicians to care for the infant may be indicated. Neonatal nursing personnel should be kept informed regarding the admission of high-risk mothers and possible pending deliveries. The pediatric surgeon should be notified of the anticipated delivery of any infants with abdominal wall defects, possible gastrointestinal anomalies or obstruction, diaphragmatic hernia, or tracheoesophageal fistula.

Table 3–4. Subjects to Discuss with Parents Before Delivery of a Sick Premature Newborn

Anticipated birth weight and gestational age
Approximate risk of death and major morbidities
Anticipated length of hospitalization
Respiratory distress syndrome, oxygen, ventilation, surfactant
Procedures: intubation, intravenous catheters, umbilical catheterization, lumbar puncture
Blood transfusion: risks, benefits, designated donations
Potential problems: patent ductus arteriosus, intraventricular hemorrhage, jaundice
Possible need for transport (if not delivered in a tertiary center)
Role of the parents in the intensive care nursery

Table 3–5. Effects of Prenatal Steroids on the Premature Newborn

Increased tissue and alveolar surfactant
Maturational effects on the lung: structural and
  biochemical
Possible maturational effects on brain,
  gastrointestinal tract, and other organs
Decreased mortality rate
Decreased incidence and severity of respiratory
  distress syndrome
?Decreased incidence of necrotizing enterocolitis
Decreased incidence of intraventricular hemorrhage
Decreased incidence of significant patent ductus
  arteriosus
Decreased length of stay and costs of hospitalization

The pediatrician can also play an important role in the appropriate prepartum management of a high-risk mother. Aggressive tocolysis and use of prenatal steroids to induce fetal lung maturity should be strongly encouraged for the mother in preterm labor. Despite the multiple postnatal benefits for prematures after prenatal steroids[9] (Table 3–5), maternal steroids are sometimes withheld in the presence of ruptured membranes, extreme prematurity, and anticipated interval of less than 24 hours before delivery. Unless there are clear contraindications to steroid treatment or proven fetal lung maturity, in the setting of anticipated premature delivery, the mother should be given steroids.[31] The pediatrician should also advocate for delivery of high-risk mothers in the most appropriate setting. The needs of the mother, the fetus, and the newborn infant must all be recognized, and the personnel, equipment, and expertise must be available to meet these needs. Certain high-risk mothers, if stable for transport, should be transferred to a perinatal center. In particular, if premature delivery is anticipated before 32 weeks' gestation, or if there are known major fetal congenital anomalies that would impact on the stabilization of the newborn, then maternal transfer to a perinatal center with an intensive care nursery is most appropriate.

◆ TRANSITION

Transition is a term used to describe a series of events that are centered around birth itself, beginning in utero and continuing into the postnatal period. The fetus is well adapted to the intrauterine environment.

However, during this intricate symbiotic relationship with the mother, the fetus must also prepare for transition to extrauterine life. This transition requires striking adaptive changes in multiple organ systems of the newborn. Some of these dynamic changes are largely completed in the first minutes to hours after birth. Others are initiated at birth, but continue to evolve over the first weeks of life. The ability of the newborn to make this transition safely and expeditiously affects both the health and survival of the infant. Recognition of the factors that may adversely impact on the transitional period allows the health professional to act promptly and judiciously for the benefit of the infant.

The most dramatic changes during transition involve the cardiovascular and respiratory systems. During fetal life, gas exchange is accomplished by the placenta, while in contrast the fetal lungs are gasless and filled with fluid. In the several days before delivery, fetal lung water begins to decrease and is accelerated by labor. Various hormones, including epinephrine and vasopressin, decrease fluid secretion into the pulmonary intraluminal space. Plasma protein levels increase with labor, and this augmented oncotic pressure likely increases pulmonary intraluminal water reabsorption. Intraluminal fluid is transported to the interstitium and removed primarily by augmented postnatal pulmonary blood flow as pulmonary artery pressure decreases. Some intraluminal fluid is transported by the lymphatics, through the mediastinal tissues, or across the pleural space. Previously, it has been suggested that thoracic compression during vaginal birth played a prominent role in the expulsion of lung fluid through the oropharynx. However, such a mechanism does not seem to have a major role in the reduction of lung water in the newborn.

Fetal breathing is episodic and occurs primarily during periods of low-voltage electrocortical activity. It likely plays a role in the conditioning of respiratory muscles and may have other effects on chest wall, lung, and muscle growth. A variety of phenomena contribute to the onset of continuous breathing, which occurs shortly after birth in relatively healthy nonasphyxiated infants. Aspects of the physical environment may play a role, such as light, sound, cutaneous stimulation, and heat loss. Cord occlusion and an increase in blood oxygen appear to be potent stimulants of continuous breathing by the newborn. The fetus prepares for air breathing by the synthesis and release of surfactant into the alveolar space. The process can be accelerated by premature rupture of fetal membrane, β-mimetic tocolysis, and the administration of steroids to the mother. Delivery of a term infant by elective cesarean section without labor may prevent maturation of this late process of surfactant production and release, resulting in an infant with respiratory distress syndrome.

The transitional changes in the cardiovascular system are primarily an adaptation to the elimination of the placental circulation and an adaptation to pulmonary gas exchange. As the lungs expand at birth, pulmonary artery pressure declines and there is a dramatic increase in pulmonary blood flow. Systemic arterial resistance increases with cord occlusion and elimination of the low resistance placental circulation. These factors combine to favor an increase in pulmonary blood flow rather than the passage of blood via the ductus arteriosus into the distal aorta. Because of the increase in pulmonary blood flow, left atrial pressure increases and functionally closes the foramen ovale, eliminating this source of previous right-to-left shunting. The right and left ventricles then function primarily in series, rather than pumping in parallel as in the fetal state. The ductus arteriosus remains open for a variable period of time, but it begins to close in response to exposure to highly oxygenated blood. It generally functionally closes by 1 to 2 days in a term infant, but frequently remains open in the premature or the seriously ill term newborn with pulmonary artery hypertension. The ductus venosus closes within 1 to 2 days (contributing to the technical difficulty of passing an umbilical venous catheter to the right atrium beyond the first day of life). Pulmonary artery pressure continues to decline through the first weeks of life. During these dramatic changes in the cardiovascular system, the sick newborn may demonstrate difficulties in making these transitions. Because of the parallel pumping systems of the fetal cardiovascular system, most infants with complex congenital heart disease are well adapted to the in utero state. However, these infants often do poorly in the transition to extrauterine life. In infants with ductal dependent cyanotic congenital heart disease, progressive cyanosis

develops as the ductus arteriosus closes. In those infants with left-sided obstructive lesions (e.g., hypoplastic left heart), acidosis and shock develop as the ductus arteriosus closes and distal aortic blood flow is lost. Infants with pulmonary artery hypertension shunt right to left at the foramen ovale or patent ductus arteriosus. Recognition of infants at risk for pulmonary artery hypertension (e.g., meconium aspiration) may lead the physician to earlier interventions (e.g., endotracheal suctioning, oxygen, ventilation) in order to reverse or prevent this problem.

The uterine environment is relatively quiet, very dark, and rather unchanging until labor and passage through the birth canal. At birth, the newborn is bombarded with stimuli, including exposure to light, different sounds, and tactile stimuli. In addition, the newborn must begin to defend its core temperature against heat loss, despite being born both wet and into a much cooler environment. These multiple stresses result in a surge of sympathetic nervous system activity. Catecholamines increase dramatically at birth. Brown fat (nonshivering) thermogenesis causes the hydrolysis of stored triglycerides and the release of fatty acids. Table 3–6 summarizes these and other events during transition.

Specific physical and behavioral changes, which occur in the healthy newborn in the hours after birth, have been described (Fig. 3–1). The healthy newborn may have some initial bradycardia or tachycardia, and cutaneous perfusion may be mottled or pale. Respirations may be initially somewhat irregular but should improve steadily and become regular and vigorous. There may be some mild transient grunting and flaring, but true respiratory distress with retractions should not be present. If the infant has made a stable transition, these parameters stabilize within the first hour of life. After birth, the healthy newborn often undergoes a quiet alert phase, which has been referred to as the *first phase of reactivity*. When placed skin to skin on the mother's chest shortly after birth, the infant often becomes quiet and exploring.[26] Rhythmic pushing movements of the lower extremities have been described as the infant searches for the mother's breast. If left undisturbed, the infant crawls and searches for the areola in an attempt to attach and suckle (Fig. 3–2). Suckling causes release of oxytocin in the

Table 3–6. Summary of Transitional Events in the Newborn

Pulmonary

Reabsorption of intraluminal fluid
Onset of continuous breathing
Expansion of pulmonary air spaces
Pulmonary gas exchange replaces placental
  circulation
Surfactant synthesis and release

Cardiovascular

Removal of the placental circulation
Decline in pulmonary artery pressure and increase in
  pulmonary blood flow
Closure of ductus arteriosus, foramen ovale, and
  ductus venosus

Glucose Homeostasis

Loss of transplacental glucose transport with decline
  in serum glucose
Increase in glucagon and decrease in insulin levels

Thermogenesis

Sympathetic nervous system activation caused by
  cold stress
Nonshivering thermogenesis (brown fat)

Hormonal and Metabolic

Shift from primarily glucose metabolism (RQ = 1) to
  glucose and fat (RQ = 0.8–0.85)
Increase in oxygen consumption
Increase in levels of epinephrine and norepinephrine
Acute increase in TSH with subsequent decline
Peak increase in T_4, free T_4, and T_3 at 48 hours
Decrease in reverse T_3

Decline in serum calcium with nadir at 24 hours and
  subsequent elevation
Increase in parathyroid hormone, 1,25 OH vitamin D,
  and calcitonin
Increase in glycerol and free fatty acids

Nervous System

Adaptive interaction with parents and environment
Movement between states
Increase in motor activity

Renal

Increase in renin production
Increase in sodium reabsorption
Onset of long-term maturational changes with
  improving glomerular filtration rate
Reduction of extracellular fluid compartment
  (diuresis)

Hematologic

Marked reduction in erythropoietin and
  erythrogenesis
Postnatal increase in blood leukocyte and neutrophil
  count
Improved vitamin K–dependent carboxylation of
  coagulation factors

Gastrointestinal

Evacuation of meconium
Induction of intestinal enzymes with feeding
Establishment of effective coordinated suck,
  swallow, breathing

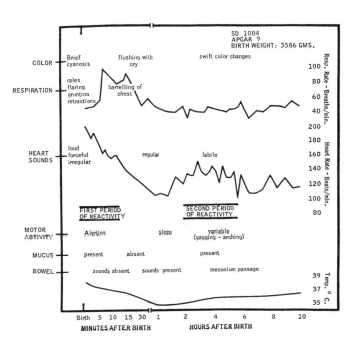

Figure 3–1. A summary of the physical findings in normal transition (the first 10 hours of extrauterine life in a representative high-Apgar-score infant delivered under spinal anesthesia without premedication). (From Desmond M, Rudolph A, Phitaksphraiwan P: The transitional care nursery. Pediatr Clin North Am 13:651, 1966.)

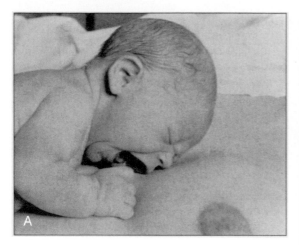

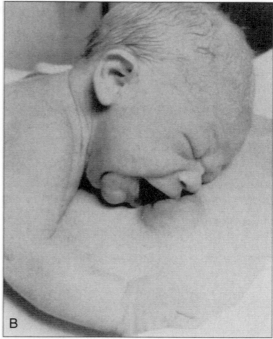

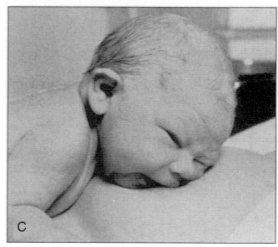

Figure 3–2. Younger than 1 hour of age, this boy crawls up the mother's body *(A)* and prepares to latch onto the breast *(B, C)* without assistance. (From Kennell JH, Klaus MH: Bonding: Recent observations that alter perinatal care. Pediatr Rev 19:7, 1998; Reprinted with permission from Lennart Righard.)

mother, stimulating milk production and uterine contractions. Sucking movements in the infant stimulate the release of multiple gastrointestinal hormones, which prepare the infant to digest enteral nutrients.[36] The warmth provided by the mother's chest maintains a stable temperature in the infant, as long as a blanket is also placed over the infant and the room is not too cold.[14] Early contact with the mother has been shown to increase the success of breast-feeding, and it is an important first step in the bonding process. Most hospital staff in birthing centers recognize the importance of this early contact between the mother and infant.

Sometimes mothers are encouraged to promptly attempt to nurse their infant immediately after birth. It may be more appropriate to quickly dry the infant and to rapidly determine that the infant is healthy and requires no immediate interventions. Then the infant can be placed upon the mother's chest, skin to skin, and allowed to have a private quiet time with the parents.

◆ PHYSICAL EXAMINATION OF THE NEWBORN

The first 24 hours of life are particularly precarious as the infant makes the transition from intrauterine to extrauterine life. During this critical period, a thorough physical examination is essential to identify problems and institute early intervention. Physicians should continually strive to improve upon their observational skills and the quality of their newborn examinations. Nothing can replace years of clinical experience with the many normal variations and abnormal findings with which a newborn may present.[18, 33]

After initial resuscitation and stabilization in the delivery room, the newborn should receive an initial examination in order to identify any significant problems or anomalies. The infant's respiratory effort and air exchange should be observed closely. An infant with persistently shallow and irregular respirations needs further resuscitation and appropriate monitoring. Symptoms of respiratory distress such as grunting, flaring, retractions, and cyanosis should be identified promptly. Particular attention should be paid to the adequacy of the infant's heart rate and clinical indicators of cardiovascular function. Pallor and poor perfusion need immediate further evaluation and possible intervention. It should be established that the infant is appropriately responsive and has good muscle tone. The extremities, facies, genitalia, abdomen, and back should be quickly inspected for any anomalies. Such a quick examination of an apparently healthy infant in the delivery room can usually be performed in 1 to 2 minutes. Any major abnormalities should be discussed with the parents as soon as feasible.

In a stable, healthy, term or near-term newborn, a more detailed examination by the physician may be deferred. However, admitting nursing personnel should perform a thorough assessment of the infant within 2 hours of birth. This allows the infant to be with the parents and to start breast-feeding. The nursing personnel should evaluate the infant for high-risk factors, review the pertinent maternal history (usually included on the labor and delivery record), and examine the infant. The physician should be notified of any high-risk factors in the history or significant findings on examination. This nursing assessment should be recorded in a standardized format. It should include measurement of weight, length, head circumference, estimate of gestational age, and vital signs. The physician should perform a complete physical examination no later than 24

hours after birth, but preferably within 12 hours of birth. The normal newborn should also be examined by the physician within the 24 hours before discharge.[8] High-risk infants, including those with respiratory distress, poor cardiac output, gestational age of less than 35 weeks, or clinical signs of asphyxia or sepsis should be assessed immediately by the nursing staff and examined by the physician.

Vital Signs, Body Measurements, and Gestational Age Assessment

The admitting nursing personnel should measure the temperature, respiratory rate, and heart rate of all newborn infants within the first hour of life. In the past, the initial measurement of temperature was commonly performed rectally in order to additionally determine patency of the anus. This practice of an initial rectal temperature has been largely abandoned by many birth centers, because of the small but real risk of bowel perforation with rectal measurement. The nurse should not only record the respiratory rate, but should observe for any signs of respiratory distress, irregularities in respiratory pattern (e.g., apnea), and the degree of work of breathing. In the first day of life most newborns have a respiratory rate of 40 to 60 breaths per minute. However, in transition, some newborns have a respiratory rate as high as 80 to 100 breaths per minute with little or no signs of distress. Heart rate should be checked by auscultation and any irregularities in rhythm noted. Healthy term newborns do not require routine blood pressure determination on admission. Any sick newborn and any premature infant (less than 35 weeks' gestational age) should have at least an initial blood pressure measurement, which is easily performed by an oscillometric technique.

Every newborn should have assessment of gestational age performed.[10] In some nurseries, the gestational age examination is performed by the nursing staff on admission of all newborns. We encourage physicians to continue to perform a gestational age assessment as part of their evaluation of a premature infant. The results of this examination should then be compared with the maternal estimated date of confinement (by ultrasound and last menstrual period). The nursing staff should record the weight (in kilograms), and the length and head circumference (in centimeters) of the infant on admission. These measurements should be plotted on the appropriate intrauterine growth curves. This facilitates the identification of infants who are small or large for gestational age, or who are microcephalic or macrocephalic. Chapter 4 addresses these areas in greater depth.

General Examination

It is useful to observe the overall condition of the infant, including major anomalies, respiratory effort, color, perfusion, activity, and responsiveness. In infants with respiratory distress, it is important to note the presence of grunting, flaring, and retractions and to assess the work of breathing. The quality and the strength of the infant's cry and overall motor activity are especially useful indicators of the infant's general condition. Such general observations are useful to quickly categorize an infant and to focus one's attention on a critically ill newborn. A vigorous, screaming, pink infant clearly does not demand the same immediate intervention required by the infant who is pale and hypotonic with labored or irregular breathing.

Edema is readily noted in any initial examination. The presenting part at birth may be edematous, bruised, and covered with petechiae. Edema of the dorsum of the feet may be seen as a focal finding in Turner syndrome, or it may be part of a more generalized picture of edema. Infants with hydrops, whether immune or nonimmune, often have generalized edema, which can include the trunk, extremities, scalp, and face. In critically ill infants who require fluid volume resuscitation, generalized edema may develop over the course of their illness. Such edema often localizes to the face and trunk, especially the flanks.

The initial examination should also include a quick survey for dysmorphic features, whether malformations or deformations. The presence of a major congenital anomaly or multiple minor anomalies may indicate the need for an aggressive investigation of other major organ defects. All nurseries should have immediate access to a standard reference book describing and illustrating common neonatal malformation and deformation syndromes.[25]

Skin

In the extremely premature infant (23 to 28 weeks' gestational age) the skin can be translucent with little subcutaneous fat and superficial veins that are easily visualized. Because the stratum corneum is quite thin, the skin of the extremely premature infant is easily injured by seemingly innocuous procedures or manipulation that result in denudation of the stratum corneum and a raw weeping surface. With advancing gestational age, the fetal skin matures as the stratum corneum thickens, subcutaneous fat increases, and the skin loses its translucent appearance. By term, the fetal skin is relatively opaque with considerable subcutaneous fat.

By 35 to 36 weeks' gestational age, the infant is covered with vernix. The vernix thins by term and is usually absent in the post-term infant. Meconium staining of the skin, nails, and cord is evident when meconium has been present in the amniotic fluid for a number of hours. The postmature infant has parchment-like skin with deep cracks on the trunk and extremities. Fingernails may be elongated, and peeling of the distal extremities is often evident in the postmature infant.

Erythema toxicum neonatorum is a benign rash seen generally in term infants beginning on the second or third day of life. It is characterized by 1- to 2-mm white papules, which may become vesicular, on an erythematous base. Wright or Giemsa stain of the lesions demonstrates large numbers of eosinophils. Milia, which are 1- to 2-mm whitish papules, are frequently found on the face of newborns. Transient neonatal pustular melanosis, which is seen predominantly in black infants, is a benign generalized eruption with a mixture of superficial pustules that progress to hyperpigmented macules. Mongolian spots are gray-blue nonraised areas of hyperpigmentation seen predominantly over the buttocks or trunk, and are seen most commonly in black, Asian, and Latino infants.

The newborn infant can have a variety of color changes in the first day of life, some of which are due to cardiovascular lability during transition. The harlequin sign is a benign transient finding in which the infant is pale on one side and flushed on the contralateral side with a distinct border in the midline. Mottling of the skin is common in the first days to weeks of life in some infants. The color and perfusion of the skin can provide information regarding cardiac output and oxygenation. Acrocyanosis is a common finding in the first 6 to 24 hours of life, but is usually of little significance by itself. Central cyanosis persisting beyond the first few minutes of life may indicate inadequate oxygen delivery and demands further evaluation. Infants can have cyanosis over just the lower half of the body in the presence of right-to-left shunting across a patent ductus arteriosus. Capillary refill time can be sluggish in the first hours of life as the infant adapts to extrauterine life. Persistent pallor and poor perfusion may reflect inadequate cardiac output as a result of perinatal hypoxia and ischemia, congenital heart disease, or sepsis. Infants with anemia may have pallor, but this is an inconsistent finding even in the presence of severe anemia. Marked plethora may occur with polycythemia, but this finding is also inconsistent. Hence, the physician must have a high index of suspicion for those infants at risk for either anemia or polycythemia. Jaundice at birth is abnormal and requires immediate investigation. Physiologic jaundice is generally not seen before 24 hours of age. Petechiae and bruising are very common on the presenting fetal parts. However, in the presence of thrombocytopenia or platelet dysfunction, petechiae are more likely to be generalized.

A careful examination of the newborn's skin should be made to identify congenital nevi, hemangiomas, areas of abnormal pigmentation, tags, and pits. A port wine stain of the face should alert the physician to the possibility of Sturge-Weber syndrome. Congenital strawberry hemangiomas should be identified and their progression monitored. Large hemangiomas of the face and neck can potentially cause airway obstruction. Massive hemangiomas of the extremities or trunk can result in large systemic shunts and high-output cardiac failure. Congenital defects in the skin are important in the identification of underlying structural problems or systemic disorders. Localized scalp defects are associated with trisomy 13. Midline posterior defects of the skin are particularly important to identify. Sacral dimples should be carefully examined to ensure that the base is clearly visualized and the possibility of a sinus tract to the spinal cord is excluded. Such dermal sinuses can communicate with the cerebrospinal fluid and result in meningitis.

Head and Scalp

The occipital-frontal head circumference should be measured and recorded for all newborns. Ideally, three careful measurements should be taken at various positions over the occipital-frontal area, and the largest measurement is then recorded. The head should be palpated carefully and visually inspected in order to detect any unusual distortions, hematomas, or caput. Because the fetal skull is molded by the delivery process, abnormal skull shapes may need to be reevaluated in 1 to 2 days. Caput succedaneum is a common and expected finding after vaginal vertex delivery. Bruising and edema caused by caput is usually soft, crosses suture lines, and does not significantly expand in size postnatally. Subperiosteal hematomas, which are common, are easily identified by their distinct margins which stop at the suture lines. Subperiosteal hematomas are generally soft and fluctuant on palpation and can give a sensation of absence of the bony skull beneath the hematoma. In contrast, subgaleal hematomas are not limited by suture margins and usually cross the midline. A rapidly expanding subgaleal hematoma can be life threatening because of the blood loss into the hematoma. Such patients require close monitoring and aggressive volume replacement.

The skull sutures should be checked to note whether they are widened or overriding. A widely open full anterior fontanelle with split sutures suggests increased intracranial pressure, which may be caused by intracranial hemorrhage, cerebral edema, or hydrocephalus. Unusual scalp hair patterns can be an indication of underlying brain dysmorphogenesis, particularly if the infant has other dysmorphic features. A midline mass protruding from the skull may be an encephalocele and requires thorough evaluation.

Eyes, Ears, Mouth, and Facial Features

The overall configuration of the face should be inspected including the profile, which helps in the detection of micrognathia. Such overview reveals areas of maxillary or mandibular hypoplasia, any distortion, or hemifacial hypoplasia. The eyes should be inspected for abnormalities in the size of the globes or orbits, and for any malposition (e.g., proptosis as in neonatal hyperthyroidism). Abnormalities of the eyebrows may be a clue to specific syndromes, such as synophrosis in Cornelia de Lange syndrome. The eyelids of the newborn may be edematous or display ecchymosis from the delivery process. Nevus flammeus is commonly noted on the upper eyelids. After vaginal delivery the conjunctivae are often injected and scleral hemorrhages may be present. The parents may need reassurance regarding these generally benign features.

Abnormal slanting of the palpebral fissures is associated with a number of syndromes. Notably an upward slant is seen in trisomy 21, whereas down-slanting eyes are a feature of Treacher Collins, Apert, and DiGeorge syndromes. Short palpebral fissures with a smooth philtrum and thin upper lip suggest fetal alcohol syndrome. Hypertelorism or inner epicanthal folds are associated with a large number of syndromes (most notably trisomy 21). Marked hypotelorism is associated with holoprosencephaly and trisomy 13. The eyes should be examined with an ophthalmoscope to check for the red reflex and the presence of cataracts. Leukocoria, or a white pupil, mandates a thorough ophthalmologic examination. Cloudiness of the cornea may be seen at birth, especially in the premature infant. The pupils should be round and equal in size. Pupillary reactivity to light is minimal beginning at 30 to 32 weeks' gestation and increases with gestational age. The lenticular pattern can be useful in gestational age assessment.

The oral cavity should be inspected using a tongue blade and a light source. Important findings to note include the presence of neonatal teeth, the arch of the palate, the integrity of both the hard and soft palate, the shape and movement of the tongue, and the presence of any oropharyngeal masses or mucosal lesions. Although cleft lip and palate are frequently isolated anomalies, the infant with these anomalies should be carefully examined for any other associated anomalies. Abnormal masses (e.g., tumors, hemangiomas) in the area of the mouth and pharynx demand prompt attention in view of their potential to cause airway obstruc-

tion. Neonatal teeth are generally a benign finding, but may be associated with several syndromes (Ellis-van Creveld, Hallermann-Streiff, and Sotos syndromes). Protrusion of the tongue from the mouth is seen in trisomy 21, or it may be due to macroglossia, which may be associated with storage diseases, Beckwith-Wiedemann syndrome, and hypothyroidism.

The position, rotation, and shape of the ears should be noted. In very premature infants, the pinna is soft, flat, and easily folded back upon itself. In term infants, the outer helix of the pinna should be well formed with a definite curvature. Infants of diabetic mothers may have unusually hairy ears. The presence of abnormally shaped or malformed (e.g., microtia) ears should prompt a careful examination of the infant for other potential dysmorphic features. In particular, low set and posteriorly rotated ears are associated with a number of syndromes. The ears are carefully inspected in order to assure patency of the external auditory canal. Otoscopy is not routinely needed in the newborn infant with normal external ear anatomy. Amniotic fluid debris and secretions often prevent easy viewing of the tympanic membrane in the first days of life.

Neck and Thorax

The neck should be supple and easily turned from side to side, and the trachea should be in the midline. Gentle extension of the neck is performed looking for any masses, cystic hygromas, or goiter. Large masses in the neck require urgent evaluation because of their potential for airway obstruction. A webbed neck or redundant skin is associated with trisomy 21, Turner, Noonan, and Zellweger syndromes. The clavicles should be palpated to check for deformities. A clavicular fracture often results in crepitance and swelling, and an asymmetric Moro reflex.

The thorax may appear to be small or malformed in a number of neuromuscular disorders, or in lung hypoplasia. With congenital disorders of generalized muscle weakness, the thorax assumes a bell-shaped appearance. In term infants, the areolae of the nipples are raised and there is an underlying breast bud with a diameter of 0.5 to 1 cm across. The nipples may be enlarged secondary to the effects of maternal hormones, and a milky discharge (so-called witch's milk) is not uncommon in both male and female infants. Mastitis, which is usually unilateral, causes swelling, erythema, warmth, and tenderness. In extremely premature infants, the areola may be quite small, flat, and difficult to identify. Abnormal displacement of the nipple or supernumerary nipples should be noted. The nipples are widely spaced in Turner syndrome, Noonan syndrome, and trisomy 18.

Respiratory System

When breathing at rest, the healthy newborn should move air easily and comfortably at a rate of 40 to 60 breaths per minute. Because most air exchange in newborns is accomplished by the effects of diaphragmatic excursion, there is considerable abdominal wall motion with breathing. Respiratory distress, whether because of lung disease or airway obstruction, is evident by the presence of subcostal or sternal retractions. Suprasternal retractions may be evident in the presence of severe respiratory distress. Audible grunting occurs as the infant expires against a partially closed glottis and is an extremely reliable indicator of any process causing alveolar collapse or atelectasis. Asymmetric movement of the chest wall with respirations occurs with a variety of unilateral lesions of the diaphragms or pleural space (e.g., pneumothorax, diaphragmatic hernia, diaphragmatic paralysis, pleural effusion). The quality of the infant's cry should be noted. A high-pitched shrill cry may suggest a central nervous system disorder. A weak cry may occur in the presence of respiratory distress or a depressed central nervous system. A hoarse or muffled cry may occur with vocal cord swelling, intratracheal narrowing, or a mass.

The lungs should be auscultated anteriorly, posteriorly, and at the sides of the chest. Comparison should be made between the two sides. The breath sounds should be checked for the amount of air exchange (whether with spontaneous or with assisted ventilation). Asymmetric breath sounds may be caused by pneumothorax (Table 3–7), an improperly placed endotracheal tube, diaphragmatic hernia, or any other space-occupying lesion in the hemithorax. Crepitant breath sounds or crackles are often heard in the initial transitional period. These sounds

Table 3–7. Signs of Tension Pneumothorax

Shift of cardiac apical impulse
Decreased breath sounds on the affected side
Asymmetric subcostal retractions and chest wall
  movement
Ballooning of the chest on the affected side
Increased halo of light with transillumination
Cardiovascular changes: hypotension, narrow pulse
  pressure, bradycardia, tachycardia

generally clear as the newborn expands the lungs and clears fluid from the pulmonary airspaces. However, crackles may be heard with respiratory distress syndrome, pneumonia, bronchopulmonary dysplasia (BPD), and various types of aspiration syndromes. Stridor occurs with a variety of causes of airway obstruction, but may be absent or difficult to appreciate in the infant who is moving little air. An audible leak during the inspiratory phase of a ventilator may be heard around the endotracheal tube of intubated infants and may obscure the quality of the breath sounds. The sounds caused by air leak are often transmitted through the mouth and are audible by the unassisted ear. These sounds, when auscultated by a stethoscope, are sometimes mistakenly attributed to wheezing caused by bronchoconstriction. True wheezing with prolonged expiratory phase is sometimes heard in infants with BPD or bronchiolitis. Coarse breath sounds or rhonchi may suggest the need for suctioning to clear secretions in the upper airway or in an endotracheal tube.

For ventilated infants, auscultation of the lungs is routinely used to confirm appropriate position of the endotracheal tube. The breath sounds should be symmetric and there should be adequate chest excursion with good air entry during the inspiratory phase of positive-pressure ventilation. Diminished breath sounds on the left may indicate that the endotracheal tube has passed into the right mainstem bronchus. In such a situation, the tube should be gradually withdrawn until the breath sounds are equal. The depth of the endotracheal tube (in centimeters from the tip) is an important part of the physical examination of an intubated infant (see Appendix I-3). Small movements of the endotracheal tube in a newborn can result in inadvertent right mainstem placement or accidental extubation. However, auscultation of breath sounds alone for confirmation of intubation is not always adequate. The small size of the neonatal chest allows for wide transmission of breath sounds. The sounds created by ventilation through an endotracheal tube inadvertently misplaced into the esophagus can transmit through the newborn's chest. Even with a properly placed endotracheal tube, chest movement and air entry may be inconsistent with positive pressure breaths if the infant is fighting the ventilator. If lung compliance is very poor, chest movement may also be diminished except with high pressures. Devices that detect exhaled CO_2 are being widely used to confirm intubation, and their routine use is highly recommended.

During high-frequency ventilation, whether by oscillation, jet, or flow interruptor, the lungs are not effectively capable of being auscultated. The amplitude of the "chest wiggle" in such infants (by visual inspection or palpation) can be a useful guide as to the effectiveness of the high-frequency pulsations. Such infants should routinely be removed from high-frequency ventilation for a brief period of time in order to auscultate the chest while the infant is given positive-pressure tidal breathing by bagging.

Cardiovascular System

The apical cardiac impulse can be appreciated by both visual inspection and palpation. A hyperdynamic precordium may occur with a large left-to-right shunt or with marked cardiomegaly. The cardiac impulse in a normally positioned heart is most prominent at the lower left sternal border. Prominence of the apical cardiac impulse at the lower right sternal border suggests dextro-rotation or dextroposition of the heart. Shift of the apical impulse is a useful sign to detect tension pneumothorax.

Auscultation of the heart should include right and left second intercostal space, right and left fourth intercostal space, the cardiac apex, and the axillae. Both the diaphragm and bell (with a good seal) of the stethoscope should be used. The infant should be as quiet as possible. It is sometimes necessary to briefly disconnect the ventilator for intubated infants who can tolerate this procedure. The quality of the heart tones (S_1 and S_2) and any clicks, murmurs, or additional heart tones (S_3, S_4) should be noted.

The heart rate in the first day of life is generally between 120 and 160 beats per minute while the infant is at rest. During quiet sleep, some term infants have a resting heart rate as low as 90 to 100 beats per minute. Normal sinus arrhythmia with breathing can be more difficult to discern because of the relatively rapid neonatal heart rate. S_1 is relatively loud in the newborn and is best heard at the apex. S_2 is loudest at the left upper sternal border. Because of the relatively fast heart rate of the newborn, it may be difficult to appreciate the splitting of S_2. With the normal postnatal decline in pulmonary artery pressure, splitting of S_2 may be easier to appreciate. A loud S_2 that is narrowly split may suggest pulmonary artery hypertension. Absence of a split S_2 may occur with various anomalies of the great vessels: aortic atresia, pulmonary atresia, transposition, and truncus arteriosus. Any murmurs should be noted with regard to timing, intensity, and location. A soft systolic murmur in a term infant during the first day of life may be due to a closing ductus arteriosus or to flow across the pulmonary valve as pulmonary resistance declines. Harsh or loud murmurs, particularly in the presence of other cardiovascular symptoms or respiratory distress, require further evaluation. The absence of a cardiac murmur does not exclude the possibility of congenital heart disease. Infants with persistent cyanosis or hypoxemia despite oxygen administration may have cyanotic congenital heart disease, primary lung disease, or pulmonary artery hypertension. Intubation and positive-pressure ventilation can sometimes distinguish an infant with pulmonary artery hypertension and lung disease from an infant with cyanotic congenital heart disease. Echocardiography should be promptly obtained in any critically ill infant with hypoxemia despite oxygen administration and ventilation. Peripheral pulmonary stenosis, which is common in premature infants during the first weeks of life, usually presents as a high-pitched soft systoloic murmur. This murmur is best heard at the cardiac base and radiates widely to the axillae and the back. Hemodynamically significant patent ductus arteriosus (PDA) in a premature infant usually has a systolic murmur best heard along the left sternal border. It is rarely a continuous murmur in the neonatal period and it may be silent. PDA with a large left-to-right shunt may further be associated with a hyperdynamic precordium, bounding pulses, low diastolic pressure, and wide pulse pressure.

The femoral and brachial pulses should be palpated and compared. Pulses may be diminished as a result of hypovolemia, depressed myocardial contractility, sepsis, or left-sided obstructive heart lesions. In left-sided obstructive heart lesions (e.g., coarctation of the aorta and hypoplastic left heart syndrome), the femoral pulses are usually diminished, but may be readily palpable if distal flow is maintained by right-to-left shunting at the ductus arteriosus. While the normal newborn does not routinely require blood pressure measurement, blood pressure should be checked by palpation or by an automated technique (e.g., oscillometric) in any unstable infant, including those infants with respiratory distress, poor perfusion, or depressed neurologic status. All premature infants admitted to an intensive care nursery should also have blood pressure monitored. The blood pressure of critically ill infants is optimally monitored continuously by a transducer connected to an indwelling umbilical or peripheral arterial catheter. Reference can be made to normal values of blood pressure by both birth weight and postnatal age (see Appendices G-11, G-12, and G-13). However, a normal blood pressure does not ensure adequate cardiac output. The quality of the pulses, skin perfusion, capillary refill time, and color are further indirect measures of cardiac output. The presence or absence of acidosis, measurement of mixed venous saturation, and the monitoring of urine output can be further useful indices of tissue perfusion.

Infants with congestive heart failure may have left-to-right shunting from congenital heart disease. Symptoms may include tachycardia, tachypnea, respiratory distress, poor feeding, and hepatomegaly. The cause of such symptoms may be obvious from echocardiography. However, more subtle etiologies of congestive heart failure may escape easy detection. The skull and abdomen (especially over the liver) should be auscultated for bruits resulting from an arteriovenous malformation. Large hemangiomas or sacrococcygeal teratomas can also cause high output failure. An enlarged thyroid gland suggests hyperthyroidism, but specific laboratory studies are needed to confirm this diagnosis.

Abdomen

The abdominal shape, size, and color should be noted. Abdominal wall defects (e.g., gastroschisis, omphalocele) are readily apparent at birth and demand immediate attention. Most newborns have a slightly protuberant abdomen, which becomes more evident as air is swallowed after birth. Bowel obstruction caused by distal atresias, stenosis, meconium plug, and Hirschsprung disease usually presents within the first 1 to 2 days of life with distention, visible loops of bowel, and emesis. In duodenal atresia, there may be only mild distention in the epigastric area resulting from an enlarged stomach. Distention is usually apparent at birth when there is massive ascites, meconium ileus, and peritonitis, or intrauterine midgut volvulus. Intestinal perforation usually gives the abdomen a bluish-gray tint, but frank abdominal wall erythema develops with the onset of peritonitis. Diaphragmatic hernia may result in a scaphoid abdomen resulting from the herniation of abdominal contents into the thorax. Visible loops of bowel suggests intestinal obstruction, particularly in the presence of bilious emesis or gastric aspirates. Bilious emesis should always be considered abnormal and requires further evaluation. In extremely premature infants, some loops of bowel may be seen through a thin abdominal wall without clinical signs of overt obstruction. In prune belly syndrome, the abdominal musculature is lax and the abdominal wall is quite thin, resulting in visible loops of bowel.

Abdominal palpation should be performed with warm hands, patience, and a quiet infant. Under such conditions, the infant's abdominal muscles generally relax after some initial resistance, thus permitting a careful palpation of the internal organs. However, if the abdomen is tense and distended, palpation may only reveal the absence or presence of tenderness. Abdominal tenderness may be obscured if the infant is obtunded, sedated with medications, or extremely premature. The size and position of the liver can be determined by a combination of percussion and palpation, but palpation is primarily used in the newborn. The liver may normally extend 1 to 2 cm below the right costal margin. A midline or left-sided liver should initiate a careful search for other anomalies and appropriate imaging studies. Hepatomegaly may be due to heart failure, congenital infection, congenital anemia, hydrops, intrahepatic tumors, hemangiomas, or hematomas. Pulmonary hyperinflation causes the liver to extend deeper into the abdomen and can give a false impression of hepatomegaly. The spleen is generally not palpable in the healthy newborn, but may be appreciated at the costal margin. Splenomegaly may occur with congenital infection, immune hemolytic disorders, and portal venous hypertension. The kidneys should be carefully palpated bilaterally with the infant relaxed. Bimanual examination can be helpful to evaluate kidney size and shape. Common causes of an enlarged kidney in the newborn include hydronephrosis, renal vein thrombosis, and multicystic renal dysplasia. Enlargement of the adrenal gland is difficult to discern from a renal mass by palpation. Causes of adrenal masses include hemorrhage and tumors (e.g., neuroblastoma). The urinary bladder is palpable only if it is distended with urine. The sick newborn can have transient urinary retention and bladder distention in the presence of a critical illness and the use of sedative drugs, particularly morphine. Reduction of an enlarged bladder by Credé's method (manual pressure) is discouraged, because it may cause ureteral reflux or bladder perforation. Infants with pathologic urinary bladder retention should undergo sterile bladder catheterization as initial management. Palpable intra-abdominal masses should be described by their location, size, shape, mobility, and consistency. It should be noted whether the mass adheres to or is contiguous with other internal organs.

Umbilicus, Cord, and Placenta

The number of arteries and veins in the cord should be noted. The presence of a single umbilical artery is associated with an increased incidence of renal anomalies. The base of the cord and umbilicus should be inspected for any herniation of intestinal contents. A short umbilical cord has been associated with an increased risk for psychomotor abnormalities,[30] cord injuries, and abruptio placentae.

Placental pathology, which may readily explain an infant's problems, is often overlooked. Abruption and infarcts of the placenta can lead to inadequate blood and oxygen delivery to the fetus. Vasa previa may lead to acute fetal blood loss. Histopathologic examination of the placenta should be performed after any complicated delivery, including multiple gestation pregnancies, premature delivery, cases of abruption or other acute blood loss, and stillbirth.

Genitalia and Inguinal Area

The physician should become familiar with the normal variations of newborn genitalia and be able to recognize those abnormalties that require evaluation. The genitalia may be abnormal as a result of primary errors in morphogenesis, but other abnormalities may result from secondary hormonal effects. Clues to underlying systemic hormonal disorders or dysmorphic syndromes may be obtained by careful examination of the genitalia. Gender assignment should never be made for the infant with ambiguous genitalia until a full assessment has been performed. The parents should be reassured that gender assignment will be made as soon as feasible.

To fully examine the female genitalia, the infant should be examined with the hips abducted while lying supine. The labia majora, labia minora, and clitoris should be inspected for size and surface characteristics. The labia majora may have some mild wrinkling, but should not have frank rugae. In the term female infant, the labia majora are more prominent than the labia minora and generally cover the latter. The female urethra may be difficult to visualize, but is found just anterior to the vaginal opening. Outpouching of the vaginal mucosa (vaginal tags) is common because of the effect of maternal hormones on the fetus. In contrast, the premature female infant may have more prominent labia minora and relative protrusion of the clitoris beyond the labial folds. Such findings are part of the normal morphogenesis of the growing fetus, but parents often need reassurance that the anatomy is normal. The groin and labia majora should be palpated for masses (gonads or herniae). Female infants often have a whitish mucous vaginal discharge. As the effects of maternal hormones subside in the first week, female infants may have a small amount of vaginal bleeding. Clitoromegaly, increased pigmentation, genital hair, and labioscrotal fusion are signs of virilization. Causes include congenital adrenal hyperplasia, virilizing tumors, and maternal androgenic medications.

In females, obstructive lesions of the genital tract, such as imperforate hymen and vaginal atresia, cause retention of secretions or blood in the uterine cavity. This condition presents as an abdominal mass or with symptoms of urinary tract obstruction.

The male infant's genitalia are also first evaluated by visual inspection. The size, color, and surface texture of the scrotum should be noted. In the term male infant, the scrotum is thin skinned, rugated, and pendulous. In the premature infant, the scrotum is thicker, smoother, and less pendulous. Superficial abrasions, ecchymosis, and swelling of the scrotum may occur after breech birth. The length and girth of the phallus are noted visually. Sometimes the phallus may appear to be small, but its true size is merely hidden by the depth of the surrounding tissues. If there is a question of micropenis, then the phallus should be palpated and stretched, so its length can be measured. Micropenis may be associated with hypothalamic dysfunction and hypopituitarism. The phallus should be observed for any unusual angulation, ventral chordee or web, and the completeness of the foreskin. If the foreskin is complete, then there is no need to retract it in order to identify the urethral opening. The urethra should be slitlike and open on the glans penis. An incomplete ventral foreskin should alert the examiner for the possibility of hypospadias. If there is hypospadias, the site of the urethral orifice(s) should be determined by inspection and, if possible, by observation of the urinary stream. Hypospadias may also be associated with bifid scrotum.

The scrotal sacs should be palpated to determine the presence of a testis on each side. The size of the testes should be noted. If the testes are undescended, then the inguinal area should be carefully palpated for incomplete descent of the testis. In the neonatal period, the testes may be very mobile between the inguinal canal and the scrotum. Torsion of a testis results in a swollen hard scrotal mass. The groin should be checked for the presence of an inguinal hernia. In male infants, it is useful to hold the testes in the scrotum while palpating the ipsilateral inguinal area in order to avoid confusing an undescended testis with a hernia. Hydroceles, a common cause of scrotal swelling, are nontender, often obscure the testis, and cause the scrotum to brightly transilluminate. If no gonads are palpable in an apparent male, then it is particularly important to examine the genitalia for other abnormalities and to exclude the possibility that the infant is a masculinized female. Observation of the urinary stream can be useful. Infants with neurogenic bladders typically "dribble" urine in small volumes with some frequency. Males with posterior urethral valves typically have a poor stream during spontaneous micturition.

Exstrophy of the bladder is evident in the suprapubic region. It is associated with a widening of the pubic symphysis, and there is epispadias or a rudimentary penis. There are often associated gastrointestinal anomalies (imperforate anus and intestinal atresia).

Anus

Determination of patency of the anus by inspection alone is usually sufficient. If there is a question of anal patency, then a small catheter should be carefully passed through the orifice. The position of the anal orifice in relation to the genitalia and the presence of fistulas or rectal prolapse should be noted. Infants with imperforate anus may pass meconium through a fistula to the genitourinary tract. Sacrococcygeal teratomas may distort the perianal anatomy, displace the anal orifice, and cause intestinal obstruction. These lesions, which can be very large and highly vascular, may rapidly enlarge after birth as a result of internal hemorrhage, causing anemia and shock. In infants with meningomyelocele or other disorders that may affect anal function, the anus should be checked for sphincter tone. An anal wink can be elicited by gently stroking the perianal area.

Back and Extremities

The back should be inspected for symmetry or any abnormal postures. The vertebral column should be palpated along its length with the fingertips. This combination is usually sufficient to detect any moderate to severe scoliosis. Vertebral anomalies may be difficult to appreciate by palpation on a routine examination. If there are clinical reasons to suspect vertebral anomalies (e.g., VATER [vertebral defects, imperforate anus, tracheoesophageal fistula, radial and renal dysplasia] syndrome), then radiographs should be obtained. If a meningomyelocele is noted, it should be carefully inspected and minimally manipulated. The size and location of a meningomyelocele should be noted, and then it should be covered with an appropriate saline-soaked sterile dressing. Once an infant is identified to have a meningomyelocele, the child should be kept in a prone or decubitus position to keep pressure off the defect. This creates a significant challenge to thoroughly perform the remainder of the physical examination. The midline of the back and sacrum should be carefully inspected for any unusual tufts of hair, dimples, or pits. Any midline palpable masses, however small, need further evaluation. Ultrasound of the spine can be very helpful in the evaluation of any vertebral or spinal cord anomaly.

Careful inspection alone usually determines whether the extremities are well formed. If there are any deformities, then careful palpation, measurements of length, and testing for range of motion may provide further information. For example, limb shortening may be visually evident in an infant with osteogenesis imperfecta. However, the bony swelling and tenderness of multiple fractures may only be evident by palpation. Fractures of long bones of the extremities are associated with swelling, distortion of shape, tenderness, and discoloration. There is often decreased spontaneous movement of the affected extremity as a result of pain. Humerus fractures may occur with birth trauma. Fractures of the femur and humerus occur spontaneously in infants with severe osteopenia of prematurity. Direct comparisons between any aspect of the right and left extremities can be very helpful to discern any abnormalities in size, shape, or function. The hands and feet of every newborn should be carefully inspected. Abnormalities of the digits, including reduction, tapering, syndactyly, polydactyly, duplication, and nail hypoplasia, can be important clues to dysmorphic syndromes. Postaxial polydactyly, which can be inherited as an autosomal dominant trait, is relatively common and is often an isolated finding. In contrast, preaxial polydactyly is more commonly associated with other anomalies. Transverse amputations or limb reductions may be a clue to amniotic band syndrome.

Circumferential girth of the extremities can be an initial clue to muscle mass, and this can be further assessed by palpation. However, marked edema (as in a hydropic infant) or increased adipose tissue (as in an infant of a diabetic mother) can make muscle palpation more difficult. Extremely premature infants have relatively little muscle mass. Observation of motor activity and muscle tone is often sufficient in a healthy term newborn. Neuromuscular disorders may be associated with a decrease in muscle mass and contractures caused by the lack of fetal movement. Infants with a high myelomeningocele can have marked muscle wasting of the lower extremities with flexion contractions of the hips and knees and clubfoot bilaterally.

The hips should be examined for range of motion, and they should be fully abducted to check for hip clicks or dislocation. Useful techniques are the Barlow and Ortolani maneuvers. Additional useful findings are discrepancies in length and asymmetric creases of the lower extremities. Maternal hormones and abnormal fetal positions (e.g., breech) can cause laxity in the newborn's hips. If findings are uncertain, then repeated examinations should be performed until the findings are clarified. If there is frank dislocation or suspicious findings, then hip ultrasound should be obtained. If there is any evidence of hip dysplasia, then orthopedic consultation should be obtained in a timely manner. Specific testing for range of motion for joints other than the hips is generally not indicated unless there are contractures or gross anomalies noted. Many aspects of joint function and range of motion are indirectly tested during the neurologic examination by passive range of motion.

Neurologic Examination

The neurologic examination of a healthy newborn is based on a combination of observations of behavior and specific testing on examination. The normal newborn certainly does not require a lengthy complete neurologic examination; however, certain aspects of neurologic function should be assessed. A more detailed neurologic examination should be performed in any infant with known neurologic disorders (seizures, intracranial hemorrhage, encephalopathy) or who is at high risk for neurologic injury.

A number of behaviors provide information about global brain function. Observations of an infant's overall responsiveness, quality of the cry, interaction with the mother, and general motor activity provide a broad useful perspective on cortical function. Although newborns sleep a great deal (18 to 20 hours per day), they do have periods of awake activity. The newborn infant goes through several states of alertness throughout each day. Chapter 17 and especially Table 17–2 describe neonatal states of alertness in more detail. The neurologic examination of the newborn is significantly affected by the state of the infant. Tone and motor activity are decreased during active or rapid eye movement (REM) sleep. Examination of an infant in this state alone may give an incomplete impression of the infant's neurologic status. Important observations can be made as to whether an infant responds to comforting or withdraws from noxious stimuli.

Tone should be assessed by observation of posture and by passive movement of the extremities. Term infants have primarily a flexion posture at the knees and elbows with the fingers generally closed. However, the term newborn spontaneously opens the hands and periodically extends the arms and legs. A term infant with tight persistent flexion of the extremities, tightly clenched fists with adducted thumbs, and hypertonia suggests that there has been a previous cortical injury. Premature infants, in contrast, have relatively more extension, especially with decreasing gestational age. At 23 to 24 weeks' gestation, the premature infant likely has fully extended extremities, relatively decreased tone, and irregular, twitchy, spontaneous motor activity as a normal finding. Head control and neck tone may be tested by gently lifting the infant by the arms slightly off the bed and assessing for head lag. Head control is generally poor in the premature infant, but some neck muscle tone is present in healthy term infants.

Motor activity of the infant should be observed to detect any asymmetry or abnormality in movement. Motor strength is assessed by the degree of resistance to passive range of motion, spontaneous movement, and active effort to restraint from the examiner. Jitteriness is very common in the newborn. In otherwise apparently healthy term infants, such jitteriness is generally benign unless the movements are particularly coarse or of a large amplitude. Occasionally, such jitteriness can be due to hypoglycemia or hypocalcemia. In an irritable, hypertonic infant, jitteriness may be due to drug withdrawal or neurologic injury.

For most infants, testing of deep tendon reflexes can be limited to the biceps and knee jerk. The ability to elicit deep tendon reflexes is dependent on the infant's activity and state, the patience of the examiner, and the effects of medications. There are a large number of elicitable reflexes in the newborn, but the physician rarely needs to test more than a few of these responses in most routine examinations. The Moro reflex is particularly useful to detect Erb palsy. The palmar reflex and asymmetric tonic neck response may reveal asymmetries in motor function or strength. Sucking can be evoked even in extremely premature infants as early as 28 weeks. Rooting is easily demonstrated in term infants by stroking the side of the mouth.

Cranial nerve function should be thoroughly and specifically evaluated in the comatose infant or as part of an assessment for brain death. However, a less formal assessment of the cranial nerves suffices in most infants. The term newborn is capable of following an object from 30 to 60 degrees. Shining a bright light into the eyes should cause the term infant to close the eyes. Pupillary response to light may be absent in the premature infant because of immaturity and cloudiness of the cornea. However, the pupils of the term or near-term infant should constrict in response to light. Eye movements should be observed for any abnormal deviation or sustained nystagmus. Conjugate gaze is often inconsistent in the newborn. Facial nerve palsy may be apparent by the observation of asymmetry during crying. The gag reflex can be checked at the same time the mouth and tongue are being evaluated as part of the general physical examination. Ineffective sucking, swallowing, and handling of oral secretions may be an indicator of cranial nerve dysfunction or central nervous system (CNS) depression. Hearing may be crudely assessed by the response to the mother's voice or sudden sounds. However, it is best to evaluate infants who are at risk for hearing loss by brainstem auditory evoked response (BAER) testing.

◆ ROUTINE EVALUATION DURING TRANSITION

The first hours of life are a period during which the newborn should be carefully monitored and evaluated. It is during this transition period that many of the problems of the high-risk infant manifest themselves. Because this is also an important period for the mother and family to bond with the infant, most of the monitoring and evaluating can be done by skilled obstetric and nursery nurses. Fortunately, most infants are healthy and require little intervention other than observation.

Where the infant is observed during the first few hours depends on the parents, the infant, and the hospital. Reasonable alternatives range from close observation of the mother and infant together in the mother's room to temporary admission to a transitional or intermediate nursery. Regardless of the setting for this transitional period, the emphasis must always be on careful observation with the ability to intervene in time to prevent significant problems.

For the high-risk infant, a number of problems may manifest themselves within the first hour. A systematic approach to these infants is important so that problems can be identified and responded to in a timely fashion, without overtreatment of infants. The most important evaluation of the infant within the first several hours is repeated physical examinations. These "mini-exams" require little intervention with the infant, but they can identify evolving problems.

Respiratory

Is there any evidence of increasing respiratory distress? All newborns have some mild grunting during the first few minutes of life. This grunting, often audible only with a stethoscope, decreases over the first 30 minutes in a healthy infant. The infant with increasing grunting at 15 to 30 minutes of age, particularly if it is associated with other signs of respiratory distress, should be considered abnormal. In the preterm infant, hyaline membrane disease is by far the most common cause of respiratory distress that increases during the first hour of life, although other processes such as pneumonia or pneumothorax may present a similar picture. In the term infant, continued grunting is most often associated with pneumonia, aspiration syndrome, or retained lung fluid.

Is there tachypnea without grunting? This is most often either a benign finding or represents transient tachypnea of the newborn. The differentiation between these two entities depends on whether the infant requires supplemental oxygen.

Is the infant pink and well saturated? In a modern nursery, all infants with any signs of respiratory distress should be placed on a pulse oximeter to more accurately assess oxygen saturation.

Cardiovascular

Is the infant well perfused? Hypoperfusion often accompanies either sepsis or significant asphyxia. Does the infant have a murmur? Although murmurs are present in a large percentage of healthy newborns during the first day of life secondary to the closing ductus arteriosus, a murmur in the presence of cyanosis, poor perfusion, or poor pulses is often associated with cardiac disease.

Neurologic

Is the infant lethargic and hypotonic, or, conversely, is the infant jittery? The former is associated with both sepsis and asphyxia, and the latter may indicate early drug withdrawal or hypoglycemia. Coarse high-amplitude jitteriness is sometimes seen in infants with hypoxic-ischemic encephalopathy.

Temperature

Temperature must be followed closely in the preterm infant who, because of a larger surface-to-volume ratio, is more likely to quickly become hypothermic. See Chapter 5 for a more detailed discussion of temperature.

Laboratory Evaluation

The two laboratory tests most commonly performed during the transition period are an assessment of blood glucose and hematocrit (or hemoglobin). Some nurseries routinely check blood glucose on all newborns. While healthy newborns without any risk factors probably do not need routine blood glucose monitoring, infants with any of the following risk factors do need glucose monitoring:

Prematurity
Respiratory distress
Suspected sepsis
Signs of hypovolemia or hypotension
Maternal diabetes

Prolonged maternal exposure to β-mimetics
Large for gestational age
Small for gestational age
Asphyxia
Signs of hypoglycemia, such as jitteriness or lethargy
Hyperviscosity syndrome

The frequency and duration of glucose monitoring depends on whether the infant has any hypoglycemia and the rate at which it resolves.

Either hematocrit or hemoglobin should be checked in newborns who fall into a high-risk group. As a minimum, all infants with the following risk factors should be tested:

Prematurity
Large for gestational age
Small for gestational age
Discordant twins
Maternal diabetes
Signs of plethora or hyperviscosity
Hypovolemia or hypotension
Maternal bleeding (abruption, previa)
Fetal or neonatal blood loss
Suspected sepsis
Pathologic jaundice

In addition to these tests, routine newborn screening is performed in many states. Typically the newborn screen includes tests for hypothyroidism, phenylketonuria (PKU), and galactosemia. In some states, routine cord blood screening for hemoglobinopathies is available. These tests are run in batches at reference laboratories and are usually not available for at least several days or weeks. Newborn screening tests should be obtained before discharge from the hospital; however, the PKU test may not be valid if performed before 12 hours of age. In most states, the hypothyroidism screen is designed to only detect primary hypothyroidism by measuring thyroid-stimulating hormone (TSH). Hypothyroidism, which is caused by hypopituitarism, is not detected by TSH screening alone. Infants with suspected secondary hypothyroidism need specific testing of free thyroxine (T_4) in order to evaluate thyroid status. Prior transfusion invalidates the results of hemoglobinopathy and galactosemia screening tests.

Routine Treatment

All newborns should receive vitamin K and ophthalmic treatment to prevent ophthalmia neonatorum resulting from gonococcal infection. We recommend the use of erythromycin, rather than silver nitrate treatment, because of the efficacy of erythromycin in treating chlamydial conjunctivitis.

Vitamin K is given as a single intramuscular dose, 1.0 mg to infants who weigh more than 2.5 kg and 0.5 mg to infants who weigh less than 2.5 kg. Whereas some studies have evaluated routine use of oral vitamin K,[21] this is not recommended for routine use at this time.[8] Failure to provide vitamin K places the newborn (especially if breast-fed) at risk for the development of hemorrhage in the first weeks of life as a result of vitamin K deficiency.

In most healthy infants, these routine treatments, like the routine monitoring of blood glucose and hematocrit, should be deferred until the infant is at least an hour old and the mother has been able to spend some private time with her infant.

◆ MANAGEMENT OF THE HIGH-RISK INFANT DURING TRANSITION

The areas that most often need to be addressed in the high-risk infant are monitoring, vascular access, oxygen and ventilatory support, and evaluation of suspected sepsis. As with most other areas of newborn care, anticipation of potential problems leads to a practical and successful plan for the care of these infants.

Monitoring

All infants who cannot be considered healthy newborns should be placed on a cardiorespiratory monitor. Because of the simplicity and noninvasive nature of these monitors, there are virtually no contraindications to their use. Similarly, blood pressure should be evaluated in all infants who require more than well-baby care. Blood pressure is easily measured with automated cuff devices, which are noninvasive and simple to use.

In any infant with an arterial catheter in place, arterial pressure should be continuously monitored, and the arterial waveform displayed on the cardiorespiratory monitor. Not only does this provide important information about the infant's cardiovascular status, but it provides important alarms in case the arterial catheter becomes disconnected. An arterial catheter that is not connected to a pressure transducer and that is not displayed with appropriate alarms could potentially cause massive undetected hemorrhage.

With the wide availability and ease of use of pulse oximetry, most nurseries have become much more aggressive about monitoring oxygenation status.[32] Essentially, any infant who requires oxygen during the transition period should be monitored with a pulse oximeter. The fact that pulse oximeters do not require correlation with a blood gas and do not require any warm-up period makes them superior to transcutaneous monitors for immediate evaluation of an infant during the transition period (see Chapter 9).

Vascular Access

The first question about vascular access is whether the infant will need ongoing blood gas monitoring. Because of the less than ideal nature of both capillary gas and arterial puncture gas monitoring, we recommend the placement of an umbilical arterial catheter in any infant who requires blood gas monitoring. Not only are the results of umbilical arterial gases more accurate than those of capillary or arterial puncture gases, but the placement of an umbilical arterial catheter is significantly less traumatic to the infant who requires repeated blood gases.

Any infant who cannot be readily weaned from supplemental oxygen with a pulse oximeter should have an umbilical arterial catheter placed. Our usual "rule of thumb" is to place a catheter in the infant who requires more than 0.30 FIO_2 at more than 30 minutes of age. Alternatives to a simple umbilical arterial catheter are catheters that continuously measure PO_2 or oxygen saturation.

The next question that needs to be answered is whether the infant will need vascular access for fluid support. In general, infants with a birth weight less than 1.5 kg do not tolerate immediate institution of entirely enteral nutrition and should be given intravenous fluids. Hypoglycemia, which is relatively common in premature and stressed infants, often requires ongoing intravenous glucose infusion until feedings can be established. Infants of diabetic mothers, who have either severe or recurrent hypoglycemia, need intravenous dextrose. Any infant with significant respiratory distress, gastrointestinal anomalies or obstruction, or suspected serious congenital heart disease needs intravenous access.

Supplemental Oxygen and Ventilatory Support

Decisions about the correct amount of supplemental oxygen to deliver are usually straightforward. Patients should receive an FIO_2 that is adequate to prevent hypoxia and hyperoxia. Usually, maintaining arterial saturation between 88% and 95% is a safe range. It is important to remember that these are the numbers for measured saturation e.g., by pulse oximeter rather than the calculated saturation that is reported by some blood gas machines. Many blood gas machines calculate saturation from measured PO_2, with the assumption that the blood measured has adult hemoglobin. Because the newborn has a high percentage of fetal hemoglobin, with a higher affinity for oxygen, the actual arterial oxygen saturation is higher than that calculated assuming that the hemoglobin is adult.

Decisions about institution of mechanical ventilation are more complex. The single unvarying rule is that ventilation should be instituted to *prevent* respiratory failure, rather than in response to it. The assessment of approaching respiratory failure is complex, depending on the infant's gestational age, postnatal age, pulmonary disease, physical examination, and blood gas measurements. General rules for instituting ventilation are as follows:

1. Inability to achieve adequate oxygenation with hood oxygen requires positive pressure. In most cases, the premature infant who requires an FIO_2 above 0.50 to 0.60 should be intubated and ventilated. Term infants who require an FIO_2 above 0.70 to 0.80 often need to be intubated and ventilated.

2. Inability to spontaneously provide adequate CO_2 exchange requires ventilation. In most cases, infants with a $PaCO_2$ between 50 and 60 should be followed up closely for potential need for ventilation. Most infants with $PaCO_2$ above 60 mm Hg during the first hours of life need mechanical ventilation.

3. Respiratory fatigue, usually manifested by markedly abnormal respiratory pattern or respiratory pauses, should be considered an indication for mechanical ventilation.

Some infants will respond to continuous positive-airway pressure (CPAP) by nasal prongs and do not need mechanical ventilation. CPAP should be instituted early, and patients should be followed closely to make sure that their respiratory failure does not progress. In our experience, the number of infants who require positive pressure but who do not need mechanical ventilation is relatively small. With the availability of surfactant, it may be prudent to proceed to intubation and surfactant administration for premature infants with respiratory distress syndrome and significant symptoms.

There is essentially no role for the use of intermittent mask ventilation to recruit alveoli and to avoid intubation and ventilation. The infant who requires intermittent ventilation should be intubated and ventilated, rather than managed with this temporizing technique. For further discussion of assisted ventilation, see Chapter 10.

Evaluation and Treatment of Suspected Sepsis

Because of the potentially lethal nature of neonatal sepsis, and because it may be difficult to detect early in its course, one should always err in the direction of over-evaluating and overtreating potential sepsis. Pneumonia in the neonate has a wide range of clinical and radiographic appearances, often mimicking either hyaline membrane disease (respiratory distress syndrome) or aspiration syndrome. For this reason, all infants with any significant degree of respiratory distress, whether from surfactant deficiency, aspiration syndrome, or an idiopathic cause, should be considered potentially septic.

No single screening test for sepsis is both sufficiently sensitive and specific. Leukocytosis and a high immature-to-mature white blood cell count may indicate sepsis, but they are often seen in normal newborns. Leukopenia is more specific for sepsis than is leukocytosis, but it is also often seen in newborns without sepsis, especially after maternal pregnancy-induced hypertension. Thrombocytopenia is a late finding that may

be seen in infants with overwhelming sepsis and disseminated intravascular coagulopathy, but it should not be seen as a screening tool for sepsis. Testing for urine bacterial antigens for group B streptococcal sepsis is not reliable and is not recommended for routine use.[39] C-reactive protein may be increased (≥ 1 mg/dL) in cases of proven bacterial sepsis at the time of initial evaluation. However, there is a significant false-negative rate at the time of presentation. C-reactive protein may be more useful to determine whether to discontinue antibiotic therapy at 48 to 72 hours after the start of treatment. It has been shown that bacterial infection is very unlikely if two sequential (24 hours apart) C-reactive protein levels are less than 1 mg/dL in the 8 to 48 hours after presentation.[11]

The minimum evaluation for sepsis includes a complete blood count with differential, platelet count, and blood culture. C-reactive protein may also be a useful test to determine the length of treatment, but its utility in the decision whether to start antibiotics remains unclear. The infant who is at more than minimal risk of sepsis should also have a lumbar puncture for cell count, glucose, protein, culture, and streptococcal antigen. However, there is considerable controversy regarding selective use of lumbar puncture in the evaluation of neonatal sepsis.[1, 17, 23, 38] Because early onset sepsis rarely presents with urinary tract infection, a urinalysis or urine culture is not part of the routine evaluation of early onset sepsis.

A number of factors are associated with an increased risk of neonatal infection:

Preterm delivery
Prolonged labor
Rupture of membranes greater than or equal to 18 hours
Maternal fever or other sign of amnionitis

It is our practice to evaluate for sepsis and treat all *asymptomatic* cases of infants who have two or more of these risk factors. Useful algorithms have also been proposed for the newborn at risk for group B streptococcal infection.[5] We would treat any case of a symptomatic infant, even without any of these risk factors. Our treatment of these infants involves a minimum of 48 hours of ampicillin and gentamicin. Antibiotics should be stopped at this point, only if the infant's blood and cerebrospinal fluid cultures are negative and if the patient is not clinically infected. Our only exception to the minimum 48-hour course of antibiotics is for the infant in whom, with no risk factors for sepsis, transient tachypnea develops and rapidly resolves. In such an infant who is clinically asymptomatic at 24 hours of age, we would not necessarily continue antibiotic treatment for 48 hours. For further discussion of antibiotics and their dosage, see Chapter 13 and Appendix A-2.

◆ BREAST-FEEDING: EFFECT OF MATERNAL ILLNESS AND DRUGS

Mothers should be encouraged and supported in their efforts to establish breast-feeding. Human milk is the preferred source of nutrition for healthy newborn infants.[29] Breast-feeding not only provides nourishment to the infant, but it also promotes the process of bonding. Human milk contains factors that support intestinal cell proliferation and bowel mucosal mass. A number of factors, including secretory IgA, lysozyme, lactoferrin, C3, C4, and maternal leukocytes, influence neonatal bacterial flora and the incidence of gastrointestinal infections. However, maternal illnesses or drugs can have adverse effects upon lactation, which may preclude the use of maternal milk or may require special precautions in its use.

Viral agents can be transmitted into human milk and result in infection in the infant. HIV is secreted into human milk and transmission to the breast-fed infant has been reported. Because about 25% (8% with prenatal, intrapartum, and postnatal zidovudine) of infants born to mothers with HIV are infected at birth, it would be prudent to not breast-feed such infants in order to prevent the transmission of HIV infection to those infants not infected at birth.[6] However, in underdeveloped countries where a safe water supply and sufficient resources for infant formula are lacking, we agree with the World Health Organization recommendation that mothers with HIV should continue to breast-feed. Herpes simplex virus has also be reported to be transmitted via maternal milk, suggesting that breast-feeding should be withheld in young infants during an episode of acute primary maternal herpes infection or if there are herpes lesions on the breasts. Mothers with recurrent cervical or oral herpes are generally allowed to breast-feed, provided good hygiene is used in order to prevent transmission.[35] Although hepatitis B virus is transmitted via human milk in mothers who are positive for hepatitis B surface antigen, these mothers are usually allowed to breast-feed. Their infants should be protected if they are given hepatitis B vaccine and hepatitis B immunoglobulin at birth, and hepatitis B vaccine again at 1 and 6 months of age. Mothers who are seropositive for cytomegalovirus (CMV) also secrete virus into human milk, but this does not appear to pose any risk to the healthy term infant. Many infants born to seropositive mothers begin to excrete CMV postnatally, whether or not they are breast-fed. For the premature infant, postnatal acquisition of CMV (via blood transfusion) has been associated with respiratory morbidity. Freezing of human milk reduces viral titers of CMV, but pasteurization may be more effective at inactivation of virus. The use of previously frozen own mother's milk in premature infants may provide some margin of safety in this situation.

Almost all maternal medications are secreted to some extent into human milk (see Appendix A-4).[2, 12, 29] Factors that affect the degree of secretion are the pKa of the drug, its lipid solubility, molecular size, and protein binding. Drugs that are small in molecular size or that are lipid soluble pass more readily into the breast milk. Drugs with a more alkaline pKa are in the non-ionized form in the plasma, permitting easier passage across membranes and into the milk. Drugs that are poorly bound to plasma proteins are more readily secreted into human milk than drugs that are tightly bound. The time of collection or feeding of human milk affects the level of the drug in the milk. Less drug is delivered to the infant if breast-feeding is performed just before the mother's dose of drug. Although the concentration of a drug in human milk provides an estimate of how much maternal drug to which an infant is exposed, the bioavailability of the drug may be limited by intestinal absorption. For example, although phenytoin is excreted into human milk, its intestinal absorption is quite poor in the newborn.

In counseling a mother regarding breast-feeding, it should be emphasized that virtually all drugs are excreted into human milk and that caution should be taken with regard to any drug. The lactating woman should always make her physician aware that she is breast-feeding when medications are prescribed for her. Although for most maternal medications, breast-feeding can be maintained, the data regarding adverse effects of drugs in infants are incomplete. Most reports about breast-feeding and maternal medications involve small numbers of infants; hence adverse effects that occur infrequently are not easily recognized. The physician is often forced to make a judgment regarding the use of a drug in a lactating woman based on incomplete data. The mother should be informed of these uncertainties when appropriate. Medications for use in a lactating woman should be chosen in such a way as to minimize any risk to the infant and yet provide a therapeutic effect for the mother. Very few maternal medications are an absolute contraindication to breast-feeding (see Appendix A-4).[2]

Maternal cocaine use during breast-feeding may cause hypertension, seizures, and other toxic effects in the infant. Maternal heroin use or other illicit intravenous drug use puts both the mother and infant at risk for HIV infection. Although breast-feeding by mothers on methadone has been reported to facilitate the control of neonatal abstinence syndrome, this may not be a sufficient reason to continue to expose the infant to such a long-acting narcotic and infectious risks (e.g., HIV infection).

◆ TRANSPORT

One of the major developments in modern neonatal care was the concept of regionalization of perinatal care. Central to this concept is transport, both of high-risk mothers and of high-risk infants, to centers that specialize in the care of these high-risk patients.[22] Although the ideal situation is to transfer the prepartum mother to a center that can provide both high-risk perinatal care to the mother and intensive care to the newborn, this is often not possible. Because of the unpredictable nature of preterm labor and of the often unexpected pathology of an infant following a normal pregnancy, high-risk infants are often born at centers that are not equipped to provide total support and therapy for them. In these situations, it is necessary to transfer the infant to a higher level center.

Nurseries are commonly classified as level I, level II, and level III. Level I nurseries are those that provide routine well newborn care and should be able to stabilize high-risk infants before transfer to a higher level center. Level II nurseries provide all of the services of a level I nursery, plus some support for smaller and sicker infants. Typically, healthy growing preterm infants, infants needing intravenous support, or infants needing hood oxygen but not prolonged mechanical ventilation, can be cared for in level II nurseries. Level III nurseries provide complete neonatal intensive care, including access to pediatric surgical support, multiple pediatric subspecialists, and all of the support services that are required to care for the smallest and sickest newborns.

A subgroup of level III nurseries, sometimes referred to as level IV nurseries, provide therapies that are new or so specialized that they are not needed at all level III nurseries. Previously, therapies such as extracorporeal membrane oxygenation (ECMO), high-frequency ventilation, and nitric oxide were available only at a level IV or regional intensive care nursery. Although ECMO will likely continue to be limited to a small number of centers, high-frequency ventilation is becoming increasingly available at most level III nurseries. Even nitric oxide, which was approved by the US Food and Drug Administration in 1999, is available at more than 500 hospitals in the United States.

Infants are transported from lower level to higher level nurseries if conditions that cannot be treated at the lower level nursery develop or if the infant is at risk for development of such conditions. The exact indications for transferring an infant often depend on multiple factors other than the degree of pathology in the infant. The skill and comfort of the physicians caring for the infant, the skill and comfort of the nursing staff, the availability of adequate numbers of skilled nurses, and the availability of ancillary services all must be considered when deciding whether to continue treating an infant at a level I or II nursery. Only if all members of the nursery team are comfortable with their ability to provide optimal care for the infant should a high-risk infant remain at a lower level center. Because the high-risk infant is often a rapidly changing patient, decisions about transferring or not transferring a given infant must be flexible. These decisions should be made in conjunction with neonatologists at the regional level III center who remain in close telephone contact with the team treating the infant.

All level III nurseries and some level II nurseries have neonatal transport teams. Whereas the composition of these teams varies widely, they should all have similar skills for stabilizing and transporting a sick newborn. The goal of a transport team is to provide total support of the newborn from the time the team arrives at the referring hospital to the time the infant is delivered to the accepting hospital. The transport team should be an extension of the intensive care nursery, and at no time should the infant be compromised by the transport process itself.

Transport teams should have the ability to rapidly and accurately assess the infant and to immediately institute appropriate therapy. This includes the ability to intubate and ventilate, gain venous and arterial access, treat pneumothoraces, treat shock, institute pharmacologic therapy for cyanotic congenital heart disease, and support the infant with congenital or surgical anomalies. In addition, the team must be able to lucidly explain the infant's condition, prognosis, and treatment plans to the parents.

Indications for instituting therapies before transport are only slightly different than the indications for instituting those therapies in an intensive care nursery. In general, because of the difficulty of instituting therapies once an infant is in an ambulance, the transport team should err on the side of early rather than late intervention. The infant who *might* need ventilation should be intubated before transport rather than risking the need to intubate and begin ventilation during the transport. Similarly, one should place a chest tube to evacuate the pneumothorax that *might* require evacuation and begin the dopamine or another pressor that *might* be needed during the transport.

The entire transport process should involve the referring physician and nursing staff, the neonatal staff at the accepting institution, the staff of the transport team, and the parents. Clearly, communication before, during, and after the transport are of paramount importance.

◆ RECOMMENDATIONS FOR CARE

Although the care of the newborn should be individualized to the needs of each infant, the perinatal service of each hospital must establish and maintain policies that ensure high quality of care for all newborns within each institution.[8] However, current practices in perinatal and neonatal care are being driven by a variety of forces. Parents, as consumers, are demanding a more comfortable, almost homelike, environment for labor and delivery of their infant. Payors are carefully scrutinizing costs and will continue to pressure hospitals to reduce both costs and patient length of stay. Health care professionals must respond to these forces of change in a careful manner so that the medical needs of the mother and infant are thoroughly met. The following general recommendations are made in light of these changes.

1. Every delivery of a newborn, whether anticipated to be routine or high risk, should be attended by a person skilled in neonatal resuscitation. This person, whether a nurse, nurse anesthetist, neonatal nurse practitioner, or physician, should be skilled in bag-and-mask ventilation, endotracheal intubation, and neonatal cardiopulmonary resuscitation. This person cannot be available just on call or standby, but should be there to immediately attend to the infant after delivery. The principles of neonatal delivery room resuscitation as outlined by the American Academy of Pediatrics and the American Heart Association should be generally followed. Health care professionals who are responsible for delivery room resuscitation should be trained in these principles. However, certification alone by the American Academy of Pediatrics/American Heart Association program of neonatal resuscitation is inadequate by itself. There is no substitute for practical experience to achieve expertise in newborn resuscitation.

2. For higher risk deliveries, a physician, a neonatal nurse practitioner, or a neonatologist may need to be present in order to immediately evaluate and, if needed, to resuscitate the newborn. Each perinatal-neonatal service should establish its own criteria for when a physician, or more specifically a neonatologist, should be called to attend a high-risk delivery. Physicians who attend high-risk deliveries and care for seriously ill newborns must be skilled in neonatal resuscitation

and certain technical procedures, including endotracheal intubation, umbilical catheterization, needle thoracentesis, and chest tube placement.

3. After delivery, a sick or premature infant should be placed on a warming table, dried, evaluated, and resuscitated as appropriate. Apgar scores are assigned at 1 and 5 minutes of age, and every 5 minutes thereafter up to 20 minutes if the child continues to require vigorous resuscitation. There should be the capability, if needed, to perform intubation, hand ventilation via the endotracheal tube, needle thoracentesis, and umbilical catheterization within the delivery room. If an infant is critically ill and further personnel are needed, assistance should be promptly called for. The sick newborn is moved from the delivery room to the intensive care nursery once the infant is initially stabilized with a patent airway, adequate ventilation, and stable heart rate.

4. The apparently stable healthy newborn can be readily evaluated in several minutes in the delivery room with careful attention to respiratory effort, heart rate, color, perfusion, and tone. A quick physical examination should be performed to ensure that there are no significant anomalies or cardiopulmonary compromise. The child should then be dried and wrapped in warm blankets and be allowed to return to the mother. The infant can be placed skin to skin on the mother's chest. This time shortly after birth is especially important to allow for the parents to be close to their infant. Such a time for private bonding between the parents and the infant should not preclude close observation of the infant. Administration of eye prophylaxis and vitamin K to the healthy newborn can generally be delayed until 1 to 2 hours of age.

5. Within the first 1 to 2 hours of life, the healthy newborn should have a full assessment performed by the nursing staff. This should include measurement of temperature, heart rate, respiratory rate, and a full physical examination. The nursing staff should pay particular attention to adequacy of the respiratory effort and observe for any signs of respiratory distress. Infants with persistent poor perfusion, poor capillary refill, cyanosis, or respiratory distress should have measurement of blood pressure. Gestational age is assessed using standard techniques such as the Dubowitz or Ballard examination. Weight, length, and occipital frontal head circumference are measured and plotted on an appropriate growth chart. The physician should be promptly notified of any significant findings or abnormalities. For stable healthy newborns, the physician should examine the infant by 12 to 18 hours of age. Infants with significant respiratory distress, major anomalies, signs of sepsis, or prematurity should be examined and evaluated promptly by the physician. The initial assessment of the apparently healthy newborn infant need not occur in the "transitional nursery" or "well newborn" nursery. When possible, the healthy infant should be evaluated in the mother's room, rather than separating her from her infant. This is particularly appropriate as labor and delivery services move to combine the care of the mother and well newborn infant, the so-called model of a mother-infant dyad. It is essential, however, that the nursing staff caring for such mother-infant dyads continue to have the training and resources they need to fully evaluate the newborn infant and to be able to expeditiously provide for the infant's needs. The newborn infant should be regularly observed with frequent measurement of the heart rate, respirations, and temperature in the first 6 hours of life to ensure that the infant has made a stable transition to extrauterine life.

6. For the sick newborn, a full assessment should be performed immediately. If an infant has respiratory distress, poor perfusion, or hypotension, signs of asphyxia, or other significant problems that require close monitoring or intervention, the child should be moved to the intensive care nursery. Infants who require intubation and ventilation for more than several hours should be transferred to an intensive care nursery that regularly ventilates newborns. Every effort should be made before transport to stabilize the infant in order to ensure a safe and expeditious transfer. A physician, neonatal nurse clinician, or other individual with the training and ability to manage an intubated and ventilated newborn should remain in attendance during the stabilization,

transport, and ongoing care of ventilated infants. Complex neonatal intensive care should remain regionalized at tertiary centers that maintain a well-organized program of services to provide the specialized care needed by critically ill newborns. Health care professionals should advocate for the best care of the newborn and not allow themselves to be forced to provide a lower quality of care in response to economic and social pressures.

7. Mothers should be encouraged and supported in their efforts to breast-feed. Nurses and physicians should be knowledgeable regarding issues of lactation support. Specialized services for lactation counseling need to be available as needed for all breast-feeding mothers.

8. Newborn infants and their mothers should be allowed to stay in hospital for at least 48 hours after birth in order to ensure a stable transition of the infant and a safe postpartum course for the mother.[4] A 48-hour stay also provides a more ample opportunity to support the mother's efforts at breast-feeding, to ensure adequate oral intake by the infant, and to evaluate the infant for significant jaundice before discharge. Outpatient follow-up plans for the infant and mother should be clearly defined before discharge.

CASE PROBLEMS

◆
Case One
A mother is in preterm labor at 30 weeks' gestation and is seen at a community hospital with a level I nursery. Ultrasound demonstrates marked polyhydramnios and an estimated fetal weight of 1250 g. The mother is given $MgSO_4$ for tocolysis. Maternal magnesium (Mg) level is 8 mg/dL. Labor progresses and vaginal delivery is anticipated soon. A single dose of betamethasone is given just 6 hours before delivery.

◆ **What factors make this a high-risk infant? What preparations should be made for the delivery?**

At 30 weeks' gestation, the anticipated survival might be 90% or more. However, this pregnancy is complicated by polyhydramnios, which raises the possibility of gastrointestinal anomalies (e.g., esophageal or duodenal atresia, diaphragmatic hernia), cardiac or central nervous system anomalies, chromosomal disorders, maternal gestational di-

abetes, or fetal anemia (wide variety of causes). The infant will be at risk for respiratory distress syndrome (RDS) because of prematurity and the short time interval between the first dose of betamethasone and delivery. The high maternal Mg level may cause hypermagnesemia and respiratory depression in the infant. If the mother had been stabilized and delivery was not expected for hours, then maternal transport to a tertiary neonatal-perinatal center should have been considered. A physician skilled at endotracheal intubation and delivery room resuscitation should attend the delivery. The infant will likely need arterial and venous access (umbilical artery catheter [UAC], umbilical venous catheter [UVC]) and surfactant administration if there is respiratory distress. Prophylactic surfactant might be indicated in view of the gestational age and the inability to complete a course of betamethasone. A nasogastric tube should be passed shortly after birth to determine whether there is esophageal atresia.

At birth, the infant has retractions and poor respiratory effort. There seems to be copious upper airway secretions. The child is intubated and ventilated with improvement in color and a decrease in retractions. An orogastric tube will not pass to the stomach. There is imperforate anus. The abdomen is becoming more distended.

◆ **What disorders does this infant likely have?**

The inability to pass an orogastric tube suggests esophageal atresia. In association with imperforate anus this child likely has VATER syndrome. The acronym has been expanded to VACTERL to include cardiac and limb anomalies. The respiratory distress may be due to RDS, the respiratory depression due to hypermagnesemia, or the pulmonary aspiration of upper airway secretions due to esophageal atresia.

◆ **What clinical and laboratory examinations should be done? What treatment should be started?**

A blood gas, glucose, complete blood count with differential, and blood culture should be sent. Radiographs of the chest and abdomen will clarify the etiology of the respiratory distress, the position of the endotracheal tube, the location of the orogastric tube in a proximal esophageal pouch, and whether there is gas in the bowel (which would suggest that a tracheoesophageal fistula is present). Other anomalies should be sought by checking for vertebral anomalies on radiographs and by obtaining an echocardiogram, cranial ultrasound, and renal ultrasound. Genetics consultation and chromosome analysis should be considered. An ultrasound should be obtained to exclude tethered spinal cord. Surfactant should be administered if there is RDS. Ampicillin and gentamicin are given pending blood culture results. Pediatric surgical consultation is needed immediately. In the presence of anal atresia and the need for positive-pressure ventilation, gastric perforation can develop in an infant with tracheoesophageal fistula. An emergency gastrostomy may be indicated, and planning should be initiated regarding the timing of repair of the esophageal atresia and tracheoesophageal fistula. The child should be transported to a level III nursery that has pediatric surgical services.

◆
Case Two

A 41 weeks' gestation, a mother is about to deliver vaginally through thick meconium-stained fluid. There have been late fetal heart rate decelerations. In the past 2 minutes, the heart rate decreased to 80 bpm. Vacuum extraction is being performed to facilitate delivery.

◆ **What considerations should be taken in preparing for the delivery of the infant? What general principles should guide the delivery room resuscitation? Are there any special risk factors for vacuum extraction?**

The obstetrician or an assistant should suction the nasopharynx and oropharynx after the delivery of the fetal head and before delivery of the shoulders in order to clear any meconium from the upper airways. Those meconium stained infants who are delivered through *thin* meconium, who have *uncomplicated* deliveries, and who are *vigorous* at birth do not require intubation and tracheal suctioning. Intubation and suctioning for meconium should be performed in this case, however, because of two factors: thick meconium and a complicated delivery. As for the method of tracheal suctioning, we prefer the use of a meconium aspirator attached to the endotracheal tube (ETT) and wall suction. The ETT is withdrawn as the suction is applied. We do not recommend the direct insertion of a suction catheter alone into the trachea. The patient should be repeatedly reintubated and suctioned as needed to remove thick or particulate meconium. However, in an infant with respira-

tory depression and a low heart rate, apnea, or poor respiratory effort, it may be necessary to proceed with resuscitation after the first suctioning of the ETT for meconium. With respect to vacuum extraction, if not applied properly, this procedure may increase the risk for intracranial and subgaleal hemorrhage.

This particular infant is critically ill with meconium aspiration syndrome, and is intubated and ventilated. The first blood gas has a pH of 7.15, Pco_2 of 40 mm Hg, Pao_2 of 40 mm Hg in 100% O_2, and mean airway pressure of 16. Blood pressure is 40/20; heart rate is 190. UAC and UVC have been placed. Chest radiograph shows the catheters and ETT in good position, and the lungs have fluffy dense infiltrates bilaterally.

◆ **The patient is in a community level I nursery. What measures might be taken immediately to help stabilize the patient for transport?**

Give volume expander 10 mL/kg (5% albumin, normal saline, lactated Ringer's solution) in repeated boluses as needed to correct hypovolemia and hypotension. After volume repletion, consider starting dopamine at 5 µg/kg/min. Correct acidosis with $NaHCO_3$, especially if it persists after volume expander has been given. Consider moderate intentional hyperventilation (Pco_2 of 30 to 40 mm Hg) to reverse pulmonary artery hypertension.

◆ **To what type of intensive care nursery should such a patient be ideally transferred?**

This patient likely has both pulmonary artery hypertension and myocardial dysfunction in addition to meconium aspiration syndrome. The patient may need high-frequency ventilation, surfactant administration, nitric oxide (NO), and possibly extracorporeal membrane oxygenation (ECMO). The patient will need an echocardiogram and cranial ultrasound before the initiation of ECMO. The patient should go to a level III nursery, preferably an ECMO center, that is capable of applying these treatments and evaluations expeditiously. Critically ill infants who are near or at ECMO criteria can be managed with high-frequency ventilation and NO in an attempt to avoid ECMO. However, application of such therapies in a non-ECMO center must allow for sufficient time to transfer the patient to an ECMO center in case the patient's clinical course deteriorates.

◆ **MATCHING**

Match the maternal medications on the left which might cause the listed neonatal problems on the right. Some of the maternal medications might cause more than one of the neonatal conditions listed.

Maternal medication or drug
1. MgSO$_4$
2. lithium
3. indomethacin
4. alcohol
5. valproic acid
6. thalidomide
7. tobacco/smoking
8. cocaine
9. phenytoin
10. heroin

Neonatal condition or disorder
a. renal failure
b. Dandy-Walker syndrome
c. limb anomalies
d. increased prematurity rate
e. reduced birth weight
f. increased risk for HIV
g. Ebstein anomaly
h. respiratory depression
i. hypoplastic nails
j. vitamin K deficiency
k. intrauterine closure of patent ductus arteriosus
l. myelomeningocele
m. decreased head circumference

Answers: 1 (h); 2 (g); 3 (a, k); 4 (c, e, i, m); 5 (l); 6 (c); 7 (d, e); 8 (d, e, m); 9 (c, i, j, m); 10 (e, h)

Match the maternal conditions or diseases on the left which might cause the listed neonatal problems on the right. Some of the maternal conditions or diseases might cause more than one of the neonatal conditions listed.

Maternal condition or disease
1. Graves disease
2. hyperparathyroidism
3. hypoparathyroidism
4. diabetes mellitus
5. pregnancy-induced hypertension
6. idiopathic thrombocytopenic purpura
7. obesity
8. systemic lupus erythematosus
9. phenylketonuria
10. chronic renal failure

Neonatal condition or disorder
a. small left colon syndrome
b. hyperthyroidism
c. intrauterine growth retardation
d. congenital heart block
e. macrosomia
f. neutropenia
g. congenital heart disease
h. thrombocytopenia
i. hypercalcemia
j. hypocalcemia
k. mental retardation
l. birth trauma

Answers: 1 (b); 2 (j); 3 (i); 4 (a, e, g, j, l); 5 (c, f, h); 6 (h); 7 (e, l); 8 (d, f, h); 9 (g, k); 10 (c)

ACKNOWLEDGMENT

Special thanks to Ed Lammer, M.D., Director of Medical Genetics, Children's Hospital Oakland, for his advice regarding Table 3–3.

REFERENCES

1. Albanyan EA, Baker CJ: Is lumbar puncture necessary to exclude meningitis in neonates and young infants: Lessons from the group B streptococcus cellulitis-adenitis syndrome. Pediatrics 102:985–986, 1998.
2. American Academy of Pediatrics: Committee on Drugs: The transfer of drugs and other chemicals into human milk. Pediatrics 93:137–150, 1994.
3. American Academy of Pediatrics: Committee on Drugs: Neonatal drug withdrawal. Pediatrics 101:1079–1088, 1998.
4. American Academy of Pediatrics: Committee on Fetus and Newborn: Hospital stay for healthy term newborns. Pediatrics 96:788–790, 1995.
5. American Academy of Pediatrics: Committee on Infectious Diseases and Committee on Fetus and Newborn: Revised guidelines for prevention of early-onset group B streptococcal (GBS) infection. Pediatrics 99:489–496, 1997.
6. American Academy of Pediatrics: Committee on Pediatric AIDS: Human milk, breastfeeding, and transmission of human immunodeficiency virus in the United States. Pediatrics 96:977–979, 1995.
7. American Academy of Pediatrics: Committee on Substance Abuse and Committee on Children with Disabilities: Fetal alcohol syndrome and fetal alcohol effects. Pediatrics 91:1004–1006, 1993.
8. American College of Obstetricians and Gynecologists: Guidelines for Perinatal Care, 4th ed. Elk Grove Village, IL: American Academy of Pediatrics, 1997.
9. Ballard PL, Ballard RA: Scientific basis and therapeutic regimens for use of antenatal glucocorticoids. Am J Obstet Gynecol 173:254–262, 1995.
10. Ballard JL, Khoury JC, Wedig K, et al: New Ballard Score, expanded to include extremely premature infants. J Pediatr 119:417–423, 1991.
11. Benitz WE, Han MY, Madan A, Ramachandra P: Serial serum C-reactive protein levels in the diagnosis of neonatal infection. Pediatrics 102:e41, 1998.
12. Briggs GG, Freeman GK, Yaffe SJ, eds: Drugs in Pregnancy and Lactation, 5th ed. Baltimore: Williams & Wilkins, 1998.
13. Centers for Disease Control: Prevention of perinatal group B streptococcal disease: A public health perspective. Morbid Mortal Wkly Rep 45(RR-7):1–24, 1996.
14. Christensson K, Siles C, Moreno L, et al: Temperature, metabolic adaptation and crying in healthy full-term newborns cared for skin-to-skin or in a cot. Acta Paediatr 81:488–493, 1992.
15. Connor EM, Sperling RS, Gelber R, et al: Reduction

of maternal-infant transmission of human immunodeficiency virus type 1 with zidovudine treatment. N Engl J Med 331:1173–1180, 1994.

16. Durand DJ, Espinoza AM, Nickerson BG: Association between prenatal cocaine exposure and sudden infant death syndrome. J Pediatr 117:909–911, 1990.

17. Fielkow S, Reuter S, Gotoff SP: Cerebrospinal fluid examination in symptom-free infants with risk factors for infection. J Pediatr 119:971–973, 1991.

18. Fletcher MA: Physical Diagnosis in Neonatology. Philadelphia: Lippincott-Raven, 1998.

19. Fulroth R, Phillips B, Durand DJ: Perinatal outcome of infants exposed to cocaine and/or heroin in utero. Am J Dis Child 143:905–910, 1989.

20. Greene MF: Prevention and diagnosis of congenital anomalies in diabetic pregnancies. Clin Perinatol 20:533–547, 1993.

21. Greer FR, Marshall SP, Severson RR, et al: A new mixed micellar preparation for oral vitamin K prophylaxis: Randomised controlled comparison with an intramuscular formulation in breast fed infants. Arch Dis Child 79:300–305, 1998.

22. Jaimovicj DG, Vidyasagar D: Handbook of Pediatric and Neonatal Transport Medicine. Philadelphia: Hanley & Belfus, 1996.

23. Johnson CE, Whitwell JK, Pethe K, et al: Term newborns who are at risk for sepsis: Are lumbar punctures necessary? Pediatrics 99:e10, 1997.

24. Jones KL: Developmental pathogenesis of defects associated with prenatal cocaine exposure: Fetal vascular disruption. Clin Perinatol 18:139–146, 1991.

25. Jones KL, ed: Smith's Recognizable Patterns of Human Malformation, 5th ed. Philadelphia: WB Saunders, 1997.

26. Kennell JH, Klaus MH: Bonding: Recent observations that alter perinatal care. Pediatr Rev 19:4–12, 1998.

27. Kohl S: Neonatal herpes simplex virus infection. Clin Perinatol 24:129–150, 1997.

28. Koren G, Pastuszak A, Ito S: Drugs in pregnancy. N Engl J Med 338:1128–1137, 1998.

29. Lawrence RA, Lawrence RM: Breastfeeding: A Guide for the Medical Profession, 5th ed. St. Louis: Mosby, 1999.

30. Naeye RL: Umbilical cord length: Clinical significance. J Pediatr 107:278–281, 1985.

31. NIH Consensus Development Panel on the effect of corticosteroids for fetal maturation on perinatal outcomes. JAMA 273:413–418, 1995.

32. Poets CF, Southall DP: Noninvasive monitoring of oxygenation in infants and children: Practical considerations and areas of concern. Pediatrics 93:737–746, 1994.

33. Rudolph AJ: Atlas of the Newborn, Vols. 1–5. Hamilton, Ontario: BC Decker, 1997.

34. Silver RK, Hageman JR, eds: Perinatal Care for Chronic Maternal Conditions. Clin Perinatol 24(2):291–521, June 1997.

35. Sweet AY, Brown EC, eds: Fetal and Neonatal Effects of Maternal Disease. St. Louis: Mosby-Year Book, 1991.

36. Uvnas-Moberg K: The gastrointestinal tract in growth and reproduction. Sci Am 261:78–83, 1989.

37. Wade NA, Birkhead GS, Warren BL, et al: Abbreviated regimens of zidovudine prophylaxis and perinatal transmission of the human immunodeficiency virus. N Engl J Med 339:1409–1414, 1998.

38. Weiss MG, Ionides SP, Anderson CL: Meningitis in premature infants with respiratory distress: Role of admission lumbar puncture. J Pediatr 119:973–975, 1991.

39. Williamson M, Fraser SH, Tilse J: Failure of the urinary group B streptococcal antigen test as a screen for neonatal sepsis. Arch Dis Child 73:F109–F111, 1995.

40. Wyszynski DF, Duffy DL, Beaty TH: Maternal cigarette smoking and oral clefts: A meta-analysis. Cleft Palate Craniofac J 34:11–16, 1997.

Classification and Physical Examination of the Newborn Infant

W. Michael Southgate
William B. Pittard, III

> There are tiny, puny infants with great vitality. Their movements are untiring and their crying lusty, for their organs are quite capable of performing their allotted functions. These infants will live, for although their weight is inferior . . . their sojourn in the womb was longer.
>
> *Pierre Budin, The Nursling*

By the early 20th century, there was debate regarding whether prematurity should be defined by gestational age or birth weight.[32] In 1935, the American Academy of Pediatrics defined prematurity as a live-born infant with a birth weight of 2500 g or less. By the 1960s, practitioners had widely accepted the concept that not all neonates weighing less than 2500 g at birth were prematurely born, and the practice of routinely classifying the newborn in terms of both his gestational age and his birth weight was established. The designation *low-birth-weight (LBW)* was applied to all infants weighing less than 2500 g at birth regardless of the duration of gestation. Subsequently, the terms *very low-birth-weight (VLBW)* and *extremely low-birth-weight (ELBW)* have been used to categorize those infants with birth weights less than 1500 and 1000 g, respectively. The classification of infants as *premature* is reserved for those having completed less than 37 weeks of gestation, whereas *term* gestation refers to those infants delivered between 37 and 42 weeks of gestation, and *post-term* indicates birth after 42 weeks. The proportion of LBW infants who are premature versus those that suffered abnormal intrauterine growth varies around the world. In developed countries, the majority of LBW babies are premature, whereas in developing nations, the major contributors to the LBW rate are undergrown term infants. As the standard of living improves in developing nations, there is a shift toward the pattern of developed nations with regard to LBW infants.

◆ DETERMINANTS OF FETAL GROWTH

Normal fetal growth requires contributions from the mother, the placenta, and the fetus. Numerous maternal metabolic adjustments are made during pregnancy, the unifying goal of which appears to be provision of an uninterrupted supply of nutrients to the developing fetus. Foremost among these are adjustments in carbohydrate metabolism. Mild fasting hypoglycemia and postprandial hyperglycemia associated with an increased basal insulin level and relative insulin resistance characterize the normal pregnancy. Maternal glucose use is attenuated, with ketones and free fatty acids increasingly serving as fuels for maternal tissues. Even though the mechanisms for these alterations are not entirely clear, the effect is the provision of a continuous supply of glucose, the primary source of fetal oxidative metabolism, to the fetus, particularly during periods of maternal fasting. During relatively extended periods of fasting, the fetus uses ketones to serve his or her energy and synthetic needs as well. Maternal serum levels of lipids increase during gestation, and, in midpregnancy, fat is stored for fetal use in late pregnancy when demands increase. These and a variety of other adjustments are so effective in supplying the fetus with required nutrients that only with severe maternal malnutrition (e.g., wartime famine), and only then if starvation occurs during the third trimester, is birth weight affected. The human placenta, in addition to its role of transmitting nutrients from mother to fetus, functions as an incredibly active endocrine organ producing an array of hormones unsurpassed in the animal kingdom. Among those products with direct growth-promoting action are growth factors and human placental lactogen (HPL), also known as chorionic somatomammotropin. HPL is produced by the syncytiotrophoblast cells of the placenta, and its growth-promoting effects are mediated by the stimulation of fetal insulin-like growth factor (IGF) production and increasing nutrient availability. The previously mentioned elevation of maternal serum lipids plays a role here as well, in that the expression of the HPL gene is regulated, in part, by apoprotein A1, the major protein component of high-density lipoprotein.[43] The fetus plays a role in his own growth by producing a variety of polypeptide IGF molecules and modulating binding proteins. These substances are produced by a spectrum of fetal tissues, with site, timing, and control of expression varying with each IGF. The biologic and clinical significance of serum levels of the various growth factors and binding proteins in the fetus and newborn is an area of active research.

◆ PATTERN AND CLASSIFICATION OF GROWTH

With the use of anthropometric measurements, including fetal weight, length, and head circumference, fetal growth standards have been determined for different reference populations from various locations.[7, 14, 62, 89] From these data, it is apparent that there are variations in "normal" weight at any given gestational age from one locale to another. This variation is related to a number of factors including sex, race, socioeconomic class, and even altitude. The Colorado data, presented by Lubchenco and colleagues[62] in the 1960s, summarized standards of intrauterine growth for white (55%), black (15%), and Hispanic (30%) newborns born between 1948 and 1961 in the vicinity of Denver. These data are unique in that each anthropometric measurement was related to gestational age. The graphic display of this relationship provides a useful and simple method for determining the appropriateness of growth with respect to gestational age. Ten years after the Colorado data were published, Brenner and colleagues[17] presented fetal weight curves based on more than

30,000 induced abortions and spontaneous deliveries, with correction factors for parity, race, and sex. Even though these and other such curves differ in details, all demonstrate nearly linear growth between 20 and 38 weeks of gestation, with slowing thereafter. In 1967, Battaglia and Lubchenco[11] used the gestational age/birth weight relationship to categorize those infants whose birth weights were less than the 10th percentile as *small for gestational age (SGA)*, those weighing more than the 90th percentile were categorized as *large for gestational age (LGA)*, and the remaining 80% were *appropriate for gestational age (AGA)* (Fig. 4–1). Nine categories of newborns were thus established. This type of classification allows clinicians to anticipate likely problems in the immediate neonatal period and potential morbidities in the long term.

When using this scheme, accuracy of the anthropometric measurements and the gestational age determination is critical. Modern scales provide nearly instantaneous, highly accurate weights of newborns. Determining the gestational age of the fetus or newborn is far less exact.

◆ ANTENATAL ASSESSMENT OF INTRAUTERINE GROWTH

Clinical Assessment of Gestational Age

Optimal management of the pregnant woman and her fetus is entirely dependent on an accurate knowledge of the age of the fetus. Knowledge of the gestational age is important for interpretation of common tests (alpha-fetoprotein), scheduling invasive procedures (amniocentesis), planning the delivery of high-risk fetuses, and determining the adequacy of fetal growth. Determination of the expected date of delivery (due date) can be made with varying degrees of certainty by history of menstrual cycles, physical examination of the pregnant woman, a variety of clinical obstetric milestones, and ultrasound examination of the developing fetus.

The average duration of pregnancy is 280 days. It is customary to determine the estimated date of delivery by adding 7 days to the date of the first day of the last normal menstrual period and counting back 3 months (Naegele's rule). This tool assumes

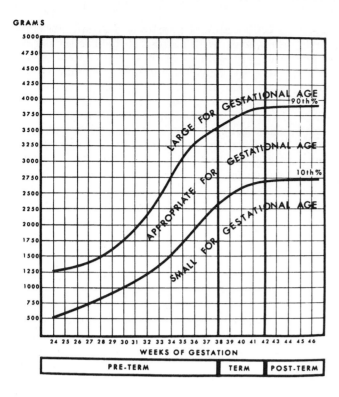

Figure 4–1. Birth weights of liveborn singleton white infants at gestational ages from 24 to 42 weeks. (From Battaglia F, Lubchenco L: A practical classification of newborn infants by weight and gestational age. J Pediatr 7:159, 1967.)

the woman has an accurate recollection of her menstrual cycle, that the menstrual cycle is not prolonged, and that ovulation occurred 14 days into the cycle. Between 18 and 32 weeks' gestation, there is good correlation between the age of the (normally growing, single) fetus in weeks and the height of the uterine fundus in centimeters when measured as the distance over the abdominal wall from the top of the symphysis pubis to the top of the fundus.[25] Physical examination estimates of gestational age are accurate within plus or minus 2 weeks in the first trimester, 4 weeks in the second trimester, and 6 weeks in the third trimester.[41] Fetal heart tones can be auscultated by 17 to 19 weeks, and fetal movements (quickening) are noted after 20 weeks.

Gestational Age Assessment by Ultrasound

Twenty percent of pregnant women have an uncertain last menstrual period, making accurate estimation of gestational age by history difficult at best. Since the 1970s, antenatal determination of gestational age using serial ultrasound studies of the fetus has been used with increasing frequency. The type of ultrasound, the parameters measured, and the accuracy of the study vary with the progression of pregnancy. In the first trimester, although it is possible to visualize the early gestational sac as early as 5 weeks, the optimal time for scanning is between 7 and 9 weeks, with measurement of the crown-rump length using a high-resolution vaginal probe. Routine ultrasound screens for dating, however, are usually carried out during the second trimester, typically between 16 and 20 weeks' gestation. The most commonly used parameters for determining estimated gestational age during the second trimester are head circumference, biparietal diameter, abdominal circumference, and femur length. Each of these measurements has its own advantages and disadvantages, but all have in common a decreasing level of accuracy with increasing gestational age, particularly after 20 weeks, because of increasing normal biologic variation with advancing gestation. To enhance the accuracy of the assessment, a composite fetal age based on the average of these four measurements is used and incorporated into the software of the ultrasound machine for instantaneous calculations. There is an approximate 8% variability throughout gestation when ultrasound is used. At 8 weeks' gestation, a precision of plus or minus 0.64 weeks can be expected, whereas at 20 and 30 weeks, accuracy decreases to a variablity of 1.6 and 2.4 weeks, respectively.[41]

In addition to determining gestational age, regular examinations of the fundal height and serial ultrasound measurements (if indicated) are used to assess the growth pattern of the fetus, perhaps the most important indicator of fetal well-being. Estimates of fetal weight and growth patterns are most accurately assessed by measuring the fetal abdominal circumference.[41] Substandard growth rates can result from a multitude of pathologic and nonpathologic processes. This abnormal pattern of fetal growth is termed *intrauterine growth restriction (retardation) (IUGR).* On the other hand, some maternal and fetal conditions may result in *fetal macrosomia.*

At times, the existence of two terms that describe less-than-desired growth (IUGR and SGA) can cause the student to be confused. Perhaps the easiest way to think about these terms is the following: IUGR is a term used by obstetricians to describe a pattern of growth over a period of time, whereas SGA is the term used by pediatricians to describe a single point on a growth curve. Although there is certainly overlap between these terms in practice, it is also possible to have an IUGR fetus that is not SGA.

Finally, the measurement of umbilical artery pulsatile blood flow by real-time ultrasonography and simultaneous Doppler analysis in the growth-restricted fetus has received attention in the past decade. Although most authorities consider *umbilical vessel velocimetry* to be of unproven benefit, some authors have demonstrated an association between abnormal umbilical blood flow in the IUGR fetus and adverse perinatal outcomes.[13, 23] Conversely, Nienhuis and colleagues[71] have concluded that this tool can be used as a cost-saving device in pregnancies complicated by IUGR by serving as a reassurance to clinicians when normal blood flow patterns are documented, thereby allowing continued outpatient management of the pregnancy.

◆ POSTNATAL ASSESSMENT OF GESTATIONAL AGE

Since the late 1960s, a variety of methods for assessing the gestational age of the newborn

infant have been developed. The complexity of these vary from observation of a few external features in the delivery room to radiographic evaluation and even nerve conduction velocity studies. Even in the most experienced hands, one can expect up to a 1- to 2-week variance in the postnatal assessment from well-established antenatal dating.

Currently, the most widely used system for the postnatal assessment of gestational age is the *New Ballard Score (NBS)* (Fig. 4–2).[8] This system, like many others, including the Dubowitz Score[29] from which the Ballard system is derived, includes both physical and neurologic characteristics. The advantages of the NBS are the relative ease with which it can be carried out, even in the newborn requiring ventilatory assistance, and the improved accuracy (within 1 week) for the extremely premature infant. Accuracy of the NBS is enhanced with experience, consideration of factors that may modify the findings, and performance of the examination within the first 12 hours of life in the infant younger than 28 weeks' gestation. The original Ballard scale is equally valid in both white and black babies, and presumably the NBS is as well.[86] Although the assessment of the gestational age is discussed separately, the student should realize that the components of the gestational age assessment are part of the general physical examination.

Technique for New Ballard Score

Neuromuscular Maturity

There is a general replacement of extensor tone by flexor tone in a cephalocaudal progression with advancing gestational age.

Posture: Observe the unrestrained infant in the supine position.
Square window: Flex the wrist and measure the minimal angle between the *ventral* surface of the forearm and the palm.
Arm recoil: With the infant supine and the head midline, hold the forearm against the arm for 5 seconds, then fully extend and release the arm. Note the time it takes for the infant to resume a flexed posture.
Popliteal angle: Flex the hips with the thighs upon the abdomen. Then, without lifting the hips from the bed surface, extend the knee as far as possible until resistance is met. (One may overestimate the

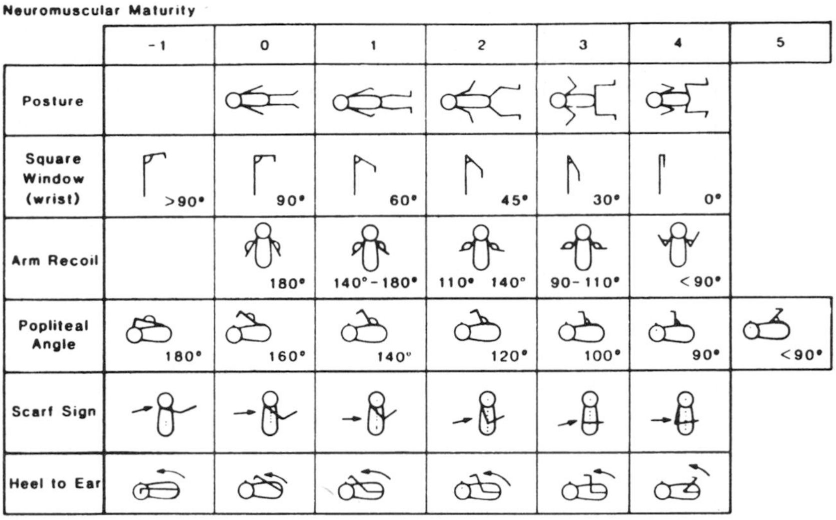

Neuromuscular Maturity

	-1	0	1	2	3	4	5
Posture							
Square Window (wrist)	>90°	90°	60°	45°	30°	0°	
Arm Recoil		180°	140°-180°	110° 140°	90°-110°	<90°	
Popliteal Angle	180°	160°	140°	120°	100°	90°	<90°
Scarf Sign							
Heel to Ear							

Physical Maturity

	-1	0	1	2	3	4	5
Skin	sticky friable transparent	gelatinous red, translucent	smooth pink, visible veins	superficial peeling &/or rash. few veins	cracking pale areas rare veins	parchment deep cracking no vessels	leathery cracked wrinkled
Lanugo	none	sparse	abundant	thinning	bald areas	mostly bald	
Plantar Surface	heel-toe 40-50mm: -1 <40mm: -2	>50mm no crease	faint red marks	anterior transverse crease only	creases ant. 2/3	creases over entire sole	
Breast	imperceptible	barely perceptible	flat areola no bud	stippled areola 1-2mm bud	raised areola 3-4mm bud	full areola 5-10mm bud	
Eye/Ear	lids fused loosely:-1 tightly:-2	lids open pinna flat stays folded	sl. curved pinna; soft; slow recoil	well-curved pinna; soft but ready recoil	formed & firm instant recoil	thick cartilage ear stiff	
Genitals male	scrotum flat, smooth	scrotum empty faint rugae	testes in upper canal rare rugae	testes descending few rugae	testes down good rugae	testes pendulous deep rugae	
Genitals female	clitoris prominent labia flat	prominent clitoris small labia minora	prominent clitoris enlarging minora	majora & minora equally prominent	majora large minora small	majora cover clitoris & minora	

Maturity Rating

score	weeks
-10	20
-5	22
0	24
5	26
10	28
15	30
20	32
25	34
30	36
35	38
40	40
45	42
50	44

Figure 4–2. New Ballard Score. (From Ballard J, Wednig K, Wang L, et al: New Ballard Score, expanded to include extremely premature infants. J Pediatr 119:417, 1991.)

extent of extension if one attempts to continue extending the knee beyond the point where resistance is first met.)

Scarf sign: Again, keeping the head in the midline, pull the hand across the chest to encircle the neck as a scarf and note the position of the elbow relative to the midline.

Heel to ear: With the infant supine and the pelvis kept on the examining surface, the feet are brought back as far as possible toward the head, allowing the knees to be positioned alongside the abdomen.

Physical Maturity

Skin: With maturation, the skin becomes thicker, less translucent and, eventually, dry and peeling.

Lanugo: This fine, nonpigmented hair is evenly distributed over the body and is most prominent at 27 to 28 weeks' gestation, then it gradually disappears, usually first from the lower back. While present over the entire body, the lanugo over the back is used for gestational age assessment.

Plantar surface: As with the hands, the presence of creases in the foot is a reflection of intrauterine activity as well as maturation. The absence of creases may indicate an underlying neurologic problem as well as immaturity. Accelerated crease development is observed when oligohydramnios was present. A new addition in the NBS is the requirement for measuring the plantar surface.

Breast: The areola development is not dependent on adequacy of intrauterine nutrition. There is no difference in male or female infants.

Ear cartilage: With maturation, the ear cartilage becomes increasingly stiff and the auricle thickens. Fold the top of the ear and assess the recoil.

Eyelid opening: Used (incorrectly) by some as a sign of nonviability. Dr. Ballard included the degree of fusion of the lids as a new assessment tool. She defined *tightly fused* as both lids being inseparable by gentle traction, and *loosely fused* as either lid being able to be partly separated by gentle traction. Tightly fused lids were observed in 20% of infants born at 26 weeks' gestation, and only 5% of babies delivered at 27 weeks. The presence of

fused eyelids alone should never be used as a sign of nonviability.

External genitalia, male: Palpate for level of testicular descent and observe the degree of rugation.

External genitalia, female. The labia minora and clitoris are prominent in the immature newborn, at times leading the inexperienced examiner to suspect clitoromegaly. With maturation, the labia majora becomes fat-filled and therefore prominent. The undernourished fetus may have relatively thin labia majora.

◆ EPIDEMIOLOGY AND ETIOLOGY OF GROWTH RESTRICTION

As previously discussed, normal fetal growth is dependent on the contributions of the mother, the placenta, and the fetus. The corollary to this is that aberrant fetal growth may result from disturbances in any of these same areas.

Race

Almost without exception, studies in the United States have demonstrated a significantly higher rate of LBW and its subcomponents IUGR and prematurity in African Americans when compared with their white contemporaries. Concomitantly, perinatal and neonatal mortality rates remain much greater in the black population. The origins of this problem remain unclear. Are black women more susceptible to other well-established risk factors such as chronic hypertension? Do socioeconomic differences between the races account for the variation? Is there a genetic basis for the delivery of LBW infants? Goldenberg et al[36] at the University of Alabama evaluated a population of more than 1500 black and white, poor, multiparous women thought to be at increased risk of delivering growth-restricted babies. In this population, the black women were generally better educated, lived in better housing, scored better on psychological testing, smoked less, and were heavier than their white counterparts. Despite these differences, which should have served to "protect" the black fetuses, white infants weighed on average 200 g more, were born later, and were less likely to be premature or LBW. In another intriguing report, David and Collins[26] attempted to answer the question of a genetic basis for the problem. Their hypothesis can be summarized as follows: If black women are more inclined to deliver LBW (premature/SGA) infants than whites, then black babies should be an intermediate group, because approximately one fourth of the genetic heritage of American blacks is European in origin. A random sample of Illinois birth certificates for a 15-year period was reviewed for infants born to three groups of women: US-born whites, US-born blacks, and African-born blacks. After controlling for a limited number of sociodemographic and reproductive risk factors, the authors discovered that babies born to US-born whites and African-born blacks were more similar than US-born and African-born blacks in terms of mean birth weight and incidence of LBW. Many questions remain unanswered.

Prior Obstetric and Family History

Women who are younger than 15 years of age, older than 45 years of age, have a history of miscarriages or unexplained stillbirths after 20 weeks' gestation, or have prior preterm deliveries are at increased risk for delivering a growth-restricted baby.[35] Familial factors appear to play a role in the birth weight of babies. Mothers of LBW infants were frequently LBW infants themselves and are more likely to have subsequent LBW babies than other mothers, as are their siblings.[30, 51, 63] This is at the heart of the debate about defining SGA/IUGR and in what circumstances the infant is truly at risk. Common sense says that some families tend to have large members whereas other families have smaller members.

Altitude

When comparing growth curves, most authors note that Lubchenco's data were generated in Denver, the "mile-high city," and that the 10th percentile thus generated is lower than the 10th percentile of data collected from centers closer to sea level. Yip[95] was able to demonstrate a "dose-dependent" effect of altitude on the LBW rate, with a two- to three-fold greater rate of LBW seen at altitudes greater than 2000 m than at sea level.

Maternal Factors Contributing to Intrauterine Growth Restriction

In developed countries, a handful of maternal characteristics and behaviors have consistently been associated with an increased risk of growth restriction. In addition to race and prior obstetric history, the list includes maternal nutritional status (pre-pregnancy weight and weight gain during pregnancy), short stature, smoking, pre-eclampsia/hypertension, multiple gestation, and female sex of the infant. In developing nations, malaria is a significant factor, but smoking is not.[4, 36, 37, 47, 53, 81]

Maternal Nutritional Status

Pre-pregnancy weight and weight gain during pregnancy, while both indicators of maternal nutritional status, are independent variables. This is an important point, in that some evidence demonstrates the potential benefits of nutritional intervention in the mother who was poorly nourished before pregnancy.[48] The effectiveness of such interventions has been questioned, however, and requires closer scrutiny.[40] Nutritional supplements provided to well-nourished women do not effect additional benefit. Finally, an obese mother is unlikely to deliver a growth-retarded baby, even if her pregnancy weight gain is low.

Smoking

Cigarette smoking, a habit practiced by 20% of pregnant Americans, has consistently been identified as a dose-dependent contributor to abruptio placentae, late fetal death, LBW, and IUGR.[19] In developed nations, it is by far the single most important contributor to LBW.[53] Rates of IUGR in smokers are 3 to 4.5 times that of nonsmokers, with average birth weights decreasing by 70 to 400 g.[68, 69] These adverse effects are particularly pronounced in babies born to older women. Elimination of smoking would diminish SGA rates by 20% to 30%.[4, 69] Multiple mechanisms may contribute to the detrimental effect of smoking during pregnancy. Nicotine and subsequent catecholamine release along with reduced synthesis of prostacycline result in placental vasoconstriction and elevated vascular resistance,

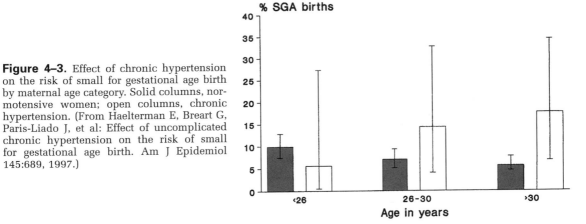

% SGA births

Figure 4–3. Effect of chronic hypertension on the risk of small for gestational age birth by maternal age category. Solid columns, normotensive women; open columns, chronic hypertension. (From Haelterman E, Breart G, Paris-Liado J, et al: Effect of uncomplicated chronic hypertension on the risk of small for gestational age birth. Am J Epidemiol 145:689, 1997.)

Age in years

decreasing delivery of nutrients and oxygen across the placenta. Levels of fetal carboxyhemoglobin are increased, further interfering with delivery of oxygen to the developing fetal tissues. Indirect effects by way of suboptimal nutritional status both before and during pregnancy have been suggested and are likely due to an increased rate of maternal metabolism rather than decreased maternal caloric intake. Smoking mothers consume more calories than their nonsmoking counterparts, and supplementing the diet of smoking mothers is ineffective in offsetting the detrimental effects on the fetus.[69, 96] If smoking mothers can be convinced to stop smoking before the third trimester, their infant's birth weight will be indistinguishable from those babies whose mothers did not smoke at all.[58]

A variety of other recreational drugs, including alcohol, marijuana, cocaine, and amphetamines, have likewise been associated with adverse fetal effects. With the exception of the fetal alcohol syndrome, the effect of these agents is not as well established or as pervasive as tobacco. Certain prescription drugs, particularly the anticonvulsants, can result in fetal growth restriction and specific malformation syndromes.[44] Finally, information from Brazil suggests that even consumption of coffee may pose a risk.[82]

Preeclampsia/Hypertension

The presence of chronic hypertension (defined as hypertension present before the 21st week of pregnancy) has been shown to be an independent risk factor for SGA infants.[42]

Once again, infants born to older mothers seem to be particularly susceptible to this effect (Fig. 4–3). Previous studies have shown that the worst perinatal outcome in hypertensive pregnancies is seen in those complicated by the superimposition of preeclampsia.[59, 94] Preeclampsia is not only a contributor to fetal growth restriction, but it is also the factor that carries the most unfavorable prognosis in terms of severity of growth deficit.[85] Both of these vascular-based problems likely produce their effects through a common placental disorder.

Multiple Gestations

The presence of more than one fetus in the uterus often results in SGA offspring. The onset of the growth restriction is determined by the number of fetuses: the more fetuses, the earlier growth restraint is observed.

Finally, a variety of other maternally related factors have been proposed to play a role in the development of an SGA infant. Chronic medical conditions that interfere with maternal nutrition (inflammatory bowel disease, short gut syndrome), fetal oxygenation caused by decreased amounts of saturated hemoglobin (sickle cell disease, cyanotic heart disease), or oxygen and nutrient delivery caused by vasculopathies (advanced diabetes mellitus, chronic renal failure) can result in IUGR. The role of psychosocial stressors in IUGR is unclear.[38, 49] A summary of the relative contributions of the various factors with direct causal impact is provided in Figures 4–4 and 4–5.

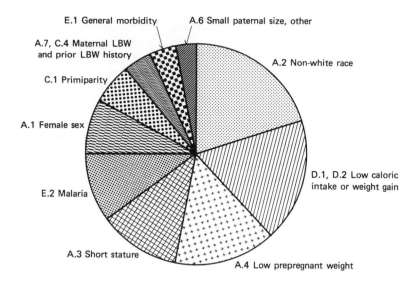

Figure 4–4. Relative importance of established factors with direct causal impacts on intrauterine growth retardation in rural, developing country. (From Kramer MS: Intrauterine growth and gestational duration determinants. Pediatrics 80:502, 1987.)

◆ PLACENTAL CONTRIBUTIONS

Placental tissue is fetal tissue. It follows that if circumstances exist that ultimately result in abnormal fetal growth, then the placenta will likewise be similarly affected. This has certainly been observed, with a significant correlation between birth weight and both placental weight and villus surface area.[2] Likewise, there are placental pathologic correlates of known causes of IUGR (intrauterine infections, chromosomal anomalies, hypertensive disorders, twins) and gross placental and cord abnormalities (chronic abruptio placentae, choriohemangioma, extensive infarction, and abnormal cord insertions), which are likely to result in restricted fetal growth. On the other hand, the majority of cases of IUGR are idiopathic, with the epidemiologic risk factors discussed earlier (e.g., previous fetal losses, extremes of maternal age, previous preterm or SGA infant, substance abuse) as the only clue. The cause of growth failure in these infants is presumed to be the result of the ill-defined *uteroplacental insufficiency*. Human and animal in vivo studies, Doppler ultrasound investigations, and pathologic evaluations have identified an array of placental abnormalities that may well shed a unifying light on these apparently disparate groups of mother-infant dyads (Table 4–1).[35, 83] As a result of these investigations, the central role of the placenta in the development of the growth-restricted baby is coming to the forefront.

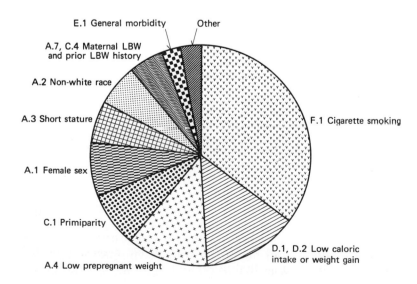

Figure 4–5. Relative importance of established factors with direct causal impacts on intrauterine growth retardation in developed country. (From Kramer MS: Intrauterine growth and gestational duration determinants. Pediatrics 80:502, 1987.)

Table 4–1. Findings in the Placenta in Idiopathic Growth Restriction

Uteroplacental blood flow
  Diminished blood flow
  Increased vascular resistance
  Absent spiral artery remodeling
  Atherosis of vessels of parietal decidua
Fetoplacental blood flow
  Diminished branching of umbilical arteries
    and veins
  Increased irregularity of luminal size
  Abnormal umbilical Doppler flow studies
  Decreased number of placental arterial vessels
  Decreased size of placental vessels
  Decreased artery to villus ratio
Interface of maternal and fetal circulations
  Cytotrophoblastic hyperplasia
  Thickened basement membrane
  Chronic villitis

◆ DIMINISHED POTENTIAL: FETAL CONTRIBUTIONS

One of several controversies that continues to be debated is, simply put: What is abnormal? As previously mentioned, Lubchenco and colleagues defined SGA as being birth weight less than the 10th percentile. By definition then, 10% of all newborns in a given population are too small. Others have proposed or have indeed used other cutoff values (e.g., the 25th, 15th, 5th, or 3rd percentile) or 2 standard deviations from the mean, which would correspond to approximately 2.5% of the population. No matter what cutoff is used, there may be multiple factors that result in a large discrepancy in absolute weights seen at the lowest "normal" percentile. Goldenberg[39] reviewed several reports wherein the 10th percentile was used as the definition of IUGR. More than a 500-g difference was noted across these studies. This observation, however, may have been a reflection of the disparate methodologic approaches among the studies. Dr. Goldenberg's plea for a concerted effort by a variety of national professional academies and federal agencies to endorse a national standard has so far gone unheeded. The approach of using *any* percentile as an absolute criteria has been thoughtfully challenged by Chard and associates[20] who point out that not only is there no statistical evidence of a subpopulation of growth-retarded babies at term, but also that, by using the 10th percentile, most cases of IUGR (defined as a failure to achieve growth potential) will be missed. Although these may be seen as interesting if somewhat arcane academic issues, the practical importance becomes apparent when one is responsible for making decisions regarding expensive and painful laboratory evaluations, the need to monitor the infant in a more costly special care nursery, and future referrals for formal developmental evaluations. In short, do you tell the mother her baby is normal or not?

With this as a preamble, it is apparent that birth weight norms vary among populations. Genetic potential for growth is inherited from both parents and is the major determinant of early fetal growth, which is subsequently modulated by environmental factors. IUGR can also result from a variety of conditions (e.g., congenital infections) in which an otherwise normal fetus is prohibited from growing normally or in which there is a genetic aberration that precludes the fetus from growing normally.

Congenital Infections

During the rubella pandemic of 1962 to 1964, IUGR was found to be the most constant characteristic of congenitally infected infants. In this episode, 60% of the affected infants were less than the 10th percentile for weight at birth and 90% were less than the 50th percentile.[22] Currently, cytomegalovirus (CMV) is the vehicle most commonly associated with IUGR, although 90% of infants congenitally infected with CMV are asymptomatic. Hepatosplenomegaly and microcephaly with paraventricular calcifications are common findings in the symptomatic infant. Diagnosis is reliably made with viral cultures of the urine obtained after birth. Human immunodeficiency virus has *not* been consistently associated with IUGR, because other confounding variables have been difficult to separate.[66] Although numerous other bacterial, protozoal, and viral pathogens are known to invade the developing fetus, most of these infants are appropriately grown.

Genetic Factors

Perhaps 8% of all SGA infants have a major congenital anomaly.[60] Conversely, the incidence of growth restriction in infants with significant congenital anomalies is 22%, nearly three times that of the general population, and a correlation exists between the number of malformations and frequency of IUGR.[50] A wide array of chromosomal aberrations (aneuploidy, deletions, translocations) have been associated with IUGR and have been seen with an unexpectedly high frequency (11%) in an "idiopathic" IUGR (less than 5th percentile) cohort.[67] The likelihood of finding a chromosomal disorder in an SGA infant with a congenital anomaly is approximately 6%.[90] A relatively recently described chromosomal disorder, uniparental disomy, wherein a pair of homologous chromosomes are both inherited from the same parent, has been associated with IUGR.[67] Single-gene disorders and inborn errors of metabolism (maternal and fetal phenylketonuria) are likewise represented in this population. A fascinating case report of an infant with severe growth restriction and subsequent postnatal growth failure as a result of a homozygous partial depletion of the IGF-1 gene represents a recent addition to the ever-expanding list of possibilities.[93] In addition there are well over 100 nonchromosomal syndromes associated with IUGR.

◆ SMALL FOR GESTATIONAL AGE INFANTS: APPEARANCE AT BIRTH AND THE SYMMETRIC/ASYMMETRIC DEBATE

When one eliminates the SGA infants who have significant congenital anomalies and infections, there is a relatively characteristic physical appearance. Their heads are often disproportionately large for their trunks, and extremities typically appear wasted. The nails are long. The facial appearance has been likened to that of a "wizened old man." The anterior fontanelle is often larger than expected, and the cranial sutures may be widened or overlapping. The umbilical cord is typically thin with little Wharton's jelly and may be meconium stained; the abdomen is scaphoid, which may mislead the examiner into considering a congenital diaphragmatic hernia. Subcutaneous fat and tissue are diminished, resulting in loose skin on the arms, legs, back, abdomen, and buttocks. Like the umbilical cord, the skin may be stained from meconium passed in utero and be unusually dry and flaky with little protective vernix caseosa present.

One physical examination feature that medical students and pediatric residents are consistently reminded to evaluate is the weight, length, and head circumference for the purpose of further classifying the SGA infant as either symmetrically growth restricted (those infants with decreased length and head circumference) or asymmetrically growth restricted (relatively normal length with relative "head sparing"). Such a distinction has been proposed as both a diagnostic tool and prognostic marker. The symmetrically growth-restricted newborn, historically representing 20% of all SGA infants, is thought to result from an injury or process (congenital infection, genetic disorders) that occurred or began in the early stages of the pregnancy, during the phase of growth primarily characterized by cellular hyperplasia. The prognosis for eventual growth and development of these infants is expected to be guarded, in large part because of the underlying etiology. The asymmetric ("wasted") SGA baby, on the other hand, has been proposed to result from a third trimester insult interfering with delivery of oxygen and nutrients (the effect of maternal hypertensive disorders, maternal starvation, advanced diabetes) during the cellular hypertrophy phase of fetal growth. This latter group has been projected to expect a much brighter future than their symmetric brethren. Various indices such as the Ponderal Index (PI = birth weight $\times$ 100/length^3) have been used to further describe or quantify the relationship between length and weight and identify these subgroups.

Whereas such an outline may appeal to one's sense of logic, more recent data have necessitated a reevaluation of this approach. Chard et al[21] demonstrated that there is a continuous relationship between the PI and weight throughout the entire range of normal birth weight. Infants in the lower half of the population have a lower PI than those in the top half. In other words, smaller infants tend to be thinner, and larger infants, fatter. Kramer and colleagues,[54] when excluding infants with evidence of major malformations and congenital infections, likewise found a direct relationship between severity of growth restriction and a decreasing PI, arguing against distinct subgroups of proportional and disproportional infants. Similarly, a normal frequency distribution of head-to-abdominal circumference ratio is seen in antenatal ultrasound assessments of growth-restricted fetuses, with increased severity of growth restriction being associated with increased asymmetry.[27] Even the relative frequency of the two groups has come under question; in some populations, symmetric SGA infants are found more frequently than asymmetric infants.[91] The concept of asymmetry serving as a diagnostic tool has been further challenged by Salafia,[83] who found that IUGR preterm infants born to mothers suffering from preeclampsia were far more likely to be symmetric than asymmetric, and David,[27] who found an equal distribution of a small number of chromosomal abnormalities between the symmetric and asymmetric populations. In summary, whereas it may well be premature to completely discard the framework of symmetry and asymmetry in intrauterine growth restriction, one should feel uncomfortable with a dogmatic approach to its use in the SGA infant.

◆ CLINICAL PROBLEMS

Perinatal and Neonatal Morbidity and Mortality

The growth-retarded fetus and newborn have been reported to be at risk for death (Fig. 4–6) and a variety of other adverse outcomes, reflecting the underlying plethora of diagnoses and chronic and acute deprivations of oxygen and nutrients. Even when those infants with major malformation syndromes and congenital infections are excluded, there remains a diverse population with a spectrum of problems that need to be anticipated and addressed by both the obstetrician and pediatrician. Before specific problems are discussed, some general issues should be addressed.

THE PREMATURE GROWTH-RESTRICTED INFANT. Animal data, as well as clinical research and experience, have led many to conclude that the growth-restricted premature infant has a more favorable respiratory prognosis than the equally premature AGA infant because of in utero stress-induced acceleration of lung maturation. Several investigations make a cogent argument against such potential complacency. Age-matched premature growth restricted neonates, in fact, appear to be at a significant *disadvantage* when compared with other premature infants (Fig. 4–7). SGA premature infants are at a greater risk of development of respiratory distress syndrome (RDS) and respiratory failure, require a longer duration of mechanical ventilation and supplemental oxygen, and are more susceptible to development of bronchopulmonary dysplasia—the chronic lung disease of premature infants. In addition, they require longer hospitalizations, are more likely to require surgical closure of their patent ductus arteriosus, and are more often found to have retinopathy of prematurity. Finally, they have a significantly higher mortality rate, whereas those infants who do survive are more likely to have a poor neurodevelopmental outcome.[10, 74, 77, 88]

ARE ALL SGA INFANTS AT THE SAME RISK? If congenital anomalies, intrauterine infections, and control for gestational age are eliminated, are all SGA infants at the same risk of short-term and long-term problems? Are there additional historical or examination criteria that might allow one to narrow the focus? There is a striking direct relationship between the degree of growth restriction and the risk of perinatal morbidity and mortality (Fig. 4–8).[55, 64, 85] On the other hand, the impact of body symmetry and asymmetry is not at all clear, with data showing increased morbidity in either or neither subgroup. There is little evidence that growth-restricted, otherwise normal infants born at term are at a significant increased risk when contrasted with AGA infants, with the exception of the severely

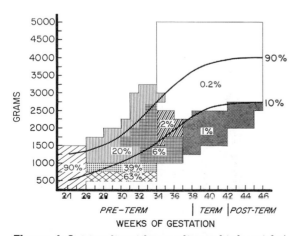

Figure 4–6. Mortality risk according to birth weight/gestational age relationship. Based on 14,413 live births at University of Colorado Health Sciences Center (1974 to 1980). (From Koops B, Morgan LJ, Battaglia FC: Neonatal mortality risk in relation to birth weight and gestational age: update. J Pediatr 101:969, 1982.)

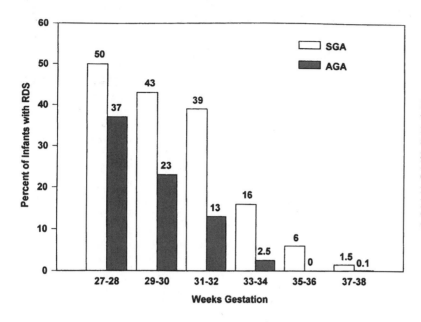

Figure 4–7. Incidence of respiratory distress syndrome in small for gestational age and appropriate for gestational age infants by gestational age. (From Tyson JE, Kennedy K, Bryles S, Rosenfeld CR: The small for gestational age infant: Accelerated or delayed pulmonary maturation? Increased or decreased survival? Pediatrics 95:534, 1995.)

Figure 4–8. Morbidity and mortality varies with degree of growth restriction. (From Kramer MS, Olivier M, McLean FH, Willis DM, Usher R: Impact of intrauterine growth retardation and body proportionality on fetal and neonatal outcome. Pediatrics 86:707, 1990.)

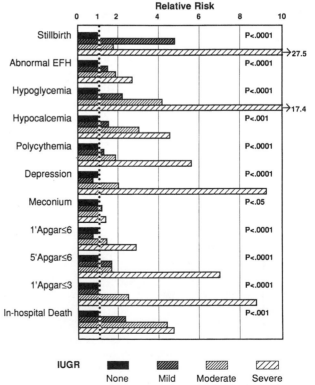

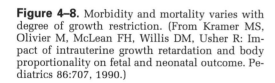

growth restricted child.[20, 46, 56, 79] Piper and colleagues[76] have suggested that the presence of preeclampsia is associated with *decreased* perinatal and neonatal mortality rates and RDS in *preterm* IUGR pregnancies, but *increased* deaths in *term* IUGR pregnancies.

Acute Neonatal Problems

Asphyxia

Perinatal asphyxia is the most significant risk for the growth-restricted fetus and newborn, who are often marginally oxygenated and have limited carbohydrate reserves; with the stresses associated with labor and delivery, fetal death or *asphyxia neonatorum* may ensue. A team of health care providers skilled in neonatal resuscitation should be present at the delivery of every IUGR infant in anticipation of a "depressed" newborn to decrease the risk of potentially preventable lifelong disabilities.

Respiratory Difficulties

In association with the relative intolerance of the stresses of labor and delivery, the passage of meconium and subsequent in utero or postpartum aspiration of this material poses a risk to the term or near-term growth-restricted infant. Meconium aspiration is best prevented by appropriate obstetric intervention before delivery. The role of the pediatrician in preventing this disease after delivery is comparatively limited. Because of concerns regarding risk of in utero fetal demise, SGA infants are more likely to be electively delivered prematurely, with the attendant risks of prematurity, including RDS.

Metabolic Concerns

HYPOGLYCEMIA AND HYPOCALCEMIA. The SGA infant is at risk of hypoglycemia during the first 48 to 72 hours of life. Hypoglycemia can result from inadequate glycogen stores, diminished gluconeogenesis, and, in some, asphyxia, polycythemia/hyperviscosity, or hypothermia. Hypoglycemia is a frequent observation in nurseries that must be given serious attention. Severe hypoglycemia can result in adverse long-term neurologic morbidity and, therefore, must be consistently sought and appropri-

ately managed. Blood glucose concentrations less than 35 to 40 mg/dL should be addressed. The ideal method of initial management is early enteral nutrition (breast milk or formula is preferable). Infusion of 10% glucose by peripheral vein can be started at a rate of 4 to 8 mg/kg/min. If the infant is symptomatic, or if the blood glucose level is very low, infusion of a "minibolus" of 2 mL/kg of 10% dextrose (200 mg/kg) followed by continuous infusion is required. *Do not use higher concentrations for boluses*, because hyperglycemia with severe rebound hypoglycemia is likely to occur. Hypocalcemia is seen less frequently, but must be considered as a possible complication in these babies (see Chapter 11).

Thermoregulation

SGA babies often have difficulty with maintaining body temperature in the normal range. This may stem from a diminished supply of glucose, diminished insulating fat, and impaired lipid metabolism. The brown adipose tissue is not consistently depleted in these infants, but, in some, this may diminish the infant's ability to respond to hypothermia. The range of thermoneutral environmental temperatures for SGA infants is narrowed when contrasted with AGA infants of the same gestational age, but wider when contrasted with more premature infants of the same birth weight.

Hematologic Issues

Spun, central venous hematocrit values greater than 65% occur in up to 40% of term or near-term SGA babies. Poor placental function with resultant relative fetal hypoxia and subsequently elevated levels of erythropoietin is thought to be the cause. Elevated levels of fetal hemoglobin and nucleated red blood cells have both been observed in SGA newborns.[9, 75] Polycythemia has been associated with a myriad of cardiopulmonary, metabolic, and neurologic effects. The need to reduce the level of red cell mass, the benefits derived, and at what level of hematocrit to intervene have been a matter of debate. Some things are certain, however: (1) the value should be believable before any corrective action is taken (the routine for many nurseries is to perform a heel-stick to routinely determine the hematocrit; a free-flowing venous sample must be obtained and a spun hematocrit determined); (2) if a partial exchange transfusion is to be carried out, saline is the diluent of choice; it is as effective and less hazardous and less expensive than any blood-derived products. Immunologic function of the growth-restricted infant may be compromised. Serum IgG concentrations are depressed in term SGA infants when compared with their AGA peers.[73] Deficiencies in lymphocyte function have been observed as well. Finally, neutropenia and thrombocytopenia are seen in some SGA infants. Infants with congenital infections and those delivered to mothers with systemic hypertension/preeclampsia are particularly at risk for these last problems.

◆ GROWTH AND LONG-TERM OUTCOME

Growth

In the immediate newborn period, all infants experience weight loss as a result of a contraction of body water. This is particularly evident for most premature newborns, in whom up to a 15% decrease from birth weight may be seen during the first several days of life. In a small group of mildly preterm SGA infants, however, Bauer et al[12] demonstrated a near absence of weight loss and body water contraction in the first week of life when compared with a more premature AGA cohort. Subsequent to the newborn period, any catch-up growth is done in the first 6 to 9 months of the SGA infant's life, whether the infant is term or preterm. Despite this period of accelerated growth for the group as a whole, a disproportionate number of SGA infants are destined to remain shorter and lighter than their AGA peers. As many as 44% of preterm and 29% of term SGA infants remain below the 5th percentile.[33] Even in this, the controversy about the importance of symmetric versus asymmetric growth restriction exists. Recent data in both term and preterm infants suggest, however, that (in nonsyndromic or congenitally infected newborns) the presence or absence of symmetry does not reliably predict poor or good growth in early childhood.[33]

Neurodevelopmental Outcome

In light of the varied causes of growth impairment, it is not surprising that the litera-ture regarding long-term neurodevelopmental outcome is contradictory and in flux. Earlier studies demonstrating generally poor outcome for SGA infants were not well controlled, included babies with disorders (congenital infections) that skewed results, were generated before modern neonatal care, and often did not consider the home environment. More recent data are less discouraging. The otherwise well term infant is likely to have a normal developmental outcome when reared in a nurturing home environment.[6, 46, 70, 92] Low and colleagues[61] reported an increased incidence of learning deficits (decreased IQ and increased behavioral problems) in a cohort of term SGA infants in the preadolescent years, whereas others have reported a statistically significant "dose response" increase of spastic cerebral palsy in severely growth retarded term and near-term babies.[15] SGA preterm infants have been found to have the same likelihood for success and failure in school as their age-matched AGA peers.[80] Although they found a relatively optimistic outlook for VLBW SGA newborns when compared with their age-matched AGA compatriots, Amin and associates[5] did note that those infants with microcephaly at birth had a much more concerning prognosis (40% with a major disability) than those with head sparing (95% without a major disability). This adds strength to earlier observations that outcomes are measurably worse with early onset of brain growth failure.[45] The debate concerning symmetry continues.

◆ FETAL MACROSOMIA

Like SGA infants, babies with excessive intrauterine growth, whose birth weight exceeds the 90th percentile for gestational age (LGA), represent a heterogeneous group. Maternal risk factors associated with fetal macrosomia include multiparity, weight of 70 kg or more at the end of pregnancy, prolonged or post-term pregnancy, abnormal glucose tolerance, and previous history of a macrosomic infant.[1, 31, 65] In one study, the overall prevalence of macrosomic infants subsequent to a previous macrosomic birth was 22%, a proportion that did not vary notably with parity or when paternity changed between successive births. Mothers with one macrosomic infant are at markedly increased risk for repeat macrosomic births.[28]

One of the more commonly recognized clinical associations with LGA infants is their increased likelihood of being delivered to diabetic women. Even in expert centers, the rates of fetal macrosomia are between 20% and 40% for offspring of women with insulin-dependent diabetes, non–insulin-dependent diabetes, and gestational diabetes.[34] Recent reports have described macrosomic infants of nondiabetic mothers who had elevated C-peptide levels in cord blood and who had significantly greater mean serum insulin levels as compared with appropriately grown infants. These manuscripts clearly document hyperinsulinemia in LGA versus AGA infants delivered to nondiabetic women.[3, 18, 78]

Because the delivery of an excessively large baby is potentially associated with significant perinatal morbidity and increased mortality rate, efforts to predict and confirm the presence of fetal macrosomia in an affected pregnancy, before labor, is beneficial.[72] This facilitates planning of appropriate management measures for the mother and infant. The neonatal morbidity anticipated among LGA infants includes birth trauma, hypoglycemia, polycythemia, and, more infrequently, congenital heart disease (in particular, transposition of the great vessels) and Beckwith-Wiedemann syndrome, all of which, when anticipated, are more likely to be detected and treated more quickly. On the other hand, although antenatal prediction of fetal macrosomia is associated with a marked increase in cesarean deliveries, there has been no significant reduction documented in the incidence of shoulder dystocia or fetal injury secondary to the surgical delivery of macrosomic infants, challenging the issue of its cost effectiveness.[16, 52, 57]

◆ **PHYSICAL EXAMINATION OF THE NEWBORN INFANT**

Preparation

Before embarking on the physical examination of the infant, the clinician must review the mother's medical and pregnancy history to help focus the examination and to ensure that no pertinent findings are overlooked. A history of maternal insulin-dependent diabetes should alert the examiner to the risk of a variety of congenital anomalies as well as aberrant growth. A history of polyhydramnios raises the suspicion of a proximal gastrointestinal obstruction or underlying neurologic problem, whereas a history of oligohydramnios may raise the question of structural renal anomalies. Both very young mothers and women older than age 35 years are at an increased risk for delivering a child with aneuploidy. Knowing that a fetus presented in breech position should lead the examiner to focus on examination of the hips. As noted in the previous sections of this chapter, the presence of IUGR should alert the examiner to search for the stigmata of intrauterine infections and various syndromes.

As with every procedure carried out in the newborn, and particularly the high-risk neonate, the physical examination introduces risks to both the infant and the clinician. Introduction of pathogenic microbes from the examiner to the baby must be prevented. To this end, the examiner must ensure that his hands and forearms are thoroughly cleaned with antibacterial soap and water and that the stethoscope to be used is cleaned with alcohol. Likewise, the examiner must practice universal precautions when examining the newborn to avoid the contraction of infectious diseases. At least until the infant has been bathed, the use of gloves after handwashing decreases the likelihood of such transmission. For all newborns, but in particular the premature or sick neonate, an examination carried out in a suboptimal thermal environment must be avoided. Attention must be given to the amount of light and noise in the examination area as well. Not only do extremes of light and the presence of noise interfere with the examination, they add unnecessary stress to the infant and interfere with the processes of stabilization and transition. Finally, attention must be given to the length of time that the examination takes. A thorough examination of the newborn should take no more than 5 to 10 minutes.

Varying Purpose of the Examination

The extent and focus of the examination varies with circumstances. There are typically three distinct periods of time during which the infant is examined: (1) a brief examination immediately after birth; (2) a complete examination in the newborn nursery or mother's room 12 to 18 hours after birth; and (3) a focused examination before discharge.

The initial examination may be carried out by the labor and delivery nurse, the newborn nursery nurse assigned to the delivery area, or the physician or nurse practitioner attending the infant, depending on the circumstances surrounding the birth. The purpose of this initial examination is two-fold: (1) to ensure that there is no evidence of significant cardiopulmonary instability that requires intervention and (2) to identify significant congenital anomalies. For the high-risk neonate, it may be advantageous to use this setting to perform as complete an examination as possible in order to forego a subsequent examination and thereby avoid an unnecessary disturbance of the baby in the intensive care nursery.

The assessment of cardiopulmonary adaptation begins as soon as the infant is delivered, and this initial evaluation is in part quantified by the Apgar score. Assessment of the presence, regularity, and effectiveness of respiratory effort is the first step in evaluating any newborn. The presence of apnea or signs of respiratory distress must be noted to determine the need for intervention. It is not unusual for a healthy newborn to require a few minutes to establish a regular respiratory pattern, and unlabored respiratory rates of 60 to 80 breaths per minute may be seen for the first 1 to 2 hours in some normal infants.

Cardiovascular adaptation is simultaneously assessed with the pulmonary adjustment to extrauterine life. The normal heart rate of a baby in the delivery area is greater than 100 beats per minute and may exceed 160 beats per minute for brief periods of time. Sustained tachycardia is not a normal finding and may indicate hypovolemia, inadequate oxygen delivery to the tissues, or, rarely, a primary tachydysrhythmia. Autonomic instability may cause an asymptomatic irregular heart beat in the first few hours of life, which is not uncommon. An oft-used indicator of perfusion is the time required to regain perfusion to the central chest after gently pressing over the sternum (capillary refill). It is important for the examiner to assess color of the infant centrally (the gums and inner lips); acrocyanosis is often present in the normal infant for the first 6 to 24 hours of life. Normal term newborns do not require a routine blood pressure evaluation. Infants who are not making a smooth transition to extrauterine life and those infants born before 35 weeks' completed gestation should have their blood pressure determined.

Once the initial cardiopulmonary assessment is complete, evaluation of muscle tone is carried out as a further indicator of the success of transition and well-being of the infant. Normal tone varies considerably with gestational age, but the finding of flaccidity, hypertonicity, or asymmetry of tone is always abnormal.

Once these initial steps are taken, an efficient survey of the face, mouth, abdomen, back, extremities, genitalia, and perineum is carried out. Major congenital anomalies must be sought while the infant is in the delivery area, and their presence and significance, and preliminary plans for their evaluation must be discussed with the family as soon as possible. Even relatively minor anomalies can precipitate strong reactions from anxious parents.

After this initial assessment, assuming the condition of the baby and mother permits, baby and parents should be provided with some private time. The baby is usually in a state of quiet alertness, facilitating parent-infant bonding. If the mother intends to breast-feed, this period will allow her to suckle her infant, an experience that has been associated with an increased likelihood of breast-feeding success. The infant and mother can be briefly assessed every 10 to 15 minutes to ensure continued stability.

Transition Period

During the initial 15 to 30 minutes of life, the *first period of reactivity*, the observed changes reflect a state of sympathetic discharge (see Fig. 3–1). In addition to the irregular respiratory efforts and relative tachycardia, the normal infant is alert and responsive, and exhibits spontaneous startle reactions, tremors, bursts of crying, side-to-side movements of the head, smacking of the lips, and tremors of the extremities. Bowel sounds, passage of meconium, and saliva production become evident as a reflection of parasympathetic discharge. Normal premature and term infants who are ill or were abnormally stressed by labor and delivery have a prolonged period of initial reactivity. During the first hour of life, the infant spends up to 40 minutes in a quiet alert state. This is often the longest period of quiet alert behavior during the first 4 days of life. After this burst of activity, the baby passes into a 1- to 2-hour period of decreased activity and sleep. A *second period of reactivity* subsequently emerges between 2 and 6 hours of age with many of the same motor and autonomic manifestations previously described for the first period of reactivity. Gagging and vomiting are often observed during this period of time. The duration of this phase is variable, lasting from 10 minutes to several hours.

The Complete Examination

The complete examination of the healthy newborn can be carried out in the nursery or in the mother's room. In the latter location, the family is more able to express their concerns about the baby's physical features and the physician is better able to observe parent-infant interactions.

The clinician needs to find a method that will enable him or her to perform a comprehensive examination while minimizing the disturbance of the baby. We use a three-stage approach that begins with an initial hands-and-stethoscope-off period, followed by a minimal disturbance segment, and concludes with a head-to-toe review.

Vital Signs

The respiratory rate and heart rate of the normal newborn vary considerably in the first few hours of life. During the remainder of the first day of life, most newborns have a respiratory rate of 40 to 60 breaths per minute and a heart rate of 120 to 160 beats per minute. The temperature of the newborn can be accurately assessed using an axillary measurement if the probe is placed firmly in the axilla with the arm held against the body until a maximum temperature is reached. A temperature between 35.5°C and 37.5°C is normal. An elevated temperature may represent a fever, but more commonly it is the result of external factors such as overbundling or ambient heat source.

Hands and Stethoscope Off

During this initial portion of the examination, the goal is for the examiner to use only his eyes and unaided ears to evaluate the baby. The baby should be undressed and observed in the bassinet, incubator, or radiant warmer.

Respiratory Effort

The respiratory effort of the newborn varies with the sleep state of the infant. During deep sleep, the infant usually has a regular breathing pattern, whereas during awake states, bursts of more rapid breathing are often observed. As a result of the newborn's compliant chest wall and almost exclusive diaphragmatic breathing, it is not unusual to observe mild subcostal and intercostal retractions, as well as paradoxical movement during inspiration, with the thorax being drawn inward accompanied by outward abdominal excursion. Even though this "see-saw" pattern is often seen in neonates with respiratory distress, in the absence of further evidence of respiratory difficulties, this movement should not cause alarm. Suprasternal and supraclavicular retractions are not normal findings. Likewise, asymmetric chest wall movement is abnormal and may indicate unilateral lesions of the diaphragm (diaphragmatic hernia or diaphragmatic paralysis associated with difficult extractions) or pleural space (effusion or pneumothorax). The normal newborn thorax is configured as an oval, with a relatively narrow anteroposterior diameter. A barrel chest appearance suggests cardiomegaly or air trapping, as may be seen with transient tachypnea of the newborn, meconium aspiration, or a pneumothorax. Audible grunting results from the infant expiring against a partially closed glottis in an effort to maintain a functional residual capacity in the face of atelectasis. This finding should be assumed to indicate a potentially significant cardiopulmonary disease until proven otherwise.

Color and Perfusion

The normal newborn is pink. The finding of other colors such as blue, purple, yellow, green; pallor; or mottling requires a closer examination. Acrocyanosis (blue discoloration of the hands, feet, and perioral area) is not unusual in the first day of life, particularly if the extremities are cool. Central cyanosis (involving the tongue and mucous membranes of the mouth) persisting beyond the first few minutes of life is always abnormal and may indicate significant cardiopulmonary disease. Occasionally, infants with polycythemia appear cyanotic despite adequate oxygenation because they have a relatively high amount of reduced hemoglobin. As noted previously, polycythemia is more likely to present in postdate, LGA, and SGA infants, and in infants of mothers with diabetes. The presenting fetal parts may be bruised during the process of birth, resulting in a localized bluish discoloration. This can be particularly striking in a face presentation or when a transient venous obstruction developed intrapartum (perhaps as the result of a nuchal cord), resulting in a purple-headed baby. To differentiate between cyanosis and bruising, apply pressure to the area. A bruise remains blue, whereas an area of cyanosis blanches. In addition, petechiae often accompany the ecchymosis. Finally, the vigorous infant may turn nearly purple as he performs a Valsalva maneuver in preparation for crying. Occasionally, the harlequin color change is observed, wherein there is a striking division into pale and red halves in an infant (typically positioned on his side), with the line of demarcation along the midline from head to foot. This finding is of no consequence outside of initial consternation in the nursery.

Even though jaundice develops in many, if not most, newborns, this finding in the first 24 hours of life is abnormal and requires investigation. Jaundice is best assessed in natural light, by applying gentle pressure and assessing the color of the underlying skin and subcutaneous tissue. The cephalopedal progression of jaundice with increasing bilirubin levels has been observed for more than a century, and the distribution of jaundice can serve as an estimate of serum bilirubin levels. Rarely, direct hyperbilirubinemia is seen in the first hours of life, providing a green cast to the infant's skin. More commonly, greenish discoloration of the skin is the result of in utero staining by meconium. Mottling may be observed in the well preterm or chilled newborn, or can be a sign of significant systemic illness. Pallor, in contrast, is never normal, and may result from poor cardiac output, subcutaneous edema, asphyxia, or anemia. Finally, a grayish hue is often associated with significant acidosis.

Position and Movement

Careful observation of an infant's position at rest (an indicator of underlying tone) and spontaneous movement provides a great deal of information about her neurologic status. Gestational age, illness, maternal medications, and sleep state influence both tone and spontaneous movements and must be considered during the evaluation. As is evident in the Ballard examination, muscle tone generally progresses in a caudocepahalad direction with advancing gestational age. In the infant of 28 weeks' gestation, there is little tone in either upper or lower extremities, and the infant generally remains in the position in which the care provider places her. By 32 weeks, the infant should have developed tone of the legs, resulting in flexion at the hips and knees. One month later, strong flexor tone is present in the lower extremities, while the arms are beginning to display some flexion. The normal, supine term infant in the quiet awake state holds all four extremities in moderate flexion suspended off the bed. Her hands intermittently open, but most often, the hands are fisted with the thumb adducted and folded (cortical thumbs). Finally, when in the prone position, the term infant should be able to briefly lift her head above the plane of her body, and often elevates the pelvis above the flexed hips and knees. As with tone, the joint mobility of the preterm infant is less than that in the term infant, a fact that seems contrary to what might be expected.

The character of normal spontaneous movements varies with gestational age. Before 32 weeks, infants demonstrate random, slow writhing movements with interspersed myoclonic activity of the extremities. This writhing quality often persists through 44 weeks' postconceptual age. By 32 weeks, flexor movements of the lower extremities begin to predominate and typically occur in unison. A month later, these movements alternate, a pattern seen more frequently in the term infant. This progression of findings is entirely dependent on postconceptual, not postnatal, age.

Normal babies of all gestational ages have symmetric tone and movements. Finding more than mild asymmetry in position and range of spontaneous movement may indicate the presence of local birth trauma (brachial plexus injury or fractures of the clavicle, humerus or femur), or, rarely, a central nervous system insult, lesion, or anomaly. Asymmetry of position may also reflect in utero positioning, which should improve with time. The finding of extremes of flexion or extension requires a more in-depth neurologic evaluation.

Face and Crying

The examiner must not become frustrated if the baby begins to cry. There is much to be gained by observing the face of both the quiet and crying baby, and then by listening to the cry. Symmetry of the mouth and eyes is the normal finding. An asymmetric mouth (the abnormal side does not "droop" with crying) with an ipsilateral eye that does not close and a forehead that does not wrinkle usually indicates an injury to the peripheral facial nerve (cranial nerve VII). This situation must be differentiated from a congenital degeneration or maldevelopment of the cranial nerve VI and VII nuclei (Möbius sequence), which is typically manifested by bilateral palsy. A palsy confined to the lower portion of the face (central facial palsy) may indicate an intracranial hemorrhage or infarct. This latter finding should be distinguished from congenital absence of the depressor anguli oris muscle, a generally benign condition, but one that may be associated with congenital cardiac anomalies.

Most reassuring to a pediatrician is the lusty cry of a newborn baby. An abnormal cry, on the other hand, often heralds underlying problems. A weak or whining cry may indicate illness, developing respiratory distress, depression from maternal narcotics, or central nervous system disturbance. Central nervous system problems may also result in persistent high-pitched crying. Hoarseness can be caused by laryngeal edema resulting from airway manipulation in the delivery room, hypocalcemia, or airway anomalies. Conditions resulting in either internal obstruction or external compression of the airway often cause stridor, which is exacerbated by crying; therefore, stridor in the newborn infant must always be considered a potentially serious finding.

Congenital Anomalies

Finally, a quick survey for dysmorphic features, whether malformations or deformations, must be undertaken. All nurseries should have immediate access to a standard reference book describing and illustrating common neonatal malformation and deformation syndromes.

Minimal Stimulation

Eyes

Dysmorphism of the eye and ocular region are the most frequently cited findings in malformation syndromes. Abnormal eyes may also indicate inborn errors of metabolism, central nervous system defects, or congenital infections. Although careful evaluation of the eyes is clearly important, it is potentially one of the most difficult aspects of the examination. The eyes of a crying baby cannot be examined. Gently rocking the infant backward and forward often prompts the baby to open his eyes.

Nevus flammeus ("angel kisses") is a common finding that disappears in a matter of weeks in most cases. The size, orientation, and position of the eyes should be noted. The diameter of the cornea and eye at term is approximately 10 mm and 17 mm, respectively. Microphthalmia is seen in a number of malformation syndromes, including trisomy 13, whereas an enlarged cornea should suggest congenital glaucoma. The eye that is positioned with the palpebral fissures slanting upward from the inner canthus is typically seen in trisomy 21, whereas Treacher Collins, Apert, and DiGeorge syndromes are characterized in part by downslanting palpebral fissures. A large number of syndromes are associated with hypertelorism (a wide interpupillary distance) (e.g., Apert syndrome and trisomy 13), whereas hypotelorism is less commonly seen (holoprosencephaly and, again, trisomy 13). Newborns often demonstrate random and, at times, disconjugate movements of the eyes. Persistent strabismus should be further evaluated. Subconjunctival hemorrhage is, at times, frightening in appearance, but it is an inconsequential common finding. The iris is blue in nearly all newborns, although some more heavily pigmented infants have dark irises at birth. Reaction of the pupil to light begins to appear by 30 weeks' gestation, but reaction may not be consistently seen for another 2 to 5 weeks. Detailed visualization of the retina is unnecessary in most infants. The goal of most funduscopic examinations is to ensure the absence of intraocular pathology and opacities of the cornea and lens by establishing the presence of a normal light reflex. Whereas the normal light reflex is red in white infants, more darkly pigmented infants have a pearly gray reflex. Patient observation of the retinal vessels passing through the examiner's field of vision is often required. The finding of a white pupillary reflex (leukocoria) can suggest the presence of a variety of ocular pathologies (cataracts, trauma, persistent hyperplastic primary vitreous, tumor, retinopathy of prematurity) and requires an urgent evaluation by an ophthalmologist.

Cardiac System

The goal of the cardiac examination generally falls into one of two categories: (1) to ensure the absence of heart disease during the routine examination and (2) to determine whether the heart is the source of the problem in the sick neonate.

The normal resting heart rate of the term newborn is between 100 and 160 beats per minute, although occasional brief fluctuations well above and below these values are expected. The premature infant's baseline heart rate tends to be slightly higher. Persistent bradycardia or tachycardia can be an indication of primary cardiac or, more commonly, other systemic processes. Normal systemic blood pressure varies with both postnatal and postconceptual age. Blood pressure in the legs is the same to slightly higher than that found in the arms. Pulse pressures likewise vary between term (25 to 30 mm Hg) and preterm (15 to 25 mm Hg) infants.

Examination of the cardiovascular system begins with an assessment of general appearance, color, perfusion, and respiratory status, as previously discussed. The presence of congenital anomalies increases the likelihood of associated congenital heart defects. Central cyanosis accompanied by a comfortable respiratory effort is suggestive of a structural heart defect with diminished pulmonary blood flow (pulmonary atresia). Because of the relative hypertrophy of the right ventricle, the point of maximal impulse (PMI) of the newborn is found just to the left of the lower sternum. In the term newborn, the precordial impulse is visible during the first few hours of life, but generally disappears by 6 hours of age. Because of the lack of subcutaneous tissue in the preterm and possibly growth retarded newborn, the PMI may be visible for a somewhat longer period of time. Abnormal persistence of the visible or easily palpated PMI is seen in both transposition of the great vessels and structural defects characterized by right-sided volume overload. Simultaneous palpation of the brachial and femoral pulses should be carried out.

Auscultation should begin with a warmed stethoscope previously cleansed with alcohol. Many students seem to believe the goal of auscultation is to rule out a murmur. Listening for murmurs should be the last priority for two reasons: (1) most babies have murmurs and the majority of them are transient and innocent, and (2) no one ever forgets to listen for a murmur, but most do forget to listen for everything else at one time or another. The first heart sound is typically single and is accentuated at birth and in conditions in which there is increased flow across an atrioventricular valve. The second heart sound is best heard at the upper left sternal border. In most infants, the second heart sound (S_2) is split, although this can be difficult for the novice to appreciate because of the relatively high heart rate. The presence of a normally split S_2 is one of the most important physical findings to determine and therefore must be mastered. The absence of a split S_2 can indicate the presence of a single ventricular valve (aortic atresia, pulmonary atresia, truncus arteriosus) or transposition of the great vessels (as a result of the orientation of the valves). Widely split S_2 is seldom indicative of increased pulmonary blood flow (atrial septal defect) in neonates, but it can be heard in total anomalous venous return and lesions characterized by an abnormal pulmonary valve. A narrowly split, accentuated S_2 is characteristic of persistent pulmonary hypertension.

The absence of a heart murmur does not eliminate the possibility of important structural heart defects, and classic murmurs ascribed to specific lesions in older children may not be present in the neonate. Even though most infants will have a heart murmur noted during their first week of life, most of these are related to ongoing circulatory adaptation to an extrauterine existence, and they are transient and inconsequential. Harsh grade 2 or 3 murmurs in the first hours of life (ventricular outflow tract obstruction), pansystolic (atrioventricular valve insufficiency), and to-and-fro, systolic-diastolic (absent pulmonary valve, valvular regurgitation) murmurs require more extensive evaluation. Finally, the disappearance of a previously noted murmur in a baby who is clinically deteriorating should make one suspect the closure of the ductus arteriosus with a ductal dependent lesion (coarctation of the aorta, tricuspid atresia, pulmonary atresia).

Respiratory System

As stated previously, the most important part of the respiratory system examination is performed while simply watching the infant breathe. The stethoscope is used to assess the quantity, quality, and equality of breath sounds (particularly in the infant receiving mechanical ventilation), to ensure the absence of bowel sounds in the chest, and to better localize the source of stridor. Alveolar pathology (atelectasis, pneumonia) may be suggested by the presence of rales at the end of the inspiratory phase, whereas crepitant sounds heard early in inspiration usually are the result of airway secretions.

Abdomen

Patience and warm hands are the key to a successful abdominal examination. In most infants, inspection reveals a rounded abdomen. A flat or scaphoid abdomen may be observed in the SGA infant or in the presence of a diaphragmatic hernia. A full upper abdomen in the presence of a flattened lower abdomen suggests a proximal bowel obstruction. Distention is usually apparent at birth when there is massive ascites, meconium ileus and peritonitis, or intrauterine midgut volvulus. Clearly visible intestinal loops are not normal in the term infant, but the thin abdominal wall of the extremely premature baby may result in easily observed loops and peristalsis. Abdominal wall defects (omphaloceles and gastroschisis) are usually readily apparent; these require urgent surgical intervention. Bowel sounds are nearly always heard, and their absence is a concerning finding.

Palpation of the abdomen is facilitated by having the infant's legs in a flexed position and allowing the infant to suckle on her own hand, a pacifier, or a gloved index finger of the examiner's hand. Palpation should begin in the lower abdomen, with the hand allowed to rest there until the infant relaxes. The kidneys are normally palpable bilaterally. Enlargement of the kidneys as a result of hydronephrosis or cystic kidney disease is the most common abdominal mass found in the newborn. The liver is usually palpable 1 to 3 cm below the right costal margin, and the left lobe extends across the midline. The liver should be smooth and its edge soft and thin. Congenital infections, cirrhosis, extramedullary hematopoiesis, tumors, hypervolemia, and a variety of inborn errors of metabolism can all result in a firm, blunt inferior margin. The spleen is less frequently palpable than the liver and should be considered abnormally large if palpable more than 1 cm below the left costal margin.

The umbilical cord normally has two umbilical arteries and one umbilical vein. A "two-vessel cord" (single umbilical artery) is usually found in an otherwise normal newborn, but the finding of other minor anomalies in a baby with a single umbilical artery should make one take notice. Infants with limited fetal activity as a result of congenital neuromuscular disorders, including Down syndrome, often have relatively short umbilical cords, which the obstetrician may note at the delivery.

Top-to-Bottom Review

Head

The scalp and size and shape of the head are next considered. Small lacerations or puncture wounds may result from the placement of the fetal scalp electrode. Use of properly placed forceps can result in superficial marks, edema, or bruising of the skin on the sides of the skull and face, whereas the vacuum extractor can leave a circumferential area of edema, bruising, and occasionally blisters. Use of either forceps or vacuum extractor is associated with an increased likelihood of injuries to the extracranial structures. Caput succedaneum is a boggy area of edema located at the presenting part of the often molded head; it is present at birth, crosses suture lines, and disappears within a few days. Cephalohematomas, present in 1% to 2% of all newborns, are subperiosteal collections of blood that do not cross suture lines. They are often bilateral, and they usually increase in size after birth. Depending on the amount of blood present, cephalohematomas may be fluctuant or tense. Cephalohematomas rarely cause problems, but they may take weeks to months to resolve. The subgaleal hemorrhage is the least common of the extracranial injuries, but is also the most dangerous. Newborns can lose tremendous amounts of blood as a result of these injuries, and they must be monitored carefully once the diagnosis is suspected. Like the caput, this swelling can cross suture lines, but, as in the cephalohematoma, it grows after birth, at times covering the entire scalp and extending into the neck.

Unusual configuration of the scalp hair, such as double or anterior whorls or prominent cowlicks, may be associated with abnormalities of the skull or brain, particularly if there are associated unusual facies. Especially unruly hair is associated with both trisomy 21 and Cornelia de Lange syndrome. A low-set posterior hairline may indicate a short or webbed neck as in Turner syndrome. Ectodermal defects, wherein a 2- to 5-cm diameter portion of the scalp appears to be totally absent, may be an isolated problem, but it is also a common finding in trisomy 13.

Accurate measurement of the head circumference is an important aspect of the physical examination. Abnormally large or small heads may indicate significant underlying neuropathology. The final configuration and even the circumference of the skull may be difficult to ascertain immediately after birth because of the molding that occurs during the birth process, and a period of time may be required before one can be sure of the presence or absence of an abnormality. Babies delivered by cesarean section without a trial of labor typically have little to no molding, whereas vaginal delivery usually results in an enhanced occipitomental dimension with a relatively narrow biparietal diameter. Those infants who were in breech presentation characteristically have an accentuation of the occipitofrontal measurement with a resultant occipital shelf and apparent frontal bossing. The effects of intrauterine positioning and birth are transient, and should recede within days. If not, underlying abnormalities should be considered. A head with a short occipitofrontal dimension (brachycephaly) is characteristic of trisomy 21. Palpation of the skull should reveal bones with mobile edges along the sagittal, coronal, and lambdoidal suture lines. Initial overlapping of the sutures is normal. A palpable ridge along suture lines should always be considered abnormal, possibly indicating premature closure of the sutures (craniosynostosis). The impact of craniosynostosis on the final configuration of the skull depends on the suture involved.

The most commonly involved is the sagittal suture, with resultant dolichocephaly ("keel head"). Even though most instances of craniosynostosis are isolated events, some syndromes (Apert, Crouzon) are characterized in part by this finding. The normal width of the various sutures of the skull is quite variable. African-American infants tend to have wider metopic and sagittal sutures. Wide lambdoidal and squamosal sutures in term infants may be a sign of increased intracranial pressure. Craniotabes, soft pliable parietal bone along the sagittal suture, is a common finding in preterm infants as well as in the term infant whose head had been resting on the pelvic brim for the last few weeks of pregnancy. As its name implies, craniotabes can be seen in congenital syphilis, but this is clearly the exception. Palpation of the anterior and posterior fontanelles should take place when the infant is relatively quiet and held in a sitting position. The normal anterior fontanelle has slight pulsations accompanying the heart beat and is flat to slightly sunken. There is a wide range of normal for fontanelle size, and racial differences have been noted. African-American babies have statistically larger fontanelles than whites. Routine measurement of fontanelles is not particularly useful and not recommended. Finally, auscultation of the head for bruits over the anterior fontanelle and temporal arteries can elucidate the cause of congestive heart failure.

Ears

Recognition of the wide variation of normal for the external ear configuration develops with experience. There are a large number of syndromes that have malformed auricles as part of their spectrum, but the findings are not pathognomonic. The "low-set ears" so often mentioned in physical examinations is usually incorrect, the result of having the head positioned at the incorrect angle or an unusual skull shape. The patency of the external ear canals should be ensured. Examination of the tympanic membrane is often difficult because of the presence of vernix and other debris in the canal soon after birth; it is not generally pursued with vigor in the routine examination. The significance of preauricular skin tags and pits is a matter of some debate in the medical literature.

Nose

The nose may appear misshapen as a result of in utero deformation, and it usually self-corrects in a few days. On the other hand, nasal asymmetry may be the result of septal displacement, which requires evaluation by an otolaryngologist. Several syndromes and teratogens have nasal manifestations including small (fetal alcohol) to large (trisomy 13) noses, and low (achondroplasia) to prominent (Seckel syndrome) nasal bridges. Patency of the nares is most readily established by alternately occluding them with gentle pressure. Fogging of a microscope slide or movement of a strand of cotton placed in front of each nare is an alternative approach and which the baby may find less objectionable. Nasal obstruction may be caused by mucus and edema resulting from well-intended suctioning in the delivery area or nursery, or it may represent true anatomic obstruction caused by tumors, encephalocele, or choanal atresia. Choanal atresia may be a unilateral or bilateral process, and may require the use of an oral airway or endotracheal intubation to maintain a patent airway. Choanal atresia is often part of the CHARGE association (*c*oloboma, *h*eart disease, *a*tresia choanae, *r*etarded growth and development and/or CNS anomalies, *g*enital anomalies and/or hypogonadism, and *e*ar anomalies and/or deafness).

Mouth

The relationship of the mandible and maxilla should be assessed. Occasionally, the mandible opens at an angle resulting from a deformation caused by in utero lateral flexion of the head on the shoulder, which can be confirmed by gently folding the infant into the fetal position and observing the shoulder pressing against the temporomandibular angle. Micrognathia is a component of many malformation syndromes, with the Pierre-Robin sequence perhaps being the most obvious example. The interior of the mouth should be evaluated with a light and tongue blade as well as a gloved finger. The frenulum labialis superior is a band of tissue that connects the central portion of the upper lip to the alveolar ridge of the maxilla. It may be prominent and be associated with a notch in the maxillary ridge where it originates. Likewise, the frenulum linguae is a band of tissue that connects the floor of the mouth to the tongue. This may extend to the tip of the tongue (tongue-tie) but does not interfere with suckling or later speech, and it does not need to be surgically clipped. Natal (present at birth) and neonatal (present in the first month of life) teeth are usually found in the mandibular central incisor region, and are bilateral approximately half of the time. White epithelial cysts on the palate known as Epstein pearls are present in most babies, and similar lesions may be seen along the gums. Clefts of the palate may be obvious to the eye, or only found by palpation (submucous cleft). This latter abnormality may be accompanied by a bifid uvula.

Face

One should be careful not to "miss the forest for the trees" during the examination. The examiner should step back and look at the face of the infant. Is there anything that just looks unusual?

Neck, Lymph Nodes, and Clavicles

The neck of the newborn is relatively short; coincidentally, it has a relatively short list of possible abnormal findings. Redundant skin along the posterolateral line (webbing) is seen in approximately half of girls with Turner syndrome (XO), whereas the neck of the infant with trisomy 21 is notable for excess skin concentrated at the base of the neck posteriorly. A variety of branchial cleft remnants are manifested by pits, tags, and cysts. The most common neck mass is a lymphangioma (cystic hygroma), which is a multiloculated cyst comprised of dilated lymphatics. Occasionally containing a hemangiomatous component, these are usually posterior to the sternocleidomastoid muscle with potential extension into the scapulae and thoracic and axillary compartments. The anterior neck should be evaluated for a midline trachea, thyromegaly, and thyroglossal duct cysts. Lymph nodes, which are usually solitary and as large as 12 mm in breadth, are palpable in one fourth of healthy newborns in the first 3 days of life. Unlike in older children, the most common location is in the inguinal area, but cervical nodes are present with some regularity. Congenital infections can also result in lymphadenopathy. Supraclavicular nodes are never normal. The clavicles are palpated for their presence or absence (cleidocranial dysostosis) and the presence of fractures, which typically manifest as an asymmetric Moro response, tenderness, and crepitus.

Chest

The chest is evaluated for size, symmetry, bony structure, musculature, and presentation of the nipples. The thorax may be malformed or small in a variety of neuromuscular disorders, osteochondrodysplasias, and processes associated with pulmonary hypoplasia. The presence of pectus excavatum (funnel chest) and carinatum (pigeon breast) can be of considerable concern to the family, and both can be associated with Marfan, Noonan, and other syndromes. Palpable pectoralis major muscle tissue in the axillae assures the presence of the muscle, the absence of which is suggestive of Poland syndrome. Supernumerary nipples, found inferomedial to the true breasts, are seen in approximately 1% of the general population, with a higher incidence in African-Americans. Renal anomalies (e.g., hydronephrosis, duplications, hypoplasia) are seen at a much higher rate than would be expected in white children with supernumerary nipples, but not in African-American infants. Breast hypertrophy, at times asymmetric, can be seen in both male and female infants in response to maternal hormones, and may be accompanied by the secretion of "witch's milk," a thin milky fluid, for a few days to weeks. Erythema and tenderness of the breasts do not accompany this normal variant.

The Back

The back is examined for the presence of abnormal curvatures and evidence of an occult dysraphic state. The presence of a tuft of hair, a subcutaneous lipoma, sinus, hemangiomata, dimples separate from the gluteal crease, aplasia cutis, or skin tag should raise suspicion regarding the possibility of an underlying occult dysraphic state. If these abnormalities are found, an ultrasound examination of the involved area of the spine should be undertaken. Finding of a structural aberration requires intervention in the neonatal period or at least in very early infancy in order to prevent the development of neurologic deficits and pain.

The Extremities

Careful inspection and palpation of the extremities alone usually determines whether the extremities are well formed. Joint contractures, asymmetries, or dislocations should be noted. Erb's palsy is manifested by an arm that is extended alongside the body with internal rotation and demonstrates limited movement. The humerus and femur are the second and third most commonly fractured bones at delivery. Abnormalities of the digits (shortening, tapering, syndactyly, polydactyly), single palmar creases, and nail hypoplasia can be important clues to dysmorphic syndromes. A variety of positional variations as a result of intrauterine positioning are seen and need to be differentiated from true equinovarus deformities. Positional deformities of the foot can usually be distinguished by the presence of a normal range of motion and ability to establish a normal appearance of the foot with gentle pressure. A careful examination of the hips of the neonate is crucial in evaluating for the presence of developmental dysplasia of the hips. This disorder is more common in females, infants with underlying neurologic abnormalities, and those presenting in the breech position. Reexamination of the hips before discharge has been shown to be the only portion of the discharge physical examination likely to pick up an abnormality not seen on the initial examination.

The Genitalia

The appearance of the genitalia is certainly one of the first, if not *the* first, areas of interest to the parents. The presence of ambiguous genitalia requires urgent evaluation and therapy at an appropriately staffed center.

MALE. The penile size, position of the meatus, appearance of the scrotum, and position of the testes must all be assessed. A penis of the term infant stretched along its length until resistance is met should be at least 2.5 cm long. It is not necessary, and potentially very painful, to retract the foreskin over the glans penis to determine the placement of the meatus. A meatal opening on the ventral surface of the penis (hypospadias) is relatively common and is readily apparent on inspection. Far less common is an epispadias, in which the meatus is present on the dorsal surface of the penis. This is usually not an isolated defect, more often being associated with exstrophy of the bladder. At the tip of the foreskin may be found a 1-mm diameter pearly white sebaceous cyst. This is of no concern and does not need to be cultured, nor should it interfere with the performance of a circumcision if requested by the parents. The testes should be palpable in the scrotum of the term infant. Approximately 2% of term infants are cryptorchid, with either one or both testes not descended. Nearly three fourths of these infants are no longer cryptorchid at 3 months of age. Premature infants are far more likely to be cryptorchid at birth than the term infant, but these differences become negligible by age 1 year. A hydrocele can usually be distinguished from a hernia by a combination of palpation and transillumination.

FEMALE. As we have seen, the appearance of the female genitalia undergoes a maturational metamorphosis. The premature infant has a prominent clitoris and labia minora, whereas in the term infant, the labia majora completely covers these other structures. The prominence of the clitoris in the premature infant is a result of this structure being fully developed by 27 weeks' gestation combined with a lack of fat in the labia majora. In the term female, outpouching of the vaginal mucosa (vaginal skin tags) is often seen at the posterior fourchette. Vaginal skin tags are inconsequential and regress within a few weeks. A mucous vaginal discharge, which is at times bloody, is usually seen and is often of concern to parents. The passage of large amounts of blood, or clots, is not normal. The hymen has some opening in the majority of females. A completely imperforate hymen may result in the development of hydrometrocolpos. This is usually heralded by the bulging hymen which is particularly prominent with crying. Virilization of the female infant consists of varying degrees of clitoral hypertrophy and labioscrotal fusion. A mass in the labia or groin may be a hernia, but consideration must be given to the possibility of an ectopic gonad, which may be either an ovary or a testis.

Anus

The presence, patency, and location of the anus should be noted. Absent (imperforate) anus should immediately bring to mind the possibility of other associated anomalies, in particular esophageal atresia (VATER association). Patency of the anus is often assessed by cautious assessment of the baby's first temperature by rectal thermometer. After this first evaluation, the benefit of rectal temperatures is likely outweighed by potential risks.

Skin

In the extremely premature infant (23 to 28 weeks' gestation) the skin can be translucent with little subcutaneous fat and easily visualized superficial veins. Because the stratum corneum is thin, the skin of the extremely premature infant is easily injured by seemingly innocuous procedures or manipulation that results in denudation of the stratum corneum and a raw weeping surface. Insensible losses of water through this immature integument can be enormous, resulting in dangerous fluid and electrolyte imbalances if measures are not taken to reduce these losses. The stratum corneum of even the extremely premature infant quickly matures so that by 1 to 2 weeks of age the insensible water losses are reduced to levels seen in the mature infant. By term, skin is relatively opaque with considerable subcutaneous fat.

By 35 to 36 weeks' gestational age, the infant is covered with the greasy vernix caseosa. The vernix thins by term and is usually absent in the post-term infant. The postmature infant has parchment-like skin with deep cracks on the trunk and extremities. Fingernails may be elongated, and peeling of the distal extremities is often evident in the postmature infant.

A variety of normal, ephemeral conditions are found in the newborn. Erythema toxicum neonatorum is a benign rash seen generally in term infants beginning on the second or third day of life. It is characterized by 1- to 2-mm white papules (which may become vesicular) on an erythematous base of varying diameter. The lesions are never found on the palms or soles, and they are relatively infrequent on the face. Wright or Giemsa stain of the lesions demonstrates large numbers of eosinophils. Milia, which are 1- to 2-mm whitish papules, are frequently found on the face of newborns. Miliaria, a result of eccrine sweat duct obstruction, are glistening vesiculopapular lesions over the forehead and on the scalp and skinfolds. Miliaria appear during the first day and disappear within the first week after birth. Transient neonatal pustular melanosis, which is seen predominantly in African-American infants, is a benign generalized eruption of superficial pustules overlying hyperpigmented macules. The pustules, which can be found on any body surface, including the palms and soles, may be removed when vernix is being wiped off or during the first bath, so that the physician may see only macules surrounded by a fine, scaly collarette. White infants may not exhibit the hyperpigmentation, making the diagnosis more difficult and possibly necessitating scraping the lesions for microscopic review. The Wright stain of pustular melanosis shows an occasional polymorphonuclear leukocyte and cellular debris. Mongolian spots are macular areas of slate-blue hyperpigmentation seen predominantly over the buttocks or trunk; they are seen most commonly in African-American, Native American, and Asian infants.

A large number of skin, nail, and hair abnormalities may be found in the newborn. Some of these are important clues in the identification of an underlying syndrome or generalized disease process. A careful examination of the newborn's skin should be made to identify any congenital nevi, hemangiomas, areas of abnormal pigmentation, tags, pits, unusual scaling, blistering, abnormal laxity, or dysplasia. The color, distribution, and texture of the body and head hair are noted. Nail hypoplasia, dysplasia, aplasia, or hypertrophy should be further investigated. Large hemangioma on the face or neck can potentially cause airway obstruction. Port wine stains, another type of congenital vascular abnormality, are usually pink macular lesions on the head, face, or neck. These may be associated with abnormalities of the choroidal vessels in the eye, which may result in glaucoma, as well as superficial cerebral and meningeal vessels and resultant seizures and neurologic abnormalities (Sturge-Weber syndrome).

CASE PROBLEMS

Case One

Baby Boy K is born at 40 weeks' gestation with a birth weight of 2200 g, a length of 46 cm, and a head circumference of 32 cm. The physical examination is remarkable for short palpebral fissures, a small jaw, a smooth filtrum, and thin upper lip.

◆ *What is this combination of features most consistent with?*
A. Trisomy 21
B. Fetal alcohol sndrome
C. Congenital cytomegalovirus infection
D. Beckwith-Wiedemann syndrome

This constellation of findings is most suggestive of (B), fetal alcohol syndrome (FAS). All but (D) can be associated with growth restriction, often "symmetric." Beckwith-Wiedemann syndrome is typically associated with macrosomia. Other physical findings suggestive of FAS include eyelid ptosis, short nose, small distal phalanges, small fifth fingernails. Long-term prognosis for these children is somewhat guarded, with the majority being developmentally delayed, often to a severe degree.

◆

Case Two

You are called to attend the delivery of Baby Girl G at uncertain gestation, who is to be delivered by emergency cesarean section after fetal distress is manifested by late fetal heart rate decelerations with uterine contractions. The fetal membranes are intact. The estimated fetal weight (determined by ultrasound during labor) is 1800 g. The mother is a 15-year-old primiparous female who had a prenatal course notable for smoking, a weight gain of 12 pounds, and infrequent visits to the clinic. She was admitted in active labor and was found to have a blood pressure of 160/110 and proteinuria. She was subsequently given magnesium sulfate for pre-eclampsia for several hours before the delivery.

◆ *What types of problems can you anticipate that you will need to address in the delivery room, and what measures will you take to be prepared?*

This is a complicated but not uncommon scenario. With a lack of regular obstetric care, the gestational age of the baby is uncertain. The baby may be preterm or term. In either case, the infant care center must be warm, and towels for drying the baby must be available. If the infant is at term, she appears to be growth restricted and has shown evidence of not tolerating the stress of labor. With the membranes intact, the presence or absence of meconium in the amniotic fluid is unknown, and one should assume that it is present. It is important to ensure that there is a suctioning device readily available for the obstetrician to use before the delivery of the body to decrease the likelihood of aspiration. The necessary supplies for airway management and suctioning must be present in the area. If the infant is preterm, meconium aspiration is less likely, but respiratory distress is still a distinct possibility, particularly in light of the evidence of distress during labor.

At delivery, there was no meconium, and the baby needed only towel drying, clearing of the airway, and a brief period of supplemental oxygen for resuscitation. In the delivery room, the following are noted: bilaterally descended testes, stiff ear cartilage, scant vernix caseosa, well-developed areola but poor breast tissue development, and decreased muscle tone. The baby's weight is 1800 g, length is 48 cm, and head circumference is 32 cm. There are no obvious anomalies on the initial examination, and the examination of the abdomen, heart, and lungs is normal.

◆ *What is your assessment of his gestational age and his classification?*

This baby is likely a term, SGA infant. The findings of the descended testes, stiff ear cartilage, lack of vernix, and well-developed areola support this contention. Those findings that seem contrary to this assessment can likely be explained on the basis of intrauterine malnutrition (poor breast development) and exposure to magnesium and a stressful intrapartum existence (decreased tone). A complete Ballard examination needs to be carried out sometime during the first 18 to 24 hours.

◆ *What problems will you be anticipating for this infant in the next 24 to 48 hours?*

As an apparently term SGA infant, he is at risk for thermoregulation difficulties, hypoglycemia, polycythemia, and possibly hypocalcemia.

◆ *Why is this baby so small?*

Several features place this baby at risk for poor growth: teenage mother, poor maternal weight during pregnancy, smoking, and apparent pregnancy-associated hypertension. How far to pursue further evaluation for other etiologies (chromosomal abnormalities, congenital infections) will vary among clinicians. The absence of obvious dysmorphology does not exclude all chromosomal aberrations in the newborn.

REFERENCES

1. Aberg A, Rydhstrom H, Kallen B, Kallern K: Impaired glucose tolerance during pregnancy is associated with increased fetal mortality in preceding sibs. Acta Obstet Gynecol Scand 76:212, 1997.
2. Aherne W, Dunnill M: Quantitative aspects of placental structure. J Pathol Bacteriol 91:132, 1966.
3. Akibini HT, Gerdes JS: Macrosomic infants of nondiabetic mothers and elevated C-peptide levels in cord blood. J Pediatr 127:481, 1995.
4. Alexander GR, Korenbrot CC: The role of prenatal care in preventing low birth weight. Fut Child 5:103, 1995.
5. Amin H, Singhal N, Sauve RS: Impact of intrauterine growth restriction on neurodevelopmental and growth outcomes in very low birth weight infants. Acta Paediatr 86:306, 1997.
6. Andersson HW, Gotlieb SJ, Nelson KG: Home environment and cognitive abilities in infants born small-for-gestational-age. Acta Obstet Gynecol Scand Suppl 165:76:82, 1997.
7. Babson S, Behrman R, Lessel R: Fetal growth: Live born birth weights for gestational age of white middle class infants. Pediatrics 45:937, 1970.
8. Ballard JL, Khoury JC, Wednig K, et al: New Ballard Score, expanded to include extremely premature infants. J Pediatr 119:417, 1991.
9. Bard H, Makowski E, Meschia E, et al: The relative rates of synthesis of hemoglobins A and F in immature red cells of newborn infants. Pediatrics 45:766, 1970.
10. Bardin C, Zelkowitz P, Papageorgiou AA: Outcome of small for gestational age and appropriate for gestational age infants born before 27 weeks gestation. Pediatrics 100:e4, 1997.
11. Battaglia FC, Lubchenco LO: A practical classification of newborn infants by weight and gestational age. J Pediatr 71:159, 1967.
12. Bauer K, Cowett RM, Howard GM, et al: Effect of intrauterine growth retardation on postnatal weight change in preterm infants. J Pediatr 123:301, 1993.
13. Berkowitz GS, Mehalek KE, Chitkara U, et al: Doppler umbilical velocimetry in the prediction of adverse outcome in pregnacies at risk for intrauterine growth retardation. Obstet Gynecol 71:742, 1988.
14. Bjerkedahl T, Bakketeig L, Lehmann E: Percentiles of birth weights of single live births at different gestation periods. Acta Paediatr Scand 62:449, 1973.
15. Blair E, Stanley F: Intrauterine growth and spastic cerebral palsy. I. Association with birth weight for gestational age. Am J Obstet Gynecol 162:229, 1990.
16. Blickstein I, Ben-Arie A, Hagay ZJ: Antepartum risks of shoulder dystocia and brachial plexus injury for infants weighing 4200 g or more. Gynecol Obstet Invest 45:77, 1998.
17. Brenner WE, Edelman DA, Hendricks CH: A standard of fetal growth for the United States of America. Am J Obstet Gynecol 126:555, 1976.
18. Carter BS: Macrosomic infants of nondiabetic mothers (letter re: J Pediatr 127:481, 1995). J Pediatr 128:439, 1996.
19. Cnattingius S: Maternal age modifies the effect of maternal smoking on intrauterine growth retardation but not in late fetal death and placental abruption. Am J Epidemiol 145:319, 1997.
20. Chard T, Yoong A, Macintosh M: The myth of fetal growth retardation at term. Br J Obstet Gynaecol 100:1076, 1993.
21. Chard T, Costeloe K, Leaf A: Evidence of growth retardation in neonates of apparently normal weight. Eur J Gynecol Reprod Biol 45:59, 1992.
22. Cooper L, Green K, Krugman S, et al: Neonatal

thrombocytopenic purpura and other manifestations of rubella contracted in utero. Am J Dis Child
110:416, 1965.

23. Craig SD, Beach ML, Harvey-Wilkes KB, et al: Ultrasound predictors of neonatal outcome in intrauterine growth restriction. Am J Perinatol 13:465,
1996.
24. Cunningham FG, et al (eds): The placental hormones. In Williams Obstetrics. 20th ed. Stamford,
CT: Appleton and Lange, 1997.
25. Cunningham FG, et al (eds): Prenatal care. In Williams Obstetrics. 20th ed. Stamford, CT: Appleton
and Lange, 1997.
26. David RJ, Collins JW: Differing birth weight among
infants of U.S.-born blacks, African-born blacks,
and U.S.-born whites. N Engl J Med 337:1209,
1997.
27. David C, Gabrielli S, Pilu G, Bovicelli L: The head
to abdomen circumference ratio: A reappraisal. Ultrasound Obstet Gynecol 5:256, 1995.
28. Davis R, Woelk G, Mueller BA, et al: The role of
previous birthweight on risk for macrosomia in a
subsequent birth. Epidemiology 6:607, 1995.
29. Dubowitz LM, Dubowitz V, Goldberg C: Clinical
assessment of gestational age in the newborn infant. J Pediatr 77:1, 1970.
30. Emanuel I, Alberman HFE, Evans SJ: Intergenera-
tional studies of human birthweight from the 1958
birth cohort, 1. Evidence for a multigenerational
effect. Br J Obstet Gynaecol 99:67, 1992.
31. Essel JK, Opai-Tetteh ET: Macrosomia—Maternal
and fetal risk factors. South Afr Med J 85:43, 1995.
32. Fischer L: Diseases of Infancy and Childhood. 7th
ed. Philadelphia: FA Davis, 1917.
33. Fitzhardinge PM, Inwood S: Long term growth in
small-for-dates children. Acta Paediatr Scand
(Suppl) 349:27, 1989.
34. Fraser R: Diabetic control in pregnancy and intrauterine growth of the fetus (editorial). Br J Obstet
Gynaecol 102:275, 1995.
35. Ghidini A: Idiopathic fetal growth restriction: A
pathophysiologic approach. Obstet Gynecol Surv
51:376, 1996.
36. Goldenberg RL, Cliver SP, Mulvihill FX, et al: Medical, psychosocial, and behavioral risk factors do
not explain the increased risk for low birth weight
among black women. Am J Obstet Gynecol
175:1317, 1996.
37. Goldenberg RL, Cliver SP, Neggers Y, et al: The
relationship between maternal characteristics and
fetal and neonatal anthropometric measurements
in women delivering at term: A summary. Acta
Obstet Gynecol Scand 165:8, 1997.
38. Goldenberg RL, Hickey CA, Cliver SP, et al: Abbreviated scale for the assessment of psychosocial status
in pregnancy: Development and evaluation. Acta
Obstet Gynecol Scand Suppl 165:19, 1997.
39. Goldenberg RL, Cutter GR, Hoffman HJ, et al: Intrauterine growth retardation: Standards for diagnosis. Am J Obstet Gynecol 161:271, 1989.
40. Graham GG: WIC—A fable for our time. Calif Pediatrician Fall:11, 1991.
41. Hadlock FP: Ultrasound determination of menstrual age. In Callen PW, ed: Ultrasonography in
Obstetrics and Gynecology. 3rd ed. Philadelphia:
WB Saunders, 1994.
42. Haelterman E, Breart G, Paris-Liado J, et al: Effect
of uncomplicated chronic hypertension on the risk
of small for gestational age birth. Am J Epidemiol
145:689, 1997.

43. Handwerger S, Richards R, Myers S: Novel regulation of the synthesis and release of human placental lactogen by high density lipoproteins—A review. Trophoblast Res 8:339, 1994.
44. Hanson J, Smith D: The fetal hydantoin syndrome.
J Pediatr 87:285, 1975.
45. Harvey D, Prince J, Burton J, et al: Abilities of
children who were small-for-dates at birth. Dev
Med Child Neurol 23:41, 1981.
46. Hawdon JM, Hey E, Kolvin I: Born too small—Is
outcome still affected? Dev Med Child Neurol
32:943, 1990.
47. Hay WW, Catz CS, Grave GD, et al: Workshop summary: Fetal growth: Its regulation and disorders.
Pediatrics 99:585, 1991.
48. Hickey CA, Cliver SP, Goldenberg RL, et al: Prenatal weight gain, term birth weight and fetal growth
retardation among high risk multiparous black and
white women. Obstet Gynecol 81:529, 1993.
49. Jacobsen G, Schei B, Hoffman HJ: Psychosocial factors and small for gestational age infants among
parous Scandinavian women. Acta Obstet Gynecol
Scand Suppl 165:76:14, 1997.
50. Khoury MJ, Erickson JD, Cordero JF, et al: Congenital malformations and intrauterine growth retardation: A population study. Pediatrics 82:83, 1988.
51. Klebanoff MA, Meirik O, Berendes HW: Second-
generation consequences of small-for-date birth.
Pediatrics 84:343, 1989.
52. Kolderup LB, Laros RK, Musci TJ: Incidence of
persistent birth injury in macrosomic infants: Association with mode of delivery. Am J Obstet Gynecol
177:37, 1997.
53. Kramer MS: Intrauterine growth and gestational
duration determinants. Pediatrics 80:502, 1987.
54. Kramer MS, McLean FH, Olivier M, et al: Body
proportionality and head and length "sparing" in
growth retarded neonates: A critical reappraisal.
Pediatrics 84:717, 1989.
55. Kramer MS, Olivier M, McLean FH, et al: Impact
of intrauterine growth retardation and body proportionality on fetal and neonatal outcome. Pediatrics
86:707, 1990.
56. Langhoff-Roos J, Lindmark G: Obstetric interventions and perinatal asphyxia in growth retarded
term infants. Acta Obstet Gynecol Scand Suppl
165:76:39, 1997.
57. Lipscomb KR, Gregory K, Shaw K: The outcome of
macrosomic infants weighing at least 4500 grams:
Los Angeles and University of Southern California
experience. Obstet Gynecol 85:558, 1995.
58. Lieberman E, Gremy F, Lang JM, Cohen AP: Low
birth weight at term and the timing of fetal exposure to maternal smoking. Am J Public Health
84:1127, 1994.
59. Lindheimer MD, Katz AI: Hypertension in pregnancy. N Engl J Med 313:675, 1985.
60. Lituania M, Passamonti U, Esposito V: Genetic factors and fetal anomalies in intrauterine growth retardation. J Perinat Med 22(Suppl 1):79, 1994.
61. Low JA, Handley-Derry MH, Burke SO, et al: Association of intrauterine fetal growth retardation and
learning deficits at age 9 to 11 years. Am J Obstet
Gynecol 167:1499, 1992.
62. Lubchenco L, Hansman C, Boyd E: Intrauterine
growth in length and head circumference as estimated from live births at gestational ages from 26
to 42 weeks. Pediatrics 37:403, 1966.
63. Magnus P, Bakketeig LS, Hoffman H: Birth weight

of relatives by maternal tendency to repeat small-for-gestational-age (SGA) births in successive pregnancies. Acta Obstet Gynecol Scand Suppl 165:35, 1997.

64. Manning FA: Intrauterine growth retardation. In Fetal Medicine. Principles and Practice. Norwalk, CT: Appleton and Lange, 1995, p 317.

65. Mello G, Parretti E, Macacci F, et al. Risk factors for fetal macrosomia: The importance of a positive oral glucose challenge test. Eur J Endocrinol 137:27, 1997.

66. Minkoff HL, Henderson C, Mendez H, et al: Pregnancy outcomes among mothers infected with human immunodeficiency virus and uninfected control subjects. Am J Obstet Gynecol 163:1598, 1990.

67. Moore GE, Ali ZA, Khan RU, et al: The incidence of uniparental disomy associated with intrauterine growth retardation in a cohort of thirty-five severely affected babies. Am J Obstet Gynecol 176:294, 1997.

68. Murphy NJ, Butler SW, Petersen KM, et al: Tobacco erases 30 years of progress: Preliminary analysis of the effect of smoking on Alaska Native birth weight. Alaska Med 38:31 1996.

69. Muscati SK, Koski KG, Gray-Donald K: Increased energy intake in pregnant smokers does not prevent human fetal growth retardation. J Nutr 126:2984, 1996.

70. Nelson KG, Goldenberg RL, Hoffman HJ, Cliver SP: Growth and development during the first year in a cohort of low income term-born American children. Acta Obstet Gynecol Scand Suppl 165:87, 1997.

71. Nienhuis SJ, Vles JSH, Gerver WJM, Hoogland HJ: Doppler ultrasonography in suspected intrauterine growth retardation: A randomized clinical trial. Ultrasound Obstet Gynecol 9:6, 1997.

72. Ogala WN, Audu LI: Predicting conception and safe delivery of a macrosomic baby. Cent Afr J Med 42:316, 1996.

73. Papadatos C, Papaevangelou G, Alexiou D, et al: Serum immunoglobulin G levels in small-for-dates newborn babies. Arch Dis Child 45:570, 1970.

74. Pena IC, Teberg AJ, Finello KM: The premature small for gestational age infant during the first year of life: Comparison by birth weight and gestational age. J Pediatr 113:1066, 1988.

75. Philip AGS, Tito AM: Increased nucleated red blood cell counts in small for gestational age infants with very low birth weight. Am J Dis Child 143:164, 1989.

76. Piper JM, Xenakis EMJ, McFarland M, et al: Do growth retarded premature infants have different rates of perinatal morbidity and mortality than appropriately grown premature infants? Obstet Gynecol 87:169, 1996.

77. Piper JM, Langer O, Xenakis EMJ, McFarland M, et al: Perinatal outcome in growth restricted fetuses: Do hypertensive and normotensive pregnancies differ? Obstet Gynecol 88:194, 1996.

78. Procianoy RS: Macrosomic infants of nondiabetic mothers and insulin levels in cord blood (letter, comment on J Pediatr 127:481, 1995). J Pediatr 129:178, 1996.

79. Robertson PA, Sniderman SH, Larcos RK Jr, et al: Neonatal morbidity according to gestational age and birth weight from five tertiary care centers in the United States, 1983 through 1986. Am J Obstet Gynecol 166:1629, 1992.

80. Robertson CMT, Etches PC, Kyle JM: Eight year school performance and growth of preterm, small for gestational age infants: A comparative study with subjects matched for birth weight or for gestational age. J Pediatr 116:19, 1990.

81. Rondo PHC, Abbott R, Rodrigues LC, Tomkins AM: The influence of maternal nutritional factors on intrauterine growth retardation in Brazil. Paediatr Perinat Epidemiol 11:152, 1997.

82. Rondo PHC, Rodrigues LC, Tomkins AM: Coffee consumption and intrauterine growth retardation in Brazil. Eur J Clin Nutr 50:705, 1996.

83. Salafia CM, Minior VK, Pezzullo JC, et al: Intrauterine growth restriction in infants of less than thirty-two weeks' gestation: Associated placental pathologic features. Am J Obstet Gynecol 173:1049, 1995.

84. Spinillo A, Capuzzo E, Piazzi G, et al: Maternal high-risk factors and severity of growth deficit in small for gestational age infants. Early Hum Dev 38:35, 1994.

85. Spinillo A, Capuzzo E, Egbe TO, et al: Pregnancies complicated by idiopathic intrauterine growth retardation. Severity of growth failure, neonatal morbidity and two-year infant neurodevelopmental outcome. J Reprod Med 40:209, 1995.

86. Stevens-Simon C, Cullinan J, Stinson S, McAnarney ER: Effects of race on the validity of clinical estimates of gestational age. J Pediatr 113:1000, 1989.

87. Strauss RS, Dietz WH: Effects of intrauterine growth retardation in premature infants on early childhood growth. J Pediatr 130:95, 1997.

88. Tyson JE, Kennedy K, Bryles S, Rosenfeld CR: The small for gestational age infant: Accelerated or delayed pulmonary maturation? Increased or decreased survival? Pediatrics 95:534, 1995.

89. Usher R, Mclean F: Intrauterine growth of liveborn caucasian infants at sea level: Standards obtained in 7 dimensions of infants born between 25 and 44 weeks of gestation. J Pediatr 74:901, 1969.

90. Van Vugt JMG, Karsdorp VHM, Van Zalen-Sprock RM, Van Geijn HP: Fetal growth retardation and structural anomalies. Eur J Obstet Gynecol Reprod Biol 42S:79, 1991.

91. Vik T, Markestad T, Gunnar Ahlsten G, et al: Body proportions and early neonatal morbidity in small-for-gestational-age infants of successive births. Acta Obstet Gynecol Scand Suppl 165:76, 1997.

92. Westwood M, Kramer MS, Munz D, et al: Growth and development of full term nonasphyxiated small-for-gestational age newborns: Follow-up through adolescence. Pediatrics 71:376, 1983.

93. Woods KA, Camacho-Hubner C, Savage M, Clark AJL: Intrauterine growth retardation and postnatal growth failure associated with deletion of the insulin-like growth factor I gene. N Engl J Med 335:1363, 1996.

94. Working Group on High Blood Pressure in Pregnancy: National High Blood Pressure Education Program Working Group report on high blood pressure in pregnancy. Am J Obstet Gynecol 103:1091, 1990.

95. Yip R: Altitude and birthweight. J Pediatr 111:869, 1987.

96. Zaren B, Cnattingius S, Lindmark G. Fetal growth impairment from smoking—Is it influenced by maternal anthropometry? Acta Obstet Scand Suppl 165:30, 1997.

5

The Physical Environment

Marshall H. Klaus
Avroy A. Fanaroff

> The foetus was no larger than the palm of his hand, but the father . . . put his son in an oven, suitably arranged . . . making him take on the necessary increase of growth, by the uniformity of the external heat, measured accurately in the degrees of the thermometer.
>
> *Laurence Sterne*

An understanding of the thermal requirements of the high-risk infant was slow to develop. Pierre Budin,[6] historically the first neonatologist, had perhaps the earliest insight into the clinical importance of the thermal environment. In 1907 in his book *The Nursling,* he emphasized the need for temperature control, after noting a markedly increased survival rate when the infant's rectal temperature was maintained (Table 5–1). He recommended an air temperature of 30°C (86°F) for the small (1 kg), fully clothed infant. Sadly, his observations were neither fully understood nor appreciated in the first 50 years of the 20th century. In addition, during this period, the clinical value of two variables (temperature and humidity) was confused.

The relative importance of incubator temperature and relative humidity was finally resolved by Silverman et al[40–42] in three sequential analyses, the design of which has become a model for further studies of the neonate. In the first study, the researchers compared high and low humidity in two groups of infants. Infants in the high humidity group had a lower mortality rate but higher rectal temperatures. In the second study, to end the confusion caused by two variables, they controlled the humidity and examined the effect of varying only environmental temperature. They noted a striking difference in survival rates. With only a 4°F increase in incubator temperature (from 85°F to 89°F), they observed a 15% increase in survival rate at the higher temperature (68.1% versus 83.5%), with the biggest difference affecting the smallest infants. In a further study, controlling environmental temperatures but varying humidity caused no difference in survival.

Hill[23, 24] in part clarified the profound effects of environmental temperature on survival observed by Silverman et al.[42] Hill, working with kittens and guinea pigs, found that, in 20% oxygen, oxygen consumption and rectal temperatures varied with the environmental temperature (Fig. 5–1). She noted *a set of thermal conditions at which heat production (measured as oxygen consumption) is minimal yet core temperature is within the normal range (neutral thermal environment).* When the animals were cooled while breathing room air, their oxygen consumption markedly increased and body temperature was maintained. However, when they were given 12% oxygen and cooled, oxygen consumption did not increase, and the animals' body temperature decreased. This, as well as the work of Bruck[5] and others, has emphasized that the human infant is a homeotherm and not a poikilotherm, as is a turtle. When the infant is cooled and not hypoxic, he or she attempts to maintain body temperature by increasing the consumption of calories and oxygen to produce additional heat. Homeotherms possess mechanisms that enable them to maintain body temperature at a constant level more or less accurately despite changes in the environmental temperature. In contrast, the body temperature of a turtle decreases if it is placed in a cool environment.

The increased survival rate in the warmer

Table 5–1. Infant's Temperature and Survival Rate

32.5°C to 33.5°C	10%
36.0°C to 37.0°C	77%

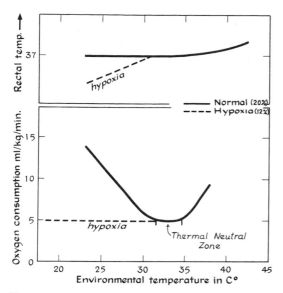

Figure 5-1. Effect of environmental temperature on oxygen consumption, breathing air, or a hypoxic mixture.

environment observed by Budin and Silverman presumably resulted from the decreased oxygen consumption and carbon dioxide production as environmental conditions approximated the neutral thermal environment. *An immature infant with a minimal ability to transfer oxygen and excrete carbon dioxide across his or her lungs has the least chance of becoming hypoxic or developing a respiratory acidosis—increased Pa_{CO_2}—if maintained in an environment that minimizes oxygen consumption or metabolic rate.*

These observations became the stimulus for intense study of temperature control. The physiologic and clinical highlights of these investigations are summarized in this chapter.

◆ PHYSIOLOGIC CONSIDERATIONS

Heat Production

The heat production within the body is a byproduct of metabolic processes and must equal the heat that flows from the surface of the infant's body and the warm air from the lungs over a given period of time if the mean body temperature is to remain constant. A characteristic of the homeothermic infant is the ability to produce extra heat in a cool environment. In the adult, additional heat production can come from (1) voluntary muscle activity, (2) involuntary tonic or rhythmic muscle activity (at high intensities, characterized by a visible tremor known as "shivering"), and (3) nonshivering thermogenesis. The latter is a cold-induced increase in oxygen consumption and heat production, which is not blocked by curare, a drug that prevents muscle movements and shivering. *In the adult, shivering is quantitatively the most significant involuntary mechanism of regulating heat production, whereas in the infant, nonshivering thermogenesis is probably most important.* From animal and human studies it can be inferred that, in the human infant, the thermogenic effector organ—brown fat—contributes the largest percentage of nonshivering thermogenesis.

Brown Fat

More abundant in the newborn than in the adult, brown fat accounts for about 2% to 6% of total body weight in the human infant. Sheets of brown fat may be found at the nape of the neck, between the scapulae, in the mediastinum, and surrounding the kidneys and adrenals.[43] Brown fat differs from the more abundant white fat. The cells are rich in mitochondria and contain numerous fat vacuoles (as compared with the single vacuoles in white fat). Brown fat contains a dense capillary network and is richly innervated with sympathetic nerve endings on each fat cell. The special property of brown fat is the uncoupling protein, which results in the oxidation of food to heat rather than energy-rich phosphate bonds. Its metabolism is stimulated by norepinephrine released through sympathetic innervation, resulting in triglyceride hydrolysis to free fatty acids (FFAs) and glycerol.

The initiation of nonshivering thermogenesis at birth depends on cutaneous cooling, separation from the placenta, and the euthyroid state. The acute surge in thyroid hormones at birth appears to be of limited importance with regard to the immediate control of thermogenesis, whereas the intracellular conversion of T_4 to T_3 and the effects of norepinephrine appear to be of greater significance.[36] Stimulation of the sympathetic nervous system by cold exposure markedly increases local norepinephrine turnover within brown adipose tissue, which may not be reflected by an increase in circulating catecholamines.[17] This results in a marked increase in oxygen consumption without any appreciable increase in physical activity.

Interesting observations made in the sheep noted that cooling of the fetus results in very small increases in FFAs and a significant decrease in body temperature. Ventilation of the fetus with increasing PO_2 resulted in a slight increase in FFAs, whereas clamping the cord resulted in a sharp increase in FFAs and glycerol. These and other observations suggest that before birth there is an inhibitor to thermogenesis, probably produced by the placenta.[16] Possible candidates for the inhibitor are adenosine or prostaglandin E_2. The nonshivering thermogenesis occurring in the brown fat during cooling can be turned off with hypoxia (see Fig. 5–1), and the sensory receptors for this are most probably the carotid body afferents.

The physiologic control mechanisms of the infant may alter the internal gradient (i.e., vasomotor) to change skin blood flow. The external gradient is of a purely physical nature. Both the large surface-to-volume ratio of the infant (especially those weighing less than 2 kg) in relation to the adult and the thin layer of subcutaneous fat increase the heat transfer in the internal gradient.

The heat transfer from the surface of the body to the environment involves four means of loss: (1) by radiation, (2) by conduction, (3) by convection, and (4) by the evaporation of water. This heat transfer is complex, and the contribution of each component depends on the temperature of the surroundings (air and walls), air speed, and water vapor pressure. Of special clinical importance to the pediatrician is the considerable increase in radiant heat loss from the infant's skin to the cold walls of incubators.

Radiant heat loss is related to the temperature of the surrounding surfaces, not air temperature. When incubators are in cool surroundings—for example, during transfer—the inner surface temperature of the single-walled incubator declines well below that of the air temperature in the incubator. In caring for the infant, this problem is easily solved by wrapping him or her in a light covering (transparent if necessary). The surrounding radiant temperature is then close to body temperature and more under the influence of the incubator air temperature.[31]

COMMENT: Because heat is transferred by four different routes, the physical characteristics of the different types of incubators and radiant heaters should be known to the doctors and nurses taking care of the infants. One should realize that the balance between the infant's heat production and heat loss is delicate. The balance may completely change when one of the parameters of the physical environment is changed. When, for example, in an incubator the air temperature is decreased from slightly above mean skin temperature to slightly below mean skin temperature, the infant's heat transfer by convection will change from heat gain to heat loss. In addition, the lower air temperature may, depending on the type of incubator, also affect heat transfer by radiation by increasing radiant heat loss if the inner wall surface temperature of the incubator is lower.

Albert Okken

In very small infants (<1500 g), evaporative heat loss is increased in the first days of life, the result of very thin skin that is unusually permeable to water (Fig. 5–2) (for further discussion, see Chapter 8).

The effect of environmental temperature on heat production (oxygen consumption) is considered in Figure 5–3. As the environmental temperature is decreased below point A (critical temperature), oxygen consumption increases. Body temperature, however, is maintained if heat production is adequate.

If cooling is severe and body temperature drops below point B, with cold paralysis of the temperature regulation center, oxygen consumption also drops—two to three times for every 10° decrease in body temperature. Homeothermy can also be abolished by sedative drugs and brain injury. Not all babies are homeotherms all the time.

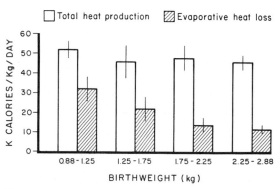

Figure 5–2. Relative role of evaporative heat loss at different birth weights.

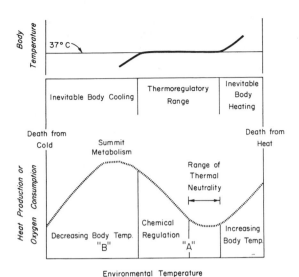

Figure 5–3. Effect of environmental temperature on oxygen consumption and body temperature. (Adapted from Merenstein G, Blackmon L: Care of the High-Risk Newborn. San Francisco: Children's Hospital, 1971.)

Figure 5–3 shows that oxygen consumption is minimal in two areas: the neutral thermal environment and severe hypothermia. The cardiac surgeon works in the latter (temperatures below point B); the neonatologist attempts to maintain the infant in a warm environment (the neutral thermal environment, or the so-called zone of thermal comfort). *It is important clinically to note that the infant may not be in a neutral thermal environment and yet the rectal temperature may be in the normal range.* As emphasized by Hey and Katz,[21] "body temperature alone fails to indicate whether a baby is subjected to thermal stress: it can only alert us to situations in which the thermal stress has been so severe that the baby's normal thermoregulatory mechanisms have been at least partially overpowered." Rectal temperature drops only when the baby's maximum effort to preserve and produce heat fails. The first mechanism to preserve heat is vasoconstriction, and this phenomenon can easily be detected by measuring skin temperature at a peripheral part of the body. A sensitive method to detect vasoconstriction is to measure both rectal and sole of the foot temperatures.[32]

Hypothermia and hyperthermia develop more rapidly in the neonate than in the adult. The infant has a lower capacity for heat storage because of the higher temperature of the body shell in relation to the environment and the larger surface-to-volume ratio. Thus, the thermoregulatory system of the homeothermic infant adjusts and balances heat production, skin blood flow, sweating, and respiration in such a way that the body temperature remains constant within a control range of environmental temperatures. The control range refers to the range of environmental temperatures at which body temperature can be kept constant by means of regulation. The control range of the infant is more limited than that of the adult because of less insulation. For the nude human adult, the lower limit of the control range is 0°C (32°F), whereas for the full-term infant it is 20°C to 23°C (68°F to 73.4°F).

The insufficient stability of body temperature in the small premature infant does not indicate an immaturity of temperature regulation, because the system is intact. As pointed out by Bruck,[5] the insufficient stability "seems to be due to the discrepancy between efficiency of the effector systems and body size." The newborn infant has a well-developed temperature regulation but a narrower control range than the adult.

COMMENT: The body surface to mass ratio of very tiny premature infants is about five times higher than in adults. The relatively very large surface area of the tiny premature is unfavorable in two ways. In a too cold environment, the infant loses heat more rapidly; in a too warm environment, it is overheated more rapidly.
Albert Okken

In Utero

While the fetus is in utero, the heat produced is dissipated through the placenta to the mother. If complete placental separation occurs in utero, the temperature of the fetus increases rapidly. Normally the temperature of the fetus is 0.6°C above the mother's temperature. When the mother's temperature increases secondary to infection or commonly with the use of an epidural analgesia for labor, the fetal temperature increases to be about 0.6°C higher than the mother's. Approximately 30% to 40% of women receiving an epidural anesthetic in early labor are noted to have a fever in late labor, the cause of which is unknown.[14] The system works well for the fetus except during periods when the mother has an increasing body temperature.

After Birth

At birth, the infant's core temperature decreases rapidly, owing mainly to evaporation from his or her moist body. The infant's small amount of subcutaneous tissue and large surface area to mass ratio compared with the adult, together with the cold air and walls of the delivery room, also result in large radiant and convective heat losses. Cold oxygen should always be warmed. Thus, under the usual delivery room conditions, deep body temperature of human newborns can decrease 2°C to 3°C unless special precautions are taken.

Although moderate to severe cooling may result in metabolic acidosis, a lower arterial oxygen level, and hypoglycemia in the newborn infant, very slight cooling of the infant may be beneficial in his or her adaptation to extrauterine life. Cooling of the skin receptors may play a significant role in initiating respiration and stimulating thyroid function. The vasoconstriction and peripheral resistance observed with mild cooling also alter systemic vascular resistance, thereby reducing the right-to-left shunting of blood through the ductus arteriosus. With severe cooling, a vicious circle can result in severe hypoxia and even death (Fig. 5–4).

The neonatologist has chosen to keep the infant warm following delivery to prevent metabolic acidosis and possibly dangerous reflex responses to cooling.

EDITORIAL COMMENT: Shortly after delivery the core temperature of low-birth-weight infants may fall precipitously, the result of significant evaporative heat loss. These infants have a relatively high surface area to volume ratio, immature epidermal barrier, and limited capacity for metabolic heat production. To prevent this fall in temperature, Vohra and colleagues conducted a prospective randomized trial wherein they demonstrated that a polyethylene wrap, applied immediately after birth, effectively prevented a fall in temperature in infants with a gestational age less than 28 weeks, when compared with unwrapped control infants. All the infants were resuscitated under a radiant warmer. Presumably the topical polyethylene film reduced evaporative water loss but still permitted penetration of infrared radiation. Furthermore, the wrapped infants had a lower mortality. All five deaths were in the nonwrap group (vs wrap, P = .04); their mean temperature was 35.1°C versus 36°C in survivors (P = .001). This is a small study that needs validation regarding the mortality; however, it once again draws our attention to the importance of thermal regulation and demonstrates that there is still a place for simple, inexpensive, low technology interventions.

◆───────

Vohra S, Frent G, Campbell V, et al: Effects of polyethylene occlusive skin wrapping on heat loss in very low-birth-weight infants at delivery: A randomized trial. J Pediatr 134:547, 1999.
Narendran V, Hoath SB: Thermal management of the low-birth-weight infant: A cornerstone of neonatology. J Pediatr 134:529, 1999.

Temperature Control in the Very Low-Birth-Weight Infant

Even though infants with a birth weight less than 1250 g make up less than 1% of the total babies born annually in the United States, they frequently constitute a significant percentage of the babies in the intensive care nursery. Very low-birth-weight (VLBW) infants' limited ability to produce heat, their increased evaporative water loss at birth,[50] secondary to extremely thin skin, as well as their small heat capacity (the result of their large surface-to-volume ratio) make them unusually susceptible to cold stress.[9, 17]

Because one of the first responses to thermal stress in these infants is a change in peripheral vasomotor tone with vasodilation when overheated and vasoconstriction with cooling, a continuous assessment of central and peripheral temperatures and their difference is clinically helpful in promptly interpreting the effect of the thermal environment on the infant.[32]

In a study of the first 5 days of life in 79

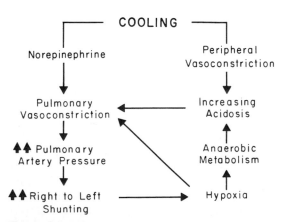

Figure 5–4. Vicious circle resulting from cooling in neonate.

infants weighing less than 1000 g and 71 infants weighing 1000 to 1500 g, central temperature (Tc) was measured with an abdominal skin probe over the liver and peripheral temperature (Tp) on the sole of the foot to calculate the central-peripheral difference (Td). The nursing care attempted to keep the abdominal skin temperature between 36.8°C and 37.2°C to maintain a Td of less than 1°C. The infants were nursed in a double-wall incubator with 80% humidity, and the nurses altered the air temperature.[28] In the heavier babies, Tc had a constant median value of 36.7°C and increased to 36.9°C for the next 4 days. During the first day, the Tc was lower than the sole of the foot nearly 20% of the time, suggesting a slow vasomotor response to cold stress in these very immature infants. To prevent cold stress in this group, Tc was greater than 37.5°C 12% of the time. The normal pattern of Tc greater than Tp was seen more commonly after the first day. In infants weighing less than 1000 g, a Td greater than 2°C can be caused by poor perfusion resulting from hypovolemic shock. In these infants, there was other evidence of hypovolemia 11% of the time (such as increasing heart rate or decreasing blood pressure). With hyperthermia, Td less than 1°C, heart rate increased. If Tc was greater than 38°C with Td greater than 1°C, the infant was investigated to rule out hypovolemia and sepsis.

For appropriate for gestational age infants weighing less than 1500 g, it is recommended that the infants be nursed in double-walled incubators, with low air velocity and additional humidity for the first week of life. Td should be maintained at less than 1°C.

COMMENT: The simultaneous measurement of two body temperatures to monitor temperature control in premature infants to me makes a lot of sense, provided that one temperature reflects core temperature and the other peripheral temperature. Don't forget that the goal of temperature regulation in the body is to keep the environment of temperature-sensitive organs such as the brain, the liver, etc., within a narrow range at the cost of a lower temperature of peripheral parts of the body.

Albert Okken

Nutrition and Temperature

As a result of the relationship between metabolic rate and body temperature, both fluid and nutritional requirements for growth are intimately linked with temperature regulation. This is especially important to the small premature infant maintained in a slightly cool environment. Caloric intake is limited by the small capacity of his or her stomach. Fewer calories would be required for maintenance of body temperature if the infant were in a warmer environment; thus, in the neutral thermal environment, caloric intake can be more effectively used for growth.

The insensible loss of water parallels the metabolic rate, with 25% of total heat produced being dissipated in this manner. Thus, an elevated metabolic rate results in elevated fluid losses and, hence, increased fluid requirements.

The neutral thermal temperature allows for small feedings and reduced caloric requirements for growth.

Glass et al[15] were able to quantitate the effect of temperature control on growth, comparing 12 matched, healthy, small infants aged 1 week and weighing between 1 and 2 kg. These infants were divided into a "warm" group (abdominal skin temperature maintained at 36.5°C [97.7°F]) and a "standard" group (abdominal skin temperature maintained at 35°C [95°F]). Both groups received 120 kcal/kg/d. Those in the warm group showed a significantly more rapid increase in body weight and length; however, their cold resistance (ability to prevent a decrease in deep body temperature in a cool environment) was diminished. Identical growth rates could be obtained by increasing caloric input in the standard group.

It is therefore difficult to decide whether the premature infant, after the early neonatal period, should be maintained in the neutral thermal environment for optimal growth or be prepared for some of the rigors of a cold apartment or house.

◆ PRACTICAL APPLICATIONS

Delivery Room

The temperature of the delivery room is frequently set for the comfort of the medical staff rather than for the comfort of the newborn. Careful and immediate drying of the infant's entire body remains critical in minimizing evaporative heat loss. Many pieces of equipment are available to warm the infant—in particular, incubators and radiant warmers. However, the warm body of the mother is well-suited to meet this need. Christensson[10] compared body temperatures over the first 90 minutes of life in healthy full-term neonates cared for skin-to-skin with their mothers. Infants were thoroughly dried immediately after birth and placed either on their mother's chest and abdomen and covered with a light blanket or wrapped in cotton blankets and placed in a cot. The infants placed skin-to-skin warmed significantly faster than those in the cot. Oxygen consumption measurement while skin-to-skin revealed that they were in a neutral thermal environment.[1] Thus, for the normal full-term infant, skin-to-skin on the mother's chest is an ideal location for the first 2 hours of life. Also, this would allow the infant to crawl to the mother's breast and begin to suckle on his or her own.

COMMENT: In most delivery rooms, radiant heaters are used to keep the infants warm. Under a radiant heater, infants gain heat by the transfer of radiant heat to the cooler skin surface. At the same time, however, the wet and naked infant loses a tremendous amount of heat by evaporation of water from the wet skin because the humidity in the delivery room is usually low. Furthermore, there are usually drafts in the busy delivery room that increase heat loss by convection. Both evaporative and convective heat loss may exceed radiant heat gain, resulting in a fall of body temperature.

Simple measures such as drying off the infant immediately after birth and covering the infant as soon as possible with a plastic cover will reduce both evaporative and convective heat losses and reduce a too great fall in body temperature.

Albert Okken

EDITORIAL COMMENT: Skin-to-skin care has been practiced in primitive and high technology cultures for body temperature preservation in neonates. Karlsson measured regional skin temperature and heat flow in moderately hypothermic term neonates (mean rectal temperature of 36.3°C) and observed that the mean rectal temperature increased by 0.7°C when placed skin-to-skin on their mothers' chests. Caution must be exercised when attempting this in very immature infants. Bauer noted no significant changes in temperature or oxygen consumption in the first postnatal week for infants between 28 and 30 weeks' gestation; however, infants of 25 to 27 weeks of gestational age lost heat during skin-to-skin contact. They recommended postponing skin-to-skin care for these infants

until week 2 of life, when their body temperature remains stable and they are more quiet during skin-to-skin contact than in the incubator.

◆

Karlsson H: Skin to skin care: Heat balance. Arch Dis Child Fetal Neonatal Ed 75:F130, 1996.

Bauer K, Pyper A, Sperling P, et al: Effects of gestational and postnatal age on body temperature, oxygen consumption, and activity during early skin-to-skin contact between preterm infants of 25–30-week gestation and their mothers. Pediatr Res 44:247, 1998.

Incubators

In the United States, most intensive care units have double-walled incubators in which the temperature of the inner wall of the incubator is not affected by a cooler room temperature. However, because single-walled incubators are still found in the United States and many countries throughout the world and because the temperature of the single walls cannot be controlled, it should be emphasized that the radiant heat loss of the infant to the wall of these incubators varies. Figure 5–5 indicates how the temperature of the inner wall of the incubator decreases with cooler room temperatures—a major disadvantage when nursing a sick infant. If the nursery is cool (23.8°C to 15.6°C [75°F to 60°F]) or if the incubator is placed near a cool window or wall, it is difficult—usually impossible—to locate and maintain the neutral thermal environment. The infant loses heat to the cold incubator wall and needlessly increases oxygen and caloric consumption in his or her efforts to stay warm. The magnitude of this loss can be predicted if room temperature is known. Hey and Katz[21] found that operative temper-

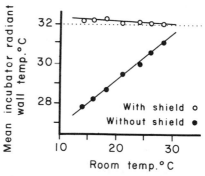

Figure 5–5. Effect of using heat shield (see Fig. 5–6) on mean incubator wall radiant temperature at varying room temperatures.

ature (true environmental temperature, taking into account radiation and convection) decreased 1°C below incubator temperature for every 7°C that incubator air exceeded room temperature. Unless the incubator, room air, and radiant surfaces have similar temperatures, innumerable thermal conditions can exist.

Different types of adaptations prevent radiant heat loss and allow a precise and controlled thermal environment. One method is to warm the nude infant with warm air and heated incubator walls (using either a layer of warm water or electrically conductive plastic paneling).

These expensive procedures have been obviated by Hey, who has developed a small clear plastic heat shield to be used within the traditional single-walled incubator (Fig. 5–6). The warm incubator air heats the plastic wall of the shield to the same temperature as the air within the incubator. The infant radiates heat only to the warm inner plastic shield, because radiant waves from the infant (2 to 9 μm) do not penetrate the plastic wall.

When the thermal conditions can be described and controlled, the neutral thermal environment for any nude infant can easily

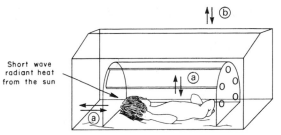

Figure 5–6. Inner heat shield provides warm inner walls to minimize radiant heat loss in cool nursery. (a) Long wave radiant exchange between baby and heat shield and between inner wall of incubator and heat shield. (b) Long wave radiant exchange between incubator walls and surroundings.

be located by using the studies of Scopes and Ahmed.[38] Generally, the thinner, smaller, and younger the infant, the higher the environmental temperature required to achieve the neutral thermal environment.[20]

Table 5–2 and Figure 5–7 are general guides for roughly locating the neutral temperature if the walls of the incubator are warm and within 1°C of the incubator air temperature. When estimating neutral temperatures in single-walled incubators, add 1°C to all the temperatures in the table for every 7°C that incubator air temperatures exceed room temperature. The abdominal

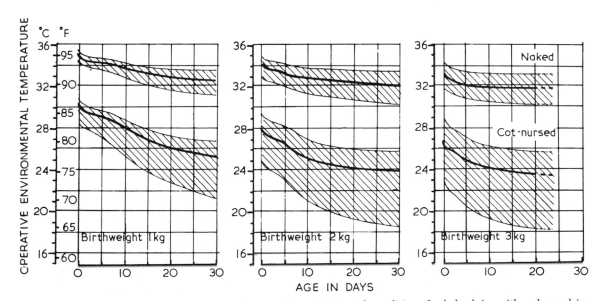

Figure 5–7. Range of temperatures to provide neutral environmental conditions for baby lying either dressed in cot or naked on warm mattress in draught-free surroundings of moderate humidity (50% saturation) when mean radiant temperature is same as air temperature. Hatched area shows neutral temperature range for healthy babies weighing 1, 2, or 3 kg at birth. *Approximately 1°C should be added to these operative temperatures to derive appropriate neutral air temperature for single-walled incubator when room temperature is less than 27°C (80°F) and more if room temperature is much less than this.*

Table 5–2. Neutral Thermal Environmental Temperatures

Age and Weight	Range of Temperature (°C)	Age and Weight	Range of Temperature (°C)
0–6 h		72–96 h	
<1200 g	34.0–35.4	<1200 g	34.0–35.0
1200–1500 g	33.9–34.4	1200–1500 g	33.0–34.0
1501–2500 g	32.8–33.8	1501–2500 g	31.1–33.2
>2500 g (and >36 wk)	32.0–33.8	>2500 g (and >36 wk)	29.8–32.8
6–12 h		4–12 d	
<1200 g	34.0–35.4	<1500 g	33.0–34.0
1200–1500 g	33.5–34.4	1501–2500 g	31.0–33.2
1501–2500 g	32.2–33.8	>2500 g (and >36 wk)	
>2500 g (and >36 wk)	31.4–33.8	4–5 d	29.5–32.6
12–24 h		5–6 d	29.4–32.3
<1200 g	34.0–35.4	6–8 d	29.0–32.2
1200–1500 g	33.3–34.3	8–10 d	29.0–31.8
1501–2500 g	31.8–33.8	10–12 d	29.0–31.4
>2500 g (and >36 wk)	31.0–33.7	12–14 d	
24–36 h		<1500 g	32.0–34.0
<1200 g	34.0–35.0	1501–2500 g	31.0–33.2
1200–1500 g	33.1–34.2	>2500 g (and >36 wk)	29.0–30.8
1501–2500 g	31.6–33.6	2–3 wk	
>2500 g (and >36 wk)	30.7–33.5	<1500 g	32.2–34.0
36–48 h		1501–2500 g	30.5–33.0
<1200 g	34.0–35.0	3–4 wk	
1200–1500 g	33.0–34.1	<1500 g	31.6–33.6
1501–2500 g	31.4–33.5	1501–2500 g	30.0–32.7
>2500 g (and >36 wk)	30.5–33.3	4–5 wk	
48–72 h		<1500 g	31.2–33.0
<1200 g	34.0–35.0	1501–2500 g	29.5–32.2
1200–1500 g	33.0–34.0	5–6 wk	
1501–2500 g	31.2–33.4	<1500 g	30.6–32.3
>2500 g (and >36 wk)	30.1–33.2	1501–2500 g	29.0–31.8

Generally speaking, the smaller infants in each weight group require a temperature in the higher portion of the temperature range. Within each time range, the younger the infant, the higher the temperature required.

Adapted from Scopes J, Ahmed I: Arch Dis Child 41:417, 1966. For their table, Scopes and Ahmed had the walls of the incubator 1°C to 2°C warmer than the ambient air temperatures.

skin temperatures in very low-birth-weight infants during the first 5 days of life are depicted in Figure 5–9B.

If an incubator is placed in the sunlight, the short wavelength radiant emission goes through the plastic wall and can overheat the infant, because long wave re-radiation through the plastic wall is prevented (the "greenhouse effect") (see Fig. 5–7).

Radiant Heaters

When radiant heat panels are placed above the infant without a complete enclosure, there is a large increase in insensible water loss. A minimal oxygen consumption can be achieved by servo-controlling the heat panel according to the abdominal skin temperature and maintaining skin temperature between 36.2°C and 36.5°C (97°F and 98°F). Darnall et al,[13] comparing radiant warmers

with an incubator, found no difference in minimal oxygen consumption, whereas LeBlanc[26] and Wheldon et al[49] found a significant increase in metabolic rate. Under a radiant warmer, radiant losses were markedly reduced, or there is a net gain, whereas convective and evaporative losses are increased. Increasing the skin temperature above a set point of 36.5°C resulted in significant hyperthermia in a minority of infants studied. Baumgart concluded that a moderate abdominal skin temperature between 36.5°C and 37°C would therefore probably best correspond to a thermal neutral zone for a naked infant supine on an open bed platform.[3] He noted that there is a risk of hyperthermia much above this level.[29] A semipermeable polyurethane membrane (Saran) used as an artificial skin resulted in significantly less radiant heat needed for infants to remain in a neutral thermal environment and also reduced evaporative water loss by 30%.[2, 25] Another concern is the effect of the infrared spectrum emanating from the radiant warmer on immature skin and eyes. To date, relatively small studies reveal no cataracts, corneal opacities, or ulcerations.[4]

Cot Nursing

An alternative approach that has been revived and studied in detail by Hey and O'Connell[22] is to care for the infant dressed (cot nursed) rather than naked. In a nude infant, the resistance to heat loss is 1.07 clo units, which is increased by 1.25 units when the infant is dressed in a shirt, diaper, and gown; additional resistance of 0.61 unit is added when a flannelette sheet and two layers of cotton blanket are added.

As emphasized by Hey, the major advantage of cot nursing is the larger latitude of safe environmental temperatures. If the incubator temperature decreases 2°C, the naked infant must increase heat production by 35% to prevent a decrease in deep body temperature, whereas a 2°C increase results in the infant becoming febrile. Similar changes in room temperature would have a negligible effect on the cot-nursed infant. Hey calculated that for the same effects in the cot-nursed infant, the room temperature must decrease to 19°C (66.2°F) or increase to 31°C (87.8°F). Lightly dressing the infant minimizes the effects of fluctuation in environmental temperature. Cot nursing is inexpensive and is clinically useful when close, continuous observation is not required. The development in full-term infants of a nighttime temperature rhythm (with a temperature decrease with sleep) first begins to be noted between 6 and 12 weeks of age.[27]

Heated Water-Filled Mattress

The 8-L polyvinylchloride heated water-filled mattress (HWM) is an effective low-cost device that has been evaluated over the last 10 years using a thermal mannequin and trials with premature infants.[37] The mattress is heated by a thermocontrolled heating plate, and the temperature display records the actual water temperature. The low electric power (50 W) makes the heating slow (4.4°C/hour) so that the mattress must be warm even when not in use. The large heat storage capacity of the water, however, results in slow cooling (several hours) in case the electric current is interrupted.[48]

A disadvantage in the use of the HWM is that the quality of the thermocontrol of the mattress must be exact because the safe temperature range is narrow, from 35°C to only 38°C. Below this range, there is cooling, with the infant losing heat by conduction to the mattress; above this range, there is the possibility of overheating and burns. In several clinical studies in which preterm infants were either in a cot with an HWM or in an air-heated single-walled incubator, the metabolic rate was lower during cot nursing with an HWM.

Hats

The relatively larger brain of the newborn is a major heat source. (The brain of the infant is 12% of body weight compared with 2% in the adult.) Studies by Stothers reveal that heat loss from the head is clinically important and can be significantly reduced with a three-layered hat made of wool and gauze.[11, 44] Figure 5–8 illustrates how the neutral thermal range is extended 1°C and oxygen consumption is reduced in a cool environment when a three-layered hat is worn by a nude 1200-g infant. A tube gauze hat had no effect. We recommend the use of

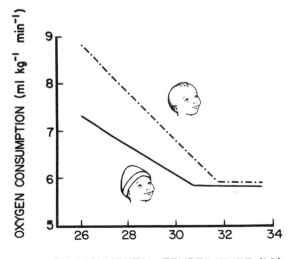

Figure 5–8. Extension of neutral thermal range and reduction of oxygen consumption in cool environment with wearing of a three-layered hat by nude 1200-g infant.

double-layered hats for all infants in home and hospital who would benefit by a controlled thermal environment.

Servo-Control

A completely different approach to caring for an infant in the neutral thermal environment is to servo-control the heating device (whether it is a heat panel or incubator) to the infant's abdominal skin temperature. If the infant's skin temperature decreases, the warming device increases its heat output. The temperature of the skin at which the incubator is servo-controlled is critical. Maintaining the abdominal skin temperature at 36.5°C (97.7°F) minimizes oxygen consumption; at an abdominal skin temperature of 35.9°C (96.6°F), oxygen consumption increases 10%.[7, 39]

Servo-control has been further refined by Perlstein et al[33] who developed a computerized system to control the heat input into the incubator. Their system was designed to maintain the infant in a thermoneutral zone, avoid wide temperature fluctuations that might induce apneic episodes, and recognize the point at which an infant can be weaned from the incubator. The use of this system led to fewer deaths, although the impact of other portions of the computer information on the infant's survival could not be separated from the effect of incubator control.

Two disadvantages of servo-controlled equipment are the increased expense and required reorientation of nurses and physicians when evaluating the infant's condition—both the infant and the incubator temperatures must be compared together, lest the infant's true condition is masked. When an infant who is under servo-control starts to become febrile, the incubator temperature drops, but there is no change in body temperature. In the other direction, when an infant who is being servo-controlled dies, his or her body temperature is maintained because the incubator temperature elevates.

◆ DISORDERS OF TEMPERATURE REGULATION

Hypothermia

Hypothermia should be anticipated in low-birth-weight infants, and the routine use of low-reading thermometers (from 29.4°C [85°F]) is advocated in their care, because temperatures less than 34.4°C (94°F) are frequently not immediately detected with the routine clinical thermometers. Hypothermia is seen particularly following resuscitation of asphyxiated premature infants. It may be an early sign of sepsis or evidence of an intracranial pathologic condition, such as meningitis, cerebral hemorrhage, or severe central nervous system (CNS) anomalies. CNS disease can also result in hyperthermia.

Neonatal Cold Injury

Neonatal cold injury following extreme hypothermia occurs under both warm and cool climatic conditions, particularly with domiciliary maternity services. Low-birth-weight infants are almost exclusively affected, except for full-term infants with problems such as intracerebral hemorrhage and major malformations of the CNS.

Clinical Features

A slight decrease in temperature may produce profound metabolic change; however, a significant decrease must occur before clinical features are evident.

The infants feed poorly, are lethargic, and feel cold to the touch. Mann and Elliott[30] describe an "aura" of coldness about the body and skin over the trunk; the periphery feels intensely cold and "corpselike." Core temperatures are depressed, often below 32.2°C (90°F).

The most striking feature is the bright red color of the infant. This red color (which may lead the physician astray, because the infant "looks so well") is due to the failure of dissociation of oxyhemoglobin at low temperatures. Central cyanosis or pallor may be present.

Respiration is slow, very shallow, irregular, and often associated with an expiratory grunt. Bradycardia occurs proportionate to the degree of temperature decrease.

Activity is lessened. Shivering is rarely observed. The CNS depression is constant, and reflexes and responses are diminished or absent. Painful stimuli (e.g., injections) produce minimal reaction, and the cry is feeble. Abdominal distention and vomiting are common.

Edema of the extremities and face is common, and sclerema is seen, especially on the cheeks and limbs. (Sclerema is hardening of the skin, associated with reddening and edema. It is observed particularly with cold injury and infection and near the time of death.)

Metabolic derangements include metabolic acidosis, hypoglycemia, hyperkalemia, elevated blood urea nitrogen, and oliguria.[30] Another problem encountered is pulmonary hemorrhage in association with a generalized bleeding diathesis (a common finding at autopsy).

Treatment

The infant should be warmed rapidly. In a study in Turkey of 60 infants with hypothermia, rewarming was much faster (1 versus 3 days) in a cot with an HWM than in the incubator, which was often affected by frequent electric failures and poorly functioning equipment. The mortality rate in the warm mattress group was 21% compared with 34% for the incubator group.[48] In areas of the world with minimal hospital budgets, the HWM may be the best solution for effectively warming the largest number of infants. This part of the traditional mode of management has been challenged by Tafari and Gentz,[45] who saw no beneficial effect in slow versus rapid rewarming of 30 cold-stressed Ethiopian infants. The use of a saline push (20 mL/kg) early in the rewarming period, however, did significantly reduce mortality rate.

In addition to the rewarming, oxygen is administered, blood sugar monitored closely, and metabolic acidosis corrected with sodium bicarbonate as required.

The infant should be fed only by intravenous (IV) infusion or gavage of dextrose solution until the temperature is 35°C (95°F). Hypothermic infants should not be permitted to feed by nipple.

Antibiotics are administered only when infection is suspected or documented.

Hypothermia as a Treatment

EDITORIAL COMMENT: There is strong experimental evidence that prolonged cerebral hypothermia initiated after a severe hypoxic-ischemic insult can reduce subsequent neuronal loss in both neonatal and adult animals.[46–48] Hypothermia induced shortly after the hypoxic-ischemic injury and prolonged up to 72 hours offers greater neuroprotection than when induced for shorter periods of time. Thoresen and Wyatt reviewed studies of six newborn animal models of hypoxia-ischemia and noted that mild to moderate hypothermia (2°C to 6°C reduction) for 3 to 72 hours initiated within 30 minutes of insult reduced brain damage by 25% to 80%. When hypothermia of 4°C was maintained for 3 hours, the neuroprotective effect was only modest (25%) by histopathologic examination (Haaland, 1997). However, 12 hours of 4°C reduction in core temperature demonstrated a greater protective effect (70% to 80%) when cerebral oxidative metabolism (adenosine triphosphate and phosphocreatine) was measured by magnetic resonance spectroscopy in the piglet model.[47] The duration of hypothermia was increased to 72 hours in another study evaluating the 14-day-old model; core temperature was reduced by only 2°C. A significant neuroprotective effect (70%) was noted on histopathologic examination of the brain. Thus, the data from animal models suggest cooling should be extended to 72 hours (Gunn, 1998a). The depth of cooling needed for neuroprotection appears to be a core temperature between 32°C and 34°C in both neonatal and adult animal models (Gunn, 1998b, 1997). Cooling to temperatures less than 32°C is less neuroprotective, whereas deep cooling to less than 30°C is associated with systemic side effects.

◆ ——————

Gunn AJ, Gluckman PD, Gunn TR: Selective head cooling in newborn infants following perinatal asphyxia: A safety study. Pediatrics 104:885, 1998a.

Gunn AJ, Gunn TR, Gunning MJ, et al: Neuroprotection with prolonged head cooling started before postischemic seizures in fetal sheep. Pediatrics 102:1098, 1998b.

Gunn AJ, Gunn TR, de Haan HH, et al: Dramatic neuronal rescue with prolonged selective head cooling after ischemia in fetal lambs. J Clin Invest 99:248, 1997.

Haaland K, Loberg EM, Thoresen M: Posthypoxic hypothermia in newborn piglets. Pediatr Res 41:505, 1997.

Thoresen M, Wyatt J: Keeping a cool head, posthypoxic hypothermia—An old idea revisited. Acta Paediatr 86:1029, 1997.

Hyperthermia

Elevation of the deep body temperature may be caused by an excessive environmental temperature, infection, dehydration, or alterations of the central mechanisms of heat control associated with cerebral birth trauma or malformations and drugs.

The question of systemic infection is invariably raised in infants with elevated deep body temperatures. Due consideration should also be given to the environmental conditions that alter heat control. It is not uncommon to find an elevated core temperature following the increased heat input with the commencement of the use of bilirubin reduction lights. This can also occur if the incubator is placed in the sun (see Fig. 5–7). A febrile baby overheated by the environment becomes vasodilated trying to lose heat, and the infant's extremities and trunk are at almost the same temperature. A septic baby is usually vasoconstricted, and the extremities become colder than the rest of the body.[35] Therefore, measuring the temperature difference between the abdominal skin (Tc) and the sole of the foot (Tp) is sometimes helpful clinically.

EDITORIAL COMMENT: Regional heat loss and skin temperature changes in 25 healthy, full-term infants were studied under controlled conditions at environmental temperatures of 28°C to 32°C (Karlsson, 1995). Mean regional skin temperatures measured at 11 body regions followed the changes in environmental tempera-tures (Fig. 5–9A). The regional dry heat losses closely followed the external temperature gradient, defined as the difference between skin and environmental temperatures. In eight of the infants, lowering the environmental temperature 3°C to 4°C induced peripheral vasoconstriction only in the feet. Many clinicians are enamored with the concept of differences in the toe-tummy temperature as an indication of sepsis. Although it is reasonable to consider sepsis, it is equally important to carefully evaluate the thermal environment if a gradient is detected between the abdominal and foot temperature.

◆ ———

Karlsson H, Hanel SE, Nilsson K, Olegard R: Measurement of skin temperature and heat flow from skin in term newborn babies. Acta Paediatr 84:605, 1995.

Asphyxia

With newborn infants, prolonged resuscitative attempts often are carried out on a damp towel, with precipitous decreases in body temperature.

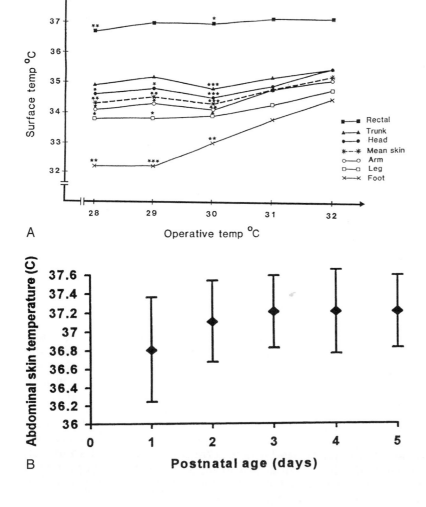

Figure 5–9. *A,* Rectal temperature, mean skin temperature, and regional skin temperatures for different body regions at different operative temperatures. Asterisk, *p* <.05; double asterisk, *p* <.01; triple asterisk, *p* <.001 compared with 32°C. (From Karlsson H, Hanel SE, Nilsson K, et al: Measurement of skin temperature and heat flow from skin in term newborn babies. Acta Paediatr 84:605–612, 1995.) *B,* Mean (standard deviation) abdominal skin temperature according to postnatal age. (From Lyon AJ, Pikaar ME, Badger P, et al: Temperature in very low birthweight infants during first five days of life. Arch Dis Child 76:F47–F50, 1997.)

Temperature responses following delivery are sometimes a guide to the state of the infant during delivery.[8] If the infant was severely asphyxiated or hypoxic, temperature control is reflexively turned off, and body temperature is often not maintained immediately after delivery.

Resuscitative procedures should be performed with due attention to heat control:

1. Evaporative losses may effectively be reduced by immediately drying the infant.
2. Conductive losses can be eliminated by laying the infant on a dry, warm towel or cloth.
3. A radiant source of heat in the form of a radiant warmer provides a heat-giving environment. This is ideal for resuscitation, because the infant can be maintained nude and is readily accessible. Abdominal skin temperature should be maintained.
4. Convection is to be controlled—no drafts in the room—and the oxygen is to be warmed.

COMMENT: It is clear that during resuscitation we should take all measures that prevent heat loss. Studies indicating that lower brain temperatures might reduce brain damage caused by asphyxia, however, may, in the future, affect this common practice.

Albert Okken

Apnea

Despite the beneficial effects of maintaining a warm environment, a possible disadvantage is its effect on respiratory control.

1. Immersing a normal infant in a bath equal to the maternal temperature sometimes stops respiration. Rapid warming is also associated with apneic episodes.
2. Observations in a group of low-birth-weight infants[12] having apneic attacks revealed that lowering the servo-controlling temperature less than 1°C significantly reduced the number of episodes.

Measuring Temperature

We suggest, therefore, that a premature infant having apneic attacks should be maintained closer to the low range of neutral thermal environment, and most importantly, temperature fluctuations should be kept to a minimum.[34]

◆ QUESTIONS

True or False

◆ *If the rectal temperature is maintained between 36.5°C and 37°C (97.7°F and 98.6°F), the infant can be considered to be in the "neutral thermal environment."*
A single measurement of temperature is of little value in defining the neutral thermal environment. The infant may have an elevated metabolic rate and be "working" to maintain normal body temperature. Therefore, the statement is false.

◆ *When trying to produce a neutral thermal environment, take into account ambient air temperature, air flow, relative humidity, and temperature of surrounding objects.*
The neutral thermal environment is that set of thermal conditions associated with minimal metabolic rate in a resting subject; thus, potential heat loss by conduction, convection, radiation, and evaporation must be considered. Therefore, the statement is true.

◆ *Swaddling the infant should not influence the temperature of the incubator when it is set to achieve neutral thermal environment.*
The use of the Scopes tables to achieve the neutral thermal environment refers to a set of specific conditions—namely, that the incubator wall temperature is 1°C higher than the air temperature and that the infants are nude. All the processes of heat exchange are altered and reduced by clothing the baby. The ambient air temperature inside the clothing is warmer than ambient incubator air, and humidity is higher, too. Therefore, the statement is false.

◆ *Overheating the infant produces no noticeable clinical effects and can only be detected by monitoring deep body temperature.*
Overheating is documented by monitoring deep body temperature. However, the infant would be flushed and panting, and the extremities and trunk would be at the same temperature. The infant would hyperventilate and initially show irritability and may have apnea. Sweating may occur but is reduced in immature infants. With prolonged hyperthermia, stupor, coma, and convulsions may occur, and brain damage may be irreversible. The statement is false.

◆ *The stimulus for an increased metabolic rate begins immediately after onset of cold stimulus, even before the deep body temperature has decreased.*

Bruck has shown that it is not necessary for body temperature to decrease before there is an increase in metabolic rate. Therefore, the statement is true. Even mild cold stress (e.g., blowing cold air on the face) may result in a significant increase in oxygen consumption. This occurs when unwarmed oxygen is blowing over the infant's face.

◆ *Maintaining an infant with respiratory distress syndrome (RDS) in the neutral thermal environment plays an insignificant part in overall management.*

Many infants with RDS have a limited capacity to transfer oxygen, and the maintenance of the neutral thermal environment is most important in their care.[19] Therefore, the statement is false.

◆ *The rate of growth in body weight and length can be influenced by environmental temperature.*

Infants kept at a warmer environment showed a significantly greater increase in body weight and length over those maintained in a cooler environment when both groups had the same caloric intake. Infants in a cooler environment require more calories to regulate body temperature and thus have fewer calories available for growth. Therefore, the statement is true.

◆ *When a fever develops in an infant who is being monitored in a servo incubator, this is reflected by an increase in incubator temperature.*

As the infant's temperature increases, the abdominal skin temperature that is controlling the infant also increases, resulting in a decrease in incubator temperature. Thus, a decrease in incubator temperature reflects an increase in the temperature of the infant and vice versa. Therefore, the statement is false.

◆ *An elevated temperature during the first month of life is common and no cause for concern.*

Too often an elevated temperature in a newborn has been attributed to environmental conditions, with disastrous consequences— for example, sepsis overlooked. A temperature elevation, particularly in infants at home, should be carefully evaluated (see Chapter 13). The answer is false.

◆ *Radiant heat losses are similar in adults and immature infants, because they are both homeotherms.*

Radiant heat loss is of less significance in adults because they are clothed and has no bearing on the question of homeothermy. A homeotherm is an animal that attempts to maintain a constant body temperature despite alterations in environment—for example, metabolic rate increases in a cool environment. Therefore, the statement is false.

◆ *The newborn infant loses equal amounts of heat per unit of body mass compared with the adult.*

Although at birth the infant's body mass is approximately 5% of that of the adult, the surface area is nearly 15%. There is also less subcutaneous tissue, resulting in a higher thermal conductance and thus a higher skin temperature at lower ambient temperatures. Bruck has estimated that, because of these facts, the heat loss of the newborn infant per unit of body mass is about four times that of the adult. Therefore, the statement is false.

◆ *Full-term infants who have been cold stressed at birth may have a normal pH and low HCO_3.*

A compensated metabolic acidosis probably secondary to lactic acid production is sometimes observed. Therefore, the statement is true.

◆ *Lowering the body temperature is beneficial in resuscitating asphyxiated newborns.*

Cooling infants during resuscitation is not beneficial and may be harmful. However, there is some evidence that cooling infants (by 2°C) in the first 6 hours for up to 72 hours following severe asphyxia may preserve brain function.[47] Therefore, the statement is false.

◆ *The duration of sleep is markedly reduced when small nude infants are exposed to an environmental temperature of only 1°C to 2°C below the lower limit of the presumed range of thermal neutrality.*

It has been suggested by some investigators that the temperature range in which the least amount of oxygen is consumed is also the temperature range of thermal comfort for the neonate. Therefore, the statement is true.

◆ *Swaddled full-term babies may not cry or otherwise call attention to the fact that they are under severe cold stress.*

This statement is true and is particularly important because the upper limit of heat production is reached for cot-nursed, full-term infants when the room temperature declines to about 10°C (50°F). In some situations at night, bedrooms get colder, and the infants become hypothermic.

◆ *The signs and symptoms of hypothermia shortly after delivery may imitate the clinical picture of RDS.*

The signs of RDS—notably grunting, acidosis, and an increased right-to-left shunt—can all be observed in a hypothermic infant. The statement is true.

CASE PROBLEMS

Case One

Baby D. O. is an 1160-g male product of a 31-week gestation. No problems are encountered in the immediate neonatal period, and the pregnancy is uncomplicated. Delivery is by forceps with the mother under caudal anesthesia. The Apgar score at 1 minute is 6. On the second day of life, the rectal temperature is noted to be 36.8°C (98.2°F). The incubator temperature at this time was 34.1°C (93.4°F).

◆ *What additional data is needed to define the neutral thermal environment?*

To define the neutral thermal environment, one also requires the temperature of the mattress with regard to conductive heat loss, the air flow in the incubator, the relative humidity, and the temperature of the inner walls of the incubator to determine the radiant heat losses that can occur to the surrounding walls of the incubator. A continuous recording of the abdominal skin temperature would permit a rough idea of whether the infant is in the neutral thermal zone. When a servo incubator is controlled to maintain an abdominal skin temperature of 36.5°C (97.7°F), oxygen consumption has been found to be minimal. In this case, the abdominal skin temperature is 34.9°C (94.8°F), the side wall of the incubator is 32.5°C (90.5°F), and the relative humidity is 80%. We can assume the temperature of the mattress to be the same as the incubator air temperature.

◆ *With these available data, is the infant in the neutral thermal environment?*

No, the infant is not in the neutral thermal environment. Our indications of this are that the abdominal skin temperature is only 34.9°C (94.8°F) even with the incubator air at 34.1°C (93.4°F). In Table 5–2, the appropriate temperature for this infant to be in the neutral thermal environment is listed as an environmental temperature of 34°C to

35°C (93.2°F to 95°F), provided that the walls are 1°C higher than the air. Note that the side wall temperature is only 32.5°C (90.5°F). The infant is losing heat by radiation.

Case Two

Baby H is delivered after a 42-week pregnancy; she weighs 1600 g. No problems are noted in the immediate neonatal period. The neurologic examination is appropriate for an infant with a 42-week gestation, except that there is diminished neck flexor tone. Head circumference is 33 cm. The infant is unable to increase her metabolic rate with cold stress.

◆ *How can the optimal thermal environment be found?*

This is a difficult question to answer because no tables are available for this age and weight. The problem may best be managed by servo-control of the incubator and maintaining the abdominal skin temperature at 36.5°C (97.7°F). Another approach is to use the "warmest" incubator possible to maintain a normal temperature in the infant.

REFERENCES

1. Acolet D, Sleath K, Whitelaw A: Oxygenation, heart rate and temperature in very low birth weight infants during skin-to-skin contact with their mothers. Acta Paediatr Scand 78:189, 1989.
2. Baumgart S: Reduction of oxygen consumption, insensible water loss and radiant heat demand with the use of a plastic blanket for low birth weight infants under radiant warmers. Pediatrics 74:1022, 1984.
3. Baumgart S: Partitioning of heat losses and gains in premature newborn infants under radiant warmers. Pediatrics 75:89, 1985.
4. Baumgart S, Knauth A, Casey FX, et al: Infrared eye injury not due to radiant warmer use in premature neonates. Am J Dis Child 147:565, 1993.
5. Bruck K: Neonatal thermal regulation. In Polin R, Fox WW, eds: Fetal and Neonatal Physiology. Philadelphia, WB Saunders, 1992, pp 488–515.
6. Budin P: The Nursling. London, Caxton Publishing, 1907.
7. Buetow K, Klein S: Effect of maintenance of "normal" skin temperature on survival of infants of low birth weight. Pediatrics 34:163, 1964.
8. Burnard E, Cross K: Rectal temperature in the newborn after birth asphyxia. BMJ 2:1197, 1958.
9. Chessex P, Blouet S, Vaucher J: Environmental temperature control in very low birth weight infants (less than 1000 grams) cared for in double-walled incubators. J Pediatr 113:373, 1988.
10. Christensson K, Sales L, Moreno A: Temperature, metabolic adaptation and crying in healthy newborns. Acta Paediatr Scand 81:488, 1992.

11. Cross KW: Review Lecture. La Chaleur Animale and the infant brain. J Physiol 294:1, 1979.
12. Dailey W, Klaus M, Meyer H: Apnea in premature infants: Monitoring, incidence, heart rate changes, and effect of environmental temperature. Pediatrics 43:510, 1969.
13. Darnall RA Jr, Ariagno RL: Minimal oxygen consumption in infants cared for under overhead radiant warmers compared with conventional incubators. J Pediatr 93:283, 1978.
14. Fusi L, Maresh JJA, Steer PJ et al: Maternal pyrexia associated with the use of epidural analgesia in labor. Lancet 333:1250, 1989.
15. Glass L, Silverman W, Sinclair J: Effects of the thermal environment on cold resistance and growth of small infants after the first week of life. Pediatrics 41:1033, 1968.
16. Gunn TR, Ball KT, Gluckman PD: Reversible umbilical cord occlusion: Effect of thermogenesis in utero. Pediatr Res 30:513, 1991.
17. Gunn TR, Ball KT, Power GG, Gluckman PD: Factors influencing the initiation of nonshivering thermogenesis. Am J Obstet Gynecol 164:210, 1991.
18. Gunn TR, Gunn AJ, deHaan HH, et al: Prolonged selective cerebral cooling prevents cytotoxic edema and improves recovery after cerebral ischemia in fetal sheep. J Clin Invest 99:248, 1997.
19. Hazan J, Maag U, Chessex P: Association between hypothermia and mortality rate of premature infants—revisited. Am J Obstet Gynecol 164:111, 1991.
20. Hey E: The relation between environmental temperature and oxygen consumption in the newborn baby. J Physiol 200:589, 1969.
21. Hey F, Katz G: The optimum thermal environment for naked babies. Arch Dis Child 45:328, 1970.
22. Hey E, O'Connell B: Oxygen consumption and heat balance in the cot-nursed baby. Arch Dis Child 45:335, 1970.
23. Hill J: The oxygen consumption of newborn and adult mammals: Its dependence on the oxygen tension in the inspired air and on environmental temperature. J Physiol 149:346, 1959.
24. Hill J, Rahimtulla K: Heat balance and the metabolic rate of newborn babies in relation to environmental temperature; and the effect of age and of weight on basal metabolic rate. J Physiol 180:239, 1965.
25. Knauth A, Gordin M, McNelis W, Baumgart S: Semipermeable polyurethane membrane as an artificial skin for the premature neonate. Pediatrics 83:945, 1989.
26. LeBlanc MH: Relative efficiency of an incubator and an open warmer in producing thermoneutrality for the small premature infant. Pediatrics 69:439, 1982.
27. Lodemore M, Petersen SA, Wailoo MP: Development of night time temperature rhythms over the first six months of life. Arch Dis Child 66:521, 1991.
28. Lyon A, Pikaar M: Temperature control in preterm infants—Effect of birth weight. In Okken A, Koch J, eds: Thermoregulation of sick and low birth weight neonates. Berlin: Springer-Verlag, 1995, pp 83–91.
29. Malin S, Baumgart S: Optimal thermal management for low birth weight infants nursed under high-powered radiant warmers. Pediatrics 79:47, 1987.
30. Mann T, Elliott R: Neonatal cold injury due to accidental exposure to cold. Lancet 1:229, 1957.
31. Okken A: Heat production and heat loss of low birth weight babies in an incubator with heated walls. Thesis. University of Groningen, The Netherlands, 1976.
32. Okken A, Koch J: Thermoregulation of sick and low birth weight neonates. Berlin: Springer-Verlag, 1995.
33. Perlstein P, Edwards N, Atherton H, et al: Computer-assisted newborn intensive care. Pediatrics 57:494, 1976.
34. Perlstein P, Edwards N, Sutherland J: Apnea in premature infants and incubator air temperature changes. N Engl J Med 282:461, 1970.
35. Pomerance JJ, Brand RJ, Meredith JL: Differentiating environmental from related fevers in the term newborn. Pediatrics 67:485, 1981.
36. Power G, Gunn TR, Johnston BM, et al: Umbilical cord occlusion but not increased plasma T_3 or norepinephrine stimulate brown adipose tissue thermogenesis in the fetal sheep. J Dev Physiol 11:171, 1989.
37. Sarnan I, Tunell R: Providing warmth for preterm babies by a heated, water-filled mattress. Arch Dis Child 64:29, 1989.
38. Scopes J, Ahmed I: Range of critical temperatures in sick and premature newborn babies. Arch Dis Child 41:94, 1973.
39. Silverman W, Agate F: Variation in cold resistance among small newborn animals. Biol Neonate 6:113, 1964.
40. Silverman W, Blanc W: The effect of humidity on survival of newly born premature infants. Pediatrics 20:477, 1957.
41. Silverman W, Agate F, Fertig J: A sequential trial of the nonthermal effect of atmospheric humidity on survival of newborn infants of low birth weight. Pediatrics 31:719, 1963.
42. Silverman W, Fertig J, Berger A: The influence of the thermal environment upon the survival of newly born premature infants. Pediatrics 22:876, 1958.
43. Silverman W, Zamelis A, Sinclair J, et al: Warm nape of the newborn. Pediatrics 33:984, 1964.
44. Stothers JK: Head insulation and heat loss in the newborn. Arch Dis Child 56:530, 1981.
45. Tafari N, Gentz J: Aspects of rewarming newborn infants with severe accidental hypothermia. Acta Paediatr Scand 63:595, 1974.
46. Thoreson M, Bägenholm R, Loberg EM: Posthypoxic cooling of neonatal rats provides protection against brain injury. Arch Dis Child 74:F3–F9, 1996.
47. Thoreson M, Penice J, Lorek A, et al: Mild hypothermia after severe transient hypoxic ischemia ameliorates delayed energy failure in the newborn piglet. Pediatric Research 37:667, 1995.
48. Tunell R: Treatment of sick newborns with heated mattress. In Okken A, Koch J, eds: Thermoregulation of sick and low birth weight neonates. Berlin: Springer-Verlag, 1995, pp 193–201.
49. Wheldon AE, Rutter N: The heat balance of small babies nursed in incubators and under radiant warmers. Early Hum Dev 6:131, 1982.
50. Wu PY, Hodgman JE: Insensible water loss in preterm infants: Changes with postnatal development and non-ionizing radiant energy. Pediatrics 54:704, 1974.

Nutrition and Selected Disorders of the Gastrointestinal Tract

Part One

NUTRITION FOR THE HIGH-RISK INFANT

Satish C. Kalhan
Pamela T. Price

The goal of nutritional support for the high-risk infant is to provide sufficient nutrients postnatally to ensure continuation of the growth at rates similar to those observed in utero. The preterm infant presents a particular challenge in that the nutritional needs must be sufficient to replenish tissue losses and permit tissue accretion. However during the early days after birth, acute illness such as respiratory distress, patent ductus arteriosus, and hyperbilirubinemia preclude maximal nutritional support. Additionally, because of the functional immaturity of the gastrointestinal tract, kidneys, and the metabolic adaptation requirements for extrauterine existence, substrate intolerances are common, limiting the nutrients available for tissue maintenance and growth.

During the last trimester of pregnancy, nutrient stores are established in preparation for birth at 40 weeks' gestation. Fat and glycogen are stored to provide ready energy during times of caloric deficit. Iron reserves accumulate to prevent iron-deficiency anemia during the first 4 to 6 months of life. Calcium and phosphorous are deposited in the soft bones to begin the mineralization process, which will continue through early adult life. However, the infant who is delivered before term has minimal nutrient stores and higher nutrient requirements per kilogram than the full-term infant.

Infants weighing less than 1.5 kg have a body composition of approximately 85% to 95% water, 9% to 10% protein, and 0.1% to 5% fat.[81, 82, 97] The fat is primarily structural and represents negligible amounts of subcutaneous fat; hepatic glycogen stores are virtually nonexistent. In the first several days of life, the sole energy source for a low-birth-weight (LBW) infant is from hypocalorie parenteral dextrose and amino acid solutions; therefore, a substantial weight loss occurs. Various authors have estimated that energy reserves of very low-birth-weight (VLBW) infants may be depleted by 8 to 12 days of life even if given 30 kcal/kg/d of a dextrose-containing intravenous (IV) fluid. The additional needed energy is primarily drawn from the catabolism of endogenous protein, probably skeletal muscle, and from limited fat stores. Therefore, insufficient exogenous protein and calories may prove to be life-threatening to the sick, preterm infant. Nutrient intake during the immediate postnatal period has been shown to impact development at 18 months. Therefore, the nutrient support of the preterm and critically ill infant is extremely important, not only for immediate survival but also for a favorable long-term outcome.

This chapter addresses the nutrient needs of the sick and LBW infant, methods for provision of nutrients both parenterally and enterally, and methods for assessing nutritional status.

◆ FLUID

In the fetus at 24 weeks' gestation, the total body water (TBW) represents more than 90% of the total body weight, with approximately 65% in the extracellular compartment, 25% in the intracellular compartment, and 1% in fat stores. The TBW and extracellular fluid volume decrease as gestational age increases; by term, the infant's TBW represents 74% of total body weight with extracellular and intracellular compartments comprising 40% and 35%, respectively.

Compared with the full-term infant, the preterm infant is in a state of relative extracellular fluid volume expansion with an excess of TBW. The dilute urine and negative sodium balance observed during the first few days after birth in the preterm infant may constitute an appropriate adaptive response to extrauterine life. In this context, the initial diuresis should be regarded as physiologic, reflecting changes in interstitial fluid volume[17] and may not be included in the calculation of fluid needs. As a result, a gradual weight loss of 15% in a VLBW infant and 5% to 10% in a larger baby during the first week of life is expected without adversely affecting urine output, urine osmolality, or clinical status.[39, 73] Provision of large volumes of fluid (160 to 180 mL/kg/d) to prevent this weight loss appears to increase the risk of the development of patent ductus arteriosus,[20] cerebral intraventricular hemorrhage,[88] bronchopulmonary dysplasia (BPD),[112, 119] and necrotizing enterocolitis (NEC).[20, 21] Therefore, a careful approach to fluid management is currently advocated in that it appears that the preterm infant can adjust water excretion within a relatively broad range of fluid intake (65 to 70 mL/kg/d to 140 mL/kg/d) without disturbing renal concentrating abilities or electrolyte balance.

Estimation of daily fluid requirements includes insensible water losses (IWLs) from the respiratory tract and skin, gastrointestinal losses (emesis, ostomy output, diarrhea), urinary losses, and losses from drainage catheters (chest tubes). IWL is a passive process and is not regulated by the infant. However, the environmental conditions in which the infant is nursed should be controlled to minimize losses (Table 6–1). The transepithelial losses are dependent on gestational age, the thickness of the skin and stratum corneum, and blood flow to the skin; the preterm infant has a high body surface area to body weight ratio with thinner, more permeable skin that is highly vascularized. These factors increase heat and fluid losses. In addition, the use of open bed platforms with radiant warmers may increase the IWL by 50% to 150%; this excessive IWL may be reduced with the use of a plastic blanket to cover the infant.[18]

Table 6–1. Factors Affecting Insensible Water Loss in Preterm Neonates

Severe prematurity	Phototherapy
Open warmer bed	Hyperthermia
Forced convection	Tachypnea

Guidelines for fluid management of the newborn infant have been reviewed[39, 87] with slightly varied regimens. The LBW infant is usually started with 80 mL/kg/d of 10% dextrose solution on the first day of life, providing approximately 6 to 8 mg glucose/kg/min. If the infant is less than 1 kg and under a radiant warmer, the fluid is liberalized to 100 to 120 mL/kg/d. On the second day of life, after renal function has been established and diuresis has begun, the fluid is increased by 20 mL/kg/d to an intake of 100 mL/kg/d and 2 to 4 mEq sodium/kg/d and 2 mEq potassium/kg/d is added to the IV fluid. Calcium may also be added at this time to provided 1 to 2 mEq calcium/kg/d (200 to 400 mg calcium gluconate/kg/d). By the third day, the fluids are increased to maintain a urine output of 2 to 3 mL/kg/h, which corresponds to an intake of 110 to 140 mL/kg/d. At this point, infants often require phototherapy; therefore, the maintenance fluid intake is increased by 30% with urine output and serum electrolyte closely monitored. If it is apparent that the infant will be unable to be on enteral feedings, parenteral nutrition is started.

The measurement of urine specific gravity is commonly used to predict urine osmolality. Although this is a reliable means of predicting hyperosmolality (urine osmolality of greater than 290 mOsm/kg water with a urine specific gravity 1.012 or greater), its reliability in predicting hypoosmolality (urine osmolality of <270 mOsm/kg water with a urine specific gravity 1.008 or less) is variable, ranging from 71% to 95% accuracy, and in predicting iso-osmolality (urine osmolality of 270 to 290 mOsm/kg water with a urine specific gravity 1.008 to 1.012), the accuracy is even less. In addition, glucose and protein in the urine may increase the urine specific gravity, giving a falsely high estimate of urine osmolality. Therefore, urine specific gravity should be checked to rule out hyperosmolar urine; a test for sugars and proteins in the urine should be conducted at the same time. The maximal concentrating capabilities in the neonate are limited compared with those in adults; thus, an infant with a urine osmolality of approximately 700 mOsm/kg water (urine specific gravity of 1.019) may be dehydrated. One can estimate the urine osmolality by determining the potential renal solute load of the infant's feeding and the fluid intake (Box 6–1). Infants at risk for high

---

♦ **Box 6–1**

Renal Solute Load Calculation

Potential renal solute load (PRSL): 4 (g protein/L) + mEq sodium/L + mEq potassium/L + mEq chloride/L = PRSL (mOsm/L)*

Example:
    Preterm formula$_{24}$ (PT$_{24}$) contains:

$$
\begin{array}{llll}
22 \text{ g protein/L} \times 4 & = & 88 \\
15.2 \text{ mEq sodium/L} \times 1 & = & 15.2 \\
26.9 \text{ mEq potassium/L} \times 1 & = & 26.9 \\
\underline{18.6 \text{ mEq chloride/L} \times 1} & = & \underline{18.6} \\
\text{PRSL} & = & 148.7 \text{ mOsm/L}
\end{array}
$$

Baby A is a 2-week-old former 32-week AGA infant weighing 1400 g now receiving 150 mL/kg/d of PT$_{24}$.

Estimated fluid losses are:
$$
\begin{array}{ll}
\text{Stool} & 10 \text{ mL/kg/d} \\
\underline{\text{Insensible water loss}} & \underline{70 \text{ mL/kg/d}} \\
\text{Total water loss} & 80 \text{ mL/kg/d}
\end{array}
$$

150 mL/kg/d intake − 80 mL/kg/d output = 70 mL/kg/d available for urine output

The PRSL of PT$_{24}$ is 148.7 mOsm/L:

$$\frac{148.7 \text{ mOsm}}{1000 \text{ ml}} = \frac{X \text{ mOsm}}{150 \text{ ml}}$$

$$22.3 \text{ mOsm} = X$$

This infant has 70 mL/kg/d to excrete 22.3 mOsm of potential renal solute.

$$\frac{22.3 \text{ mOsm}}{70 \text{ ml}} \times 1000 = X \text{ mOsm/L}$$

$$318.6 \text{ mOsm} = X$$

Therefore, the estimated osmolality of the urine is 319 mOsm/L.

---

*References 166, 167.
AGA, appropriate for gestational age.

---

urine osmolality are those who are receiving a concentrated formula and those whose fluid intake is restricted.

Water balance may be maintained with careful attention to input and output. Weight measurements should be obtained daily or twice daily with notation of any apparatus attached to the infant at the time of weighing. Meticulous records of fluid intake (with the use of accurate infusion pumps and careful measurement of enteral feedings) and output (by weighing diapers and collecting urine, ostomy output, and drainage from any indwelling catheters) are necessary to compute fluid requirements.

Serum glucose, electrolytes, blood urea nitrogen (BUN), and creatinine are monitored three to four times per day during the first 2 days and then daily or as needed thereafter. Urine glucose is routinely tested and urine specific gravity is measured every 8 hours.

♦ **ELECTROLYTES**

Often the electrolyte management of the infant is difficult due to the various sources of electrolyte input. For example, in a 600-g infant, the isotonic saline solution infused to maintain the patency of the umbilical arterial catheter may result in administration of sodium and chloride in excess of estimated daily requirements. Although VLBW infants are capable of regulating sodium balance by altering renal sodium excretion, this may not be sufficient to prevent changes in serum sodium and serum chloride concentrations. Because administration of high amounts of sodium appear to increase the risk of hypernatremia in the VLBW infant,[105] careful calculation of total intake of sodium, potassium, chloride, glucose, and water from all sources (i.e., maintenance IV fluids, flushes, medications, and bolus injections) is necessary. As fluid requirements are adjusted, recalculation should be done frequently to ensure appropriate quantities of nutrients are given.

Catheter flushes (using isotonic saline solution) may contribute significant quantities of electrolytes, including chloride, to the infant's total intake. Hyperchloremic metabolic acidosis in LBW infants has been associated with chloride loads in excess of 6 mEq/kg/d.[59] The intake can easily be decreased by substituting acetate or phosphate for chloride in the IV solution.

Sodium is required in quantities sufficient to maintain normal extracellular fluid volume (ECFV) expansion which accompanies tissue growth. In animal studies, if insufficient amounts are provided, the ECFV expansion is suppressed and there are subsequent alterations in quantitative and qualitative somatic growth.[43]

Hypochloremia has also been associated with poor growth. Supplementation with chloride to normalize serum chloride concentrations in infants with bronchopulmonary dysplasia (BPD) resulted in improved growth. Hypochloremia has been noted in infants with BPD who did not survive; however, whether this is a predictor of poor outcome or a symptom of severe illness remains to be resolved.

Potassium chloride (2 mEq/kg/d) is added to the IV fluid on the second day of life once urinary output is established and hyperkalemia is not present. The potassium dose may be adjusted dependent on urine output and use of diuretics.[40] However, it is often difficult to obtain accurate determinations of serum potassium, especially when the blood samples are from heel-sticks, which may lead to excessive red blood cell hemolysis and spuriously high serum potassium levels. If an elevated potassium concentration

is obtained, a second blood sample from venepuncture should be obtained for confirmation of the level. If infused via a peripheral vein, concentrations of potassium chloride up to 40 mEq/L are usually tolerated and do not cause localized pain. However, if higher concentrations are needed because of fluid restriction, a central vein should be used.

◆ TOTAL PARENTERAL NUTRITION

The use of parenteral nutrition to support energy and nutrition requirements began in 1968 with a single case report demonstrating normal growth and development of an infant born with multiple small bowel atresias when nourished parenterally. Subsequently, numerous reports were published documenting the feasibility of supporting normal growth with this technique.[22, 42] However, this new technology was not without problems. Several nutrient deficiency syndromes were reported including essential fatty acid deficiency[29, 54] and trace mineral deficiencies including zinc,[13] copper,[66] selenium,[72] and molybdenum; even biotin deficiency, which is rarely seen in individuals consuming normal diets, was documented in an infant receiving inadequate amounts of biotin parenterally.[84]

The various metabolic problems that have occurred as a result of the use of total parenteral nutrition (TPN) in infants has led to research that has served to define the requirements for parenterally delivered nutrients and in the development of new products and new methods of delivery designed specifically for use in the neonate.[15, 56] However, there remains a lack of agreement on the nutrient requirements of the parenterally nourished neonate. Intravenous requirements cannot be derived from the recommended dietary allowances[85] because these reflect requirements for enterally administered nutrients to healthy full-term infants. Although guidelines for certain minerals and vitamins were published in 1988[56] (Tables 6–2 and 6–3), there are no standard, universally accepted recommendations available for intravenous nutrient delivery; this results in a great variation in practice between institutions.

Supporting an infant on TPN is not without risk. This method of nutrient delivery should not be undertaken without knowl-

Table 6–2. Suggested Intake of Parenteral Vitamins in Infants and Children

Vitamin	Term Infants and Children Dose per Day	Preterm Infant Dose/kg Body Wt (Maximum Not to Exceed Term Infant Dose)	
		Current Suggestions*	Best Estimate for New Formulation†
Lipid soluble			
A (μg)‡	700	280	500
E (mg)§	7	2.8	2.8
K (μg)	200	80	80
D (μg)¶	10	4	4
(IU)	400	160	160
Water soluble			
Ascorbic acid (mg)	80	32.0	25
Thiamin (mg)	1.2	0.48	0.35
Riboflavin (mg)	1.4	0.56	0.15
Pyridoxine (mg)	1.0	0.4	0.18
Niacin (mg)	17	6.8	6.8
Pantothenate (mg)	5	2.0	2.0
Biotin (μg)	20	8.0	6.0
Folate (μg)	140	56	56.0
Vitamin B_{12} (μg)	1.0	0.4	0.3

*These represent a practical guide (40% of the currently available single dose vial MVI-Pediatric (Armour) formulation per kg body weight) which provides adequate levels of vitamins E, D, and K but low levels of retinol and excess levels of most of the B vitamins. The maximum daily dose is one single dose vial for any infant.

†Because of elevated levels of the water-soluble vitamins, the current proposal is to reduce the intake of water-soluble vitamins and increase retinol as indicated by the authors.[56]

‡700 μg retinol = 2300 international units (IU).

§7 mg alpha-tocopherol = 7 IU.

¶10 μg vitamin D = 400 IU.

edge of the potential metabolic and mechanical (or catheter-related) complications. Most complications can be avoided with careful monitoring and prompt intervention. Complication rates are minimized when parenteral nutrition is administered with strict adherence to established protocols.

Energy

Reichman and colleagues[98] demonstrated that formula-fed preterm infants receiving 150 kcal/kg/d grew at expected intrauterine rates and retained similar amounts of nitrogen; however, they deposited 2.5 times the

Table 6–3. Recommended Intravenous Intake of Trace Elements*

Element	Infant (μg/kg/d)		Children (μg/kg/d) (Maximum μg/d)	
	Preterm	Term		
Zinc	400	250 < 3 mo	50	(5000)
		100 >3 mo		
Copper†	20	20	20	(300)
Selenium‡	2.0	2.0	2.0	(30)
Chromium‡	0.20	0.20	0.20	(5.0)
Manganese†	1.0	1.0	1.0	(50)
Molybdenum‡	0.25	0.25	0.25	(5.0)
Iodide	1.0	1.0	1.0	(1.0)

*When total parenteral nutrition is only supplemental or limited to <4 wk, only Zn need be added. Thereafter, addition of the remaining elements is advisable.[56]

†Omit in patients with obstructive jaundice.

‡Omit in patients with renal dysfunction.

Available concentration of Mo and Mn are such that dilution of the manufacturer's product may be necessary. Neotrace (Lypomed Co., Rosemont, IL) contains a higher ratio of Mn to Zn than suggested in this table (i.e., Zn = 1.5 mg and Mn = 25 μg in each milliliter).

amount of fat compared to that in utero. Schulze et al[104] showed that the composition of weight gain is related to both the absolute amount and the proportion of dietary protein and energy.

Energy needs are dependent on age, weight, rate of growth, thermal environment, activity, hormonal activity, nature of feedings, and organ size and maturation[34] (Table 6–4). Measurement of a true basal metabolic rate requires a prolonged fast and cannot ethically be determined in VLBW infants; therefore, resting metabolic rate (RMR) is used to estimate energy needs, dietary-induced thermogenesis, minimum energy expended in activity, and the metabolic cost of growth.[61, 98, 121] The metabolic rate increases during the first weeks of life from an RMR of 40 to 41 kcal/kg/d during the first week to 62 to 64 kcal/kg/d by the third week of life.[61, 99, 121] The extra energy expenditure is primarily due to the energy cost of growth related to various synthetic processes.[61] The metabolic rate of the nongrowing infant is approximately 51 kcal/kg/d, which includes 47 kcal/kg/d for basal metabolism and 4 kcal/kg/d for activity.

The contribution of activity to overall energy expenditure is speculative but seems to be small, between 3 and 5 kcal/kg/d to the total energy expenditure.[99] Energy expenditure in muscular activity in immature infants is relatively small in comparison to their resting metabolism due to the large amount of time spent in the sleep state. As infants mature, they become more active; therefore, energy expenditure from activity increases.[27]

The exposure of infants to a cold environ-

ment impacts on energy expenditure with small alterations in the thermal environment making a significant contribution to energy expenditure.[28] Infants nursed in an environment just below thermal-neutrality increase energy expenditure by 7 to 8 kcal/kg/d; any handling adds to this energy loss.[53] A daily increase of 10 kcal/kg/d should be allowed to cover incidental cold stress in the preterm infant.[28] Infants who are intrauterine growth restricted, particularly the asymmetrical type, have a high RMR on a per kilogram body weight basis because of their relatively high proportion of metabolically active mass.[28] Other factors that may increase metabolic rate are speculative; the effects of fever, sepsis, and surgery on the infant's energy requirements are uncertain.

Calorie intake above maintenance is used for growth. On an average, for each 1-g increment in weight, approximately 4.5 kcal above maintenance energy need is required.[101] Therefore, to attain the equivalent of the third trimester intrauterine weight gain (10 to 15 g/kg/d), a metabolizable energy intake of approximately 45 to 70 kcal/kg/d above the 51 kcal/kg/d required for maintenance must be provided, or approximately 100 to 120 kcal/kg/d. Increasing metabolizable energy intakes beyond 120 kcal/kg/d with energy supplementation alone does not result in proportionate increases in weight gain. However, when energy, protein, vitamins, and minerals are all increased, weight gain with increases in rates of protein and fat accretion can be realized.[121] The higher the caloric intake, the greater amount of energy is expended through excretion, dietary-induced thermogenesis, and tissue synthesis. The energy cost of weight gain at 130 kcal/kg/d was reported to be 3.0 kcal/g of weight gain[61]; however, at an intake of 149 kcal/kg/d and 181 kcal/kg/d, the energy cost of weight gain was estimated to be 4.9 and 5.7 kcal/g of weight gain, respectively.[27, 28, 99]

The energy needs of the parenterally nourished infant differ from the enterally fed infant in that there is no fecal loss of nutrients. Preterm infants, who are appropriately grown for age, are able to maintain positive nitrogen balance when receiving 50 nonprotein calories (NPCs)/kg/d and 2.5 g protein/kg/d. At an NPC intake of greater than 70 NPC/kg/d and a protein intake of 2.7 to 3.5 g/kg/d, preterm infants exhibit

Table 6–4. Estimated Energy Expenditure in a Growing Preterm Infant

	kcal/kg/d
Resting energy expenditure	47
Minimal activity*	4
Occasional cold stress*	10
Fecal loss of energy (10% to 16% of total intake)	15
Growth† (includes dietary-induced thermogenesis)	45
TOTAL	121

*As an infant matures, energy expended in activities, such as crying and nursing, increases; at the same time, energy expended as a result of cold stress decreases.

†Calculated assuming 3.0 to 4.5 kcal/g weight gain at rate of gain of 10 to 15 g/kg/d.

nitrogen accretion and growth rates similar to in utero levels.[124] In LBW infants (750 to 1750 g), intrauterine weight gain (17.2 ± 5.1 g/kg/d) was achieved with 96 kcal and 2.4 g protein/kg/d, using a pediatric amino acid solution.[64]

The sources of energy for parenteral nutrition in infants is either as glucose or lipid, or a combination of the two. Although both glucose and fat provide equivalent nitrogen-sparing effects in the neonate,[92] studies have demonstrated that a nutrient mixture using intravenous glucose and lipid as the nonprotein energy source is more physiologic than supplying glucose as the only nonprotein energy source.[86] The amount of glucose required to meet the total energy needs approximates 7 mg/kg/min (10 g/kg/d). The excess glucose administered is converted to fat or triglycerides. Thus a nutrient mixture with both glucose and lipid providing NPCs as well as essential fatty acids is suggested.

Although the ideal ratio of carbohydrate to lipid is not yet known, when 60% to 63% of the NPCs given to LBW infants were derived from lipid, nitrogen retention was decreased and temperature control was adversely effected.[32] A moderate intravenous fat intake comprising approximately 35% of the NPCs is preferred.

Carbohydrate

For parenteral use, dextrose (D-glucose) is the carbohydrate of choice. It provides 3.4 kcal/g on complete oxidation. Tolerance to glucose infusions varies, especially in the VLBW infant. Infants with birth weights less than 1.0 kg should be started with glucose at 6 mg/kg/min, and infants weighing 1.0 to 1.5 kg may initially receive glucose 8 mg/kg/min. Frequent monitoring of the plasma and urine glucose levels is necessary. When plasma glucose levels exceed 150 mg/dL, glucosuria may occur, resulting in osmotic diuresis and leading to dehydration and increase in serum osmolality. Once initial glucose infusions are tolerated, stepwise increases in glucose intake of approximately 10 to 20 kcal/kg/d or 3 to 6 g dextrose/kg/d can be made. The maximum concentration of dextrose solution for parenteral nutrition should not exceed 12.5% in a peripheral vein because of high osmolality (Table 6–5). It is the rate of infusion of glucose and not the dextrose concentration in the solution

that determines the amount of dextrose provided to the infant.

Glucose intolerance, either hyperglycemia or hypoglycemia, in an infant whose rate of glucose infusion has not been recently changed and who was previously glucose tolerant may be an early sign of sepsis.

Insulin may be used to control hyperglycemia. However, plasma glucose should be monitored frequently in order to avoid serious hypoglycemia and should be started at a rate of 0.1 U/kg/h in isotonic solution.

Protein

Protein requirements of the preterm infant have been of considerable interest for many years; although better understood than many nutrients, protein needs vary depending on gestational age, disease state, and method of nutrient delivery. Excessive protein intake is poorly tolerated by the premature infant and may have adverse consequences.[55] It has been suggested that protein, rather than energy, is the most limiting nutrient for the growing infant.[124]

Protein quality, or amino acid composition, in parenteral nutrition can influence nitrogen utilization as well as the metabolic responses. Histidine is known to be necessary for protein synthesis and growth in the neonate but exact requirements are not known. Certain other amino acids are considered semiessential or conditionally essential in that the capacity to synthesize them is limited in the preterm infant. Therefore, if these conditionally essential amino acids are not exogenously available or available only in limited amounts, the infant's requirements may not be met. Three of these semiessential amino acids are cysteine, tyrosine, and taurine.

Cysteine is synthesized in vivo from methionine by the enzyme cystathionase. Because the hepatic activity of cystathionase has been found to be low or absent during fetal development and in the preterm and term neonate,[51, 63] it has been considered an essential amino acid for the infant. Zlotkin and Anderson[123] observed reduced hepatic cystathionase activity in preterm infants compared with full-term infants at the time of birth with the activity increasing in the preterm infant over the first month of life; however, mature levels were not attained until approximately 8 months. When total

Table 6–5. Characteristics of Intravenous Fluids

Type of Fluid	Cations			Anions		
	Na (mEq/L)	K (mEq/L)	Ca (mEq/L)	Cl (mEq/L)	HCO₃* (mEq/L)	Osmolarity (mOsm/L)†
Dextrose in Water Solutions						
D_5W						252
$D_{10}W$						505
$D_{20}W$						1010
$D_{50}W$						2525
Dextrose in Saline Solutions						
D_5W and 0.2% NaCl	34			34		320
D_5W and 0.45% NaCl	77			77		406
D_5W and 0.9% NaCl	154			154		559
D_5W and 0.9% NaCl	154			154		812
Saline Solutions						
1/2 NS (0.45% NaCl)	77			77		154
NS (0.9% NaCl)	154			154		308
3% (NaCl	513			513		1026
Multiple Electrolyte Solutions						
Ringer's solution	147	4	5	155		309
Lactated Ringer's	130	4	3	109	28	273
D_5W in lactated Ringer's	130	4	3	109	28	524
Lipid Emulsions						
Lipid emulsions (20%)						258–315

An easy way to *approximate* the osmolarity of an IV fluid is to consider that for each 1% dextrose there are 55 mOsm/L, for each 1% amino acids there are 100 mOsm/L, and for each 1% NaCl there are 340 mOsm/L. Therefore:

$D_{10}W$ and 0.45% NaCl (1/2 NS):

$$D_{10}W = (10 \times 55) = \qquad 550 \text{ mOsmL}$$
$$0.45\% \text{ NaCl} = (0.45 \times 340) = 153 \text{ mOsmL}$$
$$\overline{\text{Total} \qquad\qquad\qquad\quad 703 \text{ mOsm/L}}$$

12.5% dextrose and 17 g amino acids/L (or 1.7% amino acids):

$$D_{12.5}W = 12.5 \times 55 \quad = 687 \text{ mOsm/L}$$
$$1.7\% \text{ AA} = 1.7 \times 100 = 170 \text{ mOsm/L}$$
$$\overline{\text{Total} \qquad\qquad\qquad 857 \text{ mOsm/L}}$$

Parenteral nutrition solutions with an osmolarity over 900 mOsm/L should be infused through a center line.

*Or its equivalent in lactate, acetate, or citrate.
†Osmolarity of the blood is 285–295 mOsm/L.
Adapted from Wolf BM, Yamahata WI: In Zeman FJ (ed): Clinical Nutrition and Dietetics. Lexington, Massachusetts, DC Heath and Co, 1983.

cystathionase activity was estimated, which included the enzyme activity in the liver, kidneys, pancreas, and adrenal glands, he concluded that even the preterm infant has the capacity to endogenously produce adequate cysteine if adequate methionine is provided. In fact, increased parenteral methionine has been shown to increase urinary cysteine excretion. Supplementation of parenteral amino acid solutions with cysteine hydrochloride has not been shown to affect either nitrogen balance or growth in LBW infants.[64] Plasma cysteine levels were observed to be similar in infants receiving crystalline amino acid (CAA) solutions with or without cysteine.[19] Two pediatric amino acid solutions, Trophamine (McGaw, Inc., Irvine, CA) and Aminosyn-PF (Abbott Laboratories, Abbott Park, IL), are low in methionine content, 81 and 45 mg/2.5 g of amino acids, respectively, and do not contain cysteine. Therefore, supplementation with cysteine hydrochloride is recommended.

Tyrosine, which is endogenously synthesized from phenylalanine through the activity of phenylalanine hydroxylase, has also been considered an essential amino acid; however, the enzyme activity is not low during development. The low plasma tyrosine concentrations seen in infants on tyrosine-free parenteral nutrition infusates appear to be independent of the plasma phenylalanine levels and not all infants on tyrosine-free parenteral nutrition solutions have low plasma tyrosine levels.[19, 64] In addition, extremely preterm infants have been shown to convert substantial quantities of phenylalanine to tyrosine.[37] Therefore, the requirement for an exogenous source of this amino acid remains uncertain.

Taurine, which is synthesized endogenously from cysteine, is a sulfur amino acid, which is not part of structural proteins but is present in most tissues of the body; it is particularly high in the retina, brain, heart, and muscle. The biologic function of taurine in mammals includes neuromodulation, cell membrane stabilization, antioxidation, detoxification, osmoregulation, and bile acid conjugation[31]; however, its conjugation with bile acids is the only adequately documented metabolic reaction in humans. Depletion of taurine during long-term parenteral nutrition has resulted in abnormal electroretinograms in children[51] and auditory brain stem–evoked responses in preterm infants.[115] Taurine supplementation of preterm infant formula has been shown to improve fat absorption, especially saturated fats, in LBW infants.[50] Human milk is rich in taurine; infants fed human milk have higher plasma and urine concentrations of taurine than infants fed unsupplemented infant formula. Infant formulas and pediatric parenteral amino acid solutions are supplemented with taurine.

Currently, there are two kinds of CAA solutions available for use in the neonate; the standard solutions originally designed for adults are often used for infants but are not ideal. The adult products contain little or no tyrosine, cysteine, or taurine, and contain relatively high concentrations of glycine, methionine, and phenylalanine. Because the plasma amino acid patterns reflect the amino acid composition of the amino acid solution infused, the resulting abnormal plasma amino acid levels could be potentially harmful. Hyperglycinemia, for example, may have adverse effects on the central nervous system because glycine is a potent neurotransmitter inhibitor. The pediatric amino acid solutions have a greater

distribution of nonessential amino acids (particularly less glycine), greater amounts of branched-chain amino acids, less methionine and phenylalanine, and more tyrosine, cysteine, and taurine.

Studies of these products have demonstrated improved nitrogen retention and plasma aminograms resembling those of full-term breast-fed infants at 30 days of life.[63, 64] However, studies of protein turnover and urea production (protein oxidation) have not shown any difference between Trophamine and other amino acid mixtures.[16] Because of the lower pH of the pediatric CAA solutions, greater concentrations of calcium and phosphorous may be added without precipitation, which is an advantage particularly for the preterm neonate because the requirements for both minerals are quite high.[56]

Early (day 1) introduction of amino acids results in positive nitrogen balance and greater nitrogen retention. The administration of NPCs 50 kg/d and amino acids 2.5 g/kg/d results in positive nitrogen balance but no weight gain. Therefore to attain nitrogen retention similar to intrauterine rates, protein 2.7 to 3.5 g/kg/d and NPCs at least 70 kg/d should be provided.[124] However, parenteral protein intake greater than 3.0 g/kg/d may result in earlier onset and increased magnitude of cholestasis; therefore, we do not provide protein greater than 3.0 g/kg/d parenterally. The protein requirement of the sick, nongrowing VLBW infant has not been determined. The severely stressed infant may be in nitrogen equilibrium but not grow even when all nutrients are provided. In these infants, a high amino acid intake may result in a large acid load, subsequent metabolic acidosis, and elevation of plasma amino acids to potentially toxic levels. Although this is only speculative, a prudent approach to the nutritional support of such infants is to maintain the protein intake at 1.5 g/kg/d with adequate calories to maintain weight (approximately 50 NPC/kg/d) during the first few days after birth[100]; this has been shown to be well tolerated by sick preterm infants. Protein and energy intake should then be increased to 2.7 to 3.0 g protein/kg/d with 70 to 90 NPC/kg/d. Providing protein in excess of the need may result in hyperammonemia, metabolic acidosis, and elevated BUN concentrations, and may increase the risk of cholestasis.

Lipids

Although the use of intravenous lipid emulsions is currently accepted as an important component of TPN for the LBW infant, controversy related to dosage, timing of first use, and effect on lung function still exists.

Intravenous lipid emulsions are advantageous because of their high caloric density and low osmolality (Table 6–6); additionally, they reduce the need for high glucose intake and prevent essential fatty acid deficiency.

Essential fatty acid deficiency is a known complication in infants on fat-free TPN.[89] Biochemical signs of essential fatty acid deficiency become evident within 1 week of administration of fat-free TPN,[47] with the smallest infants manifesting these biochemical changes as early as the second or third day. The biochemical changes of omega-6 essential fatty acid deficiency resulting from inadequate amounts of linoleic acid are demonstrated most rapidly after CAAs are begun, perhaps because of the transition from a catabolic to a more anabolic state, requiring greater amounts of linoleic acid for tissue synthesis. This can be rapidly corrected and prevented with the use of IV lipid emulsions.

It is uncertain whether α-linolenic acid, an omega-3 fatty acid, is an essential fatty acid for infants. Omega-3 fatty acids in mammals are primarily in the form of docosahexaenoic acid, 22:6 omega-3, which is an important component of brain and retinal phospholipids, and may be essential to the developing eye and brain of the human neonate.[65, 117] Administration of low linolenic and high linoleic acid lipid emulsions with a safflower oil base has been associated with biochemical and clinical signs of omega-3 fatty acid deficiency in humans, including signs of neurologic impairment. Therefore, selecting a lipid emulsion that contains both fatty acids is optimal for the prevention of essential fatty acid deficiency (see Table 6–6); 2% to 5% of the NPCs should be provided as linoleic acid[5] and linolenic acid should be provided at 0.1 to 0.15 g/kg/d or approximately 0.54% of the calories.

Clearance of lipid emulsions depends on the hydrolysis of the cylomicron-like particles by lipoprotein lipase at the endothelial surface of the capillary walls of muscle and adipose tissue. Free fatty acids (FFAs) are used as fuel in the liver, heart, and skeletal muscle or are converted in the liver to very low-density lipoproteins. A decreased tolerance to intravenous lipid emulsions has been reported in small for gestational age infants and infants younger than 32 weeks' gestation.[11] Brans and colleagues[26] reported that lipid tolerance of the VLBW infant is improved if the lipid dose is increased slowly over several days with an hourly infusion rate of less than 0.12 g lipid/kg/h. This may be achieved by infusing lipids over a 24-hour period. A lipid-free "window," during which time no lipids are infused, is not necessary to clear lipids from the blood. A continuous 24-hour lipid infusion may be difficult to achieve if intravenous medications that are not compatible with lipids (e.g., phenytoin) also need to be administered.

Lipid emulsions are supplied as either 10% or 20% solutions providing 10 or 20 g of triglyceride/dL respectively. Both contain the same amount of egg yolk phospholipid

Table 6–6. Composition of Intravenous Lipid Emulsions

Product	Oil Base	Linoleic Acid (%)	Linolenic Acid (%)	Glycerin (%)	Osmolarity (mOsm/L)
Intralipid*	100% Soybean	50	9	2.25	260
Nutralipid†	100% Soybean	49–60	6–9	2.21	315
Soyacal‡	100% Soybean	49–60	6–9	2.21	315
Liposyn II§	50% Soybean 50% Safflower	65.8	4.2	2.5	258
Liposyn III§	100% Soybean	54.5	8.3	2.5	292

*KabiVitrum, Alameda, CA.
†McGaw, Inc., Irvine, CA.
‡Alpha Therapeutic, Los Angeles, CA.
§Abbott Laboratories, Abbott Park, IL.
Sources: *Drug Facts and Comparisons.* St. Louis: JB Lippincott, 1990.
Physicians Desk Reference. 44th ed. Oradell, NJ: Medical Economics, 1990.

emulsifier (approximately 1.2 g/dL) and glycerol (approximately 2.25 g/dL). However, each contains more phospholipid than is required to emulsify the triglyceride; the excess is formed into triglyceride-poor particles with phospholipid bilayers and is called liposomes. For any given dose of triglyceride, twice the volume of 10% emulsion must be infused compared with the 20% emulsion; therefore, for a fixed amount of triglyceride, the 10% emulsion provides at least twice and perhaps up to four times the amount of liposomes as the 20% emulsion. The 10% emulsion has been shown to be associated with higher plasma triglyceride concentrations and an accumulation of cholesterol and phospholipid in the blood of the preterm infant, probably as a result of the higher phospholipid content. LBW infants infused with lipid 2 g/kg/d of 10% emulsion had significantly higher plasma triglyceride, cholesterol, and phospholipid than infants infused with 4 g lipid/kg/d as 20% emulsion. It is speculated that the excessive phospholipid liposomes in the 10% emulsion compete with the triglyceride-rich particles for binding to lipase sites, resulting in slow triglyceride hydrolysis. It is, therefore, recommended that 20% lipid emulsions be used for the LBW and VLBW infants. More recently, 10% lipid emulsions with half the formerly used phospholipid emulsifier have become available. In a study of preterm infants, these were well tolerated without pathologic increase in triglyceride or serum cholesterol concentration.[54]

Adverse side effects of intravenous lipid emulsions have been reported including displacement of indirect bilirubin from albumin-binding sites, increasing the risk of kernicterus, suppression of the immune system, coagulase-negative staphylococcal and fungal infection,[46, 95] thrombocytopenia, and accumulation of lipid in the alveolar macrophages and capillaries, subsequently altering pulmonary gas exchange.[48, 96]

Because FFAs compete with bilirubin for binding to albumin, the use of IV lipid emulsions in jaundiced newborns has been questioned. However, it is more a theoretic concern, in that FFA concentrations do not reach high enough levels to cause displacement of bilirubin and increase free bilirubin to a very high range. Careful monitoring of plasma triglycerides has been suggested when lipids are administered to babies with hyperbilirubinemia

There may be a beneficial effect of infusing lipids. Coinfusion of lipid emulsion exerts a beneficial effect on the vascular endothelium of peripheral veins leading to longer venous patency time. Malhotra and coworkers[80] noted that hyperbilirubinemic infants given a lipid infusion of 1 to 2 g/kg/d had a significant increase in lumirubin, a water-soluble structural isomer of bilirubin that can be excreted in the bile without hepatic conjugation. Therefore, IV lipid infusions may enhance the effect of and may be a useful adjunct to phototherapy.

Suppression of immune function and increased risk of sepsis have been associated to the use of IV lipid emulsions. Diminished motility and metabolic activity of polymorphonuclear leukocytes (PMN) exposed to fat emulsion in vitro have been reported.[35] However, this could not be demonstrated in vivo in both full-term and preterm infants given lipid 0.5 to 3.0 g/kg/d over 16 hours; on the contrary, some aspects of PMN migratory properties and their oxidative metabolism improved during the study period, most likely the result of chronologic and functional maturity.[118] There have been reports of both fungal infections with *Malassezia furfur*[95] and coagulase-negative staphylococci[46] associated with lipid administration. Freeman and colleagues[46] have reported that 56.6% of all cases of nosocomial bacteremia in two neonatal intensive care units in Boston were highly correlated with lipid administration. However, they stress that the benefits derived from the lipids outweigh the apparent risk of infection.

One potential hazard of hyperlipidemia is an adverse effect on pulmonary artery pressure and the pulmonary diffusion capacity. Adult men demonstrated a transient decrease in pulmonary diffusion capacity after rapid infusion of a large dose of soybean oil emulsion. Fat droplets have been seen via electron microscopy in the pulmonary capillaries and other capillary beds of animals receiving large doses of fat emulsion. Lipid deposits have been identified at autopsy in alveolar macrophages and capillaries of LBW infants who were on intravenous lipids for 9 to 12 weeks; the effect on gaseous exchange was not established.[49] Although concerning, similar findings have been seen in infants who never received IV lipids.[111] However, no detrimental effects of lipid infusion on oxygenation in preterm infants with respiratory distress syndrome requiring ventilatory support have been reported.

Lipid emulsions should be administered to infants so that normal lipid levels are maintained. Serum triglyceride levels should be obtained during the advancement of lipid emulsion then weekly thereafter. Triglyceride levels of 150 mg/dL or lower should be maintained while bilirubin levels are elevated; otherwise, concentrations less than 200 mg/dL are acceptable. At plasma triglyceride levels of 200 to 300 mg/dL, the lipid dose should be decreased until acceptable levels are achieved.

Carnitine

Carnitine is an essential cofactor required for the transport of long-chain fatty acids (LCFAs) across the mitochondrial membrane for β-oxidation. Because the preterm infant is born with limited carnitine reserves and low plasma carnitine levels develop when parenteral nutrition is not supplemented with carnitine, several investigators have suggested adding carnitine to parenteral nutrition with lipids for preterm infants.[25, 103, 110] Addition of supplemental carnitine does increase oxidation of fat and circulating ketone body levels and results in increased tolerance to intravenous lipids. However, data on increase in weight gain and nitrogen retention are not as convincing.[109] Therefore, carnitine is recommended only for LBW infants who require prolonged (over 2 to 3 weeks) parenteral nutrition. IV carnitine has been used in doses of 50 mg/kg/day for prolonged periods[113] and in higher doses for shorter periods[67] without any observable side effects.

Parenteral Vitamins

The parenteral multivitamin guidelines proposed by the American Medical Association have been accepted for the pediatric formulation. A special committee of the American Society for Clinical Nutrition made recommendations for a new multivitamin preparation specifically for the preterm infant.[56] Although no preparation meets these guidelines, the committee recommends that MVI-Pediatric (Armour Pharmaceutical, Kankakee, IL) should be used for preterm infants

at 40% of a vial (or 2 mL) per kilogram body weight per day not to exceed a total daily dose of one vial (5 mL); infants and children should receive one vial (5 mL) daily (see Table 6–2).[56]

IV vitamins, especially vitamin A, riboflavin, ascorbic acid, and pyridoxine, may be lost through adherence to the plastic tubing or through photodegradation caused by light exposure. There is often high light intensity in a special care nursery and the TPN fluid in the tubing moves slowly; therefore, it is exposed to light for prolonged periods of time. For these reasons, vitamins are added to the TPN shortly before infusing and some nurseries have the TPN bags and infusion tubings covered with foil or opaque material to minimize light exposure.

Trace Minerals

Because the infant has minimal endogenous stores, trace minerals are added to the TPN solution (see Table 6–3). If TPN is only supplemental to enteral feeding or is limited to 1 or 2 weeks, the only trace mineral that needs to be added is zinc. If the TPN is continued beyond that period, chromium, iodine, and molybdenum should be added, and, in the absence of cholestasis, copper and manganese should be added as well. If TPN is continued for more than 4 weeks, the addition of selenium is advised. The need for iron supplementation should be evaluated. IV iron should be used with caution because excess iron can easily be given and may result in iron overload, increased risk of gram-negative septicemia, and possible increase in the requirement for antioxidants, especially vitamin E.[56]

Calcium, Phosphorus, Magnesium, and Vitamin D

Preterm infants require increased intakes of calcium and phosphorus for optimal bone mineralization. The intrauterine accretion rates for calcium in the last trimester range from 104 to 125 mg/kg/d at 26 weeks' gestation to 119 to 151 mg/kg/d at 36 weeks' gestation; phosphorus accretion rate is 63 to 86 mg/kg/d. These levels of calcium and phosphorus intake cannot be attained with conventional TPN solutions because they would be insoluble. The pediatric CAA solutions, however, have a lower pH, especially when cysteine hydrochloride is added; therefore, greater concentrations of calcium and phosphorus can remain in solution.

The sick, poorly growing VLBW infant should receive 30 mg calcium/kg/d and 40 mg phosphorus/kg/d. Otherwise the recommendation is 50 to 60 mg calcium, 40 to 45 mg phosphorus, 6 to 7 mg magnesium, and 25 IU vitamin D for each 100 mL of TPN solution, assuming a fluid intake of 120 to 150 mL/kg/d.[56] A 1.3:1 calcium-to-phosphorus ratio is suggested, although others have noted improved mineral retention with a 1.7:1 ratio. These high calcium and phosphorus infusions should be given through a central venous line and not through a peripheral line.

Practical Hints

1. During the first few days of life, provide sufficient fluid to result in urine output of 1 to 3 mL/kg/h, a urine specific gravity of 1.008 to 1.012, checking urine for sugar and protein at the same time, and a weight loss of approximately 5% or less in full-term and approximately 15% or less in VLBW infants.

2. Weigh infants twice a day the first 2 days of life then daily thereafter in order to accurately monitor input and output.

3. Use birth weight to calculate intake until birth weight is regained.

4. Keep accurate records of fluid intake, output, and weights.

5. Start TPN on the second or third day of life with 1.0 g protein/kg/d; increase dextrose and protein as tolerated. We start with a neonatal parenteral nutrition solution with 10% dextrose and 1.0 g amino acids/L (NPN I—Table 6–7). Goal for the end of the first week should be 50 NPC/kg/d and 2.5 g protein/kg/d.

6. By the third or fourth day of life, start a 20% lipid emulsion (e.g., Intralipid [KabiVitrum, Alameda, CA]) at 0.5 g lipid/kg/d at a rate not exceeding 0.12 g/kg/h. Avoid using 10% lipid emulsions because of poor tolerance.

7. If the infant is hyperbilirubinemic, provide lipid 0.5 to 1.0 g/kg/d, maintaining a serum triglyceride no greater than 150 mg/dL. Serum triglyceride should be checked before the start of the first lipid

Table 6–7. Composition of Standard Neonatal Parenteral Nutrition Solutions at Rainbow Babies' and Children's Hospital

	NPN I	NPN II*	NPN III†
Dextrose (%)	10	12.5	20
Nitrogen (g/L)	1.6	3.2	4.0
Protein (g/L)	10	20	25
Total calories (kcal/L)	380	505	780
Sodium (mEq/L)	40	40	40
Potassium (mEq/L)	25	25	25
Chloride (mEq/L)	40	40	40
Magnesium (mEq/L)	5	5	5
Calcium (mEq/L)	20	20	20
Phosphorus (mM/L)	10	10	10
Acetate (mEq/L)		Balanced by pharmacy	
Heparin (units/L)	1000	1000	1000
Trace minerals‡	+	+	+
Multivitamins§	+	+	+

*Must be infused with at least 1 g lipid/kg/d.
†Used for central venous infusion only.
‡Includes zinc, chromium, copper, manganese, and iodide.
§MVI-Pediatric Multivitamins are dosed per bag with infants weighing less than 1 kg receiving 3 mL MVI-Pediatric Multivitamins per bag, infants 1 to 3 kg receiving 5 mL MVI-Pediatric Multivitamins per bag, and infants weighing more than 3 kg receiving 5 mL MVI-Pediatric Multivitamins per bag with the size of the bag dependent on volume needed.
NPN, neonatal parenteral nutrition solution.

infusion, as lipids are being advanced, and weekly thereafter.

8. Once hyperbilirubinemia is resolved, increase lipids at a rate of 0.5 g lipid/kg/d not to exceed 3.0 g lipid/kg/d. Infuse over a 24-hour period or a rate of 0.12 g/kg/h.

9. Aim for a parenteral nutrition goal of 90 to 100 kcal/kg/d and 2.7 to 3.0 g protein/kg/d with an NPC-to-nitrogen ratio (NPC:N) of 150 to 250. NPC:N ratio can be calculated as follows:

$$\frac{\text{lipid calories} + \text{dextrose calories}}{(\text{grams of protein})(0.16)} = \frac{\text{NPC}}{1 \text{ g N}}$$

◆ ENTERAL NUTRITION

When parenteral nutrition is used exclusively for the provision of nutrients, morphologic and functional changes occur in the gut with a significant decrease in intestinal mass, a decrease in mucosal enzyme activity, and an increase in gut permeability. The changes are due primarily to the lack of luminal nutrients rather than the TPN per se.

Concerns over risks associated with feedings (e.g., aspiration pneumonia, NEC) had resulted in a more cautious approach of delaying feedings for several days to weeks. However, this practice has not resulted in a uniformly lower incidence of NEC. Early feedings, even the provision of very small enteral feedings, may impart certain benefits as a result of providing luminal nutrients to the enterocytes and by stimulating the release of enteric hormones, which exert a trophic effect on the proliferative cells of the gut.

Studies of early hypocaloric enteral feedings in sick VLBW infants have suggested that infants who are provided 12 to 24 mL of formula/kg/d (4 to 20 kcal/kg/d) starting during the first 1 to 8 days of age have better weight gain, a greater decline in serum bilirubin levels with less time spent under phototherapy, less cholestasis, lower serum concentrations of alkaline phosphatase, more rapid functional maturation of the intestine, increased serum gastrin, increased subsequent feeding tolerance, and faster attainment of full enteral feedings than infants who remain fasted during the same period of time.[38, 83]

A meta-analysis of published data on minimal enteral nutrition in parenterally fed neonates by Tyson and Kennedy concluded that the benefits from minimal enteral nutrition are not convincing because of inherent difficulty in assessing enteral feeding in high-risk infants, heterogeneity of the population, small sample size in each study, and the potential for bias in unblinded studies. Recently, Schanler et al, in a large randomized study, have shown that early gastrointestinal priming with human milk followed by bolus tube feeding, in contrast to continuous feeding, may provide the best advantage for the premature infant.[102, 114]

It is generally agreed that enteral feedings should be initiated slowly and advanced over several days; however, feeding schedules vary as to rate of advancement and type of formula used. Increases in formula intake of approximately 10 to 20 mL/kg/d are considered safe with greater volume increments associated with an increased incidence of NEC. Early introduction of 24-calorie/oz, iso-osmolar premature infant formula has been shown to be well tolerated by preterm infants. The use of dilute versus full-strength formula is an issue of debate. To date, there are no well-controlled studies that have demonstrated an advantage to the use of dilute formulas.

Carbohydrate

Carbohydrate provides 41% to 44% of the calories in human milk and most infant formulas. In human milk and standard infant formulas, it is present as lactose, which has been shown to enhance calcium absorption. In soy and other lactose-free formulas, the carbohydrate is in the form of sucrose, maltodextrins, and glucose polymers (corn syrup solids or modified starches). The three major disaccharidases responsible for the digestion of disaccharides are lactase, maltase, and sucrase-isomaltase. Maltase and sucrase-isomaltase first appear at 10 weeks' gestation, reaching approximately 70% of newborn levels at 28 weeks' gestation. However, by 28 to 34 weeks' gestation, lactase has only 30% of the activity found in the term infant; babies born before this time may have relative lactase deficiency, resulting in lactose intolerance.

When lactose is not hydrolyzed in the small intestine, bacterial fermentation of the undigested portion occurs in the colon, producing short-chain fatty acids, which enhance mineral and water absorption and may stimulate growth and cell replication in the gut lumen. Thus, colonic salvage is apparently important in disposal of unabsorbed lactose; however, its exact quantitative contribution remains unknown. Colonic bacterial fermentation of unabsorbed lactose to absorbable organic acids enables the infant to reclaim this carbohydrate energy and appears to prevent clinical symptoms of diarrhea.

Although pancreatic α-amylase, the major enzyme in starch hydrolysis, is either absent or in very low concentrations in the first 6 months of life, newborns are capable of tolerating small amounts of starch without side effects and preterm infants are able to hydrolyze glucose polymers. Several enzymes may compensate for the physiologic pancreatic amylase deficiency in infancy. Glucoamylase, an enzyme found in the brush border of the small intestine, is present in the neonate in concentrations similar to those in adults. Also, salivary and human milk amylases may provide additional pathways for glucose polymer digestion in infancy.

Because lactase is found only at the tip of the villus, it is very sensitive to mucosal injury; therefore, lactose intolerance may develop in infants with diarrhea, those suffering from undernutrition, or those recovering from NEC, necessitating temporary use of a lactose-free formula. In contrast, glucoamylase is able to survive partial intestinal atrophy because it is located at the base of the villi, thus enabling glucose polymers to be an alternative carbohydrate source when enteritis is present and lactase may be found in low concentrations.

In premature infant formulas, lactose has been partially replaced by glucose polymers, polysaccharides with chains of 5 to 10 glucose residues joined linearly by 1,4-α linkages in order to decrease the osmolality of the formula and to decrease the lactose load in the diet. Glucose polymers are well tolerated by preterm infants with glucose and insulin responses similar to those of a lactose feeding.

Protein

The protein requirement of the preterm infant is estimated to be 3.5 g/kg/d for infants weighing 1200 to 1500 g and 4.0 g/kg/d for infants weighing 800 to 1200 g.[69, 70] Protein intakes exceeding 4.0 g/kg/d may stress the metabolic capacity of the preterm infant.

Both the quality and quantity of protein that the infant receives are important. Although weight gain and growth of LBW infants fed protein intakes of 2.2 to 4.5 g/kg/d of either a casein- or whey-predominant formula have been shown to be no different from those receiving pooled human milk, the metabolic responses can be significantly different. Serum BUN, ammonia, albumin, and plasma methionine and cysteine concentrations were higher in the infants receiving high-protein formulas. Elevated levels of phenylalanine and tyrosine were seen in infants fed the casein-predominant, high-protein formula and lower concentrations of taurine were noted in infants fed casein-predominant formulas regardless of quantity. Preterm infants fed soy protein formula supplemented with methionine exhibit slower weight gain and lower serum protein and albumin concentrations than infants fed a whey-predominant formula. Thus, premature infant formulas are whey-predominant with a 60:40 whey-to-casein ratio; the use of soy protein–based formulas is not recommended for the preterm infant.[9]

Human milk is considered to have the ideal amino acid distribution for the human infant. Preterm infants fed their own mother's milk have more rapid growth than infants fed pooled, banked human milk[33, 60] with accretion of protein and fat similar to that of the fetus.[33] Human milk is lower in mineral content especially magnesium, calcium, phosphorus, sodium, chloride, and iron. To attain intrauterine growth rates, large volumes (180 to 200 mL/kg/d) of human milk must be fed.

To improve growth and bone mineralization, human milk fortifiers have been developed; VLBW infants fed their own mother's milk with human milk fortifier added have improved growth and higher serum albumin, transthyretin (prealbumin), and phosphorus concentrations than those receiving their mothers' milk unfortified. Absorption and retention of nutrients is similar to that in infants fed preterm infant formula.

Schulze and colleagues[104] studied the effect of varying energy and protein intakes on composition of weight gain in preterm infants. The energy intake varied from 113 to 149 kcal/kg/d and the protein intake was either 2.2 or 3.6 g/kg/d. The composition of new tissue reflected the proportional intakes of energy and protein. Infants receiving the lowest intake (113 kcal and 2.2 g protein/kg/d) had the smallest weight gain and nitrogen retention; infants receiving the highest calorie and protein intake (149 kcal and 3.6 g protein/kg/d) had equivalent nitrogen retention but a greater fat deposition than infants on an isonitrogenous feeding with fewer calories (115 kcal and 3.6 g protein/kg/d). Table 6–8 has advisable intakes for premature infants. The recommended dietary allowances for infants and children to age 3 years are listed in Table 6–9.

Lipids

Fat is a major source of energy for the infant, with approximately 50% of the calories in human milk derived from fat. The preterm infant has limited capacity to digest and absorb certain fats. Because of a limited bile salt pool and lower levels of pancreatic lipase, preterm infants malabsorb long-chain triglycerides (LCTs), the majority with chain lengths of 14 to 20 carbons.

Table 6–8. Enteral Intake for Premature Infants

	Advisable Intake
Calories	110–150 kcal/kg
Protein	3–4 g/kg
Fat	5–7 g/kg
Carbohydrate	10–15 g/kg
Osmolality (mOsm/kg H$_2$O)	≤300
Vitamins	
A	1400–2500 IU/d
D	400–600 IU/d
K	15 μg/kg/d
E	25 IU/d (5 IU/d after 2–4 wk)
C	60 mg/d
Thiamin	200–400 μg/d
Riboflavin	400–500 μg/d
B$_6$	250–400 μg/d
B$_{12}$	0.15 μg/kg
Niacin	6 mg/d
Folic acid	50 μg/d if <2 kg 15 μg/kg
Pantothenic acid	1.0–1.4 mg/kg
Biotin	0.6–2.3 μg/kg
Minerals	
Magnesium	20 mg/kg
Iron	2–4 mg/kg (begin 2–3 wk to 2 mo)
Iodine	1–7 μg/kg
Zinc	0.8–1.2 μg/kg
Copper	100–200 μg/kg
Chromium	2–4 μg/kg
Molybdenum	2–3 μg/kg
Selenium	1.5–2.5 μg/kg
Manganese	10 μg/kg (800–1200 g BW) 8.5 μg/kg (1200–1800 g BW)
Chloride	110 mg/kg (800–1200 g BW) 89 mg/kg (1200–1800 g BW)
Sodium	80 mg/kg (800–1200 g BW) 69 mg/kg (1200–1800 g BW)
Potassium	98 mg/kg (800–1200 g BW) 90 mg/kg (1200–1800 g BW)
Calcium (Ca)	210 mg/kg (800–1200 g BW) 185 mg/kg (1200–1800 g BW)
Phosphorus (P)	140 mg/kg (800–1200 g BW) 123 mg/kg (1200–1800 g BW)
Ca-to-P ratio	1.7–2:1

BW, body weight.

Human milk contains a bile salt–activated lipase that enhances lipid digestion in the duodenum. Standard infant formulas contain LCTs, which may be poorly digested by the premature infant, producing calcium soaps in the gut that render the calcium unavailable for absorption.

Because of the relatively poor digestion of LCTs, a theoretically attractive alternative is use of medium-chain triglycerides (MCTs), oils with a carbon chain length of 8 to 12 carbons. Unlike LCTs, MCTs do not require bile for emulsification. MCTs are rapidly hydrolyzed in the gut and pass directly to the liver through the portal circulation, whereas LCFAs must be reesterified once absorbed and are transported via the lymph system into the blood circulation where they are hydrolyzed by lipoprotein lipase. Medium-chain fatty acid (MCFA) metabolism differs from that of LCFA in that it does not require carnitine for transport into the mitochondria and is not regulated by cytosolic acyl-CoA synthetase. MCFAs enter the mitochondria directly and are rapidly oxidized. Formulas with MCTs have been shown to improve nitrogen, calcium, and magnesium absorption. Preterm infant formulas have been developed with approximately half of the fat as MCT.

Vitamin A

At birth, preterm infants less than 36 weeks' gestational age have been reported to have lower plasma retinol concentrations as compared with full-term infants, although the measured levels are quite variable with a wide range of data reported.[57, 91, 122] There is a further decrease in the plasma retinol and retinol binding protein levels during the first 2 weeks after birth, particularly when sufficient amounts of vitamin A are not provided. The measured hepatic levels of retinol expressed as μmol/g in preterm infants are reported to be the same as in infants born at term gestation but lower than those in older children and adults.[107, 108, 122] The recommended allowance for infants based on the average retinol content of human milk (40 μg/100 mL) and average daily milk consumption corresponds to 420 μg of retinol per day up to 6 months of age.

Retinol has been shown to be essential for the growth and differentiation of epithelial cells, has been suggested to have a role in prevention and repair of lung injury and vitamin A deficiency state, and is associated with histopathologic changes in the lung similar to those seen in BPD. Furthermore, infants dying of BPD were reported to have lower liver retinol ester levels.[108] For these reasons, the impact of vitamin A supplementation on chronic lung disease (BPD) in VLBW infants has been examined.[71, 90, 109, 116] In the most recent multicenter, blinded, randomized trial, the use of vitamin A 5000 IU (1.5 mg) administered intramuscularly three times per week for 4 weeks

Table 6–9. Recommended Dietary Allowances for Infants and Toddlers

	0.0–0.5 Year	0.5–1.0 Year	1–3 Years
Calories	108 kcal/kg	98 kcal/kg	102 kcal/kg
Protein	2.2 g/kg	1.6 g/kg	1.2 g/kg
Vitamins			
A	1250 IU/d	1250 IU/d	1330 IU/d
D	300 IU/d	400 IU/d	400 IU/d
E	3 IU/d	4 IU/d	6 IU/d
K	5 μg/d	10 μg/d	15 μg/d
C	30 mg/d	35 mg/d	40 mg/d
Thiamin	300 μg/d	400 μg/d	700 μg/d
Riboflavin	400 μg/d	500 μg/d	800 μg/d
B_6	300 μg/d	600 μg/d	1000 μg/d
B_{12}	0.3 μg/d	0.5 μg/d	1.7 μg/d
Niacin	5 mg/d	6 mg/d	9 mg/d
Folic acid	25 μg/d	35 μg/d	50 μg/d
Pantothenic acid	2 mg/d*	3 mg/d*	3 mg/d*
Biotin	10 μg/d*	15 μg/d*	20 μg/d*
Minerals			
Magnesium	40 mg/kg	60 mg/kg	80 mg/kg
Iron	6 mg/d	10 mg/d	10 mg/d
Iodine	40 μg/d	50 μg/d	70 μg/d
Zinc	5 mg/d	5 mg/d	10 mg/d
Copper	400–600 μg/d*	600–700 μg/d*	700–1000 μg/d*
Manganese	300–600 μg/d*	600–1000 μg/d*	1000–1500 μg/d*
Chloride	180 mg/d†	300 mg/d†	350–500 mg/d†
Sodium	120 mg/d†	200 mg/d†	225–300 mg/d†
Potassium	500 mg/d†	700 mg/d†	1000–1400 mg/d†
Calcium	400 mg/d	600 mg/d†	800 mg/d
Phosphorus	300 mg/d	500 mg/d	800 mg/d

*Safe and adequate ranges.
†Estimated *minimum* requirements for sodium, potassium, and chloride.

improved the biochemical vitamin A status, but resulted in only a marginal advantage in relation to prevention of chronic lung disease.[116] Vitamin A in such large doses was shown to have no clinically measurable toxic effects; however, long-term toxicity or any other functional abnormalities remain to be determined.

Vitamin E

Vitamin E, or tocopherol, serves as an antioxidant to protect double bonds of cellular lipids. Vitamin E requirements are increased with increasing polyunsaturated fatty acid (PUFA) intake and in the presence of oxidant stress, such as high iron intake. Vitamin E deficiency is rarely seen in infants because infant formulas are supplemented with vitamin E in proportion to the PUFA content. However, infants who are breast-fed and receiving supplemental iron should be given additional vitamin E. Preterm infants have low serum vitamin E levels and may be at increased risk for oxidative dam-

age to cell membranes. Studies to investigate the effectiveness of pharmaceutic doses of vitamin E on retinopathy of prematurity and BPD have not demonstrated benefits of this therapy. Supplemental vitamin E given during the first week of life may play a role in the prevention of intracranial hemorrhage in extremely LBW (ELBW) infants (especially those weighing 500 to 750 g).[44] Further studies need to be conducted before this becomes routine care for the ELBW infant. An increased risk of sepsis and NEC was seen in a group of VLBW infants whose serum vitamin E levels were maintained over 3.0 mg/dL.[68] According to the American Academy of Pediatrics, serum vitamin E concentrations should be maintained between 1.0 and 2.0 mg/dL.[93]

Vitamin K

Vitamin K, an important cofactor in the activation of intracellular precursor proteins to blood clotting proteins, is synthesized endogenously by bacterial flora. However, because intestinal synthesis cannot be relied upon because of a lack of gut colonization in the neonate, the American Academy of Pediatrics[4] recommends that 0.5 to 1.0 mg of vitamin K be given to all newborns as protection against hemorrhagic disease of the newborn. Preterm infants may be at particular risk for vitamin K deficiency as a result of low stores and frequent use of broad-spectrum antibiotics. In addition, asphyxiated infants have been shown to have a reduction in vitamin K–dependent coagulant proteins.

Human milk is generally low in vitamin K, and intestinal flora of breast-fed infants may produce less vitamin K than formula-fed infants. Therefore, antibiotic therapy may increase the risk of vitamin K deficiency in breast-fed infants by decreasing endogenous synthesis.

Calcium, Phosphorus, Magnesium, and Vitamin D

The amount of enteral calcium, phosphorus, and magnesium intake required to match intrauterine accretion rates is high: calcium 185 to 200 mg/kg/d, phosphorus 100 to 113 mg/kg/d, and magnesium 5.3 to 6.1 mg/kg/d. VLBW infants with minimal illness may require lower intakes.[30, 36] The American Academy of Pediatrics recommends intakes of calcium of 185 to 210 mg/kg/d, phosphorus 123 to 140 mg/kg/d, and magnesium 8.5 to 10.0 mg/kg/d.[4] However, magnesium intake at this level with such high calcium and phosphorus intake results in negative magnesium balance; therefore, a higher intake of magnesium approximately 20 mg/kg/d may be needed.[52]

The recommendation for vitamin D, which is required for normal metabolism of calcium, phosphorus, and magnesium, has ranged from 200 to 2000 IU per day for the preterm infant. VLBW infants can maintain normal vitamin D status with 400 IU/d[81]; high-dose vitamin D supplementation does not decrease the incidence of rickets in VLBW infants.

Human milk has concentrations of calcium and phosphorus that are appropriate for full-term infants. These amounts are inadequate for the VLBW infant. Breast milk should be supplemented with additional calcium, phosphorus, and vitamin D, which can easily be done with either a powdered human milk fortifier (Enfamil Human Milk Fortifier, Mead Johnson, Evansville, IN) or a liquid fortifier (Similac Natural Care, Ross Laboratories, Columbus, OH). Both yield better mineral accretion than breast milk alone, similar to that of VLBW infants fed a premature infant formula.[58]

Inadequate intakes of calcium, phosphorus, and vitamin D result in metabolic bone disease of prematurity, also called rickets of prematurity. This disease is characterized by reduced bone mineralization and, in severe cases, frank radiologic evidence of rickets and spontaneous fractures. The biochemical findings, although not highly sensitive, include an elevated alkaline phosphatase (>500 U/L), decreased serum phosphorus (<4 mg/dL), and normal serum calcium; 25-hydroxycholecalciferol (25-OH vitamin D) level is usually normal, but 1,25 dihydroxycholecalciferol (1,25-OH vitamin D) levels may be elevated as a result of increased parathyroid hormone levels and low serum phosphorus levels. The incidence of rickets was high before institution of the current nutrient practice of higher calcium and phosphorus levels in parenteral nutrient solution and early enteral feedings. The etiology of rickets remains unclear but is thought to be primarily an inadequate intake of calcium and phosphorus. Risk factors for rickets are listed in Table 6–10.

Prevention is important by using parenteral nutrition solutions containing appropriate concentrations of calcium and phosphorus. In our institution, the concentrations in the peripheral TPN were increased to 20 mEq elemental calcium/L and 10 mM phosphorus/L, which resulted in a decrease of radiographically diagnosed rickets.

Fortified human milk or premature infant formula are the preferred feedings for LBW infants. If elemental feedings are necessary for greater than 2 to 3 weeks, supplementa-

Table 6–10. Risk Factors for Metabolic Bone Disease of Prematurity

Extremely low birth weight ($\leq$1000 g)
Prolonged parenteral nutrition
Unsupplemented human milk
Use of elemental formulas and soy formulas
Chronic diuretic therapy (especially furosemide)
Chronic problems such as necrotizing enterocolitis, bronchopulmonary dysplasia, cholestasis, and acidosis

tion with calcium and phosphorus and vitamins is essential. The use of soy formulas should be avoided. If continuous infusion tube feeding is necessary, the formula should be shaken every 30 to 60 minutes to prevent precipitation of calcium and phosphorus and adherence to the tubing[12, 23, 24]; because of the precipitation of calcium and phosphorus and creaming of the fat, fortified human milk is not recommended for continuous infusion tube feedings.

Water-Soluble Vitamins

Vitamin B_{12} requires intrinsic factor for its absorption in the distal ileum; therefore, particular attention to this vitamin is necessary in infants who have had gastric resection or resection of the terminal ileum (e.g., NEC surgery). The potential neurologic complications of vitamin B_{12} deficiency are irreversible.

Serum folate levels may be low in the preterm infant. Folate is supplemented in the pediatric intravenous multivitamin preparation (MVI-Pediatric) and in infant formulas; it is not available in the infant multivitamin drops because of its instability in the liquid form. Folate plays an important role in DNA synthesis; deficiency of this vitamin may result in megaloblastic anemia, neutropenia, thrombocytopenia, and growth failure.

Iron

There has been increased interest in iron deficiency, with the data suggesting that mental and developmental test scores are lower in infants with iron deficiency anemia[10, 74, 120] and that iron therapy sufficient to correct the anemia is insufficient to reverse the behavioral and developmental disorders in many infants. This indicates that certain ill effects are persistent depending on the timing, severity, or degree of iron-deficiency anemia during infancy.

Iron deficiency develops in preterm infants weighing less than 2 kg unless they are supplemented with iron at 2 mg/kg/d. Although iron provided by human milk is highly bioavailable, the amount absorbed is inadequate for the preterm infant, resulting in lowered serum ferritin and hemoglobin concentrations by 3 months of age.

Absorption of supplementary iron by the preterm infant is a linear function of intake, suggesting immature control of iron absorption. It has been estimated that VLBW infants absorb approximately 44% of dietary iron, storing the majority (approximately 74%) for later use. After blood transfusions are given, iron absorption diminishes but may not totally inhibit absorption. Multiple blood transfusions result in high serum ferritin levels similar to those seen in iron overload. Therefore, preterm infants receiving repeated transfusions do not require iron supplementation until transfusions cease; it is then recommended that elemental iron 2 to 3 mg/kg/d be given by 2 months of age or before the infant is discharged home. There is no benefit to giving iron before 2 months except in the rare case of an infant who has had significant blood loss without red blood cell replacement. In such cases, iron therapy should begin by 2 to 4 weeks of life or when enteral feedings are tolerated. Smaller preterm infants may require greater iron dosages, with infants weighing less than 1 kg at birth perhaps needing as much as 4 mg/kg/d, with half provided by the iron-fortified formula and the remainder as iron supplementation at 2 mg/kg/d. A higher dose is also necessary for infants being given erythropoietin. Oral iron supplementation can interfere with vitamin E metabolism in the LBW infant,[10] thereby further increasing the need for vitamin E in an infant who is at risk for low serum tocopherol levels. Although premature infant formulas, both with and without iron fortification, are manufactured with ample amounts of vitamin E and a PUFA-to-E ratio of 0.6 or greater, premature infants on human milk and receiving supplemental iron should be also supplemented with 4 to 5 mg (6 to 8 IU) of vitamin E per day.

The impression that low-iron formulas are associated with fewer gastrointestinal disturbances is not supported by controlled studies. No feeding-related difficulties are seen, at least not in full-term infants receiving iron-fortified formulas. Because the bioavailability of iron from iron-fortified infant cereals is somewhat low, it is recommended that iron-fortified formulas or daily iron supplements be continued through the first year of life.[10]

Among term infants, breast-feeding usually provides adequate iron intake during the first 6 months of life and supplementation during this time is not necessary. Although the iron content of human milk is low, averaging 0.8 mg iron/L, the bioavailability is high, with a term infant absorbing about 49% of the iron content compared with 10% to 12% from iron-fortified cow's milk formula. Infants who are breast-fed exclusively can maintain normal hemoglobin and ferritin levels, and do not need iron supplementation until 6 months and perhaps even 9 months of age. However, the introduction of solid foods may interfere with the absorption of iron from human milk; therefore, when solids are introduced, they should include iron-containing foods such as infant cereals. Because preterm infants have minimal stores, the breast-fed preterm infant should receive iron supplementation at 2 mg/kg/d and 4 to 5 mg vitamin E/d by the second month as previously discussed.

Fluoride

Because human breast milk contains very low concentrations of fluoride, even if the mother resides in a community with fluoridated water, it has been suggested that infants who are completely breast-fed should receive 0.25 mg of fluoride supplementation daily. This recommendation is controversial in that there have been no published controlled clinical trials to provide guidance on this practice. Many mothers supplement breast-feeding with bottle feedings of formula mixed with city or well water and many mothers discontinue breast-feeding at 4 to 6 months. Therefore, it has been suggested that the supplementation schedule (Table 6–11) recommended by the American Academy of Pediatrics[7] and the American Dental Association be followed according to the fluoride content of the water even if the

infant is breast-fed and even though reduction in caries has been observed clinically in children raised in a naturally fluoridated community occurred without fluoride supplementation during breast-feeding.

The American Academy of Pediatrics Committee on Nutrition[7] recommends initiating fluoride supplementation 2 weeks after birth for full-term breast-fed infants, formula-fed infants if the community water is not fluoridated to 0.7 to 1.0 ppm, and infants who are receiving ready-to-feed formulas.

Method of Feeding

An important consideration in feeding the newborn is the development of sucking, swallowing, gastric motility, and emptying. Swallowing is first detected at 11 weeks' gestation and the sucking reflex is first observed at 24 weeks' gestation. However, a coordinated suck-swallow is not present until 32 to 34 weeks and even then is immature; the maturation of the swallowing reflex is related to postnatal age. Swallowing must be coordinated with respiration, in that the two processes share the common channels of the nasopharynx and laryngopharynx. The inability of the infant to coordinate this action results in choking, aspiration of feedings, and vomiting.

To evaluate the suck-swallow reflex, one should observe the number of swallows per second. An infant with a good suck-swallow reflex swallows approximately once per second. If greater than 2 per second are observed, the infant is probably not able to coordinate the swallowing. With a good suck, the temporal muscle will bulge.

When starting to introduce the nipple, a rule of thumb is to bottle feed for 20 minutes then gavage the rest. At first the infant may be offered nipple feeding once in a 24-hour period; the number of feedings are then increased as the infant becomes more able to nurse. Because of the additional work of sucking, the energy expenditure increases; therefore, an increased calorie intake may be required to maintain adequate rate of growth. Weight gain during the start of nipple feeding should be closely monitored. It is not necessary for an infant to be able to bottle feed before attempting to breast-feed. Infants who will be breast-feeding may actu-

Table 6–11. Supplemental Fluoride Dosage Schedule (mg/day)*

Age	Concentration of Fluoride in Drinking Water (ppm)		
	<0.3	0.3–0.7	>0.7
2 wk–2 y	0.25	0.0	0
2–3 y	0.5	0.25	0
3–16 y	1.0	0.5	0

*2.2 mg sodium fluoride contains 1 mg fluoride.

ally be able to nurse from the breast sooner than they will be able to coordinate bottle feeding.

If an infant's respiratory rate is 60 to 80 breaths per minute, he or she should be tube fed. With a respiratory rate of more than 80 breaths per minute, the infant should not be fed enterally because of the increased risk of aspiration.

If an infant is unable to nipple feed, he or she needs to be fed through an orogastric or nasogastric tube or, rarely, transpylorically. Intragastric tube feedings are preferable in that it allows for normal digestive processes and hormonal responses. The acid content of the stomach may impart bactericidal effects; other benefits of intragastric tube feeding include ease of insertion of tube, tolerance of greater osmotic loads with less cramping, distention, and diarrhea, and less risk of development of dumping syndrome. Continuous transpyloric feeding is rarely used in infants who cannot tolerate feedings as a result of impaired gastric emptying or who have a high risk of aspiration. However, this route of infusion has a higher risk of perforation of the gut, may not enable delivery of a large volume of feedings, and may result in inefficient nutrient assimilation because bypassing the gastric phase of digestion limits the exposure of food to acid hydrolysis and the lipolytic effects of lingual and gastric lipases.

If tube feeding is used, the decision to feed intermittently or continuously must be made. There are differences seen in the endocrine milieu between infants fed continuously as compared with those fed intermittently.[14] The significance of these differences is unclear and it is not possible to state with certainty which method is best for the prematurely born neonate. It has been suggested that the cyclic changes in circulating hormones and metabolites as seen in intermittent-bolus feeding may have quite different effects on cell metabolism,[76] gall bladder emptying, and gut development. Continuous infusion of human milk is not recommended because there is a loss of fat, and, therefore, calories, in the tubing of the pump. Additionally, at the end of the infusion, a large bolus of fat is delivered to the infant as a result of the separation of the fat during the infusion period.

Gastrostomy feedings are chosen when it becomes apparent that there will be long-term tube feeding (e.g., for a neurologically impaired infant), when there is persistent gastroesophageal reflux that is unresponsive to medical treatment, or when esophageal anomalies prevent the use of an orogastric or nasogastric tube.

Positioning of the infant during feeding is important for more efficient stomach emptying. Infants with respiratory distress fed in the supine position have delayed gastric emptying. The stomach empties more rapidly in the prone or right lateral positions; thus, these positions are preferred especially in infants with respiratory distress and in those infants who have the potential for feeding intolerance.

The evaluation of an infant's feeding tolerance is an ongoing process to determine the appropriate feeding method, type of formula to feed, and increment of feeding advancement. Vomiting, abdominal distention, significant gastric residuals, abnormal stooling patterns, and presence of reducing substances or frank or occult blood in the stool are indicators of intolerance. Sepsis and NEC may first present with one or more of these signs of feeding intolerance. Vomiting or spitting in the high-risk infant increases the risk of aspiration

Nonnutritive Sucking

Nonnutritive sucking, that is, placing a nipple or pacifier in the infant's mouth, has been related to accelerated weight gain and early hospital discharge in preterm infants. Reported benefits of nonnutritive sucking include improved oxygenation, accelerated maturation of sucking reflex, decreased intestinal transit time, and accelerated transition from gavage to oral feeding. Ernst and colleagues[41] conducted a randomized trial in medically stable infants receiving tube feedings, controlling for caloric intake, birth weight, and sex of the infant, and found no difference in growth, gastrointestinal transit time, fat excretion, or energy expenditure. Even so, providing a pacifier to a tube-fed infant may well give the infant great comfort and enable the infant to calm more quickly.

Human Milk

Although breast milk is considered the ideal food for the term infant, for the preterm infant it provides inadequate amounts of several nutrients especially protein, vitamin D, calcium, phosphorus, and sodium.[3] If given in sufficiently large volume (180 mL/kg/d), the energy content of human milk is sufficiently great to enable nearly all LBW infants to gain weight at intrauterine rates (approximately 15 g/kg/d). However, the protein content is suboptimal, especially for VLBW infants weighing less than 1500 g, resulting in lower serum albumin and transthyretin (prealbumin) levels, which have been shown to be reliable indicators of protein nutriture in preterm infants.[6, 94] The calcium and phosphorus content is low in unsupplemented human milk in comparison to that required to achieve intrauterine accretion rates, resulting in poor bone mineralization in VLBW infants.[30] In addition, the sodium content of human milk results in less sodium retention than intrauterine estimates and may result in hyponatremia.

In a large multicenter study on the short- and long-term clinical and developmental outcomes of infants randomized to different diets, Lucas and colleagues[77, 78] found that, by the time infants weighing less than 1200 g at birth who were fed unfortified human milk reached 2.0 kg, they were less than 2 standard deviations below the mean for weight for age. Infants weighing less than 1.0 kg at birth who were fed unfortified human milk would be expected to take 3 weeks longer to reach a weight of 2.0 kg than infants receiving formula. In a later study, Lucas et al[79] observed that infants receiving breast milk had a significantly higher intelligence quotient at 8 years than formula-fed infants. However, these data have not been uniformly confirmed in other studies.

The possibility that human milk may have certain nonnutritional advantages should also be considered. Human milk contains immunocompetent cellular components including secretory IgA, which has a protective effect on the intestinal mucosa. Heat treatment may adversely affect the immunoprotective components in human milk and is not recommended.

Since the composition of preterm milk varies greatly from one mother to another and the concentration of nutrients in preterm milk changes over time, it is difficult to determine the actual intake of an infant. To confer the potential nonnutritional advantages yet provide optimal nutrient intake, human milk should be supplemented,

or fortified, with protein, calcium, phosphorus, vitamin D, and sodium.

There are many practical considerations when feeding a LBW infant with his or her own mother's milk. One of the common concerns is to provide sufficient volumes of bacteriologically acceptable milk. Many mothers are unable to maintain adequate milk production even with frequent milk expression with an electric breast pump. The assistance of a health professional trained to counsel and support breast-feeding mothers may increase success rates within the hospital.

Bacterial contamination of the milk is of concern because of the greater risk of infection in the LBW infants. In some institutions, breast milk is cultured for bacterial content before its first use; weekly cultures are obtained thereafter. If a sample is unacceptable, the source of contamination is sought and the mother is counseled on proper milk expression technique. The relation between bacterial count in breast milk and sepsis in the neonate has not been confirmed, and therefore the practice of culturing human milk remains controversial. Refrigerated breast milk actually decreases in bacterial content over a 5-day period, and fresh frozen milk inoculated with bacteria demonstrated significant inhibition of bacterial growth.

◆ FORMULA TYPES

To be able to select the proper formula for feeding a sick infant, a clear understanding of the differences between formulas and unique qualities of a given formula is necessary (Table 6–12).

Premature Infant Formulas

Providing optimal nutrition to a preterm infant is complicated by a lack of a natural standard.[6] For the healthy full-term infant, human milk is considered the ideal food; therefore, it is used as the reference standard for the development of commercial infant formulas. Although milk of mothers who deliver their infants prematurely is higher in nitrogen, fatty acid content, sodium, chloride, magnesium, and iron, it is still inadequate in other nutrients, especially calcium and phosphorus. It, therefore, cannot be

Table 6–12. Comparison of Formulas

| | Formula Type | | |
	Premature	Standard	Soy
Energy*	24 kcal/oz	20 kcal/oz	20 kcal/oz
Protein	Whey-to-casein (60:40) 22–24 g protein/L	Whey-to-casein (60:40 or 18:82) 15 g protein/L	Soy protein isolate 18 g protein/L
Fat	MCT and LCT	LCT	LCT
Carbohydrate	Glucose polymers Lactose polymers	Lactose	Sucrose and/or glucose
Calcium (Ca) and phosphorus (P)	Fortified to meet needs of preterm infant Ca-to-P ratio 1.8–2:1	Not fortified to meet needs of preterm infant Ca-to-P ratio 1.3–1.5:1	Not fortified to meet needs of preterm infant Ca-to-P ratio 1.3–1.4:1
Iron	Available with or without iron fortification	Available with or without iron fortification	Available with iron fortification only

*Premature formula is available as ready-to-feed 20 kcal/oz or 24 kcal/oz. Standard cow's milk–based and soy protein–based formulas are available commercially as ready-to-feed, powder, or liquid concentrate. The powdered and liquid concentrates are less expensive and can be prepared with less water to increase the caloric concentration not to exceed 30 kcal/oz.
MCT, medium-chain triglycerides; LCT, long-chain triglycerides.

used as a standard for the development of premature infant formula. The special premature infant formulas have been developed from knowledge of the accretion rates of various nutrients relative to the reference fetus, from studies of the development of the gastrointestinal tract which have defined absorptive efficiency and function, and from metabolic studies.

Premature infant formulas have a lower lactose concentration with approximately 50% of the carbohydrate as lactose to reduce the lactose load because of relative lactase deficiency; the remainder of the carbohydrate is provided as glucose polymers, which are readily hydrolyzed by glucoamylase and result in a product with low osmolality.

The premature infant formulas are whey-predominant, which has been shown to result in less metabolic acidosis in VLBW infants. The risk of lactobezoar formation is reduced when a whey-predominant formula is used. In addition, the concentration of protein per liter is approximately 50% greater than that of standard infant formula to provide 3 to 4 g protein/kg/d. The fat is approximately 50% LCT and 50% MCT. The vitamin concentration is higher because the volume of formula consumed is significantly less in the tiny baby. The calcium and phosphorus content is greater than standard formula with variation between formula manufacturers. The calcium-to-phosphorus ratio generally is 2:1 as compared to 1.4:1 to 1.5:1

with standard infant formulas. Too high a concentration of calcium and phosphorus may result in intestinal milk bolus obstruction. As with all formulas, it is important to shake the formula before use, because precipitation may occur and the precipitate, containing high amounts of calcium and phosphorus, may remain in the bottom of the container.

Premature infant formulas have always been low in iron content (3 mg elemental iron/L) because these infants were often receiving transfusions and because the use of iron would increase the requirement for vitamin E. However, because some infants are receiving this type of formula for greater than 2 months and because the advantages of continuing a baby on premature infant formula after hospital discharge have been recognized, premature infant formulas are available both with low iron content (3 mg elemental iron/L) and with iron fortification (15 mg elemental iron/L).

The sodium content of premature infant formula is greater than human milk or standard infant formula. Because sodium requirements vary considerably between infants, this amount may be inadequate to maintain normal serum levels. Supplementation with 3% sodium chloride (0.5 mEq sodium and chloride/mL) may be necessary. Because this is a highly osmolar solution (see Table 6–5), the dose should be divided and administered several times throughout the day. One distinct advantage of premature infant formula is that, despite the high concentration of nutrients, the 24-calorie/oz premature infant formula is iso-osmolar with osmolalities ranging from 280 to 300 mOsm/kg H_2O.

The decision to supplement preterm infant formula with long-chain polyunsaturated fatty acids (LCPUFAs) has been a subject of debate.[65] Although some studies have demonstrated advantages in relation to development of visual function, particularly in preterm infants, it has not been a consistent observation. No distinct advantage of LCPUFA supplementation has been observed in full-term infants.

Standard Infant Formulas

The carbohydrate in standard infant formula is 100% lactose and the fat is all long-chain triglycerides of vegetable origin, usually soy and coconut oils. Most standard formulas are whey-predominant, with 60% of the protein whey and 40% casein. Standard formulas are available in both iron-fortified and non–iron-fortified (or "low iron") forms. Iron-fortified formula contains elemental iron 12 mg/L or approximately 2.0 mg/kg/d for an infant receiving approximately 108 kcal/kg/d. Low-iron formula contains elemental iron 1.5 mg/L or 0.2 mg/kg/d.

Most standard infant formulas are available as ready-to-feed, liquid concentrate, and powder. The concentrate and the powder provide the option of concentrating the formula to a higher caloric density. Concentrations above 1 calorie per milliliter or 30 calories per ounce is not recommended because of the high renal solute load that results from the decrease in free water intake. As the formula is concentrated, the osmolality increases to approximately the same degree as the concentration. Thus, a 20 kcal/oz formula with an osmolality of 300 mOsm/kg H_2O, if concentrated 135% or to 27 kcal/oz formula, the osmolality increases to approximately 405 mOsm/kg H_2O. If formula is to be concentrated, a written recipe should be given to the caregiver because overconcentration may be hazardous to small preterm infants.

Calorie density of a formula may also be increased by the addition of glucose polymers, which increases the osmolality of the formula, or by adding fat (e.g., vegetable oil, MCT oil). However, when an infant formula is supplemented with calories only, the intake of nutrients must be calculated and compared with recommended guidelines (see Tables 6–8 and 6–9) to ensure adequacy of intake. The distribution of calories will be affected using this method of increasing calories; therefore, the percent of calories from carbohydrate, protein, and fat should be determined. Approximately 35% to 65% of the total calories should be derived from carbohydrate, 30% to 55% from fat, and 8% to 16% from protein. LBW infants fed a formula contributing 7.8% of calories as protein grew at a significantly slower rate than infants fed formulas with either 9.4% or 12.5% of the calories from protein.

Soy Formulas

Soybean-based formulas with soy protein isolate or soybean solids with added methionine as the protein source are lactose-free and, therefore, are recommended for infants with galactosemia, with primary lactase deficiency, or recovering from secondary lactose intolerance. The carbohydrate is provided as sucrose or corn syrup solids, or as a combination of the two; the fat is provided as a vegetable oil (LCTs), usually soy and coconut oils. All soy formulas are iron-fortified. Although soy formulas have been used when cow's milk protein allergy is suspected, the American Academy of Pediatrics cautions that infants allergic to cow's milk may also develop an allergy to soy-based milk[9]; a protein hydrolysate formula should be the initial formula of choice. Infants with a family history of allergy who have not shown clinical manifestations may benefit from soy protein formula; however, such infants should be closely monitored for soy protein allergy. Soy protein formulas are appropriate for infants of vegetarian families who eat no animal products.

The use of soy protein formulas for VLBW infants is not recommended because of the low calcium and phosphorus content of these formulas. Preterm infants fed soy protein formulas have significantly lower serum phosphorus and serum alkaline phosphatase levels and an increased risk of development of osteopenia. Even when supplemented with additional calcium, phosphorus, and vitamin D, VLBW infants fed these formulas exhibit slower weight gain and lower serum protein and albumin concentrations than infants receiving a whey-predominant premature infant formula.

Protein Hydrolysate Formulas

Protein hydrolysate formulas are designed for infants who are allergic to cow's milk or soy proteins. Some protein hydrolysate formulas are also elemental with the carbohydrate in easily absorbable forms, such as glucose polymers or monosaccharides, and the fat as both medium-chain and long-chain triglycerides. These are sometimes used in the management of infants with intestinal resection or intractable diarrhea.

Follow-up Formulas

Recently, follow-up (weaning) formulas have been marketed in the United States. Their purpose is to provide a transitional milk between complete breast-feeding or formula feeding and solid food intake with cow's milk as the milk feeding.[8] The follow-up formulas are iron fortified, providing an advantage for infants taking inadequate amounts of solid foods; however, the compositional changes in protein, fat, carbohydrate, sodium, and calcium have no proven superiority over standard infant formulas or continued breast-feeding.[45]

Transition to Standard Formula

A rule of thumb for use of premature infant formula is to feed a premature infant formula to infants whose birth weight is less than 1800 g until they achieve a weight of 2000 g. Most LBW infants who are not on long-term TPN do quite well if these guidelines are followed. However, the VLBW infant may require nutrient-dense formulas for longer periods of time than is commonly practiced, beyond a weight of 2000 g. VLBW infants fed a nutrient-dense formula after they have reached 1850 g had fewer days in the hospital than those on standard infant formula with or without added mineral supplements. Former LBW infants fed premature infant formula for the first 2 months after hospital discharge were shown to have greater bone mineral content and lower serum parathyroid hormone concentration at 4 months after discharge compared with in-

fants fed standard infant formula. Although bone mineralization may be adequate in healthy preterm infants without respiratory distress syndrome and other medical complications who receive a standard infant formula, the ELBW and the sick premature infant requiring parenteral nutrition, and perhaps diuretic therapy, may need formula with greater mineral concentration. Additionally, infants on fortified human milk while in the hospital who were sent home breast-feeding had slower rates of increase of bone mineral content during the first 6 months.[1] After 6 months, when a mixed diet was consumed, the rate of increase of bone mineral content was the same as for the formula-fed infants. Therefore, by 1 year of age, the bone mineral content of former VLBW infants fed unsupplemented human milk was significantly lower than that of infants fed a standard infant formula.[2] Because the long-term effect of bone mineralization is unknown, mineral supplementation during the immediate post-hospital period should be considered if human milk is the primary feeding. This is most easily achieved by providing a premature infant formula as an alternative feeding twice a day, perhaps as the night-time feedings.

Lucas et al,[75] in a double-blind study, showed that preterm infants who were placed on a special "post-discharge" formula with higher calorie content (72 kcal/100 mL or approximately 22 kcal/ounce) had a significantly better rate of linear growth and weight gain. Since their study, others have confirmed these findings and many preterm infants are currently discharged home on the 22 kcal/ounce formula.

Practical Hints

1. Start small breast milk or formula feedings (10 to 20 mL/kg/d) as soon as possible. It is unnecessary to start with 5% glucose water.
2. Assess the infant's ability to nipple feed. Infants younger than 32 weeks' gestational age and infants with respiratory rates between 60 and 80 breaths per minute (bpm) need to be tube fed.
3. Do not feed infants who have respiratory rates in excess of 80 bpm or those who are hypothermic.
4. Use premature infant formula or fortified breast milk for infants weighing less

than 1800 g. Encourage the mother to breast-feed or pump her milk if the infant is to be tube fed. If breast milk is to be used, start feedings with unfortified breast milk until tolerance is established, then add fortifier.

5. Feed the infant every 2 hours if the infant weighs less than 1250 g; continuous feedings or hourly feedings may be necessary for infants weighing less than 800 g.

6. Monitor feeding tolerance. Vomiting, a sudden increase in abdominal girth, frank or occult blood in the stool, or large gastric residuals may be a sign of infection or NEC. The feedings should be stopped, the stomach should be aspirated, and a number 8 French nasogastric tube should be inserted for gastric decompression.

7. Keep accurate records of fluid intake, output, weight, type of feeding given, and feeding tolerance.

8. Reduce parenteral feedings proportionate to the increase of enteral feedings to provent excess fluid intake.

9. Increase feedings at a rate of 20 mL/kg/d and monitor tolerance to previous volume before increasing rate. Feed the infant in a prone position to facilitate gastric emptying and maintain better oxygenation. Once the infant is receiving 90 to 100 kcal/kg/d enterally, the TPN should be discontinued; if greater fluid volume is required, provide it as an IV glucose-electrolyte solution.

10. Aim for a goal of 110 to 130 kcal/kg/d and 3 to 4 g protein/kg/d with a weight gain of approximately 15 g/kg/d.

11. Offer a pacifier to the infant, especially while being gavage fed.

12. Encourage the parents to feed the infant after the infant is feeding well; it may be very frustrating for the parents to attempt feeding when the infant is resistant.

◆ NUTRITIONAL ASSESSMENT

An in-depth nutritional assessment requires anthropometric, biochemical, dietary, and clinical data. However, interpreting anthropometric and biochemical measurements is difficult; therefore, nutritional assessment in neonates receiving intensive care treatment is often confined to detecting fluctuations in weight gain and in caloric intake. Nonetheless, it is necessary for the clinician to be able to assess the neonate's nutritional status because of the potentially serious sequelae of malnutrition on multiple organ systems and the importance of growth (especially brain growth) on developmental outcome.

In nutritional assessment, one must consider the length of gestation and adequacy of intrauterine growth and nutrient tolerance. There should be a static assessment (current balance between intake and output) as well as a dynamic assessment (evaluation of infant's growth over time or growth velocity) of each infant. Also, the nonnutritional factors such as disease state, medication, and stress (e.g., infection and surgery) must be considered.

Weight gain is the most frequently used anthropometric measure. It is important to use the same scale, obtain weight measurements at same time each day to avoid diurnal changes, and indicate any equipment being weighed (especially arm boards and dressings); if equipment is not recorded, changes in weight may be spurious. In preterm infants, weight gain should be expressed on a gram per kilogram per day basis. Table 6–13 contains suggested weight gain goals.

When assessing weight, there are several problems to consider. In the first week of life, all newborns lose weight as a result of loss of free water and low intake; however, most preterm infants are also calorie and fluid restricted during that period as a result of illness, so that it may be difficult to separate changes in growth measurements caused by diuresis from those caused by poor protein-calorie intake. Weight gain does not necessarily reflect growth, which

Table 6–13. Approximate Daily Weight Gain for Infants

Gestational Age	g/kg/d
24–28 wk	15–20
29–32 wk	17–21
33–36 wk	14–15
37–40 wk	7–9

Corrected Age	g/d
40 wk–3 mo	30
3–6 mo	20
6–9 mo	15
9–12 mo	10
12–24 mo	6

is a deposition of new tissue of normal composition; weight increase may reflect excessive fat deposition or water retention, neither of which is truly growth.

Length measurements are the most inaccurate anthropometric measurement. Accurate technique is important in performing length measurements to detect small changes. Two trained individuals are needed to measure the infant on a measuring board containing a stationary head board, moveable foot board, and a built-in tape measure. Skeletal growth is often spared relative to weight in mildly malnourished infants; therefore, initially, linear grow is often slow or stops. Serial length measures obtained weekly are helpful in assessing nutritional status when plotted over time; length measures are especially useful in infants, such as those with BPD, whose weight fluctuates greatly. A gain in length of 1 cm per week is expected.

Increase in head circumference (HC), the measurement of the largest occipitofrontal circumference, correlates well with cellular growth of the brain in normal infants. During acute illness the velocity of head growth for the sick preterm infants is less than that of the normal fetus. During recovery, head growth parallels that of normal fetal growth and subsequently rapid "catch-up" growth in HC may occur. Normal growth does not occur until the acute illness has resolved, despite high energy intake. Preterm infants who were calorically deprived for the longest periods showed slower growth rates and longer duration of catch-up growth. In this respect, the longer these infants remain with suboptimal head size, the greater is their developmental risk.[62]

HC is usually measured once a week using a paper tape; a new tape should be used for each infant. A goal of about 0.5 to 1.0 cm per week is to be expected. If hydrocephalus is of concern, more frequent measures are warranted. The initial HC may differ from subsequent measurements because of molding of the head. Measuring HC may be difficult as a result of interfering equipment such as intravenous lines on the scalp.

Serial weight, length, and HC measurements should be plotted on an appropriate growth chart. Daily weights may be plotted on the Hall growth chart[106] or weekly on the Benda and Babson growth chart,[22] among others.

Skin fold measures of several sites have been used to estimate body fat stores and the percent body fat in children and adults. These determinations are made by using a variety of formulas that are based on the assumption that the percent of TBW and fat distribution remains constant. In the neonate, these assumptions are not valid in that the percent body water decreases with increasing gestational age and postnatal age and fat increases with increasing gestational age.

The biochemical assessment of nutritional status may be more specific than anthropometric measures and may be useful in combination with anthropometric indices for nutritional assessment of the sick neonate. Many routine tests may signal nutrition-related problems For example, an elevated alkaline phosphatase level (>500 IU) and a low serum phosphorus (<4 mg/dL) may occur during the active phase of rickets; this combination of biochemical findings indicates the need to obtain diagnostic x-ray studies. However, abnormal alkaline phosphatase levels may occur as a result of hepatic dysfunction; therefore, heat fractionation of the isoenzyme is suggested to determine its origin. As rickets begins to heal, the serum phosphorus levels normalize, whereas the alkaline phosphatase continues to be elevated during the radiographic picture of healing. Elevated alkaline phosphatase levels generally precede radiologic changes by 2 to 4 weeks.

Albumin is a serum protein commonly measured in routine laboratory tests. Although it has limited value for nutritional assessment, it may serve as an indicator of inadequate energy and protein intake. The average serum albumin concentration in infants younger than 37 weeks' gestation ranges from 2.0 to 2.7 mg/dL. This relative hypoalbuminemia of the preterm infant appears to be as a result of a more rapid turnover of a small plasma pool as opposed to a decreased rate of albumin synthesis; the half-life of albumin is approximately 7.5 days in the preterm infant as compared with 14.8 days in adults. Despite the relatively rapid turnover, serum albumin concentration changes slowly in response to nutrition rehabilitation.

To quickly assess response to nutrition support, a serum protein with a shorter half-life is necessary. Transthyretin (prealbumin), with a half-life of approximately 2 days in adults, has been shown to be a suitable marker for evaluation of nutritional status in VLBW infants.[94] Because transthyretin increases with gestational age as well as with protein and energy intake, the direction of change in serial tests may be more useful than striving for absolute values.

Because of the various metabolic, renal, respiratory, and gastrointestinal abnormalities to which VLBW infants are subject, close monitoring of blood gases, serum electrolytes, calcium, phosphorus, glucose, BUN, and creatinine is necessary.

Ongoing nutritional assessment includes careful calculation of dietary intake relative to estimated requirements, determination of fluid balance and hydration status, and tolerance to feeding method. In combination with anthropometric, clinical, and biochemical data, adjustments in intake or method of nutrient delivery can be made to achieve effective nutritional support.

CASE PROBLEMS

◆

Case One

M. J. is a former 1160-g, 28-week gestational age infant who is returning to the clinic at 5 months of age. He has gained weight at a rate of about 18 g/d over the past 2 months and currently weighs 4.0 kg. He is receiving 18 oz of 24 calorie/oz iron-fortified standard infant formula per day. His mother states he is a "good" eater; her friends advise her that he should be starting solid food. She wants to know what she should give him as his first feeding and how much she should give him.

◆ *Is this infant's growth appropriate?*

Whenever assessing the growth of a former preterm infant, one must correct for gestational age at the time of birth. To correct, simply subtract the number of weeks preterm from the chronologic age. In this example, a former 28-week gestational age infant who is now 5 months old is, in fact, only 2 months corrected age (5 months chronologic age minus 3 months premature = 2 months corrected age).

If his weight is plotted on the Benda and Babson growth chart,[22] his weight of 4.0 kg at 2 months' corrected age places him 2 standard deviations below the mean or the third percentile. His average weight gain of 18 g/d would result in a weight gain to approximately 4.5 kg in 1 month, which, if plotted at 3 months' corrected age, would drop him below the third percentile.

◆ *What is his caloric intake? Is it sufficient?*

M. J. is receiving 18 oz/d of 24-calorie/oz formula, which provides a total daily caloric intake of 432 kcal or 108 kcal/kg/day. This is an appropriate intake for a former full-term infant; however, for M. J. it is inadequate to provide for catch-up growth. A weight gain of approximately 30 g/d, equivalent to the growth rate of a 2-month-old infant at the fiftieth percentile, would result in accelerated growth and weight gain of 900 g in the next month, which would place him above the third percentile at 3 months. Additional calories and protein need to be given to enable this kind of weight gain. Therefore, if the infant's intake can be increased to 21 oz each day or the caloric concentration is increased to 27 calories/oz, an intake of 122 calories/kg/d would result, or an additional 56 calories/d. Because 1 g of mixed tissue growth requires approximately 4.5 extra calories,[101] in theory, it should result in an additional weight gain of 12 g/d.

◆ *What other information would you like to know?*

An accurate measure of linear growth using an infant measuring board and an occipito-frontal HC measurement is necessary for a more complete assessment of growth. HC should catch up by 8 months' corrected age, even if the weight and length are still suboptimal.[62]

Information on vitamin supplementation also would be helpful. A vitamin supplement should be provided to infants whose enteral intake is less than 750 mL of 20-calorie/oz formula or the equivalent in concentrated formula. This infant is receiving 540 mL/day of formula concentrated 120% (24 kcal/20 kcal = 1.2 × 100 = 120%) or the equivalent of the nutrients found in 648 mL of 20-kcal/oz formula (18 oz × 30 mL/oz × 1.2 = 648 mL). If no vitamin supplements have been used, there may have been a period of inadequate vitamin intake; therefore, a supplement should be started and used over the next month. If one has been used and if the formula is to be concentrated 135% to 27 kcal/oz or the total volume per day increased to 21 oz of 24 kcal/oz formula, this will provide the equivalent of approximately 750 mL of 20-kcal/oz formula and the supplement may be stopped.

◆ *Should the mother start solid foods?*

An infant at 2 months has low concentrations of pancreatic amylase and may not completely digest the starch present in cereal; the developmental readiness for solids is not yet present. The infant will still have a strong tongue thrust, which would push solid foods out of the month instead of to the back of the month in preparation for swallowing. Therefore, it should be recommended to this mother that she wait until the infant is 4 to 6 months' corrected age or 7 to 9 months' chronologic age before solids are begun. Some infants develop feeding aversions after extended periods of parenteral nutrition, tube feeding, and ventilatory support; in these infants, the introduction of solids should occur at 4 months' corrected age to provide the infant with ample time to learn to accept the spoon. An occupational or speech therapist may need to become involved to teach the caregivers techniques to use to stimulate feeding readiness.

REFERENCES

1. Abrams SA, Schanler RJ, Garza C: Bone mineralization in former very low birth weight infants fed either human milk or commercial formula. J Pediatr 112:956, 1998.
2. Abrams SA, Schanler RJ, Tsang RC, et al: Bone mineralization in former very low birth weight infants fed either human milk or commercial formula: One-year follow-up observation. J Pediatr 114:1041, 1989.
3. American Academy of Pediatrics, Committee on Nutrition: Commentary on breast-feeding and infant formulas, including proposed standards for formulas. Pediatrics 57:278, 1976.
4. American Academy of Pediatrics, Committee on Nutrition: Vitamin and mineral supplement needs in normal children in the United States. Pediatrics 66:1015, 1980.
5. American Academy of Pediatrics, Committee on Nutrition: Use of intravenous fat emulsions in pediatric patients. Pediatrics 68:738, 1981.
6. American Academy of Pediatrics, Committee on Nutrition: Nutritional needs of low-birth-weight infants. Pediatrics 75:976, 1985.
7. American Academy of Pediatrics, Committee on Nutrition: Fluoride supplementation. Pediatrics 77:758, 1986.
8. American Academy of Pediatrics, Committee on Nutrition: The use of whole cow's milk in infancy. Pediatrics 89:1105, 1992.
9. American Academy of Pediatrics, Committee on Nutrition: Soy protein-based formulas: Recommendations for use in infant feeding. Pediatrics 101:148, 1990.
10. American Academy of Pediatrics, Committee on Nutrition: Iron fortification of infant formulas. Pediatrics 104:119, 1999.
11. Andrew G, Chan G, Schiff D: Lipid metabolism in the neonate. I. The effects of Intralipid on plasma triglyceride and free fatty acid concentrations in the neonate. J Pediatr 88:273, 1976.
12. Antonson DL, Smith JL, Nelson RD, et al: The stability of vitamin and mineral concentrations of a low-birth-weight infant formula during continuous enteral feeding. J Pediatr Gastroenterol Nutr 2:617, 1983.
13. Arakawa T, Tamura T, Igarashi Y, et al: Zinc deficiency in two infants during total parenteral alimentation for diarrhea. Am J Clin Nutr 29:197, 1976.
14. Aynsley-Green A, Adrian TE, Bloom SR: Feeding and the development of enteroinsular hormone secretion in the preterm infant: Effects of continuous gastric infusions of human milk compared with intermittent boluses. Acta Paediatr Scand 71:379, 1982.
15. Baeckert PA, Greene HL, Fritz I, et al: Vitamin concentrations in very low birth weight infants given vitamins intravenously in a lipid emulsion: Measurement of vitamins A, D, and E and riboflavin. J Pediatr 113:1057, 1988.
16. Battista MA, Price PT, Kalhan SC: Effect of parenteral amino acids on leucine and urea kinetics in preterm infants. J Pediatr 128:130, 1996.
17. Bauer K, Bovermann G, Roithmaier A, et al: Body composition, nutrition, and fluid balance during the first two weeks of life in preterm neonates weighing less than 1500 grams. J Pediatr 118:615, 1991.
18. Baumgart S: Reduction of oxygen consumption, insensible water loss, and radiant heat demand with use of a plastic blanket for low-birth-weight infants under radiant warmers. Pediatrics 74:1022, 1984.
19. Bell EF, Filer LJ Jr, Wong AP, Stegink LD: Effects of a parenteral nutrition regimen containing dicarboxylic amino acids on plasma, erythrocyte, and urinary amino acid concentrations of young infants. Am J Clin Nutr 37:99, 1983.
20. Bell EF, Warburton D, Stonestreet BS, et al: High-volume fluid intake predisposes premature infants to necrotizing enterocolitis. Lancet 2:90, 1979.
21. Bell EF, Warburton D, Stonestreet BS, et al: Effect of fluid administration on the development of symptomatic patent ductus arteriosus and congestive heart failure in premature infants. N Engl J Med 302:598, 1980.
22. Benda GIM, Babson SG: Peripheral intravenous alimentation of the small premature infant. J Pediatr 79:494, 1971.
23. Bhatia J, Fomon SJ: Formulas for premature infants: Fate of the calcium and phosphorus. Pediatrics 72:37, 1983.
24. Bhatia J: Formula fixed (letter). Pediatrics 75:800, 1985.
25. Bonner CM, DeBrie KL, Hug G, et al: Effects of parenteral L-carnitine supplementation on fat metabolism and nutrition in premature neonates. J Pediatr 126:287, 1995.
26. Brans YW, Andrew DS, Carrillo DW, et al: Tolerance of fat emulsions in very-low-birth-weight neonates. Am J Dis Child 142:145, 1988.
27. Brooke OG, Alvear J, Arnold M: Energy retention, energy expenditure, and growth in healthy immature infants. Pediatr Res 13:215, 1979.
28. Brooke OG: Energy expenditure in the fetus and neonate: Sources of variability. Acta Paediatr Scand Suppl 319:128, 1985.
29. Caldwell MD, Jonsson HT, Othersen HB: Essential fatty acid deficiency in an infant receiving pro-

longed parenteral alimentation. J Pediatr 81:894, 1972.

30. Chan GM, Mileur L, Hansen JW: Calcium and phosphorus requirements in bone mineralization of preterm infants. J Pediatr 113:225, 1988.

31. Chesney RW: Taurine: Its biological role and clinical implications. In Barness LA, ed: Advances in Pediatrics. 32nd ed. Chicago: Year Book Medical Publishers, 1985, p 1.

32. Chessex P, Gagne G, Pineault M, et al: Metabolic and clinical consequences of changing from high-glucose to high-fat regimens in parenterally fed newborn infants. J Pediatr 115:992, 1989.

33. Chessex P, Reichman BL, Verellen GJE: Quality of growth in premature infants fed their own mothers' milk. J Pediatr 102:107, 1983.

34. Chessex P, Reichman BL, Verellen GJE, et al: Influence of postnatal age, energy intake, and weight gain on energy metabolism in the very-low-birth weight infant. J Pediatr 99:761, 1981.

35. Cleary TG, Pickering LK: Mechanisms of intra-lipid effect on polymorphonuclear leukocytes. J Clin Lab Immunol 11:21, 1983.

36. Decsi T, Fekete M: Follow-up of calcium and phosphorus homeostasis in preterm infants who are not extremely ill. Am J Dis Child 144:1183, 1990.

37. Denne SC, Karn CA, Ahlrichs JA, et al: Proteolysis and phenylalanine hydroxylation in response to parenteral nutrition in extremely premature and normal newborns. J Clin Invest 97:746, 1996.

38. Dunn L, Hulman S, Weiner J, et al: Beneficial effects of early hypocaloric enteral feeding on neonatal gastrointestinal function: Preliminary report of a randomized trail. J Pediatr 112:622, 1988.

39. Ekblad H, Kero P, Takala J, et al: Water, sodium and acid-base balance in premature infants: Therapeutical aspects. Acta Paediatr Scand 76:47, 1987.

40. Engle WD, Arant BS Jr: Urinary potassium excretion in the critically ill neonate. Pediatrics 74:259, 1984.

41. Ernst JA, Rickard KA, Neal PR, et al: Lack of improved growth outcome related to nonnutritive sucking in very low birth weight premature infants fed a controlled nutrient intake: A randomized prospective study. Pediatrics 83:706, 1989.

42. Filler RM, Eraklis AJ, Rubin VG, et al: Long-term parenteral nutrition in infants. N Engl J Med 281:589, 1969.

43. Fine BP, Ty A, Lestrange N, et al: Sodium deprivation growth failure in the rat: Alterations in tissue composition and fluid spaces. J Nutr 117:1623, 1987.

44. Fish WH, Cohen M, Franzek D, et al: Effect of intramuscular vitamin E on mortality and intra-cranial hemorrhage in neonates of 1000 grams or less. Pediatrics 85:578, 1990.

45. Fomon SJ, Sanders KD, Ziegler EE: Formulas for older infants. J Pediatr 116:690, 1990.

46. Freeman J, Goldmann DA, Smith NE, et al: Association of intravenous lipid emulsion and coagulase-negative staphylococcal bacteremia in neonatal intensive care units. N Engl J Med 323:301, 1990.

47. Friedman Z, Danon A, Stahlman MT, et al: Rapid onset of essential fatty acid deficiency in the newborn. Pediatrics 58:640, 1976.

48. Friedman Z, Lamberth EL, Stahlman MT, et al: Platelet dysfunction in the neonate with essential fatty acid deficiency. J Pediatr 90:439, 1977.

49. Friedman Z, Marks KH, Maisels J, et al: Effect of parenteral fat emulsion on the pulmonary and reticuloendothelial systems in the newborn infant. Pediatrics 61:694, 1978.

50. Galeano NF, Darling P, Lepage G, et al: Taurine supplementation of a premature formula improves fat absorption in preterm infants. Pediatr Res 22:67, 1987.

51. Gaull G, Sturman JA, Raiha NCR: Development of mammalian sulfur metabolism: Absence of cystathionase in human fetal tissue. Pediatr Res 6:538, 1972.

52. Giles MM, Laing IA, Elton RA, et al: Magnesium metabolism in preterm infants: Effects of calcium, magnesium, and phosphorus, and of postnatal and gestational age. J Pediatr 117:147, 1990.

53. Glass L, Silverman WA, Sinclair JC: Effect of the thermal environment on cold resistance and growth of small infants after the first week of life. Pediatrics 41:1033, 1968.

54. Gohlke BC, Fahnenstich H, Kowalewski S: Serum lipids during parenteral nutrition with a 10% lipid emulsion with reduced phopholipid emulsifier content in premature infants. J Pediatr Endocrinol Metab 10:505, 1997.

55. Goldman HI, Goldman JS, Kaufman I, et al: Late effects of early dietary protein intake on low birth weight infants. J Pediatr 85:764, 1974.

56. Greene HL, Hambidge KM, Schanler R, et al: Guidelines for the use of vitamins, trace elements, calcium, magnesium, and phosphorus in infants and children receiving total parenteral nutrition: Report of the Subcommittee on Pediatric Parenteral Nutrient Requirements from the Committee on Clinical Practice Issues of The American Society for Clinical Nutrition. Am J Clin Nutr 48:1324, 1988.

57. Greene HL, Phillips BL, Franck L, et al: Persistently low blood retinol levels during and after parenteral feeding of very low birth weight infants: Examination of losses into intravenous administration sets and methods of prevention by addition to a lipid emulsion. Pediatrics 79:894, 1987.

58. Greer FR, McCormick A: Improved bone mineralization and growth in premature infants fed fortified own mother's milk. J Pediatr 112:961, 1988.

59. Groh-Wargo S, Ciaccia A, Moore J: Neonatal metabolic acidosis: Effect of chloride from normal saline flushes. J Parenter Enteral Nutr 12:159, 1988.

60. Gross SJ, Gabriel E: Vitamin E status of preterm infants fed human milk or infant formula. J Pediatr 106:635, 1985.

61. Gudinchet F, Schutz Y, Micheli JL: Metabolic cost of growth in very low-birth-weight infants. Pediatr Res 16:1025, 1982.

62. Hack M, Breslau N: Very low birth weight infants: Effects of brain growth during infancy on intelligence quotient at 3 years of age. Pediatrics 77:196, 1986.

63. Heird WC, Gomez MR: Parenteral nutrition in low-birth-weight infants. Ann Rev Nutr 16:471, 1996.

64. Heird WC, Hay W, Helms RA, et al: Pediatric parenteral amino acid mixture in low birth weight infants. Pediatrics 81:41, 1988.

65. Heird WC, Prager TC, Anderson RE: Docosahexa-

enoic acid and the development and function of the infant retina. Current Opin Lipidol 8:12, 1997.

66. Heller RM, Kirchner SG, O'Neill JA Jr, et al: Skeletal changes of copper deficiency in infants receiving prolonged total parenteral nutrition. J Pediatr 92:947, 1978.

67. Helms RA, Maure EC, Hay WW Jr, et al: Effect of intravenous L-carnitine on growth parameters and fat metabolism during parenteral nutrition in neonates. J Parenter Enteral Nutr 14:448, 1990.

68. Johnson L, Bowen FW, Abbasi S, et al: Relationship of prolonged pharmacologic serum levels of vitamin E to incidence of sepsis and necrotizing enterocolitis in infants with birth weight 1,500 grams or less. Pediatrics 75:619, 1985.

69. Kashyap S, Forsyth M, Zucker C, et al: Effects of varying protein and energy intakes on growth and metabolic response in low birth weight infants. J Pediatr 108:955, 1986.

70. Kashyap S, Schulze KF, Forsyth M, et al: Growth, nutrient retention, and metabolic response of low-birth-weight infants fed supplemented and unsupplemented preterm human milk. Am J Clin Nutr 52:254, 1990.

71. Kennedy KA, Stoll BJ, Ehrenkranz RA, et al: Vitamin A to prevent bronchopulmonary dysplasia in very-low-birth-weight infants: Has the dose been too low? Early Human Dev 49:19, 1997.

72. Kien CL, Ganther HE: Manifestations of chronic selenium deficiency in a child receiving total parenteral nutrition. Am J Clin Nutr 37:319, 1983.

73. Lorenz JM, Kleinman LI, Kotagal UR, et al: Water balance in very low-birth-weight infants: Relationship to water and sodium intake and effect on outcome. J Pediatr 101:423, 1982.

74. Lozoff B, Brittenham GM, Wolf AW, et al: Iron deficiency anemia and iron therapy effects on infant developmental test performance. Pediatrics 79:981, 1987.

75. Lucas A, Bishop NJ, King FJ, et al: Randomised trial of nutrition for preterm infants after discharge. Arch Dis Child 67:324, 1992.

76. Lucas A, Bloom SR, Aynsley-Green A: Metabolic and endocrine consequences of depriving preterm infants of enteral nutrition. Acta Paediatr Scand 72:245, 1983.

77. Lucas A, Gore SM, Cole TJ, et al: Multi-centre trial on feeding low birthweight infants: Effects of diet on early growth. Arch Dis Child 59:722, 1984.

78. Lucas A, Morley R, Cole TJ, et al: Early diet in preterm babies and developmental status at 18 months. Lancet 335:1477, 1990.

79. Lucas A, Morley R, Cole TJ, et al: Early diet in preterm babies and developmental status in infancy. Arch Dis Child 64:1570, 1989.

80. Malhotra V, Greenberg JW, Dunn LL, et al: Fatty acid enhancement of the quantum yield for the formation of lumirubin from bilirubin bound to human albumin. Pediatr Res 21:530, 1987.

81. Mayfield SR, Uauy R, Waidelich D: Body composition of low-birth-weight infants determined by using bioelectrical resistance and reactance. Am J Clin Nutr 54:296, 1991.

82. McMillan JA, Landaw SA, Oski FA: Iron sufficiency in breast-fed infants and the availability of iron from human milk. Pediatrics 58:686, 1976.

83. Meetze W, Valentine C, McGuigan J, et al: Gastrointestinal (GI) priming prior to full enteral nutrition in very low birthweight (VLBW) infants. Pediatr Res 29:300A, 1991.

84. Mock DM, DeLorimer AA, Liebman WM, et al: Biotin deficiency: An unusual complication of parenteral alimentation. N Engl J Med 304:820, 1981.

85. National Research Council: Recommended Dietary Allowances. 10th ed. Report of the Subcommittee on the Tenth Edition of the RDAs, Food and Nutrition Board, Commission of Life Sciences. Washington, DC: National Academy Press, 1989.

86. Nose O, Tipton JR, Ament ME, et al: Effect of the energy source on changes in energy expenditure, respiratory quotient, and nitrogen balance during total parenteral nutrition in children. Pediatr Res 21:538, 1987.

87. Oh W: Renal function and fluid therapy in high risk infants. Biol Neonate 53:230, 1988.

88. Papile L, Burstein J, Burstein K, et al: Relationship of intravenous sodium bicarbonate infusions and cerebral intraventricular hemorrhage. J Pediatr 93:334, 1978.

89. Paulsrud JR, Pensler L, Whitten CF, et al: Essential fatty acid deficiency in infants induced by fat-free intravenous feeding. Am J Clin Nutr 25:897, 1972.

90. Pearson E, Bose C, Snidow T, et al: Trial of vitamin A supplementation in very low birth weight infants at risk for bronchopulmonary dysplasia. J Pediatr 121:420, 1992.

91. Peeples JM, Carlson SE, Werkman SH, et al: Vitamin A status of preterm infants during infancy. Am J Clin Nutr 53:1455, 1991.

92. Pineault M, Chessex P, Bisaillon S, et al: Total parenteral nutrition in the newborn: Impact of the quality of infused energy on nitrogen metabolism. Am J Clin Nutr 47:298, 1988.

93. Poland RL: American Academy of Pediatrics, Committee on Fetus and Newborn: Vitamin E: What should we do? Pediatrics 77:787, 1986.

94. Polberger SKT, Fex GA, Axelsson IE, et al: Eleven plasma proteins as indicators of protein nutritional status in very low birth weight infants. Pediatrics 86:916, 1990.

95. Powell DA, Aungst J, Snedden S, et al: Broviac catheter-related *Malassezia furfur* sepsis in five infants receiving intravenous fat emulsions. J Pediatr 105:987, 1984.

96. Prastersom W, Phillipos EZ, Van Aerde JE, et al: Pulmonary vascular resistance during lipid infusion in neonates. Arch Dis Child 74:F95, 1996.

97. Raghavan CV, Super DM, Chatburn RL, et al: Estimation of total body water in very low birthweight (VLBW) infants using bioelectric impedance and [^{18}O] labeled water. Am J Clin Nutr 68:668, 1998.

98. Reichman BL, Chessex P, Putet G, et al: Diet, fat accretion, and growth in premature infants. N Engl J Med 305:1495, 1981.

99. Reichman BL, Chessex P, Putet G, et al: Partition of energy metabolism and energy cost of growth in the very low-birth-weight infant. Pediatrics 69:446, 1982.

100. Rivera A Jr, Bell EF, Stegink L, et al: Plasma amino acid profiles during the first three days of life in infants with respiratory distress syndrome: Effect of parenteral amino acid supplementation. J Pediatr 115:465, 1989.

101. Roberts SB, Young VR: Energy costs of fat and protein deposition in the human infant. Am J Clin Nutr 48:951, 1988.

102. Schanler RJ, Shulman RJ, Lau C, et al: Feeding

strategies for premature infants: Randomized trial of gastrointestinal priming and tube-feeding method. Pediatrics 103:434, 1999.

103. Schmidt-Sommerfeld E, Penn D: Carnitine and total parenteral nutrition of the neonate. Biol Neonate 58:81, 1990.

104. Schulze KF, Stefanski M, Masterson J, et al: Energy expenditure, energy balance, and composition of weight gain in low birth weight infants fed diets of different protein and energy content. J Pediatr 110:753, 1987.

105. Shaffer SG, Meade VM: Sodium balance and extracellular volume regulation in very low birth weight infants. J Pediatr 115:285, 1989.

106. Shaffer SG, Quimiro CL, Anderson JV, Hall R: Postnatal weight changes in low birth weight infants. Pediatrics 79:702, 1987.

107. Shenai JP, Chytil F, Stahlman MT: Liver vitamin A reserves of very low birth weight neonates. Pediatr Res 19:892, 1985.

108. Shenai JP, Chytil F, Stahlman MT: Vitamin A status of neonates with bronchopulmonary dysplasia. Pediatr Res 19:185, 1985.

109. Shenai JP, Kennedy KA, Chytil F, et al: Clinical trial of vitamin A supplementation in infants susceptible to bronchopulmonary dysplasia. J Pediatr 111:269, 1987.

110. Shortland GJ, Walter JH, Stroud C, et al: Randomised controlled trial of L-carnitine as a nutritional supplement in preterm infants. Arch Dis Child Fetal Neonatal Ed 78:F185, 1998.

111. Shulman RJ, Langston C, Schanler RJ: Pulmonary vascular lipid deposition after administration of intravenous fat to infants. Pediatrics 79:99, 1987.

112. Spahr RC, Klein AM, Brown DR, et al: Fluid administration and bronchopulmonary dysplasia. Am J Dis Child 134:958, 1980.

113. Sulkers EJ, Lafeber HN, Degenhart HJ, et al: Effects of high carnitine supplementation on substrate utilization in low-birth-weight infants receiving total parenteral nutrition. Am J Clin Nutr 52:889, 1990.

114. Tyson JE, Kennedy KA, Cochrane Neonatal Collaborative Review Group, 24/07/1997: Minimal enteral nutrition in parenterally fed neonates. http://www.nichd.nih.gov/cochraneneonatal/tyson/tyson.htm.

115. Tyson JE, Lasky R, Flood D, et al: Randomized trial of taurine supplementation for infants <1300 gram birth weight: Effect on auditory brain-stem evoked responses. Pediatrics 83:406, 1989.

116. Tyson JE, Wright LL, Oh W, et al: Vitamin A supplementation for extremely-low-birth-weight infants. N Engl J Med 340:1962, 1999.

117. Uauy RD, Birch DG, Birch EE, et al: Effect of dietary omega-3 fatty acids on retinal function of very low birth weight neonates. Pediatr Res 28:485, 1990.

118. Usmani SS, Harper RG, Usmani SF: Effect of a lipid emulsion (Intralipid) on polymorphonuclear leukocyte functions in the neonate. J Pediatr 113:132, 1988.

119. Van Marter LJ, Leviton A, Allred EN, et al: Hydration during the first days of life and the risk of bronchopulmonary dysplasia in low birth weight infants. J Pediatr 116:942, 1990.

120. Walter T, DeAndraca I, Chadud P, et al: Iron deficiency anemia: Adverse effects on infant psychomotor development. Pediatrics 84:7, 1989.

121. Whyte RK, Bayley HS, Sinclair JC: Energy intake and the nature of growth in low birth weight infants. Can J Physiol Pharmacol 63:565, 1985.

122. Zachman RD: Retinol (vitamin A) and the neonate: Special problems of the human premature infant. Am J Clin Nutr 50:413, 1989.

123. Zlotkin SH, Anderson GH: The development of cystathionase activity during the first year of life. Pediatr Res 16:65, 1982.

124. Zlotkin SH, Bryan MH, Anderson GH: Intravenous nitrogen and energy intakes required to duplicate in utero nitrogen accretion in prematurely born human infants. J Pediatr 99:115, 1981.

Part Two

SELECTED DISORDERS OF THE GASTROINTESTINAL TRACT

Avroy A. Fanaroff

Anomalies of the gastrointestinal tract[51, 67] may involve any part of the primitive tube from the hypopharynx to the anal dimple. The most common lesions are atresias, stenoses, duplications, and functional obstructions. Vascular occlusions, sometimes resulting from rotational anomalies and intussusceptions, may be in utero factors in atresias and stenoses. Presenting findings include the following:

- History of hydramnios
- Increased salivation, cyanosis, and choking with feedings
- Large gastric aspirate (>25 mL) in delivery room
- Vomiting, especially bile stained
- Abdominal distention with or without visible peristalsis
- Failure to pass a stool or delayed passage of stool

Definitions

Atresia. Complete luminal discontinuity of the gastrointestinal tract, ranging from the shortest segment web to complete loss of a major segment of bowel and mesentery. Multiple atresias may occur throughout the intestinal tract, especially in the jejunoileal segments.

Stenosis. A narrowing that may involve the entire thickness of the bowel wall or may be merely a partial web.

Duplications. May vary from simple cystlike

projections into the mesentery to complete replication of any length of the gastrointestinal tube, with or without luminal continuity with the in-line segment. They may occur anywhere along the gastrointestinal tract and present as obstructions, as perforations, or simply as a palpable mass.

Functional obstructions. Those obstructions not associated with anatomic malformation. They include achalasia, pyloric stenosis, and aganglionic megacolon, all of which have some component of myoneural dyscoordination in their etiologies. Other functional obstructions, such as meconium ileus and meconium plug syndrome, are caused by abnormalities of intraluminal contents.

Understanding of the basic entities and familiarity with some essential principles help to differentiate the lesions. The following basic principles are helpful when considering neonatal and infant bowel problems:

- Intestinal obstruction may be anticipated in 1 of every 1000 births. Multiple anomalies occur frequently.
- Lesions producing obstruction of the upper gastrointestinal tract may be associated with maternal hydramnios and large gastric aspirates at birth.
- Green vomitus should be considered an indication of bowel obstruction until proven otherwise.
- The clinical features of intestinal obstruction include vomiting, abdominal distention, visible peristalsis, and delayed passage of meconium. With upper gastrointestinal obstruction, meconium may be passed but no transitional stool is seen.
- Gastrointestinal obstruction between the pylorus and the ligament of Treitz is malrotation until proven otherwise.
- Once the continuity of the gastrointestinal tract is clearly demonstrated postnatally by the passage of "transitional stools" or air or contrast medium administered from above, congenital atresia has been excluded as the cause of the obstruction. Note that meconium may be passed from bowel distal to a complete obstruction.
- Colonic obstruction may present with the same constellation of symptoms as

upper gastrointestinal obstruction. Particular note is taken of delayed passage of meconium (Hirschsprung disease, meconium plug syndrome).
- In patients younger than 2 years, it is hazardous to attempt to differentiate large from small bowel on the basis of plain abdominal radiographs, particularly because the frequent errors in this evaluation may lead to delay in diagnosis and therapy for an obstructive bowel lesion.
- An entity that can obstruct the bowel may also lead to perforation and the resulting signs and symptoms of peritonitis. Thus, when peritonitis is the presenting symptom, an obstructing lesion must be sought and corrected.

Imaging plays a major role in most neonatal gastrointestinal emergencies. The role varies from helping to establish a diagnosis to evaluating associated abnormalities and planning surgical solutions or therapy for such conditions as meconium ileus and meconium plug syndrome. Plain radiographs and bowel contrast examinations serve as primary imaging modalities with ultrasound, computed tomography (CT) scan, and magnetic resonance imaging (MRI) playing roles in more complex cases.

Ultrasound can help correctly identify meconium ileus and meconium peritonitis and is useful in the diagnosis of enteric duplication cysts. In malrotation and anorectal anomalies, CT and MRI can provide superb anatomic detail and added diagnostic specificity. Intestinal duplications manifest as an abdominal mass at radiography, contrast enema examination, or ultrasound. On CT scan, most duplications manifest as smoothly rounded, fluid-filled cysts or tubular structures with thin, slightly enhancing walls. On MRI scan, the intracystic fluid has heterogenous signal density on T1-weighted images and homogeneous high signal intensity on T2-weighted images. Familiarity with these gastrointestinal abnormalities is essential for correct diagnosis and appropriate management

EDITORIAL COMMENT: Lilien et al accumulated a series of 45 newborns, initially thought to be normal, who had green vomiting in the first 72 hours of life; 20% required surgical intervention, 11% had nonsurgical obstruction (meconium plug, left microcolon), and 60% had idiopathic bilious vomiting. The last group of infants had a benign course. Of note, 56% of infants with surgical lesions had negative plain films of the abdomen and required contrast studies to establish the diagnosis. Lilien et al concluded that, whereas isolated green vomiting in an otherwise normal neonate is not invariably a surgical problem, a thorough investigation including contrast studies is warranted. We concur.

Lilien LD, Srinivasan G, Pyati SP, et al: Green vomiting in the first 72 hours in normal infants. Am J Dis Child 140:662, 1986.

With these principles in mind, the following illustrative cases deal with approaches to some serious and frequently seen gastrointestinal anomalies.

CASE PROBLEMS

Case One

Pregnancy complicated by hydramnios. A full-term male infant presents with increased salivation and chokes with feedings. Vomitus is never bile stained. Subsequently, respiratory distress develops. On physical examination, the infant is noted to be blue when crying and salivating excessively. The abdomen is distended. No obvious external malformation is noted. The x-ray film from the referring hospital is reported to demonstrate aspiration pneumonia.

AUTHOR'S COMMENT: With a history of hydramnios and increased salivation, the most likely diagnosis is esophageal atresia. The presence of abdominal distention suggests that atresia is associated with a fistula. The absence of bile staining of the vomitus indicates obstruction proximal to the entry of the common duct into the duodenum.

Diagnostic Maneuver

Pass a radiopaque nasogastric tube until it stops and obtain an x-ray film, including neck, chest, and upper abdomen. When passing a nasogastric tube for a diagnostic maneuver in suspected esophageal atresia, use as large a tube as will pass the nares. A small tube may enter the larynx and pass down the trachea, through the fistula to the esophagus, and into the stomach, giving the false impression of esophageal continuity. A large tube will not be tolerated in the larynx. If the tube passes through the esophagus to the stomach, esophageal atresia is ruled out.

Contrast medium should not be used in this evaluation until continuity of the esophagus has been demonstrated, because the inhalation of contrast medium from a blind esophageal pouch may produce pneumonia.

X-ray Findings in Esophageal Atresia

- There is a wide, air-filled pouch in the neck or upper mediastinum.
- The nasogastric tube is seen to stop in the upper mediastinum at about T3.
- Aspiration pneumonia may be noted, usually in the right upper lobe.
- Visible parts of the abdomen show air in the intestines (often as excess amount).
- Often skeletal anomalies are present (vertebrae/ribs).

EDITORIAL COMMENT: The VATER association is a nonrandom association of vertebral defects, imperforate anus, and esophageal atresia with tracheoesophageal fistula. The association may be broadened by the inclusion of cardiac defects, limb abnormalities, renal dysplasia, and single umbilical artery. These associated defects should be looked for.

Management Considerations in Esophageal Atresia[1, 18, 29, 30, 37, 59, 62, 63, 68]

More than 90% of all patients with esophageal atresia have the common variety of blind upper esophagus with the lower segment entering into the membranous posterior portion of the trachea above the carina as a fistula. This connects the acid-filled stomach to the tracheobronchial tree. A small percentage have esophageal atresia without tracheoesophageal fistula, in which case the abdomen is airless. From the first suspicion that a fistula exists until complete separation of the esophagus from the trachea is achieved, proper management is essential to prevent the fatal complication of aspiration pneumonia. Aspiration from the proximal pouch into the larynx is prevented by withholding all feedings and continuously aspirating the pouch with a sump tube. Reflux of gastric juice into the fistula is more damaging and more difficult to prevent but can be offset by attention to optimal positioning and by early surgical intervention. The child should be maintained in the prone, head-elevated position, which allows the stomach to fall anteriorly away from the esophagus and provides an inclined esophagus as a retardant to reflux of gastric juice.

Once the diagnosis is confirmed, rapid evaluation of the child for tolerance of surgical correction should be undertaken. Our criteria for primary repair (transthoracic extrapleural fistula ligation and end-to-end esophageal anastomosis) include the following:

- Chest clear to auscultation and on radiograph
- No life-threatening cardiac anomalies
- PaO_2 of 60 mm Hg or better in room air (usually from an established arterial catheter, such as umbilical)

If these criteria cannot be immediately satisfied, immediate gastrointestinal decompression by tube gastrostomy performed with the patient under local anesthesia should be achieved, and intensive respiratory care should be instituted. Established aspiration pneumonitis may require 2 to 3 weeks of intensive therapy to clear. If improvement is not rapid, tracheostomy may be an essential therapeutic component, because the fistula may interfere with effective coughing.

If prolonged preoperative care is required, nutritional support by total parenteral nutrition (TPN) will be essential. Feedings by gastrostomy are rarely tolerated as long as the tracheoesophageal fistula remains.

Cervical esophagostomy in esophageal atresia when initial repair cannot be made makes sham feeding necessary. This teaches the child the mechanics of swallowing as well as supporting the oral gratification so essential in this period for later motor development. An interposition procedure using colon or stomach will be required but is usually delayed until after 6 months of age.

EDITORIAL COMMENT: Spitz and associates reported on the outcome of 148 infants with esophageal atresia encountered over 5 years at the Hospital for Sick Children, Great Ormond Street, the regional referral center in London. The results were outstanding, with deaths predominantly resulting from associated congenital cardiac anomalies. They reported that endoscopy provided valuable information in planning the surgery, which should be delayed if there is aspiration pneumonia. They recommended immobilization and mechanical ventilation of the infants for 5 days after the operative repair.

Choudhury and colleagues have confirmed these excellent results even in infants with birth weights less than 1500 g. Death is associated with complex cardiac and chromosomal anomalies.

◆

Choudhury SR, Ashcraft KW, Sharp RJ, et al: Survival of patients with esophageal atresia; influence of birth weight, cardiac anomaly and late respiratory complications. J Pediatr Surg 34:70, 1999.

Spitz L, Kiely E, Brereton RJ: Esophageal atresia: Five year experience with 148 cases. J Pediatr Surg 22:103, 1987.

◆ DUODENAL OBSTRUCTION[21, 46, 67]

Obstruction of the duodenum may be complete or partial and due to extrinsic (malrotation, annular pancreas) or intrinsic lesions (duodenal atresia, duodenal stenosis). Malrotation is the most common extrinsic lesion obstructing the duodenum and because of the potential for vascular compromise to the bowel constitutes a true emergency in the neonate. Vomiting is the predominant presenting symptom and, if the obstruction is below the second part of the duodenum, it will be bile stained. Duodenal atresia is commonly associated with trisomy 21.

The diagnosis of duodenal atresia is made with a plain x-ray film of the abdomen revealing a "double-bubble," that is, the air- and fluid-filled stomach and duodenum. The presence of air bubbles beyond the second part of the duodenum suggests incomplete obstruction. An upper gastrointestinal series is indicated if malrotation is suspected.

◆ JEJUNOILEAL ANOMALIES[67]

Atresia is more common than stenosis, and ileal lesions are more common than jejunal lesions. It has been postulated that these lesions arise from intrauterine bowel ischemia.

Anomalies that produce obstruction of the small intestine may present with bilious vomiting, abdominal distention, and obstipation. The combination of bilious vomiting and passage of blood by rectum signifies vascular compromise of the intestine, necessitating immediate operative intervention. Atresias and stenoses must be differentiated from meconium ileus and meconium peritonitis as described later.

Plain radiographic studies may show nonspecific bowel dilation. It is extremely difficult to distinguish small bowel from colon in the neonatal period. Contrast enemas may show a microcolon together with one or more focal small bowel narrowings.

EDITORIAL COMMENT: Dalla Vecchia et al encountered 277 neonates with intestinal atresia and stenosis between 1972 and 1997. The level of obstruction was duodenal in 138 infants, jejunoileal in 128, and colonic in 21. Of the 277 neonates, 10 had obstruction in more than one site. Duodenal atresia was associated with prematurity (46%), maternal polyhydramnios (33%), Down syndrome (24%), annular pancreas (33%), and malrotation (28%). Jejunoileal atresia was associated with intrauterine volvulus (27%), gastroschisis (16%), and meconium ileus (11.7%). Operative mortality for neonates with duodenal atresia was 4%; with jejunoileal atresia, 0.8%; and with colonic atresia, 0%. Cardiac anomalies (with duodenal atresia) and ultra-short-bowel syndrome (<40 cm) requiring long-term total parenteral nutrition, which can be complicated by liver disease (with jejunoileal atresia), are the major causes of morbidity and mortality. The long-term survival rate for children with duodenal atresia was 86%; with jejunoileal atresia, 84%; and with colon atresia, 100%.

◆────────

Dalla Vecchia LK, Grosfeld JL, West WK, et al: Intestinal atresia and stenosis: A 25-year experience with 277 cases. Arch Surgery 133:490, 1998.

◆ MALROTATION/VOLVULUS[6, 43, 56, 58]

Incomplete rotation and fixation of the embryonic intestine as it returns to the fetal abdominal cavity from its embryonic extracoelomic position is referred to as malrotation. The normal alignment of the gut has the distal duodenum crossing to the left of the vertebral column to join the jejunum at a normally positioned ligament of Treitz with the cecum in the right lower quadrant. With malrotation, the cecum is undescended and situated in the right hypochondrium, abnormally fixed by bands crossing the second part of the duodenum.

Fetal bowel obstruction has a prevalence of 1 in 3000 to 5000 live births. Ultrasonographic diagnosis is made by demonstrating distended loops of bowel, fetal ascites, or echogenic bowel. Echogenic bowel, defined as small bowel more echogenic than liver or bone, in addition to bowel obstruction, has also been associated with congenital infections, cystic fibrosis, and chromosomal abnormalities.

Malrotation may be associated with other gastrointestinal lesions, including duodenal atresia, small intestinal atresia, gastroschisis, omphalocele, and congenital diaphragmatic hernia as well as cardiac, renal, and other major anomalies. Malrotation may present with bile-stained vomiting and abdominal distention. The obstruction may be intermittent. On the other hand, there may be a dramatic presentation with bile-stained vomiting, abdominal distention, possibly an abdominal mass, shock, pallor, and bloody stools. This presentation signifies a volvulus, that is, a strangulation obstruction with occlusion of blood flow to the gut.

Plain films of the abdomen may reveal a double bubble, with air patterns visible beyond the duodenum. Malrotation or volvulus must be diagnosed with upper gastrointestinal contrast studies, because the diagnosis is missed on plain films. The major purpose of the study is to establish the anatomic relationships and that the duodenum crosses the midline. A sharp cutoff with curved narrowing of the distal duodenum is characteristic of an obstruction secondary to a volvulus. If there is any doubt concerning the diagnosis, an exploratory laparotomy is mandatory, because the integrity of the bowel may be rapidly compromised by vascular occlusion.

EDITORIAL COMMENT: Volvulus of the bowel can be a fulminant and even fatal condition. Rapid diagnosis and prompt surgical intervention are mandatory to maintain the integrity of the bowel. The traditional approach to a suspected volvulus was a barium enema examination; however, this only provided indirect evidence of a volvulus if the cecum was not in the right lower quadrant. Volvulus of the small bowel may occur with a normal rotation and position of the colon. Therefore, an upper gastrointestinal approach has been adopted to establish the diagnosis. Both the site of obstruction and often the cause can be identified in this manner. Concerns about the contrast medium above the obstruction have proven to be unfounded. If the obstruction is complete, surgery is indicated and the contrast can be removed during the operative procedure.

Ultrasound is an additional means of evaluating infants with suspected upper gastrointestinal obstruction. Cohen and colleagues, using a fluid-aided ultrasound evaluation of the stomach and duodenum, were able to obtain a dynamic view of duodenal rotation and anatomy and correctly identify a number of lesions.

◆───

Cohen HL, Haller JO, Mestel AL, et al: Neonatal duodenum: Fluid-aided US examination. Radiology 164:805, 1987.

◆ MECONIUM ILEUS[32, 42]

Meconium ileus is a luminal obstruction of the distal small intestine by abnormal meconium, in contrast to meconium plug syndrome, which is a colonic obstruction. Meconium ileus is seen exclusively in patients with cystic fibrosis. The infants present with bile-stained vomiting and abdominal distention, and the meconium-filled loops have a doughy feel.

Radiographic evidence exists of complete obstruction with a characteristic soap bubble appearance produced by the air trapped in the thick meconium. Intrauterine perforation (meconium peritonitis) with the passage of sterile meconium into the peritoneal cavity may be reflected by calcification and predisposes to intestinal obstruction from adhesive bands.

The diagnosis may be confirmed with a water-soluble diatrizoate enema, which may also be therapeutic because it facilitates passage of the tenacious meconium. The study is contraindicated if signs of peritonitis or pneumoperitoneum are present.

◆ MECKEL DIVERTICULUM[5]

The omphalomesenteric duct usually obliterates spontaneously during embryonic development. Umbilical anomalies arise from fetal structures such as the omphalomesenteric duct or urachus, or from failure of closure of the umbilical fascial ring. Persistence of the omphalomesenteric duct may lead to several anomalies including umbilical sinus, umbilical cyst, Meckel diverticulum, or patent omphalomesenteric duct. A patent omphalomesenteric duct is usually associated with the ileum, but rarely may be with the cecum or appendix. If the duct remains patent at the umbilicus, the umbilicus is constantly moist from intestinal secretions, whereas persistence of a blind duct produces a "strawberry" tumor at the umbilicus. Persistence at the ileal end is noted in 2% of the population and results in Meckel diverticulum, which often also contains ectopic gastric and pancreatic tissue. Meckel diverticulum is rarely significant in the neonatal period but may present with painless rectal bleeding (the result of ulceration caused by gastric secretions) or obstruction. The diverticulum may also serve as the point for an intussusception.

◆ COLONIC LESIONS

Meconium Plug Syndrome[32]

Infants with meconium plug syndrome fail to pass meconium in the first 24 hours of life and present with clinical and radiologic features of intestinal obstruction. Rectal examination may prompt passage of meconium with a characteristic white plug; otherwise, a radiographic contrast enema is indicated. This may serve a dual function, that is, diagnosis and therapy. Inspissated meconium may be documented in the distal colon with dilation above. The contrast examination may precipitate passage of the meconium plug and relieve the symptoms. It is important to recognize that a meconium plug may be associated with cystic fibrosis and Hirschsprung disease. Hence, if the symptoms persist or recur, the infant should have a sweat chloride test and rectal mucosal biopsy.

Failure of a small premature newborn to adequately evacuate meconium for days or weeks has been attributed to probable necrotizing enterocolitis (NEC), or "microcolon of prematurity." Extremely premature infants may also present with intestinal obstruction and perforation secondary to inspissated meconium in the absence of cystic fibrosis.

Krasna[39] reported a series of 20 babies with birth weights between 480 and 1500 g who appeared to have an unusual type of "meconium plug syndrome," which required a contrast enema or Gastrografin upper gastrointestinal series to evacuate the plugs and relieve the obstruction. Many of the mothers were on magnesium sulfate or had eclampsia. The plugs were diagnosed late rather than shortly after birth, and the plugs were significant, extending to the right colon.

Greenholz[23] identified 13 patients who underwent treatment for intestinal obstruction secondary to inspissated meconium. The average birth weight was 760 g. Prenatal and postnatal risk factors included intrauterine growth retardation, maternal hypertension, prolonged administration of tocolytics, patent ductus arteriosus, hyaline membrane disease, and intraventricular hemorrhage.

Stooling was absent or infrequent during the first 2 weeks of life. The infants had abdominal distention or perforation between days 2 and 17 of life. Twelve patients required operative intervention. Findings invariably included one or more obstructing meconium plugs with proximal distention, and the dilated segments were frequently necrotic. None of the patients had cystic fibrosis. The markedly premature infant is at risk for obstruction and eventual perforation secondary to meconium plugs, presumably formed in conjunction with intestinal dysmotility. This entity must be distinguished from spontaneous intestinal perforation, which occurs in the absence of plugs (see later text). Prompt diagnosis and timely intervention require a high index of suspicion, including close attention to stooling patterns, careful abdominal examinations, and screening radiographs when indicated.

EDITORIAL COMMENT: The sonographic findings associated with meconium peritonitis in utero include polyhydramnios, ascites, dilatation of the bowel, hyperechoic bowel, and the tell-tale sign of intraabdominal calcification, which is considered to be pathognomonic of meconium ileus.

Neonatal Small Left Colon

Small left colon is a rare entity encountered predominantly among infants of diabetic mothers. The presenting features characteristically include delayed passage of meconium. Radiographic evidence includes dilation of the proximal colon, a clearly delineated transition zone, usually the splenic flexure, and narrowing of the distal colon. Resolution of the problem may be anticipated in the first month of life. Management is expectant.

Congenital Aganglionic Megacolon (Hirschsprung Disease)[65, 67]

Congenital aganglionic megacolon occurs in approximately 1 in 5000 births and is the most common cause of large-bowel obstruction in the newborn. It is a potentially serious and life-threatening entity that should be considered in any neonate with intestinal obstruction. It is more common in males, infants with trisomy 21, and siblings of children with the disorder. Hirschsprung dis-

ease is thought to result from defective migration of neural crest cells to the distal colon, leaving a segment of bowel aganglionic and dysfunctional.

Only 10% to 20% of patients with this disorder are first seen in the newborn period. In the infant, symptoms may present as acute obstruction, abdominal distention, vomiting, and delay in passing or failure to pass meconium. Constipation is a prominent feature. Irritability, poor feeding, and failure to thrive are other presenting features. Rectal examination or rectal stimulation such as with a rectal thermometer may produce an explosive gush of gas, and meconium may obscure the diagnosis; however, in the absence of rectal stimulation, no stools are passed.

Radiographic findings include nonspecific obstructive features, such as dilated loops of bowel and multiple fluid levels with the absence of air in the rectum. Barium studies should be performed without prior cleansing enemas. The findings include proximal dilation and distal narrowing in the aganglionic segment. Note, however, that the transition zone may not be clearly defined in the neonate and the barium may be retained for more than 24 hours. The diagnosis is established by biopsy, which must be of adequate depth to confirm the absence of ganglia in the nerve plexus.

Surgical treatment is mandated in the newborn. Generally a colostomy in a segment of normally innervated bowel is required. Definitive correction had usually been deferred until the end of the first year of life. Hirschsprung disease can now be successfully treated in the neonatal period with a one-stage pull-through. The short- and long-term results are as good as those with the three-stage procedure, with the child usually benefiting by having a shorter hospital stay and not requiring a stoma.

◆ ABDOMINAL WALL DEFECTS[5, 7, 15, 45, 69]

Omphalocele and gastroschisis are major defects of the abdominal wall resulting in parts of the gastrointestinal tract remaining outside the abdominal cavity. An omphalocele is covered by peritoneum and is frequently associated with other anomalies (congenital heart disease, trisomy 13 or 18, urinary tract anomalies, and Beckwith-Wiedemann syndrome, which includes macrosomia, macroglossia, omphalocele, and hypoglycemia; see Chapter 11). Malrotation is invariable with an omphalocele. The pentalogy of Cantrell refers to an omphalocele accompanied by defects in the diaphragm, sternum, heart, and pericardium.

Gastroschisis is a cleft in the abdominal wall to the right of the umbilicus. The extruded loops of bowel are thickened and covered by a fibrinous peel that develops in the latter part of the third trimester. Atresias, strictures, adhesions, and stenoses of the bowel accompany gastroschisis, but other malformation syndromes are unusual. The atretic areas are considered to be secondary to vascular insults.

Both lesions may be identified relatively early in gestation through alpha-fetoprotein screening (see Chapter 1) and the lesions accurately delineated with antenatal ultrasound. Delivery should take place at a tertiary center, because these cases represent complex management problems. The mode of delivery is determined by obstetric factors; vaginal delivery has not been proven to increase morbidity, mortality risk, or length of stay. Thermal regulation, fluid and electrolyte management, nutritional support, and measures to prevent infection are needed to complement the surgical team.

◆
Case Two

An infant takes initial feedings and then vomits bile-stained material. He is otherwise asymptomatic. Examination may or may not reveal abdominal distention. The anus is patent, and meconium is usually passed.

Any gastrointestinal obstruction distal to the entry of the common duct into the duodenum can lead to bile-stained vomiting. As a general rule (but not an infallible one), the earlier the onset of bile-stained vomiting, the higher the level of obstruction. Lower-level obstructions usually present initially with distention and failure to pass meconium with bile-stained vomiting occurring hours to days later.

X-ray findings vary with the level and type of obstruction. They may be clearly diagnostic, as is the case with complete obstruction of the duodenum (double bubble; duodenal atresia, annular pancreas, occasionally malrotation), or they may be equivocal, as in meconium ileus or Hirschsprung disease.

Eventual diagnosis is forthcoming in every case, given enough time and persistence. In the interim, effective nasogastric decompression and parenteral fluid, electrolyte, and nutritional support by vein sustain most of these infants, even if significant time lapses before diagnosis and definitive therapy. Only those lesions that may lead to catastrophe require urgent diagnosis and treatment, so attention should be directed to recognizing these entities rapidly. These entities include malrotation, neonatal perforations, and aganglionic megacolon.

◆
Case Three

Bilious vomiting, usually with some abdominal distention, occurs in a baby who passed normal meconium and has an open anus. X-ray films may show duodenal obstruction and usually show some gas throughout the abdomen.

Diagnosis: Malrotation

Malrotation is the most malevolent lesion of infancy because of its propensity toward volvulus with resultant strangulation of the superior mesenteric artery. This catastrophe can lead to total destruction of the digestive-absorptive segment of the intestinal tract—the jejunoileum. Furthermore, compared with any other single anomaly, this lesion is quite common. It must, therefore, always be in the differential diagnostic forefront to be rapidly ruled in or out. The most direct method for doing so is by upper gastrointestinal contrast study, which demonstrates obstruction of the duodenum. If obstruction is incomplete, the study reveals that the duodenal C loop fails to complete its normal course to a position in the left upper quadrant behind the stomach—the ligament of Treitz.

Contrast enemas, frequently recommended for diagnosis of malrotation in the past, may be confusing. The high-riding cecum with malpositioned appendix is diagnostic if clearly present, but often the cecal position is equivocal and difficult to locate clearly. Reflux of dye into the ileum may mask the position of the cecum. Therapeutic delay is intolerable here. One should quickly intervene operatively in any duodenal obstruction not *clearly* caused by an entity other than malrotation.

EDITORIAL COMMENT: Intestinal malrotation is

a common cause of upper gastrointestinal obstruction and presents with duodenal obstruction caused by volvulus of the midgut loop. Patients are at risk of catastrophic midgut infarction and malrotation is a more frequent cause of duodenal obstruction in infants than duodenal atresia. Bilious vomiting and bloody stools are the two most common clinical presentations in neonates. Rectal bleeding is an ominous sign; most patients manifesting such bleeding having gangrenous bowel. Urgent upper contrast studies are necessary. Ultrasound may also be helpful as a characteristic pattern of echogenic ascites, thickened bowel wall, dilated, fluid-filled bowel lumen, and lack of peristalsis may be seen in children with gangrenous bowel.

◆ BLOOD IN STOOL[2, 67]

Blood in the stool is a frequent problem confronting the neonatal team. Whether gross blood is present, streaks of blood are on the outside of an otherwise normal-appearing stool, or only occult blood is present, a prompt and diligent search for the cause is mandatory. In many instances no cause will be found; however, major pathologic disorders accounting for the blood in the stool must be ruled out.

Disorders resulting in the presence of frank blood in the stool range from swallowed maternal blood, an inconsequential problem, to life-threatening disorders, including NEC, malrotation with volvulus, disturbances of coagulation, ulcerative disorders, and infections. Blood-streaked stools are most commonly seen with an anal fissure or following trauma to the rectum with temperature probes and thermometers. Occult blood may signify blood swallowed during breast-feeding, upper gastrointestinal disorders, milk intolerance, hemorrhagic disorders, or NEC.

Gastrointestinal bleeding in the newborn must be differentiated from swallowed maternal blood caused by antepartum hemorrhage, the episiotomy, or cracked, bleeding nipples. The Apt test distinguishes maternal from fetal red blood cells, in that the fetal cells are resistant to alkali denaturation (addition of sodium hydroxide). Hence a solution containing maternal blood changes from pink to brown. Other laboratory tests include a complete blood count with a differential and smear; platelet count; coagulation studies such as partial thromboplastin time, prothrombin time, and fibrinogen level; blood culture; and a plain film of the abdomen. These tests should point to the cause of the bleeding, which can then be managed appropriately.

◆ SPONTANEOUS INTESTINAL PERFORATION

A new disorder has emerged amongst the ELBW infants. It has been designated *spontaneous intestinal perforation* and may be indistinguishable from NEC. Spontaneous perforation, however, occurs much less frequently than NEC in preterm infants. The infants may have dramatic abdominal distention often associated with blue discoloration of the abdominal wall. Obvious clinical signs of bowel perforation are infrequent with spontaneous intestinal perforation.

Infants with spontaneous perforation were smaller and born more prematurely when compared with infants who had NEC.[3, 50] The onset of illness was earlier and was associated with antecedent hypotension, leukocytosis, and a gasless appearance on abdominal radiograph. Infants with spontaneous perforations are more likely to have received postnatal steroids or to have systemic candidiasis. Conditions associated with fetal or neonatal hypoxia are important antecedents for this emerging distinct clinical entity. Other factors implicated in the etiology include indomethacin therapy, patent ductus arteriosus, and intraventricular hemorrhage. Peritoneal drainage alone may be considered definitive therapy for intestinal perforation in the majority of extremely immature infants.

Part Three

NECROTIZING ENTEROCOLITIS[33–35, 53, 55]

Deanne Wilson-Costello
Robert M. Kliegman
Avroy A. Fanaroff

NEC remains the major gastrointestinal cause of morbidity and mortality among the neonatal intensive care population. The incidence varies among countries and among units. Uauy et al,[64] reporting on behalf of the National Institute of Child Health and

Development Neonatal Multicenter Research Network, noted that 10% of 2681 infants with birth weights between 501 and 1500 g had proven NEC (Bell stage II and beyond; Table 6–14). Using data from a nationwide survey, Sweet[60] had estimated an occurrence rate of 22 per 1000 admissions. Most infants with NEC have a low birth weight, are appropriately grown, and are immature.

Although patent ductus arteriosus, low Apgar scores, and umbilical catheters have been implicated in the etiology, matched studies did not identify these as risk factors. Nonetheless, the odds ratio for NEC increased with antepartum hemorrhage, pro-

longed rupture of membranes beyond 36 hours, and 5-minute Apgar scores below 7.

The age of onset for NEC varies inversely with gestation.[53] In approximately half of the term infants with NEC, symptoms present in the first day of life. Specific risk factors for NEC among term infants include cyanotic heart disease, polycythemia, and twin gestation. Whereas sporadic cases of endemic NEC occur throughout the year, temporal and geographic epidemic clusters are associated with gastrointestinal illness among nursery staff.

Infection plays a prominent role and the disease occurs in clusters with various outbreaks reported from *Escherichia coli* and

Table 6–14. Modified Bell's Staging Criteria for Neonatal Necrotizing Enterocolitis

Stage	Systemic Signs	Intestinal Signs	Radiologic Signs	Treatment
IA—Suspected NEC	Temperature instability, apnea, bradycardia, lethargy	Elevated pregavage residuals, mild abdominal distension, emesis, guaiac-positive stool	Normal or intestinal dilation, mild ileus	Nothing by mouth, antibiotics for 3 d pending cultures
IB—Suspected NEC	Same as above	Bright red blood from rectum	Same as above	Same as above
IIA—Definite NEC: mildly ill	Same as above	Same as above, *plus* diminished or absent bowel sounds with or without abdominal tenderness	Intestinal dilation, ileus, pneumatosis intestinalis	Nothing by mouth, antibiotics for 7–10 d if examination is normal in 24–48 h
IIB—Definite NEC: moderately ill	Above *plus* mild metabolic acidosis and mild thrombocytopenia	Above *plus* definite abdominal tenderness, with or without abdominal cellulitis or right lower quadrant mass, absent bowel sounds	Same as stage IIA with or without portal vein gas, with or without ascites	Nothing by mouth, antibiotics for 14 d $NaHCO_3$ for acidosis
IIIA—Advanced NEC: severely ill, bowel intact	Same as IIB *plus* hypotension, bradycardia, severe apneas, combined respiratory and metabolic acidosis, disseminated intravascular coagulation, neutropenia, anuria	Above *plus* signs of generalized peritonitis, marked tenderness, distension of abdomen, and abdominal wall erythema	Same as stage IIB, definite ascites	Same as above *plus* 200 ml/kg/d fluids, fresh frozen plasma, inotropic agents; intubation, ventilation therapy; paracentesis; surgical intervention if patient fails to improve with medical management within 24–48 h
IIIB—Advanced NEC: severely ill, bowel perforation	Same as stage IIIA	Same as stage IIIA	Same as stage IIB *plus* pneumoperitoneum	Same as above *plus* surgical intervention

Klebsiella, Salmonella, and *Clostridium* species. Viruses have also been implicated. Recent reports suggest significant alterations in the gastrointestinal flora colonizing critically ill neonates. A review of peritoneal cultures from infants undergoing surgery for NEC reveals a predominance of *Klebsiella* and *Enterobacter* species (63%), frequent *E. coli* (21%), coagulase-negative *Staphylococci* (30%), occasional anaerobes (6%) and *Candida* isolates (10%).[47] Clinical classifications and the pathogenesis of the disease are outlined in Tables 6–14 and 6–15 and Figure 6–1. The inciting event may be hypoxemia, sepsis, low cardiac output, or factors within the bowel such as hypertonic feeding. Although feeding precedes the onset of symptoms in most cases, delayed feeding does not lower the incidence of NEC and, in fact, may promote its occurrence.[40] It remains unclear whether the major factor is the formula itself, the volume of formula, the rate at which feeding is advanced, or the effect of the bacteria on the formula.

Gut ischemia is a potential risk factor for NEC. Intrauterine growth retarded infants with aberrant fetal Doppler blood flow velocity waveforms[26] and infants born to cocaine-abusing mothers show increased rates of NEC.[14, 61] In addition, cocaine-exposed infants with NEC are more likely to require

Table 6–15. Clinical Classification of Neonatal Enterocolitis*

Classic NEC
  Endemic
  Epidemic
    Identifiable organism
    No organism identified
Benign NEC (pneumatosis coli)
NEC following exchange transfusion
NEC following mucosal injury
  Hypertonic feeding
  Allergic enteritis
  Nonspecific diarrhea
  Polycythemia
Primary bowel pathologic findings
  Spontaneous bowel perforation
  Congenital intestinal obstruction
Neonatal appendicitis
Neonatal pseudomembranous colitis

Adapted from Kliegman RM, Fanaroff AA: Necrotizing enterocolitis. N Engl J Med 310:1093, 1984.
*Each category is a distinct clinical and pathologic entity. The inclusive heading of neonatal enterocolitis includes classic idiopathic NEC (I, II), NEC associated with other factors (III, IV), and those newborn diseases that clinically resemble NEC (V, VI, VII). These disease processes may be distinguished from each other by history, clinical course, laboratory tests, and pathologic examination.

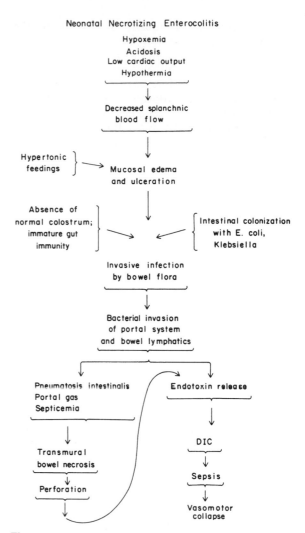

Figure 6–1. Possible factors in etiology and outcome of neonatal necrotizing enterocolitis. DIC, disseminated intravascular coagulation. (From Burrington JD: Clin Perinatol 5:30, 1978.)

surgical intervention, have massive gangrene, or die.[14]

The role of cytokines in the pathogenesis of NEC has emerged. Caplan et al[13] reported a small series of patients with NEC in whom both tumor necrosis factor and platelet activating factor (which synergistically can produce an injury pattern in the rat gut resembling NEC) were elevated. In an experimental model of asphyxiated rats, pretreatment with enteral platelet activating factor (PAF) acetylhydrolase (a PAF-degrading enzyme) significantly reduced the incidence of NEC.[12] Preliminary work suggests that nitric oxide, a vasodilator produced by endothelium, may have a protective role in regulating intestinal vascular tone. Administration of a reversible nitric oxide blocker increases swine intestinal vascular resistance.[49] Mucosal irritation, leading to damaged endothelial cells with reduced levels of nitric oxide, has been suggested as a possible mechanism for NEC. Any consideration of the pathogenesis of NEC must, therefore, include the interrelationships among ischemia, immaturity, infection, immunity, and nutrition.[42]

In summary, NEC is a multifactorial disorder with a delicate balance between bowel perfusion, enteric organisms, and nutritional intake.[37] The disorder was reduced by the prenatal administration of steroids,[27] although larger series have not confirmed this, or possibly by the postnatal administration of immunoglobulin A.[17] Breast milk is also protective, as shown by Lucas and Cole[44] in a multicenter study addressing the role of diet in NEC. Furthermore, pasteurizing the milk did not reduce its effectiveness and the combination of breast milk and formula was less likely to be associated with NEC than was formula alone. Breast milk contains bifidus factor, which enhances gut colonization with lactobacillus. In an experimental rat model, bifidobacterial supplementation significantly reduced the incidence of NEC.[11] Mothers should therefore be encouraged to provide breast milk for their own infants during their sojourn in the intensive care unit.

Prophylactic oral antibiotics confer protection against NEC in preterm infants and have been associated with a 50% reduction in its incidence.[57] However, widespread implementation of prophylactic antibiotics is not recommended because of the danger of emergence of resistant organisms. The use of prophylactic oral antibiotics should be restricted to high-risk nurseries for short time periods.

◆ CLINICAL FEATURES[36]

The clinical features of NEC are variable, and the signs and symptoms may not be specific. Most often, temperature instability, lethargy, abdominal distention, and retention of feedings develop. Occult blood is present in the stools, which may sometimes be frankly bloody. Reducing substances are often detected before the onset of NEC.[9] Apnea may be a prominent feature as well as bilious vomiting, increased abdominal distention, acidosis, and disseminated intravascular coagulation. The characteristic x-ray features are pneumatosis intestinalis, with bubbles or layers of gas in the wall of the bowel as well as portal venous gas. Free air within the peritoneum is associated with perforation of a viscus. Engel et al[19] demonstrated that about 30% of the gas in the wall of the bowel is hydrogen, the product of bacterial fermentation of formula.

Medical management includes nasogastric suction, IV fluids, and broad-spectrum systemic antibiotics[20] (Appendix A-2). Frequent abdominal examinations as well as determination of abdominal girth and cross-table lateral x-ray films are important to detect free air. We maintain the infants on a regimen of nothing per os for up to 2 weeks while they receive all nutritional support intravenously. The main indication for surgery is perforation, which is demonstrated by free air in the peritoneum.[22] However, surgery may also be considered for infants with worsening clinical status, refractory disseminated intravascular coagulation, or acidosis. The discovery of an abdominal mass and gas in the portal venous system is not necessarily an indication for surgery. Some infants may require surgery at a later stage because of the development of strictures. With present vigorous medical and surgical management as outlined earlier, 75% of infants should survive. Developmentally, at follow-up these infants usually do extremely well. Many complications relate to short bowel syndrome or infections and metabolic complications related to TPN.

Current research efforts concentrate on early identification of the severity of NEC. Edelson et al[16] reported that intestinal fatty acid binding protein in the blood of infants with NEC is a specific marker for severe NEC.

COMMENT: NEC is an entity that has emerged as a prominent factor in neonatal morbidity with the advent of neonatal intensive care. It is also known that the entity is seen in many neonatal intensive care centers and not observed at all in others. The phenomenon strongly suggests the multifactorial and perhaps iatrogenic nature of the disease. The incidence or occurrence depends on the presence or absence of the factors and nursery routines enumerated by the authors in the previous paragraph.

CASE PROBLEMS

◆ ─────────────────────────────

Case One

C. K. weighs 1300 g at 32 weeks' gestation; his Apgar scores were 4 at 1 minute and 6 at 5 minutes. Respiratory distress syndrome (RDS) develops on the first day of life, an arterial catheter is placed at the level of T10, and 60% oxygen but no assisted ventilation is used. The RDS resolves by 48 hours of life, and the catheter is removed. Standard formula is first fed on the third day of life. On the eighth day, abdominal tenderness and distention are observed, and the nurses reported guaiac-positive stools, 5 mL residual from the last feeding, and a higher incubator temperature required to maintain body temperature.

◆ *What is the most likely preliminary diagnosis?*
1. *Meconium plug syndrome*
2. *Necrotizing enterocolitis*
3. *Septicemia*
4. *Malrotation*
5. *Hirschsprung disease*

Any neonate with a triad of abdominal distention, Hematest- or guaiac-positive stools, and retention of gastric formula should be suspected of having NEC and should be immediately evaluated for such. The initial manifestation of NEC may be indistinguishable from septicemia, and a positive blood culture is obtained from 30% of infants with NEC. The answer is 2, necrotizing enterocolitis.

◆ *Initially, how should this patient be evaluated?*
1. *Culture of blood, urine, cerebrospinal fluid, and stool*
2. *Complete blood count and clotting profile*
3. *Barium swallow*
4. *Gastrografin enema*
5. *Anteroposterior and lateral film of abdomen*
6. *Blood gases and serum electrolytes*

1. Because sepsis is present in many if not all of these patients and many investigators believe that infection is directly related to the pathogenesis of the disease, blood, urine, stool, and cerebrospinal fluid cultures should be obtained.
2. A complete blood count, blood smear, and clotting profile should be ordered and the type and cross-match sent to the blood bank. Take specific note of fragmented red cells (disseminated intravascular coagulation), neutropenia (margination of white cells), and thrombocytopenia.

3. Barium swallow is not indicated immediately. If there is evidence of obstruction without pneumatosis on the flat film, then a barium swallow may be necessary to exclude malrotation.
4. Gastrografin enema may be curative if there is a meconium plug but is contraindicated in this case because the hyperosmolar contrast medium may produce further damage to already compromised bowel and result in perforation.
5. Abdominal x-ray films, both KUB (kidney, ureter, and bladder) and cross-table lateral, should be ordered to detect the presence of pneumatosis intestinalis, hepatic portal gas, or free intraabdominal gas, indicating a perforated viscus. If no free air is seen initially but there is pneumatosis present, the cross-table lateral x-ray film should be repeated every 4 to 6 hours or sooner if there is clinical deterioration.
6. It is important to evaluate acid-base status and serum electrolytes in infants with suspected gastrointestinal disturbances. Correction of these metabolic derangements is crucial before submitting these precarious infants to major surgery.

The x-ray films reveal pneumatosis intestinalis with no air in the liver or free intraperitoneal air. The blood pressure is 55/35; blood gases pH 7.32, Pao_2 65, and Pco_2 40; bicarbonate 20; serum sodium 132; potassium 4.8; chloride 105; BUN 10; hematocrit 38%; white blood cell count 14,900 with 70% segmented cells; platelets adequate; clotting profile normal. Pediatric surgeons were consulted, and together with the nursery staff, they managed the case.

◆ *The following treatments should be instituted (true or false):*
1. *Nasogastric suction, IV fluids, and nothing per os (NPO)*
2. *Systemic and orogastric antibiotics*
3. *Laparotomy*
4. *Exchange transfusion*
5. *Placement of central hyperalimentation line*

1. True. It is imperative to decompress the abdomen with a large oral or nasogastric tube. Carefully record all intake and output, weigh the baby twice daily, and measure abdominal girth frequently. IV fluid therapy must take into consideration significant third-space losses. We keep patients with documented NEC NPO for at least 10 days.
2. True. The patient was started on appro-

priate doses of IV *piperacillin* and an *aminoglycoside.* We no longer administer antibiotics via nasogastric tube because this has not proved to be efficacious.

3. False. There is no clear-cut indication for a laparotomy at this stage. Whereas surgery is clearly indicated for intestinal perforation, some units operate when medical management fails to correct the shock-acidosis; if there is persistent cellulitis of the anterior abdominal wall or if radiologically a single dilated loop of bowel persists.

4. False. With normal clotting studies and no evidence of bleeding or significant hyperbilirubinemia, exchange transfusion is not indicated.

5. False. TPN is going to be necessary for this infant. However, with septicemia likely, it is advisable to wait until the sepsis has been controlled and the general condition stabilized before placing a central line for IV nutrition. Some centers provide all nutritive support with peripheral lines, using glucose–amino acid mixtures supplemented with IV fat.

One hour later, the blood pressure drops from 55/35 to 40/0. The urine output decreases to less than 1 mL/h, and the abdomen is more distended, edematous, and tender. On physical examination, the infant is pink with a wide pulse pressure, tachycardia, and warm extremities. Repeat complete blood count reveals white blood cell count of 3.1, with 10% segmented cells and 10% bands.

◆ *These data should be interpreted as (true or false):*
1. *Septic shock*
2. *Perforated abdominal viscus*
3. *Patent ductus arteriosus with congestive heart failure*
4. *Pneumothorax*
5. *Third-space loss*

1. and 5. True. The patient as described—pink with wide pulse pressure, tachycardia, and warm extremities—has the classic features of warm shock. When such cases are untreated, the blood pressure decreases further and vasoconstriction predominates, transforming the "warm" shock to "cold" shock. A major factor contributing to shock in patients with NEC is the massive third space that develops in the abdomen, which results from the inflammatory response and bowel necrosis. These large fluid and

protein losses result in hypovolemia and require urgent therapy. The mainstay of treatment is to elevate the blood pressure by supporting the intravascular space with sufficient blood, plasma, or crystalloid to maintain the blood pressure and urine output. Whole blood is preferred because it remains in the intravascular space, whereas other fluids leak through the damaged capillaries and contribute to intestinal edema. Large volumes of crystalloid may be required. Neutropenia may be documented in NEC without bacteremia. Margination of neutrophils is assumed, because marrow reserves are not depleted.

2. False. Although the sudden deterioration is suggestive of perforation and evaluation by transillumination and an x-ray film is certainly indicated, no perforation was present at this time. The wide pulse pressure is not usually detected at the time of perforation.

3. False. Tachycardia, edema, and wide pulse pressure are present with patent ductus arteriosus and congestive heart failure. However, the striking abdominal findings, together with the diminished blood pressure, suggest that this is not the primary problem. Patent ductus arteriosus, however, is found frequently in infants with NEC.

4. False. This is unlikely, given the complete picture, particularly with a pink baby and wide pulse pressure.

Two hours later, x-ray films show increased distention and no evidence of free air but the appearance of bowel "floating" in the abdomen.

◆ *What is the significance of this finding?*
Bowel floating in the abdomen in a patient with sepsis and a distended tender abdomen indicates ascites caused by peritonitis. Because many cases of "intraabdominal sepsis" are caused by anaerobic bacteria, anaerobic antimicrobial coverage should be started following paracentesis. (Clindamycin is instituted for infants with suspected NEC and perforation.)

On surgically introducing a drain into the left lower quadrant, 10 mL of purulent fluid is removed. The cell count shows 90,000 white blood cells with 75% PMNs. Gram stain shows both gram-positive and gram-negative rods.

The patient is noted to have blood oozing from venipuncture sites, with petechiae and a falling hematocrit despite multiple blood transfusions.

Laboratory data

CBC Hct = 28; platelets 5000; smear shows fragmented red blood cells and burr cells

Prothrombin time = patient, 50 seconds; control, 10 seconds

Partial thromboplastin time = patient, 180 seconds; control, 30 seconds

Fibrinogen = 50 mg/dL (normal 200 mg/dL)

Fibrin split products = 4+ (normal not present)

Disseminated intravascular coagulation has complicated the picture, and therefore an exchange transfusion with fresh blood is performed (see Chapter 16).

Blood pressure, urine output, and activity are normal for 3 days. The abdomen is softer, but there is still some edema of the abdominal wall. Repeated x-ray films fail to reveal free intraabdominal air. After 5 days of relative stability, the patient becomes acutely distended with signs of respiratory embarrassment.

◆ *Which of the following management options is appropriate?*

1. *Repeat clotting profile and exchange transfusion.*
2. *Percuss abdomen and then transilluminate while awaiting x-ray film.*
3. *Repeat blood cultures and change antibiotics.*
4. *Measure blood gas and increase environmental oxygen.*

1. This acute episode following a period of stability cannot entirely be attributed to disseminated intravascular coagulation.
2. This acute change is probably due to intestinal perforation. Abdominal percussion used to demonstrate the absence of hepatic dullness and positive transillumination may confirm suspicions before the cross-table lateral x-ray film has been developed. The film in this instance demonstrated free air.
3. Blood culture should be repeated, but there is no reason to change antibiotics at this time.
4. This is only symptomatic management. The basic cause for the abdominal distention and respiratory embarrassment must be determined. The blood gas will indicate the need for ventilatory support.

The child is brought to the operating room where the perforated area of ileum is resected and an ileostomy and colostomy are performed. Two days postoperatively a central IV catheter is placed in the operating room and TPN is administered via this route for 21 days. After this period of being NPO, he was started on breast milk and did well.

◆
Case Two

M. P. is born at 34 weeks' gestation, weighing 1200 g. His perinatal course is complicated by intrauterine growth retardation, hyperbilirubinemia, and polycythemia, requiring a single volume exchange transfusion done through an umbilical venous catheter. At 8 days of age, abdominal distention, hematochezia, acidosis, and hypotension develop. NEC is diagnosed and is treated with medical management. He recovers and begins enteral feedings 14 days after the onset of acute NEC.

M. P. is discharged home at 6 weeks of age, having tolerated full volume enteral feedings for 2 weeks. Three weeks after discharge, he has acute abdominal distention, vomiting, and hematochezia. Abdominal examination reveals guarding and tenderness.

◆ *What is the most likely diagnosis?*
1. **Clostridium difficile** *infection*
2. *Intestinal stricture*
3. *Anal fissure*
4. *Milk protein allergy*

Intestinal stricture. Strictures are one of the most common complications of NEC, occurring in 10% to 35% of all survivors.[52, 66] They result from healing and cicatricial scarring of an ischemic area of bowel.[38] Signs include hematochezia, vomiting, abdominal distention, and sudden bowel obstruction.[10] Strictures usually present in the first 2 months following acute NEC, but may present as late as 6 months afterward.[10]

◆ *Which of the following management options is appropriate?*
1. *Perform stool culture and start oral antibiotics*
2. *Change infant to soy formula feedings*
3. *Obtain abdominal x-ray, do barium enema, and consult pediatric surgery*
4. *Reassure mother that rectal bleeding is common, and send child home with office follow-up in 1 to 2 days.*

Any neonate with past history of NEC followed by the onset of hematochezia and vomiting should undergo evaluation to rule out strictures. Recent reports have suggested that clinical observation alone is associated with significant morbidity in this population. Failure to rapidly detect and manage stricture complications has resulted in intestinal perforation and life-threatening sepsis.[28] The proper management includes abdominal x-rays, barium enema, and pediatric surgical evaluation.

Abdominal x-rays reveal acute intestinal obstruction. Barium enema demonstrates multiple strictures of the ileum, transverse and descend-

ing colon, and rectosigmoid region, as well as perforation with intraperitoneal contrast extravasation.

Emergency ileostomy is performed. Postoperatively, M. P. has a rocky course, complicated by multiple episodes of sepsis and feeding intolerance. He is given several courses of antibiotics and nearly 3 weeks of hyperalimentation nutrition.

Approximately 1 month after surgery, M. P. is noted to have direct hyperbilirubinemia, poor growth, hepatomegaly, and elevated liver function tests. Workup includes a negative hepatitis panel, normal hepatic and gallbladder ultrasound, negative sepsis, TORCH (toxoplasmosis, rubella, cytomegalovirus, and herpes simplex) workups, and a normal newborn screen.

◆ *What is the most likely diagnosis?*
1. *Biliary atresia*
2. *TPN cholestasis*
3. *α_1-Antitrypsin deficiency*
4. *Cystic fibrosis*

Although all of the above are possible, the most likely diagnosis is TPN cholestasis. It typically develops after 2 or more weeks of enteral fasting with TPN providing the sole nutritional support. With initiation of trophic feeding to enhance bile flow, TPN cholestasis gradually resolves over 1 to 3 months.[22] If persisting despite enteral feeding, a full diagnostic workup is indicated.

By 6 weeks after operation, M. P. has advanced to full-volume enteral feedings with slow resolution of the TPN cholestasis. However, he continues to demonstrate poor growth and develops increasing stool output through the ileostomy. He undergoes a second surgery to reanastomose the bowel. Following reanastomosis, M. P.'s nutritional status improves and he is discharged to home. At 10 months of age, he is tolerating a normal diet, although he remains at the third percentile for all growth parameters.

REFERENCES

1. Abrahamson J, Shandling B: Esophageal atresia in the underweight baby: A challenge. J Pediatr Surg 7:608, 1972.
2. Abramo TJ, Evans JS, Kokomoor FW, et al: Occult blood in stools and necrotizing enterocolitis: Is there a relationship? Am J Dis Child 142:451, 1988.
3. Adderson EE, Pappin A, Pavia AT: Spontaneous intestinal perforation in premature infants: A distinct clinical entity associated with systemic candidiasis. J Pediatr Surg 33:1463, 1998.
4. Amoury RA, Beatty EC, Wood WG, et al: Histology of the intestine in human gastroschisis—relationship to intestinal malfunction: Dissolution of the "peel" and its ultrastructural characteristics. J Pediatr Surg 23:950, 1988.
5. Amoury RA: Meckel's diverticulum. In Welch KJ, Randolph JG, Ravitch MM, et al, eds: Pediatric Surgery. Chicago: Year Book, 1986.
6. Berdon W, Baker D, Bull S, et al: Midgut malrotation and volvulus: Which films are most helpful? Radiology 96:375, 1970.
7. Bethel CAI, Seashore JH, Touloukian RJ: Cesarean section does not improve outcome in gastroschisis. J Pediatr Surg 24:1, 1989.
8. Bond SJ, Harrison MR, Filly RA, et al: Severity of intestinal damage in gastroschisis: Correlation with prenatal sonographic findings. J Pediatr Surg 23:520, 1988.
9. Book L, Herbst J, Jung A: Carbohydrate malabsorption in necrotizing enterocolitis. Pediatrics 57:201, 1976.
10. Brown EG, Sweet AY: Neonatal necrotizing enterocolitis. Pediatr Clin North Am 29:1149, 1982.
11. Caplan MS, Miller-Catchpole R, Kaup S, et al: Bifidobacterial supplementation reduces the incidence of necrotizing enterocolitis in a neonatal rat model. Gastroenterology 117:577, 1999.
12. Caplan MS, Lickerman M, Adler L, et al: The role of recombinant platelet-activating factor acetyl hydrolase in a neonatal rat model of necrotizing enterocolitis. Pediatr Res 42:779, 1997.
13. Caplan MS, Sun X-M, Hsueh W, et al: Role of platelet activating factor and tumor necrosis factor-alpha in neonatal necrotizing enterocolitis. J Pediatr 116:960, 1990.
14. Czyrko C, Del Pin CA, O'Neill JA, et al: Maternal cocaine abuse and necrotizing enterocolitis: Outcome and survival. J Pediatr Surg 26:414, 1991.
15. de Vries PA: The pathogenesis of gastroschisis and omphalocele. J Pediatr Surg 15:245, 1980.
16. Edelson MB, Sonnino RE, Bagwell CE, et al: Plasma intestinal fatty acid binding protein in neonates with necrotizing enterocolitis: A pilot study. J Pediatr Surg 34:1453, 1999.
17. Eibl MM, Wolf HM, Furnkranz H, et al: Prevention of necrotizing enterocolitis in low-birth-weight infants by IgA-IgG feeding. N Engl J Med 319:1, 1988.
18. Ein S, Therman T: A comparison of the results of primary repair of esophageal atresia with tracheoesophageal fistulas using end-to-side and end-to-end anastomosis. J Pediatr Surg 8:641, 1973.
19. Engle R, Virnig N, Hunt C, et al: Origin of mural gas in necrotizing enterocolitis. Pediatr Res 7:292, 1973.
20. Faix RG, Polley TZ, Grasela TH: A randomized, controlled trial of parenteral clindamycin in neonatal necrotizing enterocolitis. J Pediatr 112:271, 1988.
21. Fomon S: Infant Nutrition. Philadelphia: WB Saunders, 1967.
22. Freeman RB, Lloyd DJ, Miller SS, et al: Surgical treatment of necrotizing enterocolitis: A population-based study in the Grampian Region, Scotland. J Pediatr Surg 23:942, 1988.
23. Greenholz SK, Perez C, Wesley JR, Marr CC: Meconium obstruction in markedly premature infant. J Pediatr Surg 31:117, 1996.
24. Grosfeld JL, Molinari F, Chaet M, et al: Gastrointestinal perforation and peritonitis in infants and children: Experience with 179 cases over ten years. Surgery 120:650, 1996 (discussion, 655).
25. Haber BA, Lake AM: Cholestatic jaundice in the newborn. Clin Perinatol 17:483, 1990.
26. Hackett GA, Campbell S, Gamru H, et al: Doppler studies in the growth retarded fetus and prediction

of neonatal necrotizing enterocolitis, hemorrhage and neonatal morbidity. BMJ 294:13, 1987.

27. Halac E, Halac J, Begue EF, et al: Prenatal and postnatal corticosteroid therapy to prevent neonatal necrotizing enterocolitis: A controlled trial. J Pediatr 117:132, 1990.

28. Hartman GE, Drugas GT, Shochat SS: Post-necrotizing enterocolitis strictures presenting with sepsis or perforation: Risk of clinical observation. J Pediatr Surg 23:562, 1988.

29. Holder TM, Ashcraft KW, Sharp RJ, Amoury RA: Care of infants with esophageal atresia, tracheoesophageal fistula, and associated anomalies. J Thorac Cardiovasc Surg 94:828, 1987.

30. Holder T, Cloud D, Lewis J Jr, et al: Esophageal atresia and tracheoesophageal fistula: A survey of its members by the Surgical Section of the American Academy of Pediatrics. Pediatrics 34:542, 1964.

31. Jassani MN, Gauderer MW, Fanaroff AA, et al: A perinatal approach to the diagnosis and management of GI malformations. Obstet Gynecol 59:33, 1982.

32. Jhaveri MK, Kumar SP: Passage of the first stool in very low birth weight infants. Pediatrics 79:1005, 1987.

33. Kliegman RM: Models of pathogenesis of necrotizing enterocolitis. J Pediatr 117:S2, 1990.

34. Kliegman RM, Fanaroff AA: Necrotizing enterocolitis. N Engl J Med 310:1093, 1984.

35. Kliegman RM, Horn M, Jones P, et al: Epidemiologic study of necrotizing enterocolitis among low birth weight infants. J Pediatr 100:440, 1982.

36. Kliegman RM, Walsh M: Neonatal necrotizing enterocolitis: Pathogenesis, classification and spectrum of disease. Curr Prob Pediatr 17:215, 1987.

37. Koop C, Hamilton J: Atresia of the esophagus: Factors affecting survival in 249 cases. Z Kinerchir 5:319, 1968.

38. Kosloske AM, Musemeche CA: Necrotizing enterocolitis of the neonate. Clin Perinatol 16:97, 1989.

39. Krasna IH, Rosenfeld D, Salerno P: Is it necrotizing enterocolitis, microcolon or prematurity, or delayed meconium plug? A dilemma in the tiny premature infant. Pediatr Surg 31:855, 1996.

40. LaGamma EF, Ostertag SG, Birenbaum H: Failure of delayed oral feeding to prevent necrotizing enterocolitis. Am J Dis Child 139:385, 1985.

41. Lake A, Walker W: Neonatal necrotizing enterocolitis: A disease of altered host defense. Clin Gastroenterol 6:463, 1977.

42. Lloyd DA: Meconium ileus. In Welch KJ, Randolph JG, Ravitch MM, eds: Pediatric Surgery. Chicago: Year Book, 1986.

43. Louw J, Barnard C: Congenital intestinal atresia. Observations on its origin. Lancet 2:1065, 1955.

44. Lucas A, Cole TJ: Breast milk and neonatal necrotizing enterocolitis. Lancet 336:1519, 1990.

45. Meller JL, Reyes HM, Loeff DS: Gastroschisis and omphalocele. Clin Perinatol 16:113, 1989.

46. Miro J, Bard H: Congenital atresia and stenosis of the duodenum: The impact of a prenatal diagnosis. Am J Obstet Gynecol 158:555, 1988.

47. Mollitt DL, Tepas JJ, Talbert JL: The microbiology of neonatal peritonitis. Arch Surg 123:176, 1988.

48. Nair R, Hadley GP: Intestinal malrotation—experience with 56 patients. S Afr J Surg 34:73, 1996.

49. Nowicki P, Edwards R: Effect of N^G-monomethyl-L-arginine on postnatal intestinal vascular resistance (Abstract). Pediatr Res 31:64A, 1992.

50. Raghuveer G, Speidel B, Marlow N, Porter H: Focal intestinal perforation in preterm infants is an emerging disease. Acta Paediatr 85:237, 1996.

51. Reyes HM, Vidyasagar D, eds: Clinics in Perinatology, Neonatal Surgery. Vol 16. Philadelphia: WB Saunders, March 1989.

52. Ricketts RR, Jerles ML: Neonatal necrotizing enterocolitis: Experience with 100 consecutive surgical patients. World J Surg 14:600, 1990.

53. Ross Symposium on Pediatric Research: Necrotizing enterocolitis in the newborn infant. Columbus, Ohio, Ross Laboratories, 1975.

54. Russell MB, Russell CA, Niebuhr E: An epidemiologic study of Hirschsprungs's disease and additional anomalies. Acta Paediatr 83:68, 1994.

55. Santulli T, Schullinger J, Heird W, et al: Acute necrotizing enterocolitis in infancy: A review of 64 cases. Pediatrics 55:376, 1975.

56. Simpson A, Leonidas J, Krasna I, et al: Roentgen diagnosis of midgut malrotation: Value of upper gastrointestinal radiographic study. J Pediatr Surg 7:243, 1972.

57. Siu YK, Ng PC, Fung SC, et al: Double blind, randomized, placebo controlled study of oral vancomycin in prevention of necrotising enterocolitis in preterm, very low birth weight infants. Arch Dis Child 79:F105, 1998.

58. Smith EI: Malrotation of the intestine. In Welch KJ, Randolph JG, Ravitch MM, et al, eds: Pediatric Surgery. Chicago: Year Book, 1986.

59. Spitz L, Kiely E, Brereton RJ: Esophageal atresia: Five year experience with 148 cases. J Pediatr Surg 22:103, 1987.

60. Sweet AY: Personal communication (Abstract). 1982.

61. Telsey AM, Merrit TA, Dixon SD: Cocaine exposure in a term neonate-necrotizing enterocolitis as a complication. Clin Pediatr 27:547, 1988.

62. Touloukian R, Pickett L, Spackman T, et al: Repair of esophageal atresia by end-to-side anastomosis and ligation of the tracheoesophageal fistula: A critical review of 18 cases. J Pediatr Surg 9:305, 1974.

63. Ty T, Brunet C, Beardmore H: A variation in the operative technique for the treatment of esophageal atresia with tracheoesophageal fistula. J Pediatr Surg 2:118, 1967.

64. Uauy R, Fanaroff A, Korones S, et al: Necrotizing enterocolitis in very low birth weight infants: Biodemographic and clinical correlates. J Pediatr 119:630, 1991.

65. Vaos GC, Lister J: Anatomic evidence for coexistence of cholinergic and adrenergic neurons in the developing human intestine. New aspects in the pathogenesis of developmental neuronal abnormalities. J Pediatr Surg 23:231, 1988.

66. Weiss NJ: Necrotizing enterocolitis: Pathophysiology and prevention. JPEN J Parenter Enteral Nutr 23:S13, 1999.

67. Welch, KJ, Randolph JG, Ravitch MM, et al, eds: Pediatric Surgery. 4th ed. Chicago: Year Book, 1986.

68. Wise WE Jr, Caniano DA, Harmel RP Jr: Tracheoesophageal anomalies in Waterston C neonates: A 30 year perspective. J Pediatr Surg 25:526, 1987.

69. Yaster M, Buck JR, Dudgeon DL, et al: Hemodynamic effects of primary closure of omphalocele/gastroschisis in human newborns. Anesthesiology 69:84, 1988.

Care of the Parents

Marshall H. Klaus
John H. Kennell

> Unfortunately . . . a certain number of mothers abandon the babies whose needs they have not had to meet, and in whom they have lost all interest. The life of the little one has been saved, it is true, but at the cost of the mother.
>
> *Pierre Budin,* The Nursling

A renewed interest in the first minutes, hours, and days of life has been stimulated by several provocative behavioral and physiologic observations in both mother and infant. These assessments and measurements have been made during labor, birth, the immediate postnatal period, and the beginning breast-feedings. They provide a compelling rationale for major changes in care in the perinatal period for both mother and infant. Surprisingly, these findings form a novel way to view the mother-infant dyad.

To understand how these observations fit together, it is necessary to appreciate that the time period of labor, birth, and the ensuing several days can probably best be defined as a "sensitive period." During this time, the mother and probably the father are especially open to changing their later behavior with their infant depending on the quality of their care during the sensitive period.

Winnicott[74] also described this period. He reported a special mental state of the mother in the perinatal period that involves a greatly increased sensitivity to, and focus upon, the needs of her baby. He indicated that this state of "primary maternal preoccupation" starts near the end of pregnancy and continues for a few weeks after the birth of the baby. A mother needs nurturing support and a protected environment to develop and maintain this state. This special preoccupation and the openness of the mother to her baby is probably related to the bonding process. Winnicott wrote that "Only if a mother is sensitized in the way I am describing, can she feel herself into her infant's place, and so meet the infant's needs." In the state of "primary maternal preoccupa-

tion," the mother is better able to sense and provide what her new infant has signaled, which is her primary task. If she senses the needs and responds to them in a sensitive and timely manner, mother and infant will establish a pattern of synchronized and mutually rewarding interactions. It is our hypothesis that as the mother-infant pair continues this dance pattern day after day, the infant will more frequently develop a secure attachment, with the ability to be reassured by well-known caregivers and the willingness to explore and master the environment when caregivers are present.

This chapter describes studies of the process by which a parent becomes attached to the infant, and the physiologic and behavioral components in the newborn, and suggests applications of these findings to the care of the parents of a normal infant, a premature or malformed infant, and a stillbirth or neonatal death.

◆ PREGNANCY

A mother's and father's actions and responses toward their infant are derived from a complex combination of their own genetic endowment, the way the infant responds to them, a long history of interpersonal relations with their own families and with each other, past experiences with this or previous pregnancies, the absorption of the practices and values of their cultures, and probably most importantly, how each was raised by his or her own mother and father. The parenting behavior of each woman and man, his or her ability to tolerate stresses, and his or her need for special attention differ

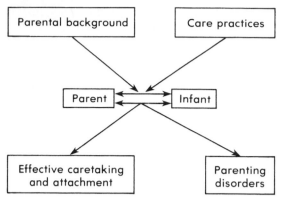

Figure 7–1. Major influences on parent-infant attachment and resulting outcomes.

greatly and depend on a mixture of these factors. Figure 7–1 is a schematic diagram of the major influences on paternal and maternal behavior and the resulting disturbances that we hypothesize may arise from them.

Included under *parental background* are the parent's care by his or her own mother, endowment or genetics of parents, practices of the culture, relationships within the family, experiences with previous pregnancies, and planning, course, and events during pregnancy. Strong evidence for the importance of the effect of the mother's own mothering on her caretaking comes from an elegant 35-year study by Engel et al[16] that documented the close correspondence between how Monica (an infant with a tracheoesophageal fistula) was fed during the first 2 years of life, how she then cared for her dolls, and how as an adult she fed her own four children.

Included under *care practices* are the behavior of physicians, nurses, and hospital personnel, care and support during labor, first days of life, separation of mother and infant, and rules of the hospital.

Included under *parenting disorders* are the vulnerable child syndrome,[21] child abuse,[24, 38] failure to thrive,[62] and some developmental and emotional problems in high-risk infants.[30] Other determinants—such as the attitudes, statements, and practices of the nurses and physicians in the hospital, whether the mother is alone for short periods during her labor, whether there is separation from the infant in the first days of life, the nature of the infant, his or her temperament, and whether he or she is healthy, sick, or

malformed—will affect parenting behavior and the parent-child relationship.

The most easily manipulated variables in this scheme are the separation of the infant from the mother and the practices in the hospital during the first hours and days of life. It is here, during this period, that studies have in part clarified some of the steps in parent-infant attachment.

A wide diversity of observations are beginning to piece together some of the various phases and time periods that are helpful for this process (Table 7–1).

Pregnancy for a woman has been considered a process of maturation,[5] with a series of adaptive tasks, each dependent on the successful completion of the preceding one.

Many mothers are initially disturbed by feelings of grief and anger when they become pregnant, because of factors ranging from economic and housing hardships to interpersonal difficulties. However, by the end of the first trimester, the majority of women who initially rejected pregnancy have accepted it. This initial stage as outlined by Bibring[5] is the mother's *identification of the growing fetus as an "integral part of herself."*

The second stage is *a growing perception of the fetus as a separate individual,* usually occurring with the awareness of fetal movement. After quickening, a woman generally begins to have some fantasies about what the baby may be like; she attributes some human personality characteristics, and develops a sense of attachment and value toward the baby. At this time, further acceptance of the pregnancy and marked changes in attitude toward the fetus may be observed; unplanned, unwanted infants may

Table 7–1. Steps in Attachment

Before pregnancy
  Planning the pregnancy
During pregnancy
  Confirming the pregnancy
  Accepting the pregnancy
  Experiencing fetal movement
  Beginning to accept the fetus as an individual
Labor
Birth
After birth
  Touching and smelling
  Seeing the baby
  Breast-feeding
  Caring for the baby
  Accepting the infant as a separate individual

seem more acceptable. Objectively, the health worker usually finds some outward evidence of the mother's preparation in such actions as the purchase of clothes or a crib, selecting a name, and arranging space for the baby.

The increased use of amniocentesis and ultrasound has appeared to affect parents' perceptions of babies in a rather unexpected fashion. Many parents have discussed with us the disappointment they experienced when they discovered the sex of the baby. Half of the mystery was over. Everything was possible, but once the amniocentesis was done and the sex of the baby known, the range of the unknown was considerably narrowed. However, the tests have the beneficial result of removing some of the anxiety about the possibility of the baby having an abnormality. We have noted that, following the procedure, the baby is sometimes named, and parents often carry around a picture of the very small fetus. This phenomenon requires further investigation to understand the significance of these reactions to the bonding process.

Cohen[10] suggests the following questions to learn the special needs of each mother:

- How long have you lived in this immediate area, and where does most of your family live?
- How often do you see your mother or other close relatives?
- Has anything happened to you in the past (or do you currently have any condition) that causes you to worry about the pregnancy or the baby?
- What was the father's reaction to your becoming pregnant?
- What other responsibilities do you have outside the family?

When planning to meet the needs of the mother, it is important to inquire about how the pregnant woman was mothered—did she have a neglected and deprived infancy and childhood or grow up with a warm and intact family life?

◆ LABOR AND DELIVERY

Newton and Newton[48] noted that those mothers who remain relaxed in labor, who are supported, and who have good rapport with their attendants are more apt to be pleased with their infants at first sight.

In five[25, 31, 32, 36, 64] separate randomized controlled studies of a total of 1809 mothers, women who had continuous social support during labor and birth had labors that were significantly shortened compared with the control group. Likewise, in the experimental group, perinatal interventions including cesarean deliveries and maternal drugs were significantly reduced compared with those used in the control subjects. A meta-analysis of these five randomized trials revealed that women who received continuous support in labor with a doula had a 25% reduction in the length of labor, greater than 50% reduction in cesarean deliveries, and required significantly less oxytocin, medication, and operative vaginal deliveries.[61] This low-cost intervention may be a simple way to reduce the length of labor and perinatal problems for women and their infants during childbirth.

◆ EFFECTS OF SOCIAL AND EMOTIONAL SUPPORT ON MATERNAL BEHAVIOR

This short but highly significant time in a woman's life has been explored in depth because the care during labor appears to affect a mother's attitudes, feelings, and responses to her family, herself, and especially her new baby to a remarkable degree. In a well-conducted trial of continuous social support in South Africa, both mothers with and without doula support were interviewed immediately after delivery and 6 weeks later.[26, 75] Women who had doula support during labor had significantly increased self-esteem, believed they had coped well with labor, and thought the labor had been easier than they had imagined. Women who received this support reported being less anxious 24 hours after birth compared with mothers without a doula. Doula-supported mothers were significantly less depressed 6 weeks postpartum, as measured on a standard depression scale, than mothers who had no doula. Also, doula-supported mothers had a significantly greater incidence of breast-feeding without supplements (52% versus 29%), and they breast-fed for a longer period of time.

The supported mothers said it took them an average of 2.9 days to develop a relationship with their babies compared with 9.8 days for the nonsupported mothers. This feeling of attachment and readiness to fall in love with their babies made them less willing to leave their babies alone. They also reported picking up their babies more frequently when they cried than did nonsupported mothers. The doula-supported mothers were more positive on all dimensions describing the specialness of their babies than were the nonsupported mothers. A higher percentage of supported mothers not only considered their babies beautiful, clever, healthy, and easy to manage but also believed their infants cried less than other babies. The supported mothers believed that their babies were "better" when compared with a "standard baby," whereas the nonsupported mothers perceived their babies as "almost as good as" or "not quite as good as" a "standard baby." "Support group mothers also perceived themselves as closer to their babies, as managing better, and as communicating better with their babies than control group mothers did," the study reported. A higher percentage of the doula-supported mothers indicated that they were pleased to have their babies, found becoming a mother was easier than expected, and thought that they could look after their babies better than anyone else could. In contrast, the nonsupported mothers perceived their adaptation to motherhood as more difficult and believed that others could care for their baby as well as they could.

A most important aspect of emotional support during childbirth may be the most unexpected internalized one—that of the calm, nurturing, accepting, and holding model provided for the parents by the doula during labor. Maternal care needs modeling; each generation is influenced from the care received by the earlier one. Social support appears to be an essential ingredient of childbirth that was lost when birthing moved from home to hospital.

◆ THE DAY OF DELIVERY

Mothers after delivery appear to have common patterns of behavior when they begin to care for their babies in the first hour of life. Filmed observations[35] reveal that when a mother is presented with her nude, full-term infant in privacy, she begins with fingertip touching of the infant's extremities and within a few minutes proceeds to massaging, encompassing palm contact of the infant's trunk. Mothers of premature infants also follow this sequence but proceed at a much slower rate. Fathers go through some of the same routines.[58]

A strong interest in eye-to-eye contact has been expressed by mothers of both full-term and premature infants. Tape recordings of the words of mothers who had been presented with their infants in privacy revealed that 73% of the statements referred to the eyes. The mothers said, "Let me see your eyes" and "Open your eyes and I'll know you love me." Robson[56] has suggested that eye-to-eye contact appears to elicit maternal caregiving responses. Mothers seem to try hard to look "en face" at their infants—that is, to keep their faces aligned with their baby's so that their eyes are in the same vertical plane of rotation as the baby's. Complementing the mother's interest in the infant's eyes is the early functional development of his visual pathways. The infant is alert, active, and able to follow during the first hour of life if maternal sedation has been limited and the administration of eye-drops or ointment is delayed.

Additional information about this early period was provided by Wolff,[76] who described six separate states of consciousness in the infant, ranging from deep sleep to screaming. (See Chapter 17 for further details of infant states.) The state in which we are most interested is state 4, the quiet, alert state. In this state, the infant's eyes are wide open, and she is able to respond to her environment. She may only be in this state for periods as brief as a few seconds. However, Emde et al[15] observed that the infant is in a wakeful state on the average for a period of 38 minutes during the first hour after birth. It is currently possible to demonstrate that an infant can see, that he has visual preferences, that he has a memory for his mother's face at 4 hours of age, that he will turn his head to the spoken word, and that he moves in rhythm to his mother's voice in the first minutes and hours of life—a beautiful linking and synchronized dance between the mother and infant. After this, however, he goes into a deep sleep for 3 to 4 hours.

Therefore, during the first 60 to 90 minutes of his life, the infant is alert, responsive, and especially appealing. In short, he is ideally equipped to meet his parents for the first time. The infant's broad array of sensory and motor abilities evokes responses from the mother and begins the communication that may be especially helpful for attachment and the initiation of a series of reciprocal interactions.

Observations by Condon and Sander[11] reveal that newborns move in rhythm with the structure of adult speech. Interestingly, synchronous movements were found at 16 hours of age with both of the two natural languages tested, English and Chinese.

Mothers also quickly become aware of their infant. Kaitz and colleagues[28, 29] demonstrated that after only 1 hour with their infants in the first hours of life, mothers are able to discriminate their own baby from other infants. Parturient women know their infant's distinctive features after minimal exposure using olfactory and tactile cues (touching the dorsum of the hand), whereas discrimination based on sight and sound takes somewhat longer to develop.

◆ WHEN DOES LOVE BEGIN?

The first feelings of love for the infant are not necessarily instantaneous with the initial contact.

MacFarlane et al[44] helped to answer this question by asking 97 mothers "When did you first feel love for your baby?" The replies were as follows: during pregnancy—41%, at birth—24%, first week—27%, and after the first week—8%.

In another study of two groups of primiparous mothers[57] (n = 112, and n = 41), 40% recalled that their predominant emotional reaction when holding their babies for the first time was one of indifference. The same response was reported by 25% of 40 multiparous mothers. In both groups, 40% felt immediate affection.

◆ CARE OF THE NORMAL INFANT AND PARENTS FOLLOWING BIRTH

After birth, the newborn should be thoroughly dried with warm towels so as not to lose heat, and once it is clear that he has good color and is active and appears normal (usually within 5 minutes), he can go to his mother. At this time, the warm and dry infant can be placed between the mother's breasts or on her abdomen or, if she desires, next to her.

When newborns are kept close to their mother's body or on their mother, the transition from life in the womb to existence outside the uterus is made much easier for them. The newborn recognizes his mother's voice[13] and smell,[69] and her body[9] warms his to just the right temperature. In this way, the infant can experience sensations somewhat similar to what he felt during the last several weeks of uterine life.

In the past, many caretakers believed that the newborn needs help to begin to nurse. So, often, immediately after birth the baby's lips are placed near or on the mother's nipple. In that situation, some babies do start to suckle, but the majority just lick the nipple or peer up at the mother. They appear to be much more interested in the mother's face, especially her eyes, even though the nipple is right next to their lips. They most commonly begin, when left on their own, to move toward the breast 30 to 40 minutes after birth.

The Breast Crawl

One of the most exciting observations made is the discovery that the newborn has the ability to find his mother's breast all on his own and to decide for himself when to take his first feeding. In order not to remove the taste and smell of the mother's amniotic fluid, it is necessary to delay washing the baby's hands. The baby uses the taste and smell of amniotic fluid on his hands to make a connection with a certain lipid substance on the nipple related to the amniotic fluid.

The infant usually begins with a time of rest and quiet alertness, during which he rarely cries and often appears to take pleasure in looking at his mother's face. Around 30 to 40 minutes after birth, the newborn begins making mouthing movements, sometimes with lip smacking, and shortly after, saliva begins to pour down onto his chin.[73] When placed on the mother's abdomen, babies maneuver in their own ways to reach the nipple. They often use stepping motions of their legs to move ahead, while horizontally moving toward the nipple, using small push-ups and lowering one arm first in the direction they wish to go. These efforts are interspersed with short rest periods. Sometimes babies change direction in midstream.

These actions take effort and time. Parents find patience well worthwhile if they wait and observe their infant on his first journey.

In Figure 7–2, one newborn is seen successfully navigating his way to his mother's breast. At 10 minutes of age, he first begins to move toward the left breast, but 5 minutes later he is back in the midline. Repeated mouthing and sucking of the hands and fingers is commonly observed. With a series of push ups and rest periods, he makes his way to the breast completely on his own, placing his lips on the areola of the breast. He begins to suckle effectively and closely observes his mother's face.

In one group of mothers who did not receive pain medication and whose babies were not taken away during the first hours of life for a bath, vitamin K administration, or application of eye ointment, 15 of 16 babies placed on their mother's abdomen were observed to make the trip to their mother's breast, latch on their own, and begin to suckle effectively.[55]

This sequence is helpful to the mother as well, because the massage of the breast and suckling induce a large oxytocin surge into her bloodstream, which helps contract the uterus, expelling the placenta and closing off many blood vessels in the uterus, thus reducing bleeding. The stimulation and suckling also helps in the manufacture of prolactin, and the suckling enhances the closeness and new bond between mother and baby. Mother and baby appear to be carefully adapted for these first moments together.

To allow this first intimate encounter, we strongly urge that the injection of vitamin K, application of eye ointment, washing, and any measuring of the infant's weight, height, and head circumference be delayed for at least 1 hour. More than 90% of all full-term infants are normal at birth. In a few moments they can be easily evaluated to ensure that they are healthy. They can then, after thorough drying, be safely placed on their mother's chest if the parents wish.

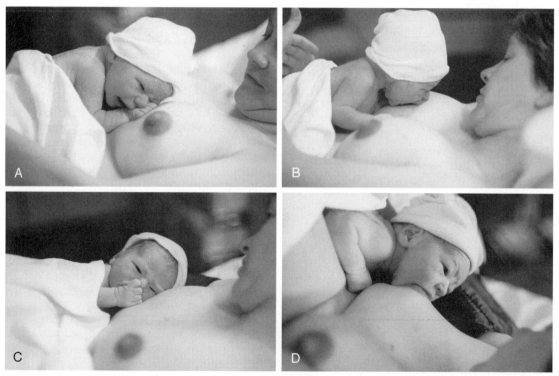

Figure 7–2. *A,* At 10 minutes of life, this newborn male infant, after thorough drying but sparing the hands, was placed between the mother's breasts at the nipple line. He looks at the left nipple. *B,* However, at 30 minutes, with a series of push-ups and letting his left arm down first, he moves toward the right nipple. *C,* He frequently takes time out to suck on his fingers. His hands were never washed or dried with a towel. If washed, this frequent hand-sucking disappears.[68] *D,* At 50 minutes, the baby is sucking easily on the areola and mother and baby look at each other en face for long periods. If kept with the mother throughout the hospital stay, he will nurse every 45 to 90 minutes. It should be noted that this baby did not have any eye ointment, vitamin K injection or bath. At 1½ hours, he received the eye ointment and vitamin K only. (With permission of the photographer, Elaine Siegel.)

The odor of the nipple appears to guide a newborn to the breast.[53, 69] If the right breast is washed with soap and water, the infant will crawl to the left breast, and vice versa. If both breasts are washed, the infant will go to the breast that has been rubbed with the amniotic fluid of the mother. The special attraction of the newborn to the odor of *his* mother's amniotic fluid may reflect the time in utero when, as a fetus, he swallowed the liquid. It appears that amniotic fluid contains some substance that is similar to some secretion of the breast, albeit not the milk. Amniotic fluid on the infant's hands probably also explains part of the interest in sucking the hands and fingers seen in the photographs. This early handsucking behavior is markedly reduced when the infant is bathed before the crawl. With all these innate programs, it almost seems as if the infant comes into life carrying a small computer chip with these instructions.

At a moment such as childbirth, we come full circle to our biologic origins. Many separate abilities enable a baby to do this. Stepping reflexes help the newborn push against his mother's abdomen to propel him toward the breast. Pressure of the infant's feet on the abdomen may also help in the expulsion of the placenta and in reducing uterine bleeding. The ability to move his hand in a reaching motion enables the baby to claim the nipple. Taste, smell, and vision all help the newborn detect and find the breast. Muscular strength in neck, shoulders, and arms helps newborns bob their heads and do small push-ups to inch forward and side to side. This whole scenario may take place in a matter of minutes, most often it occurs within 30 to 60 minutes, but it is within the capacity of the newborn. It appears that young humans, like other baby mammals, know how to find their mother's breast.

When the mother and infant are resting skin-to-skin and gazing eye-to-eye, they begin to learn about each other on many different levels. For the mother, the first minutes and hours after birth are a time when she is uniquely open emotionally to respond to her baby and to begin the new relationship.

A Sensitive Period?

Many studies have focused on whether additional time for close contact of the mother and infant alters the quality of attachment.[3,]
[35, 37] These studies have addressed the question of whether there is a sensitive period for parent-infant contact in the first minutes, hours, and days of life that may alter the parents' later behavior with their infant. In many biologic disciplines, these moments have been called *sensitive periods.* However, in most of the examples of a sensitive period in biology, the observations are made on the young of the species rather than the adult. Evidence for a sensitive period comes from the following series of studies. Note that in each study increasing mother-infant time together or increased suckling improves caretaking by the mother.

In six of nine randomized trials of only early contact with suckling (during the first hour of life), both the number of women breast-feeding and the length of their lactation were significantly increased for early contact mothers compared with women in the control group.

In addition, studies of Brazelton[6] and others have shown that if nurses spend as little as 10 minutes helping mothers discover some of their newborn infant's abilities, such as turning to the mother's voice and following the mother's face, and assisting mothers with suggestions about ways to quiet their infants, the mothers become more appropriately interactive with their infants face-to-face and during feedings at 3 and 4 months of age.

O'Connor and colleagues[50] carried out a randomized trial with 277 mothers in a hospital that had a high incidence of parenting disorders. One group of mothers had their infants with them for 6 additional hours on the first and second day, but no early contact. The routine care group began to see their babies at the same age but only for 20-minute feedings every 4 hours, which was the custom throughout the United States at that time. In follow-up studies, 10 children in the routine care group experienced parenting disorders, including child abuse, failure to thrive, abandonment, and neglect during the first 17 months of life compared with two children in the experimental group who had 12 additional hours of mother-infant contact. A similar study[62] in North Carolina that included 202 mothers during the first year of life did not find a statistically significant difference in the frequency of parenting disorders; 10 infants failed to thrive or were neglected or abused in the control group compared with seven in the group that had extended contact. When the results of these two studies are combined in a meta-analysis ($\rho = .054$), it appears that simple techniques, such as adding additional early time for each mother and infant to be together, such as continuous rooming-in, may lead to a significant reduction in child abuse. A much larger study is necessary to confirm and validate these relatively small studies.

Swedish researchers[9] have shown that the normal infant, when dried and placed nude on the mother's chest and then covered with a blanket, will maintain his or her body temperature as well as when elaborate, high-tech heating devices that usually separate the mother and baby are used. The same researchers found that when the infants are skin-to-skin with their mothers for the first 90 minutes after birth, they cry hardly at all compared with infants who were dried, wrapped in a towel, and placed in a bassinet. It is likely that each of these features—the crawling ability of the infant, the decreased crying when close to the mother, and the warming capabilities of the mother's chest—are adaptive features that have evolved to help preserve the infant's life.

When the infant suckles from the breast, it stimulates the production of oxytocin in both the mother's and the infant's brains, and oxytocin in turn stimulates the vagal motor nucleus, releasing 19 different gastrointestinal hormones, including insulin, cholecystokinin, and gastrin.[65] Five of the 19 hormones stimulate growth[68] of the baby's and mother's intestinal villi and increase the surface area and the absorption of calories with each feeding. The stimuli for this release are touch on the mother's nipple and the inside of the infant's mouth. The increased gut motility with each suckling may help remove meconium with its large load of bilirubin.

These research findings may explain some of the underlying physiologic and behavioral processes and provide additional support for the importance of 2 of the 10 caregiving procedures that the United Nations International Children's Emergency Fund (UNICEF) is promoting as part of its Baby Friendly Initiative to increase breast-feeding: (1) early mother-infant contact, with an opportunity for the baby to suckle in the first hour, and (2) mother-infant rooming-in throughout the hospital stay.

Following the introduction of the Baby Friendly Initiative in maternity units in several countries throughout the world, an unexpected observation was made. In Thailand,[8] in a hospital where a disturbing number of babies are abandoned by their mothers, the use of rooming-in and early contact with suckling significantly reduced the frequency of abandonment from 33 in 10,000 births to 1 in 10,000 births a year. Similar observations have been made in Russia, the Philippines, and Costa Rica where early contact and rooming-in were also introduced.

These reports are additional evidence that the first hours and days of life are a sensitive period for the human mother. This may be due in part to the special interest that mothers have shortly after birth in hoping that their infant will look at them and to the infant's ability to interact in the first hour of life during the prolonged period of the quiet alert state. There is a beautiful interlocking at this early time of the mother's interest in the infant's eyes and the baby's ability to interact and to look eye-to-eye.

A possible key to understanding what is happening physiologically in these first minutes and hours comes from investigators who noted that, if the lips of the infant touch the mother's nipple in the first hour of life, a mother will decide to keep her baby 100 minutes longer in her room every day during her hospital stay than another mother who does not have contact until later.[72] This may be partly explained by the small secretions of oxytocin (the "love hormone") that occur in both the infant's and mother's brains when breast-feeding occurs. In sheep,[34] dilation of the cervical os during birth releases oxytocin within the brain, which, acting on receptor sites, is important for the initiation of maternal behavior and for the facilitation of bonding between mother and baby. In humans, there is a blood–brain barrier for oxytocin, and only small amounts reach the brain via the bloodstream. However, multiple oxytocin receptors in the brain are supplied by de novo oxytocin synthesis in the brain. Increased levels of brain oxytocin result in slight sleepiness, euphoria, increased pain threshold, and feelings of increased love for the infant. It appears that, during breast-feeding, elevated blood levels of oxytocin are associated with increased brain levels; women who exhibit the highest plasma oxytocin concentration are the most sleepy.

Measurements of plasma oxytocin levels in healthy women who had their babies skin-to-skin on their chests immediately after birth reveal significant elevations compared with the prepartum levels and a return to prepartum levels at 60 minutes. For most women, a significant and spontaneous peak concentration was recorded about 15 minutes after delivery, with expulsion of the placenta.[49] Most mothers had several peaks of oxytocin up to 1 hour after delivery. The vigorous oxytocin release after delivery and with breast-feeding not only may help contract the uterine muscle to prevent bleeding, but may also enhance bonding of the mother to her infant. These findings may explain an observation made in France in the 19th century when many poor mothers were giving up their babies. Nurses recorded that mothers who breast-fed for at least 8 days rarely abandoned their infants. We hypothesize that a cascade of interactions between the mother and baby occurs during this early period, locking them together and ensuring further development of attachment. The remarkable change in maternal behavior with just the touch of the infant's lips on the mother's nipple, the effects of additional time for mother-infant contact, and the reduction in abandonment with early contact, suckling, and rooming-in, as well as the elevated maternal oxytocin levels shortly after birth in conjunction with known sensory, physiologic, immunologic, and behavioral mechanisms all contribute to the attachment of the parent to the infant.

Early and Extended Contact for Parents and Their Infant

Although debate continues on the interpretation and significance of some of the research studies regarding the effects of early and extended contact for mothers and fathers on bonding with their infants, both sides agree that all parents should be offered such contact time with their infants. Thompson and Westrich,[66] in their extensive critical review of obstetric and neonatal care, reached the following conclusions regarding a sensitive period:

We have been unable to find any evidence suggesting that the restriction of early postnatal mother-infant interaction, which has been such a common feature of the care of women giving birth in hospitals, has any beneficial effects; on the contrary, the available evidence suggests that the effects that these restrictive policies have are undesirable. The data suggest the plausible hypothesis that women of low socioeconomic status may be particularly vulnerable to the adverse effects of restricting contact. It may be thought surprising that disruption of maternal-infant interaction in the immediate postnatal period may set some women on the road to breast-feeding failure and altered subsequent behavior towards their children. Pediatricians, psychologists, and others have indeed debated this issue. This skepticism does not, however, constitute grounds for acquiescing in hospital routines which lead to unwanted separation of mothers from their babies. In the light of the evidence that such policies may actually do harm, they should be changed forthwith.

It is hoped that, as we become better acquainted with the biology of both the mother and infant, their perinatal care will become more appropriate to their physiology.

On the basis of our observations and the reports of parents, we believe that every parent has a task to perform during the postpartum period. The mother in particular must look at and "take in" her real live baby and then reconcile the fantasy of the infant she imagined with the one she actually delivered.

Evidence suggests that many of these early interactions also take place between the father and his newborn child. Parke[52] in particular has demonstrated that when fathers are given the opportunity to be alone with their newborns, they spend almost exactly the same amount of time as mothers in holding, touching, and looking at them.

How strongly should physicians and nurses emphasize the importance of parent-infant contact in the first hour and extended visiting for the rest of the hospital stay? Despite a lack of early contact experienced by many parents in hospital births in the past, almost all these parents became bonded to their babies. The human is highly adaptable, and there are many fail-safe routes to attachment. Sadly, some parents who missed the bonding experience have felt that all was lost for their future relationship. This was (and is) completely incorrect, but it was so upsetting that we have tried to speak more moderately. It is unfortunate that we find that this had led some skeptics to discontinue the practice of early and extended contact or to make a slapdash, rushed charade of the parent-infant contact, often without attention to the details necessary to the experiences provided for mothers in the studies. There are still large hospitals that have never provided for early and extended contact, and the mothers who miss out are often those at the limits of adaptability[43] and who may benefit the most—the poor, the single, the unsupported, the teenage mothers.

We believe that at least 60 minutes of early contact in privacy should be provided if possible for parents and their infant to enhance the bonding experience. If the health of the mother or infant makes this impossible, then discussion, support, and reassurance should help the parents appreciate that they can become as completely attached to their infant as if they had the usual bonding experience. The infant should only be with the mother and father if she is known to be physically normal and if appropriate temperature control is used. We also strongly urge that the baby remain with the mother as long as she wishes throughout the hospital stay so that she and the baby can get to know each other. This permits both mother and father more time to learn about their baby and to gradually develop a strong tie in the first weeks of life.

From these many recent findings, we make the following recommendations for changing the perinatal period for mother and infant.

1. Every mother should have continuous physical and emotional support during the entire labor by a knowledgeable, caring woman (e.g., doula, obstetric nurse, or midwife) in addition to her partner, as recommended by the Oxford Perinatal Study Group in England and the Royal Canadian Obstetrical Society.
2. Child birth educators and obstetric caregivers should discuss the newly discovered information in this chapter with every pregnant woman so that she will be aware of the advantages of an unmedicated labor to avoid interference with the infant's ability to interact, self-attach, and successfully breast-feed.
3. Immediately after birth and a thorough drying, an infant who has a good Apgar score and appears normal should be offered to the mother for skin-to-skin contact, with warmth provided by her body and a light blanket covering the baby. The baby should not be removed for a bath, footprinting, or administration of vitamin K or eye medication until after the first hour. The baby thus can be allowed to decide when to begin his first feeding.
4. The central nursery should be closed. All babies should room-in with their mothers throughout the short hospital course unless this is prevented by illness of mother or infant. A small nursery area can be available for infants of mothers who are ill or who require a short observation period.
5. Early and continuous mother-infant contact appears to decrease the incidence of abandonment and increase the length and success of breast-feeding. All mothers should begin breast-feeding in the first hour, nurse frequently, and be encouraged to breast-feed for at least the first 2 weeks of life, even if they plan to go back to work. Early frequent breast-feeding has many advantages, including earlier removal of bilirubin from the gut as well as aiding in mother-infant attachment.

◆ THE SICK OR PREMATURE INFANT

Although parental visiting has been permitted in the intensive care nursery, a number of studies[4, 23, 45, 47] have revealed that most parents continue to suffer severe emotional stress. Harper et al[23] noted that, even when parents have close contact with their infants in the intensive care nursery, they experience prolonged stress.

Newman[47] described "coping through commitment" as an intense yet variable involvement in the care of a low-birth-weight infant. In contrast, "coping through distance" was a slower acquaintance process in which the parents expressed fear, anxiety, and at times denial before they accepted the surviving infant.

Highly interacting mothers visit and telephone the nursery more frequently while the infants are hospitalized and stimulate their infants more at home. Mothers who stimulate their infants very little in the nursery also visit and telephone less frequently and provide only minimal stimulation to them at home. Most perceptively, Minde et al[46] noted that mothers who touched and fondled their infants more in the nursery had infants who opened their eyes more often. He and his associates observed the contingency between the infant's eyes being open and the mother's touching and between gross motor stretches and the mother's smiling. They could not determine to what extent the sequence of touching and eye opening was an indication of the mother's primary contribution or whether it was initiated by the infant. Thus, Newman,[47] and Minde et al[46] predict that mothers who become involved with, interested in, and anxious about their infants in the intensive care nursery will have an easier time when the infant is taken home.

Field[18] has demonstrated the close connection between what a mother does and her infant's arousal level. Whereas most mothers of full-term babies adopt a moderate level of activity that is associated with optimal arousal in their babies, some mothers of "preemies" either overreact or underreact. Field found that mothers of premature infants who were overreactive during early face-to-face interactions were more likely to be overprotective and overcontrolling during interactions with their infants 2 years later.[18]

◆ INTERVENTIONS FOR FAMILIES OF PREMATURE INFANTS

Transporting the Mother to Be Near Her Small Infant

With the development of high-risk perinatal centers, there has been an increasing number of mothers who are transported to the maternity division of hospitals with a neonatal intensive care nursery just before delivery or shortly after. If there is not sufficient time to arrange for her transport before she gives birth, we strongly recommend that the mother be moved during her early postpartum period.

Transporting the Healthy Premature Infant to the Mother

Rather than bringing mothers into the neonatal intensive care unit, with its frightening sounds, strange equipment, and unfamiliar faces, the baby may be brought to the mother in her own room in the maternity division of the hospital. In this way, the mothers have an opportunity to become acquainted with their premature newborns under circumstances similar to those experienced by mothers of full-term infants.

We include healthy infants whose birth weight is between 1.5 and 2.1 kg, whose gestational age is between 32 and 36 weeks, and whose medical status during the first days permits the infant to stay with the mother (e.g., no continuing respiratory distress or hypoglycemia).

The early contact consists of 0.5 to 1 hour of mother-infant interaction on each of the first, second, and third days after birth. A nurse brings the baby to the mother's room in a transport incubator and stays with the mother. The baby, clothed only in a diaper, is placed in the mother's bed with a radiant heat panel overhead. The nurse is present during the visit but is seated out of the mother's view above the head of her bed. During the visit, the nurse observes the infant's condition, particularly color and respirations. Resuscitation equipment is carried on the transport incubator for use in case of apnea.

We monitor the babies' temperatures frequently. With the use of a heat panel and transport incubator, there have been no significant problems with temperature control. In addition, we have had no episodes of apnea, bradycardia, vomiting, or other unusual behavior. We appreciate that there may be times when difficulties with premature babies occur, so the nurses continue to monitor them closely.

Rooming-In for the Parent of a Premature Infant

When Tafari and Ross[65] in Ethiopia permitted mothers to live within their crowded premature unit 24 hours each day, they were able to care for three times as many infants in their premature nursery, and at the end of 1 year, the number of surviving infants had increased 500%. Mother-infant pairs were discharged when the infants weighed an average of 1.7 kg, and most infants were breast-fed. Previous to this, most of the infants had gone home and were bottle-fed, and usually died of intercurrent respiratory and gastrointestinal infections. When the cost of prepared milk amounts to a high proportion of the parents' weekly income, policies in support of the mother rooming-in and breast-feeding in premature nurseries have a direct impact on infant mortality. In several other countries throughout the world, including Argentina, Brazil, Estonia, and South Africa, mothers of premature infants live in a room adjoining the premature nursery or they room in. This arrangement appears to have multiple benefits. It allows the mother to continue producing milk, permits her to take on the care of the infant more easily, greatly reduces the caregiving time required of the staff for these infants, and allows a group of mothers of premature infants to talk over their situation and gain from discussion and mutual support. This procedure is probably appropriate for 50% of the world.

Torres,[67] in a special care unit in the slums of Santiago, Chile, achieved excellent, low perinatal mortality and morbidity rates by placing special care units for low-birth-weight infants in the maternity unit, thus maintaining babies under professional observation for only as long as necessary.

At a general hospital in High Wycombe, England, a 20-bed special infant care unit can accommodate eight mothers at a time and 250 admissions each year. No matter how seriously ill they may be, some 70% of the babies have their mothers with them from the first few days of life. Six of the mothers' rooms open directly into the infant special care unit so that the parents can easily see or care for their infants.

Nesting

In the United States, James and Wheeler[27] first described the successful introduction of a care-by-parent unit to provide a homelike caretaking experience. Before discharge, nursing support was available for parents of premature infants.

For several years we have studied "nesting"—namely, permitting mothers to live in with their infants before discharge. When babies reached 1.72 to 2.11 kg, each mother was given a private room with her baby where she provided all caregiving. Impressive changes in the behavior of these women were observed clinically. Even though the mothers had fed and cared for their infants in the intensive care nursery on many occasions before living-in, eight of the first nine mothers did not sleep during the first 24 hours in order to learn more about their infant's behavior. However, in the second 24-hour period, the mothers' confidence and caretaking skills improved greatly. At this time, mothers began to discuss the proposed early discharge of their infants and, often for the first time, began to make preparations at home for their arrival. Several insisted on taking their babies home earlier than planned.

We suggest that early discharge, preceded by a period of isolation of the mother and infant, may help to normalize mothering behavior in the intensive care nursery. Encouraging the increasing possibilities for mother-infant interaction and total caretaking may reduce the incidence of mothering disorders among mothers of small or sick premature infants.

Parent Groups

A number of neonatal intensive care units have formed groups of parents of premature infants who meet once each week or more often for 1- to 2-hour discussions. Documented clinical reports from these centers suggest that parents find both support and considerable relief in being able to talk with each other and to express and compare their inner feelings.

Minde and colleagues,[45] in a controlled study of a self-help group, reported that parents who participated in the group visited their infants in the hospital significantly more often than did parents in the control group. The self-help parents also touched, talked, and looked at their infants more in the en face position and rated themselves as more competent than the control group on infant care measures. The mothers in the group continued to show more involvement with their babies during feedings and were more concerned about their general development 3 months after their discharge from the nursery.

Kangaroo Baby Care

Allowing a mother to hold the infant skin-to-skin for prolonged periods of time in the hospital has salutary effects (Fig. 7–3). Several trials have noted that, if the usual precautions are taken, such as hand washing, there is no increase in the infection rate or problems in oxygenation, apnea, or temperature control. The most significant medical benefit appears to be a significant increase in the mother's milk supply and success at nursing.[70, 71] Several studies noted that the mother's own confidence in her caretaking improved along with an eagerness for discharge, and many women reported feeling an increased closeness to the infant compared with a control group of mothers. At the first skin-to-skin experience, the mother is usually tense, so it is best for the nurse to stay with her to answer questions and make any necessary adjustments in position and ensure that warmth is maintained. A few mothers find that one such experience is enough. However, most mothers find repeated kangaroo care experiences especially pleasurable. We believe, however, that there is not adequate information to support discharge of appropriate for gestational age (AGA) infants weighing less than 1700 g on solely kangaroo care without daily nursing visits.

Early Discharge

Derbyshire[14] and associates have studied discharging premature infants when they weighed about 2 kg and found no deleterious effects associated with this early discharge. To make this workable and to prevent complications, experienced personnel should visit the home to organize the families and, after discharge, to help supervise infant care. Recent studies of early discharge have not revealed any adverse effects on the physical health of the infants.

Another approach for the mother with emotional distress after the birth of a small premature infant is to alter the responses of the developing infant, an area of intense study by Als and associates[2]. In a series of creative studies, they demonstrated that individualized nursing care plans for high-risk, low-birth-weight infants involving their behavioral and environmental needs remarkably altered their outcome. Their requirements for light, sound, position, and detailed nursing were only developed after a sensitive, detailed behavioral assessment.

In four randomized trials using the preceding procedure, infants receiving individualized behavioral management required shorter stays on a respirator and fewer days on supplemental oxygen, their average daily waking time increased, they were discharged earlier, and they had a lower incidence of intraventricular hemorrhage. In addition, following discharge, their behavioral development progressed more normally and their parents more easily developed ways of sensing their needs and responding and interacting with them in a pleasurable fashion. Parents have an easier time adapting to premature infants who are more responsive.

Further emphasizing the importance of the home and family in the final result is a very large, randomized, well carried out trial (985 premature infants) in eight centers in the United States.[22] The study demonstrated that a comprehensive program with weekly home visits in the first year of life, group meetings for mothers during all 3 years, and daily attendance by the child at a developmental center from 1 to 3 years of age re-

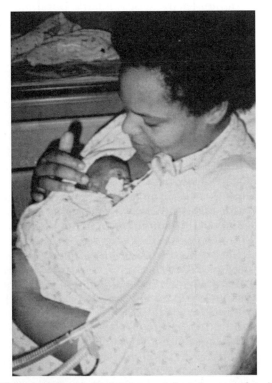

Figure 7–3. Small immature infant (on ventilator) skin-to-skin with his mother.

sulted in a significant improvement in intelligence quotient (IQ) scores as well as reports by mothers of fewer developmental problems.

In assessing the effects of any intervention following discharge from the hospital, it is important to remember that more than half the variance in IQ can be accounted for by social conditions that include parental occupation, education, minority status, anxiety, and mental illness. As the social conditions for the entire population are improved, so will the outcome for the low-birth-weight infant.

Practical Hints for Parents of Sick or Premature Infants

1. The obstetrician of a high-risk mother should consult the pediatrician early and continue to involve him in decisions and plans for the management of the mother and baby.
2. If the baby must be moved to a hospital with an intensive care unit, we have found it helpful always to give the mother a chance to see and touch her infant, even if he has respiratory distress and is in an oxygen hood. The house officer or the attending physician stops in the mother's room with the transport incubator and encourages her to touch her baby and look at him at close hand. A comment about the baby's strength and healthy features may be long remembered and appreciated.

   We encourage the father to follow the transport team to the hospital so he can see what is happening with his baby. He uses his own transportation so that he can stay in the premature unit for 3 to 4 hours. This extra time allows him to get to know the nurses and physicians in the unit, to find out how the infant is being treated, and to talk with the physicians about what they expect will happen with the baby in the succeeding days. We ask him to help act as a link between us and his family by carrying information back to his wife and request that he come to our unit before he visits his wife so that he can let her know how the baby is doing. We suggest that he take a Polaroid picture, even if the infant is on a respirator, so that he can show and describe to his wife in detail

how the baby is being cared for. The mothers often tell us how valuable the picture is in allowing them to maintain some contact with the infant, even while physically separated.

3. Transporting the mother and baby together to the medical center that contains the intensive care nursery should be encouraged for its immediate and long-term benefits.
4. The intensive care nursery should be open for parental visiting 24 hours each day and should be flexible about visits from others such as grandparents, supportive relatives, and sometimes siblings. If proper precautions are taken, infection transmission will not be a problem.
5. Communication is essential. The health care workers should communicate with the mother about her condition and about the baby's condition. This is important before, during, and after the birth of the baby, even if the information is brief and incomplete.

   Clinically, we have been impressed and disturbed by the devastating and lasting untoward effects on the mothering capacity of women who have been frightened by a physician's pessimistic outlook about the chance of survival and normal development of an infant. For example, when the newborn infant is a 3-pound (1360 g) premature baby who is doing well but the mother is told by a physician that there is a reasonable chance the baby may not survive, the mother will often show evidence of mourning (as if the baby were already dead) and reluctance to "become attached" to her baby. We have repeatedly observed that such mothers may refuse to visit or will show great hesitation about any physical contact. When discussing such a situation with the physician who has spoken pessimistically with the mother, we have often been told that it is important to share all worries with her so that she will be prepared in case of a bad outcome. If there is a close and firm bond between the mother and infant (which occurs after an infant has been home for several months), there is no reason for the physician to withhold concern. However, while the ties of affection are still forming, they can be easily retarded, altered, or possibly permanently damaged. Physicians should not be untruthful because parents will quickly sense their true feelings, but they must base their statements on the current situation (infant mortality in low-birth-weight nurseries has decreased steadily year by year), not on past high mortality figures from the period during which they were being trained. Today, the vast majority of these infants will live.

We find it best to describe what the infant looks like to us and how the infant will appear physically to the mother. We do not talk about chances or survival rates or percentages but stress that most babies survive despite early and often worrisome problems. We do not emphasize problems that may occur in the future. We do try to anticipate common developments (e.g., the need for bilirubin reduction lights for jaundice in small premature infants).

6. If possible, mother and infant should be kept near each other in the same hospital and on the same floor.

7. It is useful to talk with the mother and father together. When this is not possible, it is often wise to talk with one parent on the telephone in the presence of the other. At least once each day we discuss how the child is doing with the parents; we talk with them at least twice each day if the child is critically ill. It is essential to find out what the mother believes is going to happen or what she has read about the problem. We move at her pace during any discussion.

The physician should not relieve his anxiety by adding his worries to those of the parents. If there is a possibility, for example, that the child has Turner syndrome, it is not necessary to share this with the parents while the infant is still acutely ill with other problems and while affectional bonds are still weak. If the physician is worried about a slightly high bilirubin level, it is not necessary to dwell on kernicterus. Once mentioned, the possibility of death or brain damage can never be completely erased.

8. Before the mother comes to the neonatal unit, the nurse or physician should describe in detail what the baby and the equipment will look like. When she makes her first visit, it is important to anticipate that she may become distressed when she looks at her infant. We always have a stool nearby so that she can sit down, and a nurse stays at her side during most of the visit, describing in detail the procedures being carried out, such as the monitoring of respiration and heart rate. The nurse should be nearby so that she may answer questions and give support during the difficult period when the mother first sees her infant.

9. It is important to remember that feelings of love for the baby are often elicited through contact. Therefore, we turn off the lights and remove the eye patches from an infant under bilirubin lights, so that the mother and infant can see each other.

10. When the immature infant has passed the acute phase, both the father and the mother should be encouraged to touch, massage, and interact with their infant. This helps the parents get to know her, reduces the number of breathing pauses (if this is a problem), increases weight gain, and hastens the infant's discharge from the unit. Initially, if the infant is acutely ill, touching and fondling her sometimes results in a decrease in the level of blood oxygen; therefore, parents should begin this contact when the infant is stable and the nurse or physician agrees that the infant is ready. Firm massage of preterm infants 15 minutes three times a day results in markedly improved growth, less stress behavior, improved performance on the Brazelton Neonatal Behavior Assessment scale, and better performance on a developmental assessment at 8 months.[60]

11. We believe that the mother and father can receive feedback from their baby in response to their caregiving. If the infant looks at their eyes, moves in response to them, quiets down, or shows any behavior in response to their efforts, the parents' feeling of attachment is encouraged. Practically speaking, this means that the mother must catch the baby's glance and be able to note that some maneuver on her part, such as picking up the baby or making soothing sounds, actually triggers a response or quiets the baby. We suggest to parents, therefore, that they think in terms of trying to send a message to the baby and of picking one up from him or her in return. Some

parents think we are joking. We then explain that small premature infants do see and are especially interested in patterned objects, that they can hear as well as adults, and that evidence suggests they will benefit greatly from receiving messages.

12. We should continue to study interventions such as rooming-in, nesting, and early discharge as well as transporting a healthy premature infant to be with his mother. It is necessary to test these various interventions in different hospital settings and to evaluate their ability to reduce the severe anxiety that many parents experience during the prolonged hospitalization and the early days following discharge.

13. In all these interventions, it is critical that nurses take mothers under their wing, especially supporting and encouraging them during these early days and weeks.[1] The nurse's guidance in helping a mother with simple caretaking tasks can be extremely valuable in helping her to overcome anxiety. In this sense, the nurse assumes the role of the mother's own mother and contributes much more than teaching her basic techniques of caretaking.

14. To begin an intervention with parents early, it is necessary to identify high-risk parents who are having special difficulties in adapting. Generally these parents visit rarely and for short periods,[17] appear frightened, and do not usually engage the medical staff in any questioning about the infant's problems. Sometimes the parents are hostile or irritable and show inappropriately low levels of anxiety.

15. As we develop a further understanding of the process by which normal mothers and infants interact with each other during the first months and year of life, it appears that some recommendations for stimulation may be detrimental to normal development. Rather than suggesting stimulation, it may be important for a mother naturally and unconsciously to use imitation to learn about and get to know her own infant.

It is possible that, in the future, several of these interventions will be combined so that a mother may have early contact with her premature infant if he is healthy and have the baby brought to her bedside in the maternity unit on several occasions early in the course of the infant's stay in the hospital. In addition, she will be a member of a parent group, and she will be living-in with the baby for 3 or 4 days before early discharge. For further discussion of parents of premature infants see Cases One and Three.

◆ CONGENITAL MALFORMATIONS

The birth of an infant with a congenital malformation presents complex challenges to the physician who will care for the affected child and his family. Although previous investigators agree that the child's birth often precipitates major family stress,[59] relatively few have described the process of family adaptation during the infant's first year of life.[59] Solnit and Stark's conceptualization of parental reactions[63] emphasized that a significant aspect of adaptation is the mourning that parents must undergo for the loss of the normal child they had expected. Observers have also noted pathologic aspects of family reactions, including the chronic sorrow that envelops the family of a defective child.[51] Less attention has been given to the more adaptive aspects of parental attachment to children with malformations.

Parental reactions to the birth of a child with a congenital malformation appear to follow a predictable course. For most parents, initial shock, disbelief, and a period of intense emotional upset (including sadness, anger, and anxiety) are followed by a period of gradual adaptation, which is marked by a lessening of intense anxiety and emotional reaction (Fig. 7–4). This adaptation is characterized by an increased satisfaction with and ability to care for the baby. These stages in parental reactions are similar to those reported in other crisis situations, such as occur with terminally ill children. The shock, disbelief, and denial reported by many parents seem to be an understandable attempt to escape the traumatic news of the baby's malformation, news so at variance with their expectations that it is impossible to register except gradually.

The intense emotional turmoil described by parents who have produced a child with a congenital malformation corresponds to a period of crisis (defined as "upset in a state of equilibrium caused by a hazardous event which creates a threat, a loss, or a challenge

Figure 7–4. Hypothetical model of normal sequence of parental reactions to birth of malformed infant. (Adapted from Drotar D, Baskiewicz A, Irwin et al: Pediatrics 51:710, 1975. Reproduced by permission of Pediatrics. Copyright 1975.)

for the individual"). A crisis includes a period of impact, an increase in tension associated with stress, and finally a return to equilibrium. During such crisis periods, a person is at least temporarily unable to respond with his or her usual problem-solving activities to solve the crisis. Roskies[59] noted a similar "birth crisis" in her observations of mothers of children with limb defects caused by thalidomide.

With the birth of a child with a malformation, the mother must mourn the loss of her expected normal infant.[63] In addition, she must become attached to her actual living, damaged child (Fig. 7–5). However, the sequence of parental reactions to the birth of a baby with a malformation differs from that following the death of a child in another respect. Because of the complex issues raised by the continuation of the child's life

and hence the demands of his physical care, the parents' sadness, which is initially important in their relationship with the child, diminishes in most instances once they take over the physical care. Most parents reach a point at which they are able to care adequately for their child and to cope effectively with disrupting feelings of sadness and anger. The mother's initiation of the relationship with her child is a major step in the reduction of anxiety and emotional upset associated with the trauma of the birth. As with normal children, the parents' initial experience with their infant seems to release positive feelings that aid the mother-child relationship following the stresses associated with the news of the child's anomaly and, in many instances, the separation of mother and child in the hospital. Lampe et al[39] noted a significantly greater amount of

Figure 7–5. Change in mental image that mother with malformed baby must make following delivery. Normal mental portrait must be changed to real baby.

MOTHER'S
MENTAL IMAGE
(during pregnancy)

REAL BABY

HAPPY
BEAUTIFUL
ACTIVE BOY
(BLUE EYED)

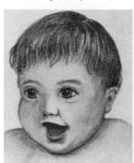
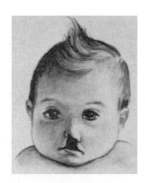

visiting if an infant with an abnormality had been at home for a short while before surgery for a cleft lip repair.

Practical Suggestions for Parents of Malformed Infants

1. If medically feasible, it is far better to leave the infant with the mother and father for the first 2 to 3 days or to discharge them. If the child is rushed to the hospital where special surgery will eventually be done, the mother and father will not have enough opportunity to become attached to him. Even if immediate surgery is necessary, as in the case of bowel obstruction, it is best to bring the baby to the mother first, allowing her to touch and handle him, and to point out to her how normal he is in all other respects.
2. The parents' mental picture of the anomaly may often be far more alarming than the actual problem. Any delay greatly heightens their anxiety and causes their imaginations to run wild. Therefore, we suggest that it is helpful to bring the baby to both parents when they are together as soon after delivery as possible.
3. We believe that parents should not be given tranquilizers, which tend to blunt their responses and slow their adaptation to the problem. However, a sedative at night is sometimes helpful.
4. Parents who are adapting reasonably well often ask many questions and indeed at times appear to be almost overinvolved in clinical care. We are pleased by this and are more concerned about the parents who ask few questions and who appear stunned or overwhelmed by the problem. Parents who become involved in trying to find out what the best procedures are and who ask many questions about care are sometimes annoying but often adapt best in the end.
5. Many anomalies are frustrating to the physicians and nurses as well. There is a temptation for the physician to withdraw from the parents who ask many questions and then appear to forget and ask the same questions again and again.
6. We have found it best to move at the parents' pace. If we move too quickly, we run the risk of losing the parents along the way. It is beneficial to ask the parents how they view their infant.
7. Each parent may move through the process of shock, denial, anger, guilt, and adaptation at a different pace. If the parents are unable to talk with each other about the baby, their own relationship may be disrupted. Therefore we use the process of early crisis intervention and meet several times with the parents. During these discussions we ask the mother how she is doing, how she feels the father is doing, and how he feels about the infant. We then reverse the questions and ask the father how he is doing and how he thinks his wife is progressing. Many times a parent is surprised by the responses of his or her partner. The hope is that the parents not only will think about their own reactions but also will begin to consider each other's. For further discussion see Case Two.
8. Most maternity units are designed for the care of healthy mothers and babies. Therefore, when a baby is born with a problem such as a congenital malformation, the mother's mood and needs are out of step with the routines of the floor. Usually there is no special provision to meet the needs of the small group of parents with babies with malformations. They suffer from the assembly-line routines set up to provide care for the large volume of parents with husky and fully intact newborns. Physicians and nurses may cheerfully burst into the room and ask how the baby is doing, forgetting that he has been kept in the nursery because of the problem or has been transferred to another hospital or division. We try to assign a specific nurse to the mother of such an infant. This nurse needs to have the ability to sit for long periods with the mother and just listen to her cry and tell about her powerful reactions, which are often disturbingly critical and negative.
9. One of the major goals of postpartum discussions is to keep the family together both during this early period and in subsequent years. This is best done by working hard to bring out issues early and by encouraging the parents to talk about their difficult thoughts and feelings as they arise. It is best for them to share their problems with each other. Some couples who do not seem to be close

previously may move closer together as they work through the process of adaptation. As with any painful experience, the parents may be much stronger after they have gone through these reactions together. It is helpful when the father stays with his partner during the hospitalization.

◆ STILLBIRTH OR DEATH OF A NEWBORN

Despite the advances in obstetric and neonatal care, many mothers encounter a great disappointment with an early abortion or the perinatal loss of an infant. Until recently, it was not appreciated that a mourning reaction in both parents after the death of a newborn is universal.[33] Whether the baby lives 1 hour or 2 weeks, whether the baby is a nonviable 500 g or weighs 4000 g, whether or not the baby was planned, and whether or not the mother has had physical contact with her baby, clearly identifiable mourning will be present. Mothers and fathers who have lost a tiny newborn show the same mourning reactions as those reported by Lindemann,[42] who studied survivors of the Coconut Grove fire.

Lindemann has concluded that normal grief is a definite syndrome. It includes the following aspects:

- Somatic distress with tightness of the throat, choking, shortness of breath, need for sighing, and an empty feeling in the abdomen, lack of muscular power, and an intense subjective distress described as tension or mental pain
- Preoccupation with the image of the deceased
- Feelings of guilt and preoccupation with one's negligence or minor omissions
- Feelings of hostility toward others
- Breakdown of normal patterns of conduct

Although originally we believed that loss of an infant was similar to the loss of a close relative, we believe now, based on clinical studies and observations, that it fits far more closely with the concepts proposed by Furman[20] and Lewis.[41] Furman eloquently notes these reactions:

Internally, the mourning process consists of two roughly opposing mechanisms. One is the generally known process of detachment, by which each memory that ties the family to the person who is deceased has to become painfully revived and painfully loosened. This is the part of the process that involves anger, guilt, pain, and sadness. The second process is commonly called "identification." It is the means by which the deceased or parts of him are taken into the self and preserved as part of the self, thereby soothing the pain of loss. In many instances, a surviving marriage partner takes over hobbies and interests of the deceased spouse. These identifications soothe the way and make the pain of detachment balanced and bearable.

For the surviving parents, the death of a newborn is special in several ways. Because mourning is mourning of a separate person, the process can apply only to that small part of the relationship to the newborn that was characterized by the love of a separate person, but there has not been time to build up strong ties and memories of mutual living. It is also not possible for parents—adults functioning in the grown-up world—to take into themselves any part of a helpless newborn and make it adaptively a part of themselves; the mechanism of identification does not work. But what about the part of the newborn which was still part of the self and that cannot be mourned? To understand this part, one has to look at the different process by which individuals cope with a loss of a part of the self, for example, amputation or loss of function. Insofar as the newborn remains a part of the parent's self, the death has to be dealt with as would the amputation of a limb or the loss of function of the parent's body. Detachment is the mechanism with which the victim deals with such tragedies, but it is detachment of a different kind. Acceptance that one will never ever again have that part of oneself is very different from the detachment that

deals with the memories of living together with a loved one. The feelings
that accompany this detachment are
similar in kind and intensity: anger,
guilt, fury, helplessness, and horror. In
the case of the loss of a part of the self,
however, they are quite unrelieved by
identification.

Next, with such a tragedy there must
be a readjustment in one's self-image.
It is, however, altogether different to
have to readjust to thinking of oneself
as an imperfect human being, a human
being that cannot walk or cannot see.
That is a pain of a different kind, and
the feelings that accompany it are emp-
tiness, loss of self-esteem, and feeling
low. Because the internal self never
materialized in those arms and has not
had a chance to be detached, it is very
different from the process of mourning.

These feelings are made particularly
difficult because people around the
parents are not there to help. At a conscious level, people say they simply do
not understand about losing part of the
self, and indeed they do not. Unconsciously they understand it all too
well. It fills them with fear the way an
amputee fills many people with fear
and anxiety and makes them shun him.
This is the treatment that parents of
dead newborns get. They are shunned,
and they cannot rely on the sympathy
that is usually accorded the bereaved.

This grief syndrome may appear immediately after a death or may be delayed or
apparently absent. Those who have studied
mourning responses have indicated that a
painful period of grieving is a normal and
necessary response to the loss of a loved one
and the absence of a period of grieving is not
a healthy sign but rather a cause for alarm.

Without any therapeutic intervention, a
tragic outcome for the mother has been
shown in one third of the perinatal deaths.
Cullberg[12] found that 19 of 56 mothers studied 1 to 2 years after the deaths of their
neonates had developed severe psychiatric
disease (psychoses, anxiety attacks, phobias,
obsessive thoughts, and deep depressions).
Because of the disastrous outcome in such a
high proportion of mothers, it is necessary
to examine in detail how to care for the
family following a neonatal death.

In observations of parents who have lost
newborns, the disturbance of communication between the parents has been a particularly troublesome problem. A father and
mother who have communicated well before
the birth of a baby often have such strong
feelings after an infant's death that they are
unable to share their thoughts and therefore
have an unsatisfactory resolution to their
grieving. In the United States it is expected
that men will be strong and not show their
feelings, so a physician should encourage a
father and mother to talk together about the
loss and advise them not to hold back their
responses—"Cry when you feel like crying."
Unless told what to expect, their reactions
may worry and perplex them, and this may
tend further to disturb the preexisting father
and mother relationship.

At the time of the baby's death, it is important to tell the parents *together* about the
usual reactions to the loss of a child and the
length of time these last. It is desirable to
meet a second time with both parents before
discharge to go over the same suggestions,
which may not have been heard or may have
been misunderstood under the emotional
shock of the baby's death. The pediatrician
or social worker should plan to meet with
the parents together again 3 or 4 months
after the death to check on the parents' activities and on how the mourning process is
proceeding. At the same time, he or she can
discuss the autopsy findings and any further
questions presented by the parents. At this
visit, the pediatrician or social worker
should be alert for abnormal grief reactions,
which, if present, may guide the physician
to refer the parents for psychiatric assistance. It is important that these recommendations not become an exact prescription for
every parent. As noted by I. Leon,[40] "Such
protocols can lead to a regimented assembly-line approach—which impedes attempts
to attune to parents individually and
empathetically—the very essence of providing support."

Lindemann noted that pathologic mourning reactions represent distortion of normal
grief. On the basis of his observations, he
lists 10 such reactions.

- Overactivity without a sense of loss
- Acquisition of symptoms belonging to
  the last illness of the deceased
- Psychosomatic reactions such as ulcerative colitis, asthma, or rheumatoid arthritis

◆ Alterations in relation to friends and relatives
◆ Furious hostility against specific persons
◆ Repression of hostility against specific persons
◆ Repression of hostility, leading to a wooden and formal manner resembling schizophrenic pictures
◆ Lasting loss of patterns of social interaction
◆ Activities detrimental to one's own social and economic existence
◆ Agitated depressions

For further discussion see Case Four.

EDITORIAL COMMENT: Cullberg's report about the severe psychiatric reactions in Swedish mothers was published in 1966. The practices in the United States following a stillbirth or neonatal death, at that time, were similar to those in Sweden. Following other reports about parents' turbulent and prolonged mourning reactions, similar changes in the care of bereaved families were introduced in both countries. Valuable new information for counseling parents has recently come from a large study in Sweden that found a more favorable long-term adjustment.

In a systematic study of 380 women following a stillbirth, Rädestad[54] observed that mothers of stillborn infants had a diminished risk of symptoms 3 years after the death if there was a short time between diagnosis of death and initiation of the delivery, if the mother was allowed to meet and say farewell to her child as long as she wished, and if there was a collection of tokens of remembrance (hand or footprints, lock of hair, and photograph). They noted that mothers living alone may have special needs for support.

CASE PROBLEMS

The clinical relevance of this subject can best be appreciated by the following case examples and the questions they raise. The words chosen in any discussion depend on the needs and problems of individual patients at that moment. We have not given our answers as a specific formula but rather so that the reader may have an idea of how we approach parents.

◆

Case One

Mrs. W had a normal pregnancy until 32 weeks' gestation, when she unexpectedly went into labor and delivered a 2 lb 15 ounce (1332 g) female infant in a community hospital. The baby cried promptly but then moderate respiratory distress developed requiring arterial catheterization, prompt intubation, surfactant administration, and ventilator care up to and during transfer to a tertiary level neonatal intensive care unit (NICU) at the medical center.

The following questions should be answered when caring for this mother, father and infant.

◆ *What is the ideal method of communicating with both parents?*
The best method of communicating with both parents is to have them sit down with you in a quiet, private room. You will be most effective if you can listen to the parents, let them express their worries and feelings, then give simple, realistically optimistic explanations.

◆ *How should advice be given when discussing the situation with the parents? What should they be told about their infant and her chances for survival?*
When first discussing the situation with the parents, advice should be given promptly, simply, and optimistically. As soon as possible after the birth, the mother and father can be told that the baby is small but well formed. When it is clear that the baby has respiratory distress, you can explain to the parents that the baby has a common problem of premature infants ("breathing difficulty") caused by the complex adjustments she must make from life in utero to life outside. This is called respiratory distress syndrome (RDS). In addition, it should be stated that because this condition is common, the neonatologists at the tertiary NICU in a medical center know best how to treat it, and their results with this weight infant are quite good.

◆ *What should the mother and father be told about the ventilator?*
Some of the parents' anxiety can be relieved by pointing out that the ventilator is augmenting the baby's breathing; that is, the baby is still able to breathe, but this is helping. Explaining that the baby is not able to cry audibly when an endotracheal tube is present relieves another common concern.

◆ *Can the parents see the baby before transfer?*
Yes! You can explain that the mother, father, and siblings will be given time and an opportunity to see and touch the baby in the transport incubator with a nurse or neonatologist present to monitor and support the

baby, siblings, and parents. Pictures of the baby will be obtained before the transfer.

◆ **Is it wise to discuss breast-feeding and the value of breast milk for a baby that will be transferred?**

Yes, emphasizing the importance of pumping milk right away will increase the odds that Mrs. W will be able to provide breast milk for her baby. Discussing breast-feeding at this time when the parents are extremely anxious about whether the baby will live, conveys to the parents that you expect Baby Girl W to do well. You can explain that the staff will help the mother start pumping her breasts because her breast milk will be an essential part of the treatment for her daughter, not only for her nutrition but also to decrease the risk of infection and to improve the baby's brain development. It will also enhance the mother's bonding with her daughter, particularly when Mrs. W begins to directly breast-feed her daughter and repeatedly experiences the let-down reflex.

◆ **What other arrangements should be made before the baby is transferred?**

Communication with both the referring and receiving centers and the obstetrician is necessary. Most obstetricians want to know whether a baby is transferred. They can help the family by arranging for the early discharge of the mother so she can go to her baby in the medical center. Sometimes mother and baby can both be transferred.

Checking that the baby is sent to the correct hospital that accepts the family's insurance is crucial.

◆ **Baby Girl W is transported by helicopter to the NICU at the medical center. She receives surfactant and gradually begins to wean off the ventilator. After 4 hours, the ventilator settings have decreased to FiO_2 60%, peak inspiratory pressure 26 mm Hg, positive end-expiratory pressure 5 mm Hg, rate 25. An ABG reveals pH 7.33; $PaCO_2$ 41 mm Hg; PaO_2 62 mm Hg. When the mother and father arrive, the neonatologist meets with them in her office.**

The physician asks "Would you please tell me what the doctors at the community hospital told you and what you understand about your daughter's condition?" After hearing the answer, she explains that the baby tolerated the transfer well and that they are beginning to wean their daughter off the ventilator. She agrees with the diagnosis of RDS and comments that "RDS often runs a course of increasing symptoms for a day or two and then the breathing gradually becomes easier. With RDS there is stress on the whole baby, so, as the lungs improve,

other organs, such as the intestines, may show problems. Distention or fullness of the abdomen may develop and it may be necessary to progress slowly with feedings. Throughout the first few days, routine blood tests, ultrasound, x-rays, and other studies may be obtained repeatedly to be certain that the diagnosis and treatment are correct and to check that no other problem such as infection has developed. The outlook for your daughter is good for complete recovery after several days."

The physician says she will be giving their daughter routine care for a premature infant. She says "When I have had time to complete more tests and observations, if there is any change in what I have told you, I will call you. I will keep you posted on the baby's progress. I would like you to call at other times if you have questions. I am pleased that you both came in together. In the next days if one of you is here and I have something new to report, I will plan to talk to one of you on the telephone while the other is in the office with me.

"I would like you to come to the nursery as often as you can. I want you to become well acquainted with your daughter and her care. Your milk will be a very important part of her treatment and you may find your milk flows more abundantly when you are with your baby, particularly when you are skin-to-skin in kangaroo care. I will tell you more about this when I think the baby is ready."

◆ **Can the nurses help the mother adapt to the premature infant?**

The nurses can aid the mother in adapting to the premature infant by standing with her and explaining the equipment being used for the baby, by welcoming the mother by name and with personalized comments at each visit and encouraging her to come back soon, by carefully considering the mother's concerns and feelings, by explaining to her that the baby will benefit from her visits, and by showing her how she can gradually assume more of the baby's care and do the mothering better than the nurses. Together they may identify events such as loud noises and bright lights that appear to be stressful to the baby as well as environmental changes that appear to relax her. Then they can plan modifications in positioning, feeding, and times for medications as well as environmental adjustments to increase the amount of time when the baby appears to be free of stress.

◆ *What are the normal processes that a mother goes through when she delivers a premature infant and how can the physicians and nurses assist her?*

The premature delivery often occurs before a mother is thoroughly ready to accept the idea that she is going to have an infant. Such a mother is faced with a baby who is thin, scrawny, and very different from the ideal full-sized baby she has been picturing in her mind. She may have to grieve the loss of this anticipated ideal baby as she adjusts to the reality of the premature baby with all her problems and special needs.

All of the equipment and activities of a premature nursery are new and may be frightening to a mother. The tubes, the flashing lights, the beepers, and other instruments used in a premature nursery are disturbing. If the functions of these items are explained to the mother, her concern will decrease. For example, "The two wires on the baby's chest and the beeping instrument tell us if the baby slows down in her respirations so we can rub her skin to remind her to keep breathing. This is frequently necessary during the first few days with a tiny infant." It may be helpful for the mother and infant to be together as much as possible in the early days. The mother's guilt and anxiety, and the fear that touching the infant will harm her, sometimes leads her to turn down an offer to visit the infant. No mother should be forced to visit her infant against her wishes; however, it is important for the hospital personnel to reassure her and encourage her visits, but always to move at the mother's pace.

◆ *What should the mother be told when she asks, "How is the baby doing?"*

It is a common reflex in physicians and nurses to prepare patients for a possible poor outcome and to think in a problem-oriented manner. It is of great importance to provide encouragement to the mother so that mother-infant affectional ties develop as easily as possible, so it is desirable to approach this question in an optimistic but realistic manner. It is wise to start out by asking the mother how *she* thinks the baby is doing.

◆ *When should these parents take the baby home?*

At 2 weeks, Baby Girl W developed an episode of suspected sepsis with abdominal distention that responded to nothing-by-mouth and antibiotics. The cultures were negative. At 4 weeks, Baby Girl W weighs 3 pounds 14 ounces (1758 g).

The baby has been breast-feeding one or two times a day for the past 4 days and taking breast milk from the bottle. She is gaining weight and has good temperature control without an incubator. There is no infection in the home. Shortly after the baby responded to the sepsis treatment, Mrs. W called to say she was sick with the flu and would not come to the NICU. She called each day for 10 days and her husband brought in the breast milk she had pumped. In this case, the timing of going home depends on the mother whose visiting pattern was regular until the last week. At that time, Baby Girl W's nurse suggested that the mother spend 3 or 4 hours with her baby, give her a bath, and feed her. Mrs. W agreed, enjoyed this, and spent 6 to 8 hours caring for her baby girl over the next 3 days. Mrs. W has a bassinet and equipment to care for her daughter at home and her husband has canceled his out-of-town trips for the next 3 weeks.

Baby Girl W went home in the winter so the parents were advised to avoid contact with children with colds. Baby Girl W was given the first injection of Synagis to be followed by injections monthly until April to protect her against respiratory syncytial virus infection.

◆

Case Two

Mrs. J, a 25-year old primiparous mother, delivered a full-term infant after a 12-hour uneventful labor. The infant was found to have a cleft lip and palate. The following questions should be answered concerning the care of this infant and mother.

◆ *Should the father be told about this before the mother has returned to her room?*

Every effort should be made to tell the mother and father together about this problem; however, this is such an obvious defect that the father will notice it and the mother will at least sense that something is wrong. If this is the case, the doctor should indicate that there is a problem but that he wants to check the baby over thoroughly and will then tell both parents about the problem and what will be done about it. It is popularly believed that the father is in much better condition to learn about difficulties right after delivery than the mother, but often a woman is better able to accept news about an illness or abnormality in her baby—in an emotional sense—than the father. Any plan to give one bit of news or a different shading about the prognosis to one parent and not the other interferes with the communication between the parents. It is extremely important to support and encourage this communication. The infant should be brought to the parents as soon as the mother and the infant are in satisfactory condition and after the caregiving physician (obstetrician or pediatrician) has the details of the baby's problem clearly in mind and is aware of the baby's health status. The baby should be kept in the delivery room for the examinations and then brought to the mother's bed. The appearance of a baby with an uncorrected cleft palate and lip is grotesque and shocking for anyone who has not seen this before. Allowing the parents time to observe, react, and ask questions will be necessary. Fantasies about what can be seen are common, for example, that there is an open connection to the brain. Therefore, the experienced physician or nurse will point out the underlying structures, emphasize that they are basically normal, and demonstrate how the surgeon will pull the skin edges of the cleft together to cover the exposed underlying tissue. Before and after pictures of surgically repaired infants are helpful and may enable parents to appreciate why the physician has been so optimistic about the baby's future appearance and normal developmental potential. It is worthwhile to repeat and emphasize the general good health and well-being of the baby.

◆ **Who should tell the mother: the obstetrician, the pediatrician, the nurse, or the father?**
The obstetrician, whom the mother has known for many months, is usually the best person to tell the mother. He or she needs information from a pediatrician about the nature of the problem and the general health of the baby. Even better, the obstetrician and the pediatrician may go together to tell the parents about the problem. If the obstetrician can speak briefly and calmly to the mother, then the pediatrician can continue with a brief explanation about the problem. Under most circumstances, neither the nurse nor the father will be in a position to provide enough reassurance to the mother to make this first encounter progress optimally.

◆ **How should the problem be presented to the parents?**
It is desirable whenever possible to emphasize to the parents the normal healthy features of the baby. For example, "Mr. and Mrs. Jones, you have a strong 8-pound baby

boy who is kicking, screaming, and carrying out all the normal functions of a healthy baby. There is one problem present that fortunately we will be able to correct, so it will not be a continuing problem for your son. As far as I can tell, the baby is completely well otherwise. I would like to show the baby and this problem to you."

◆ **Should the baby be present?**
Yes. As ugly as a cleft palate and lip may appear to a mother, exposure to the reality of the problem is important and is usually less disturbing than the mother's fantasies.

◆
Case Three
At birth, the male infant of a white 28-year-old mother was scrawny with decreased subcutaneous fatty tissue and axillary and gluteal skin folds. At 35 weeks' gestational age, the weight was 3 lbs 4–1/2 oz (1480 g), more than 2 standard deviations below the mean and fiftieth percentile for 31 weeks. The length was in the low normal range and the head circumference was at the 2 percentile line. The baby breathed and cried promptly. The mother was upset with his thinness, saying her two previous babies were full-term and "filled out." When blood was drawn and an intravenous (IV) line with glucose started, the infant was noted to be jittery. Glucose, calcium, electrolytes, and blood counts were normal. Examination showed no malformations.

◆ **What other causes should be considered?**
The previous record of the mother was not found. When asked about prenatal care, she indicated that she had attended two prenatal visits with an obstetrician at the medical center. She said she had planned to deliver there but when labor pains started she had thought it best to go to the nearby community hospital. This was an unusual course of action. Obstetric patients do not often change obstetrician and hospital with onset of labor.

Shortly after delivery, a well-dressed, polite father arrived and immediately inquired which laboratory tests had been sent on his wife and son. The father remained with his wife during all postnatal care, often answering questions for her. Upon seeing his newborn son attached to an IV line, he insisted, "My child is perfectly well, just small and cold. I want both my wife and son discharged today."

Perplexed by the excessive anxiety of the family as well as the continued jitteriness of the baby, the neonatologist sent infant urine and stool toxicology screens, which were positive for cocaine. The laboratory technician said that (in 1999) these tests were very rarely obtained on an infant in this hospital and that this was the first positive test.

At this point the father picked up the baby, and with his wife, started to leave. Security personnel were called and stopped the father. He had a gun in his pocket. Emergency custody for the baby was obtained.

In retrospect, the neonatologist wished that he had told Security before he told the parents. He realized that he should have notified the Department of Human Services that he was suspicious and was going to test and tell the parents.

◆ *What other concerns should be checked when a baby is positive for cocaine?*
This is often just the tip of an iceberg. Spouse abuse, human immunodeficiency virus infection, and the safety of other children in the home must be seriously considered.

When the mother was examined, there were large bruises on her trunk. When asked in privacy, she said her husband hit her. She agreed to go into treatment for her cocaine addiction. As an adult, she could not be kept in the hospital if she did not wish to stay. Photographs of the mother and her bruises were taken before she left, and she was told that these and the records of what she said would be kept if she needed them in the future. Custody of the baby was given to the maternal grandmother. Later, the mother said she came to this community hospital because she thought there would be no testing for cocaine.

As a result of this incident, the hospital has installed surveillance cameras. Some hospitals have coded bracelets for the baby's arms or ankles, or umbilical tags that set off an alarm if a baby is taken. Others have a hospital public address code for a missing baby, e.g., "Baby White."

◆
Case Four
A 1-pound, 15 ounce (880 g) infant of a 29-year-old mother with 2-year-old and 4½-year-old children died suddenly at 26 hours. The pregnancy was planned. The mother had not held or touched her baby.

◆ *What are the processes this mother and father will go through?*
The parents in this situation will go through intense mourning reactions. It will help the parents to see and hold the baby after the death. They may wish to bathe or undress and dress the baby. There should be no restriction on the time with their infant. The mother and father may desire to have a nurse with them or to be alone and may want relatives or friends or the two siblings to see the baby. If the parents can cry together, they themselves can best help each other. The use of drugs, except for a night's sleep, is therefore not indicated. Even though the mother did not handle the infant, she and the father will be expected to show strong mourning responses, which will be intense for 1 or 2 months, and under optimal circumstances will be decreased by 6 months. In the United States, where the expression of emotion is not encouraged, the father will often force himself to hold back his emotions to provide "strong support" for the mother. This is actually harmful, because a free and easy communication between the parents about their feelings is highly desirable for the resolution of mourning. On the basis of the studies that have been carried out, the stronger the mourning reaction in the early days and weeks, the more favorable the outcome.

◆ *How can the physician help them?*
It is important for the physician to describe the details of the baby's death to both parents together within a few hours of the death of the baby. At that time, he should explain the type of mourning reaction they will go through. Then, as a minimum, the physician should again meet with the parents 3 or 4 days later, or after the funeral, to find out how they are managing, to go over the details once more, and to indicate availability for any questions or problems. At the postpartum checkup, the obstetrician should take time to ask how the parents are managing and should evaluate the normality of their mourning and their communication. When there are other children in the family, the pediatrician should inquire about their responses. Parents are in emotional pain and are distracted with their own thoughts after a perinatal loss. It is desirable to have someone else—a grandparent or a friendly neighbor—be attentive to the surviving children and to listen to their questions and concerns. It should be explained (if appropriate) that changes in the appearance or behavior of their parents are because they feel so badly about the death. This "surrogate parent" should reassure the siblings that the baby died because of its premature

birth and that nothing they thought or did caused the baby to be sick or to die.

Three or four months after the death of the baby, the physician should set aside a period of time to meet with both parents to present and discuss the autopsy results, review the present status of the parents and their children, and go over what has occurred since the death, their understanding of the death, and the normality of their reactions. If the mourning response is pathologic, the physician should then refer the parents for additional assistance. Using these procedures, Forrest et al[19] noted significantly less depression and anxiety in parents compared with control subjects. Also, they noted that an early pregnancy (<6 months after the loss) was strongly associated with high depression and anxiety scores at 14 months.

This short enumeration of guidelines may incorrectly convey the impression of a mechanical quality to these discussions, which is not at all our intent. Parents appreciate evidence of human concern and reactions in a physician at times such as these, so we would encourage physicians to show the sadness they feel and to allow the parents to express their pent-up feelings by making a statement such as "I know you both must feel very sad and upset."

◆ SUMMARY

In most instances, the hospital determines the events surrounding birth and death, stripping these two most important events in life of the long-established traditions and support systems established over centuries to help families through these transitions.

Because the newborn baby completely depends on his parents for his survival and optimal development, it is essential to understand the process of attachment. Although we are only beginning to understand this complex phenomenon, those responsible for the care of mothers and infants would be wise to reevaluate the hospital procedures that interfere with early, sustained parent-infant contact and to consider measures that promote parents' experiences with their infant.

REFERENCES

1. Achenbach M, Phares V, Howell CT, et al: Seven-year outcome of the Vermont Intervention Program for Low-Birthweight Infants. Child Dev 61:1772, 1990.
2. Als H, Lawhon G, Duffey FH, et al: Individual developmental care for the very low-birth weight preterm infant. JAMA 272:853, 1994.
3. Anisfeld E, Lipper E: Early contact, social support, and mother-infant bonding. Pediatrics 72:79, 1983.
4. Barnett C, Leiderman P, Grobstein R, et al: Neonatal separation: The maternal side of interactional deprivation. Pediatrics 45:197, 1970.
5. Bibring G: Some considerations of the psychological processes in pregnancy. Psychoanal Study Child 14:113, 1959.
6. Brazelton TB, Cramer B: The Earliest Relationship. Reading, MA: Addison-Wesley, 1990.
7. Budin P: The Nursling. London: Caxton, 1907.
8. Buranasin B: The effects of rooming-in on the success of breast-feeding and the decline in abandonment of children. Asia-Pacific J Public Health 5:217, 1991.
9. Christenson K, Siles L, Moreno A, et al: Temperature, metabolic adaptations, and crying in healthy newborn's cared for skin-to-skin or with a cot. Acta Paediatr Scand 81:488–493, 1992.
10. Cohen R: Some maladaptive syndromes of pregnancy and the puerperium. Obstet Gynecol 27:562, 1966.
11. Condon W, Sander L: Neonate movement is synchronized with adult speech: Interactional participation and language acquisition. Science 183:99, 1974.
12. Cullberg J: Mental reactions of women to perinatal death. In Morris N, ed: Psychomatic Medicine in Obstetrics and Gynecology. New York: S Karger, 1972.
13. De Casper A, Fifer WF: Of human bonding: Newborns prefer their mothers' voices. Science 208:1174, 1980.
14. Derbyshire F, Davies DP, Baeco A: Discharge of preterm babies from neonatal units. BMJ 284:233, 1982.
15. Emde R, Swedberg J, Suzuki B: Human wakefulness and biological rhythms after birth. Arch Gen Psychiatry 32:780, 1975.
16. Engel GL, Reichsman F, Harvay VT: Infant feeding behavior of a mother gastric fistula fed as an infant: A 30 year longitudinal study of enduring effects. In Anthony EJ, Pollack GH, eds: Parental Influences in Health and Diseases. Boston, Little Brown, 1985, p 29.
17. Fanaroff A, Kennell J, Klaus M: Follow-up of low-birth-weight infants—The predictive value of maternal visiting patterns. Pediatrics 49:287, 1972.
18. Field TM: Effects of early separation, interactive deficits and experimental manipulations on infant-mother face-to-face interaction. Child Dev 48:763, 1977.
19. Forrest GC: Care of the bereaved after perinatal death. In Chalmers I, Enkin M, Keirse MJNC, eds: Effective Care in Pregnancy and Childbirth. Oxford: Oxford University Press, 1989.
20. Furman EP: The death of a newborn: Care of the parents. Birth Fam J 5:214, 1978.
21. Green M, Solnit A: Reactions to the threatened loss of a child: A vulnerable child syndrome. Pediatrics 34:58, 1964.
22. Gross R, et al: Enhancing the outcomes of low birth-weight premature infants. JAMA 263:3035, 1991.

23. Harper RG, Sia C, Sokal M: Observations on unrestricted parental contact with infants in the neonatal intensive care unit. J Pediatr 89:441, 1976.
24. Helfer R, Kempe C, eds: The Battered Child. Chicago: University of Chicago Press, 1997.
25. Hodnett ED, Osborne RW: Effects of continuous intrapartum professional support on childbirth outcomes. Res Nurs Health 12:289, 1989.
26. Hofmeyer GJ, Nikodem VC, Wolman NL: Companionship to modify the clinical birth environment. Br J Obstet Gynecol 98:756, 1991.
27. James VL Jr, Wheeler WE: The care-by-parent unit. Pediatrics 43:488, 1969.
28. Kaitz M, Good A, Rokem AM, et al: Mother's and father's recognition of their newborn's photographs during the postpartum period. J Dev Behav Pediatr 9:223, 1988.
29. Kaitz M, Good A, Rokem AM, Eidelman AI: Mothers' recognition of their olfactory cues. Dev Psychobiol 20:587, 1987.
30. Kennell J, Rolnik A: Discussing problems in newborn babies with their parents. Pediatrics 26:832, 1960.
31. Kennell J, Klaus M, McGrath S, et al: Continuous emotional support during labor in a U.S. hospital. JAMA 265:2197, 1991.
32. Kennell JH, McGrath SK: Labor support by a doula for middle-income couples. Pediatric Res 33:12A, 1993.
33. Kennell J, Slyter H, Klaus M: The mourning response of parents to the death of a newborn. N Engl J Med 283:344, 1970.
34. Keverne EB, Kendrick KM: Maternal behavior in sheep and its neuroendocrine regulation. Acta Paediatr Scand 83:47, 397, 1994.
35. Klaus M, Kennell J: Parent-Infant Bonding. St. Louis: CV Mosby, 1982.
36. Klaus MH, Kennell JH, Robertson SS, et al: Effects of social support during parturition on maternal and infant morbidity. BMJ 293:585, 1986.
37. Klaus M, Jerauld R, Kreger N, et al: Maternal attachment: Importance of the first post-partum days. N Engl J Med 286:460, 1972.
38. Klein M, Stern L: Low birth weight and the battered child syndrome. Am J Dis Child 122:15, 1971.
39. Lampe J, Trause M, Kennell J: Parental visiting of sick infants: The effects of living at home prior to hospitalization. Pediatrics 59:294, 1977.
40. Leon I: Perinatal loss: Choreographing grief on an obstetrical unit. Am J Orthopsychiatry 62:7, 1992.
41. Lewis E: Inhibition of mourning by pregnancy: Psychopathology and management. BMJ 2:27, 1979.
42. Lindemann E: Symptomatology and management of acute grief. Am J Psychiatry 101:141, 1994.
43. Lozoff B, Brittenham G, Trause M, et al: The mother-newborn relationship: Limits of adaptability. J Pediatr 91:1, 1977.
44. MacFarlane JA, Smith DM, Garrow DH: The relationship between mother and neonate. In Kitzinger S, Davis JA, eds: The Place of Birth. New York: Oxford University Press, 1978.
45. Minde K, Shosenberg B, Marton P, et al: Self-help groups in a premature nursery—A controlled evaluation. J Pediatr 96:933, 1980.
46. Minde K, Trehub S, Corter C, et al: Mother-child relationships in the premature nursery: An observational study. Pediatrics 61:373, 1978.
47. Newman LF: Parents' perceptions of their low birth weight infants. Pediatrician 9:182, 1980.
48. Newton N, Newton M: Mothers' reactions to their newborn babies. JAMA 181:206, 1962.
49. Nissen E, Lilja G, Widstrom AM: Elevation of oxytocin levels in early postpartum women. Acta Obstet Gynecol Scand 74:530, 1995.
50. O'Connor S, Vietze PM, Sherrod KB, et al: Reduced incidence of parenting inadequacy following rooming-in. Pediatrics 66:176, 1980.
51. Olshansky S: Chronic sorrow: A response to having a mentally defective child. Social Casework 43:190, 1962.
52. Parke R: Fatherhood. Cambridge: Harvard University Press, 1996.
53. Porter RH, Makin JW, Davis LB, et al: Breast-fed infants respond to olfactory cues from their own mother and unfamiliar lactating females. Infant Behav Dev 15:85, 1992.
54. Rädestad I, Steineck G, Nordin C, Sjögren B: Psychological complications after stillbirth—Influence of memories and immediate management: Population-based study. BMJ 3112:1505–1508, 1996.
55. Righard L, Blade MO: Effect of delivery routines on success of first breast-feed. Lancet 336:1105, 1990.
56. Robson K: The role of eye-to-eye contact in maternal-infant attachment. J Child Psychol Psychiatry 8:13, 1967.
57. Robson K, Kumar R: Delayed onset of maternal affection after childbirth. Br J Psychiatry 136:347, 1980.
58. Rodholm M: Father-infant interaction at the first contact after delivery. Early Hum Dev 3:21, 1979.
59. Roskies E: Abnormality and Normality: The Mothering of Thalidomide Children. New York: Cornell University Press, 1972.
60. Scafidi F, Fields T, Schonberg, et al: Massage stimulates growth in premature infants: A replication. Infant Behav Dev 13:167, 1990.
61. Scott K, Berkowitz G, Klaus M: A comparison of intermittent and continuous support during labor: A meta-analysis. Am J Obstet Gynecol 180:1054, 1999.
62. Siegel E, Bauman KE, Schaefer ES, et al: Hospital and home support during infancy: Impact on maternal attachment, child abuse and neglect, and health care utilization. Pediatrics 66:183, 1980.
63. Solnit A, Stark M: Mourning and the birth of a defective child. Psychoanal Study Child 16:523, 1961.
64. Sosa R, Kennell J, Klaus M, et al: The effect of a supportive companion on perinatal problems, length of labor, and mother-infant interaction. N Engl J Med 303:597, 1980.
65. Tafari N, Ross SM: On the need for organized perinatal care. Ethiop Med J 11:93, 1973.
66. Thompson M, Westreich R: Restriction of mother-infant contact in the immediate postnatal period. In Chalmers I, Enkin M, Kierse MJNC, eds: Effective Care in Pregnancy. Oxford: Oxford University Press, 1989, p 1328.
67. Torres J: The Sotero del Rio Hospital, Santiago, Chile. In Davis JA, Richards MPM, Roberton WRC, eds: Premature Infants. Burrell Row, Kent: Croom Helm Ltd, Provident House, 1983.
68. Uvnäs-Moberg K: The gastrointestinal tract in growth and reproduction. Scientific American 261:78, 1989.
69. Varendi H, Porter RH, Winberg J: Attractiveness and amniotic fluid odor: Evidence of prenatal learning? Acta Paediatrica 85:1223, 1996.

70. Whitelaw A: Kangaroo baby care: Just a nice experience or an important advance for preterm infants? Pediatrics 85:604, 1990.
71. Whitelaw A, Heisterkamp G, Sleath K, et al: Skin to skin contact for very low birthweight infants and their mothers. Arch Dis Child 63:1377, 1988.
72. Widstrom AM, Wahlberg V, Matthiesen AS, et al: Short-term effects of early suckling and touch of the nipple on maternal behavior. Early Hum Dev 21:153, 1990.
73. Widstrom AM, Ransjo-Arvidson AB, Christensson K, et al: Gastric suction in healthy newborn infants: Effects on circulation and developing feeding behavior. Acta Pediatr Scand 76:566, 1987.
74. Winnicott DW: Primary maternal preoccupation. In Collected Papers: Through Pediatrics to Psychoanalysis. New York: Basic Books, 1958.
75. Wolman WL, Chalmers B, Hofmeyer G, et al: Postpartum depression and companionship in the clinical birth environment: A randomized, controlled study. Am J Obstet Gynecol 168:1388, 1993.
76. Wolff P: The Development of Behavioral States and the Expression of Emotions in Early Infancy. Chicago: University of Chicago Press, 1987.

Nursing Practice in the Neonatal Intensive Care Unit

Linda Lefrak
Carolyn Houska Lund

The planning and delivery of nursing care to critically ill neonates is a complex process that necessitates thorough, ongoing evaluation to determine effectiveness of both nursing and medical therapies. This unique evaluation takes into account (1) the frequent introduction of new treatment modalities, (2) the lack of verbal communication with the patient, (3) the narrow margin between safe and adverse responses to therapy, (4) the lack of disease-specific symptoms because of immature development, and (5) the patient's extreme vulnerability, particularly in the most premature or sick infants.

Neonatal nursing involves a variety of unique functions, skills, and responsibilities that are essential in assessing, understanding, and safely supporting the newborn infant and family during this critical time. Neonatal intensive care unit (NICU) nurses must anticipate problems and systematically evaluate the infant and all the support systems to identify any new problems as early as possible. Each nurse completes the following head-to-toe assessment and prepares the associated documentation at least every 8 to 12 hours:

1. Observes physical characteristics such as color, tone, skin integrity, perfusion, and edema
2. Assesses organ systems, including chest auscultation, peripheral pulses, heart sounds, urine output, bowel sounds, and presence of reflexes
3. Checks patency and function of all intravascular devices and security of endotracheal tubes and other invasive devices
4. Verifies presence and appropriate function of all respiratory equipment and monitors
5. Assesses neurobehavioral activity, in-cluding level of pain or discomfort in relation to treatment
6. Describes parental contact and attachment behaviors.

Thorough assessment by the NICU nurse is followed by the identification of specific patient problems that require either nursing or medical intervention. Once problems are identified, the process of planning and implementing of interventions is undertaken.

EDITORIAL COMMENT: Nurses also make innumerable subconscious assessments of each infant they manage. Any physician who does not take into consideration a nurse's objective as well as subconscious observations courts disaster. The signs and signals that nurses perceive may be the first indication that a major problem is beginning.

The nurse is also responsible for the safe and appropriate use of technical equipment in the care of these critically ill newborns. Since the 1970s, the number of electrical devices used for a single patient has steadily increased, beginning with the use of a single warming device (the incubator) and progressing to the current standard use of 10 to 12 devices per patient. The nurse is responsible for using these devices with a level of expertise such that problems can be recognized. An essential component of the nursing role involves the relationship between the nurse and the parents and family of each infant. Because initial phases of attachment develop during this time of crisis, the whole family is in a vulnerable position as members begin to establish their relationship with the baby. The neonatal nurse assists the parents in beginning to know and appreciate their baby in a highly technical environment where touching and holding are sometimes difficult to accomplish (see Chapter 7). The modeling of communication and interaction with fragile newborns is a particularly effective method of assisting parents with this process. The explanation of the treatments and continual reinforcement of information provided by the infant's physicians regarding current condition and prognosis are necessary during this crisis. Nurses often become a major source of social support, especially during long or complicated hospitalizations.

EDITORIAL COMMENT: As the nurse cares for both the infant and the family, there is a delicate balance to achieve to prevent the mother from feeling excessively jealous as well as inept. A positive comment by the nurse describing a caretaking task in which the mother was successful will certainly improve her self-esteem. Interviews of mothers following discharge from the premature nursery often describe both jealousy of the nurses caring for their infants and pleasure at how devoted and skilled the nursing staff was.

Neonatal nurses play a major role as protector, advocate, and, at times, nurturer to the infant in the NICU. Because the nurse's scope of responsibility is limited to a small number of patients at any given time (generally two to three), and because she needs to be almost constantly present at the bedside of these patients, the nurse's observations and evaluations often guide any interventions. For example, an observation regarding an infant's adverse reaction to noise or handling may guide the team to alter their intervention or physical examination. Nurses provide a vital link between the patient and the health care team through their knowledge, proximity to the patient, and skill at interpreting physiologic, behavioral, and technical information. The following discussion provides an overview of the range of nursing practice that currently exists in the NICU, touching on four areas: developmental care, skin care, venous access, and iatrogenic complications.

◆ DEVELOPMENTAL CARE

A significant aspect of providing nursing care to infants in the NICU is to create an environment that reduces noxious stimuli, promotes positive development, and minimizes the negative effects of illness, early delivery, and separation from parents. Neo-natal nurseries have become increasingly concerned about the negative effects of the NICU environment and have begun to identify preventive strategies and integrate changes in this highly technical, overstimulating environment. Interventions are focused on protecting the delicate, immature central nervous system of premature and ill newborns; the term *developmental care* is used to describe this process.

Studies using the NIDCAP (Newborn Individualized Developmental Care and Assessment Program) have shown improved developmental and medical outcomes for premature infants cared for in a developmentally supportive environment with caregivers specially educated in assessing premature infant behavior and modifying care practices to reduce negative or stressful responses.[3, 4, 11, 20, 34] The NIDCAP examination involves in-depth observation and objective scoring of the individual infant's responses to caregiving, with nursing and medical interventions tailored to each infant's needs. Outcomes such as fewer days on ventilation, earlier oral feedings, shorter stays in the hospital with reduced costs, and improved neurodevelopmental behavioral performance have all been described by these studies, as well as in a large, unpublished, multisite study. Despite ongoing skepticism and critique of developmental research,[8, 73] the modern NICU appears quite different than its predecessor: for example, dimmed lights, crib covers, swaddling and supported positioning, and decibel meters are becoming familiar sights. Future research to better understand the effects and contributions of each intervention will shed more light on this area of neonatal nursing care.

This section addresses the effects of noise, light, positioning, and handling during routine care, and it suggests modifications in each area that can reduce the detrimental effects.

Noise in the Neonatal Intensive Care Unit

Much of the technology used to support the newborn in the NICU generates a significant amount of noise and activity. Excessive noise can stimulate the premature or ill term newborn and lead to agitation and crying. This agitation has been shown to cause decreased oxygenation, increased intracranial pressure, and elevated heart and respiratory rates.[62, 107, 108] Noise also disrupts the sleep–wake cycle and may delay recovery and the ability to have positive interactions with parents and caregivers because of fatigue and overwhelming overstimulation.[86]

Noise levels in the NICU are noted to range from 50 to 80 decibels; inside the incubator, measurements from 55 to 88 decibels, with peak levels of 117, have been reported.[100] Damage to delicate auditory structures has been associated with prolonged exposure to over 90 decibels in adults; in neonates, the decibel levels that result in hearing damage have not been identified. However, immature auditory structures may be more susceptible to damage because of the combination of noise and ototoxic medications that are frequently used in NICU patients.

Incubator motors generate an average of 55 to 60 decibels; equipment and activity inside or around the incubator can add an additional 10 to 40 decibels.[100] Routine care activities such as placing glass formula bottles on the bedside table, closing storage drawers, or opening packaged supplies have been recorded at sound levels from 58 to 76 decibels; alarms from intravenous (IV) pumps and cardiorespiratory monitors have also measured 57 to 66 decibels.[30] Noise from staff talking, radios, and monitors can add to this cacophony.[62] Use of ear muffs and other similar devices has been studied,[108] but long-term effects of sensory deprivation are needed before routine use is recommended.

The American Academy of Pediatrics Committee on Environmental Health has concluded that exposure to environmental noise in the NICU may result in cochlear damage and may disrupt normal growth and development. Its recommendations include monitoring decibel readings and providing interventions to keep levels less than 45 decibels.[5]

Interventions to Reduce Noise Levels

1. Modify staff behaviors such as loud talk and playing radios near radiant warmers and incubators.
2. Institute "quiet hours" several times each day when noise-producing activities are curtailed and lights are dimmed.
3. Measure decibel levels to identify baseline sounds as well as any problem areas and times.
4. If possible, avoid overhead paging systems.
5. Remove loud devices from patient care areas.
6. Observe carefully individual infant's responses to auditory stimulation such as music boxes and tape recorders.
7. Consider offering only one sensory stimulus at a time, such as talking or singing without visual, tactile, or vestibular stimuli.
8. Gently open and close isolette doors.
9. Pad doors and drawers of storage closets.
10. Design ceilings with noise-absorbing materials.

Light in the Neonatal Intensive Care Unit

The effect of continuous light exposure is another topic of interest when providing an environment that is developmentally supportive for babies in the NICU. Although constant light exposure in adult ICUs may result in patient disorientation, this finding is not easy to evaluate in newborns. Other concerns about continuous light exposure include the effects on eye structures such as the retina and the visual cortex, and the overall behavioral state modulation.

Attempts to provide more normal lighting conditions have resulted in several studies on the effects of cycling light by alternating periods of bright light and dimmed light. Such studies have found that infants subjected to the cycled lighting conditions spend more time in sleep states and have increased weight gain,[68] lower motor activity levels, and lower heart rates.[17] Thus, cycling of light periods should be considered in nurseries to help infants begin their regulation of sleep–wake periods.

Concerns about the effects of light on infants in the NICU have also focused on the possible damaging effects on the developing optic structures already at risk for retinopathy of prematurity (ROP) and the effects of constant exposure on diurnal rhythms. Glass et al[43] found a reduced incidence of ROP in infants weighing less than 2000 g when their incubators were covered with a plastic gel that reduced light intensity from 60 to 25 footcandles (ftc). A later study failed to find a change in the incidence of ROP when incubators were covered with a blanket, even when light levels were similarly reduced.[1] A large randomized, controlled trial of 409 premature infants weighing less than 1251 g found no difference in the incidence of ROP in infants who wore goggles that reduced visible light exposure by 97% and ultraviolet light by 100%.[88]

Safe levels of light in NICU have not yet been established and further research is needed to define the optimal approaches for lighting the immediate environment for the NICU patient. However, shielding infants from light in incubators or on warming tables is relatively easy and may prove beneficial in promoting rest, behavioral stability, and recovery.

Interventions to Reduce Light Levels

1. Shade head of table, crib, or incubator whenever possible using cloth crib covers, blankets, or quilts; tenting over the head can be used if constant visual observation of the infant is needed.
2. When infants are stable, consider markedly reducing nursery light levels for 12-hour periods each day.
3. Consider individual lighting over each bedside with a dimmer switch to control light intensity and individualize lighting needs.

Positioning

Because body alignment is known to affect many physiologic and neurobehavioral parameters, the positioning of neonates is important. Proper positioning can prevent postural deformities such as hip abduction and external rotation, ankle eversion, retracted and abducted shoulders, increased neck hyperextension and shoulder elevation, and cranial molding, or dolichocephaly, and improve neuromuscular development.[22, 64, 103] Positioning can also alter respiratory physiology. Placing an infant in the prone position increases oxygenation, tidal volume, and lung compliance, and reduces energy expenditure when compared with the supine position.[16, 60, 70] Side-lying seems to have no significant effect on either oxygenation or carbon dioxide exchange.[19]

Body position affects gastric emptying and skin integrity as well as neurobehav-

ioral development. Activities such as hand-to-mouth ability, midline orientation, flexion, and self-soothing and self-regulatory abilities can be enhanced through facilitating body positions. In terms of prevention of intracranial hemorrhage or extension of existing head bleeds, maintaining unobstructed venous return from the head is a concern when selecting body position; head in midline or side-lying is best for this.

Gestational age, degree of illness, and use of neuromuscular blocking medications all influence positioning decisions. Global hypotonia in infants younger than 30 weeks' gestation requires significant intervention. Critically ill premature and term infants cannot expend any energy to move and require assistance to attain any body position. Infants receiving neuromuscular blocking agents, such as pancuronium, must receive positioning assistance to maintain basic physiologic stability. Thus, selecting an appropriate body position and assisting the patient into it are important considerations for nurses in the NICU.

Interventions to Position Neonates

1. Change the infant's position every 2 to 3 hours for extremely ill or immature infants.
2. Promote hand-to-mouth behavior by allowing the hands to be free when the caregiver is present; side-lying positioning also assists in this goal.
3. Attempt to "nest" the infant with blanket rolls or other positioning aids (Fig. 8–1).
4. Place rolls under the infant's hips when the infant is prone to prevent hip abduction.
5. Roll the infant's shoulders gently forward with soft rolls when both prone and supine to prevent shoulder extension.
6. Use water- or air-filled pillows under the infant's head to minimize cranial molding; frequent position changes (every 2 to 3 hours) from side to side and midline also facilitate this goal.
7. Support the infant's soles of feet with rolls to prevent ankle extension.
8. Swaddle the infant with blankets or buntings when the infant is stable to promote flexion and self-regulatory behavior.
9. Consider gentle massage to promote

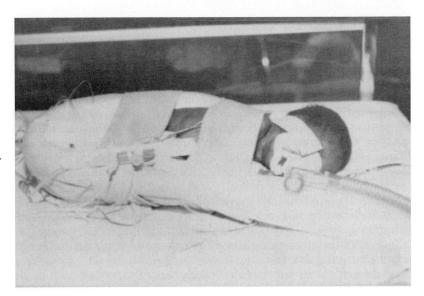

Figure 8–1. Nesting the infant.

skin blood flow in infants on neuromuscular blocking agents; reposition the infant every 2 hours to prevent pressure sores.

10. Position infants with right side down or prone to promote gastric emptying. Prone position is best for minimizing effects of gastroesophageal reflux. In preterm infants, it improves oxygenation.

11. Elevate head of bed after feedings to reduce pressure of full stomach against the diaphragm and improve respiratory capacity.

12. Hold stable infants, even when on the ventilator; holding may be soothing and provides vestibular stimulation similar to fetal experience.

Handling During Procedures

Premature and seriously ill neonates are continually bombarded by procedures to improve their physiologic status or monitor their condition. When it became possible to continuously monitor the effects of routine procedures on oxygenation (including heel-stick blood sampling, intubation, suctioning the endotracheal tube, chest physical therapy, weighing, bathing, changing diapers, and even social interaction), it was observed that procedures often resulted in significant and prolonged reductions in oxygenation.[32, 62, 63, 72, 82, 83, 104, 107] The extent of hypoxemia and overall distress can be dramatically reduced when personnel modify their caregiving according to the infant's responses. The monitoring of oxygenation and behavioral reactions suggests that caregiving practices can result in significant stress for hospitalized neonates and that awareness of such, followed by changes in practices, can reduce the amount of stress the infant experiences.

Supporting the infant's body position can also reduce the stressful effects of procedures and other interventions. Swaddling, rolls, and the use of other containment techniques have been shown to improve physiologic and behavioral organization during weighing,[77] suctioning, and heel-sticks,[30, 98] and provide comfort from pain.[26] The positive effects of infant massage techniques in the NICU include improved weight gain and longer rest periods,[33] but they should be used with careful observation of the infant's reactions to this form of stimulation and avoided in infants with physiologic instability.

Pain Management in the Neonate

Nurses collaborate with medical and surgical staff to determine the treatment of pain in neonates. The assessment tools, both behavioral and physiologic, are relatively new and most difficult to use in the preterm infant.[51, 57, 97] The attitudes of staff and parents continue to have an impact on the use of pharmacologic interventions. Barriers include but are not limited to (1) disagreement about whether an infant is having pain, (2) fear of side effects of the treatment, (3) concern over dependence on pain medications, (4) pharmacologic and individual differences of the drug used to treat pain, and (5) lack of agreement about the adverse effects of pain.[15, 51, 52, 99] Research and reason have made it clear that even the most immature infant perceives pain and that there are real and ongoing physiologic consequences of untreated pain.[6, 7, 53, 84]

Currently some neonatal units are considering treatment guidelines for infants undergoing common surgical procedures in the NICU.[39] These protocols include an initial postoperative bolus of an opiate with a continuous drip of opiate for a variable period of time and then a change to a non-opiate pain medication. Procedural pain management remains problematic because of the need to plan for premedication with possibly no previous experience with the infant to guide determination of the dose or drug that will have the best effect.[9, 14, 55, 87, 97] Neonatal staff continue to have fears and concerns about adverse effects of procedural pain dosing in the nonintubated infant and in those with low blood pressure. This issue can be handled by titrating the dose to effect, using a higher dose in infants on assisted ventilation, and using volume or vasopressors to treat low blood pressure. Opiates are readily reversed if the infant becomes apneic or hypotensive after the drug is given, which is uncommon when doses of 0.1 mg/kg of morphine sulfate are used in neonates.[99] There are clear individual differences among infants in their reaction to medications, and a consistent caregiver for each infant can guide future procedural pain medication dosing.

A difficult area of pain management involves day-to-day concerns about the infant undergoing invasive procedures. The frequency of painful procedures makes individual medication dosing problematic. Procedures such as heel-stick, endotracheal suctioning, IV placement, venipunctures, and adhesive removal are clearly painful. Intubation and position restriction are additionally uncomfortable. Rutter[90] encourages the practitioner of neonatal units to question the need for each and every painful invasive procedure, citing a descriptive study that showed that infants younger than 31 weeks' gestation averaged a mean of 142 painful

procedures during their NICU stay. Other interventions such as containment and offering a pacifier have been shown to reduce overall crying time and behavioral response to pain.[26, 96, 98] Oral sucrose has been shown to reduce crying when offered during a painful procedure, such as heel-stick blood sampling, in newborns.[18] Dipping a pacifier in sucrose or sterile water was also shown to significantly reduce pain responses in premature infants.[96] The use of oral sucrose for premature infants undergoing repeated painful procedures has not been studied.

Pain management in neonates should include use of pain medication with anesthesia during surgical procedures to blunt the global stress response.[2] Postoperative pain relief may be achieved through the use of epidural administration and, when feasible, continuous drip, or intermittent bolus, of opiates.[13, 92] These practices must be regularly assessed for adequacy in individual infants. Dependence develops in most infants after 5 to 9 days of opiate use and, therefore, the drug must be tapered with Abstinence Scoring after this time or else withdrawal will occur in these infants just as it does in those prenatally exposed to opiates because of maternal addiction (Fig. 8–2).[37] Infants undergoing painful procedures should be premedicated with systemic or local agents with enough time to allow for assessment of adequacy and the need for more drug. These procedures include but are not limited to intubation, chest tube insertion, central line insertion, peripheral arterial line insertion, and spinal tap.

Interventions to Reduce Negative Responses to Caregiving

1. Assess each infant for signs of stress during procedures, and note each patient's threshold for stress in the care plan.
2. Identify infants' stress responses before physiologic compromise; these include increased motor activity, mottling or pallor, splaying of the fingers, eyes lidded or shut, extension of extremities, hyperalert facial reaction, and hiccoughs.
3. Document interventions that minimize hypoxemia or other physiologic stress symptoms during procedures such as suctioning, weighing, diaper changes, IV insertions, and position changes.
4. Observe infants for up to 10 minutes after

Analgesia/Sedation Orders (Drug/Dose/Frequency)   **Addressograph**

Date											
Drug											
Administration time											
Dose ↑ or ↓ or frequency											

Time:

Choose one: Crying/agitated 25–50% of interval	2											
Crying/agitated >50% of interval	3											
Choose one: Sleeps ≤25% of interval	3											
Sleeps 26–75% of interval	2											
Sleeps >75% of interval	1											
Choose one: Hyperactive Moro	2											
Markedly hyperactive Moro	3											
Choose one: Mild tremors, disturbed	1											
Moderate/Severe tremors, disturbed	2											
Increased muscle tone	2											
Temperature 37.2–38.4°C	1											
Temperature >38.4°C	2											
Respiratory rate >60 (extubated)	2											
Suction > twice/interval (intubated)	2											
Sweating	1											
Frequent yawning (>3–4/interval)	2											
Sneezing (>3–4/interval)	1											
Nasal stuffiness	1											
Emesis	2											
Projectile vomiting	3											
Loose stools	2											
Watery stools	3											
Total score												
Adjusted score												
Initials of person scoring												

Directions: Score every 2–4 hours per guideline. Score greater than 8–12 may indicate withdrawal.

Figure 8–2. Assessment form for drug withdrawal: opiate weaning flowsheet. (Adapted from Finnegan LP, Connaughton JF Jr, Kron RE, et al: Neonatal abstinence syndrome: Assessment and management. Addict Dis 2:141–158, 1975. Version 1/94.)

procedures to determine the effects of stress.

5. Use self-regulation—promoting activities to assist infants through painful procedures including swaddling, nonnutritive sucking, and containing limbs and comforting infant; use analgesia or sedation when needed.

6. Consider allowing infants time to recover after each intervention, rather than performing all interventions during the same period.

7. Since even positive social interaction can be stressful, observe infant after visual, auditory, tactile, or vestibular stimulation to determine tolerance; educate parents about the need to approach their infant in terms of tolerance and observe for stressful reactions; consider offering only one sensory modality at a time until the infant appears able to process multiple interactions (e.g., hold infant, but do not talk or look at him; stroke infant, but do not make eye contact or talk at the same time).

◆ SKIN CARE

Protection and preservation of the skin of term and premature newborns are significantly important, considering that this organ acts as a barrier against infection and is a major contributor to temperature control. It is a challenge to maintain the integrity of this delicate organ when providing care to premature infants in the NICU. Trauma to skin can occur when life support or monitoring devices that have been securely attached to the skin are removed or replaced, or when procedures such as blood sampling and chest tube insertion penetrate the skin's barrier. Repair of the skin after tissue injury also requires a large consumption of energy. When the skin is damaged, evaporative heat loss and the risk of toxicity from topically applied substances are increased. In addition, there is an increased portal of entry for microorganisms including common skin flora such as coagulase-negative *Staphylococcus* and *Candida*. Thus, significant morbidity and even death can potentially be attributed to practices that cause trauma or alterations in normal skin function.

Developmental Variations in Premature Skin

The term infant has a well-developed epidermis, with the stratum corneum structured similar to that of the adult. The premature infant has fewer layers of stratum corneum, and it has been described histologically as thinner, with the cells of all strata more compressed.[47] This results in increased permeability and transepidermal water loss. Clinical implications of these differences include increased evaporative heat loss, increased fluid requirement, and risk of toxicity from topically applied substances. Despite research indicating acceleration in the maturation of the stratum corneum during the first 10 to 14 days of life in premature infants,[45] other studies report higher transepidermal water losses and decreased barrier function lasting up to 28 days[94] or until the infants reached 30 to 32 weeks postconceptional age, regardless of the postnatal age.[54]

In premature infants, the numerous fibrils connecting the epidermis to the dermis are fewer and more widely spaced than in the term infant.[47] Thus, premature infants are more vulnerable to blistering and a tendency toward stripping of the epidermis when adhesives are removed because the adhesives may be more firmly attached to the epidermis than the epidermis is to the dermis.

The functional capacity of the skin to form an "acid mantle" also differs. Normally in both adults and children, skin surface pH is less than 5. In the term newborn, the pH immediately after birth is alkaline, with a mean pH of 6.34, with a decline to 4.95 within 4 days.[12] Premature infants have been shown to have a pH greater than 6 on the first day of life, decreasing to 5.5 over the first week and gradually declining to 5 by the fourth week.[36] An acid skin surface is credited with bacteriocidal qualities against some pathogens and serves in the defense against infection. A shift in skin surface pH from acidic to neutral can result in an increase in total numbers of bacteria, a shift in the species present, and an increase in transepidermal water loss.[106]

Skin Care Practices

Skin care practices performed daily by nurses in the NICU include bathing, lubrication with moisturizers, antimicrobial skin preparation, and affixation of adhesives for life support and monitoring devices. These activities have the potential for causing trauma and altering the skin pH, thus disrupting the barrier function of the skin.

Bathing

The daily bath is traditionally administered to all hospitalized patients, including newborns in the NICU. Newborns are bathed to remove waste materials, improve general aesthetic qualities, and reduce microbial colonization. This latter purpose has been studied the most extensively. Bathing with hexachlorophene, although effective in reducing colonization with *Staphylococcus aureus* strains, has been abandoned in nurseries because of toxicity from absorption, particularly in premature infants.[56, 91] Chlorhexidine and povidone-iodine soaps are used in many newborn nurseries for the first bath but are effective in reducing colonization only for a 4-hour period after bathing.[29] Although absorption of chlorhexidine occurs in both term and premature infants,[27] toxicity from chlorhexidine has not been reported. In clinical practice, many NICUs are reluctant to risk even potential toxicity from antimicrobial bathing in very small premature infants, so bathing once or not at all in the first days is typical practice.

Cleansers that are used for routine bathing include "baby" soaps, neutral pH synthetic detergents, and superfatted and even deodorant-type cleansers that contain antimicrobial properties. All soaps are at least mild irritants to the skin, and frequent soaping increases the irritant effect.[38, 102] Bathing infants has been shown to cause an increase in the skin's pH and a decrease in its fat content, most significantly with alkaline soap.[41a] Although most children without dermatologic disease can tolerate bathing with soap without adverse effects,[75] this may not be true in the smallest premature infants. To reduce alterations in skin pH, dryness, and irritation, it may be prudent to limit soap bathing to two to three times per week, and to cleanse with warm water baths at other times until the skin becomes more mature.

Moisturizers

The degree of hydration in the stratum corneum is related to the capacity of this layer to absorb and retain water. Moisturizers improve skin function by restoring intercellular lipids in dry or injured stratum corneum. These are products such as emollient creams, lanolin, mineral oil, or lotions; many include petrolatum as an ingredient because of its excellent hydrating and healing qualities.[42, 105]

The beneficial effects of routine emollient use in premature infants younger than 33 weeks' gestation were reported from a randomized, controlled trial of 60 infants. Improved barrier function and reduced transepidermal water loss was seen in infants treated with a petrolatum-based, water miscible emollient, and there was no increase in bacterial or fungal colonization and no evidence of altered skin temperature or burns when used under a radiant heater or concurrently with phototherapy.[78]

Routine use of an emollient to prevent or treat excessive drying, skin cracking, or fissures is recommended. It is also prudent to select products that are free of perfumes or dyes that can be absorbed and may result in later sensitization or toxicity.[24]

EDITORIAL COMMENT: Prophylactic application of emollient ointment decreased transepidermal water loss, dermatitis severity, and the risk of suspected sepsis and proven sepsis.[1, 2] Preliminary reports from a large multicenter randomized trial have not confirmed the benefits of the routine use of an emollient, Aquaphor. Although the skin appeared to be healthier, there were more systemic infections with coagulase negative staphylococci.

◆

1. Lane AT, Drost SS: Effects of repeated application of emollient cream to premature neonates' skin. Pediatrics 92:415, 1993.

2. Nopper AJ, Horii KA, Sookdeo-Drost S, et al: Topical ointment therapy benefits premature infants. J Pediatr 128:660, 1996.

Skin Disinfectants

Decontamination of the skin before invasive procedures such as blood sampling or placement of vascular access devices is common practice in the NICU. Anecdotal reports of harmful effects from some of the solutions used include skin necrosis, blistering, burns, and both alcohol and iodine toxicity.[46, 49, 93] Prospective studies of povidone-iodine use in nurseries further document that iodine is absorbed readily from the skin of premature infants and that toxicity in the form of altered thyroid function occurs.[59, 74, 80, 95] No toxicity from chlorhexidine has yet been reported in any of these studies.

Efficacy of solutions is also a consideration. Povidone-iodine proved better than 70% isopropyl alcohol in reducing skin colonization in a study of pediatric patients.[25] A prospective, randomized study comparing isopropyl alcohol, povidone-iodine, and 2% aqueous chlorhexidine solutions in skin preparation and central line site care in 668 adults showed chlorhexidine to significantly reduce catheter-related infections.[67] A sequential study of 254 premature and term infants in the NICU found IV catheter colonization to be reduced in sites prepared with 0.5% chlorhexidine in alcohol solution compared with povidone-iodine.[40]

When any of the skin disinfectant solutions are used, it is necessary to remove the preparation completely when the procedure is finished. Water or saline is preferred for removing disinfectants to reduce the risk of further skin injury from these caustic preparations.

Adhesive Application and Removal

The traumatic effects of adhesive removal have been documented for premature infants and include reduced barrier function, increased transepidermal water loss, increased permeability, erythema, and skin stripping.[45, 66] Skin barrier function has also been shown to be altered in adults with tape removal, but requires repeated strippings.[61] Solvents have been used in hospitals for a number of years to remove tape and adhesives. Although effective, these products should not be used in the premature infant because of the risk of toxicity from absorption and because of the potential for skin irritation and injury.[48] Bonding agents that increase the adherence of adhesives may also cause more skin stripping and damage, because they form a stronger bond between the adhesive and the epidermis than the fragile bond between epidermis and dermis, especially in the premature infant.

Skin barriers made from pectin and methylcellulose are used between skin and adhesive; they mold well to curved surfaces and maintain adherence in moist areas. Although studies initially described less visible trauma to skin with pectin barriers,[31, 65, 71] a study using evaporimeter measurement of skin barrier function found that pectin caused a similar degree of trauma as commonly used plastic tape.[66]

Preventing trauma from adhesives can be accomplished by minimizing use of tape when possible, dabbing cotton on tape to reduce adherence, using hydrogel adhesives for electrodes, and delaying tape removal for more than 24 hours when the adhesive attaches less well to skin. Removal can be facilitated by applying warm water or an emollient or mineral oil if reapplication of adhesives at the site is not necessary.

Transparent adhesive dressings made from a polyurethane are impermeable to water and bacteria but allow the free flow of air, thus enabling the skin to "breathe." Uses for transparent dressings include securing IV catheters, percutaneous catheters and central venous lines, nasogastric tubes, and nasal cannulas. They can also be used to prevent skin breakdown over areas that have the potential for friction burns or pressure sores, such as the knees, elbows, or sacrum, or as a dressing over surface injuries.

Skin Care Recommendations

Bathing: Use neutral pH cleansers on infants. Bathe the infant with cleansers infrequently—two to three times per week; at other times, use warm water baths. For infants with very immature skin, less than 32 weeks' gestation, give warm sterile water baths for the first week.

Moisturizers: Use a petrolatum-based, water miscible emollient that does not contain perfume or dyes for premature infants less than 32 weeks' gestation. Apply moisturizer sparingly to body surfaces twice daily for the first 2 to 4 weeks of life; apply emollient to cracked or fissured areas in all newborns. If the infant's skin is colonized with *Candida*, use antifungal ointment instead of petrolatum-based ointment.

Antimicrobial skin preparation: Use povidone-iodine or chlorhexidine solution before any invasive procedure that penetrates the skin surface; remove the solution completely with water or saline. Avoid the use of isopropyl alcohol to remove skin disinfectants.

Adhesives and adhesive removal: Limit the amount of tapes and adhesives used to secure equipment as much as possible. Do not use solvents to remove tape; remove tape with water-soaked cotton balls. Tincture of benzoin is not routinely recommended for very immature infants, because this can create a stronger bond of adhesive to the epidermis than the bond between epidermis and dermis. Consider use of pectin barriers between tape and skin for better adherence. Use hydrogel adhesives for electrodes, soft gauze wraps for pulse oximeter probes, and transparent adhesive dressings to secure IV catheters and to protect skin that is prone to excoriation such as on the knees and sacrum. Use transparent adhesive dressings over excoriations that are not infected to promote healing.

◆ VENOUS ACCESS

The provision of vascular access in the NICU is essential. The numerous options for vascular access are associated with significant risks as well as benefits.

Peripheral Access

Although stainless steel "butterfly" needles are still found in most NICUs, studies reveal that they remain in place about half as long as Teflon-coated catheters, primarily because of the incompatibility of the needle with the vessel leading to infiltration; the mean time to infiltration is about 16 hours.[50] Although scalp vein needles are useful for collecting arterial or venous blood samples, they are not the best choice for indwelling IV use.

The mean catheter life of Teflon-coated catheters in several studies, when used for peripheral venous access, varied from 31 to 48 hours.[89] Although these catheters appear similar, they may vary in terms of ease of insertion, biocompatibility, smoothness, and presence of flaws. Flaws and smoothness can be ascertained, when evaluating a specific brand of catheter, using a magnifying glass. When IV access is needed, the time of the therapy, size of the infant, general vein numbers, and ease of cannulation must be considered and discussed for the individual infant. Infants such as those born to diabetic mothers and those with trisomy 21 may have veins in which peripheral access is difficult to establish; in such cases, central venous access may need to be immediately considered. When peripheral veins are used for intravenous fluids or medications, hourly assessment of sites must occur and protocols must be in place for the use of Wydase and Regitine to reduce tissue damage if infiltration occurs.[85] Tissue damage from peripheral IV infiltration should be a rare occurrence in the NICU.

Long, small-bore percutaneous catheters can be threaded into peripheral veins through larger (19- to 20-gauge) needles and left in place as either central lines or peripheral catheters after the needle is removed. These catheters are soft, very flexible, and made of either silicone or polyurethane, both with reduced risk of tissue reaction. Although the cost of both materials and insertion of these catheters may be somewhat higher than for Teflon-coated catheters, the catheter lasts longer (5 days) even when left in a peripheral vein. This type of catheter is considered a peripheral access device if the tip is located in the smaller vessels of the leg, arm, or scalp, and it is considered a central access device if the tip is threaded to one of the vessels close to the heart. These larger, higher flow veins include the subclavian, innominate vein, iliac vein, superior vena cava, and inferior vena cava. The vessels are a gradient from small to large as they approach the heart and that coupled with infant size determines the relative safety of infusing concentrated solutions and the risk of extravasation. Both peripheral and central tip locations should be carefully documented and monitored to prevent complications such as extravasation; simple observation of the insertion site of such devices is inadequate.

Peripheral IV Access Recommendations

1. Select a biocompatible IV catheter that comes in 24- and 22-gauge sizes and does not fray, crack, or break during insertion. Teflon, silicone, and polyurethane are preferred.
2. Develop a training program for nurses that includes knowledge, skill, and documentation related to IV therapy.
3. Have experienced senior staff nurses supervise new nurses learning IV insertion.
4. Secure devices with transparent occlu-

sive dressings for ease of site visualization.

5. Tape devices to minimize compromise to venous return or overall restriction of circulation; for example, if the device is placed in a hand vein, secure by taping the fingers and elbow, not the forearm. This results in reduced swelling from obstruction and increases the space in which extravasated IV fluid can collect, thus reducing the risk of tissue damage from extravasation.

6. Check insertion site hourly for signs of swelling, redness, pallor, other discoloration, and change in temperature.

7. When trying to determine whether an IV catheter is infiltrated, consider the following: swelling; circumference of arm or leg compared with baseline; ease of flushing; infant's reaction to flushing including crying, grimacing, presence or absence of blood return, temperature of site, color differences (especially erythema or blanching); and a second opinion from a staff member who has not been observing the site continuously.

8. Change questionable IV catheters if the infusates are potentially damaging to tissue, such as calcium-containing solutions or other medications known to cause significant vein damage and irritation (e.g., nafcillin and erythromycin).

9. Select infusion pumps that detect air in the line and occlusion.

10. Develop a protocol for the use of hyaluronidase (Wydase) and phentolamine (Regitine) when extravasation has potential of tissue damage. To prevent tissue necrosis, administer hyaluronidase within 1 hour of the extravasation and removal of the device. Hyaluronidase is an enzyme that breaks down the interstitial fluid barrier, resulting in the diffusion of the extravasated fluid over a large surface area. The dose for treating extravasated fluid injuries in neonates is 15 units diluted to 1 ml administered in five sites around the extravasation. Hyaluronidase is not recommended if the extravasation contains a vasoactive drug such as dopamine, because spreading out the medication would further compromise circulation to the skin. The antidote for dopamine extravasation is phentolamine (Regitine), which directly counteracts the action of dopamine. It is administered in the same manner as hyaluronidase. The dose is 0.5 mg diluted to 1 ml.[109]

11. To assist in problem identification, consider quality assurance audits or other types of follow-up on all infiltrates that meet established criteria to assist in problem identification.

12. If restarting peripheral IVs occurs with frequency and is not achieved on the first stick, then central venous access should be discussed, particularly if tissue damage results from extravasation.

Central Venous Access

Central venous access for sick newborns has several advantages over peripheral access. One of the most compelling advantages is the ability to deliver higher glucose and protein concentrations, resulting in higher caloric density of the fluid and allowing for relative fluid restriction while meeting nutritional goals. Most NICUs limit the glucose content to 12.5% and protein to 2% amino acids when using peripheral access. Under these circumstances, it is impossible to provide adequate parenteral calories and protein for growth and repair of tissues unless fluids are delivered at excessive rates, near 180 ml/kg/day. Central access has other advantages that include providing a steady system for infusion of fluids and medications, reducing painful procedures, and allowing the infant to be cared for in more comfortable positions, because boards and restraints are not necessary. Multiple attempts at peripheral access can disrupt the skin barrier and create a potential portal of entry for pathogenic organisms.

The primary reported risk of central venous access is infection. There is considerable debate about the incidence, definition, and risk of sepsis in the neonate with a central venous access device.[101] The method of insertion, percutaneous or surgical, has not been shown to influence the risk of infection. Another risk, accidental disconnection of the IV line, resulting in blood loss, can be reduced by the use of Luer-locking connectors, high-grade plastic adapters that are unlikely to break or crack, and occlusive dressings over insertion sites with additional tape to prevent dislodgment.

Infants with central venous catheters in place must be monitored for all complications, including infection. Because many infants have other potential sources for infection, the vascular device should be considered along with other causes of infection and not immediately removed when a positive blood culture is obtained. Some authors have reported success in clearing bloodstream infection with the catheters left in place.

Central venous access is possible by many routes.[21, 69] One of the most readily available is the umbilical venous catheter. In the past, reported complications with umbilical venous catheters were high and many units either stopped using them or removed them after only a few days. However, with the increasing number of infants weighing less than 1000 g, this method of access has once again become popular, and one study does not support the high rate of infection.[44] Modern catheters are made of either silicone or polyurethane, which reduce the risk of thrombus formation. There are also double- and triple-lumen devices that can be used for infants who require frequent blood sampling or continuous medication infusions along with amino acid solutions and IV fat administration. When silicone catheters are used, it is essential to avoid clamping catheters with clamps that have "teeth" or grooves to prevent catheter rupture.

Another option for central venous access utilizes percutaneously inserted Silastic or polyurethane catheters. The percutaneous catheter, which is currently in widespread use, has dramatically reduced the need for surgically placed devices such as Broviac catheters.[23, 28, 41, 58, 76, 79] Several companies manufacture percutaneous catheters in a variety of small sizes including 1.2, 1.9, and 2 French. They are inserted through a 19-, 20-, or 24-gauge needle or introducer that "breaks away" or is removed from the system before the catheter is secured for long-term use. Advantages to the percutaneously placed central venous lines are many and include decreased risk of effusion, thrombus, or emboli; no permanent vein ligation; and no need for anesthesia during insertion. The use of a peripheral insertion site has the added benefits of avoiding periclavicular insertion with its hemothorax and pneumothorax complications and having a "cleaner" insertion site owing to the lower bacterial counts on extremity insertion sites compared with the neck and upper chest. In addition, there are lower costs associated

with the insertion procedure. Another distinct advantage is that the small size makes insertion feasible in even the smallest premature infant at a time when vascular access is most needed. One disadvantage is that the small size does not work well for blood sampling, although blood may be drawn for culture if catheter-associated sepsis is a concern. There may, however, be hemolysis of red blood cells for other laboratory specimens and a risk of lumen occlusion and fibrin formation that is thought to harbor bacteria and yeast.

Percutaneous Central Line Recommendations

1. Place lines early in the course of hospitalization, before peripheral veins have been damaged.
2. Basilic and cephalic veins in the arm are veins of choice for insertion because of decreased risk of complication during insertion and direct vascular route to the superior vena cava.
3. Use transparent occlusive dressings over insertion site and inspect for security of adhesion daily.
4. When feasible, catheter tips should optimally be located in superior or inferior vena cava to decrease the risk of effusions.
5. Do not routinely draw blood from 1.9- or 2-French catheters, because they may occlude during the process, thus increasing the risk of infection.
6. Do not administer medications known to be at high risk for precipitation such as Dilantin through central lines because of the risk of precipitates causing occlusion.
7. Consider adding 0.5 units of heparin to each milliliter of IV fluid infused through central lines.
8. Educate all nursing staff about how to repair and avoid leaks in catheters or connectors and how to clear occluded lines.
9. Keep track of all central line complications in a log, or audit to assist in education of staff and quality assurance.
10. Use radiopaque catheters for easy monitoring for tip location over time.

In conclusion, regardless of the type of IV device used, it is essential that all practices, policies, procedures, and protocols as well as complications be regularly reviewed and all practices updated and scrutinized. As vascular devices continue to improve, it is imperative for each NICU to be aware of the new technology and to evaluate it critically and carefully, introducing new devices if they can be useful in patient care.

◆ IATROGENIC COMPLICATIONS

In light of the serious emotional, biologic, and social burdens that complications of therapy can lead to, it is imperative that nurses collaborate with other members of the medical team to identify and reduce complications. Reducing errors can only occur through comprehensive programs that address the spectrum of what can go wrong.

The first aspect of reducing complications by caregivers involves the planning and organization of several "routine" aspects of nursing care delivery. These include initial and ongoing education of nursing staff; development of written policies, procedures, and protocols; unit-specific medication reference manuals; a system for reporting and evaluating complications; and a commitment by the nursing and medical leadership to address complications in a timely and comprehensive manner.

Education of nursing staff should address the development of core content knowledge and skill required by the newest nursing staff to safely deliver care. New nurses require many months of close supervision, because skill mastery usually precedes the integration of rationale for care delivery, the mastery of pathophysiology and the intuitive knowledge about a finding that may lead to an early detection of illness. The educational needs of staff who continue to work in the NICU should also be evaluated and planned so that content addresses new therapies and identifies problem areas.

The development of policies, procedures, and protocols can also assist in the reduction of nursing complications. Although these documents may be interchangeable in many settings, it is generally accepted that *procedures* refer to a list of psychomotor skills required to complete a task, such as performing a bladder catheterization. *Policies* state what does and does not happen in a particular NICU related to nursing practice; for example, a policy may be written that two nurses must check all narcotic medications before administration. *Protocols* are sets of instructions or information about how to care for a patient receiving a particular therapy, such as how to care for an infant with an external ventricular drain. Nursing care that differs from the identified standard can be justified and, at times, in the patient's best interest, modified with supportive documentation. Nursing procedures that are associated with complications should be regularly reevaluated. Such procedures include airway suctioning, weighing the infant, securing life support devices (e.g., endotracheal tubes, umbilical catheters, and central venous lines), sampling body fluids, giving IV therapy, delivering medication, and delivering enteral nutrients.

Equipment Evaluation

The care of critically ill newborns is increasingly dependent on technology. Nurses are in a unique position to assist in evaluating equipment and are often first to detect failure or unusual events related to the equipment's use or adverse interaction. Therefore, they must maintain an active role in the selection and evaluation process, and a continued commitment to problem identification.

Several standards can assist in error reduction because of faulty or misused equipment and supplies, including the following:

1. Select a multidisciplinary group in each unit that formally conducts an evaluation before purchasing new durable medical equipment and supplies such as IV tubing, suction catheters, and stopcocks.
2. Select at least one member of the nursing staff to participate on the hospital-wide product evaluation committee so that the needs of the neonatal patients are addressed before any product changes occur.
3. Plan a formal evaluation for all new equipment and supplies, including any changes in brands or models. Plan an evaluation of 1 to 3 months for large purchases so that staff has adequate time to try the equipment.
4. Never assume a product will perform as promised, and consider every item as having the potential to cause harm to the patient.

5. Teach all nurses that equipment may fail and cause complications; develop a system to report equipment failures.
6. Develop a system to report adverse patient impact from equipment and supplies in compliance with the Safe Medical Device Act. This law requires that health care facilities report failure or adverse patient outcome owing to medical devices, both to the department of Health and Human Services and the manufacturer of the device within 10 working days.

Another way to reduce the complications related to new equipment and supplies is to create a list of "critical qualities" that are necessary before even considering an evaluation of a product. For example, before evaluating a new umbilical vessel catheter, a list might be formulated with the following "critical qualities":

Biocompatibility (Silastic or polyurethane preferred)
Radiopaque
Appropriate range of sizes (3.5-, 4-, 5- French)
Available with more than one lumen
Centimeter markings
Accuracy in transducing blood pressure
End or side hole preference
High-grade plastic hub with Luer-locking capability that adapts to all stopcocks
Ease of insertion
Cost

This list contains some of the qualities that concern most users. If a catheter does not meet these minimum standards, it is not worth the effort of an evaluation. Critical qualities for evaluation are best generated in a group setting, which allows for a better interchange with sales personnel. This activity also saves time by reducing the number of inferior products selected for evaluation.

Another crucial area to address is the suitability of the manufacturer. Questions that assist with this concern are the following: How long has the manufacturer been making this product? Can the manufacturer provide written information about the product including data from clinical trials? Will the manufacturer provide training and support a 1- to 6-week trial? Will the manufacturer provide names of other clinicians who currently use the product?

If these questions are answered satisfactorily and a product meets a critical quality list, then it is reasonable to proceed with product evaluation. Evaluation may still yield information that a product is not suitable. For example, a stopcock may look promising initially but when used by staff it may be too hard to turn without creating tension on peripheral arterial lines. In this example, all other critical qualities are noted because the evaluations should be stopped. It is essential that a mechanism be in place for reporting problems related to equipment and supplies. The potential for even the smallest item to cause patient harm exists, and nurses must be constantly on the alert and committed to the process of early detection.

The era of managed care and cost containment has placed many nurseries in a position of being part of buying cooperatives and standardization. These practices often place supplies and equipment at the bedside that are substandard or not suited for infants and can lead to care delivery complications. Clear and timely reporting of the adverse patient impact resulting from a product can facilitate prompt removal from the area and the purchase of a product that meets patient care delivery needs safely.

Medication Administration

Once an NICU medication administration reference manual is developed or purchased along with written policies and procedures, a program should be developed to report, review, and reduce complications from medication errors. A reporting mechanism must exist for all detected medication errors so that errors can be tabulated and categorized over time (Table 8–1). For example, all errors related to a wrong dose being given, a wrong route, or omitted doses could be examined at monthly or quarterly intervals.[10] A mechanism to determine all of the factors that led to the error can be used. Tools can be used to quantify the significance of the error and therefore guide the amount of time spent on each review. At this point, the nurse managers can discuss the error with the nurses or physicians involved in a comprehensive manner.

A denominator is used to tabulate and compare error rate over time, so that specific trends or interventions that reduce errors

Table 8–1. Medication Errors: Causes, Prevention, and Risk Management

Types of Errors
A. Adverse Reaction
B. The Wrong
   drug
   patient
   dosing
   time
   route
   documentation
   not given
C. Pharmacy-related
   dispensing error
   change in supplier, labeling confusion, etc.
   education deficit
D. Human-related
   zeros and decimal points
   handwriting
   ambiguous or incomplete orders
   phone, verbal order communication
   education deficit
   "simple human," confirmation bias, etc.
E. Error Reduction
   user friendly, nonpunitive-based error-reporting
      system
   rate collection method
   access to national reporting database problems
      and solutions
   intradisciplinary review process
   identification of causes
   improvement or change in contributing factors
   evaluation of intervention
   planning for intervention when error occurs

Cohen MR (ed): Medication Errors: Causes, Prevention, and Risk Management. Jones & Bartlett: Sudbury, MA, 1999.

can be meaningfully interpreted. The number of medication doses dispensed for a given unit each month is a suitable denominator for reviewing medication errors. There should be an agreement that all medications are dispensed in standard strengths and that no new medications or changes in medication packaging are dispensed without notification and an attached warning about the changes. The pharmacy must also accept the responsibility of screening all medications for the types of preservatives used and the appropriateness for neonates.

Many units find that a neonatal pharmacy liaison has a profound effect on the safe and timely administration of medication.[35] Regular education for nursing staff on pharmacology is necessary because of the rapidly expanding list of medications being used in this very vulnerable population and the lack of pharmacokinetics to guide the monitoring of neonates' responses to many of the newer drugs.

Some nurseries have found it beneficial to develop drug administration algorithms for medications that are frequently used or have potential for complication. Examples include protocols or algorithms for commonly used medications such as dexamethasone or indomethacin.

Interdisciplinary Quality Improvement

Because the NICU involves the complex interaction of various health professionals in the care of critically ill newborns, there is a need for ongoing quality improvement that includes all disciplines. Many units have organized committees with a variety of names, including the *NICU operating committee* and *NICU interdisciplinary quality improvement committee*. The membership may include physicians, nurse managers, clinical nurse specialists and practitioners, staff nurses, respiratory therapists, pharmacists, biomedical engineers, and others directly involved in daily operations. Unusual occurrence reports are reviewed in this setting. Additional forms or reports are developed where potential patient harm existed but did not occur as a result of early detection or luck. In addition, routine practices (e.g., initiation and advancing of total parenteral nutrition) can be scrutinized according to approved practices and updated through the collaboration of all disciplines involved in the practice.

It is apparent that, in the increasingly complicated technologic environment of the NICU, all professionals must participate in the ongoing evaluation and monitoring of care so that safety is achieved and the risk of complications minimized. The impact of managed care has resulted in small or newly developed NICU units being encouraged to keep more complicated infants. Complications of care occur in nurseries because of the vulnerability of the patient, the severity of the affliction being treated, and the burden of the treatment. Even in the most experienced setting, patient harm from therapy can occur. Small centers must develop close professional relationships with larger tertiary centers to obtain consultation when such complications occur to provide the best possible treatment to the patient affected.

CASE STUDIES

Case One

An infant born at 26 weeks' gestation weighing 680 g is admitted to the neonatal intensive care unit. His skin is extremely translucent in appearance, and there is already an area of skin excoriation on the right side of the chest where an ECG electrode has been removed.

◆ **What is the recommended treatment for the area of excoriation?**

This area can be covered with a transparent adhesive dressing to promote healing and reduce the risk of infection through the site, or coated with petrolatum-based emollient. The best option for the ECG electrodes is hydrogel adhesive.

◆ **What are the best ways to approach bathing and moisturization?**

Areas of the skin that become soiled (with blood or stool) can be cleansed with warmed sterile water and cotton balls for the first 2 weeks. After this time, twice weekly baths with neutral pH cleanser are begun, with warm water baths given on alternating days. Twice daily application of petrolatum-based emollient promotes better skin barrier function.

◆ **What is the safest way to prepare the skin surface before invasive procedures?**

The skin is prepped with povidone-iodine or chlorhexidine solution before any procedure and the disinfectant is then removed entirely with sterile water after the procedure. Isopropyl alcohol is to be avoided until the skin matures because it causes drying and can be absorbed. It has been reported to cause burns in the very low-birth-weight infant.

Case Two

B. N. is born at 32 weeks' gestation after an uncomplicated delivery. She recovers from her respiratory distress syndrome (RDS) and is on room air by 5 days of age. At 12 days, she is taking full enteral feeds, but necrotizing enterocolitis (NEC) develops and she requires resection of 13 cm of terminal ileum. Postoperatively, she is managed on peripheral total parenteral nutrition (TPN). An intravenous (IV) infiltrate is found, and the site, the left foot, is white and cool to the touch.

◆ **What is the recommended treatment of the site?**

Treatment is with hyaluronidase (Wydase), 15 units injected subcutaneously in four or five sites surrounding the area of infiltrate. The 15 units is divided into 0.2 ml injections,

◆ **Within what time frame should the treatment occur?**

The treatment should occur as soon as possible but is felt to be of benefit if instituted within 1 hour of identifying the extravasation.

◆ **What is a logical alternate IV access in this infant?**

For this preterm infant needing TPN until the bowel has rested and feedings are established, a percutaneous central venous line is recommended. This access would allow the infant to receive a high-calorie, high-protein solution that would optimize wound healing and growth. It would also provide long-term access that would reduce time and pain associated with intermittent IV insertion. This method has additional benefits in that it does not require an incision, does not require vein ligation, and costs less to insert than surgically placed venous catheters.

REFERENCES

1. Ackerman B, Sherwonit E, Williams J: Reduced incidental light exposure: effect on the development of retinopathy of prematurity in low birth weight infants. Pediatrics 83:958, 1985.
2. Acute pain management in infants, children, and adolescents: operative and medical procedures. Quick Reference Guide for Clinicians. AHCPR Pub. No. 92-0020. Rockville, MD: Agency for Health Care Policy and Research, Public Health Service, U.S. Department of Health and Human Services, 1992.
3. Als H, Lawhon G, Duffy FH, et al: Individualized behavioral and environmental care for the very low birth weight preterm infants at high risk for bronchopulmonary dysplasia: neonatal intensive care unit and developmental outcome. Pediatrics 78:1123, 1986.
4. Als H, Lawhon G, Duffy FH, et al: Individualized developmental care for the very low birth weight preterm infant: medical and neurofunctional effects. JAMA 272:853, 1994.
5. American Academy of Pediatrics, Committee on Environmental Health: Noise: a hazard for the fetus and newborn. Pediatrics 100:724, 1997.
6. Anand KJ, Phil D, Hickey PR: Halothane-morphine compared with high-dose sufentanil for anesthesia and postoperative analgesia in neonatal cardiac surgery. N Engl J Med 326:1, 1992.
7. Anand KJS, Hickey PR: Pain and its effects in the human neonate and fetus. N Engl J Med 317:1321, 1987.
8. Ariagno R, Thoman E, Boeddiker M, et al: Developmental care does not alter sleep and develop-

ment of premature infants. Pediatrics 100:e9. 1997.

9. Bauchner H, May A, Coates E: Use of analgesic agents for invasive medical procedures in pediatric and neonatal intensive care units. J Pediatr 121:647, 1992.

10. Bechtel GA: A continuous quality improvement approach to medication administration. J Nurs Care Qual 7:28, 1993.

11. Becker P, Grunwald P, Moorman J, et al: Outcomes of developmentally supportive nursing care for very low birth weight infants. Nurs Res 40:150, 1991.

12. Behrendt H, Green M: Patterns of Skin pH from Birth Through Adolescence. Springfield: Charles C Thomas, 1971.

13. Bell SG: The national pain management guideline: Implications for neonatal intensive care. Neonatal Network 13:9, 1994.

14. Bhat R, Abu-Harb M, Chari G, et al: Morphine metabolism in acutely ill preterm newborn infants. J Pediatr 120:795, 1992.

15. Bildner J, Kretchel SW: Increasing staff nurse awareness of postoperative pain management in the NICU. Neonatal Network 15:11, 1996.

16. Bjornson K, Deitz J, Blackburn S, et al: The effect of body position on the oxygen saturation of ventilated preterm infants. Pediatr Phys Ther 4:109, 1992.

17. Blackburn S, Patteson D: Effects of cycled light on activity state and cardiorespiratory function in preterm infants. J Perinat Neonatal Nurs 4:47, 1991.

18. Blass EM, Hoffmeyer LB: Sucrose as an analgesic for newborn infants. Pediatrics 87:215, 1991.

19. Bozynski ME, Naglie R, Nicks J, et al: Lateral positioning of the stable ventilated very-low-birth-weight infant: Effect on transcutaneous oxygen and carbon dioxide. Am J Dis Child 142:200, 1988.

20. Buehler D, Als H, Duffy F, et al: Effectiveness of individualized developmental care for low-risk preterm infants: Behavioral and electrophysiologic evidence. Pediatrics 96:923, 1995.

21. Carey B: Major complications of central lines in neonates, Neonatal Network 7:17, 1989.

22. Cartlidge P, Rutter N: Reduction of head flattening in preterm infants. Arch Dis Child 63:755, 1988.

23. Cathas MK, Paton JB, Fisher DE, et al: Percutaneous central venous catheterization. Am J Dis Child 144:1246, 1990.

24. Cetta F, Lambert G, et al. Newborn chemical exposure from over-the-counter skin care products. Clin Pediatr 30:286, 1991.

25. Choudhuri M, McQueen R, et al. Efficiency of skin sterilization for a venipuncture with the use of commercially available alcohol or iodine pads. Am J Infect Control 18:82, 1990

26. Corff K, Seideman R, Venkataraman P, et al: Facilitated sucking: A nonpharmacologic comfort measure for pain in preterm infants. J Obstet Gynecol Neonatal Nurs 24:143, 1995.

27. Cowen J, Ellis S, et al: Absorption of chlorhexidine from the intact skin of newborn infants. Arch Dis Child 54:379, 1979.

28. Crowley JJ, Pereira JK, Harris LS, et al: Peripherally inserted central catheters: Experience in 523 children. Pediatr Radiol 204:617, 1997.

29. Davies J, Babb J, et al: The effect on the skin flora of bathing with antiseptic solutions. J Antimicrob Chemother 3:473, 1977.

30. DePaul D, Chambers S: Environmental noise in the neonatal intensive care unit: Implications for nursing practice. J Perinat Neonatal Nurs 8:71, 1995

31. Dollison EJ, Beckstrand J: Adhesive tape vs. pectin-based barrier use in preterm infants. Neonatal Network 14:35, 1995.

32. Evans J: Reducing the hypoxemia, bradycardia, and apnea associated with suctioning in low birthweight infants. J Perinatol 12:137, 1992.

33. Field T, et al: Tactile/kinesthetic stimulation effects on preterm neonates. Pediatrics 77:654, 1986.

34. Fleisher B, VandenBerg K, Constantinou J, et al: Individualized developmental care for very low birth weight premature infants. Clin Pediatr 34:523, 1995.

35. Folli HL, Poole RL, Benitz WE, et al: Medication error prevention by clinical pharmacists in two children's hospitals. Pediatrics 79:718, 1987.

36. Fox C, Nelson D, Wareham J: The timing of skin acidification in very low birth weight infants. J Perinatol 18:272, 1998.

37. Franck LS, Vilardi J, Durand D, et al: Opioid withdrawal in neonates after continuous infusions of morphine or fentanyl during extracorporeal membrane oxygenation. Am J Crit Care 7:364, 1995.

38. Frosch P, Kligman A: The soap chamber test. J Am Acad Dermatol 1:35, 1979.

39. Furdon SA, Eastman M, Benjamen K, et al: Outcome measures after standardized pain management strategies in postoperative patients in the neonatal intensive care unit. JPNN 12:58, 1998.

40. Garland J, Buck R, Maloney P, et al: Comparison of 10% povidone-iodine and 0.5% chlorhexidine gluconate for the prevention of peripheral intravenous catheter colonization in neonates: A prospective trial. Pediatr Infect Dis J 14:510, 1995.

41. Geidel-Oellrich R, Murphy MR, Goldberg LA, et al: The percutaneous central venous catheter for small or ill infants. MCN Am J Matern Child Nurs 16:92, 1991.

41a. Gfatter R, Hackl P, Braun F: Effects of soap and detergents on skin surface pH, stratum corneum hydration and fat content in infants. Dermatology 195:258, 1997.

42. Ghadially RL, Halkier-Sorensen, et al: Effects of petrolatum on stratum corneum structure and function. J Am Acad Dermatol 26:387, 1992.

43. Glass P, Avery G, Kolinjavada N, et al: Effect of bright light in the hospital nurseries on the incidence of retinopathy of prematurity. N Engl J Med 313:401, 1985.

44. Green C, Yohannan MD: Umbilical arterial and venous catheters: placement, use and complications. Neonatal Network 17:23, 1998.

45. Harpin V, Rutter N: Barrier properties of the newborn infant's skin. J Pediatr 102:419, 1983.

46. Harpin V, Rutter N: Percutaneous alcohol absorption and skin necrosis in a preterm infant. Arch Dis Child 57:825, 1982.

47. Holbrook KA: A histological comparison of infant and adult skin. In Maibach H, Boisits ER, eds: Neonatal Skin: Structure and Function. New York: Marcel Dekker, 1982, pp 3–31.

48. Ittman P, Bozynski ME: Toxic epidermal necrolysis in a newborn infant after exposure to adhesive remover. J Perinatol 13:476, 1993.

49. Jackson H, Sutherland R: Effect of povidine-iodine on neonatal thyroid function. Lancet 2:992, 1981.

50. Johnson RV, Donn SM: Life span of intravenous cannulas in a neonatal intensive care unit. AJDC 142:968, 1988.

51. Johnston CC, Stevens BJ, Yang F, et al: Differential response to pain by very premature neonates. Pain 61:471, 1995.

52. Johnston CC, Stevens BJ: Experience in a neonatal intensive care unit affects pain response. Pediatrics 98:925, 1996.

53. Jones MO, Pierro A, Hammond P, et al: The metabolic response to operative stress in infants. J Pediatr Surg 28:1258, 1993.

54. Kalia YN, Nonato LB, Lund CH, et al: Development of skin barrier function in premature infants. J Invest Dermatol 111:320, 1998.

55. Koehntop DE, Rodman JH, Brundage DM, et al: Pharmacokinetics of fentanyl in neonates. Anesth Analg 65:227, 1986.

56. Kopelman AE: Cutaneous absorption of hexachlorophene in low-birth weight infants. J Pediatr 82:972, 1973.

57. Krechel SW, Bildner J: CRIES: A new neonatal postoperative pain measurement score; initial testing of validity and reliability. Paediatr Anaesth 5:53, 1995.

58. Leike-Rude MK: Use of percutaneous Silastic intravascular catheters in high-risk neonates. Neonatal Network 9:17, 1990.

59. Linder N, Davidovitch N, et al: Topical iodine-containing antiseptics and subclinical hypothyroidism in preterm infants. J Pediatr 131:434, 1997.

60. Lioy J, Manginello F: A comparison of prone and supine positioning in the immediate post extubation period of neonates. J Pediatr 112:982, 1988.

61. Lo J, Oriba H, et al: Transepidermal potassium ion, chloride ion, and water flux across delipidized and cellophane tape-stripped skin. Dermatologica 180:66, 1990.

62. Long J, Lucey J, Philip A: Noise and hypoxemia in the intensive care nursery. Pediatrics 65:143, 1980.

63. Long J, Philip A, Lucey J: Excessive handling as a cause of hypoxemia. Pediatrics 65:203, 1980.

64. Long T, Soderstrom E: A critical appraisal of positioning infants in the neonatal intensive care unit. Phys Occup Ther Pediatr 15:17, 1995.

65. Lund CH, Kuller JM, Tobin K, et al: Evaluation of a pectin-based barrier under tape to protect neonatal skin. J Obstet Gynecol Neonatal Nurs 15:39, 1986.

66. Lund CH, Nonato LB, Kuller JM, et al: Disruption of barrier function in neonatal skin associated with adhesive removal. J Pediatr 131:367, 1997.

67. Maki D, Ringer M, et al: Prospective randomised trial of povidone-iodine, alcohol, and chlorhexidine for prevention and infection associated with central venous and arterial catheters. Lancet 338:330, 1001.

68. Mann N, Haddow R, Stokes L, et al: Effect of day and night on preterm infants in the newborn nursery: randomized trial. BMJ 293:1265, 1986.

69. Marcoux C, et al: Central venous access devices in children. Pediatr Nurs 16:123, 1990.

70. Masterson J, Zucker C, Schulze K. Prone and supine positioning effects on energy expenditure and behavior of low birth weight infants. Pediatrics 5:689, 1988.

71. McLean S, Kirchhoff K, et al: Three methods of securing endotracheal tubes in neonates: A comparison. Neonatal Network 11:17, 1992.

72. Medoff-Cooper B: The effects of handling on preterm infants with bronchopulmonary dysplasia. Image 20:132, 1988.

73. Merenstein G: Individualized developmental care: An emerging new standard for neonatal care units? (editorial). JAMA 272:890, 1994.

74. Mitchell I, Pollock C, et al: Transcutaneous iodine absorption in infants undergoing cardiac operation. Ann Thorac Surg 52:1138, 1991.

75. Morelli J, Weston W: Soaps and shampoos in pediatric practice. Pediatrics 80:634, 1987.

76. Nakamura KT, Sato Y, Erenberg A: Evaluation of a percutaneously placed 27-gauge central venous catheter in neonates weighing < 1200 grams. JPEN J Parenter Enteral Nutr 14:295, 1990.

77. Neu M, Browne J: Infant physiologic and behavioral organization during swaddled versus unswaddled weighing. J Perinatol 17:193, 1997.

78. Nopper AJ, Horii KA, et al: Topical ointment therapy benefits premature infants. J Pediatr 128:660, 1996.

79. Oellrich R, Murphy M, Goldbergh L, et al: The percutaneous central venous catheter for small premature infants. MCN Am J Matern Child Nurs 16:921, 1991.

80. Parravicini E, Fontana C, et al: Iodine, thyroid function, and very low birth weight infants. Pediatrics 98:730, 1996.

81. Peck S, Botwinick J: The buffering capacity of infants' skin against an alkaline soap and neutral detergent. J Mt Sinai Hospital 31:134, 1964.

82. Peters K: Bathing the premature infant: Physiologic and behavioral consequences. Am J Crit Care 7:90, 1998.

83. Peters K: Does routine nursing care complicate the physiologic status of the premature neonate with respiratory distress syndrome? J Perinat Neonatal Nurs 6:67, 1992.

84. Peters K: Neonatal stress reactivity and cortisol. J Perinat Neonatal Nurs 11:45, 1998.

85. Petit J, Huges K: Intravenous extravasation: Mechanisms, management, and prevention. J Perinat Neonatal Nurs 6:69, 1993.

86. Philbin M: Some implication of early auditory development for the environment of hospitalized preterm infants. Neonatal Network 15:71, 1996.

87. Pokela ML: Pain relief can reduce hypoxemia in distressed neonates during routine treatment procedures. Pediatrics 93:379, 1994.

88. Reynolds J, Hardy R, Kennedy K, et al: Lack of efficacy of light reduction in preventing retinopathy of prematurity. N Engl J Med 338:1572, 1998.

89. Reynolds J: Comparison of percutaneous venous catheters and Teflon catheters for intravenous therapy in neonates. Neonatal Network 12:33, 1993.

00. Ruttor N, Barker DP: Invasive procedures in a newborn intensive care unit. Pediatric Pain Symposium 1995, Abstract 196.

91. Sarkany I, Arnold L: The effect of single and repeated applications of hexachlorophene on the bacterial flora of the skin of the newborn. Br J Dermatol 82:261, 1970.

92. Sartorelli KH, Abajian JK, Kreutz JM, et al: Improved outcome utilizing spinal anesthesia in high risk infants. J Pediatr Surg 27:1258, 1992.

93. Schick JB, Milstein JM: Burn hazard of isopropyl alcohol in the neonate. Pediatrics 68:587, 1981.

94. Sedin G, Hammarlund K, et al: Measurements of transepidermal water loss in newborn infants. Clin Perinatol 12:79, 1985.

95. Smerdely P, Boyages S, et al: Topical iodine-containing antiseptics and neonatal hypothyroidism in very-low-birthweight infants. Lancet 16:661, 1989.

96. Stevens B, Johnston C, Franck L, et al: The efficacy of developmentally sensitive interventions and sucrose for relieving procedural pain in very low birth weight neonates. Nurs Res 48:35, 1998.

97. Stevens B, Johnston C, Petryshan P: Premature infant pain profile: Development and initial validation. Clin J Pain 12:13, 1996.

98. Taquino L, Blackburn S: The effects of containment during suctioning and heelsticks on physiological and behavioral responses of preterm infants. Neonatal Network 13:55, 1994.

99. Tholl DA, Wager MS, Sajous CH, et al: Morphine use and adverse effects in a neonatal intensive care unit. Am J Hosp Pharm 51:2801, 1994.

100. Thomas K: How the NICU environment sounds to a preterm infant. MCN Am J Matern Child Nurs 14:249, 1989.

101. Trotter CW: Percutaneous central venous catheter-related sepsis in the neonate: An analysis of the literature from 1990–1994. Neonatal Network 15:15, 1996.

102. Tupker RA, Pinnagoda J, et al: Evaluation of detergent-induced irritant skin reactions by visual scoring and transepidermal water loss measurement. Dermatol Clin 8:33, 1990.

103. Updike C, Schmidt R, Macke C, et al: Positional support for premature infants. Am J Occup Ther 40:712, 1986.

104. White-Traut R, Nelson M, Silvestri J, et al: Responses of preterm infants to unimodal and multimodal sensory intervention. Pediatr Nurs 23:169, 1997.

105. Wigger-Alberti W, Elsner P: Petrolatum prevents irritation in a human cumulative exposure model in vivo. Dermatology 194:247, 1997.

106. Wilhelm K, Maibach H: Factors predisposing to cutaneous irritation. Dermatol Clin 8:17, 1990.

107. Zahr L, Balian S: Responses of premature infant to routine nursing interventions and noise in the NICU. Nurs Res 44:179, 1995.

108. Zahr L, de Traversay J: Premature infant responses to noise reduction by earmuffs: Effects on behavioral and physiologic measures. J Perinatol 15:448, 1995.

109. Zenk K: Management of intravenous extravasations. Infusion 5:77, 1981.

Respiratory Problems

Richard J. Martin
Ilene Sosenko
Eduardo Bancalari

When one considers the complexity of the pulmonary and hemodynamic changes occurring after delivery, it is surprising that the vast majority of infants make the transition from intrauterine to extrauterine life so smoothly and uneventfully. Nonetheless, the staff working in the intensive care nursery spends a lion's share of their time in caring for neonates with respiratory problems, diseases that are still responsible for much of the morbidity and mortality in this period.

◆ PHYSIOLOGIC CONSIDERATIONS
Normal Developmental Changes

Before birth, the lung is a fluid-filled organ receiving 10% to 15% of the total cardiac output. Within the first minutes of life, a large portion of the fluid is absorbed or expelled, the lung fills with air, and the blood flow through the lung increases 8- to 10-fold. This considerable increase results from a decrease in pulmonary arterial tone and other physiologic changes that convert the circulation from a parallel arrangement to a series circuit.

The high vascular resistance in the fetal lung is due to pulmonary arterial vasoconstriction. The pulmonary arterial vasodilation observed following delivery results in part from the large increase in oxygen tension, from the small decrease in CO_2 tension and corresponding increase in pH, biochemical changes such as elevated prostaglandins, and from the mechanical effect of lung inflation.[34]

At the same time, an adequate functional residual capacity (FRC = volume of air in the lungs at end expiration) is quickly attained. High opening pressures are not a prerequisite to lung expansion during the first breaths.[102] At 1 hour, the distribution of air with each breath in the newborn is already similar to that observed in later life. Specific lung compliance (*change* in lung volume expressed in mL of air/cm of H_2O pressure *change*/mL of lung volume) and vital capacity increase briskly in the first hours of life, reaching values proportional to those in the adult.

Chemical control of respiration is, in general, similar in the newborn infant and the adult. As inspired (and arterial) PCO_2 is increased, both infants and adults increase their ventilation, although the neonatal ventilatory response is smaller. The ventilation of the newborn is also transiently increased when inspiring gas mixtures containing less than 21% oxygen; this response suggests that the carotid body chemoreceptors are active at birth. The infant, however, differs from the adult in that if hypoxic exposure continues beyond about 1 minute, respiration is depressed during the first weeks of life.[90] Hypoxia thus appears to depress the respiratory center, negating the hypoxic stimulation via peripheral chemoreceptors. This hypoxic respiratory depression in the newborn appears to depend on the presence of suprapontine structures in the brain.[95] Even though hypoxic respiratory depression may be useful to the fetus (who maintains a normal PaO_2 of 20 to 25 mm Hg), persistence of this phenomenon into postnatal life may enhance vulnerability of neonatal respiratory control.

The effects of pulmonary stretch receptor activity on the timing of respiration (Hering-Breuer reflex) are more readily elicited in the newborn than in the adult. In infants, a sustained increase in FRC causes a marked slowing of respiratory rate by prolonging expiratory time.[92] In the first days of life, a brisk lung inflation causes a deep gasp

(Head paradoxic gasp reflex) followed by apnea, which is again a manifestation of the Hering-Breuer inflation reflex. The deep gasp observed in the first day of life with low inflation pressures may explain the clinical observation that very low pressures (10 to 15 cm H_2O) are often effective in resuscitating the apneic newborn at birth by stimulating a gasp reflex.

The partial pressure of carbon dioxide (Pco_2) reflects the ability of the lung to remove CO_2. The HCO_3 concentration is controlled by the kidney. When the pH and CO_2 are determined, the HCO_3^- can be calculated by using the Henderson-Hasselbach equation:

$$pH = 6.1 + \log \frac{HCO_3}{Pco_2 \times sol}$$

If only the pH is measured, the cause of the acidosis or alkalosis cannot be determined. With metabolic acidosis, HCO_3 is decreased. To compensate for this, the infant hyperventilates, lowering arterial Pco_2. With respiratory acidosis resulting from pulmonary disease, apnea, or hypoventilation, the arterial Pco_2 increases. The kidney attempts compensation by retaining HCO_3 and excreting hydrogen ions. Only by measuring the Pco_2 and pH and calculating HCO_3 can the cause of an abnormality in acid-base balance be determined. The normal newborn quickly regulates his or her pH to near adult values, although HCO_3^- may be lower than normal adult values.

Oxygen Delivery

Oxygen is carried in the blood in chemical combination with hemoglobin and also in physical solution. The oxygen taken up by both processes depends on the partial pressure of oxygen (Po_2).

At ambient pressures, the amount of dissolved oxygen is only a small fraction of the total quantity carried in whole blood (0.3 mL O_2/dL plasma/100 mm Hg at 37°C). Most of the oxygen in whole blood is bound to hemoglobin (1 g of hemoglobin combines with 1.34 mL of oxygen at 37°C). The quantity of oxygen bound to hemoglobin depends on the partial pressure and is described by the oxygen dissociation curve (Fig. 9–1).

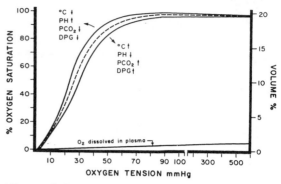

Figure 9–1. Factors that shift oxygen dissociation curve of hemoglobin. (Fetal hemoglobin is shifted to left as compared with that of adult.) (From Fanaroff AA, Martin RJ, eds: Neonatal-Perinatal Medicine. 6th ed. St. Louis: Mosby–Year Book, 1997.)

The blood is almost completely saturated* at an arterial oxygen tension (Pao_2) exceeding 90 mm Hg.

As an example, if the arterial Po_2 is 50 mm Hg, saturation is 90%, and hemoglobin (Hb) is 10 g/dL, then 9.0 g Hb is bound to oxygen. Thus, the oxygen content of this 100-mL sample is 12.06 mL O_2 bound to Hb (1.34 × 9) + 0.15 mL O_2 (0.3 × 50/100) dissolved in plasma for a total of 12.21 mL O_2. Naturally, if the hemoglobin is doubled, then for the same saturation the O_2 transported by hemoglobin is also doubled (1.34 × 18 = 24.12 mL O_2) without changing the amount dissolved. The dissociation curve of fetal blood is shifted to the left and, at any Pao_2 less than 100 mm Hg, fetal hemoglobin binds to more oxygen. The shift is the result of the lower affinity of fetal Hb for diphosphoglycerate (DPG). In contrast, the dissociation curve is shifted to the right by increasing acidosis and temperature. Thus, oxygen delivery to the tissues is determined by a combination of cardiac output, total hemoglobin concentration, and hemoglobin oxygen affinity in addition to arterial Po_2.

Figure 9–2 illustrates that, at an alveolar Po_2 of 100, the three different blood samples have very similar saturations and O_2 contents. However, if a tissue Po_2 of 30 is as-

---

*The arterial oxygen saturation is the actual oxygen bound to hemoglobin divided by the capacity of hemoglobin for binding oxygen.

$$\% \ sat. = \frac{mL \ O_2 \ combined \ with \ Hb}{Hb \ (g) \times 1.34} \times 100$$

1.0 g of hemoglobin can maximally bind to 1.34 mL of O_2.

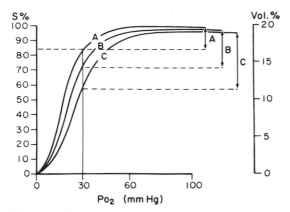

Figure 9–2. Effect of three different oxygen dissociation curves of hemoglobin on oxygen delivered at tissue Po_2 of 30 mm Hg. (From Duc G: Assessment of hypoxia in the newborn: Suggestions for a practical approach. Pediatrics 48:469, 1971.)

sumed, each sample will unload different amounts of oxygen/dL of plasma (A—3.0 mL, B—5.0 mL, C—7.0 mL) to the tissues. The clinical significance of this is that the sick neonate's blood (fetal) will take up more oxygen at an alveolar Po_2 of 40, but the tissue Po_2 will need to decrease to a very low level to unload adequate amounts of oxygen.[37]

The shift in dissociation curve induced by fetal hemoglobin makes clinical recognition of hypoxia (insufficient amount of oxygen molecules in the tissues to cover the normal aerobic metabolism) more difficult, because cyanosis is observed at a lower oxygen tension. Cyanosis is first observed at saturations from 75% to 85%, which correspond to oxygen tensions of 32 to 42 mm Hg on the fetal dissociation curve. Cyanosis in the adult is observed at higher tensions. The flattening of the upper portion of the S-shaped dissociation curve makes it almost impossible to monitor oxygen tensions above 60 to 80 mm Hg by following arterial oxygen saturation. Although the shape of the oxygen dissociation curve limits the usefulness of pulse oximetry to detect high Pao_2 values, keeping saturation measured via pulse oximeter under 92% to 95% is one of the most effective and practical ways of reducing the risk of hyperoxemia.

The partial pressure of oxygen in arterial blood not only depends on the ability of the lung to transfer oxygen but also is modified by the shunting of venous blood into the systemic circulation through the heart or lungs. Breathing 100% oxygen for a pro-

longed time partially corrects desaturation resulting from alveolar hypoventilation, diffusion abnormalities, or ventilation/perfusion inequality. Measurements of Pao_2 while breathing 100% oxygen are therefore useful diagnostically in determining whether arterial desaturation is caused by an anatomic right-to-left shunt, in which case oxygenation will fail to improve the condition (hyperoxia testing).

After birth, Pao_2 increases to between 60 and 90 mm Hg. During the first days of life, 20% of the cardiac output is normally shunted from right to left, in either the heart or lungs. When the normal adult breathes 100% oxygen, Pao_2 increases to 600 mm Hg as compared with approximately 300 to 500 mm Hg in healthy neonates, which results from the substantial shunting in infants.

At the end of the first hour of life, perfusion of the lung is distributed in proportion to the distribution of ventilation. The effects of this rapid adaptation on the blood gases are illustrated in Figure 9–3, which shows the mean arterial pH, Pao_2, $Paco_2$, and bicarbonate in normal full-term infants during the early hours and days of life. The speed with which pulmonary ventilation and per-

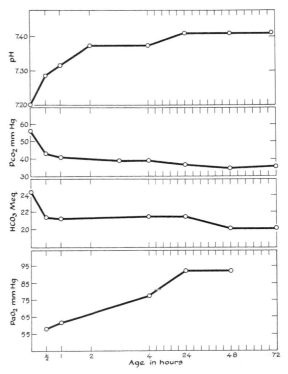

Figure 9–3. Arterial Pco_2, HCO_3, pH, and Pao_2 during first hours and days of life.

fusion are uniformly distributed is an indication of the remarkable adaptive capacities of the newborn infant for the maintenance of homeostasis.

◆ PRACTICAL CONSIDERATIONS
Oxygen Therapy

Oxygen supplementation is critical for the survival of many infants with respiratory problems. Previous restricted use resulted in an increase not only in mortality rate but also in neurologic handicaps.[68] Additionally, a recognition of the toxic effects of excessive or prolonged oxygen therapy is imperative when treating sick newborn infants. Therefore, oxygen administration must be performed with great precision, while carefully monitoring arterial oxygen tension or assessing oxygenation via the various available noninvasive techniques.

Oxygen Administration

For spontaneously breathing infants, use of a small hood prevents fluctuations in inspired oxygen when opening the incubator (Fig. 9–4). The inspired gas must be humidified and the temperature must be warmed to that of the incubator and monitored continuously. The flow into the hood must be at least 5 L/min to prevent CO_2 accumulation. Because improper oxygen administration can be disastrous for the small preterm infant, the following practical considerations should be highlighted:

1. *Peripheral* cyanosis may be present in a neonate with a normal or high arterial oxygen tension.
2. Environmental (or inspired) oxygen should be continuously monitored in all infants receiving supplementary oxygen or assisted ventilation.
3. Oxygen therapy without concurrent assessments of arterial oxygen tension is dangerous. A noninvasive monitoring device to measure oxygen saturation by pulse oximetry or transcutaneous P_{O_2} should be used continuously in preterm infants receiving any supplemental oxygen. In the presence of an arterial line during the acute phase of illness, measure Pa_{O_2} at least every 4 hours if the infant is receiving oxygen.
4. In preterm infants, arterial oxygen tension should be maintained between 50 and 80 mm Hg during the acute phase of respiratory failure.
5. The development of retinopathy of prematurity (ROP) is related to high arterial oxygen tension levels, and these may rise above the normal range even with relatively low inspired oxygen concentrations.
6. When infants receiving supplemental oxygen require mask-and-bag ventilation, both oxygen concentration and inflating pressures must be monitored closely.
7. Use of a nasal cannula for prolonged oxygen therapy allows greater mobility for the infant and enables oral feeding without manipulating oxygen concentration. Both inspired oxygen concentration and flow rate are precisely adjusted and the infant's oxygenation closely monitored, typically via pulse oximetry. Administration of oxygen by nasal cannula requires close monitoring because in active infants the cannula is easily displaced from the nose. Also, changes in respiratory pattern may entrain different amounts of room air around the prongs, changing the true inspired oxygen concentration. Finally, high gas flows through the prongs can produce positive airway pressure if the prongs are fitted tightly.
8. When the infant with respiratory distress syndrome (RDS) is improving, environmental oxygen should be lowered in small decrements while continuously monitoring oxygenation.
9. Any inspired oxygen concentration above room air can be damaging to pulmonary tissue if maintained over several days. Oxygen therapy is continued only if necessary.

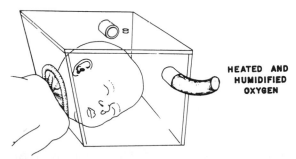

HEATED AND
HUMIDIFIED
OXYGEN

Figure 9–4. Plastic hood for oxygen administration.

10. Premature infants receiving additional oxygen for extended periods of time should be examined by an experienced ophthalmologist by 4 to 6 weeks after birth to screen for treatable ROP.

Assessment of Oxygen Tension and Saturation

Direct measurements of arterial oxygen tension are usually based on intermittent sampling of blood from indwelling arterial catheters. In infants who have no arterial line because of mild respiratory disease or prolonged (weeks to months) oxygen requirement, indirect measurements of oxygenation are available. These techniques also allow *continuous* Po_2 monitoring, making them an invaluable adjunct to intermittent arterial sampling during the acute course of respiratory disease. Transcutaneous (tc) Po_2 electrodes employ a heated electrode that is easily attached to the skin and measures oxygen tension of the gas that has diffused from the arterialized capillary bed to the skin surface and through an O_2-permeable membrane. There is typically an excellent correlation between $tcPo_2$ and Pao_2 in normal and sick neonates with respiratory disease at Pao_2 values below 90 mm Hg.[94] As Pao_2 exceeds 90 mm Hg, $tcPo_2$ underestimates Pao_2, and the scatter between these two parameters increases.[94] A major contribution of $tcPo_2$ monitoring has been the realization that excessive and vigorous handling of sick infants results in hypoxemia and that procedures such as lumbar punctures, when necessary, must be performed under optimal conditions (Fig. 9–5).[55] It should be noted that noninvasive measurements of arterial blood gases remain an adjunct to and not a substitute for intermittent blood sampling in the very sick neonate.

Measurement of $tcPo_2$ does not accurately assess Pao_2 during severe hypotension with tissue hypoperfusion, which markedly alters skin blood flow.[135] The electrode is repositioned every 4 hours; transient areas of erythema, usually disappearing within hours, can be expected at the electrode site especially in shocked or very low-birth-weight (<1 kg) infants. Transcutaneous Pco_2 ($tcPco_2$) electrodes have been combined with those for $tcPo_2$, although $tcPco_2$ responds more slowly than $tcPo_2$ to changes in arterial blood gases. During profound hypoperfusion or shock, the normal elevation of $tcPco_2$ levels over the simultaneously measured $Paco_2$ is further increased, presumably as a result of CO_2 accumulation in tissues.[20]

Because poor perfusion, hyperoxemia, and advancing postnatal age may make $tcPo_2$ somewhat unreliable as a measure of Pao_2,[135] the technique of continuous noninvasive measurement of arterial hemoglobin O_2 saturation has gained general acceptance.[38] This typically employs a microprocessor-based *pulse oximeter* comprising a light-emitting probe attached to the distal extremity of the infant. Oxygen saturation is computed from the light absorption characteristics of the pulsatile flow (containing both oxygenated and nonoxygenated hemoglobin) as it passes beneath the probe. The resultant monitor readings closely correlate with saturation measurements obtained from arterial samples.[63]

The major disadvantage of pulse oximetry is that changes in saturation are very small

Figure 9–5. Transcutaneous oxygen and carbon dioxide measurement during various stages of spinal tap performed in lateral flexed position in preterm infant. Performing proce dure with infant in upright position can minimize detrimental effect on blood gases. (From Gleason CA, Martin RJ, Anderson JV, et al: Optimal position for a spinal tap in preterm infants. Pediatrics 71:31, 1983.)

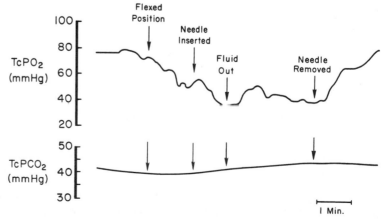

and difficult to evaluate on the flat portion of the hemoglobin dissociation curve at values of PaO_2 above about 50 to 60 mm Hg. This is less of a problem in infants beyond 1 month of age with chronic lung disease when PaO_2 is generally maintained in the 50 to 70 mm Hg range (comparable to an oxygen saturation in the low to mid-90% range).[133] If saturation is less than 95% hyperoxia is extremely unlikely.[17, 117, 143]

Oxygen Toxicity

Although high concentrations of oxygen at atmospheric pressures can adversely affect the stability of cells in many organ systems, serious toxicity may contribute to major clinical problems in the lung and retina of the premature infant.

The Retina

ROP only occurs in those infants (typically of very low birth weight) whose retinal vessels have not yet completed their centrifugal growth from the optic disc. Hyperoxia is one of several events that appears to disrupt this natural progression. The effect of oxygen on the retinal vessels depends on (1) the stage of development of the retinal vessels, (2) the length of the exposure to oxygen, and (3) the partial pressure of oxygen in the arterial blood. The vasoconstricting effects of very short periods of hyperoxia are reversible. If the vasoconstriction (first stage) is prolonged, it may not be reversible, and, for unknown reasons, disrupted growth of primitive vessels proceeds. This is not observed when the retina is fully vascularized.

The second stage is the proliferative phase, in which new vessels grow from the capillaries and sprout through the retina into the vitreous. These vessels are usually permeable, and hemorrhages and edema sometimes follow. Organization of the hemorrhages that enter the vitreous can produce traction on the retina and may result in detachment and blindness.

EDITORIAL COMMENT: The international classification has now gained general acceptance in describing retinopathy of prematurity. The disease is reported by location within the retina and by the extent of the developing vasculature involved (Fig. 9–6). Three zones of retinal involvement are recognized moving from the optic nerve (zone I) to the periphery (zone III).

Zone III is the last zone vascularized and therefore is most often involved with retinopathy. The extent is specified according to the hours of the clock. The disease is further categorized according to the progression, commencing with stage I, the presence of a demarcation line; stage II, a ridge; stage III, a ridge with extraretinal fibrovascular proliferation; and stage IV, retinal detachment. Plus disease refers to the situation wherein the posterior veins are enlarged and the arterioles tortuous and the condition progresses rapidly. In general, the more posterior the disease and the more extensive the involvement of the retinal tissue, the more serious the disease.

Gestational age and birth weight have been related inversely to the risk of ROP in all available studies. Other predisposing factors include prolonged oxygen administration or ventilatory support and complexity of the infant's neonatal course.[87, 144] It has been proposed that the arterial oxygen tension must be kept below the level that stimulates vasoconstriction, although the exact concentration that is toxic is unknown and ROP can develop in premature infants with cyanotic congenital heart disease despite persistent hypoxemia. Other factors such as the volume of replacement blood transfusions and multiple birth have been associated with an increased risk of ROP. Myopia frequently develops in infants with ROP. For the sick infant, the general practice is to maintain the PaO_2 between 50 and 80 mm Hg. Recent experimental data suggest that lower levels of arterial oxygen tension may also increase the risk for severe ROP.[49] This makes it even more important to continuously monitor oxygenation in these infants to maintain the levels of PaO_2 within a narrow safe range.[49, 116]

Continuous monitoring of oxygen tension in very low-birth-weight infants has not reduced the incidence of ROP when compared with standard techniques of intermittent blood gas sampling.[7] Preliminary studies suggested that the administration of the antioxidant vitamin E may reduce the incidence of ROP. Subsequent studies have confirmed a modest benefit of vitamin E in decreasing the incidence of severe ROP, although current risk-to-benefit data are insufficient to justify routine prophylactic treatment of infants at risk.[120] Cryotherapy or laser therapy effectively slows the progression of ROP of moderate severity.[27] Therefore, high-risk infants should have initial ophthalmologic

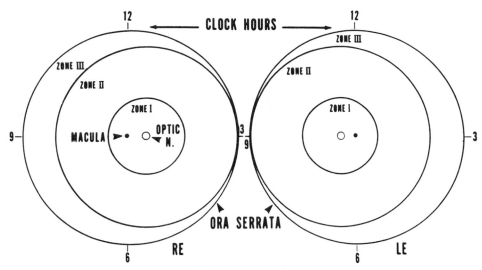

Figure 9–6. Scheme of retina of right eye (RE) and left eye (LE) showing zone borders and clock hours employed to describe location and extent of retinopathy of prematurity. (From an international classification of retinopathy of prematurity. Pediatrics 74:127, 1984. Reproduced by permission of Pediatrics. Copyright 1984.)

evaluations at 4 to 6 weeks, with repeat examinations until vascularization is complete to decide whether an ablation procedure is indicated.[69, 72]

The Lung

The lung is the organ exposed directly to the highest partial pressure of inspired oxygen. Although oxygen itself is essentially nonreactive, its potential for toxicity is derived from the formation of reactive oxygen species during normal cell metabolism, and even more so during exposure to high concentrations of oxygen.[46] These oxygen-free radicals are cytotoxic because of their potential for interaction with all of the principal cellular components, resulting in inactivation of enzymes, lipid peroxidation in cellular and organelle membranes, and damage to DNA.[46] Pathologically, hyperoxic lung damage consists of edema and destruction to alveolar epithelium, with replacement of alveolar type I cells by type II cells, and vulnerability of the vascular endothelium.[74] The precise concentration of oxygen that is toxic to the lung probably depends on a large number of variables, including maturation, nutritional and endocrine status, and duration of exposure to oxygen and other oxidants. A safe level of inspired oxygen has not been established; it is even possible that exposure of the extremely immature lung to 21% oxygen may represent a cytotoxic challenge.

To combat the detrimental effects of oxygen toxicity, cells have evolved a complex system of antioxidant defenses to scavenge and detoxify reactive oxygen-free radicals. These antioxidant defenses include both chemical antioxidants, such as vitamin E, ascorbate and glutathione, and the antioxidant enzyme system, consisting mainly of superoxide dismutase, catalase, and glutathione peroxidase.[64] Studies have demonstrated a late gestational developmental pattern of pulmonary antioxidant enzyme maturation in numerous species.[44] Therefore, experimental animals, and presumably the human infant as well, if delivered prematurely, would be denied late gestational increases in antioxidant enzyme activities. This could partially explain the vulnerability of the premature infant to oxidant lung damage. Similarly, studies in rabbits have shown that the preterm rabbit is not capable of inducing a protective increase in antioxidant enzymes in response to hyperoxia exposure,[45] which may offer an additional explanation for the vulnerability of the premature infant to hyperoxic exposure.

Although neonatal chronic lung disease (CLD) is multifactorial in etiology, several lines of evidence suggest that oxygen-free radicals play a role in its etiology. Studies have linked free radical formation or antioxidant indices with prematurity and CLD. For example, when free radical–mediated lipid peroxidation rate was studied in premature infants by measuring expired ethane and pentane, these measurements suggested that lipid peroxidation correlated with low gestational age and birth weight.[140] Furthermore, infants with the highest expired ethane and pentane had an increased risk of dying or acquiring CLD.[140] Using a different marker of free radical generation, namely plasma allantoin concentration, investigators found an increase within the first 24 to 48 hours after birth in premature infants who required significant oxygen exposure and in whom CLD subsequently developed.[109]

Additional factors may contribute to the negative influence of hyperoxia on the neonatal lung. When the lung is continuously exposed to high O_2, an influx of polymorphonuclear leukocytes containing proteolytic enzymes such as elastase occurs. Bruce et al[19] have observed that the antiproteinase defense system is significantly impaired in infants exposed to greater than 60% inspired O_2 for 6 or more days, and, therefore, proteolytic damage of structural elements in alveolar walls may be an important pathogenetic factor. Loss of mucociliary function may be an additional pathogenetic component, in that exposure to 80% oxygen has resulted in a cessation of ciliary movement after 48 to 96 hours in cultured human neonatal respiratory epithelium.[15] Finally, lung growth and development appear to be highly sensitive to oxygen exposure. When postmortem examinations of lungs from infants dying of CLD were compared with those of infants dying without lung disease, results revealed a significant reduction in total alveolar number and lung internal surface area, as well abnormal alveolar architecture in the CLD infants.[89]

Studies designed to enhance antioxidant capabilities in the human infant have yet to show any sustained benefit in terms of lung protection, although some show considerable promise. Clinical trials of vitamin E failed to demonstrate a lung protective effect; more recently, however, vitamin A has been shown to modestly reduce the primary outcome variable, death or CLD (55% vs. 62%, vitamin A vs. control respectively).[138] In addition, administration of antioxidant enzymes, particularly superoxide dismutase, premixed with a commercially available surfactant preparation might prove to provide protection of the lung from oxidant damage.[106] Other agents that could potentially be protective include such iron-bind-

ing agents as deferoxamine or transferrin, which could function via reduction of iron-catalyzed free radical formation.[43, 62]

Nonetheless, epidemiologic data suggest that CLD may not primarily relate to oxidant lung damage. Specifically, CLD has been found to occur with significant frequency in very low-birth-weight infants without preceding RDS, and with minimal early supplemental oxygen exposure.[125] Therefore, antioxidant augmentation alone may not be adequate to completely eradicate CLD from premature infant populations.

◆ NEONATAL PROBLEMS

Diagnosis

The initial objective is to establish an etiologic diagnosis for any observed respiratory symptoms. A major error in care can easily be made if other organ systems are not considered initially. *Not every cyanotic, rapidly breathing infant has respiratory distress syndrome or even respiratory disease.* Hypovolemia, hyperviscosity (polycythemia), anemia, hypoglycemia, congenital heart disease, hypothermia, metabolic acidosis of any etiology, or even the effects of drugs or drug withdrawal may all mimic primary respiratory disorders. Appropriate care depends on the diagnosis. For example, rewarming should rapidly relieve respiratory symptoms in a mildly hypothermic infant; otherwise, sepsis must be strongly considered.

A working classification of some of these disorders is presented in Table 9–1. Whenever faced with these respiratory symptoms, the next steps (following a history and physical examination) should be to obtain the following:

Chest x-ray film
White blood cell count with differential and hematocrit (peripheral hematocrits can be 25% higher than intravascular hematocrits)
Blood sugar
Assessment of blood gas status via an arterial stick or noninvasive techniques

The decision to catheterize the umbilical artery depends on the infant's condition (see Appendix I-2). The umbilical artery and/or vein may need to be catheterized during the first 15 minutes of life if significant meta-

Table 9–1. Differential Diagnosis of Neonatal Respiratory Distress

Pulmonary Disorders

Respiratory distress syndrome
Transient tachypnea
Meconium aspiration syndrome
Pneumonia
Air leak syndromes
Pulmonary hypoplasia

Systemic Disorders

Hypothermia
Metabolic acidosis
Anemia/polycythemia
Hypoglycemia
Pulmonary hypertension
Congenital heart disease

Anatomic Problems Comprising Respiratory System

Upper airway obstruction
Airway malformations
Space-occupying lesions
Rib cage anomalies
Phrenic nerve injury
Neuromuscular disease

bolic acidosis or blood loss is suspected or if the infant remains severely distressed (as defined by continued hypoxemia and severe respiratory distress). On the other hand, if the infant has tachypnea and grunting with retractions but is active and pink, it may be possible to withold catheterization unless there is deterioration as manifested by marked respiratory distress and an oxygen requirement exceeding 40% to 50%.

Although the newborn has a relatively larger cardiac output and a lower peripheral resistance and blood pressure than the older child and adult, measurements of blood pressure in this low-resistance circuit must be routine. (In the low-resistance circuit of the newborn kitten, the blood volume must be reduced by 40% before blood pressure is observed to decline.) Nonetheless, it has been shown that hypotension in sick preterm infants need not be associated with hypovolemia.[9] Hypothermia or acidemia results in severe peripheral vasoconstriction and will confound blood volume estimates from measurement of blood pressure. In a hypovolemic infant, blood pressure often declines only after acidemia and hypoxemia are corrected. Blood pressure can be measured with a blood pressure cuff of correct size placed on one or all extremities (if coarctation of the aorta is suspected), employing either oscillometric or Doppler ultrasound techniques. Alternatively, direct arterial measurements may be made via indwelling catheters. Normal blood pressures and ranges are found in Figure 9–7.

If the initial hematocrit is less than 30% without blood incompatibility or if blood pressure is reduced, it is reasonable to assume blood loss (e.g., an acute fetomaternal hemorrhage) and consider immediate correction of blood volume. Saline is initially used and blood requested, starting with a push infusion of 10 mL/kg, observing blood pressure, heart rate, and the infant's general condition. One must be extremely careful with rapid infusions of any solution in the critically ill premature infant because of the risk of increasing the incidence of intraventricular hemorrhage (IVH) by rapid volume expansion.[9]

Once a diagnosis has been made, it is necessary to determine whether the neonatal unit has all of the facilities that might be needed during the course of the illness.

The ability to predict the course of the respiratory disease permits the physician to

Figure 9–7. Blood pressure ranges in premature infants over first week of life. (From Hegyl T, Anevar M, Carbone MT, et al: Blood pressure ranges in premature infants: II. The first week of life. Pediatrics 97:336–342, 1996.)

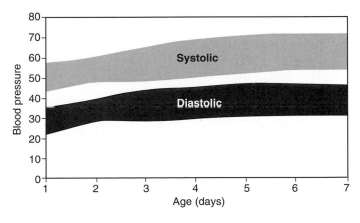

determine which infant will require special respiratory therapy and therefore be transferred. Unfortunately, this is not always possible.

A low PaO_2 while breathing high O_2 concentrations combined with a respiratory acidosis usually means severe disease. We recommend transfer to a special center where all facilities are available while the infant is in reasonable physical condition before becoming damaged or moribund.

The following section discusses RDS in great depth, because this is the major neonatal respiratory disorder and has been the primary model for understanding pathophysiology and management of neonatal respiratory disease.

Respiratory Distress Syndrome (Hyaline Membrane Disease)

RDS is still probably the most common initial problem in the intensive care nursery.[114] The disease is observed in roughly 10% of all premature infants, with the greatest incidence in those weighing less than 1500 g. In infants of less than 1000 g, typically intubated for assisted ventilation in the delivery room and given intratracheal surfactant, the characteristic clinical course for RDS may not be apparent. In fact, without a characteristic radiographic appearance of RDS, the clinical diagnosis may be controversial in extremely low-birth-weight infants, and other terms, such as *respiratory insufficiency of prematurity,* have been proposed.

The following lists give the common symptoms, the physiologic abnormalities, and the pathologic findings.

Signs and Symptoms

- Difficulty in initiating normal respiration. The disease should be anticipated if the infant is premature and the mother is bleeding or has diabetes or if the infant has suffered perinatal asphyxia.[124]
- Expiratory grunting or whining—observed when the infant is not crying (caused by closure of the glottis), a most important sign that sometimes may be the only early indication of disease; a decrease in grunting may be the first sign of improvement.
- Sternal and intercostal retractions (sec-

ondary to decreased lung and increased rib cage compliance).
- Nasal flaring.[21]
- Cyanosis (if supplemental O_2 is inadequate).
- Respirations—rapid (or slow when seriously ill).
- Extremities edematous—after several hours (altered vascular permeability).
- X-ray film showing reticulogranular, ground-glass appearance with air bronchograms.

Physiologic Abnormalities

- Lung compliance reduced to as much as one fifth to one tenth of normal (Fig. 9–8).
- Large areas of lung not ventilated (right-to-left shunting of blood).[134]
- Large areas of lung not perfused.[24]
- Decreased alveolar ventilation and increased work of breathing.
- Reduced lung volume.

These changes result in hypoxemia, often hypercarbia, and, if hypoxemia is severe, a metabolic acidosis.

Pathologic Findings (Anatomic, Biophysical, Biochemical)

- Gross—the lung is collapsed, firm, dark red, and liverlike.
- Microscopic—alveolar collapse, with overdistention of the dilated alveolar ducts, pink-staining membrane on alveolar ducts (composed of products of the infant's blood and destroyed alveolar

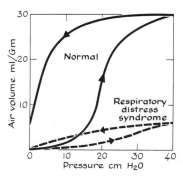

Figure 9–8. Air pressure volume curves of normal and abnormal lung. Volume is expressed as milliliters of air per gram of lung. Lung of infant with respiratory distress syndrome (RDS) accepts smaller volume of air at all pressures. Note that deflation pressure volume curve follows closely inflation curve for the RDS lung.

cells); muscular coat of pulmonary arteriolar walls thickened; small lumen; distended lymphatic vessels.

- Electron microscopic—damage and loss of alveolar epithelial cells (especially type II cells); disappearance of lamellar inclusion bodies.
- Biophysical and biochemical—deficient, or absent pulmonary surfactant,[70] especially phospholipid (surface tension lowering) component; abnormal pressure volume curve, as shown in Figure 9–8.

Etiology

The distal respiratory epithelium responsible for gas exchange features two distinct cell types in the mature infant lung. Type I pneumocytes cover most of the alveolus, in close proximity to capillary endothelial cells. Type II cells have been identified in the human fetus as early as 22 weeks' gestation but become prominent at 34 to 36 weeks of gestation. These highly metabolically active cells contain the cytoplasmic lamellar bodies that are the source of pulmonary surfactant. The autonomic nervous system and its mediators appear to influence the rate of surfactant secretion or turnover. Surfactant synthesis is a complex process that requires an abundance of precursor substrates, such as glucose, fatty acid, and choline, and a series of key enzymatic steps that are regulated by various hormones, including corticosteroids.

Phosphatidylcholine is the dominant surface tension–lowering component of surfactant. In addition surfactant-specific proteins have been characterized and their functions partially elucidated. Of particular interest is surfactant protein B (SP-B), which is critical for minimizing surface tension and whose absence results in the phenotypic expression of lethal RDS at term.[79] Following secretion from lamellar bodies within the type II alveolar cells, the key phospholipid and protein components of surfactant are conserved by recycling and subsequent regeneration of surfactant. Exogenously administered surfactant appears to contribute to this recycling program by increasing surfactant pool size without inhibiting endogenous surfactant production.[70]

It is widely accepted that RDS is the result of a primary absence or deficiency of this highly surface-active alveolar lining layer (pulmonary surfactant). Surfactant, a complex lipoprotein rich in saturated phosphatidylcholine molecules, binds to the internal surface of the lung and markedly lessens the forces of surface tension at the air-water interphase, thereby reducing the pressure tending to collapse the alveolus. By equalizing the forces of surface tension in alveolar units of varying size, it is a potent antiatelectasis factor and is essential for normal respiration. Alteration or absence of the pulmonary surfactant would lead to the sequence of events shown in Fig. 9–9; this results in decreased lung compliance (stiff lung) and thus an increase in the work of breathing. The additional work would soon tire the infant, leading to a sequence of reduced alveolar ventilation, atelectasis, and alveolar hypoperfusion.

Asphyxia would induce pulmonary vasoconstriction; blood would bypass the lung through the fetal pathway (patent ductus, foramen ovale), lowering pulmonary blood flow; and a vicious circle would be promoted. The resulting ischemia would be an added insult and may further reduce lung metabolism and surfactant production.

General Preventive Measures

A major effort in treating this disease should continue to focus on its prevention, including the result of elective cesarean deliveries performed without adequate documentation of pulmonary maturity from amniotic fluid testing.[61] The prolongation of pregnancy with bed rest or drugs that inhibit premature labor, as well as the induction of pulmonary surfactant with maternally administered steroids, plays an important role in reducing the incidence of this disease (see Chapter 1).

Antenatal steroids not only enhance surfactant production but also may improve pulmonary function (e.g., tissue elasticity) by nonsurfactant mechanisms.[121] Therefore, the combined use of prenatal corticosteroids and postnatal surfactant therapy is complementary.[71] Antenatal steroids also reduce the incidence of periventricular hemorrhage in preterm infants, possibly secondary to enhanced vascular integrity in the germinal matrix.[83] Concern about the possibility of increased infection with antenatal steroids in mother or infant appears unfounded. In the United States, antenatal steroids are administered to about 75% of mothers delivering infants of less than 1.5 kg.[107] Thyroid

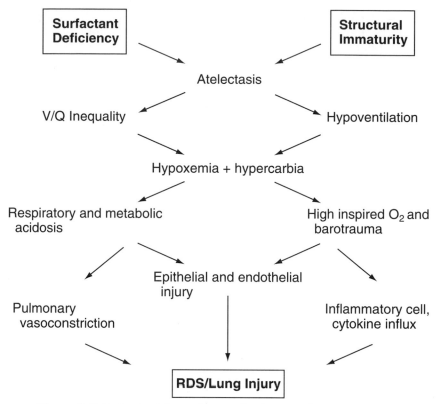

Figure 9–9. Pathophysiology of neonatal respiratory distress syndrome.

hormones enhance surfactant production; however, maternally administered thyrotropin-releasing hormone (TRH) combined with antenatal steroids failed to offer any advantage over glucocorticoids alone.[5]

Surfactant Therapy

Since the discovery that surfactant deficiency was a prominent feature of the pathophysiology of RDS, investigators have attempted to administer artificial aerosolized phospholipids to these infants.[4] Only limited therapeutic success was encountered in these early studies. In contrast, animal models in which natural surfactant compounds were used yielded more promising results. This stimulated Fujiwara et al[47] to develop a mixture of both natural and synthetic surface-active lipids for use in humans. The goal was to achieve alveolar stability with less potential risk for a reaction to foreign protein than would be the case with exclusively natural surfactant. When administered to an initial group of 10 preterm infants with severe RDS who were not improving despite artificial ventilation, a single 10-mL dose of surfactant instilled into the endotracheal tube resulted in a dramatic decrease in inspired oxygen and ventilator pressures. Other studies confirmed this initial success, employing calf and pig lung extract, pooled human surfactant obtained from amniotic fluid, and purely synthetic phospholipid preparation.[98, 104]

Subsequent collaborative multicenter trials employed multiple doses of purely synthetic and mixed natural/synthetic preparations and confirmed clinical efficacy, leading in the 1990s, to the widespread introduction of exogenous surfactant therapy into neonatal care. A protein containing extract of minced calf lung supplemented with dipalmitoyl phosphatidylcholine, tripalmitin, and palmitic acid and marketed as Survanta is widely used in North America.[141] Both prevention (delivery room administration) and rescue (administration for established RDS) protocols have their advocates.[75] Of particular interest, as summarized in Table 9–2, is the ability of surfactant to decrease the number of deaths in low-birth-weight infants without significantly reducing the incidence of bronchopulmonary dys-

Table 9–2. Surfactant Therapy for Respiratory Distress Syndrome

Resolved	Unresolved
Greatest benefit when combined with antenatal corticosteroids	Ideal preparation: role of surfactant proteins in improving respiratory function
Major surface tension–lowering ingredient: phosphatidylcholine	Risk of pulmonary hemorrhage: role of indomethacin in its prevention and continued surfactant treatment
Administration of fluid suspension requires endotracheal tube	Role of ventilatory strategy in optimizing surfactant response—rapid wean to nasal CPAP
Improvement in arterial oxygenation	Effect on incidence and severity of chronic lung disease
Surfactant proteins enhance speed of action	Effect on immune mechanisms, especially in septic infants
Exogenous surfactant enhances rather than inhibits endogenous surfactant synthesis	Role of surfactant therapy in other neonatal respiratory disorders: meconium aspiration, pneumonia, pulmonary hypoplasia, congenital diaphragmatic hernia
Decrease in incidence of air leaks	Appears beneficial for severe meconium aspiration and pneumonia
Improved mortality rate	
Prevention more effective than rescue up to <29 weeks	

Adapted from Martin RJ, Fanaroff AA: The respiratory distress syndrome and its management. In Martin RJ, Fanaroff AA, eds: Neonatal-Perinatal Medicine. 6th ed. St. Louis: Mosby–Year Book, 1997.

plasia (BPD) in the smallest infants. The latter may be a consequence of the enhanced survival caused by surfactant administration to very preterm infants or to the multifactorial etiology of BPD.

Surfactant therapy currently requires the presence of an endotracheal tube, and multiple doses are usually needed for optimal benefit. The dramatic improvement in oxygenation is not accompanied by an immediate improvement in $Paco_2$ or lung compliance unless ventilator settings are rapidly weaned.[33] These data suggest that an increase in lung volume, rather than improved alveolar ventilation, is the primary mechanism whereby surfactant dramatically improves Pao_2 in preterm infants with RDS. In the usual dose, 4 to 5 mL/kg, hypotension and bradycardia may occur acutely during surfactant therapy, and pulmonary hemorrhage has been reported following surfactant instillation.[119] Therefore, caution must be exercised when using this treatment to avoid potential iatrogenic complications.

Since the genes that code for the surfactant proteins have been characterized, recombinant DNA technology will make production of modified human surfactant proteins possible. In combination with synthetic phospholipids, this will allow the widespread availability of a protein-containing artificial surfactant. Although no adverse immunologic consequences of foreign tissue protein administration have yet been reported in the recipients of natural surfactant therapy, close follow-up of these high-risk survivors of neonatal intensive care is always imperative.

General Clinical Management

The same principles of basic care for RDS can be applied to infants with many other neonatal pulmonary problems. During the acute phase, every maneuver is directed to ensuring the infant's survival with minimal risk of chronic morbidity. The infant is placed in a neutral thermal environment (see Chapter 5) to reduce oxygen requirements and CO_2 production. To meet fluid and partial caloric requirements (dependent on environmental conditions, maturity, renal function, risk for patency of the ductus arteriosus, and hydration), the infant is typically begun at 60 to 80 mL/kg/d of a 10% dextrose solution. This is increased to 120 to 160 mL/kg/d by the fifth day, recognizing that there is a high risk for either fluid overload or dehydration if clinical status, fluid balance, and electrolytes are not closely monitored in the smallest infants with RDS, who may require up to 200 mL/kg/d. Administration of an amino acid solution should begin over the first days, supplemented by small volume feeds as respiratory status stabilizes. To meet the immediate and changing oxygen and ventilatory requirements of the infant, we monitor color, activity, heart rate, and skin or rectal temperature at least hourly and pH, $Paco_2$, Pao_2, and HCO_3 at least every 4 hours. Respiration, heart rate, blood pressure,[142] and oxygenation (via noninvasive techniques) are monitored continuously.

Most important in the prescription is skilled nursing and physician management. Vital signs must be noted and observations made in such a fashion as not to disturb the infant continually, yet the patient must always be observed. Modern electronic monitoring of heart rate, respiration, temperature, and oxygenation makes gentler care easier to administer. Noninvasive monitoring of oxygenation has confirmed the importance of minimizing simple maneuvers[84] such as taking a rectal temperature, vigorous oral, pharyngeal, or endotracheal suctioning, and vigorous auscultation of the chest.[84] The real skills of a unit can be tested by noting attentiveness to small details in neonatal respiratory management. Is the environmental oxygen at the correct percentage, temperature, and flow rate? Is the arterial oxygen permitted to go too high or too low for a prolonged period? Is the unit anticipating the future needs of the infant or always treating complications? As an example, if during the acute phase, an infant with RDS has an apneic episode, it usually signifies that the infant's condition is deteriorating and urgent intervention is indicated. Waiting for a PaO$_2$ of 30 mm Hg and a severe respiratory and metabolic acidosis before beginning ventilatory therapy is not adequate anticipation. While basic care is being arranged (metabolic rate minimized, fluid and electrolyte needs met), the essentials of care involve maintaining an adequate PaO$_2$ and pH and closely observing for a change in the infant's state.

Our general plan is to maintain the PaO$_2$ in the abdominal aorta between 50 and 80 mm Hg, PaCO$_2$ in the 40 to 55 mm Hg range, and pH above 7.25. Because clinical differentiation from group B streptococcal (or other bacterial) pneumonia is not possible, a blood culture should be obtained and antibiotics begun for at least 48 hours. It is equally important to discontinue broad-spectrum antibiotics as soon as the possibility of infection is ruled out to prevent nosocomial fungal and bacterial infections.

Correction of severe metabolic acidosis with alkali has many physiologic benefits. With normalization of pH, myocardial contractility is increased, pulmonary vascular resistance is reduced, and the length of survival with asphyxia is prolonged. However, the rapid injection of hypertonic solutions such as NaHCO$_3$ is associated with a marked change in osmolality. Studies have revealed that excessive and rapid NaHCO$_3$ administration may be associated with an increased incidence of intracranial hemorrhage.[40, 130] Therefore, the following general guidelines for its use should be considered:

1. To reduce the corrosive effects of hypertonic solutions, use NaHCO$_3$ solutions diluted with equal parts of distilled H$_2$O.
2. To prevent the toxic effects from large changes in osmolality, attempt to limit alkali to 8 mEq/kg/d. In practice, much less should be needed.
3. Because other substances can also contribute to a significant increase in osmolality, closely monitor glucose. (Each 18 mg/dL of glucose results in an osmolar rise of 1 mOsm/L.) Glucose intolerance may signify sepsis.
4. Do not correct a respiratory acidosis with alkali, because administered NaHCO$_3$ is converted to CO$_2$ and is dependent on the lung for its removal.[110] Respiratory acidosis is due to retention of CO$_2$ and its relief can be accomplished only by reduction of the CO$_2$ levels, usually with some form of controlled or assisted ventilation.
5. The specific amount of bicarbonate cannot be determined from any of the widely used "recipes"; rather, treatment is empirical, with NaHCO$_3$ administration determined by serial blood gas studies.
6. When an infant is severely asphyxiated, it may be necessary to administer alkali before the pH and HCO$_3$ measurements have been completed (usually 2 mEq/kg NaHCO$_3$).

Many infants with RDS require further ventilatory support in the form of either continuous positive airway pressure (CPAP) or respirator treatment. For a complete discussion of mechanical ventilation and CPAP, see Chapter 10. Requirement for a high concentration of inspired oxygen (70% to 100%) is an indication for assisted ventilation before hypoxemia ensues.

Other criteria for a ventilator include a respiratory acidosis with a pH of less than 7.20 (and possibly 7.25) and apnea complicating the course of RDS.

After 72 hours of age (or earlier after surfactant therapy), most infants with classic

RDS start the recovery phase. Respiratory rate and retractions decrease, and PaO_2 increases without evidence of further CO_2 retention.

COMMENT: This recovery phase is preceded by a period of spontaneous diuresis during which there is improved gas exchange, lung compliance, and functional residual capacity. Since the improved pulmonary function occurs after diuresis, it is important that the clinician anticipate the recovery phase and reduce ventilatory support to prevent barotrauma.

Waldemar Carlo

During this phase, expertise in oxygen management is required. PaO_2 should be kept to less than 80 mm Hg, but if environmental oxygen is decreased too rapidly and PaO_2 is not closely monitored, a larger than expected decrease in PaO_2 may occur when the ambient oxygen is lowered, and the PaO_2 does not return to the original level when the ambient oxygen is again increased. We rarely decrease ambient oxygen faster than 10% every hour, carefully monitoring O_2 saturation before each decrease in ambient oxygen.

In infants of very low birth weight, even in the absence of severe RDS over the first few days, recovery may be prolonged. This may be attributed to impaired respiratory drive or respiratory muscle failure, persistent atelectasis not related to surfactant deficiency, nutritional compromise, intercurrent infection, congestive heart failure, or some combination of these interrelated factors.

In the absence of assisted ventilation, oral feedings can begin during the recovery phase, when bowel sounds are present, the ambient oxygen has declined to below 30%, and the umbilical arterial catheter has been removed. Many very low-birth-weight infants require prolonged assisted ventilation and even more prolonged supplemental oxygen. Small volume gavage feeds of breast milk or formula can begin when respiratory status has stabilized, despite continuing ventilatory support. This is a valuable adjunct to amino acid–glucose IV alimentation. As the infant recovers, apneic periods may be observed, but they do not have the ominous significance as when observed in the acute phase.[22]

The complications of RDS may occur spontaneously or result from well-intended therapeutic interventions. Major problems may be a consequence of arterial catheter placement, oxygen administration, mechanical ventilation, and the use of endotracheal tubes, as discussed in Chapter 10. As the number of very low-birth-weight survivors grows, the time and effort devoted to preventing and treating the complications of RDS and its management steadily increase.

During or following the recovery phase of RDS, cardiac failure secondary to a large left-to-right shunt through the patent ductus arteriosus may occur as pulmonary vascular resistance declines. This may initially manifest as inability to wean oxygen or ventilator support. Bounding pulses, a wide pulse pressure, and a systolic murmur are most useful in making a clinical diagnosis. In most cases, conservative medical management with cautious fluid administration and diuretics will control the congestive heart failure, and the patent ductus arteriosus will close as the infant grows.[12] Although the patent ductus arteriosus will close spontaneously in most cases, early intervention to close it and reduce the risk of chronic pulmonary overflow, edema, and BPD is recommended.

Although cardiomegaly is often noted on x-ray examination, an enlarged liver and edema are not usually found with cardiac failure. Further evaluation of the magnitude of shunting by echocardiography is usually indicated before initiating either pharmacologic or surgical closure of the ductus[149] (see Chapter 14; for further details, see Table 9–3). Indomethacin therapy enhances ductal closure when given either concurrently with or after failure of usual medical therapy.[54] Although prophylactic indomethacin administration appears to reduce the frequency of large left-to-right ductal shunts, there is no clear evidence that routine early indomethacin therapy reduces longer-term morbidity in susceptible infants.[88] An additional benefit of prophylactic indomethacin may be to decrease the incidence of intraventricular hemorrhage, although this does not necessarily translate into improved long-term neurodevelopmental outcome.[97] The case problems and questions in this chapter further illustrate the care of these infants.

Persistent Pulmonary Hypertension

Persistent pulmonary hypertension (PPHN) rather than the previous nomenclature, per-

Table 9–3. Supportive Care for Infants with Respiratory Distress Syndrome

Treatment	Logic
1. (a) Trained staff nurses (ratio of 1:2), respiratory therapists, and monitoring equipment. (b) Available trained physicians, nurse practitioners.	1. Early management of complications and notification of change in course (e.g., apnea, bleeding from catheter).
2. Precise temperature control to maintain infant in neutral temperature (includes oxygen hood—see Chapter 5).	2. Maintains minimal oxygen consumption and carbon dioxide production.

3. (a) pH, Pao_2, $Paco_2$, and HCO_3^- measurements at least every 4 h. Maintain Pao_2 at 50–80 mm Hg. *Continuous* Pao_2 or Sao_2 is optimal.
   (b) Monitor blood pressure.
   (c) Attempt to keep pH >7.25. If $Paco_2$ >60 or Pao_2 <50 mm Hg, change treatment.
   (d) Lower environmental oxygen slowly when RDS infant is still ill.
   (e) Limit $NaHCO_3$ to 8 mEq/kg/d.
	3. (a) To determine requirements for oxygen and additional HCO_3^-. Permits continual assessment of infant's condition and limits toxic effects of oxygen.
	   (b) Recognize hypoperfusion, hypovolemia, patent ductus arteriosus.
	   (c) Same as (a).
	   (d) Prevents greater than expected decrease in Pao_2 when environmental oxygen is reduced (right-to-left shunt etiology?).
	   (e) Prevents hypernatremia with possible brain damage.

4. Surfactant therapy (requires endotracheal tube).	4. Therapeutic approach to underlying etiology of RDS.
5. IV glucose 60 mL/kg 1st day, 80–100 mL/kg 2nd day with body weight determination for small infants to calculate if larger amounts of H_2O required. May require 150 mL/kg or more.	5. Need to balance fluid and partial caloric requirements while minimizing the risk of fluid overload problems (e.g., patent ductus arteriosus).
6. Controlled oxygen administration: warmed and humidified, using a hood.	6. Prevents large swings in environmental oxygen concentration and temperature and decreases water requirements.
7. Continually monitor respiration, heart rate, and temperature as well as blood pressure, 3(b).	7. Prevents hypoxemia and acidemia with apneic episodes.
8. Frequent determinations of blood sugar and hematocrit (Na, K, and Cl every 12–24 h).	8. Necessary for calculating general metabolic requirements.
9. Transfuse if central hematocrit <35 during acute phase of illness.	9. For adequate oxygen-carrying capacity.
10. Record all observations (laboratory, nurse's notes, etc.) on single form.	10. Permits immediate correlation of many variables.
11. Urinary output, blood urea nitrogen, creatinine, and when indicated urinary pH, electrolytes, and osmolality.	11. Evaluation of renal function and blood flow to the kidney. An increase in output occurs as the infant starts to improve.
12. Obtain blood culture; treat with ampicillin and gentamicin until cultures available.	12. Cannot radiographically separate RDS from group B streptococcal (or other) pneumonia.[82]
13. Minimize routine procedures such as suctioning, handling, and auscultation.	13. Prevents iatrogenic decreases in Pao_2.

sistent fetal circulation (PFC), more aptly describes the syndrome characterized by pulmonary hypertension resulting in severe hypoxemia secondary to right-to-left shunting through the foramen ovale and ductus arteriosus in the absence of structural heart disease. Pulmonary hypertension in these infants is thought to result from pulmonary vasospasm presumably as a result of altered pulmonary vasoreactivity and, at times, may be accompanied by an increase in muscle mass in the pulmonary

vascular bed. The increase in pulmonary arterial smooth muscle tone may develop in response to intrauterine stress, whereas a decrease of a circulating (or local) pulmonary vasodilator such as endothelium-derived relaxing factor (found to be endogenous nitric oxide, NO) at the time of birth or an increase in the amount of circulating (or local) pulmonary vasoconstrictors such as endothelin during intrauterine or postnatal life may be responsible for altered vasoreactivity.

This syndrome was initially described in term infants with respiratory distress and cyanosis without demonstrable cardiac, pulmonary, hematologic, or central nervous system (CNS) disease.[53] However, this same hemodynamic pattern can occur in both preterm and term infants with primary pulmonary disease (such as surfactant deficiency, pneumonia, or meconium aspiration syndrome), polycythemia, or pulmonary hypoplasia (such as congenital diaphragmatic hernia), or following neonatal asphyxia. Sometimes no clear etiology for the PPHN or underlying lung disease can be assigned. The end result is cyanosis, tachypnea, and acidemia, which can superficially resemble cyanotic congenital heart disease, primary pulmonary disease, or cardiomyopathy. The initial roentgenographic descriptions of PPHN stressed the absence of pulmonary parenchymal disease; however, it is presently recognized that the chest x-ray study may instead reflect the concurrence of underlying pulmonary disease such as meconium aspiration or pneumonia. Echocardiography is invaluable as a guide to assessing elevated pulmonary artery pressure and pulmonary vascular resistance and more importantly as a means of excluding most anatomic cardiac malformations[123] (see Chapter 14). Before the advent of echocardiography, cardiac catheterization (which presently is rarely, if ever, required) revealed normal cardiac structure, pulmonary hypertension, and evidence of right-to-left shunting at the level of the foramen ovale and ductus arteriosus.

The management of PPHN can be complex and very difficult, because the severe hypoxemia may be poorly responsive to high oxygen therapy or pulmonary vasodilators. Every attempt should be made to anticipate and possibly prevent the development of PPHN in patients with severe meconium aspiration syndrome or neonatal pneumonia, and early and aggressive treatment of hypoxemia should be provided. These babies are exquisitely sensitive to changes in environmental oxygen. Most require an environmental oxygen approaching 100% and may show little improvement without mechanical ventilation. Some infants benefit from modest alkalinization, brought about by hyperventilation or the administration of $NaHCO_3$ which may relieve the intense pulmonary vasospasm and allow oxygenation to improve.[36] Similarly PaO_2 is maintained

at the upper recommended levels (80 to 100 mm Hg or greater) to minimize hypoxic pulmonary vasoconstriction. Polycythemia, hypoglycemia, hypocalcemia, and hypotension should be treated if present. In fact, maintenance of systemic blood pressure at the high range of normal is often required to exceed excessively high pulmonary artery pressures and thereby counteract right-to-left shunting. Pharmacologic pressor support (e.g., dopamine or dobutamine) may be preferable to volume expansion, because excessive fluids are poorly tolerated. Adequate sedation and, at times, muscle paralysis may be necessary to combat the hypoxemia associated with agitation.

Historically, tolazoline (Priscoline) was the only pharmacologic vasodilator available to treat infants with PPHN. Its efficacy was blunted by its concurrent vasodilatory effect on the systemic circulation, thereby producing systemic hypotension; additional complications include gastrointestinal hemorrhage and renal insufficiency. The use of tolazoline has not been demonstrated to change the survival statistics of infants with PPHN. A major breakthrough in the treatment of PPHN has been the use of inhaled NO at doses of 20 ppm or less to produce pharmacologic selective pulmonary vasodilatation without producing significant systemic hypotension. Inhaled NO has been reported to significantly reduce the need for extracorporeal membrane oxygenation (ECMO), shorten duration, and reduce cost of hospitalization in PPHN.[42a, 105a] Nonetheless, ECMO remains a lifesaving treatment modality in infants who fail to respond to ventilatory and pharmacologic management of severe PPHN.

Meconium Aspiration Syndrome

Meconium is present in the amniotic fluid in 10% of all births, and its presence suggests that the infant may have suffered some asphyxial episode in utero. Evidence for this is derived from studies such as postmortem data demonstrating severe structural abnormalities in the muscular walls of the pulmonary arterial vascular bed, suggesting chronic in utero hypoxia, in infants with fatal meconium aspiration.[105] It is doubtful that amniotic fluid alone can produce any airway obstruction. However, pulmonary disease is definitely observed in infants who have aspirated meconium (Fig. 9–10), and mortality and morbidity are significant without immediate aggressive management. Interestingly, the passage and subsequent aspiration of meconium are almost never seen before 34 weeks' gestation.

In order to prevent the significant morbidity and mortality associated with meconium aspiration, studies[23, 60, 137] strongly indicate that every infant with frank meconium staining of the amniotic fluid requires the following preventive measures:

1. Immediate suctioning of the nasopharynx by the obstetrician as soon as the head appears on the perineum.
2. If there is cardiorespiratory depression, immediately after delivery, visualization of the cords by laryngoscopy and direct suctioning of the trachea through an endotracheal tube. This endotracheal suctioning should be done before stimulation of the infant or positive pressure ventilation.

Because asphyxia is often the basis for the presence of meconium in the amniotic fluid, the infant who aspirates meconium at birth is often depressed and requires some resuscitation. Positive pressure resuscitation should be delayed in these infants if possible until adequate laryngotracheal toilet has been performed, to prevent pushing meconium farther into the small airways. Most recommendations do not include aggressive laryngotracheal suctioning in vigorous infants with "light" or "thin" meconium, in whom the oropharynx has been suctioned at delivery.[148] In support of a conservative approach to such infants, no morbidity from meconium aspiration was observed in a group of meconium-stained infants with Apgar scores above 8 at 1 minute who underwent only oropyaryngeal suctioning immediately after the infant's head had been delivered.[113] Recently, obstetricians have applied transcervical amnioinfusion in labor when meconium-stained amniotic fluid is present; however, a conclusive positive effect on neonatal outcome remains to be demonstrated.[139]

EDITORIAL COMMENT: A multicenter, multinational trial to assess whether intubation and suctioning of apparently vigorous, meconium-stained neonates would reduce the incidence of meconium-aspiration syndrome (MAS) enrolled 2094 neonates. Compared with expectant management, intubation and suctioning of the apparently vigorous meconium-stained infant did not result in a decreased incidence of MAS or

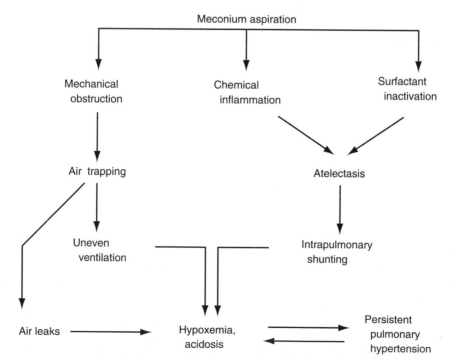

Figure 9–10. Pathophysiology of cardiorespiratory problems accompanying meconium aspiration syndrome.

other respiratory disorders. There were few and only short-lived complications of intubation. Hence there is no justification for routine intubation of the VIGOROUS meconium stained neonate.[147]

Meconium aspiration syndrome is characterized by respiratory distress ranging from tachypnea to gasping respirations. Rales and wheezing may be heard. The infant may appear barrel-chested with an increase in the anteroposterior diameter of the chest. A chest x-ray film shows areas of increased density and areas of overexpansion irregularly distributed throughout the lung; differentiation from pneumonia and retained lung fluid may be difficult.

The lung can remove meconium rapidly. Studies with puppies in which meconium was instilled into the trachea revealed that it quickly moved to the periphery of the lung.[56] Infants with mild cases usually recover after 48 hours of life. However, in sicker infants, respiratory compromise may be severe, with mechanical obstruction, hyperinflation and atelectasis producing severe gas maldistribution with ventilation-perfusion mismatching. One complication of partially blocked, overexpanded areas of lung, occurring in 20% to 50% of infants with meconium aspiration syndrome, is the development of air leaks, such as pneumothorax. Pneumothorax should be suspected if the clinical status of the infant deteriorates suddenly. Additional pulmonary pathology occurring as a result of meconium aspiration includes chemical pneumonitis and interstitial edema and surfactant inactivation. Frequently, PPHN with severe superimposed hypoxemia develops in infants with significant meconium aspiration syndrome. Respiratory failure is associated with a significant mortality rate in these infants. Several studies have demonstrated that surfactant replacement therapy improves oxygenation, reduces pulmonary air leak, reduces the need for ECMO, and improves outcome in infants with meconium aspiration syndrome.[42, 86] Nevertheless, severe respiratory failure and hypoxemia may require additional treatment modalities such as high frequency ventilation and nitric oxide administration, with ECMO therapy for those who fail to respond.

Pneumothorax

Pulmonary air leaks comprise a spectrum of disorders that includes pneumomediasti-

num, pneumopericardium, pulmonary interstitial emphysema and pneumothorax. An asymptomatic pneumothorax is found in approximately 1% of all routine newborn chest radiographic examinations. Considering the high negative intrathoracic pressures recorded during the first minutes of life, it is surprising that pneumothorax is not a more frequent occurrence. When air leak occurs, air from the ruptured alveolus dissects up the vascular sheath into the mediastinum and from there into the pleural space. In some series, as many as one half of the symptomatic patients had aspirated meconium or blood. This suggests that obstruction with a ball-valve action may be the basis for the rupture. A pneumothorax frequently develops in infants with pulmonary interstitial emphysema, in whom there is a tracking of air from ruptured alveoli into the perivascular pulmonary tissues, usually during prolonged assisted ventilation. Before the advent of exogenous surfactant therapy, the incidence of pulmonary air leak in infants with birth weights less than 1000 g was reported to be as high as 40%.[150] However, multiple studies of various exogenous surfactant preparations have demonstrated a significant reduction in pneumothorax among surfactant-treated infants.[67, 77] Prognostically, the development of air leak in very low-birth-weight infants requiring mechanical ventilation increases the risk of death or chronic lung disease.[118] In addition, pneumothorax presenting with concurrent hypotension is associated with increased risk of intraventricular hemorrhage.[96]

Pneumothorax should be suspected in any newborn with respiratory distress or in a baby on a respirator whose condition suddenly worsens. In infants with RDS, a pneumothorax may develop when the severity of disease is decreasing and lung compliance is increasing. Bilateral pneumothoraces are often observed in infants with the hypoplastic lungs accompanying renal agenesis (Potter syndrome), other forms of renal dysplasia, or congenital diaphragmatic hernia. In fact, the presence of otherwise unexplained extrapulmonary air in the early neonatal period should raise the question of an underlying renal or pulmonary malformation.

A high-intensity transilluminating light, using a fiberoptic probe, is especially helpful in quickly diagnosing a pneumothorax.[80] If the infant's clinical condition is relatively stable, it is wise to check the diagnosis radiographically before treatment. An antero-posterior film may underestimate the size of a large anterior pneumothorax, in which case a horizontal-beam lateral film of the supine infant is helpful.

Clinical findings include cyanosis, tachypnea, grunting, nasal flaring, or intercostal retractions. If the pneumothorax is unilateral and under tension, the cardiac impulse may be shifted away from the affected side and ipsilateral breath sounds may be decreased. A distended abdomen with an easily palpable liver or spleen pushed down by the diaphragm is often a useful clinical feature signifying a tension pneumothorax. This may be useful in differentiating a left-sided tension pneumothorax presenting in the delivery room from a (typically left-sided) congenital diaphragmatic hernia. Both are characterized by mediastinal shift to the right hemithorax; however, in the hernia patient, a scaphoid (rather than distended) abdomen is a presenting feature.

If the pneumothorax causes only minor symptoms, no specific therapy is necessary, but the infant's color, heart rate, respiratory rate, blood pressure, and oxygenation should be monitored. If severe respiratory distress is noted or the infant has underlying pulmonary disease, a thoracostomy tube should be placed to evacuate the pneumothorax with the application of continuous suction of 10 to 20 cm H_2O. Lung perforation has been described at autopsy following chest tube replacement, and thus a trocar should not be used to guide the catheter into the pleural space.[103] Damage to the lung may be avoided by disconnecting the patient from the ventilator during the insertion of the chest tube into the pleural space. The catheter should be placed in the pleural space anterior to the lung. This is best achieved by insertion near the third intercostal space just lateral to the anterior axillary line. To achieve resolution of the pneumothorax, it is usually necessary to maintain suction on the chest tube for 24 to 72 hours. In the report of Bhatia and Mathew,[14] 83% of pneumothoraces had resolved by 168 hours with thoracostomy drainage. Occasionally, with a large area of rupture or bronchopleural fistula, significantly more time is required. Fibrin glue instillation into the pleural space has been reported to successfully treat prolonged persistent pneumothorax in premature infants.[13]

Pneumomediastinum does not require intervention, and asymptomatic pneumopericardium should also be managed conservatively. Pneumopericardium may, however, present with profound hypotension if there is accompanying gas tamponade, and pericardiocentesis will be lifesaving. Both pneumopericardium and pulmonary interstitial emphysema (PIE) are almost invariably complications of assisted ventilation. In an attempt to avoid air leak and to manage air leak when present, mechanical ventilatory pressures should be kept at a safe minimum. The use of high-frequency ventilation appears to be effective in treating air leak and may actually reduce the risk of development of air leak in preterm infants with severe respiratory failure.[66]

Transient Tachypnea of the Newborn

Transient tachypnea of the newborn (TTN) often follows an uneventful delivery at (or close to) term. The major presenting symptom is a persistently high respiratory rate.[3] Cyanosis may be present but is usually not of major significance, with few infants requiring more than 35% to 40% oxygen to remain pink. Air exchange is good and therefore rales and rhonchi, expiratory grunting and intercostal retractions are minimal, and arterial pH and $PaCO_2$ measurements are usually within normal limits. The chest x-ray study reveals central perihilar streaking because fluid remains in the peri-arterial tissue, often with fluid in the interlobar fissure and occasionally there is a small pleural effusion; the cardiac silhouette may be slightly enlarged. If the radiologic picture includes patchy infiltrates, which probably reflect liquid-filled lobes, then TTN probably cannot be initially distinguished from infiltrates associated with meconium aspiration or bacterial pneumonia. The clinical picture of increased respiratory rate improves gradually during the first 5 days of life.

The pathogenesis appears to involve delayed resorption of fetal lung fluid and may also be associated with abnormal epithelial ion transport.[58] In experimental situations, catecholamines have been found to stimulate fetal lung fluid resorption. Infants delivered by cesarean delivery without antecedent labor are found to have decreased catecholamine levels and an increased likelihood of development of transient tachypnea.[59] Infants of diabetic mothers are also at increased risk of transient tachypnea, thought to be due to the interference by insulin on the β-adrenergic response of the lung.[31]

The presence of unabsorbed lung fluid produces decreased lung compliance, whereas the infant's increased respiratory rate attempts to minimize respiratory work. Positioning infants in the prone and head elevated position has been demonstrated to decrease tachypnea, thought to be related to improved FRC with decreased diaphragmatic impingement by the abdomen.[127] The syndrome appears to be self-limited, and there have been no reported complications. The use of diuretics such as furosemide has not been found to be effective in decreasing the symptoms or duration of illness.[148]

Pulmonary Hemorrhage

The spectrum of pulmonary hemorrhage ranges from blood-tinged tracheal or pharyngeal secretions to massive intractable bleeding. Most studies define significant pulmonary hemorrhage as bright red blood from the endotracheal tube in amounts that increase the need for ventilatory support or produce chest x-ray changes. Historically, pulmonary hemorrhage was associated with intrapartum asphyxia, infection, hypothermia, and defective hemostasis. Although occasionally presenting in low-birth-weight infants who have previously appeared well, it more often affects infants who are already suffering from other life-threatening abnormalities or illnesses. The composition of the lung effluent in infants with massive pulmonary hemorrhage in most cases is a filtrate of plasma with a small admixture of whole blood, producing a hemorrhagic edema fluid, presumably formed as a result of increased pulmonary capillary pressure. Factors that might predispose infants to development of hemorrhagic pulmonary edema included those favoring filtration of fluid (hypoprotcinemia, overtransfusion), those causing damage to lung tissue (infection, RDS, and mechanical ventilation in high inspired oxygen) abnormalities of coagulation, as well as left-to-right shunting through a patent ductus arteriosus.

More recently pulmonary hemorrhage has been associated with respiratory distress syndrome in premature infants treated with exogenous surfactant therapy. Pathologically, infants who died of pulmonary hemorrhage before the introduction of surfactant therapy were found to have pulmonary interstitial hemorrhage in contrast to extensive intra-alveolar hemorrhage in infants dying with hemorrhage associated with surfactant therapy.[112] The mechanism by which pulmonary hemorrhage develops in certain surfactant-treated infants remains uncertain. Natural surfactants were associated with a higher incidence of pulmonary hemorrhage than synthetic surfactants by meta-analysis, and treatment strategy and lower birth weight significantly increased relative risk of pulmonary hemorrhage.[119] In a retrospective cohort study, pulmonary hemorrhage was associated with the presence of a clinically significant patent ductus arteriosus before, or at the time of, the hemorrhage.[48] In vitro studies suggest that surfactant preparations may actually have some degree of cytotoxicity, producing evidence of hemolysis and cell damage.[41] Surfactant-treated infants with pulmonary hemorrhage were not found to have a generalized bleeding diathesis.[85] Most recently, pulmonary hemorrhage has been seen in several neonates following treatment with extracorporeal life support.[57]

Pulmonary hemorrhage occurs most commonly on the second to fourth days of life. The usual mode of presentation is the development of bradycardia, apnea, or slow gasping respirations and peripheral vasoconstriction. Blood-stained hemorrhagic edema fluid is then seen welling from the trachea. By comparison with hemorrhagic pulmonary edema, frank bleeding into the lung seems relatively unusual and probably occurs only in association with profound hemostatic failure, severe pneumonia, or direct trauma. Pulmonary hemorrhage can often be successfully treated by mechanical ventilation employing extra positive end-expiratory pressure (PEEP) and transfusion of fresh blood; occasionally, high-frequency ventilation may be required. Exogenous surfactant therapy has been found to produce respiratory improvement in infants with profound respiratory deterioration secondary to pulmonary hemorrhage.[111]

Bronchopulmonary Dysplasia/ Neonatal Chronic Lung Disease

In 1967, Northway et al[108] first described BPD, a clinical syndrome associated with the use of assisted ventilation and high concentrations of oxygen. Their patients had been on respirators using greater than 70% oxygen for longer than 5 to 6 days. During the prolonged recovery, the infants exhibited persistent respiratory difficulty and a characteristic radiographic progression that resulted in cystic lung changes. Increased concentrations of oxygen were required for several weeks before slow improvement was noted. Autopsy of those infants who died revealed that their lungs were diffusely involved with areas of emphysema and collapse, interstitial fibrosis, and changes in the airway's epithelium.

The radiographic sequence initially described by Northway et al is no longer commonly seen, and stage I is essentially indistinguishable from uncomplicated RDS. Dense parenchymal opacification, as seen in stage II BPD, may commonly simulate another process, such as congestive heart failure from a patent ductus arteriosus or an infection. The bubbly pattern of stage III BPD is not necessarily seen, and when it does appear, it may not follow a period of parenchymal opacity. Finally, roentgenographic development of chronic lung disease (stage IV) may be more insidious than originally described. The characteristic picture of chronic lung disease ultimately ap-

pears at around 20 or 30 days of age. The major features of stage IV disease include hyperinflation and nonhomogeneity of pulmonary tissues, together with multiple fine, lacy densities extending to the periphery.

Since Northway et al's original description of BPD, the problem of chronic respiratory disease in infants has steadily increased, because of more aggressive respiratory management and increased survival of very low-birth-weight infants.[8] In the absence of clear diagnostic criteria for BPD, the following definitions for BPD are in current use: (1) the criteria of Northway et al as described previously, (2) oxygen dependence beyond 28 days of age with persistent chest x-ray changes after mechanical ventilation, and (3) oxygen dependence beyond 36 weeks' corrected postnatal gestational age.[129] BPD has been correlated with subsequent abnormal pulmonary findings at follow-up. It has been proposed that the more nonspecific term *neonatal chronic lung disease* be employed for the large number of very low-birth-weight infants who fall under the second definition of BPD (Fig. 9–11). These infants may never have had severe RDS, with high inspired oxygen or ventilator requirements. The term *Wilson-Mikity syndrome* has been used in the past to describe some of these infants.[146]

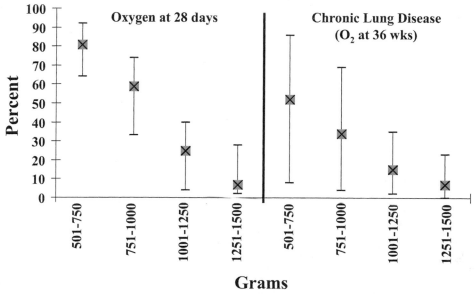

Figure 9–11. Incidence of chronic neonatal lung disease in inborn infants by birth weight. Data from the neonatal centers comprising the NICHD Neonatal Research Network (1/95–12/96). Data are presented as mean and range among centers. (From Lemons, et al: Very-low-birth-weight (VLBW) outcomes of the NICHD Neonatal Research Network, January 1995 through December 1996. Pediatrics, in press.)

Pathophysiologic and Clinical Features

Controversy surrounds the individual contributions of immaturity, inhaled oxygen, ventilator pressures, endotracheal tube injury, infection, and nutritional deficiencies to the overall pathologic picture of BPD (Fig. 9–12). The cellular basis for oxygen toxicity in these infants is discussed earlier.

Abnormal pulmonary function is characterized by decreased lung compliance resulting from areas of fibrosis, overdistention, and atelectasis and increased pulmonary resistance resulting from airway damage.[51] Wheezing may be episodic and markedly contribute to the increased work of breathing and oxygen requirement. Chronic respiratory acidosis is accompanied by elevated bicarbonate and close to normal pH. This increase in serum bicarbonate is frequently exaggerated by chronic diuretic therapy.

Pulmonary edema is a prominent complication of BPD, largely caused by the increased pulmonary vascular pressure and permeability. Hypoxic pulmonary vasoconstriction and injury to the pulmonary vascular bed appear to be involved. Exacerbations of congestive heart failure may present with wheezing, fluid retention, and hepatomegaly. The underlying disease may mask the chest x-ray changes of pulmonary edema including cardiomegaly.

Infection and the resultant inflammatory response frequently complicate the clinical course of chronic neonatal lung injury. Inflammatory mediators released by either infection (or high inspired oxygen) may aggravate the bronchoconstriction and vasoconstriction to which the lungs of these infants are predisposed.

Nutritional deficiencies and inadequate

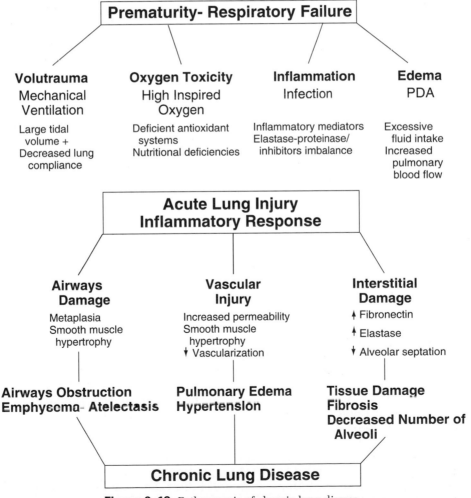

Figure 9–12. Pathogenesis of chronic lung disease.

caloric intake can interfere with normal alveolar development and with the repair process of injured lung tissue. It can also negatively affect the antioxidant mechanisms. The problem is compounded by these infants' elevated oxygen consumption, contributed to by the increased work of breathing.[81, 145]

Management

With skillful and patient management, most of these infants will recover, although abnormalities in pulmonary function may persist into childhood.[132] Furthermore, prolonged need for supplemental oxygen over several months is associated with a greater incidence of neurodevelopmental disorders when compared with infants with less severe lung disease.[131] The key to survival for infants with severe lung disease depends on close attention to details such as vigorous treatment of right-sided heart failure, precise fluid balance, use of diuretics, and gradual weaning from mechanical ventilation and raised environmental oxygen. The latter may need to occur in decrements of 1% to 2% of inspired oxygen. Oxygenation is typically monitored via pulse oximetry, and oxygen saturation is maintained in the low to mid-90s. Furosemide (Lasix), 1 to 2 mg/kg/d, is the most widely used diuretic, although prolonged use has been associated with nephrocalcinosis and impaired hearing.

These infants need to be closely watched for early signs of infection because pneumonia generally results in a setback. Bronchodilators are of benefit especially when there are clinical signs of acute bronchospasm. They may be administered as systemic theophylline or as β-agonist inhalation therapy.[73, 126]

Controlled trials of both diuretic therapy and bronchodilator inhalation have revealed encouraging short-term improvements in airway resistance, even in the absence of wheezing.[32]

Steroids administered systemically or by inhalation have also been used either to ameliorate BPD or to assist in weaning these infants from the ventilator. Although many reports are encouraging, more clinical trials are needed to define the optimal dose, timing, and outcome of this intervention.[6, 25, 28] Reports of an increased incidence of cerebral palsy after postnatal systemic steroid use for BPD are of concern.

EDITORIAL COMMENT: There is considerable tension in differentiating the benefits and risks of postnatal corticosteroids. The potential reduction of mortality and chronic lung disease is counterbalanced by the short- and long-term complications that include hyperglycemia, hypertension, hypertrophic cardiomyopathy, gastric hemorrhage, gastric perforation, and cerebral palsy. Corticosteroids should at present be reserved for critically ill ventilator-dependent infants. Short courses or pulses using low dose regimens are recommended.

◆————

Halliday HL, Ehrenkranz RA: Moderately early (7–14 days) postnatal corticosteroids for preventing chronic lung disease in preterm infants. Cochrane Database Syst Rev. (2):CD001144, 2000. Review.

Halliday HL, Ehrenkranz RA: Early postnatal (<96 hours) corticosteroids for preventing chronic lung disease in preterm infants. Cochrane Database Syst Rev. (2):CD001146, 2000. Review.

Halliday HL, Ehrenkranz RA: Delayed (>3 weeks) postnatal corticosteroids for chronic lung disease in preterm infants. Cochrane Database Syst Rev. (2):CD001145, 2000. Review.

Doyle L, Davis P: Postnatal corticosteroids in preterm infants: systematic review of effects on mortality and motor function. J Paediatr Child Health 36:101–107, 2000.

Many of these infants require prolonged hospitalization, and a well-organized program of infant stimulation may help the child achieve maximum potential. Parents must be encouraged to assume some of the responsibility for medical procedures, such as chest physiotherapy, and, where possible, a consistent medical team should oversee the infant's care and be available for continuing parental support. Finally, adequate nutritional management is very important because malnutrition delays somatic growth and the development of new alveoli in these high-risk, labile infants.

Apnea in the Immature Infant

Periodic breathing (short, recurring pauses in respiration) of 5 to 10 seconds' duration is common in the immature infant and should be considered a normal respiratory pattern at this age. Apnea, on the other hand, has been defined as either (1) a given time period with complete cessation of respiration (typically >15 to 20 seconds) or (2) the time without respiration after which functional changes are noted in the infant, such as a decrease in heart rate to about 80 per minute or oxygen saturation to about 80%. Although the use of a standard, set time period appears to simplify routine nursery management, some small infants (usually <1000 g) appear to desaturate if the apneic period extends beyond as little as 10 seconds. The problem increases substantially in both incidence and severity with decreasing gestational age.

The relationship between apnea, desaturation, and bradycardia is not simple, as summarized in Figure 9–13. Decreased central respiratory drive is the usual initiating event, with reflex bradycardia presumably triggered by the resultant desaturation. Excitation of inhibitory reflexes may also occasionally precipitate both apnea and bradycardia.[91] A particularly perplexing problem is the frequent occurrence of desaturation and bradycardia in intubated, ventilated very low-birth-weight infants. In such infants, hypoventilation is probably the initiating event associated with impaired lung function and ineffective ventilation.[16, 35]

Hypoglycemia, fluid and electrolyte imbalance, temperature fluctuations, sepsis, anemia with or without a patent ductus arteriosus, and severe brain lesions can be heralded by apneic spells and should be ruled out when apneic episodes first begin.[115] In a small number of infants, usually close to term, apneic spells may be the manifestation of a seizure disorder. However, the vast majority of apneic periods occur in infants who are immature and have no organic disease.

An exception is an apneic episode in an infant with severe RDS, which usually indicates the presence of hypoxia and acidemia or sepsis and is a clear indication for immediate intervention, such as assisted ventilation.[22]

The premature infant in whom specific causes for apnea have been reasonably excluded may be considered to have true idiopathic apnea of prematurity. Although no single physiologic or neurochemical explanation completely describes these apneic spells, Table 9–4 lists factors that singly or together make the immature infant more susceptible to apnea.[100]

Treatment

Because prolonged apnea may result in clinically significant hypoxemia, and because these spells occur so commonly, all premature infants weighing less than 1750 g or younger than 34 weeks' gestation should be routinely and continuously monitored until no significant apneic episode has occurred for up to 5 to 7 days. Because heart rate does not regularly decrease in all infants with apnea, respiration monitors must not depend solely on a change in heart rate to signal an alarm.[29] Conversely, because apnea with an obstructive component (so-called mixed apnea) may not trigger a respiration alarm, simultaneous heart rate must always be monitored. In these infants, oxygen saturation is a useful adjunct to cardiorespiratory monitoring. Most episodes of 15 to 20

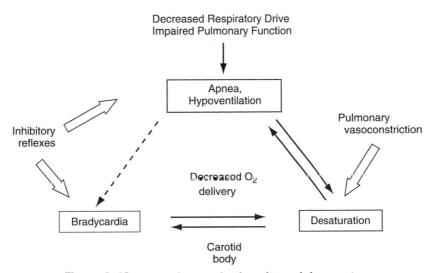

Figure 9–13. Neonatal apnea, bradycardia, and desaturation.

Table 9–4. Factors Related to Apnea in the Immature Infant

Observation	Explanation
Hypoxemia causes respiratory depression and results in hypoventilation in neonate instead of sustained hyperventilation as in adult.[90]	Hypoxemic depression of respiration in young infant is centrally mediated and appears to override stimulation from peripheral chemoreceptors.[90, 122]
Hypercapnia causes hyperventilation as in adult, with diminished response in apneic versus nonapneic infants.	Decreased hypercapnic ventilatory response in apneic infants is probably secondary to immature central neural mechanisms.[50]
Obstructed inspiratory efforts may occur during apnea and may be misdiagnosed as primary bradycardia when breathing movements persist.[136]	Pharyngeal hypotonia and failure of upper airway respiratory muscles (genioglossus, alae nasi) to contract during inspiration may compromise upper airway patency.[18]
Apnea is more common during active sleep.[93]	During active sleep, respiration is irregular, lung volume and oxygenation may decrease.[65]

seconds' duration of apnea resolve spontaneously. Most of the remainder stop with gentle diffuse cutaneous stimulation. However, a mask and bag should be set up near every monitored infant, to be used if breathing does not begin promptly after stimulation. Inspired oxygen concentration depends on the infant's prior oxygen requirement.

A marked reduction in apnea has been noted with a low continuous positive airway pressure and respiratory stimulants such as theophylline or caffeine.[1, 76, 99, 128] Table 9–5 illustrates principles in the management of idiopathic apnea. The order in which these therapeutic steps are undertaken is based on the assessment of each individual patient.

A reasonable principle is to commence with a therapy that carries a low potential for short- or long-term side effects. Nasal CPAP at 3 to 5 cm of water is particularly effective in treatment of apneic episodes with an obstructive component.[99] The most probable mechanisms for the beneficial effect of CPAP include maintenance of upper airway patency, increase in FRC and Pao_2, and stabilization of the chest wall. The use

Table 9–5. Management of Idiopathic Apnea

Diagnosis and treatment of specific causes (e.g., hypoglycemia, anemia, sepsis)
Nasal continuous positive airway pressure (4 cm H_2O).[99]
Xanthine (caffeine or theophylline) therapy, commencing with a loading dose followed by maintenance therapy, and serum level monitoring, especially for theophylline.
Increased environmental oxygen only as necessary to maintain adequate baseline oxygen saturation. Often associated with treatment of anemia.
Assisted ventilation if all else fails.

of xanthines (theophylline, caffeine) is widespread in the management of neonatal apnea. Theophylline is metabolized to caffeine in substantial amounts in neonates, although the precise mechanism whereby either of these xanthines decreases apnea remains unclear.[52] Proposed mechanisms include generalized enhancement of central respiratory drive via adenosine receptor antagonism, more efficient diaphragmatic contraction, and reversal of hypoxic respiratory depression.[101] Although long-term sequelae from xanthine use have not appeared, care must be taken to avoid short-term side effects such as tachycardia and diuresis, probably more so with theophylline than caffeine as the latter appears to have a greater margin of safety.

Resolution of Neonatal Apnea

Apnea may persist longer in preterm infants than was generally acknowledged. Such episodes may be accompanied by desaturation and/or bradycardia and often persist beyond 40 weeks of age in infants delivered before 28 weeks' postconceptional age.[39] Persistent apnea may also be asymptomatic in a large proportion of very low-birth-weight infants.[10] Prolonged apnea, often manifesting as bradycardia in these very low-birth-weight infants, is associated with chronic neonatal lung disease, but not with significant CNS lesions as determined by ultrasound. Persistence of symptomatic apnea and bradycardia prolongs the hospitalization of very premature infants, and raises questions about the margin of safety for their discharge[30] as well as about the indications for, and utility of, home apnea monitoring. Data still support the traditional belief that discharge is appropriate after the infant has been free of symptomatic apnea for approximately 5 to 7 days.

What is the overall significance of these events in former preterm infants? Because evidence does not link the persistence of these events to sudden infant death syndrome (SIDS), the tendency is to dismiss them as clinically insignificant. Persistence of these cardiorespiratory events may be part of the spectrum of normal postnatal maturation. However, this assumption may be incorrect, and the possibility exists that they represent a subtle marker for neurodevelopmental or sleep disturbances, or other disorders of childhood.[101]

◆ QUESTIONS

True or False

◆ *As long as the arterial PaO_2 remains less than 100 mm Hg, there will be no retinal damage when using high concentrations of oxygen ($>$40%) for the treatment of RDS.*

When PaO_2 is measured every 4 hours and is less than 100 mm Hg, retinal damage still develops in some very low-birth-weight infants. Therefore the statement is false. There are several possible explanations: (1) a large right-to-left ductal shunt is directed to a sampling site in the lower aorta, while retinal vessels receive blood with a higher PaO_2; (2) PaO_2 constantly fluctuates between arterial measurements; and (3) factors other than PaO_2 are involved in retinal injury. Continuous monitoring should detect (2) and should detect (1) if a skin PO_2 electrode or pulse oximeter is sited over the right upper thorax (preductal blood) and compared with postductal PaO_2. Nevertheless, even with continuous monitoring of the oxygen level, retinopathy of prematurity still occurs.

◆ *Sensory stimulation in the form of multiple examinations, measurements of pulse, rectal temperature, and heart rate, and noninvasive studies such as echocardiograms and head ultrasounds may destabilize an infant with severe RDS.*

Continuous monitoring has revealed striking declines in oxygenation with standard nursing manipulations. This has caused minimal handling to be recommended in many infants, especially in the presence of PPHN. Therefore the statement is true. Although gentleness and avoidance of unnecessary trauma are mandatory, minimal handling must not be allowed to become an excuse for failure to initiate diagnostic studies and carefully apply adequate therapy when indicated.

◆ *B. W. is a 2-day-old, 1200-g male infant with moderate RDS. During the first 2 days of life he has not been apneic and has maintained a reasonable pH, $PaCO_2$, and PaO_2 in 40% oxygen. However, the most recent PaO_2 measurement has decreased to 35 mm Hg (breathing 40% oxygen). This environmental oxygen concentration should be left the same, because raising it beyond 40% predisposes to oxygen toxicity.*

A decrease in PaO_2 to 35 mm Hg suggests worsening of the infant's condition. His condition may deteriorate rapidly if he remains in 40% oxygen. If the arterial oxygen is monitored closely (continuously or at least every 4 hours), elevating the inspired oxygen concentration to maintain the PaO_2 between 50 and 80 mm Hg should not predispose to lung or retinal injury. Therefore the statement is false. The oxygen concentration should be increased.

◆ *The occurrence of 20 apneic periods (no respiration for more than 10 to 15 seconds) during the first 10 days of life in a premature infant without respiratory distress is commonly associated with brain damage.*

In years past, when respiration was not closely monitored and apneic episodes were not promptly terminated with either stimulation or short-term mask-and-bag ventilation, frequent apneic periods were associated with brain damage. Currently, this should not occur. Although there may be a slightly increased incidence of neurologic impairment, this is unproven and most of them do quite nicely. Therefore, the statement is false. If there is no specific cause for the apnea, intervention with CPAP or a xanthine is probably indicated.

◆ *If apneic periods are noted after several oral feedings at 34 weeks' gestation, it is recommended that oral feeding be stopped.*

Apneic periods are more commonly noted after feedings and are not an indication to stop feedings if the infant is otherwise well. Therefore, the statement is false, although manipulating the quantity and frequency of the feedings and the position of the infant may help. It is not clear whether such apneic episodes following feedings represent a vagal reflex or hypoventilation in response to swallowing.

◆ *Maintaining the arterial PaO_2 between 50 and 80 mm Hg will prevent pulmonary oxygen toxicity.*

Pulmonary oxygen toxicity is related to the inspired concentration of oxygen, not the arterial oxygen concentration. Therefore the statement is false.

CASE PROBLEMS

When studying each case, refer to the blood gas record sheet (Box 9–1).

◆ ───────────────────────────

Case One

A. B. is a 1500-g, growth-retarded female with meconium aspiration pneumonia. At 8 hours of age, she is in oxygen concentration of 70% and an umbilical arterial catheter has been placed. She has meconium-stained nails and a good urine output.

◆ **At 8 hours, the baby's left leg turns white. What should be done?**
If the blanching does not quickly disappear with warming of the contralateral extremity, remove the umbilical artery catheter without delay.

◆ **If the catheter is removed, how is the infant's environmental oxygen concentration managed?**
There is no substitute for the combination of continuous oxygen monitoring (via continuous $tcPo_2$ or pulse oximeter) and intermittent arterial blood sampling via an indwelling arterial catheter in an acutely ill infant. Placement of an arterial line in an extremity (e.g., radial artery line) should therefore be attempted for intermittent arterial sampling, because the infant has a respi-

---

◆ **Box 9–1**
Blood Gas Record Sheet

Start _____
      Date   Time

Finish _____
       Date   Time

	Time	Age (hr)	O_2 conc.	Temperature (°C) Hood / Inc	Skin / Rectal	BP (M)	P	R	Hct / Hgb	Dext	#	pH	Po_2	Pco_2	HCO_3
Case One	8	70	34 / 34	36⁶ / 37¹	53	130	80			5	7.16	50	60	
Case Two	½	40	33⁶ / 33⁶	33 / 32	39	160	60	43	>90	1	7.14	30	35	11.4
	1	70	33⁶ / 33⁶	34 / 33	22	120	70	43		2	7.28	90	36	16.4
Case Four	3	70	33⁶ / 33⁶	36⁵ / 36⁷	40	120	50	54	>90	2	7.36	280	40	22.2
	4½	60	33⁶ / 33⁶	36⁵ / 36⁷	39	120	45			4	7.35	250	42	22.8
	5	40	33⁶ / 33⁶	36⁶ / 36⁷	39	140	65			5	7.36	30	43	23.9
	5½	60	33⁶ / 33⁶	36⁵ / 36¹	38	130	60			6	7.37	70	33	18.7
Case Five	6	100	34 / 34	36 / 36.5	54	140	80	52	>90	4	7.4	32	29	19

ratory acidosis, and pH and P_{CO_2} should be measured in addition to P_{O_2}.

When arterial catheterization is impossible, heel-stick or venous blood sampling can be used to monitor pH and Pa_{CO_2} but not Pa_{O_2}. Noninvasive oxygen monitoring is needed to control ambient oxygen.

With respiratory acidosis and borderline oxygenation at high oxygen requirement, this infant requires endotracheal intubation and mechanical ventilation.

◆
Case Two

C. D. is a 2100-g male who has been grunting since birth. X-ray film shows no pneumothorax but is of poor quality. See blood gases at 30 minutes.

◆ *What are this infant's obvious problems?*
(1) Hypothermia, (2) hypoxemia, and (3) metabolic acidosis. He may have been resuscitated without good thermal control, which hastened his decrease in body temperature. Infants with prenatal asphyxia have been noted to have a greater decrease in body temperature during the first hours of life. His Pa_{CO_2} is not elevated, but he is not making a respiratory adjustment for the metabolic acidosis as one might expect in the "normal" infant.

◆ *How should these problems be handled?*
Provide an increased oxygen concentration, treat with bicarbonate (2 mEq/kg), and repeat the blood gas. Many would be more comfortable intubating this hypoxic infant before administering bicarbonate. We concur.

◆ *What problem is noted at 1 hour?*
The blood pressure has decreased but the hematocrit has not. Note: caregivers elected not to intubate, and blood gas status is adequate despite shock, persistent hypothermia, and increase in supplemental O_2.

◆ *What is the explanation for what happened?*
Hypoxemia or acidemia alone or in combination may result in an elevation of blood pressure. Partial correction of the metabolic acidosis and elevating the Pa_{O_2} probably reduced the increased peripheral vascular resistance. The low blood pressure suggests a severely reduced blood volume, which should be expanded. Antibiotics are needed after appropriate cultures in this hypothermic, hypotensive infant.

◆
Case Three

B. S. is a 900-g female delivered at 27 weeks' gestation. Her Apgar scores are 1 and 6 at 1 and 5 minutes, respectively. She is intubated and mechanically ventilated and has a chest x-ray film compatible with RDS. Blood gases at age 1 hour in Fi_{O_2} 80% on ventilator 20/5 at rate of 30 are pH 7.40, Pc_{O_2} 32 mm Hg, Pa_{O_2} 60 mm Hg, and HCO_3 19.5.

◆ *Should surfactant therapy be administered?*
Because surfactant has improved survival, reduced the incidence of air leaks, and probably reduced the severity and incidence of chronic lung disease in infants with respiratory distress, this approach is definitely warranted. In fact this should already have occurred within the first 20 to 30 minutes of life.

◆ *What are the complications of surfactant therapy?*
Significant desaturation occurs in a small percentage of infants shortly after receiving surfactant therapy. There have also been concerns about pulmonary hemorrhage associated with surfactant administration. This appears to be more of a problem in the most immature infants, those weighing less than 750 g and younger than 25 weeks' gestation. Close monitoring for a patent ductus arteriosus and aggressive means to close it have been recommended by some investigators.

◆ *At 8 hours of age, the infant is weaned from an Fi_{O_2} of 80% to 40% and blood gases are pH 7.38, Pa_{O_2} 62, Pc_{O_2} 38, and HCO_3 22. Should surfactant dose be repeated?*
There has been a great deal of flexibility with regard to the redosing with surfactant. Multiple doses have proven superior to single-dose regimens, and despite the improvement, this infant may further benefit from repeating the surfactant therapy.

◆
Case Four

G. H. is a 2000-g male who has been grunting since birth. His x-ray film reveals questionable RDS. He is placed in 70% oxygen.

◆ *At 3 hours, what should be done, if anything?*
Decrease environmental oxygen to 60% immediately and, if possible, start tcP_{O_2} monitoring or pulse oximetry for rapid weaning. Inspired oxygen should then be lowered in steps of 2% to 5% at least every 15 minutes during continuous P_{O_2} monitoring and a re-

peat blood gas obtained when tcPo$_2$ approaches 90 mm Hg or pulse oximeter is around 96%. This is a dangerous level of oxygen.

◆ **What happened at 5 hours? What now?**

This patient demonstrated a greater than expected decrease in PaO$_2$ when environmental oxygen was decreased. This can generally be avoided with continuous Po$_2$ monitoring. First, return the baby to an oxygen concentration of 60% to 70%. Second, transilluminate the chest to rule out the possibility of pneumothorax. Determine another blood oxygen tension in 15 to 20 minutes after the environmental oxygen has been increased.

◆ **What is the explanation for what happened between 4½ and 5½ hours of life?**

There is not a complete physiologic explanation underlying this phenomenon. It is assumed that, in some infants, the pulmonary vessels are particularly sensitive to changes in oxygen tension, and lowering the environmental oxygen results in pulmonary vasoconstriction and an increased right-to-left shunt. Under these circumstances, the PaO$_2$ decreases out of proportion to what might ordinarily be expected when the environmental oxygen is reduced.

◆

Case Five

M. L. weighs 3000 g at 41 weeks' gestation and is covered with thick meconium. Apgar scores are 2 and 5 in the delivery room. Immediate suctioning via endotracheal tube produces thick meconium from the trachea. Chest x-ray film at 2 hours shows bilateral patchy infiltrates.

◆ **What is the main problem at 6 hours?**

The infant has marked hypoxemia in 100% O$_2$. It would be unusual for such a degree of hypoxemia without CO$_2$ retention to be attributable to meconium pneumonitis alone in a well-resuscitated infant. If appears that persistent pulmonary hypertension secondary to neonatal asphyxia has complicated the course of this infant.

◆ **How should this be handled?**

The response of the hypoxemia to ventilatory support in such an infant is variable; nonetheless, assisted ventilation should be administered and a mild respiratory alkalosis (pH ~ 7.4) induced if oxygenation fails to improve. The outcome for infants with PPHN and meconium aspiration syndrome has improved remarkably with the availability of surfactant therapy and inhaled nitric oxide. ECMO should be reserved for these infants who do not respond to maximal conservative management.

REFERENCES

1. Aranda J, Sitar D, Parsona W, et al: Pharmacokinetic aspects of theophylline in premature newborns. N Engl J Med 295:413, 1976.
2. Avery GB, Fletcher AB, Kaplan M, et al: Controlled trial of dexamethasone in respirator-dependent infants with bronchopulmonary dysplasia. Pediatrics 75:106, 1985.
3. Avery M, Gatwood O, Brumley G: Transient tachypnea of newborn: Possible delayed resorption of fluid at birth. Am J Dis Child 111:380, 1966.
4. Avery M, Mead J: Surface properties in relation to atelectasis and hyaline membrane disease. Am J Dis Child 97:517, 1959.
5. Ballard RA, Ballard PL, Cnaan A, et al. The North American trial of antenatal thyrotropin-releasing hormone (TRH) for the prevention of lung disease in the preterm infant. N Engl J Med 338:493–498, 1998.
6. Bancalari E: Corticosteroids and neonatal chronic lung disease. Eur J Pediatr 157:S31–S37, 1998.
7. Bancalari E, Flynn J. Goldberg RN, et al: Influence of transcutaneous oxygen monitoring on the incidence of retinopathy of prematurity. Pediatrics 79:663, 1987.
8. Bancalari E, Gerhardt T: Bronchopulmonary dysplasia. Pediatr Clin North Am 33:1, 1986.
9. Barr PA, Bailey PE, Sumners J, et al: Relation between arterial blood pressure and blood volume and effect of infused albumin in sick preterm infants. Pediatrics 60:282, 1977.
10. Barrington KJ, Finer N, Li D: Predischarge respiratory recordings in very low birth weight newborn infants. J Pediatr 129:934–940, 1996.
11. Behrman R: Persistence of fetal circulation. J Pediatr 89:636, 1976.
12. Bell EF, Warburton D, Stonestreet BS, et al: Effect of fluid administration on the development of symptomatic patent ductus arteriosus and congestive heart failure in premature infants. N Engl J Med 302:598, 1980.
13. Berger JT, Gilhooly J: Fibrin glue treatment of persistent pneumothorax in a premature infant. J Pediatr 122:958–960, 1993.
14. Bhatia J, Mathew OP: Resolution of pneumothorax in neonates. Crit Care Med 13:417–419, 1985.
15. Boat FF, Kleinerman JI, Fanaroff AA, et al: Toxic effects of oxygen on cultured human neonatal respiratory epithelium. Pediatr Res 7:607, 1973.
16. Bolivar JR, Gerhardt T, Gonzalez A, et al: Mechanisms for episodes of hypoxemia in preterm infants undergoing mechanical ventilation. J Pediatr 127:767–773, 1995.
17. Brockway J, Hay WW Jr: Prediction of arterial partial pressure of oxygen with pulse oxygen saturation measurements. J Pediatr 133:63–66, 1998.
18. Brouillette RT, Thach BT: A neuromuscular mechanism maintaining extrathoracic airway patency. J Appl Physiol 46:772, 1979.
19. Bruce M, Boat T, Martin RJ, et al: Proteinase inhib-

itors and inhibitor inactivation in neonatal airways secretions. Chest 81(Suppl):44, 1982.

20. Brunstler I, Enders A, Versmold HT: Skin surface P_{CO_2} monitoring in newborn infants in shock: Effect of hypotension and electrode temperature. J Pediatr 100:454, 1982.

21. Carlo WA, Martin RJ, Abboud EF, et al: Alae nasi activation (nasal flaring) decreases nasal resistance in preterm infants. Pediatrics 72:338, 1983.

22. Carlo WA, Martin RJ, Versteegh FGA, et al: The effect of respiratory distress syndrome on chest wall movements and respiratory pauses in preterm infants. Am Rev Respir Dis 126:103, 1982.

23. Carson B, Losey R, Bowes W, et al: Combined obstetric and pediatric approach to prevent meconium aspiration syndrome. Am J Obstet Gynecol 126:712, 1976.

24. Chu J, Clements J, Cotton E, et al: Neonatal pulmonary ischemia. Pediatrics 40:709, 1967.

25. Collaborative Dexamethasone Trial Group: Dexamethasone therapy in neonatal chronic lung disease: An international placebo-controlled trial. Pediatrics 88:421, 1991.

26. Cross K: Cost of preventing retrolental fibroplasia. Lancet 2:954, 1973.

27. Cryotherapy for Retinopathy of Prematurity Cooperative Group: Multicenter Trial of Cryotherapy for Retinopathy of Prematurity: Preliminary results. Pediatrics 81:697–706, 1988.

28. Cummings JJ, D'Eugenio DB, Gross SJ: A controlled trial of dexamethasone in preterm infants at risk for bronchopulmonary dysplasia. N Engl J Med 320:1505, 1989.

29. Daily W, Klaus M, Meyer H: Apnea in premature infants: Monitoring, incidence, heart rate changes, and an effect of environmental temperature. Pediatrics 43:510, 1969.

30. Darnall RA, Kattwinkel J, Nattie C, et al: Margin of safety for discharge after apnea in premature infants. Pediatrics 100:795–801, 1997.

31. Davis DJ, Hickman JM, Lefebvre CA, Lyon ME: Insulin inhibits beta-adrenergic responses in fetal rabbit lung in explant culture. Am J Physiol 263:L562–L567, 1992.

32. Davis JM, Sinkin RA, Aranda JV: Drug therapy of bronchopulmonary dysplasia. Pediatr Pulmonol 8:117–125, 1990.

33. Davis JM, Veness-Meehan K, Notter RH, et al: Changes in pulmonary mechanics after the administration of surfactant to infants with respiratory distress syndrome. N Engl J Med 319:476, 1988.

34. Dawes G: Foetal and Neonatal Physiology. Chicago, Year Book Medical, 1968.

35. Dimaguila MA, DiFiore JM, Martin RJ, et al: Characteristics of hypoxemic episodes in very low birth weight infants on ventilatory support. J Pediatr 130:577–583, 1997.

36. Drummond WH, Gregory GA, Heymann MA, et al: The independent effects of hyperventilation, tolazoline, and dopamine on infants with persistent pulmonary hypertension. J Pediatr 98:603, 1981.

37. Duc G: Assessment of hypoxia in the newborn: Suggestions for a practical approach. Pediatrics 48:469, 1971.

38. Durand M, Ramanathan R: Pulse oximetry for continuous oxygen monitoring in sick newborn infants. J Pediatr 109:1052, 1986.

39. Eichenwald EC, Aina A, Stark AR: Apnea frequently persists beyond term gestation in infants delivered at 24 to 28 weeks. Pediatrics 100:354–359, 1997.

40. Finberg L: The relationship of intravenous infusions and intracranial hemorrhage: A commentary. J Pediatr 91:77, 1977.

41. Findlay RD, Taeusch HW, David-Cu R, Walther FJ: Lysis of red blood cells and alveolar epithelial toxicity by therapeutic pulmonary surfactants. Pediatr Res 37:26030, 1995.

42. Findlay RD, Taeusch HW, Walther FJ: Surfactant replacement therapy for meconium aspiration syndrome. Pediatrics 97:48–52, 1996.

42a. Finer NN, Barrington KJ: Nitric oxide for respiratory failure in infants born at or near term. Cochrane Database Syst. Rev. CD000399. Review. 2000.

43. Frank L: Hyperoxic inhibition of newborn rat lung development: Protection by deferoxamine. Free Rad Biol Med 11:341–348, 1991.

44. Frank L, Sosenko IRS: Prenatal development of lung antioxidant enzymes in four species. J Pediatr 110:106–110, 1987.

45. Frank L, Sosenko IRS: Failure of premature rabbits to increase antioxidant enzymes during hyperoxic exposure: Increased susceptibility to pulmonary oxygen toxicity compared to term rabbits. Pediatr Res 29:292–296, 1991.

46. Freeman BA, Crapo JD: Biology of disease. Free radicals and tissue injury. Lab Invest 47:412–426, 1982.

47. Fujiwara T, Maeta H, Chide S, et al: Artificial surfactant therapy in hyaline membrane disease. Lancet 1:55, 1980.

48. Garland J, Buck R, Weinberg M: Pulmonary hemorrhage risk in infants with a clinically diagnosed patent ductus arteriosus: A retrospective cohort study. Pediatrics 94:719–723, 1994.

49. Gaynon MW, Stevenson DK, Sunshine P, et al: Supplemental oxygen may decrease progression of prethreshold disease to threshold retinopathy of prematurity. J Perinatol 17:434–438, 1997.

50. Gerhardt T, Bancalari E: Apnea of prematurity: Lung function and regulation of breathing. Pediatrics 74:58, 1984.

51. Gerhardt T, Hehre D, Feller R, et al: Serial determination of pulmonary function in infants with chronic lung disease. J Pediatr 110:448, 1987.

52. Gerhardt T, McCarthy J, Bancalari E: Effect of aminophylline on respiratory center activity and metabolic rate in premature infants with idiopathic apnea. Pediatrics 63:537, 1979.

53. Gersony W, Duc G, Sinclair J: "PFC" syndrome (persistence of fetal circulation). Circulation 39:111, 1969.

54. Gersony WM, Peckham GJ, Ellison RC, et al: Effects of indomethacin in premature infants with patent ductus arteriosus: Results of a national collaborative study. J Pediatr 102:895, 1983.

55. Gleason CA, Martin RJ, Anderson JV, et al: Optimal position for a spinal tap in preterm infants. Pediatrics 71:31, 1983.

56. Gooding G, Gregory G, Taber P, et al: An experimental model for the study of meconium aspiration of the newborn. Radiology 100:137, 1971.

57. Goretsky MJ, Martinasek D, Warner BW: Pulmonary hemorrhage: A novel complication after extracorporeal life support. J Pediatr Surg 31:1276–1281, 1996.

58. Gowen CW Jr, Lawson EE, Gingras J, et al: Electrical potential difference and ion transport across nasal epithelium of term neonates: Correlation with mode of delivery, transient tachypnea of the newborn, and respiratory rate. J Pediatr 113:121–127, 1988.

59. Greenough A, Lagercrantz H: Catecholamine abnormalities in transient tachypnea of the premature newborn. J Perinatal Med 20:223–226, 1992.

60. Gregory G, Gooding C, Phibbs R, et al: Meconium aspiration in infants—A prospective study. J Pediatr 85:848, 1974.

61. Hack M, Fanaroff A, Klaus M, et al: Neonatal respiratory distress following elective delivery: A preventable disease? Am J Obstet Gynecol 126:43, 1976.

62. Hallman M, Chundu V, Barsotti M, Bry K: Transferrin modifies surfactant responsiveness in acute respiratory failure: Role of iron-free transferrin as an antioxidant. Pediatric Pulmonol 22:14–22, 1996.

63. Hay WW Jr, Thilo E, Curlander JB: Pulse oximetry in neonatal medicine: Clin Perinatol 18:441–471, 1991.

64. Heffner JE, Repine JE: Pulmonary strategies of antioxidant defense. Am Rev Respir Dis 140:531–554, 1989.

65. Henderson-Smart D, Read D: Depression of intercostal and abdominal muscle activity and vulnerability to asphyxia during active sleep in the newborn. In Guilleminault C, Dement WC, eds: Sleep Apnea Syndromes. New York: Alan R Liss, 1978.

66. HiFO Study Group. Randomized study of high-frequency oscillatory ventilation in infants with severe respiratory distress syndrome. J Pediatr 122:609–619, 1993.

67. Horbar JD, Soll RF, Sutherland JM, et al: A multi-centered randomized placebo-controlled trial of surfactant therapy for respiratory distress syndrome. N Engl J Med 320:959–965, 1989.

68. James L, Lanman J, eds: History of oxygen therapy and retrolental fibroplasia (supplement). Pediatrics 57:591, 1976.

69. Javitt J, Dei Cas R, Chiang Y: Cost-effectiveness of screening and cryotherapy for threshold retinopathy of prematurity. Pediatrics 91:859–866, 1993.

70. Jobe AH: Lung development. In Fanaroff AA, Martin RJ, eds: Neonatal-Perinatal Medicine. 6th ed. St. Louis: Mosby, 1997.

71. Jobe AH, Mitchell BR, Gunkel JH: Beneficial effects of the combined use of prenatal corticosteroids and postnatal surfactant on preterm infants. Am J Obstet Gynecol 168:508–513, 1993.

72. Joint Statement of the American Academy of Pediatrics, the American Association for Pediatric Ophthalmology and Strabismus, and the American Academy of Ophthalmology: Screening examination of premature infants for retinopathy of prematurity. Pediatrics 100:273–274, 1997.

73. Kao L, Warburton D, Platzker A, et al: Effect of isoproterenol inhalation on airway resistance in chronic bronchopulmonary dysplasia. Pediatrics 73:509, 1984.

74. Kaplan H, Robinson F, Kapanci Y, et al: Pathogenesis and reversibility of the pulmonary lesions of oxygen toxicity in monkeys. I. Clinical and light microscopic studies. Lab Invest 20:94, 1969.

75. Kattwinkel J, Bloom BT, Delmore P, et al: Prophylactic administration of calf lung surfactant extract is more effective than early treatment of respiratory distress syndrome in neonates of 29 through 32 weeks' gestation. Pediatrics 92:90–98, 1993.

76. Kattwinkel J, Nearman H, Fanaroff A, et al: Apnea of prematurity: Comparative therapeutic effects of cutaneous stimulation and continuous positive airway pressure. J Pediatr 86:588, 1975.

77. Kendig JW, et al: Surfactant replacement therapy at birth: Final analysis of a clinical trial and comparisons with similar trials. Pediatrics 82:756–762, 1988.

78. Kennaugh JM, Kinsella JP, Abman SH, et al: Impact of new treatments for neonatal pulmonary hypertension on extracorporeal membrane oxygenation use and outcome. J Perinatol 17:366–369, 1997.

79. Klein JM, Thompson MW, Snyder JM, et al: Transient surfactant protein B deficiency in a term infant with severe respiratory failure. J Pediatr 132:244–248, 1998.

80. Kuhns L, Bednarek R, Wyman M, et al: Diagnosis of pneumothorax or pneumomediastinum in the neonate by transillumination. Pediatrics 56:355, 1975.

81. Kurzner SI, Garg M, Bautista DS, et al: Growth failure in bronchopulmonary dysplasia: Elevated metabolic rates and pulmonary mechanics. J Pediatr 112:73, 1988.

82. Leonidas J, Hall R, Beatty E, et al: Radiographic findings in early onset neonatal group B streptococcal septicemia. Pediatrics 59:1006, 1977.

83. Leviton A, Kuban KC, Pagano M, et al: Antenatal corticosteroids appear to reduce the risk of postnatal germinal matrix hemorrhage in intubated low birth weight newborns. Pediatrics 91:1083–1088, 1993.

84. Long JG, Philip AGS, Lucey JF: Excessive handling as a cause of hypoxemia. Pediatrics 65:203, 1980.

85. Long W, Corbet A, Allen A, et al: Retrospective search for bleeding diathesis among premature newborns with pulmonary hemorrhage after synthetic surfactant treatment. J Pediatr 120:S45–S48, 1992.

86. Lotze A, Mitchell BR, Bulas DI, et al: Multicenter study of surfactant use in the treatment of term infants with severe respiratory failure. J Pediatr 132:40–47, 1998.

87. Lucey JF, Dangman B: A Reexamination of the role of oxygen in retrolental fibroplasia. Pediatrics 73:82–96, 1984.

88. Mahony L, Cladwell RL, Girod DA, et al: Indomethacin therapy on the first day of life in infants with very low-birthweight. J Pediatr 106:801, 1985.

89. Margraf LR, Tomashefski JF Jr, Bruce MC, Dahms BB: Morphometric analysis of the lung in bronchopulmonary dysplasia. Am Rev Respir Dis 143:391–400, 1991.

90. Martin RJ, DiFiore JM, Jana L, et al: Persistence of the biphasic ventilatory response to hypoxia in preterm infants. J Pediatr 132:960–964, 1998.

91. Martin RJ, Fanaroff AA, eds: Neonatal apnea, bradycardia, or desaturation: Does it matter? J Pediatr 132:758–759, 1998.

92. Martin RJ, Okken A, Katona PG, et al: Effect of lung volume on respiratory time in the newborn infant. J Appl Physiol 45:18, 1978.

93. Martin RJ, Okken A, Rubin D: Arterial oxygen tension during active and quiet sleep in the normal neonate. J Pediatr 94:271, 1979.
94. Martin RJ, Robertson SS, Hopple MM: Relationship between transcutaneous and arterial oxygen tension in sick neonates during mild hyperoxemia. Crit Care Med 10:670, 1982.
95. Martin-Brady RL: Brain transections demonstrate the central origin of hypoxic ventilatory depression in carotid body-denervated rats. J Physiol 407:41, 1988.
96. Mehrabani D, Gowen CW Jr, Kopelman AE: Association of pneumothorax and hypotension with intraventricular hemorrhage. Arch Dis Child 66:48–51, 1991.
97. Ment LR, Vohr B, Oh W, et al: Neurodevelopmental outcomes at 36 months' corrected age of preterm infants in the multicenter indomethacin intraventricular hemorrhage prevention trial. Pediatrics 98:714–718, 1996.
98. Merritt TA, Hallman M, Berry C, et al: Randomized, placebo-controlled trial of human surfactant given at birth versus rescue administration in very low birth weight infants with lung immaturity. J Pediatr 118:581, 1991.
99. Miller MJ, Carol WA, Martin RJ: Continuous positive airway pressure selectively reduces obstructive apnea in preterm infants. J Pediatr 106:91, 1985.
100. Miller MJ, Fanaroff AA, Martin RJ: Respiratory disorders in preterm and term infants. In Fanaroff AA, Martin RJ, eds: Neonatal-Perinatal Medicine. 6th ed. St. Louis: CV Mosby, 1997.
101. Miller MJ, Martin RJ: The pathophysiology of apnea of prematurity. In Polin RA, Fox WW, eds: Fetal and Neonatal Physiology. 2nd ed. Philadelphia: 1998, pp 1129–1143.
102. Milner Ad, Vyas H: Lung expansion at birth. J Pediatr 101:879, 1982.
103. Moessinger AC, Driscoll JM, Wigger HT: High incidence of lung perforation by chest tube in neonatal pneumothorax. J Pediatr 92:635, 1978.
104. Morley CJ, Greenough A, Miller NG, et al: Randomized trial of artificial surfactant (ALEC) given at birth to babies from 23 to 34 weeks gestation. Early Human Dev 17:41, 1988.
105. Murphy J, Vawter G, Reid LH: Pulmonary vascular disease in fatal meconium aspiration. J Pediatr 104:758–762, 1984.
105a. The Neonatal Inhaled Nitric Oxide Study Group (NINOS): Inhaled nitric oxide in term and near-term infants with hypoxic respiratory failure. N Engl J Med 336:597, 1997.
106. Nieves-Cruz B, et al: Clinical surfactant preparations mediate SOD and catalase uptake by type II cells and lung tissue. Am J Physiol (Lung) 270:L659–L667, 1996.
107. NIH Consensus Statement: Effect of corticosteroids for fetal maturation on perinatal outcomes. Am J Obstet Gynecol 173:246–252, 1995.
108. Northway W, Rosan R, Porter D: Pulmonary disease following respirator therapy. N Engl J Med 276:357, 1967.
109. Ogihara T, et al: New evidence for the involvement of oxygen radicals in triggering neonatal chronic lung disease. Pediatr Res 39:117–119, 1996.
110. Ostrea E, Odell G: The influence of bicarbonate administration on blood pH in a "closed system": Clinical implications. J Pediatr 80:671, 1972.
111. Pandit PB, Dunn MS, Colucci EA: Surfactant therapy in neonates with respiratory deterioration due to pulmonary hemorrhage. Pediatrics 95:32–36, 1995.
112. Pappin A, Shenker N, Hack M, Redline RW: Extensive intraalveolar pulmonary hemorrhage in infants dying after surfactant therapy. J Pediatr 124:621–626, 1994.
113. Peng TCC, Gutcher GR, Van Dorsten JP: A selective aggressive approach to the neonate exposed to meconium-stained amniotic fluid. Am J Obstet Gynecol 175:296–301, 1996.
114. Perelman RH, Farrell PM: Analysis of causes of neonatal death in the United States with specific emphasis on fatal hyaline membrane disease. Pediatrics 70:570, 1982.
115. Perlstein P, Edwards H, Sutherland J: Apnea in premature infants and incubator-air temperature changes. N Engl J Med 282:461, 1970.
116. Phelps DL, Rosenbaum AL: Effects of marginal hypoxemia on recovery from oxygen-induced retinopathy in the kitten model. Pediatrics 73:1–6, 1984.
117. Poets CF, Wilken M, Seidenberg J, et al: Reliability of a pulse oximeter in the detection of hyperoxemia. J Pediatr 122:87–90, 1993.
118. Powers WF, Clemens JD: Prognostic implications of age at detection of air leak in very low birth weight infants requiring ventilatory support. J Pediatr 123:611–617, 1993.
119. Raju TN, Langenberg P: Pulmonary hemorrhage and exogenous surfactant therapy: A metaanalysis. J Pediatr 123:603–610, 1993.
120. Raju TNK, Langenberg P, Bhutani V, et al: Vitamin E prophylaxis to reduce retinopathy of prematurity: A reappraisal of published trials. J Pediatr 131:844–850, 1997.
121. Rider ED, Jobe AH, Ikegami M, et al: Antenatal betamethasone dose effect in preterm rabbits studied at 27 days gestation. J Appl Physiol 68:1134, 1990.
122. Rigatto H, Brady J: Periodic breathing and apnea in preterm infants. II. Hypoxia as a primary event. Pediatrics 50:219, 626, 1977.
123. Riggs T, Hirschfeld S, Fanaroff A, et al: Persistence of fetal circulation syndrome: An echocardiographic study. J Pediatr 91:626, 1977.
124. Robert M, Neff R, Hubbell J, et al: Association between maternal diabetes and the respiratory distress syndrome in the newborn. N Engl J Med 294:357, 1976.
125. Rojas M, et al: Changing trends in the epidemiology and pathogenesis of neonatal chronic lung disease. J Pediatr 126:605–610, 1995.
126. Rooklin AR, Moomjian As, Shutack JG, et al: Theophylline therapy in bronchopulmonary dysplasia. J Pediatr 95:882, 1979.
127. Sconyers GM, Ogden BE, Goldberg HS: The effect of body position on the respiratory rate of infants with tachypnea. J Perinatol 7:118–121, 1987.
128. Shannon D, Gotay F, Stein I, et al: Prevention of apnea and bradycardia in low birthweight infants. Pediatrics 55:589, 1975.
129. Shennan AT, Dunn MS, Ohlsson A, et al: Abnormal pulmonary outcomes in premature infants: Prediction from oxygen requirement in the neonatal period. Pediatrics 82:527, 1988.
130. Simmons M, Adcock E, Bard H, et al: Hypernatremia and intracranial hemorrhage in neonates. N Engl J Med 291:6, 1974.

131. Skidmore MD, Rivers A, Hack M: Increased rate of cerebral palsy among very low-birthweight infants with chronic lung disease. Dev Med Child Neurol 32:325, 1990.

132. Smyth JA, Tabachnik E, Duncan WJ, et al: Pulmonary function and bronchial hyperreactivity in long-term survivors of bronchopulmonary dysplasia. Pediatrics 68:336, 1981.

133. Solimano AJ, Smyth JA, Mann TK, et al: Pulse oximetry advantages in infants with bronchopulmonary dysplasia. Pediatrics 78:844–849, 1986.

134. Strang L, MacLeish M: Ventilatory failure and right-to-left shunt in newborn infants with respiratory distress. Pediatrics 28:17, 1961.

135. Task Force on Transcutaneous Monitors: Report of a consensus meeting. Pediatrics 83:122, 1989.

136. Thach BT, Stark AR: Spontaneous neck flexion and airway obstruction during apneic spells in preterm infants. J Pediatr 94:295, 1979.

137. Ting P, Brady J: Tracheal suction in meconium aspiration. Am J Obstet Gynecol 122:767, 1975.

138. Tyson JE, Ehrenkranz RA, Stoll BJ, et al: Vitamin A supplementation for extremely low birth weight infants. N Engl J Med 340:1968, 1999.

139. Usta IM, Mercer BM, Aswad NK, Sibai BM: The impact of a policy of amnioinfusion for meconium-stained amniotic fluid. Obstet Gynecol 85:237–241, 1995.

140. Varsila E, et al: Immaturity-dependent free radical activity in premature infants. Pediatr Res 36:55–59, 1994.

141. Vermont-Oxford Neonatal Network: A multicenter, randomized trial comparing synthetic surfactant with modified bovine surfactant extract in the treatment of neonatal respiratory distress syndrome. Pediatrics 97:1–6, 1996.

142. Versmold HT, Kitterman JA, Phibbs RH, et al: Aortic blood pressure during the first 12 hours of life in infants with birth weight 610 to 4,220 grams. Pediatrics 67:607, 1981.

143. Walsh MC, Noble LM, Carlo WA, et al: Relationship of pulse oximetry to arterial oxygen tension in infants. Crit Care Med 15:1102, 1987.

144. Weakley DR, Spencer R: Current concepts in retinopathy of prematurity. Early Human Development 30:121–138, 1992.

145. Weinstein MR, Oh W: Oxygen consumption in infants with bronchopulmonary dysplasia. J Pediatr 99:958, 1981.

146. Wilson M, Mikity V: A new form of respiratory disease in premature infants. Am J Dis Child 99:489, 1960.

147. Wiswell TE, Gannon CM, Jacob J, et al: Delivery room management of the apparently vigorous meconium-stained neonate: Results of The Multicenter, International Collaborative Trial. Pediatrics 105:1–7, 2000.

148. Wiswell TE, Rawlings JS, Smith FR, Goo ED: Effect of furosemide on the clinical course of transient tachypnea of the newborn. Pediatrics 75:908–910, 1985.

149. Yeh TF, Luken JA, Thalji A, et al: Intravenous indomethacin therapy in premature infants with persistent ductus arteriosus—a double-blind controlled study. J Pediatr 98:137, 1981.

150. Yu VY, Wong PY, Bajuk B, Szymonowicz W: Pulmonary air leak in extremely low birth weight infants. Arch Dis Child 61:239–241, 1986.

Assisted Ventilation

Waldemar A. Carlo

> But that life may, in a manner of speaking, be restored to the animal, an opening must be attempted in the trunk of the trachea, into which a tube or reed or cane should be put; you will then blow into this so that the lung may rise again and the animal take in air. Indeed, with a single breath in the case of this living animal, the lung will swell to the full extent of the thoracic cavity and the heart become strong and exhibit a wondrous variety of motions . . . when the lung long flaccid has collapsed, the beat of the heart and arteries appears wavy, creepy, twisting, but when the lung is inflated, it becomes strong again and swift and displays wondrous variations . . . as I do this, and take care that the lung is inflated at intervals, the motion of the heart and arteries does not stop.
>
> *Andreas Vesalius*
> *De Humani Corporis Fabrica (1543)*

The primary objective of assisted ventilation is to support breathing until the patient's respiratory efforts are sufficient to sustain adequate gas exchange and oxygenation. Ventilation may be required during immediate care of the depressed or apneic infant, before evaluation and final treatment, or for prolonged periods of treatment for respiratory failure. Appropriately trained personnel and equipment for emergency ventilation should be available in every delivery room and newborn nursery. Bag-and-mask ventilation effectively stabilizes most infants who require resuscitation.

This chapter is an introduction to assisted ventilation. Before undertaking assisted ventilation of any form, it must be recognized that the techniques demand time, resources, and experienced personnel. Prolonged ventilation should only be used in special units where expert nursing, respiratory therapy, and medical care are continuously available.

◆ RESPIRATORY FAILURE

Hypercapnic respiratory failure is the inability to remove CO_2 by spontaneous respiratory efforts and results in an increasing arterial P_{CO_2} (Pa_{CO_2}) and a decreasing pH. Assisted ventilation is most commonly needed to treat hypercapnic respiratory failure. Hypoxemia is usually (but not invariably) present; in many instances, arterial oxygenation can be normalized if the inspired oxygen is increased. Infants with hypoxemic respiratory failure have a predominant problem of oxygenation, usually the result of right-to-left shunt or severe ventilation-perfusion mismatch. Respiratory failure can occur because of disease in the lungs, the thorax, the airways, the respiratory muscles, or the central nervous system (Table 10–1). Assisted ventilation is usually required when severe respiratory failure ensues (Table 10–2). Depending on many clinical considerations (e.g., very low birth weight), assisted ventilation may be initiated earlier.

Clinical Manifestations of Respiratory Failure in the Newborn

The following are findings that should make the clinician suspect respiratory failure:

1. Increase or decrease in respiratory rate
2. Increase or decrease in respiratory efforts
3. Periodic breathing with increasing prolongation of respiratory pauses
4. Apnea

Table 10–1. Causes of Respiratory Failure in Neonates

Pulmonary
    Respiratory distress syndrome
    Aspiration syndrome
    Pneumonia
    Transient tachypnea of the newborn
    Persistent pulmonary hypertension
    Pneumothorax
    Pulmonary hemorrhage
    Pulmonary edema
    Bronchopulmonary dysplasia
    Diaphragmatic hernia
    Tumors
    Pleural effusion
    Congenital lobar emphysema
Airway
    Laryngomalacia
    Tracheomalacia
    Choanal atresia/stenosis
    Pierre Robin syndrome
    Micrognathia
    Tumors and cysts
Respiratory muscles
    Phrenic nerve palsy
    Spinal cord injury
    Myasthenia gravis
Central nervous system
    Apnea of prematurity
    Drugs: sedatives, analgesics, magnesium
    Seizures
    Birth asphyxia
    Hypoxic encephalopathy
    Central nervous system hemorrhage
    Ondine's curse
Miscellaneous
    Cyanotic heart disease
    Patent ductus arteriosus
    Congestive heart failure
    Anemia/polycythemia
    Postoperative state
    Asphyxia neonatorum
    Tetanus neonatorum
    Extreme immaturity
    Shock
    Sepsis

5. Cyanosis unrelieved by oxygen
6. Decreasing blood pressure with tachycardia associated with pallor, circulatory failure, and ultimately bradycardia

Cardiac Versus Pulmonary Disease

The clinician may frequently need to distinguish between cardiac and pulmonary dis-

Table 10–2. Indications for Assisted Ventilation

Respiratory acidosis with pH less than 7.20 to 7.25
Hypoxemia while on 100% oxygen or continuous
    positive airway pressure with 60% to 100% oxygen
Severe apnea

ease in the sick newborn infant. Cyanotic heart disease may mimic a respiratory disease. One possible way to differentiate between the two is to obtain an arterial Po_2 (PaO_2) after about 10 minutes of inhalation of 100% oxygen or ventilation. In infants with pulmonary disease, PaO_2 usually increases more than 100 mm Hg, whereas infants with cyanotic heart disease show little change in PaO_2. The hyperoxia test, although useful diagnostically, may be misleading. In infants with severe pulmonary hypertension and right-to-left shunt, PaO_2 may not elevate with 100% oxygen, and PaO_2 may increase more than 100 mm Hg early in life in infants with forms of cyanotic heart disease that have high pulmonary blood flow (e.g., total anomalous pulmonary venous return). Usually, echocardiography can be used to make a definitive diagnosis of the cause of severe hypoxemic respiratory failure.

COMMENT: Use of a transcutaneous oxygen monitor during the test can be helpful in improving both the interpretation and the safety of the test.

John Kattwinkel

◆ ENDOTRACHEAL INTUBATION

Most infants should be ventilated with a bag-and-mask plus 100% oxygen before attempting endotracheal intubation. This improves oxygenation and decreases $PaCO_2$, decreasing the likelihood of cardiac arrest during endotracheal intubation. Bag-and-mask ventilation is impractical for prolonged periods of time but can be used for the following:

* Immediate resuscitation
* Stabilization following endotracheal intubation
* Ventilation in infants whose condition is deteriorating without obvious cause
* Ventilation during transport to intensive care facilities when mechanical ventilation is unavailable

Mechanical ventilation is not warranted when there is no reasonable chance of intact survival, as in the following diagnoses: anencephaly, trisomy 13 or 18, Werdnig-Hoffmann disease, Potter syndrome, intracranial hemorrhage with marked cerebral extension, or hypoxic encephalopathy without reflexes or cerebral blood flow.

Endotracheal Tube Size

It is preferable to use relatively small endotracheal tubes to prevent tracheal damage. The endotracheal tube should fit loosely enough to allow a leak of gas between tube and trachea when 10 cm H_2O inspired pressure is generated. Tube size can be related to infant size or gestational age. Recommended sizes are as follows:

Gestational Age (wk)	Endotracheal Tube Size (mm internal diameter)
<30	2.5
30–34	3.0
>35	3.5

Intubation

Insertion of an endotracheal tube should be performed with universal precautions under a radiant heat lamp to keep the infant warm. Free flow oxygen should be administered as required.

The infant should be ventilated with a bag-and-mask and high oxygen concentration between attempts. The tip of the tube should be placed midway between the carina and the glottis.[28] The length of insertion of the endotracheal tube is shown in Figure 10–1. The following measurements can be used for endotracheal tube placement:

Infant Weight (g)	Endotracheal Tube Insertion Length (tip to lip, cm)
1000	7
2000	8
3000	9
4000	10

At these lengths, the distal end of the endotracheal tube should be at the midtrachea. Gas entry should be equal bilaterally. It is easy to inadvertently pass the tube into the right mainstem bronchus. The position should be checked radiographically at the completion of the procedure. The tube should be secured so that movement of the head and neck will not dislodge it. Lightweight plastic connectors can be used to prevent kinking the tube. Adapters with narrow tips should not be used, as the resistance is increased.

Oral Intubation

The advantages of oral intubation are the relative ease of insertion and that a stylet can be used to aid insertion. Oral tubes should always be used in emergencies. The disadvantages are the increased tube mobility if the tube is inadequately taped to the upper lip, the greater difficulty in keeping the tube in position, and the tendency to distort the hard palate following prolonged oral intubation, which may cause dental problems later in life.

A laryngoscope with a Miller number 0 or 1 blade inserted in the vallecula is used to pull upward to visualize the glottis while leaving the head in a neutral position. It is important not to traumatize the gums and tooth buds. The heart rate should be monitored continuously with auditory and visual signals during attempts at intubation. Continuous O_2 saturation or transcutaneous P_{O_2} monitoring is invaluable because oxygenation can worsen abruptly. Intubation at-

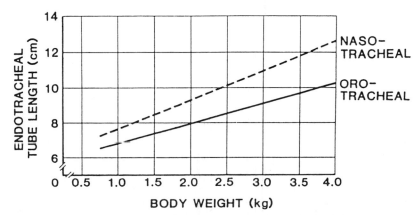

Figure 10–1. Graph for determination of length of insertion of endotracheal tubes. The tip of the endotracheal tube is aimed at the midtrachea. (From Lough MD, Carlo WA: Clinical Care Techniques. In Carlo WA, Chatburn RL, eds: Neonatal Respiratory Care. Chicago: Year Book Medical Publishers, 1988, p 122.)

tempts should be limited to 20 seconds. It is helpful if the tube has been previously curved. Cooling of the endotracheal tube or a stylet may be used to stiffen the tube for orotracheal intubation.

Nasal Intubation

The advantage of nasal intubation is the improved stability with the reduced likelihood of slippage into the right mainstem bronchus or accidental extubation. The disadvantages are trauma to the nares and nasal septum, greater difficulty in insertion of the tube, possibility of an increased number of gram-negative nasal superinfections, and potential trauma to the developing eustachian tubes and sinuses. Nasotracheal intubation should always be performed as an elective procedure and should not be done in emergencies.

Using a laryngoscope blade, the lubricated endotracheal tube is inserted through the nares until visualized in the oropharynx. The McGill forceps is used to guide the tube into the glottis. It is helpful if the endotracheal tube has been previously lubricated with a nontoxic, water-soluble lubricant. A stylet is never used for nasotracheal intubation.

Suctioning

If necessary, suctioning can be done every 1 to 2 hours if there are copious amounts of secretions or every 4 to 8 hours if the amount of secretions is sparse. A strict sterile technique with disposable gloves and suction tubes is necessary. The infant should be allowed to recover between episodes of suctioning by increasing the inspired oxygen concentration by 10% to 20% and by reexpanding the lung with 10% to 20% more pressure than used for routine ventilation. Saline instillation is done to facilitate removal of secretions when secretions are thick or when meconium or blood has been aspirated.

Although necessary, suctioning is potentially dangerous, because it may result in a hypoxic episode resulting from discontinuation of ventilation, extraction of gas from small airways, or atelectasis. It may also produce lesions in the trachea at the site of the suction catheter tip. Use of a special endotracheal tube connector that allows continuation of mechanical ventilation during suctioning may prevent or reduce some of these problems.

COMMENT: suctioning of the endotracheal tube will decrease oxygenation and pulmonary function. I would advocate increasing inspired oxygen concentration by 10% to 15% immediately before and following the period of suctioning and avoiding the practice of "routine" suctioning except as secretions warrant.
John Kattwinkel

Changing an Endotracheal Tube

An endotracheal tube change is only required if the tube becomes dislodged or occluded or if the infant outgrows it. Routine change is not indicated.

◆ APPLIED PULMONARY MECHANICS

The following principles are helpful in understanding mechanical ventilation. A pressure gradient between the airway opening and alveoli must exist in order to drive the flow of gases during both inspiration and expiration. The pressure gradient required to inflate the lungs is determined largely by the compliance and the resistance of the lungs.

Compliance

Compliance is a property of elasticity or distensibility (e.g., of the lungs and chest wall) and is calculated from the change in volume per unit change in pressure:

$$\text{Compliance} = \frac{\Delta \text{ Volume}}{\Delta \text{ Pressure}}$$

Therefore, the higher the compliance, the larger the delivered volume per unit of pressure. Compliance in babies with normal lungs ranges from 0.003 to 0.005 L/cm H_2O. Compliance in infants with respiratory distress syndrome (RDS) ranges from 0.0005 to 0.001 L/cm H_2O.

Resistance

Resistance is a property of the inherent capacity of the gas-conducting system (e.g., airways, endotracheal tube, and lung tissue) to oppose airflow and is expressed as the change in pressure per unit change in flow:

$$\text{Resistance} = \frac{\Delta\,\text{Pressure}}{\Delta\,\text{Flow}}$$

Resistance in babies with normal lungs ranges from 25 to 50 cm H_2O/L/s. Resistance is not dramatically altered in infants with RDS but is increased in intubated infants and ranges from 50 to 100 cm H_2O/L/s.

Time Constant

Time constant is a measure of the time (expressed in seconds) necessary for 63% of a step change (e.g., airway pressure gradient) toward equilibration. A step change in airway pressure occurs at the beginning and at the end of a machine-delivered inspiration (during pressure-limited, time-cycled ventilation). The product of compliance and resistance determines the time constant of the respiratory system:

$$\text{Time constant} = \text{Compliance} \times \text{Resistance}$$

For example, in an infant with normal lungs:

One time constant
= 0.005 L/cm H_2O × 25 cm H_2O/L/second
= 0.125 second

In an intubated infant with RDS:

One time constant
= 0.001 L/cm H_2O × 50 cm H_2O/L/second
= 0.050 second

It takes three time constants to achieve 95% of the pressure change to be equilibrated throughout the lungs; it takes five time constants for a 99% change to equilibrate. Thus, to allow for a fairly complete inspiration and expiration, inspiratory and expiratory times set on the ventilator should last about three to five time constants. In this example, the duration of three to five time constants is 0.150 to 0.250 second. A very short inspiratory time can lead to inadequate tidal volume because ventilatory pressures may not equilibrate throughout the lungs (Fig. 10–2). A very short expiratory time can lead to gas trapping because exhalation may not be completed. Very long inspiratory or expiratory times are also not beneficial (see Fig. 10–2).

◆ CONTINUOUS DISTENDING PRESSURE

Respiration can also be assisted by expansion of the lungs with continuous dis-

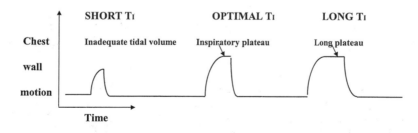

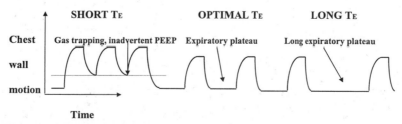

Figure 10–2. Estimation of optimal inspiratory (T_I) and expiratory (T_E) times. Inspiratory and expiratory times are optimal when inspiration and expiration are complete but the times are not too prolonged. See text for further details.

tending pressure. This technique is valuable when respiratory drive is normal and pulmonary disease is not overwhelming. Continuous distending pressure can be applied with a continuous positive airway pressure (CPAP) or a continuous negative pressure around the chest wall. Because of the ease of delivery, CPAP has become the usual mode of delivery of continuous distending pressure.

Studies by Gregory and colleagues[18] demonstrated that gas exchange can be improved in infants with RDS by applying CPAP. Frequently, CPAP is the first method used to assist ventilation in many infants with RDS (Fig. 10–3). Early use of CPAP in infants with RDS decreases the need for high oxygen concentration and endotracheal intubation.[4]

Because of surfactant deficiency in RDS, alveoli tend to collapse easily. The resulting atelectatic areas of the lungs are the sites of right-to-left shunting. When alveoli are prevented from closing by maintaining a continuous positive transpulmonary pressure throughout the respiratory cycle, functional residual capacity increases. In addition, ventilation of perfused areas of the lung increases, which reduces intrapulmonary shunt.

A simple system for CPAP was described by Gregory et al.[18] A suitable air-oxygen mixture passes through a humidifier. Gas passes the tubing, which is attached to an endotracheal tube. The screw clamp on the reservoir controls the flow of gas and maintains a constant positive pressure within the system, as indicated on the pressure manometer. The side arm acts as an underwater safety valve by ending under a column of water (15 cm). Nasal CPAP is simple and effective, and can be applied by endotracheal tube, head box, nasal prongs, or nasopharyngeal prongs (Table 10–3). CPAP prevents the need for endotracheal intubation in many premature infants with RDS. Problems with CPAP are similar to those with a ventilator. Nursing and medical care are similar to those undertaken during mechanical ventilation.

EDITORIAL COMMENT: There has been a shift back to greater use of CPAP with efforts to minimize mechanical ventilation. Intubation for a brief period to instill surfactant followed by nasal CPAP has been successfully employed for larger preterm infants.

General Guidelines for Continuous Positive Airway Pressure

1. In most centers, use of CPAP is indicated in infants with RDS when Pao_2 is less than 50 to 60 mm Hg while the infant is breathing more than 40% to 70% oxygen or when the infant has recurrent apnea.

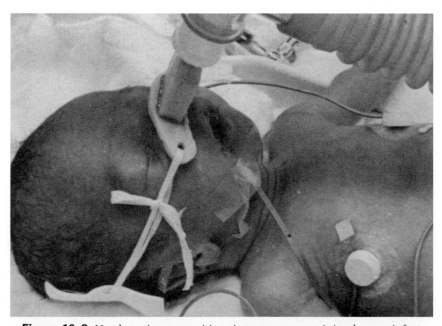

Figure 10–3. Nasal continuous positive airway pressure unit in place on infant.

Table 10–3. Techniques of Applying Continuous Distending Pressure

Method	Advantages	Effective for Infants <1500 g	Disadvantages
Endotracheal	Effective	Yes	Requires intubation; nursing and medical skills as for ventilator
Head box	Noninvasive	No	Neck seal a problem; suction difficult; nerve palsies
Face mask	Simple, inexpensive	Yes	Abdominal distention, pressure on face and eyes, CO_2 retention, cerebellar hemorrhage
Nasal prongs	Simple	No	Trauma to turbinates and septum, excessive crying, variation in FIO_2, increased work of breathing
Nasopharyngeal prongs	Relatively simple, fixation easy	Yes	May become blocked or kinked
Face chamber	Good seal, minimal trauma to face	Yes	Expensive; baby inaccessible

2. Initially, nasal CPAP of 6 cm H_2O or endotracheal CPAP of 4 cm H_2O is used. If there is no improvement, the pressure can be increased in 2-cm H_2O increments up to 8 to 12 cm H_2O. Very high CPAP levels may overdistend the lungs and decrease their compliance.
3. Arterial blood gases should be measured within 20 minutes of each change of pressure. Continuous measurement of transcutaneous PO_2 and PCO_2 or oxygen saturation with a pulse oximeter are of great value and can decrease the need for frequent blood gas measurements.
4. Because these positive pressures are not completely transmitted to the pleural space as a result of reduced lung compliance, venous return and cardiac output are usually not compromised. However, if $PaCO_2$ increases and PaO_2 decreases, a reduction in CPAP pressure should be considered.
5. Inspired oxygen should be increased in 5% to 10% increments if PaO_2 remains less than 50 mm Hg at pressures of 8 to 12 cm H_2O.

COMMENT: Because low levels of CPAP (e.g., <6 cm H_2O) probably have little effect on cardiac output, we tend to use CPAP earlier than previously recommended. If a baby clearly has decreased pulmonary compliance (he is grunting and/or retracting), we will begin nasal CPAP when only 40% O_2 is required. If the baby is extremely preterm (e.g., 29 weeks' gestation or less), we may begin nasal CPAP even earlier. Thoracic wall elastic recoil is almost nonexis-

tent in such babies, so that the resting volume of the lung is very close to the collapsed volume. Also, the compliant chest wall tends to collapse as the diaphragm descends, resulting in an ineffective tidal volume. Early use of CPAP may improve the efficiency of ventilation in these very immature babies.

John Kattwinkel

Weaning from Continuous Positive Airway Pressure

1. Inspired oxygen can be reduced by 2% to 5% when the PaO_2 exceeds 70 mm Hg.
2. CPAP can be reduced when the PaO_2 is more than 70 mm Hg and the inspired oxygen is less than 40%.

COMMENT: With small babies (<1500 g), if recurrent apneic spells are a problem, we may continue low-pressure CPAP (<6 cm H_2O) until inspired oxygen concentrations have been reduced to 21% to 30%.

John Kattwinkel

See Chapter 9 for a discussion of the use of CPAP for apnea of prematurity.

◆ MECHANICAL VENTILATION

Mechanical ventilation is one of the most important breakthroughs in the history of neonatal care. Mechanical ventilation allows the survival of previously nonviable infants, stimulating the development of a new era in neonatology. Technologic advances in mechanical ventilators and improved concepts of ventilatory management continue to result in better outcomes.[9, 29, 38]

Mechanical ventilators achieve a pressure gradient between the airway opening and lungs, producing a flow of gas into the lung. This is usually created by intermittently building up a positive pressure in the proximal airway. Ventilators for infants are usually one of the following types:

1. *Pressure-controlled ventilators.* A constant flow of gas passes through the ventilator. Intermittently, the expiratory relief valve closes and the gas flows to the infant. Pressure is limited to the desired magnitude. When the expiratory relief valve has been closed for the preset period of time, the valve opens, and inspiration ceases. Pressure-controlled ventilation is usually used with the technique of intermittent mandatory ventilation, which allows spontaneous breathing between ventilator breaths. Examples of pressure-controlled ventilators include the Bear Cub, Dragger, Healthdyne, Infant Star, and Sechrist-100B.
2. *Volume-controlled ventilators.* A preset volume of gas is delivered to the system (patient and ventilator circuit). When this gas has been delivered by the piston, inspiration is terminated. Examples of this type of ventilator include the Bird VIP, Newport Breeze, and Siemens Servo 300.

Pressure-controlled ventilators are the most frequently used types in neonates, but volume-controlled neonatal ventilators are being used more.[39] The clinician is advised to learn about and understand one or two ventilators and circuits, rather than using several.

Ventilators have the following features:

1. Gas mixer, to allow easy adjustment of the inspired oxygen concentration between 21% and 100%.
2. Inspiratory-expiratory time adjustment, to allow altering of the inspiratory time. This permits prolongation of inspiratory time in patients with a long inspiratory time constant or widespread atelectasis as well as its shortening if the time constant is short (see Fig. 10–2). Expiratory time should be prolonged when gas trap-

ping is present or the expiratory time constant is long. Expiratory time can be shortened when the respiratory time constant is short.
3. Expiratory relief valve, to limit the peak inspiratory pressure. When used in combination with the inspiratory time adjustment, it allows the peak pressure to be held, generating a pressure plateau (see Fig. 10–2). A very long plateau is not beneficial. This valve also allows one to limit the peak pressure to reduce the likelihood of volutrauma or barotrauma.
4. Pressure gauge, to measure the applied airway pressures accurately. An adequate pressure monitor must be placed close to the endotracheal tube in order to measure correct peak inspiratory and positive end-expiratory pressures.
5. Alarms, to warn of inadvertent disconnections, pressure loss, high pressures, and failure of the ventilator to cycle at the proper time.
6. Humidification or nebulization, to saturate the inspired gases with water at 34°C to 37°C. The temperature of the inspired gas close to the endotracheal tube should be measured continuously and used to servo-control the humidification system.
7. Positive end-expiratory pressure (PEEP), to maintain functional residual capacity. It should be adjustable between 0 and 10 cm H_2O, although end-expiratory pressure of 3 to 6 cm H_2O is usually used in neonates.
8. Exhalation assist, to reduce the end-expiratory pressure to desired levels when rapid rates are used. Inadvertent PEEP can be a problem with some pediatric ventilators because of a high expiratory resistance.

◆ ALTERNATIVE MODES OF MECHANICAL VENTILATION

Technologic advances including improvement in flow delivery systems, breath termination criteria, guaranteed tidal volume delivery, stability of PEEP, air leak compensation, prevention of pressure overshoot, online pulmonary function monitoring, and triggering systems have resulted in better ventilators.[38] Patient-initiated mechanical ventilation, patient-triggered ventilation, and synchronized intermittent mandatory ventilation are increasingly being used in neonates.

1. *Patient-triggered ventilation.* Pressure-controlled conventional ventilation is the most commonly used mode of assisted ventilation in neonates. With pressure-controlled ventilation, the ventilator breath is time-triggered at a preset frequency, but the patient can take other spontaneous breaths. In contrast, patient-triggered ventilation (also called assist/ control) uses spontaneous respiratory efforts to trigger the ventilator. With pressure-triggered ventilation airflow, chest wall movements, airway pressure, and esophageal pressure are used as indicators of the onset of the inspiratory effort. Once the ventilator detects an inspiratory effort, it delivers a ventilator breath of predetermined settings (peak inspiratory pressure, inspiratory duration, flow). Although improved oxygenation has been observed, patient-triggered ventilation frequently may have to be discontinued in some very immature infants because of weak respiratory effort.[31] A backup rate may be used to reduce this problem.

2. *Synchronized intermittent mandatory ventilation.* This mode of ventilation achieves synchrony between the patient and the ventilator breaths. Synchrony easily occurs in most neonates because strong respiratory reflexes during early life elicit relaxation of respiratory muscles at the end of lung inflation. Furthermore, inspiratory efforts usually start when lung volume is decreased at the end of exhalation. Synchrony may be achieved by nearly matching the ventilator frequency to the spontaneous respiratory rate or by simply ventilating at relatively high rates (60 to 120 breaths/ min). Triggering systems can be used to achieve synchronization when synchrony does not occur with these maneuvers. Synchronized intermittent mandatory ventilation is as effective as conventional ventilation but no major benefits were observed in a large randomized, controlled trial.[5]

3. *Proportional assist ventilation.* Ventilators reduce work of breathing. Both modes of patient-initiated mechanical ventilation discussed earlier (patient-triggered ventilation, synchronized intermittent mandatory ventilation) are designed to synchronize the onset of the inspiratory support. In contrast, proportional assist ventilation matches the onset and duration of both inspiratory and expiratory support. Furthermore, ventilatory support is in proportion to the volume or flow of the spontaneous breath. Thus, the ventilator can selectively decrease the elastic or resistive work of breathing. The magnitude of the support can be adjusted depending on the patient's needs. When compared with conventional and patient-triggered ventilation, proportional assist ventilation reduces ventilatory pressures while maintaining or improving gas exchange.[36] Randomized clinical trials are needed to determine whether proportional assist ventilation leads to major benefits when compared with conventional mechanical ventilation.

4. *Tracheal gas insufflation.* The added dead space of the endotracheal tube and the ventilator adapter that connects to the endotracheal tube contributes to the anatomic dead space. With smaller infants and with increasing severity of pulmonary disease, this added dead space that does not participate in gas exchange becomes the largest proportion of tidal volume. Delivery of gas to the distal part of the endotracheal tube during exhalation (tracheal gas insufflation) washes out this dead space and the accompanying CO_2. Tracheal gas insufflation results in a decrease in $PaCO_2$ or peak inspiratory pressure.[13] If proven safe and effective, tracheal gas insufflation should be useful in reducing tidal volume and the accompanying volutrauma, particularly in very premature infants.

◆ CARBON DIOXIDE ELIMINATION

CO_2 elimination depends largely on the amount of gas that passes in and out of the alveoli (Fig. 10–4). The total amount of gas that passes in and out of the lungs (including alveoli and airways) is called *minute ventilation*. Minute ventilation may be calculated from the product of the tidal volume and respiratory frequency. Thus, increases in either tidal volume or frequency increase minute ventilation, increase CO_2 elimination, and decrease $PaCO_2$. Some of the tidal volume distributes to parts of the lungs

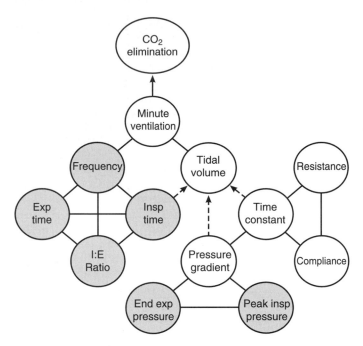

Figure 10–4. Determinants of CO_2 elimination during pressure-limited, time-cycled ventilation. Circles depicting ventilator-controlled variables are shaded. The relations between the circles that are joined by solid lines are described by simple mathematical equations. (Adapted from Chatburn RL, Lough MD: Mechanical ventilation. In Lough MD, Doerschuck C, Stern R, eds: Pediatric Respiratory Therapy. 3rd ed. Chicago: Year Book Medical Publishers, 1985, p 161.)

(dead space) that are not involved in gas exchange (e.g., airways).

Tidal volume may be increased by increasing the pressure gradient between inspiration and expiration. This may be accomplished by increasing peak inspiratory pressure or by decreasing PEEP. Tidal volume is usually independent of inspiratory and expiratory times. However, depending on the time constant of the respiratory system, very short inspiratory times may limit tidal volume delivery.[8, 37]

Frequency is the other major determinant of minute ventilation. In addition to the frequency set on the ventilator, the infant may take spontaneous breaths because neonatal ventilators provide a continuous flow of gas during the expiratory phase.

Hypercapnia can be caused by ventilation-perfusion ($\dot{V}/\dot{Q}$) mismatch or hypoventilation.[14] Optimal $\dot{V}/\dot{Q}$ matching occurs when the ratio of alveolar ventilation and alveolar perfusion is approximately one. $\dot{V}/\dot{Q}$ mismatch is probably the most important mechanism of gas-exchange impairment in infants with respiratory failure of various causes including RDS. Hypoventilation is another important cause of hypercapnia. Hypercapnia occurs when alveolar ventilation decreases. Hypercapnia caused by hypoventilation is easily managed with mechanical ventilation. Hypercapnia second-

ary to severe $\dot{V}/\dot{Q}$ mismatch may be difficult to manage with mechanical ventilation.

◆ OXYGENATION

In infants with RDS, oxygenation depends largely on the inspired oxygen concentration and the mean airway pressure (Fig. 10–5). Oxygenation increases linearly with increases in mean airway pressure, largely because functional residual capacity can be optimized with mean airway pressure adjustments.[8] Mean airway pressure is a measure of the average pressure to which the lungs are exposed during the respiratory cycle. Mean airway pressure may be calculated from the area under the curve divided by the duration of the cycle (Fig. 10–6). The equation is as follows:

Mean airway pressure =
$$\text{K (PIP} - \text{PEEP)} \frac{\text{(Ti)}}{\text{(Ti + Te)}} + \text{PEEP}$$

where K is a constant that depends on the rate of increase of the airway pressure curve, PIP is peak inspiratory pressure, PEEP is positive end-expiratory pressure, Ti is inspiratory time, and Te is expiratory time. Therefore, mean airway pressure is in-

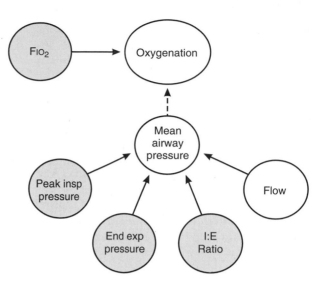

Figure 10–5. Determinants of oxygenation during pressure-limited, timed-cycle ventilation. Circles depicting ventilation-controlled variables are shaded. Solid lines represent mathematical relationships.

creased by increasing any of the following (see Fig. 10–6):

1. PEEP
2. Peak inspiratory pressure
3. Inspiratory to expiratory (I/E) ratio/inspiratory time
4. Rate
5. Inspiratory flow (increases K)

Although a direct relationship usually exists between mean airway pressure and oxygenation, there are several limitations:

1. For the same change in mean airway pressure, increases in peak inspiratory pressure and PEEP enhance oxygenation more than increases in I/E ratio.
2. Increases in PEEP are not as effective once an elevated level (more than 5 to 6 cm H_2O) is reached.

3. Very high mean airway pressure may cause lung overdistention, right-to-left shunting in the lungs (by redistribution of blood flow to poorly ventilated areas), or decreased cardiac output.
4. Long inspiratory times increase the risk for pneumothorax.

Hypoxemia can be due to $\dot{V}/\dot{Q}$ mismatch, shunting, diffusion abnormalities, and hypoventilation.[6] $\dot{V}/\dot{Q}$ mismatch is a major cause of hypoxemia in infants with RDS and in neonates with other causes of respiratory failure. In these patients, the alveoli are poorly ventilated relative to their perfusion. In neonates with persistent pulmonary hypertension or congenital cyanotic heart disease, shunting is the predominant mechanism that leads to hypoxemia. Diffusion abnormality, typical of interstitial lung disease and other diseases that affect the alveo-

INTERVENTIONS

1. Increase PEEP
2. Increase PIP
3. Increase I/E or T_I
4. Increase Rate
5. Increase Flow

Figure 10–6. Methods to increase airway pressure. PEEP, positive end expiratory pressure; PIP, peak inspiratory pressure; I/E, inspiratory-to-expiratory ratio; T_I, inspiratory time; T_E expiratory time.

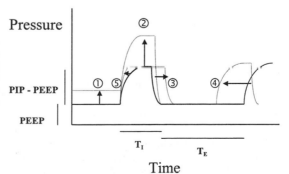

lar-capillary interface, is not prominent in neonates with RDS and does not cause severe hypoxemia. Hypoventilation usually causes mild hypoxemia unless severe hypercapnia ensues.

Unlike other causes of hypoxemia, shunting usually is unresponsive to oxygen supplementation and mechanical ventilation unless the shunt is reversed. Hypoxemia resulting from $\dot{V}/\dot{Q}$ mismatch can be difficult to manage, but may be resolved if an increase in airway pressure reexpands atelectatic alveoli. Hypoxemia caused by impaired diffusion or hypoventilation usually responds to oxygen supplementation and mechanical ventilation.

◆ LUNG INJURY AND GENTLE VENTILATION

Recently, emphasis has been placed on the possibility that lung injury is dependent on the ventilatory strategies used. In a consensus conference, experts concluded that mechanical ventilation might lead to many adverse consequences.[40] They recommended that clinicians should consider using more gentle ventilatory strategies in which gas trapping and alveolar overdistention are minimized while blood gas targets are modified to accept higher than "normal" Pa_{CO_2} and lower than "normal" Pa_{O_2}. Strategies that reduce volutrauma and lung overinflation such as decreased tidal volume, gentle ventilation, permissive hypercapnia, and optimization of conventional ventilation may reduce the risk of lung injury.[16, 26, 30, 46] Determination of the optimal ventilatory strategies is dependent on the pathophysiology of the respiratory disorder. Gentle ventilation has been suggested as a ventilatory strategy to optimize conventional mechanical ventilation. Nonetheless, the etiology of lung injury is known to be multifactorial and other risk factors appear to be the degree of prematurity (with its related pulmonary immaturity), the presence and severity of RDS, duration and intensity of oxygen supplementation and positive pressure mechanical ventilation, nutritional deficiency, patent ductus arteriosus, fluid overload, infection, and air leak.[1, 3, 12, 15]

◆ VENTILATOR SETTING CHANGES AND GAS EXCHANGE

From the earlier discussion, the effects of the changes in individual ventilator settings on blood gases can be extrapolated. The major effects are summarized in Table 10–4. Although effects may vary, and trial and error may be used at times, these basic principles should serve as guidelines. However, when faced with an abnormal blood gas result, several alternative ventilator setting changes may be acceptable. Controversy still exists as to the optimal way to ventilate infants. It is generally preferred to provide an adequate tidal volume and then adjust the frequency to achieve sufficient CO_2 elimination. Mean airway pressure can then be changed to optimize oxygenation. The use of very high frequencies in which short inspiratory time decreases tidal volume delivery or short expiratory time causes gas trapping and inadvertent PEEP is not advocated.

Thus, in summary, major concepts of gas exchange in infants with RDS are that CO_2 elimination is proportional to minute ventilation and that oxygenation is related directly to mean airway pressure. Based on these concepts, ventilatory strategies may be combined into a flow chart. This approach should provide an organized, logical, and consistent means of achieving desired blood gas results, supporting the clinician in the ventilator management decisions. Studies in neonates with RDS managed with such an algorithm revealed more frequent correction of blood gas derangements and more appropriate efforts to wean the infant from ventilatory assistance.[10]

◆ GENERAL CONSIDERATIONS

The respiratory pattern can be described by the duration of the inspiratory gas flow, the tidal volume, and the pressure required to produce them. They are interrelated:

Compliance = Δ Volume/Δ Pressure
Resistance = Δ Pressure/Δ Flow
Volume = Flow × Time

Pressure-controlled ventilators deliver a tidal volume by altering the pressure in the airway relative to atmospheric pressure. The respiratory cycle generated consists of four

Table 10–4. Effect of Ventilator Setting Changes on Blood Gases

	Change	$PaCO_2$	PaO_2	Comments
PIP	↑	↓	↑	Use of high PIP increases risk of barotrauma (e.g., pneumothorax, interstitial emphysema)
	↓	↑	↓	
PEEP	↑	↑	↑	Adequate PEEP prevents alveolar collapse and improves ventilation/perfusion relationship. A PEEP of 2 to 3 cm H_2O is physiologic.
	↓	↓	↓	High PEEP decreases compliance and may cause CO_2 retention. Very high PEEP (e.g., >6 cm H_2O) is not very effective in increasing PaO_2.
Frequency	↑	↓	—	High ventilator frequencies may allow the use of low PIP and reduce the risk of pneumothorax. If I/E ratio is kept constant, frequency changes do not alter mean airway pressure and do not substantially affect PaO_2.
	↓	↑	—	
I/E Ratio	↑	—	↑	I/E ratio changes do not usually alter tidal volume or CO_2 elimination unless inspiratory time or expiratory time, or both, are too short.
	↓	—	↓	
Flow	↑	± ↓	± ↑	The effects of flow changes on blood gases have not been well studied in infants.
	↓	± ↑	± ↓	

PIP, peak inspiratory pressure; PEEP, positive end-expiratory pressure; I/E ratio, inspiratory to expiratory ratio.

elements: inspiration, inflation hold, expiration, and the pressure at end-expiration.

Setting Up the Ventilator

It is essential that the clinician understand the circuit, the humidification system, the ventilator capabilities, and the ventilatory strategies that can be used to optimize ventilation. Before starting mechanical ventilation, the following steps should be taken:

1. Check that the circuit to be used is leak-proof. This may be done by cycling the ventilator with a finger over the patient outlet. At this time, set the pressure relief valve to the peak inspiratory pressure desired.
2. Ensure that the nebulization of inspired gas is adequate and that the heated nebulizer is functioning. Temperature gradients between the air outside the infant's incubator and inside the incubator tend to result in condensation of water in respirator tubing. This should be caught in a water trap. Excessive condensation suggests that the gas delivered may be losing too much water and may be insufficiently humidified. Keep the volume of tubing outside the incubator minimal. Heat the tubing to avoid condensation.
3. Understand the effect of every ventilator knob.
4. Select ventilator settings suitable for the patient. There are no absolute rules. Although there has been little assessment of the effect of altering ventilator settings on gas exchange, the following guidelines are generally useful.

Volume-Controlled Ventilator

The tidal volume delivered by the ventilator must be adequate to normalize arterial oxygen and carbon dioxide. Important considerations are as follows:

- Infant's tidal volume (4 to 8 mL/kg)
- Compression loss in the ventilator tubings (if ventilator tubing volume is large, this may be appreciable)
- Volume losses by leaks from the tubing system around the endotracheal tube

Pressure-Controlled Ventilator

The peak inspiratory pressure depends largely on the desired tidal volume and the compliance of the lungs. Suggested initial ventilator settings are as follows:

	Normal lungs	RDS lungs
PIP (cm H_2O)	12–10	20–25
PEEP (cm H_2O)	2–3	4–5
Rate (per min)	10–20	20–60
I/E ratio	1:2–1:10	1:1–1:3

Independent of the type of ventilator used, inspired oxygen should initially correspond to the oxygen necessary to maintain an adequate PaO_2 (50 to 70 mm Hg). Watch for an elevated PaO_2 after starting mechanical ventilation because effective mechanical ventilation may result in a sudden reduction in oxygen requirements.

COMMENT: It is important to consider the disease process when deciding on initial ventilator settings. If the disease process involves alveolar collapse (e.g., RDS), the need for higher PEEP should be anticipated. If airway disease and gas trapping are predominant (e.g., meconium aspiration syndrome), expiratory time should be long and PEEP kept relatively low. If pulmonary vascular resistance is high (e.g., persistent pulmonary hypertension of the newborn), high cycling frequencies may be required to achieve alkalosis and hence pulmonary vasodilation.

John Kattwinkel

Care of the Ventilator

After ventilator use, ensure the following:

1. Adequate sterilization (ideally by soaking detachable tubings in bactericidal solution or by gas sterilization of ventilator unit)
2. Maintenance by an experienced technician
3. Routine cultures to check sterilization and mode of storage

◆ MONITORING THE INFANT DURING MECHANICAL VENTILATION

During mechanical ventilation the clinician undertakes the responsibility for the infant's gas exchange. Hence, monitoring the patient's condition is vital and requires continuous observation. Frequent arterial blood gas estimations should be performed as follows:

- Within 20 minutes of initiating mechanical ventilation
- After 20 minutes of a major alteration of ventilator settings
- Immediately, if the infant's condition changes markedly
- Otherwise, every 4 to 8 hours during the acute stage

The goal should be to maintain PaO_2 between 50 and 70 mm Hg, $PaCO_2$ at more than

40 mm Hg, and pH between 7.25 and 7.40. Continuous monitoring with a pulse oximeter or transcutaneous PCO_2 and PO_2 electrodes or a catheter electrode is invaluable during intubation, stabilization procedures, or weaning, as oxygenation can worsen abruptly.

Changes in Blood Gas Status: A Practical Approach

1. *A sudden decrease in PaO_2 accompanied by an increase in $PaCO_2$ associated with rapid clinical deterioration of the infant.* To differentiate whether the problem is with the ventilator or the infant, disconnect the ventilator from the infant and manually inflate the infant's lungs.

   If the infant's condition improves, the problem is with the ventilator. Check the following:

   - Concentration of inspired oxygen going to the ventilator
   - Presence of leaks or disconnected tubing
   - Mechanical or electrical failure

   If the infant shows no clinical improvement with manual inflation, the problem is with the infant. Check gas entry bilaterally by auscultation, listen over the stomach, and determine the position of the heart and trachea. If gas entry is diminished bilaterally, look for the cause:

   - Tube displaced into nasopharynx. There may be gas entry heard over stomach, and gas may be visibly escaping at the mouth or via a nasogastric tube with the end placed under water. Action—Replace the tube.
   - Tube blocked. Tube blockage occurs especially after a few days of ventilation and afterward because of the increased accumulation of secretions. Action—Suction tube briefly. If this has no effect, replace the tube.
   - Tension pneumothorax. Diminished breath sounds are heard on the affected side and there may also be abdominal distention and an easily palpable liver and spleen; the condition is usually critical. Action—Emergency relief of tension pneumothorax by inserting a chest tube or a 22-gauge catheter

attached to a three-way stopcock and a 20-mL syringe into the third intercostal space at the midclavicular line or the fourth or fifth intercostal space at the anterior axillary line. Remove gas until the condition improves. Insert a chest tube and check its position with a chest radiograph.

If gas entry is diminished unilaterally, ascertain the cause:

◆ Tube in mainstem bronchus. It is usually in the right mainstem bronchus, producing decreased gas entry on the left. Action—Verify endotracheal tube measurement at the lip level. Withdraw tube 0.5 to 1 cm. Immediate improvement in gas entry will result. Recheck position by x-ray study.
◆ Unilateral pneumothorax. Radiologic confirmation of clinical diagnosis is obtained if the condition of the infant warrants a delay in initiating therapy. If not, treat as for tension pneumothorax.

If gas entry is not diminished and the infant does not improve with manual lung inflation, this suggests a nonrespiratory cause such as intraventricular hemorrhage, pneumopericardium, convulsions, hypoglycemia, hypotension, or overwhelming sepsis. The incidence of intraventricular hemorrhage is greatly increased in infants who have a pneumothorax. The occasional occurrence of pneumoperitoneum, as a result of forcing gas through the diaphragm in the periaortic spaces, can seriously mislead the clinician into the assumption that a ruptured viscus has occurred and abdominal surgery is indicated.

COMMENT: Airway sounds are easily transmitted across a small chest, and therefore evaluation of breath sounds can be terribly misleading in small infants. Even with "adequate" breath sounds I would transilluminate the chest, check the placement of the endotracheal tube with a laryngoscope, and perhaps replace the endotracheal tube before attributing the problem to a nonrespiratory etiology.

John Kattwinkel

2. *Gradual decrease in PaO$_2$ accompanied by an increase in PaCO$_2$ associated with gradual deterioration of the infant.* This suggests inappropriate ventilator set-

tings. A decrease in PaO$_2$ suggests increasing intrapulmonary shunting resulting from progressive atelectasis.

To improve PaO$_2$, consider the following measures:

◆ Increase peak inspiratory pressure (PIP)
◆ Increase PEEP
◆ Increase the I/E ratio or the inspiratory time

The responses to these maneuvers may vary, and blood gas analyses must be obtained.

3. *Gradual increase in PaCO$_2$ without gross changes in PaO$_2$.* A gradual increase in PaCO$_2$ is usually due to insufficient alveolar ventilation (insufficient tidal volume or frequency, or both). A gradual increase in PaCO$_2$ can also be due to increased "anatomic" (i.e., airways, tubing) or "physiologic" (i.e., nonventilated but perfused alveoli) dead space. An increase in PaCO$_2$ is an indication for an increase in alveolar ventilation by increasing PIP or decreasing PEEP during pressure-controlled ventilation, by increasing tidal volume during volume-controlled ventilation, or by increasing cycling frequency. A reduction of anatomic dead space (e.g., shortening the endotracheal tube) may relieve hypercapnia.

To improve PaCO$_2$, increase minute ventilation by the following measures:

◆ Increase PIP by 2 to 5 cm H$_2$O (pressure-cycled ventilator)
◆ Increase tidal volume by 1 to 2 mL/kg (hence increasing PIP; volume-cycled ventilator)
◆ Increase ventilator rate by 10 breaths/min

4. *A decrease in PaCO$_2$ caused by overventilation.* A decrease in PaCO$_2$ is potentially dangerous, because it produces a respiratory alkalosis and an elevation in pH. Alkalosis is associated with decreases in cardiac output, cerebral blood flow, and tissue oxygen delivery, especially if the infant is also hypotensive. The lungs may be subjected to volutrauma if the low PaCO$_2$ is the result of ventilation with large tidal volumes. Hence, a low PaCO$_2$ is an indication for a reduction in overall alveolar ventilation, preferably. The insertion of artificial dead space to increase

"dead space ventilation" is unnecessary and potentially harmful. It should always be possible to reduce total ventilation until $Paco_2$ returns to normal or the infant is extubated.

5. *Increase in Pao_2 unaccompanied by changes in $Paco_2$.* This suggests a decrease in intrapulmonary shunting and reduction in degree of atelectasis. Because of the toxic effect of high inspired oxygen on lung tissue but the benefits of maintaining lung inflation, it is generally better to reduce the concentration of inspired oxygen to less than 40% to 70% before attempting to markedly reduce ventilator parameters.

Routine Care of the Infant

Monitoring of blood gases and respiratory status represents only one aspect of supportive treatment. Due attention must also be paid to temperature control, caloric and fluid intake, and metabolic balance. Clinicians should avoid excessive and unnecessary handling of the infant.

◆ SPECIAL INSTANCES
Pulmonary Interstitial Emphysema

Infants with severe RDS and those who have pulmonary interstitial emphysema (PIE) on x-ray film may respond better to a rapid ventilating rate (60 to 150 breaths/min), low peak pressure, low PEEP, and high-frequency ventilation.

Pulmonary Hypertension/Meconium Aspiration Syndrome

Infants with severe pulmonary hypertension with or without meconium aspiration syndrome may benefit from inhaled nitric oxide, a selective pulmonary vasodilator. Nitric oxide reduces the need for extracorporeal membrane oxygenation (ECMO) in neonates with pulmonary hypertension.[33] Alkalosis appears to be of value in reducing the severe pulmonary vasoconstriction in these infants and may result in an increase in Pao_2. If hyperventilation is used, the pH and $Paco_2$ should be kept at 7.45 to 7.55 or higher and at 25 to 30 mm Hg, respectively.

High distending pressures (PIP 30 to 40 and PEEP 4 to 6 cm H_2O) and rapid ventilating rates (60 to 100/min) may be necessary. Other therapies used have included sedation, analgesia, paralysis, and inotropic support.[42]

Neonatal Surgery

Intubation of the very low-birth-weight infant in the intensive care nursery and use of a ventilator during surgery are preferable. In this way, inspired oxygen and inspired gas temperature can be carefully controlled. The anesthetic can be "bled" into the nebulizer in low concentrations. However, it may not be possible to ventilate patients adequately with a pressure-controlled ventilator during abdominal or thoracic surgery because they may not be able to compensate for the changes in lung and chest compliance that can occur. The only solution is to use a modified Ayres T-piece. Arterial blood gas analyses are done frequently throughout surgery to maintain the infant in acid-base balance and Pao_2 within normal limits. Oxygen saturation or transcutaneous Po_2 should be monitored continuously. The infant is slowly weaned after surgery (see Weaning from Ventilator).

Drug Therapy

The use of muscle paralysis with curare, pancuronium bromide (Pavulon), or metocurine may be invaluable in infants who "fight" the ventilator when $Paco_2$ is increasing and Pao_2 is decreasing on "maximum" ventilation. Curare may cause relaxation of the pulmonary vascular bed, resulting in increased oxygenation and improvement in gas exchange. A marked improvement in oxygenation may be observed, particularly in infants with pulmonary hypertension.

COMMENT: Muscle paralysis for babies on ventilators must be viewed with caution. The histamine-releasing effect of competitive neuromuscular blocking agents (particularly curare) can cause hypotension and, rarely, bronchospasm. Some patients may require higher ventilator settings after paralysis as their own respiratory efforts are eliminated. Also, a system failure (e.g., extubation, tubing disconnection) in a paralyzed patient will be rapidly fatal.

John Kattwinkel

Sedatives and analgesics are increasingly being used in the care of neonates requiring assisted ventilation. These agents may be used in combination with muscle paralysis. However, when it is desirable to preserve the patient's own respiratory effort, sedatives or analgesics may be used without muscle paralysis. Fentanyl and morphine sulfate are commonly used sedatives/analgesics. Sedatives and analgesics may decrease respiratory drive and should be used carefully.

Antibiotics should be used whenever a bacterial infection is suspected. A Wright stain for neutrophils and cultures of endotracheal tube secretions may be useful in recognizing superinfection. However, the appearance of neutrophils is also a sign of early bronchopulmonary dysplasia.

Preextubation systemic corticosteroids and postextubation racemic epinephrine reduce airway resistance when there is laryngeal edema. However, if the endotracheal tube is not too large, is well positioned, and is not mobile during ventilation, it is rare to have problems with the glottis following extubation.

Weaning from Ventilator

Ventilator weaning should be attempted when the concentration of inspired oxygen is 40% or less. The PIP is gradually reduced as is the ventilator rate to allow the patient to contribute more to his or her ventilation. When the ventilator breaths elicit minimal chest rise and the ventilator frequency is less than or around 10/min, the infant is placed in a concentration of oxygen 5% higher than that used during ventilation and is allowed to breathe spontaneously through the endotracheal tube at a CPAP level of 2 to 4 cm H_2O. The infant should not be stressed just before weaning. Extubation is done when CPAP has been reduced to 2 to 4 cm H_2O and the patient has been breathing spontaneously for 1 to 2 hours without clinically important changes in blood gases or clinical condition. After extubation, a brief period of manual inflation with a face mask or mask ventilation may be helpful.

Often, extremely low-birth-weight infants do not tolerate endotracheal CPAP because the resistance of the 2.5-mm tube is too high. They should be weaned to a low pressure around 12/2 cm H_2O (PIP/PEEP) and rates of less than 10 breaths per minute before extubation.

COMMENT: In my experience, babies can be weaned from the ventilator much sooner if they are placed on nasal CPAP rather than directly in an oxygen hood. The resistance to gas flow and therefore inhibition of spontaneous ventilation through a small endotracheal tube may be too great for some babies. Any baby with an endotracheal tube should be given at least 2 cm H_2O CPAP, since glottic closure and grunting are prohibited by the tube. In selected babies who are particularly difficult to wean (e.g., with bronchopulmonary dysplasia), administration of theophylline may help, perhaps by lessening diaphragmatic fatigue.

John Kattwinkel

EDITORIAL COMMENT: When weaning any infant from assisted ventilation—respirator, bagging, or CPAP—change one variable at a time and check blood gases. For example, do not reduce oxygen concentration and respirator pressure at the same time. Our practice is to reduce environmental oxygen until it is 40% and then reduce pressure.

◆ HIGH-FREQUENCY VENTILATION

Even though conventional mechanical ventilation has contributed to a substantial reduction in neonatal mortality, morbidity in the form of pulmonary air leaks and bronchopulmonary dysplasia (BPD) occurs in about 20% to 40% of ventilated infants. Although the precise pathophysiologic mechanisms underlying these forms of lung injury have not been determined, high ventilatory pressures and the resultant volutrauma are thought to be contributing factors.

High-frequency ventilation encompasses modes of assisted ventilation that employ smaller tidal volumes and higher frequencies than conventional techniques. Because of its potential to reduce volutrauma, there has been a surge of interest in high-frequency ventilation in the past few years. The characteristics of the various high-frequency ventilators overlap (Table 10–5). Furthermore, clinicians may employ widely varying ventilatory strategies. High-frequency ventilation may improve blood gases because, in addition to the gas transport by convection, other mechanisms may become active at high frequencies. For example, variable velocity profiles of gas during inspiration and exhalation, gas exchange between

Table 10–5. Techniques for High-Frequency Ventilation

	HFPPV	Jet Ventilation	Flow Interruption	Oscillatory Ventilation
Tidal volume	> Dead space	> or < Dead space	> or < Dead space	< Dead space
Expiration	Passive	Passive	Passive	Active
Airway pressure waveform	Variable	Triangular	Triangular	Sine wave
Frequency	60–150/min	60–600/min	300–900/min	300–900/min

HFPPV, high-frequency positive pressure ventilation; <, smaller; >, larger.

parallel lung units, increased turbulence, and diffusion may improve blood gases.

High-frequency positive-pressure ventilators employ standard ventilators modified with low-compliance tubing and connectors so that an adequate tidal volume may be delivered despite very short inspiratory times. High-frequency jet ventilation is characterized by the delivery of gases from a high-pressure source through a small-bore injector cannula. It is possible that the fast flows out of the cannula produce areas of relative negative pressure that entrain gases from their surroundings. High-frequency flow interruption also delivers small tidal volumes by interrupting a flow of pressure source, but in contrast to jet ventilation, it does not use an injector cannula. High-frequency oscillatory ventilation delivers very small volumes (even smaller than dead space) at extremely high frequencies. Oscillatory ventilation is unique because exhalation is actively generated, as opposed to other forms of high-frequency ventilation, in which exhalation is passive.

Respiratory Distress Syndrome

There has been extensive clinical use of the various high-frequency ventilators in neonates with RDS. Controlled trials with high-frequency positive pressure using rates of 60 breaths/min (versus 30 to 40 breaths/min for conventional mechanical ventilation) reported a decreased incidence of air leaks.[34, 35] Small randomized trials suggest that BPD may be prevented with high-frequency jet ventilation,[23] but results are inconclusive.[7, 22] The largest randomized trial of high-frequency ventilation revealed that early use of high-frequency oscillatory ventilation did not improve outcome.[20] Although various randomized, controlled trials show heterogeneous results, a meta-analysis confirms the original results.[19] However, there are trends toward decreases in BPD/chronic lung disease but increases in severe intraventricular hemorrhage and in periventricular leukomalacia as well as small increases in air leaks with high-frequency oscillatory ventilation or high-frequency flow interrupters.[19, 32, 41]

Air Leaks

In addition to the possible prevention of pneumothorax, high-frequency ventilation has been used to treat established air leaks. Use of jet ventilation in neonates with pulmonary interstitial emphysema may accelerate resolution of the air leak,[22] whereas in those with bronchopleural fistula, flow through the fistula may be decreased.[17] However, air leaks may be increased by oscillatory ventilation.[19, 20, 41]

Other Potential Uses

High-frequency oscillatory ventilation is a safe alternative for infants who fail conventional ventilation and are candidates for ECMO.[11] High-frequency oscillatory ventilation may increase the effectiveness of inhaled nitric oxide in these patients.[24] Neonates with impaired cardiac function may improve if the high ventilatory pressures are reduced with high-frequency ventilation.[43] Because of reduction of respiratory excursions, high-frequency ventilation may be beneficial in patients undergoing airway/thoracic surgery or bronchoscopy.

COMMENT: The technique of high-frequency ventilation requires major changes in the concept of gas flow in the lung. Currently it is believed that by vibrating the gas column, gas exchange is promoted by a process of facilitated diffusion rather than by convection, which is the predominant mechanism of conventional ventilation. Early studies suggest that high-frequency ventilation may improve ventilation/perfusion matching throughout the respiratory cycle, thus permitting lower peak inflation pressures and lower inspired oxygen concentrations. Both high pressure and high oxygen have been implicated in the development of bronchopulmonary dysplasia. Although high-frequency ventilation is an exciting new concept, technical problems (e.g., provision of adequate humidification) and physiologic questions (e.g., what is the effect of pulmonary and cerebral blood flow) remain. Many investigative studies are required before this technique is ready for widespread use.

John Kattwinkel

◆ COMPLICATIONS OF ASSISTED VENTILATION

Despite major improvements in equipment and increased expertise in the applications of assisted ventilation, the care of smaller and sicker infants has maintained a high rate of complications (Table 10–6). Pulmonary air leaks are one of the most common complications and occur in approximately 25% of ventilated patients. Pneumothorax may result from the use of high peak inspiratory pressure and inspiratory time, particularly in infants who "fight" the ventilator. However, spontaneous pneumothoraces are commonly observed, even in healthy neonates. Transillumination of the chest is extremely useful for immediate diagnosis, but radiographic confirmation should be obtained if the patient's status is not life threatening. PIE, usually secondary to the use of high airway pressures, is associated with gas trapping and impaired gas exchange.

BPD, a form of chronic lung disease that occurs in neonates, is one of the most important complications associated with assisted ventilation. Although its precise pathophysiology remains obscure, volutrauma appears to be important. The increasing incidence of BPD is largely due to improving survival rate of small immature infants. The incidence of BPD varies widely and may be as high as 50% in infants weighing less than 1500 g who require assisted ventilation from birth. Management of these patients must be multidimensional, with particular emphasis on prevention of further lung injury, maintenance of adequate oxygenation and nutrition, and prevention of bronchospasm, infection, and fluid overload. Comparison of the incidence of BPD in eight centers in North America suggests that optimal respiratory management of very low-birth-weight infants may decrease the incidence of BPD.[2] Evaluation of this hypothesis awaits confirmation in clinical trials.

Liquid Ventilation

Various fluids have been used to transport gases as an alternative to gas ventilation. Perflubron liquids, which dissolve large quantities of respiratory gases, have been extensively used in immature animals.[45] In these studies liquid ventilation resulted in improved gas exchange and higher lung compliance. Immature animals unable to survive with gas ventilation have maintained appropriate gas exchange using liquid ventilation. Small clinical studies that demonstrate improved gas exchange are encouraging,[27] but large clinical trials are required to determine safety and efficacy.

◆ EXTRACORPOREAL MEMBRANE OXYGENATION

ECMO is a technique that allows drainage of blood from the patient followed by the

Table 10–6. Complications of Assisted Ventilation

Pulmonary air leaks	Pneumothorax, pneumomediastinum, pneumoperitoneum, pulmonary interstitial emphysema, pneumopericardium, pulmonary venous air embolism
Airway injury	Erosion, granuloma, palatal groove, subglottic stenosis, necrotizing tracheobronchitis
Endotracheal tube related	Dislodgement, extubation, atelectasis, occlusion, tracheal stenosis, vocal cord paralysis
Infection	Pneumonia, septicemia, meningitis
Miscellaneous	Volutrauma, bronchopulmonary dysplasia, hyperinflation, impaired cardiac output, intracranial hemorrhage, patent ductus arteriosus, retinopathy of prematurity

passage of this blood through a membrane for extracorporeal exchange of oxygen and carbon dioxide. ECMO is particularly useful in neonates with transient pulmonary artery hypertension and severe hypoxemia resulting from a right-to-left blood shunt. Common conditions associated with pulmonary hypertension include meconium aspiration syndrome, RDS, idiopathic pulmonary hypertension of the neonate, pneumonia/sepsis, asphyxia, and congenital diaphragmatic hernia. Neonates with these and other conditions are considered candidates for ECMO if they have severe impairment of oxygenation. The alveolar to arterial oxygen gradient (A-aDo$_2$) is frequently used to evaluate impairment of oxygenation. An alveolar-arterial oxygenation gradient of 600 to 620 for 8 to 12 hours despite maximal therapy is usually considered to be an indication for ECMO. In the past, predicted survival rate for infants with such severe respiratory failure was as low as 20%. In marked contrast to the poor outcome that predated ECMO, survival currently approximates 85% in these infants.[21]

Complications during ECMO may be related to the primary disease or to technical aspects of the circuit. Intracranial hemorrhage and infarction, hemodynamic alterations, and hematologic disturbances occur occasionally. The improved survival rate has not been accompanied by an increase in permanent morbidity.

Inhaled Nitric Oxide

High pulmonary artery resistance is common in infants with pulmonary disease. Pulmonary artery vasodilators have been used in treatment of these infants, but the systemic vasodilatory effects have precluded efficacy and widespread use. Nitric oxide, an endogenous gas in the lungs, regulates pulmonary artery tone in utero and after birth. Exogenous nitric oxide reduces pulmonary vascular resistance during the perinatal period. Inhaled nitric oxide has been shown to improve oxygenation and reduce the need for ECMO in well-designed, large, randomized, controlled trials[14, 25, 33, 44] in neonates with severe hypoxemic respiratory failure.

◆ SUMMARY

Survival of very low-birth-weight infants has dramatically improved with the intro-

duction of techniques of assisted ventilation. Meticulous care is necessary with the following: strategies to optimize conventional ventilation; placement of endotracheal tubes; frequent blood gas determinations; continuous monitoring of oxygen saturation, transcutaneous Po$_2$, and transcutaneous Pco$_2$; and, fluid, caloric, and thermal balance. However, most of the difficulty with adequately ventilating small infants resides not in the ventilator, but in the infant's lungs and airways. The clinician should identify and correct atelectasis, increased dead space, and gas trapping. He or she should look for a way to correct the patient's pulmonary problems rather than look for a better ventilator. Long-term morbidity associated with mechanical ventilation is still a major problem. Assisted ventilation is a critical part of neonatal intensive care. A thorough understanding of pulmonary mechanics and gas exchange as well as knowledge of the techniques and alternative modes of ventilation are essential to optimize their use.

◆ QUESTIONS
True or False

◆ *If you set a pressure-limited safety valve on a volume-controlled ventilator at 30 cm H$_2$O, a pneumothorax will not occur.*
Although pneumothorax is particularly associated with high inflation pressures, it can occur at any time during either mechanical or spontaneous ventilation. Therefore, the statement is false.

◆ *The larger the volume of ventilator tubings, the less the compression volume at any given pressure.*
During ventilation, a proportion of the gas delivered by the pump ("compression volume") does not reach the alveoli. The larger the volume of ventilator tubings, the greater the compression volume. Hence, ventilator tubings should be low volume and nondistensible. The statement is false.

◆ *Condensation of water in ventilator inspiratory tubings can be reduced by placing as much tubing as possible inside the incubator.*
A temperature gradient exists between air outside and inside the incubator. Water vapor condenses at lower temperatures, and droplets appear in tubing exposed to low temperatures. If water condensation occurs in the tubing, the gas delivered to the infant

will have a water saturation lower than gas coming out of the humidifier. Therefore the statement is true.

◆ *If a small leak develops between the trachea and the endotracheal tube during pressure-controlled ventilation, there will be adequate compensation by the ventilator.*

A pressure-controlled ventilator delivers gas until a preset pressure is attained. Hence, it is possible to compensate for a small leak (e.g., around the endotracheal tube); a large leak may cause failure to reach the desired peak inspiratory pressure. Therefore the statement is true.

◆ *During mechanical ventilation with 80% oxygen (for RDS), an increase in peak inspiratory pressure may increase the PaO_2 by 200 mm Hg without altering $PaCO_2$ significantly.*

When breathing a high concentration of oxygen, a low PaO_2 indicates venous admixture or shunting. This shunting is thought to occur primarily through areas of atelectatic lung. Effective ventilation may open some of these atelectatic areas, reducing the degree of shunting, with an ensuing increase in PaO_2. However, a large right-to-left shunt may not increase $PaCO_2$ markedly because the arteriovenous difference for CO_2 is only 4 mm Hg. Therefore, resolution of the shunt may not decrease $PaCO_2$, so the statement is true.

◆ *During mechanical ventilation, pH remains constant as long as the $PaCO_2$ does not change.*

The pH depends on both the $PaCO_2$ and the bicarbonate level. Metabolic and respiratory factors are often closely associated (e.g., a period of apnea is associated with both an increase in $PaCO_2$ and a decrease in PaO_2, the latter leading to tissue anoxia and anaerobic metabolism). However, they may operate quite independently. Therefore the statement is false.

CASE PROBLEMS

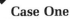

Case One

Before mechanical ventilation using a pressure-limited ventilator, the PaO_2 is 30 mm Hg and the $PaCO_2$ is 60 mm Hg in 100% oxygen. Thirty minutes after initiating therapy, a blood gas analysis is performed.

◆ *PaO_2 has risen to only 35 mm Hg, and $PaCO_2$ is still 60 mm Hg. It is advisable to switch to a volume-controlled ventilator, because the lungs are too stiff to be adequately ventilated by a pressure-controlled machine. True or false?*

The statement is false. The initial ventilator settings were probably somewhat subjective

and should now be adjusted to the infant's requirements. The high PCO_2 indicates hypoventilation, and an attempt should be made to increase minute ventilation by increasing PIP. The increase in PIP should also improve oxygenation. If oxygenation is unresponsive, PaO_2 can be increased by raising end-expiratory pressure 1 or 2 cm H_2O or by increasing inspiratory time. Adjustments should be made every 10 minutes, checking blood gases until PaO_2 is higher than 50 mm Hg and $PaCO_2$ is less than 50 mm Hg.

◆ *PaO_2 is only 35 mm Hg and $PaCO_2$ is 35 mm Hg. It might be helpful to try adding positive end-expiratory pressure before increasing PIP further. True or false?*

A positive expiratory pressure of 5 to 6 cm H_2O will help to prevent small airway closure. This may prevent atelectasis and hence reduce the degree of right-to-left shunt. Therefore the statement is true.

◆ *The PaO_2 has risen to 140 mm Hg. This is a dangerous level, and the concentrations of inspired oxygen should be reduced at once. True or false?*

In immature infants, arterial oxygen tensions in that range have been associated with retinopathy of prematurity. The high inspired oxygen concentration can damage the lungs. Therefore, the statement is true. Priority should be given to reducing the concentration of inspired oxygen in this situation rather than altering other ventilator settings. We decrease environmental oxygen 5% to 10% every 10 to 15 minutes and perform continuous or intermittent blood gas measurement after each change.

COMMENT: A decrease of 5% to 10% every 10 to 15 minutes may be too fast or too slow. A pulse oximeter or transcutaneous oxygen monitor can be very useful for titrating the appropriate FIO_2 to PaO_2. A blood gas determination should then be made once the continuous monitor shows that a steady state has been reached.

John Kattwinkel

Case Two

A blood gas analysis is performed during mechanical ventilation in 80% oxygen. There has been no change in the clinical condition of the infant since the previous estimation.

◆ *It is found that $PaCO_2$ has changed from 36 to 24 mm Hg and pH has risen from 7.38 to 7.56. This is a sign that the infant is recovering and ventilator settings should remain unchanged. True or false?*

A $PaCO_2$ of 24 mm Hg suggests overventilation. The resulting alkalosis is dangerous, because it causes a reduction in cerebral blood flow and may be associated with lung injury. The Pa_{CO_2} should be brought back to a more physiologic range by reducing minute ventilation (i.e., by reducing peak inspiratory pressure, tidal volume, or cycling frequency). The statement is therefore false.

◆ *The arterial oxygen tension is 39 mm Hg, pH is 7.36, and Pa_{CO_2} is 35 mm Hg. The ventilator should not be changed. True or false?*

Pa_{CO_2} and pH are satisfactory, but oxygenation is unsatisfactory. PEEP can be increased to increase mean airway pressure. The statement is false.

◆ *The arterial oxygen tension is 46 mm Hg, pH is 7.30, and Pa_{CO_2} is 26 mm Hg on low ventilator settings. Although the pH is within normal range, there is metabolic acidosis, which should be corrected with intravenous sodium bicarbonate. True or false?*

Spontaneous hyperventilation on the ventilator may be due to compensation for a metabolic acidosis. Correction of metabolic acidosis is indicated with intravenous bicarbonate. Therefore, the statement is true. A search should be made for the etiology of the acidosis, such as reduced cardiac output, patent ductus arteriosus, or pneumothorax. FI_{O_2} should also be increased.

◆

Case Three

During mechanical ventilation, an infant becomes cyanotic. He is noted to be making very vigorous respiratory efforts with considerable intercostal and sternal retractions out of phase with the ventilator.

◆ *This is a good indication for sedation and attempting to adjust the ventilator to accommodate the infant's respiratory pattern. True or false?*

Although "out of phase" respiration could account for this clinical picture, an obstructed airway must first be excluded. Vigorous respiratory efforts with cyanosis suggest an obstructed endotracheal tube. Therefore, the statement is false.

◆ *Gas entry is diminished over the left lung field. The diagnosis is pneumothorax, which should be relieved immediately. True or false?*

Diminution of gas entry over the left lung field may be due to (1) the endotracheal tube slipping into the right mainstem bronchus or (2) pneumothorax. The steps should be to check the endotracheal tube length of insertion (at the lip) and, if necessary, to withdraw the endotracheal tube slightly. If this fails to improve the infant's condition, a chest x-ray film is indicated unless the infant is deteriorating rapidly and the left side of the chest is tympanic, transillumination is positive, and the heart is displaced. Emergency relief of a pneumothorax is then indicated. Therefore the statement is false.

◆ *A blood sample for gas estimation is obtained immediately and resuscitative measures started. When the blood sample is analyzed 1 hour later, the results show Pa_{O_2} to be 127 mm Hg and Pa_{CO_2} to be 8 mm Hg. This suggests that the infant had been crying before this cyanotic spell. True or false?*

The most likely explanation for these bizarre blood gas findings is that an air bubble was left in the syringe and equilibration has occurred between gas in the blood and gas in the air. The values tend to approximate the Pa_{O_2} and Pa_{CO_2} of room air. (Samples drawn for blood gases must be bubble free, capped, iced, and analyzed immediately.) The statement is false.

◆ *Following prolonged mechanical ventilation and extubation, an infant may have some stridor and copious secretions. The stridor usually decreases spontaneously. True or false?*

Despite the use of nontoxic nasotracheal tubes, there can be some laryngeal edema. This, together with large quantities of secretions and lack of tracheal cilia, may lead to some degree of upper airway obstruction, which decreases in 2 to 3 days. Therefore, the statement is true.

◆

Case Four

A 1500-g male infant delivered after 31 weeks' gestation had signs of respiratory distress at birth. Apgar scores were 4 and 7 at 1 and 5 minutes, respectively. Analysis of amniotic fluid revealed a lecithin/sphingomyelin (L/S) ratio of 1.5:1 with no phosphatidylglycerol present. At initial assessment, the infant was tachypneic (60 breaths/min) and had nasal flaring and retractions. Breath sounds were equal but diminished bilaterally. Dubowitz examination was consistent with maternal dates. Immediate chest x-ray film showed diffuse granularity and air bronchograms. Blood sugar was 45 mg/dL, hematocrit 43%, blood pressure 50/32 (mean 40 mm Hg), and temperature 36.3°C. In 35% oxygen by hood, arterial blood gas values from umbilical catheter were as follows: pH 7.15, PCO_2 55, and PO_2 80. The infant was intubated, given surfactant, and placed on a pressure-limited ventilator at peak inspiratory pressure (PIP) of 22 cm H_2O, positive end-expiratory pressure (PEEP) of 4 cm H_2O, frequency (rate) of 20 breaths/min, I/E ratio of 1:3, and FI_{O_2} of 35%. The patient initially responded well, but 2 hours later arterial blood *gas values were as follows: pH 7.40, P_{CO_2} 36, and P_{O_2} 35.*

NOTE: There may be several arterial blood gases and ventilator changes between each situation presented. Assume good breath sounds, chest rise, and blood pressure throughout, unless otherwise stated. Attempting to answer questions by looking at data subsequently presented is only confusing.

Select the **best** answer, although more than one answer may be acceptable.

◆ *What is the most appropriate ventilator setting change at this time?*
  1. Increase PIP
  2. Increase PEEP
  3. Increase frequency
  4. Decrease I/E ratio (e.g., 1:3 to 1:3.5)
  5. Increase F_{IO_2}

The patient has hypoxemia with adequate ventilation and relatively low F_{IO_2}. Therefore the best answer is to increase F_{IO_2}.

◆ *At 12 hours of age, the ventilator settings and blood gas values are pressure 26/4 cm H_2O, frequency 25 breaths/min, I/E ratio 1:3.5, F_{IO_2} 80%, pH 7.16, P_{CO_2} 55 mm Hg, and P_{O_2} 135 mm Hg. What is the most appropriate change at this time?*
  1. Decrease PIP and decrease F_{IO_2}
  2. Increase PEEP and decrease F_{IO_2}
  3. Increase frequency and decrease F_{IO_2}
  4. Increase I/E ratio and decrease F_{IO_2}
  5. Decrease I/E ratio and decrease F_{IO_2}

The patient has hyperoxemia and mild respiratory acidosis. Of the alternatives given, increasing frequency is the most effective way to increase minute ventilation and resolve the respiratory acidosis. F_{IO_2} should be decreased.

◆ *At 18 hours of age, the ventilator settings and blood gas values are pressure 28/4 cm H_2O, frequency 60 breaths/min, I/E ratio 1:1.5, F_{IO_2} 90%, pH 7.19, P_{CO_2} 52 mm Hg, and P_{O_2} 50 mm Hg. What is the most appropriate change at this time?*
  1. Increase PIP
  2. Increase PEEP
  3. Increase frequency
  4. Increase I/E ratio
  5. Increase F_{IO_2}

Respiratory acidosis is still present but is now accompanied by hypoxemia. Increasing peak PIP is the best choice because the resultant increase in minute ventilation and mean airway pressure should improve Pa_{CO_2} and Pa_{O_2}. Increasing frequency is also an acceptable alternative.

REFERENCES

1. Abman SH, Groothuis JR: Pathophysiology and treatment of bronchopulmonary dysplasia. Pediatr Clin North Am 41:277, 1994.
2. Avery ME, Tooley WH, Keller JB, et al: Is chronic lung disease in low birth weight infants preventable? A survey of eight centers. Pediatrics 74:26, 1987.
3. Bancalari E: Pathogenesis of BPD. An Overview. In Bancalari E, Stocker JT, eds: Bronchopulmonary Dysplasia. Washington, DC: Hemisphere Publishing, 1988, p 3.
4. Bancalari E, Sinclair JC: Mechanical Ventilation. In Sinclair JC, Bracken MD, eds: Effective Care of the Newborn Infant. New York: Oxford University Press, 1992.
5. Bernstein G, Mannino FL, Heldt GP, et al: Randomized multicenter trial comparing synchronized and conventional intermittent mandatory ventilation in neonates. J Pediatr 128:453, 1996.
6. Boynton BR, Hammond MD: Pulmonary Gas Exchange: Basic principles and the effects of mechanical ventilation. In Boynton BR, Carlo WA, eds: New Therapies for Neonatal Respiratory Failure: A Physiological Approach. New York: Cambridge University Press, 1994.
7. Carlo WA, Chatburn RL, Martin RJ: Randomized trial of high frequency jet ventilation versus conventional ventilation in respiratory distress syndrome. J Pediatr 110:275, 1987.
8. Carlo WA, Greenough A, Chatburn RL: Advances in Conventional Mechanical Ventilation. In Boynton BR, Carlo WA, eds: New Therapies for Neonatal Respiratory Failure: A Physiological Approach. New York: Cambridge University Press, 1994.
9. Carlo WA, Martin RJ: Principles of neonatal assisted ventilation. In Polin RA, Fox WW, eds: The Newborn I. Pediatr Clin North Am 33:221, 1986.
10. Carlo WA, Pacifico L, Chatburn RL, et al: Efficacy of computer-assisted management of respiratory failure in neonates. Pediatrics 78:139, 1986.
11. Clark RH, Dykes FD, Bachman TE, et al: Intraventricular hemorrhage and high-frequency ventilation: A meta-analysis of prospective clinical trials. Pediatrics 98:1058, 1996.
12. Cotton RB: Contribution of the patent ductus arteriosus to lung injury. In Merrit TA, Northway WH, Boynton BR, eds: Bronchopulmonary Dysplasia. Boston: Blackwell Scientific, 1988, p 235.
13. Danan C, Dassieu G, Janaud J-C, et al: Efficacy of dead-space washout in mechanically ventilated premature newborns. Am J Respir Crit Care Med 153:1571, 1996.
14. Davidson D, Barefield ES, Kattwinkel J, et al: Inhaled nitric oxide for the early treatment of persistent pulmonary hypertension of the term newborn: A randomized, double-masked, placebo-controlled, dose-response, multicenter study. Pediatrics 101:325, 1997.
15. DeLemos RA, Coalson JJ: The contribution of experimental models to our understanding of the pathogenesis and treatment of bronchopulmonary dysplasia. Clin Perinatol 19:521, 1992.
16. Garland JS, Buck RK, Allred EN, et al: Hypocarbia before surfactant therapy appears to increase bronchopulmonary dysplasia risk in infants with respiratory distress syndrome. Arch Pediatr Adolesc Med 149:617, 1995.

17. Gonzalez F, Harris T, Black P, et al: Decreased gas flow through pneumothoraces in neonates receiving high-frequency jet versus conventional ventilation. J Pediatr 110:464, 1987.
18. Gregory GA, Kitterman JA, Phibbs RH, et al: Treatment of the idiopathic respiratory distress syndrome with continuous positive airway pressure. N Engl J Med 284:1333, 1971.
19. Henderson-Smart DJ, Bhuta T, Cools F, et al: Elective high frequency oscillatory ventilation vs conventional ventilation in preterm infants with acute pulmonary dysfunction. Cochrane Collaboration, http://silk.nih.gov/SILK/COCHRANE/COCHRANE.htm, 1998.
20. The HIFI Study Group: High-frequency oscillatory ventilation compared with conventional ventilation in the treatment of respiratory failure in preterm infants. N Engl J Med 320:88, 1989.
21. Ichiba S, Bartlett RH: Current status of extracorporeal membrane oxygenation for severe respiratory failure. Artif Organs 20:120, 1996.
22. Keszler M, Donn SM, Bucciarelli RL, et al: Multicenter controlled trial comparing high-frequency jet ventilation and conventional mechanical ventilation in newborn infants with pulmonary interstitial emphysema. J Pediatr 119:85, 1991.
23. Keszler M, Modanlou HD, Brudnos DS, et al: Multicenter controlled clinical trial of high-frequency jet ventilation in preterm infants with uncomplicated respiratory distress syndrome. Pediatrics 100:593, 1997,
24. Kinsella JP, Truog WE, Walsh WF, et al: Randomized, multicenter trial of inhaled nitric oxide and high-frequency oscillatory ventilation in severe, persistent pulmonary hypertension of the newborn. J Pediatr 131:55, 1997.
25. Kinsella JP, Truog WE, Walsh WF, et al: Randomized, multicenter trial of inhaled nitric oxide and high-frequency oscillatory ventilation in severe, persistent pulmonary hypertension of the newborn. J Pediatr 131:55, 1997.
26. Kraybill EN, Runyun DK, Bose CL, et al: Risk factors for chronic lung disease in infants with birth weights of 751 to 1000 grams. J Pediatr 115:115, 1989.
27. Leach CL, Greenspan JS, Rubenstein SD, et al: Partial liquid ventilation with perflubron in premature infants with severe respiratory distress syndrome. N Engl J Med 335:761, 1996.
28. Lough MD, Carlo WA: Clinical care techniques. In Carlo WA, Chatburn RL, eds: Neonatal Respiratory Care. Chicago: Year Book Medical Publishers, 1988.
29. Mammel MC, Bing DR: Mechanical ventilation of the newborn: An overview. Clin Chest Med 17:603, 1996.
30. Mariani G, Cifuentes J, Carlo WA: Randomized controlled trial of permissive hypercapnia in preterm infants. A pilot study. Pediatr Res 41:163A, 1997.
31. Mitchell A, Greenough A, Hird M: Limitations of patient-triggered ventilation in neonates. Arch Dis Child 64:924, 1989.
32. Moriette G, Walti H, Salanave B, et al: Prospective randomized multicenter comparison of high-frequency oscillatory ventilation (HFOV) and conventional ventilation (CV) in preterm infants < 30 weeks gestational age (GA) with RDS. Pediatr Res 45:1247, 1998.
33. The Neonatal Inhaled Nitric Oxide Study Group: Inhaled nitric oxide in full-term and nearly full-term infants with hypoxic respiratory failure. N Engl J Med 336:597, 1997.
34. Oxford Region Controlled Trial of Artificial Ventilation (OCTAVE) Study Group: Multicenter randomized controlled trial of high against low frequency positive pressure ventilation. Arch Dis Child 66:770, 1991.
35. Pohlandt F, Saule H, Schroder H, et al: Decreased incidence of extra-alveolar air leakage or death prior to air leakage in high versus low rate positive pressure ventilation: Results of a randomized seven-center trial in preterm infants. Eur J Pediatr 151:905, 1992.
36. Schulze A, Gerhardt T, Musante G, et al: Proportional assist ventilation (PAV): A new strategy for mechanical ventilation in low birth weight infants. Pediatr Res 41:1038, 1997.
37. Simbruner G, Gregory GA: Performance of neonatal ventilators: The effects of changes in resistance and compliance. Crit Care Med 9:509, 1981.
38. Sinha SK, Donn SM: Advances in neonatal conventional ventilation. Arch Dis Child 75:F135, 1996.
39. Sinha SK, Donn SM, Gavey J, et al: Randomized trial of volume controlled versus time cycled, pressure limited ventilation in preterm infants with respiratory distress syndrome. Arch Dis Child 77:F202, 1997.
40. Slutsky AS: Mechanical ventilation. ACCP consensus conference. Chest 104:1833, 1993.
41. Thome U, Kossel H, Lipowsky G, et al: Randomized comparison of high frequency ventilation with high rate intermittent positive pressure ventilation in preterm infants with respiratory failure. J Pediatr 35:39, 1999.
42. Walsh-Sukys MC, Cornell DJ, Houston LN, et al: Treatment of persistent pulmonary hypertension of the newborn without hyperventilation: An assessment of diffusion of innovation. Pediatrics 94:303, 1994.
43. Weiner JH, Chatburn RL, Carlo WA: Ventilatory and hemodynamic effects of high-frequency jet ventilation following cardiac surgery. Respir Care 32:332, 1987.
44. Wessel DL, Adatia I, Van Marter LJ, et al: Improved oxygenation in a randomized trial of inhaled nitric oxide for persistent pulmonary hypertension of the newborn (abstract). Pediatrics Electronic Pages, www.pediatrics.org. 1999.
45. Wolfson MR, Greenspan JS, Shaffer TH: Liquid-assisted ventilation: An alternative respiratory modality. Pediatr Pulmonol 26:420, 1998.
46. Wung JT, James LS, Kilchevsky E, et al: Management of infants with severe respiratory failure and persistence of the fetal circulation, without hyperventilation. Pediatrics 76:488, 1985.

Problems in Metabolic Adaptation: Glucose, Calcium, and Magnesium

Robert M. Kliegman

These infants are remarkable not only because like foetal versions of Shadrach, Meshach and Abednego, they emerge at least alive from within the fiery metabolic furnace of diabetes mellitus, but because they resemble one another so closely that they might well be related. They are plump, sleek, liberally coated with vernix caseosa, full-faced and plethoric. . . . They convey a distinct impression of having had such a surfeit of both food and fluid pressed upon them by an insistent hostess that they desire only peace so that they may recover from their excesses. And on the second day their resentment of the slightest noise improves the analogy while their trembling anxiety seems to speak of intrauterine indiscretions of which we know nothing.

James W. Farquhar*

The newborn emerges from a uterine environment where glucose, calcium, and magnesium have been continuously provided and fetal plasma levels are closely regulated, in part by maternal metabolic homeostasis, placental exchange, as well as fetal regulatory mechanisms. Abrupt termination of supply at birth requires profound changes in energy and mineral metabolism, depending on the provision of exogenous nutrients and the mobilization of endogenous fuel and mineral stores. The result is the potential for rapid changes in plasma glucose and calcium during the first days of life. The infant who is premature, growth retarded, stressed, or born to a diabetic mother is at increased risk for problems with homeostasis, and hypoglycemia or hypocalcemia can develop.

Broad surveys with modern analytic methods have demonstrated that glucose and calcium problems are common, frequently asymptomatic, and thus often unrecognized in high-risk infants. Subsequently, changing routines of care, with prevention, early identification, and metabolic support of the sick newborn have made severe hypoglycemia and hypocalcemia infrequent problems.

---

*Farquhar JW: The child of the diabetic woman. Arch Dis Child 34:76, 1959.

◆ GLUCOSE

Fetal and Neonatal Energy Metabolism[2, 3, 11, 24, 27, 36, 55]

A composite picture of fetal and neonatal fuel metabolism has emerged from studies in animals[3] and humans. Fetal energy consumption is high, deriving from growth needs and energy storage as well as metabolic maintenance. The fetus receives energy continuously as glucose, lactate, free fatty acids, ketones, and surplus amino acids. Hepatic gluconeogenesis from lactate may occur in utero and is certainly active at birth. Gluconeogenesis from alanine has been reported shortly after birth. Neither fatty acids nor ketones supply significant energy in utero in normal states of maternal nutrition. Essential fatty acids are predominantly used for tissue growth.

COMMENT: In isolated, perfused placentae, differential transfer of free fatty acids has been noted. Short-chain free fatty acids are transferred 1000 times more rapidly than palmitic acid. Thus mother contributes few long-chain fatty acids to the embryo.

Cynthia Bearer

Energy is stored rapidly near term. Fat storage exceeds 100 calories/d in the ninth month. Glycogen stores, a vital source of energy in the first hours of life, increase toward term to reach about 5% by weight in liver and muscle and up to 4% in heart muscle. These energy stores are compromised by prematurity and by intrauterine growth retardation (IUGR). Acute perinatal distress or chronic fetal hypoxia can particularly diminish glycogen stores and predispose the infant to hypoglycemia after birth.

Insulin appears in the fetal pancreas and plasma by 12 weeks' gestation. There is a poor insulin response to glucose infusion very early in gestation and a blunted response near term. Insulin does not usually cross the placenta unless it is bound to antibodies in diabetic mothers.

In the normal fetus, insulin is permissive in the accumulation of hepatic glycogen stores. The presence of maternal hyperglycemia and fetal hyperinsulinemia as seen in the infant of a diabetic mother (IDM) is associated with macrosomia and elevated liver glycogen and total body fat stores. Macrosomia in the presence of fetal hyperinsulinemia without maternal hyperglycemia is seen with Beckwith-Wiedemann syndrome and in the rare infant with hyperinsulinemic hypoglycemia (nesidioblastosis), suggesting that fetal insulin and *not maternal hyperglycemia* may be the important growth-promoting factor. Furthermore, infants born with pancreatic aplasia and those with transient neonatal diabetes mellitus have little or no insulin present and demonstrate severe IUGR, suggesting that insulin is an important hormone for fetal growth.

COMMENT: Insulin is one of a family of homologous hormones that includes insulin-like growth factor I (IGF-I) and insulin-like growth factor II (IGF-II). IGF-I is also called somatomedin-C and is a primary regulator of growth hormone. For example, the difference between standard and miniature poodles is the amount of IGF-I produced. IGF-II binds to the cation-independent mannose-6-phosphate receptor. High levels of IGF-II are found in fetal rats, but the role of IGF-II is unclear.

Cynthia Bearer

At birth, cold stress, work of respiration, and muscle activity all cause increased energy demands. The newborn must call on stored fuels to maintain blood glucose levels.

The first response is rapid glycogenolysis; hepatic glycogen falls to low levels within 24 hours. Because the newborn has a two-fold greater basal fasting glucose utilization than the adult, gluconeogenesis must supplement glycogenolysis. Lipolysis begins at birth, and plasma free fatty acids treble, subsequently remaining high. The respiratory quotient then decreases to less than 0.8 during the first day as most tissues switch to burning fat. High growth hormone, glucagon, and catecholamine levels may help fat mobilization and gluconeogenesis. Metabolism of free fatty acids and ketones stabilizes blood glucose levels by (1) sparing glucose utilization in heart, liver, muscle, and brain (ketones) and (2) supporting hepatic gluconeogenesis by producing NADH.

COMMENT: Glucose is taken up into cells by molecules called glucose transporters. Some tissues have insulin-dependent glucose transporters. The transporter molecules are moved to the cell surface in response to insulin. The glucose transporters in the brain are insulin independent. Therefore glucose uptake of the brain is a function of the glucose concentration of the blood.

Cynthia Bearer

The brain requires continued glucose supply. Hepatic glucose production in fasted healthy newborns is 4 mg/kg/min. The additional energy to support oxygen consumption comes from fat metabolism. Brain metabolism may be supported only in part by the oxidation of ketones and lactate.

Blood glucose at birth, transported across the placenta by facilitative diffusion, is 60% to 70% of the simultaneous maternal level. Glucose then normally decreases over 1 to 2 hours, stabilizes at a minimum of 40 to 45 mg/dL, and increases by 6 hours at 50 to 60 mg/dL in healthy unstressed newborns (Fig. 11–1). The current practice of early oral or intravenous (IV) alimentation avoids the many instances of neonatal hypoglycemia previously reported when neonates fasted for 24 hours (Fig. 11–2).

COMMENT: Healthy newborns are well equipped to stabilize their blood glucose concentration. Remember the infants in Mexico City who survived 6 days while buried in rubble following an earthquake.

Cynthia Bearer

Methodology—A Few Pitfalls
Sampling Problems

Capillary samples from unwarmed heels may lead to underestimation of venous glu-

FUEL METABOLISM IN INFANTS OF "CONTROLLED" DIABETIC MOTHERS

Figure 11–1. Glucose, free fatty acids (FFA), β-hydroxybutyrate (βOHB) in normal infants (o---o) and infants of diabetic mothers (IDM) (•—•). Note that not only does blood glucose decline more abruptly in the IDM, but FFA and ketones increase less. With more time, the blood glucose spontaneously increases over the next 4 to 6 hours. (From Persson B, Gentz J, Kellum M, et al: Metabolic observations in infants of strictly controlled diabetic mothers. II. Plasma insulin, FFA, glycerol, betahydroxybutyrate during intravenous glucose tolerance test. Acta Paediatr Scand 65:1, 1976.)

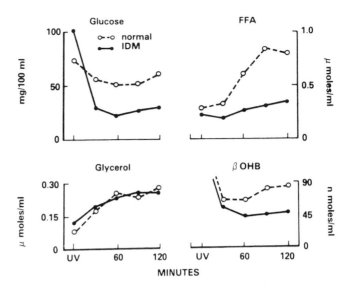

cose because of stasis. Glucose level declines as much as 18 mg/dL/h at room temperature while awaiting analysis. Thus, all samples should be immediately placed on ice. Plasma glucose exceeds whole blood glucose by 15%, more when hematocrit is very high.

Dextrostix

Used with the Eyetone Reflectance Meter, Dextrostix achieves a generally satisfactory precision for *screening* and following newborn glucose levels, *if* they are fresh, the instrument properly functioning and calibrated, the blood spot generous, and the operator experienced and careful. Used otherwise, Dextrostix can give disastrous false reassurance. At least one or two laboratory glucose determinations should be done to confirm any established glucose problem.

COMMENT: Certainly, clinical suspicion should make one wary of an unexpected normal Dex-

Figure 11–2. Plot of mean blood glucose as a function of age in both intravenous and fasted groups. Bars indicate range of 1 standard deviation. (From Mamunes P, Baden M, Bass J, et al: Early intravenous feeding of low birth weight neonate. Pediatrics 43:241–250, 1969. Reproduced by permission of Pediatrics. Copyright 1969.)

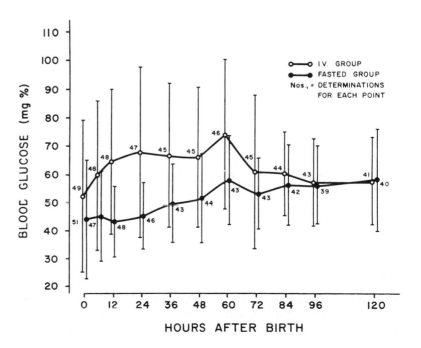

trostix value. One's clinical judgment should be used rather than relying on a single test result.

Cynthia Bearer

Hypoglycemia[2, 10, 27, 30, 45, 55, 68]

Definition

Prior definitions of hypoglycemia were population-based statistical values rather than functional values and resulted in very low cutoff levels of blood glucose: 20 and 30 mg/dL for preterm and term infants, respectively. Current recommendations are based in part on statistical analysis of ranges of blood glucose levels *and* adverse neurodevelopmental outcomes caused by hypoglycemia of infants with varying blood glucose levels.[10, 28, 33] Blood glucose levels should be maintained at more than 40 mg/dL in infants of all ages. The risk of hypoglycemia-induced neurodevelopmental sequelae may be related to the duration and the depth of the blood glucose level. Nonetheless, all blood glucose levels less than 40 mg/dL require treatment. Furthermore, compatible manifestations, relieved by glucose administration at blood glucose levels of more than 40 mg/dL, should also be considered as caused by hypoglycemia.

EDITORIAL COMMENT: In a position paper on the definition of hypoglycemia, Cornblath and associates commented, "The definition of clinically significant hypoglycemia remains one of the most confused and contentious issues in contemporary neonatology." They commented further, "Significant hypoglycemia is not and can never be defined by a number that can be applied universally to every individual patient . . . . It can be defined as the concentration of glucose in the blood or plasma at which the individual demonstrates a unique response to the abnormal milieu caused by inadequate delivery of glucose to a target organ (for example the brain). At present, no simple bedside measures exist that can determine these values and hence provide an absolute indication for an intervention in any individual patient." Hence, clinicians should be alerted to neonates at risk and intervene if the plasma glucose remains below 36 mg/dL (2.0 mmol/L).

◆————

Cornblath M, Hawdon JM, Williams AF, et al: Controversies regarding definition of neonatal hypoglycemia: Suggested operational thresholds. Pediatrics 105:1141, 2000.

Symptoms

Hypoglycemia in newborns is often asymptomatic but can cause jitteriness, convul- sions, apathy, hypotonia, coma, refusal to suck, apnea, congestive heart failure, cyanosis, high-pitched cry, abnormal eye movements, or temperature instability with hypothermia. In small sick infants, symptoms may easily be missed (Table 11–1).

Many newborns with one or more of these symptoms are normoglycemic and have another problem (Table 11–2). Hypoglycemia must therefore always be confirmed chemically and by response to treatment.

Transient Neonatal Hypoglycemia[2, 10, 27, 55]

Transient neonatal hypoglycemia is the most common type of hypoglycemia in a well baby nursery and an intensive care nursery. It occurs in low-birth-weight infants, particularly in those with IUGR. Males are more susceptible. The smaller of discordant twins is frequently affected. Maternal preeclampsia, perinatal asphyxia, hypothermia, and respiratory distress all increase the incidence. It may occur early, within 1 to 2 hours of birth, or classically later between the second and fourth day of life. Asymptomatic patients exceed those with symptoms by about 10 to 1.

The pathogenesis involves multiple factors affecting glucose supply and demand: low total body energy reserves; high energy requirement—particularly a large, glucose-requiring brain; and inordinate energy demands imposed by disease. There is an association with central nervous system (CNS) injury or anomaly, which may reflect a subtle control problem (see Table 11–1).

Table 11–1. Neonatal Symptomatic Hypoglycemia in 56 Infants

Clinical Manifestations	No.	Presenting Sign
Tremors ("jitteriness")	42	20
Cyanosis	43	19
Convulsions	29	9
Apnea, irregular respiration	23	6
Apathy	16	2
Cry—high pitched or weak	10	1
Limpness	13	4
Refusal to eat	5	1
Eye rolling	2	2

Age of Onset (h)

<6	6–24	24–48	48–72	>72
8	6	18	18	6

From Cornblath M, Pildes R, Schwartz R, et al: Hypoglycemia in infancy and childhood. J Pediatr 83:692, 1973.

Table 11–2. Differential Diagnosis in Neonates with Episodes of Tremors, Cyanosis, Convulsions, Apnea, Irregular Respiration, Apathy, High-Pitched or Weak Cry, Limpness, Refusal to Feed, Eye Rolling

Central nervous system
  Congenital defects
  Hypoxic-ischemic encephalopathy
  Meningitis-encephalitis
  Bilirubin encephalopathy—kernicterus
Sepsis
Heart disease
  Congenital
  Acquired
  Arrhythmias
Iatrogenic
  Drugs to mother or infant; withdrawal
  Overheating
Adrenal hemorrhage
Congenital adrenal hyperplasia
Polycythemia
Metabolic
  Hypocalcemia
  Hyponatremia
  Hypernatremia
  Pyridoxine dependency
  Magnesium deficiency
  Hyperammonemias
  Organic acidemias
Neonatal symptomatic hypoglycemia

From Cornblath M, Pildes R, Schwartz R, et al: Hypoglycemia in infancy and childhood. J Pediatr 83:692, 1973.

Hypoglycemia should be *anticipated* and is preventable in this large group of infants, which includes all admissions to the intensive care nursery. Providing caloric support with early feeding or IV glucose by 1 to 2 hours of age and maintaining continuous energy supply through the neonatal period dramatically reduce the incidence of hypoglycemia. Such support should provide, at a minimum, glucose at rates normally generated by the liver of a healthy newborn: 4 to 8 mg/kg/min. Therapeutic measures that reduce energy needs also help. These include a neutral thermal environment and reduction of evaporative heat loss.

With such support, hypoglycemia is uncommon, but high-risk infants should still be screened for hypoglycemia at intervals of 1 to 2 hours initially and then 2 to 4 hours until their condition is definitely stabilized.

Hyperinsulinemic Hypoglycemia

Infants of Diabetic Mothers[1, 6, 9, 11, 14–16, 25, 26, 39, 42–44, 51–54, 56, 65]

Hypoglycemia occurs regularly in infants of diabetic mothers soon after birth, with the nadir at 1 to 2 hours of age being as low as 10 mg/dL (see Fig. 11–1). Spontaneous increase in glucose usually follows, reaching acceptable levels by 4 to 6 hours of age. Few IDMs become symptomatic. Infants of gestational diabetic mothers have a less dramatic decline in glucose.

Fluctuating maternal hyperglycemia results in fetal hyperglycemia, pancreatic β-cell hyperplasia, and hyperinsulinism. After birth, hyperinsulinemia persists, as evidenced by accelerated use of exogenous glucose and diminished endogenous glucose production. Furthermore, free fatty acids and ketones are low (see Fig. 11–1).

Careful metabolic control of pregnant diabetic women during pregnancy and prevention of hyperglycemia in labor ameliorates excess fetal weight and helps prevent perinatal deaths and reduces the incidence of neonatal hypoglycemia. Early oral feeding is both prophylactic and therapeutic. Poor feeding, respiratory distress, or additional problems (congenital anomalies) may require IV glucose.

Additional problems of the IDM are listed in Table 11–3.

Other Syndromes[10, 45, 47, 48, 62]
(Table 11–4)

Erythroblastosis

Infants with erythroblastosis show islet cell hyperplasia, increased cord blood insulin, and hypoglycemia both shortly after birth and reactively following exchange transfusion. The severity of the problem relates inversely to cord hemoglobin level.

COMMENT: It is thought that reduced glutathione released from massive hemolysis of red cells stimulates insulin production with resultant hypoglycemia.

Cynthia Bearer

Familial and Nonfamilial Hyperinsulinemic Hypoglycemia (Nesidioblastosis)[2, 13, 30, 41, 67–69]

Hypoglycemia tends to be profound, symptomatic, unremitting, resistant to medical management, and best handled by surgical removal of most or all abnormal islet tissue. Hyperinsulinemia may be temporarily managed with diazoxide or the long-acting somatostatin analog octreotide. Hyperinsulinemia may be difficult to document. Plasma ketones, free fatty acids, branch-chain amino acids, and the insulin/glucose ratio may help establish the diagnosis.

Table 11–3. Pathophysiology of Morbidity and Mortality of IDM

Problem	Pathophysiology
Fetal demise	Acute placental failure?
	Hyperglycemia—lactic acidosis—hypoxia?
Macrosomia	Hyperinsulinism
Respiratory distress syndrome	Insulin antagonism of cortisol
	Variant surfactant biochemical pathways
Wet lung syndrome	Cesarean delivery
Hypoglycemia	↓ Glucose and fat mobilization
Polycythemia	Erythropoietic "macrosomia"
	Mild fetal hypoxia?
	↓ O_2 delivery to fetus—HbA_{1c}?
Hypocalcemia	↓ Neonatal parathyroid hormone
	↑ Calcitonin?
	↓ Magnesium
Hyperbilirubinemia	↑ Erythropoietic mass
	↑ Bilirubin production
	Immature hepatic conjugation?
	Oxytocin induction
Congenital malformations (central nervous system, heart, skeletal)	Hyperglycemia
	Genetic linkage?
	Insulin as teratogen?
	Vascular accident?
Renal vein thrombosis	Polycythemia
	Dehydration
Neonatal small left colon syndrome	Immature gastrointestinal motility?
Cardiomyopathy	Reversible septal hypertrophy
	↑ Glycogen
	↑ Muscle?
Family psychologic stress	High-risk pregnancy
	Fear of diabetes in infant
Subsequent development of insulin-dependent diabetes	Genetic HLA markers; risk is greater for infant of diabetic father (type I diabetes)

Adapted from Kliegman RM, Fanaroff AA: Developmental metabolism and nutrition. In Gregory GA, ed: Pediatric Anesthesiology. New York: Churchill Livingstone, 1983.

Familial hyperinsulinemic hypoglycemia (nesidioblastosis) may be an autosomal recessive disease characterized by excessive fetal growth and severe neonatal hypoglycemia. This severe form is due to defects in either of the two components of the islet β-cell K_{ATP} channel (either the sulfonylurea receptor or the Kir6.2 inward rectifier K^+ channel). A milder autosomal dominant form with delayed onset has an unknown etiology. Familial or sporadic hyperammonemic hyperinsulinemia is due to a mutation of the glutamate dehydrogenase gene (increased glutamate oxidation in the β-cell releases insulin). Activating mutations of the glucokinase gene may also produce hyperinsulinemic hypoglycemia.

Beckwith-Wiedemann Syndrome (Hyperplastic Fetal Visceromegaly)

Beckwith-Wiedemann syndrome (BWS) is an overgrowth syndrome associated with macrosomia, macroglossia, abdominal wall defects, usually an omphalocele, hypoglycemia in the neonatal period, and embryonal cancers of infancy and early childhood. The frequency of hypoglycemia in BWS is between 30% and 50%. The hypoglycemia may be asymptomatic and usually resolves within the first 3 days of life. Less than 5% will have hypoglycemia beyond the neonatal period requiring either continuous feeding or rarely partial pancreatectomy. Hyperinsulinemia has been implicated as the cause of hypoglycemia. The genes associated with BWS and the genotype of persistent hyperinsulinemic hypoglycemia of childhood are both in the 11p15 region, which may provide a molecular basis for hypoglycemia in BWS, particularly for the occasional patients with hypoglycemia requiring a partial pancreatectomy.[12]

Maternal Drugs (e.g., β-Sympathomimetics, β-Blockers, Chlorpropamide)

In chlorpropamide treatment, hypoglycemia may be prolonged for days; exchange transfusion may be helpful.

Table 11–4. Classification of Neonatal Hypoglycemia

Neonatal-Transient Hypoglycemia

Associated with inadequate substrate or enzyme function	Associated with hyperinsulinemia
Prematurity	Infants of diabetic mothers
Asphyxia	Infants with erythroblastosis fetalis
Small for gestational age	Infants with intrauterine growth retardation
Smaller of twins	Infants with improper position of umbilical artery catheter infusions
Infants with severe respiratory distress	Infants exposed to maternal β-mimetic agents
Infant of toxemic mother	Infants exposed to maternal oral hypoglycemic agents

Neonatal-Infantile Persistent Hypoglycemia

Hyperinsulinemic states	Other enzyme defects
Familial hyperinsulinemia	Galactosemia; galactose-1-phosphate uridyl transferase deficiency
Hyperammonemic hyperinsulinism	Fructose intolerance; fructose-1-phosphate aldolase deficiency
β-Cell adenoma	Disorders of fat (alternate fuel) metabolism
Leucine sensitivity	Primary carnitine deficiency
Beckwith-Wiedemann syndrome	Secondary carnitine deficiency
Hormone deficiency	Carnitine palmitoyl transferase deficiency
Panhypopituitarism	Long-, medium-, short-chain fatty acid acyl-CoA dehydrogenase deficiency
Isolated growth hormone deficiency	Amino acid and organic acid disorders
Adrenocorticotropic hormone deficiency	Maple syrup urine disease
Adrenal insufficiency	Propionic acidemia
Glucagon deficiency	Methylmalonic acidemia
Epinephrine deficiency	Tyrosinosis
Glycogen storage disease	Glutaric aciduria
Glucose-6-phosphatase deficiency	3-Hydroxy-3-methylglutaric aciduria
Amylo-1, 6-glucosidase deficiency	Systemic disorders
Liver phosphorylase deficiency	Sepsis
Glycogen synthetase deficiency	Hepatic failure
Disorders of gluconeogenesis	Heart failure
Hyperglycinemia	Hyperviscosity-polycythemia
Fructose-1, 6-diphosphatase deficiency	
Pyruvate carboxylase deficiency	
Phosphoenolpyruvate carboxykinase deficiency	

Modified from Sperling M, Chernausek S: Endocrine disorders. In Behrman R, Kliegman R, eds: Nelson Essentials of Pediatrics. Philadelphia, WB Saunders, 1990.

Hyperviscosity

An increased rate of glucose disposal without hyperinsulinemia is part of the syndrome of hyperviscosity; it responds to exchange transfusion to reduce hematocrit.

Failure of Glycogen Storage or Release, Gluconeogenic Blocks, Galactose or Fructose Intolerance, Carnitine Deficiency, Fatty Acid Oxidation Defects, Congenital Heart Disease, and Endocrine Deficiencies

These disorders are all very rare. Clues to the diagnosis include lactic acidosis, excessive or reduced ketonuria, persistent emesis and coma despite correction of hypoglycemia, hepatomegaly, family history, and elevated liver function tests (e.g., ammonia, direct bilirubin). Medium chain acyldehydrogenase deficiency, a cause of hypoglyce-mia in toddlers, has been reported in neonates.

Infusion of glucose through an incorrectly placed umbilical artery catheter located near T11–12 may produce hyperinsulinemic hypoglycemia. In addition, some hypoglycemic infants with IUGR demonstrate transient mild to moderate hyperinsulinemia.

COMMENT: One should also consider "mechanical" errors such as infiltrated IV site, malfunctioning IV pump, or incorrectly calculated dextrose concentration or infusion rate when considering unexplained hypoglycemia.

Cynthia Bearer

Treatment of Hypoglycemia[2, 11, 13, 31, 33]

Prophylactic care (to be instituted as soon as an infant is determined "at risk") consists of early oral or enteral tube breast milk or formula feeding if appropriate or 10% dex-

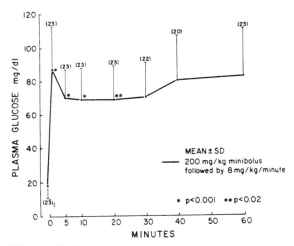

Figure 11-3. Minibolus therapy of neonatal hypoglycemia achieves euglycemia without excessively high glucose levels, which may further stimulate insulin release and later result in rebound hypoglycemia. (From Lilien L, Pildes R, Srinivasan G, et al: Treatment of neonatal hypoglycemia with minibolus and intravenous glucose infusion. J Pediatr 97:295, 1980.)

trose and water IV, 70 to 80 mL/kg in the first 24 hours increasing to 100 to 120 ml/kg/24 h thereafter (4 to 5 mg, increasing glucose to 7 to 8 mg/kg/min). Glucose infusion should be continuous and steady, by pump, and continued until replaced calorically by enteral feeding.

Treatment is indicated for all hypoglycemic infants. Asymptomatic infants with transient hypoglycemia and *no* other medical illness may be given enteric formula or breast milk. Blood glucose should be monitored every 30 minutes to determine a response. If glucose measurement does not increase or if enteric alimentation is contraindicated, IV glucose, 4 to 8 mg/kg/min, should begin. If symptoms other than seizures are present, a "minibolus" of 2 mL/kg (4 mL/kg for seizures) of $D_{10}W$ should be infused to prevent excessive hyperglycemia and rebound hypoglycemia (Fig. 11-3). This should be followed by 8 mg/kg/min of glucose together with vigilant blood glucose monitoring. The minibolus and infusion should be adequate for almost all infants. However, on rare occasions refractory hypoglycemia may require as much as 20 mg/kg/min in addition to hydrocortisone, 10 mg/kg/d in two divided doses. More severely ill patients may require diazoxide, nifedipine, or somatostatin plus glucagon replacement to alleviate hyperinsulinemic hypoglycemia.

Additional Management

- ◆ Reduce energy needs: for example, correct acidosis, place infant in neutral thermal environment.
- ◆ Monitor treatment at least every half hour until the infant's condition is stable.
- ◆ Titrate glucose infusion. Consider sepsis. Avoid iatrogenic hyperinsulinism from umbilical arterial glucose infusion into the pancreatic artery and rebound hypoglycemia following rapid IV boluses of hypertonic glucose.

COMMENT: The use of a constant infusion pump is extremely efficacious. If hypoglycemia persists, check pump function and IV site infiltration, and recheck calculations before considering further therapy.

Cynthia Bearer

COMMENT: My bias is that it is relatively easy to maintain normoglycemia with early intervention. When an infant of a diabetic mother has serum glucose concentrations that fall below 40 mg/dL, early institution of constant glucose infusion of 4 to 8 mg/kg/min is very effective. If the serum glucose is not raised in 30 minutes with 4 mg/kg/min, the dose is raised to 6 mg/kg/min; if that does not increase the serum glucose in another 30 minutes, it can be raised to 8 mg/kg/min. It is rare, with this management, to need any "bolus" glucose infusions or other therapeutic agents. Prevention or early intervention appears to be the key in this equation.

Reginald Tsang

Prognosis

Symptomatic and prolonged or recurrent hypoglycemia causes specific CNS damage. It commonly occurs in sick small infants with other factors affecting outcome, such as anoxia or severe intrauterine malnutrition. Infants with hypoglycemia with seizures have the poorest outcome.

Survivors of symptomatic neonatal hypoglycemia have shown a 30% to 50% incidence of neurologic impairment and a 10% incidence of recurrent hypoglycemia. Infants with asymptomatic hypoglycemia do well. Infants with hyperinsulinemic hypoglycemia or with inborn metabolic errors have a prognosis related to their primary illness.

Prompt diagnosis and treatment of hypoglycemia should prevent CNS injury from this cause.

Hyperglycemia[17, 38]

Hyperglycemia (glucose greater than 150 mg/dL) is a common, serious, iatrogenic problem of very immature infants receiving IV support. One cause appears to be the reduced insulin secretion to glucose characteristic of extreme immaturity. Hepatic glucose release also may fail to decrease when exogenous glucose is given. Most affected infants are also stressed by respiratory, infectious, or other metabolic problems. Thus, catecholamines may further elevate glucose levels and inhibit glucose use and insulin release. In anticipating hyperglycemia, four factors are paramount.

1. Immaturity: infant almost always less than 30 weeks' gestation and 1.0 kg birth weight
2. Age: usually less than 3 days, most often 1 day
3. Glucose infusion rates: exceed 8 mg/kg/min (equivalent to 10% glucose at 100 mg/kg/24 h)
4. Septicemia: bacterial and fungal

Hyperglycemia can cause at least two serious secondary problems. Osmotic changes (glucose 450 mg/dL equivalent to an additional 24 mOsm/L) can cause brain volume change because of fluid shifts and may cause intraventricular hemorrhage. Glycosuria may increase renal water and electrolyte losses.

Treatment and prevention are effected by adjusting the glucose infusion rate to that tolerated by each individual infant. Rates of 4 to 8 mg/kg/min, previously suggested, are *usually* tolerated. D_5W may be needed. Occasionally, insulin infusion of 0.001 to 0.01 U/kg/min is indicated. Monitoring (Dextrostix, urine glucose) is crucial.

COMMENT: It is important to stress the use of glucose calculations expressed as mg/kg/min, since variations in either volume or sugar content result in variations in actual delivery of glucose to the infant. Many iatrogenic effects of hyperglycemia and hypoglycemia in small infants have been caused by alterations in fluid volume delivery or glucose content without realizing the impact on actual glucose delivery to the infant.

To use $D_{2\frac{1}{2}}W$, one has to be very careful about osmolarity, since this solution is hypoosmolar and newborn red cells may be more fragile and susceptible to hemolysis. Use of this solution therefore requires the use of concomitant saline correction for osmolar defects. Because of concern for hypo-osmolar hemolysis, I prefer to avoid the use of this solution and either reduce the volume of delivery or, in unusual circumstances of intractable hyperglycemia, institute concomitant insulin infusion. However, with infusion rates described above and careful monitoring of serum glucose measurements, fortunately the incidence of hyperglycemia is markedly reduced.

Reginald Tsang

Transient Neonatal Diabetes[17, 38]

Transient neonatal diabetes is a rare disorder. Most infants are at or near term, with marked intrauterine malnutrition. Weight loss, dehydration, hyperglycemia, and occasional ketosis appear at a few days of age. Treatment is with insulin, with a usual daily dose of 2 to 6 units. The diabetic state resolves in a few days to weeks, glucose metabolism is subsequently normal, and prognosis is good.

EDITORIAL COMMENT: Transient neonatal diabetes (TND) is a rare type of diabetes that presents soon after birth, resolves by 18 months, and predisposes to diabetes later in life. An abnormality of chromosome 6 can be identified in approximately 70% of sporadic TND cases and in all familial cases. Genotypically they include paternal uniparental isodisomy of chromosome 6 or duplication involving chromosome band 6q24. Most patients are severely small for gestational age at birth, and present within a few days of birth and recover within three months. However they may develop diabetes later in life.

◆————

Temple IK, Gardner RJ, Mackay DJ, et al: Transient neonatal diabetes: Widening the understanding of the etiopathogenesis of diabetes. Diabetes 49:1359, 2000.

◆ CALCIUM

Fetal and Neonatal Calcium Metabolism[20–22, 35, 46, 57]

The placenta actively transports calcium to the fetus and maintains fetal total and ionized calcium levels about 1 mg/dL above the respective maternal levels. Between 28 weeks' gestation and term, fetal weight triples, but calcium content quadruples as bone mineral density progressively increases (Fig. 11–4). Fetal acquisition of calcium averages 150 mg/kg/d throughout this period.

Placental active transport allows fetal bone calcification to proceed normally. The calcium drain causes a modest decrease in maternal calcium levels near term. Maternal parathyroid activity, 1,25-dihydroxyvitamin D, calcium absorption, and calcium mobilization from bone are all increased. Parathyroid hormone and calcitonin do not cross the placenta, whereas 25-hydroxyvitamin D does.

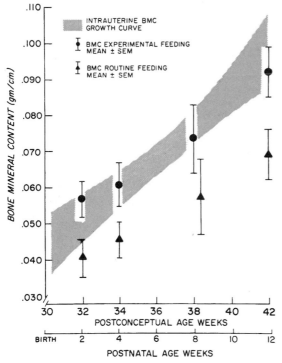

Figure 11–4. Hatched area is in utero rate of bone mineral content, depicting progressive bone mineralization during gestation until term. The triangles represent premature infants fed Similac 20 who have diminished bone mineral accumulation in contrast to infants (circles) fed formula with calcium (1260 mg/L), phosphorus (630 mg/L), and vitamin D (1000 U/L) who have intrauterine rates of bone mineralization. These latter infants received calcium, 220 to 250 mg/kg/d, and phosphorus, 110 to 125 mg/kg/d. The calcium intake exceeds the in utero rate of calcium accumulation (150 mg/kg/d), possibly as a result of fecal losses. (From Steichen J, Gratton T, Tsang R, et al: Osteopenia of prematurity: The cause and possible treatment. J Pediatr 96:528–534, 1980.)

At birth, the constant calcium supply is interrupted. Although the premature baby has skeletal reserves of calcium, the maintenance of serum calcium requires rapid changes in endocrine function and in the equilibrium between serum and bone. The factors affecting calcium in the neonate can be summarized as follows:

1. Parathyroid hormone mobilizes calcium from bone, promotes calcium absorption from the gut, and increases renal phosphate excretion. Levels are low in cord blood, suppressed by the mild hypercalcemia caused by placental transport. Postnatally, even with hypocalcemia as a stimulus, parathyroid hormone remains low for the first 2 days and for longer in premature infants. Parathyroid response usually becomes effective by about 3 to 4 days. Parathyroid secretion and function require magnesium.
2. Vitamin D is required for effective parathyroid hormone action on both bone and gut. Newborn stores are usually adequate, unless there is significant maternal dietary inadequacy. Levels of 25-hydroxyvitamin D vary directly with gestational age, and conversion of 25-hydroxyvitamin D to 1,25-dihydroxyvitamin D may be slow in premature infants.
3. Calcitonin inhibits calcium mobilization from bone. Levels are high in neonates and are further elevated by asphyxia and prematurity.
4. Serum phosphate increases after birth, even more so after birth asphyxia.
5. "Stress" factors introduced by perinatal illness are discussed later in relation to early neonatal hypocalcemia.

EDITORIAL COMMENT: The human calcium-sensing receptor (CaSR) is a 1078-amino-acid cell surface protein which is expressed in the parathyroid glands, thyroid gland, and kidney and is a member of the family of G protein-coupled receptors. The CaSR allows regulation of parathyroid hormone (PTH) secretion and renal tubular calcium reabsorption in response to alterations in extracellular calcium concentrations. The human CaSR gene is located on chromosome 3q13.3-q21, and loss of function CaSR mutations have been reported in the hypercalcemic disorders of familial benign (hypocalciuric) hypercalcaemia (FBH) and neonatal severe primary hyperparathyroidism. In addition, gain of function CaSR mutations have been observed in a novel familial syndrome of hypocalcemia with hypercalciuria. The human CaSR gene on chromosome 3q13.3-q21 is likely to be one of several, as two other loci for FBH have been located on chromosome 19p and 19q13. Cloning and characterization of these genes will help to further elucidate the mechanisms regulating extracellular calcium.

◆───

Thakker RV: Disorders of the calcium-sensing receptor. Biochim Biophys Acta 1448:166, 1998.

There is normally a decrease in serum calcium in the first hours after birth, continuing for 24 to 48 hours and then stabilizing. Levels of total and ionized calcium (particularly in preterm infants) are then about 8.0 to 9.0 and 3.5 to 4.0 mg/dL, respectively, and subsequently increase gradually. By 1 week of age, breast-fed infants achieve a total calcium of 10.0 ± 1.0 mg/dL and phosphorus of 6.5 ± 1.0 mg/dL. In contrast, infants fed commercial formulas show calcium levels 1 mg/dL lower, phosphorus levels 1 to 2 mg/dL higher, and a greater variability in both values than the breast-fed group.

COMMENT: Studies of placental involvement in fetal calcium metabolism are intriguing. Homogenates of human placental villus (fetal tissue) synthesize 1,25-dihydroxyvitamin D from 25-hydroxyvitamin D. Calcium pump activity also has been studied in vesicles prepared from the microvillus brush border of the human placental syncytiotrophoblast. It is always a source of amazement to observe the complex functions that the placenta undertakes during a critical period of fetal life, and calcium and vitamin D metabolism appears to be no exception to this rule.

The ability of preterm infants to convert vitamin D to 25-hydroxyvitamin D and 1,25-dihydroxyvitamin D has been demonstrated in preterm infants of 32 to 37 weeks' gestation.

Reginald Tsang

Methodology

Serum total calcium, as routinely reported by clinical laboratories, represents the sum of protein-bound calcium, diffusible but complexed calcium (e.g., citrate bound), and free ionized calcium. Only the ionized calcium fraction, normally 4.4 to 5.4 mg/dL,

is physiologically active, transported across membranes, or regulated homeostatically. When ionized calcium is determined directly with a calcium electrode,* values show reliable clinical correlation, with symptoms appearing at levels less than 2.5 to 3.0 mg/dL.

Variations in the two inert calcium fractions occur commonly with such conditions as alteration in serum protein, pH change, and citrate load postexchange and make correlation of total and ionized calcium difficult. Use of the McLean-Hastings nomogram to estimate "ionized calcium" has not correlated well with direct measurements. The Q-oTc interval, derived from the electrocardiogram, has been shown to correlate with low ionized calcium.

Direct determination of ionized calcium is currently an option, but when not possible, ionized calcium usually follows values for total calcium.

COMMENT: Ionized calcium electrodes have come of age, and it is now possible to determine ionized calcium accurately and reproducibly using fairly small volumes of blood. In a prospective study of normal term infants with no perinatal risk factors that may alter calcium metabolism, the nadir of serum ionized calcium concentrations at 24 hours of age was 4.4 to 5.4 mg/dL (95% confidence limits). Using these data, neonatal values below 4.4 mg/dL should be considered abnormal.

Reginald Tsang

◆───

Loughead JL, Mimouni F, Tsang RC: Serum ionized calcium concentrations in normal neonates. Am J Dis Child 142:516, 1988.

Symptoms and Definition[8, 20, 27, 32, 40, 46, 58, 63]

Hypocalcemia is often asymptomatic but causes twitching, "hyperalertness," increased tone, jitteriness, and convulsions. Cyanosis, vomiting or intolerance of feedings, and high-pitched cry have also been noted. None of these symptoms is specific for hypocalcemia, and all are common in high-risk infants generally. Chvostek's sign does not have value in premature infants but occurs in 20% of hypocalcemic term or

───

*Orion Research Corp, Cambridge, MA. Not generally in use.

older infants and is frequently seen also in normal infants. Hypocalcemia, therefore, can only be suspected and must be confirmed both by the laboratory and by response to specific treatment.

COMMENT: Seizures secondary to both hypoglycemia or hypocalcemia may be either focal, unilateral, or general. The presence of any sign of seizure activity should initiate a complete workup, including glucose, calcium, magnesium, and electrolyte determinations.

Cynthia Bearer

Serum calcium should be determined daily for all infants at risk for hypocalcemia and supportive treatment considered when low levels are encountered. The differential diagnosis of hypocalcemia is noted in Table 11–5.

Early Neonatal Hypocalcemia[5, 8, 27, 40, 46, 64]

Early neonatal hypocalcemia represents an exaggeration of the physiologic decrease in serum calcium during the first 2 days of life. In 30% to 40% of all low-birth-weight infants, chemical hypocalcemia develops, which is less than 7 mg/dL and less than 3.0 to 3.5 ionized, at this time. A smaller

Table 11–5. Etiology of Neonatal Hypocalcemia

Hypoparathyroidism
  Transient early neonatal
  Transient late neonatal
  Maternal hyperparathyroidism
  Maternal hypercalcemic hypocalciuria
DiGeorge syndrome: permanent gland hypoplasia or
    aplasia
  With maternal ^{131}I treatment and congenital
    hypothyroidism
  Familial X linked
  Familial autosomal dominant
  Inactive hormone (pseudoidiopathic)
  Hormone unresponsiveness
    (pseudohypoparathyroidism)
Vitamin D deficiency (rickets)
  Diet
  ↓ Hepatic synthesis
  ↓ Renal synthesis
  Malabsorption
  Anticonvulsant drugs
  End-organ resistance (vitamin D dependent)
  Transient resistance to 1,25 dihydroxyvitamin D
    (infants <1250 g birth weight)
Hypomagnesemia
Hyperphosphatemia

number of infants become symptomatic. The following factors identify infants at high risk:

- Male sex; delivery in early spring (low maternal vitamin D)
- Prematurity
- Obstetric trauma, fetal distress, or abnormal presentation
- Neonatal asphyxia, metabolic acidosis requiring IV bicarbonate
- Neonatal illness—respiratory distress syndrome (RDS), cerebral injury, hypoglycemia, and sepsis
- Maternal diabetes, which exaggerates neonatal parathyroid immaturity

The pathogenesis is a failure of homeostatic control of the calcium partition between bone and serum. Interruption of calcium supply, parathyroid hypofunction, calcitonin excess, and unknown effects of acid-base balance shifts and cerebral injury all may contribute. The serum phosphorus is usually normal but may be elevated. Magnesium may be low.

In anticipation of hypocalcemia, serum calcium should be determined daily for high-risk infants. Hypocalcemia may be prevented by 24 mg/kg/d of elemental calcium IV or 75 mg/kg/d by enteric routes. Calcium and bicarbonate cannot be mixed in infusion solutions.

Classic Neonatal Tetany[8, 46, 58]

Less commonly, hypocalcemia occurs at 5 to 7 days of age in association with hyperphosphatemia. Three factors are important in the pathogenesis.

1. Formula with a high phosphorus content and a low calcium-to-phosphorus ratio. Breast milk contains 150 mg phosphorus per liter and has a Ca-to-P ratio of 2.3. In contrast, some formulas have 310 to 600 mg phosphorus per liter and Ca-to-P ratios of 1.3 to 1.4.
2. Immaturity of parathyroid vitamin D and renal function, causing phosphorus retention, hyperphosphatemia, and inability to support calcium levels. Factors associated with "early" hypocalcemia are present in 50% of infants with classic tetany and include high parity, Asian mothers, male sex, low socioeconomic

status, and borderline maternal vitamin D deficiency.

3. With current commercial formulas, classic neonatal tetany has become quite rare. With breast milk feeding, it should not occur at all. At present, therefore, infants with hypocalcemia after 5 days of age must be observed for possible parathyroid disease.

COMMENT: An additional pathogenetic mechanism for hypocalcemia in the very low-birth-weight infant (less than 1250 g) appears to be resistance to 1,25-dihydroxyvitamin D action. 1,25-Dihydroxyvitamin D is necessary for mobilization of calcium from bone, but even when extremely large doses of 1,25-dihydroxyvitamin D_3 are given to very low-birth-weight infants, serum calcium is not raised, in contrast to the positive response in larger preterm infants.

Infants fed "humanized" commercial cow milk formula with phosphate content intermediate between cow and human milk can still have neonatal tetany, often dismissed by house staff as "idiopathic seizures" and treated with phenobarbital. In observing a group of such infants we have found that the serum parathyroid hormone concentrations remain significantly elevated for 6 months beyond the levels in breast-fed infants. This sequence would support the contention that even a moderate increase in phosphate load to term infants results in a "metabolic stress," and infants compensate for this stress by increasing parathyroid hormone production.

Reginald Tsang

◆————

Venkataraman PS, Buckley D, Neumann V, et al: Profound neonatal hypocalcemia in very low birth weight infants with unresponsive parathyroid glands, refractory to 1,25-dihydroxyvitamin D_3. Pediatr Res 17:340A, 1983.

Venkataraman PS, Greer FR, Noguchi A, et al: "Late" infantile tetany and secondary hyperparathyroidism in infants fed "humanized" cow milk formula. J Am Coll Nutr 1:123, 1983.

EDITORIAL COMMENT: These problems are rarely encountered with the modern versions of humanized formulas. The topic remains of historical importance.

Hypoparathyroidism[46, 57]

Maternal Hyperparathyroidism

Exposure to hypercalcemia in utero can cause persisting neonatal parathyroid suppression. Vague maternal symptoms, a history of pancreatitis or renal stones, or a history of a previous infant with neonatal

tetany may be present. The mother's disease is frequently clinically silent. Calcium and phosphorus determinations should be obtained for the mother whenever neonatal hypocalcemia is prolonged or resistant to treatment.

COMMENT: There are several maternal hypercalcemic states that may lead to neonatal transient hypoparathyroidism, including maternal hyperparathyroidism and maternal familial "benign" hypercalcemic hypocalciuria. A high degree of suspicion and an inquisitive mind may lead one to a diagnosis benefiting both mother and infant.

Cynthia Bearer

Transient Congenital Idiopathic Hypoparathyroidism

Transient congenital idiopathic hypoparathyroidism is a benign, self-limited hypoparathyroid state persisting from 1 to 14 months and responding to calcium or moderate vitamin D supplements. The mother is euparathyroid.

Permanent Hypoparathyroidism

Hereditary and sporadic forms of hypoparathyroidism are described. They may be accompanied by absent thymus, immunodeficiency, micrognathia, and aortic arch anomalies (DiGeorge syndrome) (see Table 11–5).

EDITORIAL COMMENT: CATCH 22 is a medical acronym for Cardiac defects, Abnormal facies, Thymic hypoplasia, Cleft palate, Hypocalcemia, and a variable deletion on chromosome 22. The deletion within the chromosome region of 22q11 may occur in patients with three well-described dysmorphologic/cardiologic syndromes: DiGeorge syndrome, velocardiofacial syndrome, and conotruncal anomaly face syndrome. In patients with 22q11 microdeletion, there is a high incidence of hypocalcemia. Indeed hypocalcemia and hypoparathyroidism may be the presenting features. On the other hand, many patients are asymptomatic or present with late onset hypocalcemia. It is advisable to perform genetic analysis of the 22q11 region in patients with late onset or recurrent hypoparathyroidism and to systematically include serum calcium in the survey of patients with known 22q11 microdeletion, especially during the neonatal period if the infants become septic, as well as prior to and during cardiac surgery.

◆————

Garabedian M: Hypocalcemia and chromosome 22q11 microdeletion. Genet Couns 10(4):389–394, 1999.

Other Hypocalcemic Syndromes

Severe maternal calcium and vitamin D deficiency can cause rickets in infants and neonatal hypocalcemia.

Hypocalcemia can occur with uremia, hypoproteinemia (ionized calcium normal; no tetany), furosemide treatment, and magnesium deficiency (see Table 11–5).

Treatment of Hypocalcemia[5, 7, 27, 40, 46, 49]

If desired, supportive treatment may be given to asymptomatic infants at risk. Calcium, 24 to 35 mg/kg/24 h, is added to the IV infusion solution. Calcium Gluceptate Injection (Lilly), 18 mg calcium per mL, or 10% calcium gluconate USP, 9 mg calcium per mL, may be used. Infusion rate should be regulated by pump. Calcium may not be mixed with bicarbonate. Calcium has also been given by slow IV bolus injection every 6 to 8 hours, but this is more difficult.

COMMENT: Calcium infusions should be given preferably through a central line whenever possible. Peripheral administration may result in skin sloughs from IV solution infiltration. The use of hyaluronidase injected subcutaneously around IV infiltrates has dramatically decreased the morbidity associated with this complication.
Cynthia Bearer

Treatment for Symptomatic Hypocalcemia

Stat Treatment

A slow calcium push is hazardous but indicated with seizures or extreme irritability as a therapeutic trial while awaiting laboratory confirmation. Use established IV line and monitor pulse or electrocardiogram continuously for bradycardia. Calcium gluconate, 10%, is injected over 10 minutes to a maximum dose of 4 mL/kg, stopping when clinical response is obtained. Hypocalcemia unresponsive to parenteral therapy should suggest hypomagnesemia (see later text).

Continued Treatment

PARENTERAL. Calcium infusion, as just described, but with a dose of 75 mg calcium/kg/24 h, is indicated. Pulse must be checked frequently, serum calcium checked at least daily, and extravasation avoided. Calcium infusion is hazardous and is rarely required longer than 3 days.

ENTERAL. Dietary calcium therapy is indicated in prolonged or late-onset ("classic") hypocalcemia. Low phosphorus formula (Similac PM 60/40 [Ross], phosphorus 190 mg/L, Ca-to-P of 2.0) or breast milk is used. Calcium supplement as calcium lactate (13% calcium), calcium gluconate (9% calcium), or calcium glubionate (Neo-Calglucon [Dorsey], 23 mg/mL) is added to elevate the fed Ca-to-P ratio to between 4.0 and 6.0. This requires 35 to 70 mg supplemental calcium per deciliter of feeding. Enteric supplementation should not increase gastric tonicity and thus should be mixed with appropriate volumes of formula to avoid necrotizing enterocolitis.

Enteral treatment can usually be tapered after 2 to 4 weeks. With severely depressed parathyroid function, however, treatment may need to be prolonged beyond this period, and therapy with dihydrotachysterol or 1,25-dihydroxyvitamin D may be necessary.

The hazards of IV calcium injection include bradycardia, cardiac arrest, cutaneous necrosis, cerebral calcifications, and intestinal gangrene. Care should be employed to ensure patency of IV lines, with labels to avoid inadvertent flushing. Intraarterial calcium should be avoided.

COMMENT: Enteric calcium salts can be used to treat or prevent neonatal hypocalcemia at 75 mg/kg/d, divided into six equal doses. Enteric calcium salts are much safer than IV calcium salts and can be given to large numbers of sick neonates. The preferred approach at the Cincinnati neonatal intensive care units (ICUs) is early detection of neonatal hypocalcemia followed by prompt enteric calcium supplementation for 2 to 3 days (2 days full supplementation, or 1 day full dose followed by stepwise tapering doses for 2 days). Neo-Calglucon has a syrup base and high osmolality; apart from frequent stools its use might be a disadvantage in infants prone to necrotizing enterocolitis.
Reginald Tsang

Prognosis

Hypocalcemia with seizures may present an immediate threat to life in an infant with other problems with which to contend. However, unlike with hypoglycemia, there seems to be no structural damage to the CNS. Thus, hypocalcemia alone has a good prognosis. If hypocalcemia is complicating other serious conditions such as asphyxia, the prognosis is determined by the other problems.

Hypercalcemia[19, 21, 34, 37]

Often hypercalcemia is iatrogenic, but it may be due to (1) primary hyperparathyroidism, (2) maternal hypoparathyroidism, (3) massive idiopathic fat necrosis, (4) vitamin D toxicity, or (5) aluminum toxicity. Other etiologies are noted in Table 11–6. Specific treatment is directed to the underlying disorder, while calcium excretion may be enhanced with fluids and diuretics.

COMMENT: Another cause of hypercalcemia is the use of thiazide diuretics in the neonatal ICU. Neonatologists have been limiting the use of furosemide because of its calciuric effect. Thiazides reduce renal calcium excretion but raise serum calcium concentrations. Another common cause of hypercalcemia in the nursery is the use of human milk feedings, which results in hypophosphatemia and secondary hypercalcemia.

Reginald Tsang

Table 11–6. Etiology of Hypercalcemia

Neonatal hyperparathyroidism (transient versus permanent)
Maternal hypoparathyroidism
Excessive calcium supplementation including continued feeding of premature formula to babies >36 wk
Excessive vitamin D supplementation
Williams syndrome (↑ 1,25-dihydroxyvitamin D)
Familial hypocalciuric hypercalcemia (autosomal dominant)
Phosphate depletion
Hypervitaminosis A
Thiazide diuretics
Hyperthyroidism
Adrenal insufficiency
Idiopathic subcutaneous fat necrosis
Aluminum toxicity
Hypophosphatasia
Primary chondrodystrophy (metaphyseal dysplasia)

◆ MAGNESIUM

Fetal and Neonatal Magnesium Metabolism[8, 20, 27, 35, 59]

Magnesium is actively transported from mother to fetus. Unlike calcium, this transfer is adversely affected both by placental insufficiency and by maternal magnesium deficiency caused by poor diet or disease. Fifty percent of total body magnesium (versus 1% of calcium) is in soft tissue and plasma. Hypomagnesemia consequently reflects a true magnesium deficiency in the newborn rather than a disturbance in homeostasis with bone.

Parathyroid function has a small direct effect on serum magnesium levels. Magnesium, on the other hand, is critically necessary for normal parathyroid function.

Normal newborn serum magnesium is 1.5 to 2.8 mg/dL and relates directly to the mother's level. Through the first week of life, magnesium levels show small variations, correlating directly with changes in serum calcium and inversely with phosphorus.

Hypomagnesemia

Magnesium levels less than 1.5 mg/dL are encountered in the following conditions:

- In fetal growth retardation of any cause, including multiple birth, or with malnourished or hypomagnesemic mothers
- In infants of diabetic mothers, correlating with the severity of the mother's disease
- With hyperphosphatemia and following exchange transfusion (Magnesium, like calcium, is subject to citrate complexing.)
- In hypoparathyroidism
- In older infants secondary to diarrhea or malabsorption states
- Rarely, with a specific magnesium malabsorption syndrome
- Secondary to renal losses (primary or drug induced, e.g., amphotericin B)

Hypomagnesemia can cause symptoms similar to those caused by hypocalcemia but is unresponsive to calcium therapy.

Coexistence of Hypomagnesemia and Hypocalcemia

Hypomagnesemia and hypocalcemia, two metabolic problems, frequently coexist. They have common antecedents, such as maternal diabetes, hypoparathyroidism, malabsorption, exchange transfusion, and excess dietary phosphorus.

Magnesium deficiency causes failure of parathyroid hormone release and of parathyroid hormone's effect on serum calcium. Magnesium appears crucial for normal bone-serum calcium homeostasis. Magnesium therapy alone may elevate serum calcium in classic neonatal tetany.

COMMENT: One needs to be aware that treatment of hypomagnesemia-induced hypocalcemia with calcium may worsen the hypocalcemia. The additional calcium may compete with magnesium at sites of uptake, thus reducing magnesium availability further.

Cynthia Bearer

EDITORIAL COMMENT: Hypocalcemia is common in IDMs and may be caused by secondary hypoparathyroidism related to hypomagnesemia. A prospective randomized trial demonstrated that the administration of intramuscular magnesium sulfate to IDMs with low cord magnesium <0.74 mM (1.8 mg/dL) does not reduce the incidence of hypocalcemia in infants of well-controlled diabetic mothers.

◆───

Mehta KC, Kalkwarf HJ, Mimouni F, et al: Randomized trial of magnesium administration to prevent hypocalcemia in infants of diabetic mothers. J Perinatol 18:352, 1998.

Therapy

Hypomagnesemia with tetany is treated with magnesium sulfate, 25 to 50 mg/kg (of elemental magnesium) per dose intramuscularly (IM) every 6 to 8 hours. Serum magnesium should be checked every 24 hours. Hypermagnesemia with hypotonia may occur with overtreatment. Alternatively, magnesium may be given with feedings. The sulfate, gluconate, chloride, or citrate salt may be used in an initial dose of 100 to 200 mg magnesium/kg/d given every 6 hours. Excessive doses have a laxative effect.

COMMENT: For any newborn with symptomatic hypocalcemia, intravenous replacement is indicated. Oral therapy may be compromised by vomiting, poor absorption, or diarrhea and is inadequate for reversal of symptoms.

Cynthia Bearer

Hypermagnesemia

Magnesium crossing the placenta following treatment for toxemia may produce hypotonia, flaccidity, respiratory depression, poor suck, and decreased gastrointestinal motility. Treatment is expectant, because magnesium levels decline by 48 hours. If severe symptoms are present, calcium may reverse these effects, whereas forced diuresis may speed magnesium excretion.

COMMENT: Hypermagnesemia may also occur in the neonatal ICU from overdosage during hyperalimentation and is often overlooked because serum magnesium measurements are not routinely made. Preterm infants are less able to excrete any magnesium excess. Curiously, magnesium treatment in mothers, which is associated with neonatal hypermagnesemia, results in elevation of neonatal serum calcium concentrations in spite of suppression of neonatal parathyroid function.

Reginald Tsang

◆───

Donovan EF, Tsang RC, Steichen JJ, et al: Neonatal hypermagnesemia: Effect on parathyroid hormone and calcium homeostasis. J Pediatr 96:305, 1980.

◆ OSTEOPENIA—RICKETS OF PREMATURITY[4, 18, 22, 23, 29, 32, 50, 66]

Bone mineralization in utero increases to term (see Fig. 11–4). In contrast, prematurely born infants demonstrate diminished rates of bone mineralization. These infants are usually very low-birth-weight (less than 1.0 kg); have chronic problems (bronchopulmonary dysplasia [BPD], necrotizing enterocolitis [NEC], cholestasis, acidosis); require calciuric drugs (Lasix) or bicarbonate; have diminished calcium, phosphorus, or vitamin D intake; and are fed a soy-based formula or receive excess aluminum.

Osteopenia may be asymptomatic or show classic rickets at 1 to 4 months of age with undermineralized bone, pathologic fractures, craniotabes, rachitic rosary, hypocalcemia, hypophosphatemia, elevated parathyroid hormone, increased alkaline phosphatase, and increased 1,25-dihydroxyvitamin D levels (if not caused by vitamin D deficiency). Copper deficiency must be ruled out. Treatment requires adequate calcium supplementation. Phosphate therapy is indicated for the presence of hypophosphatemia (rare). In the presence of cholestasis or suspected malabsorption of vitamin D, treatment is usually effective with 1000 to 4000 U of vitamin D or lesser amounts of 1,25-dihydroxyvitamin D. In utero rates of bone mineralization may be achieved with formula containing calcium (1200 to 1400 mg/L), phosphorus (630 to 750 mg/L), and vitamin D (1000 to 1200 U/L) (see Fig. 11–4). The fat-lactose-calcium interaction is also important in intestinal absorption in that older formula resulted in only 40% calcium absorption, whereas newer formula and breast milk result in 70% or greater absorption.

COMMENT: The major factor in osteopenia and rickets of prematurity is mineral deficiency. Thus significant efforts should be made to enhance mineral delivery, either parenterally or enterally. Parenteral fluids containing 60 mg/dL of calcium and 45 mg/dL of phosphate have been used with success even with minimal vitamin D intake. High enteral calcium and phosphorus intake can be achieved with modern preterm formulae or preterm human milk fortifiers with high calcium and phosphorus content.

In general it is not necessary to "overtreat" the infant with vitamin D because most studies indicate that the premature infant is able to hydroxylate vitamin D well in both the liver and kidney.

Reginald Tsang

◆————

Koo WWK, Tsang RC, Succop P, et al: Minimal vitamin D and high calcium, phosphorus needs for preterm infants receiving parenteral nutrition. J Pediatr Gastroenterol Nutr 8:225, 1989.

Steichen JJ, Gratton TL, Tsang RC: Osteopenia of prematurity: The cause and possible treatment. J Pediatr 96:528, 1980.

◆ QUESTIONS

◆ *A 1.2-kg premature infant is noted to have a serum calcium level of 14.5 mg/dL on the 20th day of life. The child is receiving all nutrients by hyperalimentation fluid. There is no evidence of subcutaneous fat necrosis, and prior serum calcium levels obtained 10 days earlier were normal. The hyperalimentation fluid formulation should be checked to determine the child's intake of which of the following:*
1. *Vitamin D*
   2. *Vitamin A*
   3. *Calcium*
   4. *Phosphorus*
   5. *Vitamin B$_{12}$*

Excessive intake of vitamins A and D and calcium may produce iatrogenic hypercalcemia, whereas reduced intake of phosphate may produce similar laboratory results with concomitant hypophosphatemia. Answers 1 to 4 are correct.

◆ *Match the statements with the following conditions and state reasons:*
1. *Hypoglycemia*
2. *Hypocalcemia*
3. *Both*
4. *Neither*

◆ *A maternal history of three miscarriages*

A history of excessive fetal wastage can mean maternal gestational diabetes with a risk of neonatal hypoglycemia and hypocalcemia. Fetal wastage is also seen with hyperparathyroidism. Therefore the answer is 3.

◆ *An infant, 22 hours old, birth weight 1200 g, 29 weeks' gestation, type I respiratory distress with mixed acidosis treated with IV bicarbonate*

This infant has multiple risk factors for hypocalcemia. His risk of hypoglycemia is not great, especially if he is receiving IV fluid and caloric support, as he should be with prematurity and respiratory distress. The answer is, therefore, 2.

COMMENT: Current management in our nursery includes the addition of calcium to D$_{10}$W solutions. If umbilical venous access is unavailable, a percutaneous central line is placed as soon as possible. Thus the risk to this infant is equal for both hypoglycemia and hypocalcemia and depends on pump function, IV infusion rate, and proper mixing of IV solution.

Cynthia Bearer

◆ *Following exchange transfusion for erythroblastosis*

Hypoglycemia may occur following exchange transfusion as a rebound effect precipitated by the glucose added to the donor unit. Citrate complexes calcium and causes a severe decrease in the ionized fraction, which may, in turn, cause symptoms. The answer is 3.

COMMENT: Since the decrease in calcium during "exchange" blood transfusion is in the ionized fraction, the total calcium may not be decreased. In fact, if calcium supplementation is given during the exchange transfusion, total calcium concentrations will be elevated, especially if the last calcium supplement has been given shortly before the determination of serum calcium was made.

Reginald Tsang

◆ *Irritability, jitteriness, and seizures*

These symptoms may mean either hypoglycemia or hypocalcemia. The answer is 3. Drug withdrawal should also be considered.

◆ May be a clue to significant undiagnosed disease in the mother

In a large-for-dates infant, early hypoglycemia should be sought (Dextrostix at 2 hours) and may indicate unsuspected maternal diabetes. Neonatal hypocalcemia may be a clue to a maternal parathyroid adenoma. The answer is 3.

◆ May be precipitated by medication taken during pregnancy

Hypoglycemia of the newborn may be severe and prolonged if a mother is treated with oral hypoglycemics. Exchange transfusion may be necessary to remove the drug from the infant. Although much less likely, a mother with milk-alkali syndrome or vitamin D intoxication with hypercalcemia could have a hypocalcemic infant. The answer is 3.

◆ A 2600-g newborn with a hemoglobin of 26 g/dL

Hypoglycemia is frequent in plethoric infants. A high hemoglobin level may be a factor in hypoglycemia in infants of diabetic mothers and with Beckwith-Wiedemann syndrome. A pair of parabiotic twins has been described in which the larger and more plethoric twin had hypoglycemia while his sibling did not. The answer is 1.

◆ A 3400-g, 53-cm long infant with desquamation and meconium-stained nails and cord, estimated gestation 43 weeks, Apgar scores 9 and 9

Postmaturity per se is not associated with hypocalcemia. When postmaturity is associated with placental insufficiency and signs of intrauterine malnutrition, hypoglycemia may be a problem after birth. The answer, in this infant, is 1. He should be fed early and watched closely.

◆ A jittery and twitchy 4200-g infant 2 hours old

This infant is too young to be hypocalcemic. He is at a typical age for the early hypoglycemia of an infant of a diabetic mother. Of course, the problem might also be an anoxic insult at birth or CNS injury. The answer is 1.

CASE PROBLEMS

Case One

You are called to see a 5-day-old infant because of irritability and jerking movements of the left arm and leg. He was the product of a full-term pregnancy, birth weight 2.8 kg. Pregnancy was complicated by third trimester bleeding. Delivery was by cesarean because of placenta previa. One-minute Apgar score was 6; 5-minute Apgar was 9. Evaporated milk formula was begun at 16 hours of age, and he did very well until a few hours ago when he became tremulous and fed poorly. Intermittent convulsions were noted. Examination reveals irritability but no other abnormalities. However, as the examination ends, the child convulses.

◆ What diagnostic tests and procedures would you perform initially?

The symptoms shown by this baby are nonspecific. CNS injury or infection is possible, and a lumbar puncture must be done. There is nothing in the case history to suggest hypoglycemia as a *probable* cause of the seizures, but some less common hypoglycemic syndromes (inborn error of metabolism, islet adenoma) may present this way, and Dextrostix testing should be performed. Serum should be drawn for electrolytes, calcium, blood urea nitrogen (BUN), and glucose.

Several features of this case suggest the possibility of hypocalcemia, notably stormy obstetric course, milk feedings, the age of onset of symptoms after the initially benign course, and irritability and tremulousness as cardinal symptoms. These features justify a trial with parenteral calcium after initial studies are done.

The therapeutic infusion is 2 mL/kg of 10% calcium gluconate at 1 mL/min into an established IV line with ECG monitoring.

COMMENT: I would just like to emphasize the importance of drawing blood for initial studies *before* administration of parenteral calcium, because the calcium-regulating hormones are directly affected by calcium status in the blood. Hence, if one is trying to determine the cause of the condition, it is extremely important to be able to draw the sample before any intervention, presumably at the time of low calcium concentrations. Subsequent to the intervention, when the serum calcium concentrations have returned to normal, another blood sample should be drawn. The relationship between calcium-regulating hormones and calcium status is dynamic. For example, if parathyroid hormone concentration is measured at the time of severe hypocalcemia and found to be low, this would support the contention that the parathyroids of the infant are not able to mount an adequate response to the hypocalcemia and imply a parathyroid insufficient state. If serum parathyroid hormone concentrations are markedly elevated at the time when serum calcium concentrations are low, this would imply an appropriate response of the parathyroids and would suggest that the low calcium is related to some other disturbance; in this circumstance when the calcium concentrations are restored to normal, the parathyroid hormone concentrations in blood should then fall to the normal range too.

Reginald Tsang

Subsequent to immediate evaluation and treatment, the laboratory reports a calcium of 5.8 mg/dL and phosphorus of 11.5 mg/dL.

◆ *What factors may be important in pathogenesis of the hypocalcemia?*

The high serum phosphorus indicates that dietary phosphorus load, relative hypoparathyroidism, and renal immaturity with retention of phosphate are important factors in the hypocalcemia. Maternal vitamin D status or neonatal vitamin D metabolism may be the cause.

◆ *What further tests are indicated?*

Calcium and phosphorus should be determined in the mother. If hypocalcemia proves resistant to treatment, serum magnesium should be determined in the infant.

◆ *What management should be instituted?*

Low phosphorus formula or formula with a favorable Ca-to-P ratio: PM 60/40, or breast milk. Calcium supplementation: 62 mg calcium added to each 4-oz bottle of formula (10% calcium gluconate, 7 mL; Neo-Calglucon syrup, 2.7 mL; calcium lactate, 470 mg). This will make the fed Ca-to-P ratio 5.0.

◆ *What is the prognosis?*

Excellent. Supplemental calcium may be tapered and withdrawn at 3 to 4 weeks of age. Serum calcium should be monitored at this time to be sure hypocalcemia does not recur. There should be no long-term sequelae.

COMMENT: This case study describes very accurately the consequences of feeding a high-phosphate formula to an infant ill-equipped to handle the load. Prevention of this condition is more effective and economical than treatment. As providers of health care to newborns, we should make it our responsibility to educate parents and staff members that breast milk remains the formula of choice with humanized formulae an alternative.

Cynthia Bearer

◆
_____

Case Two
You attend the delivery at 36 weeks by cesarean section of a 24-year-old juvenile-onset diabetic woman. The infant boy weighs 3.8 kg, is ple-thoric, appears cushingoid, and has moderate hepatomegaly and splenomegaly and a respiratory rate of 60 without retractions or grunting. His Dextrostix at 15 minutes of age reads 90 mg/dL. At 2 hours of age, all seems well. A capillary blood glucose sample is obtained. An hour later, the laboratory reports a value of 12 mg/dL.

◆ *How would you proceed at this point?*

Many infants of diabetic mothers (IDMs) reach glucose levels as low as 12 mg/dL in the first 2 hours, and most rebound satisfactorily (see Fig. 11–1). Check the baby. If he is symptomatic, treat after drawing another sample. If symptoms are absent, draw a sample and feed milk immediately. If he is tachypneic, begin IV glucose at 4 to 8 mg/kg/min.

COMMENT: I have usually advocated a more aggressive approach. IV dextrose solutions are now so readily administered that it is a great deal more practical to start IV dextrose solutions with any sign of hypoglycemia, especially in an infant of an insulin-dependent diabetic mother. Certainly I will start IV dextrose when serum glucose concentrations are below 20 mg/dL, because it is my experience that these infants just do not do well when they have such severe hypoglycemia. Enteric treatment with glucose is erratic in my experience and leads to more prolonged hypoglycemia than necessary. At my institution I standardize the drawing of blood sugars in IDMs to 0 hour, ½ hour, 1 hour, and 2 hours in order to pick up the early drop in sugar, and it is very rare now to see prolonged hypoglycemia. Using early intervention with IV dextrose solutions, we do not even need the initial bolus of sugar but simply place the child on 5 to 8 mg/kg/min of glucose infusion.

Reginald Tsang

◆ *The laboratory reported the second sample as 27 mg/dL. At 4 hours, blood glucose was 34 mg/dL. What next?*

Early feeding may be continued if clinical condition is good. Also repeat glucose values until stable and greater than 40 mg/dL.

At 24 hours of age, the baby is reported as irritable. Feedings have been started and are taken very slowly. Examination reveals that the Moro reflex and tone are reduced. Color is good, pulse is 120/minute, and respirations are 65 breaths/minute without retractions. Chvostek sign is elicited. Blood glucose is 35 mg/dL. Serum calcium is 7.8 mg/dL.

◆ *What is the management?*

This behavior calls for careful evaluation and observation for complications (venous thromboses, anomalies) found in these babies. Blood glucose is borderline low and more persistently depressed in the presence of symptoms; 2 mL/kg of 10% dextrose followed by IV infusions of 8 mg/kg/min is indicated. Furthermore, because calcium may continue to decline over the next 24 hours, calcium supplementation should begin.

Case Three

A 2-month-old infant has increasing respiratory distress and an "incidental" finding on chest x-ray film. He was a 27-week, 0.8 kg infant and has had RDS necessitating 1 month of respirator and 1 month of continuous positive airway pressure care. Multiple episodes of cor pulmonale requiring chronic diuretics and failure to establish enteral alimentation necessitated total parenteral alimentation. Direct reacting hyperbilirubinemia was evident at 1 month.

◆ *Figure 11–5 demonstrates what important observations?*

In addition to chronic lung disease and cardiomegaly, metabolic bone disease is evident. Poorly mineralized bone, in addition to rachitic rosary and pathologic fractures, is present.

◆ *What common deficiency may be present?*

Congenital rickets in the neonate is almost always due to severe maternal vitamin D deficiency. This patient has acquired nutritional rickets and may be deficient in calcium, phosphorus, or vitamin D.

◆ *What therapy should be started?*

Maximize calcium intake by oral and parenteral routes. If hypophosphatemia is present, maximize intake of phosphorus. In the presence of hepatic dysfunction (cholestasis) or suspected malabsorption, vitamin D (1000 U/day) should be added.

COMMENT: I have found that it is usually not necessary to even increase the vitamin D dosage. A liver hydroxylation defect in vitamin D metabolism occurs only in very serious liver disease. Most infants are easily capable of hydroxylating vitamin D in the neonatal period. Thus the major emphasis should be toward increasing the calcium and phosphorus intake. Parenteral calcium and phosphorus intake can be maximized by careful consultation with the pharmacist in designing a fluid that is appropriate for the infant according to the guidelines recently established. Thiazide diuretics may be used in place of furosemide to minimize the losses of calcium and the possibility of nephrocalcinosis. If sufficient parenteral calcium and phosphorus are administered, the vitamin D intake becomes much less important, since the major action of vitamin D is to increase calcium and phosphorus absorption through the gut.

Reginald Tsang

Greene HL, Hambridge KM, Schanler R, Tsang RC: Guidelines for the use of vitamins, trace elements, calcium, magnesium, and phosphorus in infants and children receiving total parenteral nutrition: Report of the Subcommittee on Pediatric Parenteral Nutrient Requirements from the Committee on Clinical Practice Issues of the American Society for Clinical Nutrition. Am J Clin Nutr 48:1324, 1988.

◆ *Why did this patient have pulmonary deterioration?*

Rachitic muscle weakness or rib cage dysfunction may result in pulmonary insufficiency. Alternative approaches employ supplementation with calcium and phosphorus to enhance postnatal bone mineralization.

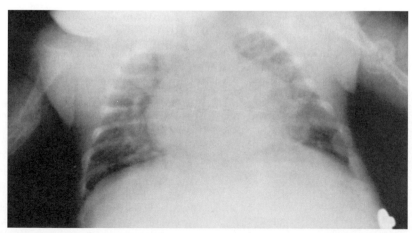

Figure 11–5. Respiratory distress and incidental radiographic findings in a 2-month-old, 800-g infant (Case Three).

Calcium, 250 mg/kg/d (elemental), and phosphorus, 125 mg/kg/d, may prevent this osteopenia and may be easily obtained from newer formulas containing calcium (1400 mg/L), phosphorus (750 mg/L), and vitamin D (1200 U/L).

◆ *A similar patient also demonstrates periosteal bone elevation, anemia, and neutropenia. What rarer nutritional deficiency is present?*

In infants receiving prolonged hyperalimentation, trace mineral deficiency may occur. In this particular infant, copper intake was deficient.

◆

Case Four

A 4500-g infant born to a 23-year-old primiparous breast-feeding mother was found unresponsive at 24 hours of age. The infant's initial sepsis workup revealed a normal complete blood count and electrolytes. The cerebrospinal fluid profile was protein, 120 mg/dL; glucose, 10 mg/dL; 9 leukocytes, 30 red blood cells, and a negative Gram stain.

◆ *The most likely diagnosis is*
A. Congenital herpes simplex encephalitis
B. Group b streptococcal meningitis
C. Hyperglycinemia
D. Hypoglycemia

On further history, the mother has had a normal weight gain during pregnancy and a normal glucose tolerance test. The family history is positive for a niece who died suddenly on the third day of life in 1985.

◆ *A blood sample drawn at the same time as the lumbar puncture revealed a blood glucose of 15 mg/dL. The best approach to treatment is to*
A. Have the mother pump her milk and feed the infant by nasogastric tube
B. Administer glucagon
C. Administer an intravenous 2- to 4-mg/kg bolus of glucose
D. Administer an intravenous 2- to 4-mg/kg bolus of glucose and begin a glucose infusion at 6 to 8 mg/kg/min
E. Administer 2 mL/kg of $D_{50}W$

The administration of a minibolus (2 to 4 mg/kg) of glucose should bring the blood glucose level into the normal range. The infusion keeps the blood glucose level in the normal range in most circumstances. This is usually true regardless of the cause of the neonatal hypoglycemia. The answer is D.

◆ *After giving the minibolus, the child's mental status improves. Nonetheless, despite a glucose infusion rate of 10 mg/kg/min, hypoglycemia recurs. The most likely diagnosis is:*
A. Glycogen storage disease
B. Medium-chain acyl CoA dehydrogenase deficiency

C. Carnitine deficiency
D. Mitochondrial disorder of energy metabolism
E. Hyperinsulinism

Hyperinsulinism is suggested by the high rate of glucose infusion needed to keep the blood glucose level normal. Despite this high rate, the hypoglycemia recurred. Additional clues to hyperinsulinism include absent ketonuria (uncommon in the first day in neonates; may also be absent in fatty acid oxidation disorders), and normal but inappropriately high serum insulin in the presence of hypoglycemia.

◆ *Despite a glucose infusion rate of 18 mg/kg/min delivered through the umbilical vein, the patient remains hypoglycemic. The next therapeutic step is to begin*
A. Glucagon
B. Diazoxide
C. Somatostatin
D. Prednisone
E. Anti-insulin antibodies

Diazoxide is the next treatment of choice because it inhibits pancreatic insulin secretion with relatively few acute side effects (rarely hypotension is seen).

This patient has familial hyperinsulinemic hypoglycemia and, because of persistence of hypoglycemia, eventually needed a 95% pancreatic resection.

REFERENCES

1. Anonymous: Congenital abnormalities in infants of diabetic mothers. Lancet 1:1313, 1988.
2. Antunes JD, Geffner ME, Lippe BM, et al: Childhood hypoglycemia: Differentiating hyperinsulinemic from nonhyperinsulinemic causes. J Pediatr 116:105, 1990.
3. Battaglia F, Meschia G: Principal substrates of fetal metabolism. Physiol Rev 58:499, 1978.
4. Bishop N: Bone disease in preterm infants. Arch Dis Child 64:1403, 1989.
5. Brown D, Steranka B, Taylor F: Treatment of early onset neonatal hypocalcemia: Effects on serum calcium and ionized calcium. Am J Dis Child 135:24, 1981.
6. Centers for Disease Control: Perinatal mortality and congenital malformations in infants born to women with insulin-dependent diabetes mellitus—United States, Canada, and Europe, 1940–1988. Morbid Mortal Weekly Rep 39:363, 1990.
7. Changaris DG, Purohit DM, Balentine JD, et al: Brain calcification in severely stressed neonates receiving parenteral calcium. J Pediatr 104:941, 1984.
8. Cockburn F, Brown J, Belton N, et al: Neonatal convulsions associated with a primary disturbance of calcium, phosphorus, and magnesium metabolism. Arch Dis Child 48:99, 1973.
9. Cordero L, Treuer SH, Landon MB, et al: Manage-

ment of infants of diabetic mothers. Arch Pediatr Adolesec Med 152:249, 1998.

10. Cornblath M, Schwartz R, Aynsley-Green A, et al: Hypoglycemia in infancy: The need for a rational definition. Pediatrics 85:834, 1990.

11. Coustan DR: Pregnancy in diabetic women. N Engl J Med 319:1663, 1988.

12. DeBaun MR, King AA, White N: Hypoglycemia in Beckwith-Wiedemann syndrome. Semin Perinatol 24:164, 2000.

13. DeClue TJ, Malone JI, Bercu BB: Linear growth during long-term treatment with somatostatin analog (SMS 201-995) for persistent hyperinsulinemic hypoglycemia of infancy. J Pediatr 116:747, 1990.

14. Deorari AK, Saxena A, Singh M, et al: Echocardiographic assessment of infants born to diabetic mothers. Arch Dis Child 64:721, 1989.

15. Diamond MP, Salyer SL, Vaughn WK, et al: Reassessment of White's classification and Pedersen's prognostically bad signs of diabetic pregnancies in insulin-dependent diabetic pregnancies. Am J Obstet Gynecol 156:599, 1987.

16. Drexel H, Bichler A, Sailer S, et al: Prevention of perinatal morbidity by tight metabolic control in gestational diabetes mellitus. Diabetes Care 11:761, 1988.

17. Dweck H, Cassady G: Glucose intolerance in infants of very low birth weight. Pediatrics 53:189, 1974.

18. Evans JR, Allen AC, Stinson DA, et al: Effect of high-dose vitamin D supplementation on radiographically detectable bone disease of very low birth weight infants. J Pediatr 115:779, 1989.

19. Garabedian M, Jacqz E, Guillozo H, et al: Elevated plasma 1,25-dihydroxyvitamin D concentrations in infants with hypercalcemia and an elfin facies. N Engl J Med 312:948, 1985.

20. Giles MM, Laing IA, Elton RA, et al: Magnesium metabolism in preterm infants: Effects of calcium, magnesium, and phosphorus, and of postnatal and gestational age. J Pediatr 117:147, 1990.

21. Harris SS, D'Ercole AJ: Neonatal hyperparathyroidism: The natural course in the absence of surgical intervention. Pediatrics 83:53, 1989.

22. Holland PC, Wilkinson AR, Diez J, et al: Prenatal deficiency of phosphate, phosphate supplementation, and rickets in very-low-birthweight infants. Lancet 335:697, 1990.

23. Horsman A, Ryan SW, Congdon PJ, et al: Osteopenia in extremely low birthweight infants. Arch Dis Child 64:485, 1989.

24. Huang MME, Kliegman RM, Trindade C, et al: Allocation of systemic glucose output to cerebral utilization as a function of fetal canine growth. Am J Physiol 254(Endocrinol Metab 17):E579, 1988.

25. Keller JD, Metzger BE, Dooley SL, et al: Infants of diabetic mothers with accelerated fetal growth by ultrasonography: Are they all alike? Am J Obstet Gynecol 163:893, 1990.

26. Kjos SL, Walther FJ, Montoro M, et al: Prevalence and etiology of respiratory distress in infants of diabetic mothers: Predictive value of fetal lung maturation tests. Am J Obstet Gynecol 163:898, 1990.

27. Kliegman RM: Fetal and neonatal medicine. In Behrman RE, Kliegman RM, eds: Nelson Essentials of Pediatrics. 3rd ed. Philadelphia: WB Saunders, 1998.

28. Koh THHG, Aynsley-Green A, Tarbit M, et al: Neu-ral dysfunction during hypoglycaemia. Arch Dis Child 63:1353, 1988.

29. Koo WWK, Sherman R, Succop P, et al: Serum vitamin D metabolites in very low birth weight infants with and without rickets and fractures. J Pediatr 114:1017, 1989.

30. Kukuvitis A, Deal C, Arbour L, et al: An autosomal dominant form of familial persistent hyperinsulinemic hypoglycemia of infancy, not linked to the sulfonylurea receptor locus. J Clin Endocrinol Metab 82:1192, 1997.

31. Lilien L, Pildes R, Srinivasan G, et al: Treatment of neonatal hypoglycemia with minibolus and intravenous glucose infusion. J Pediatr 97:295, 1980.

32. Lucas A, Brooke OG, Baker BA, et al: High alkaline phosphatase activity and growth in preterm neonates. Arch Dis Child 64:902, 1989.

33. Lucas A, Morley R, Cole TJ: Adverse neurodevelopmental outcome of moderate neonatal hypoglycaemia. BMJ 297:1304, 1988.

34. Marx SJ, Attie MF, Spiegel AM, et al: An association between neonatal severe primary hyperparathyroidism and familial hypocalciuric hypercalcemia in three kindreds. N Engl J Med 306:257, 1982.

35. McGuinness G, Weinstein M, Cruikshank D, et al: Effect of magnesium sulfate treatment on perinatal calcium metabolism. II. Neonatal responses. Obstet Gynecol 56:595, 1980.

36. Menon RK, Cohen RM, Sperling MA, et al: Transplacental passage of insulin in pregnant women with insulin-dependent diabetes mellitus. N Engl J Med 323:309, 1990.

37. Miller RR, Menke JA, Menster MI: Hypercalcemia associated with phosphate depletion in the neonate. J Pediatr 105:814, 1984.

38. Milner R, Ferguson A, Naidu S: Aetiology of transient neonatal diabetes. Arch Dis Child 46:724, 1971.

39. Mimouni F, Miodovnik M, Whitsett JA, et al: Respiratory distress syndrome in infants of diabetic mothers in the 1980s: No direct adverse effect of maternal diabetes with modern management. Obstet Gynecol 69:191, 1987.

40. Nerves C, Shott R, Bergstrom W, et al: Prophylaxis against hypocalcemia in low birth weight infants requiring bicarbonate infusion. J Pediatr 87:439, 1975.

41. Nestorowicz A, Inagaki N, Gonoi T, et al: A nonsense mutation in the inward rectifier potassium channel gene, Kir6.2 is associated with familial hyperinsulinism. Diabetes 46:1743, 1997.

42. Perrine SP, Greene MF, Faller DV: Delay in the fetal globin switch in infants of diabetic mothers. N Engl J Med 312:334, 1985.

43. Persson B, Gentz J, Kellum M, et al: Metabolic observations in infants of strictly controlled diabetic mothers. II. Plasma insulin, FFA, glycerol, betahydroxybutyrate during intravenous glucose tolerance test. Acta Paediatr Scand 65:1, 1976.

44. Philipson EH, Super DM: Gestational diabetes mellitus: Does it recur in subsequent pregnancy? Am J Obstet Gynecol 160:1324, 1989.

45. Phillip M, Bashan N, Smith CPA, et al: An algorithmic approach to diagnosis of hypoglycemia. J Pediatr 110:387, 1987.

46. Pitkin RM: Calcium metabolism in pregnancy and the perinatal period: A review. Am J Obstet Gynecol 151:99, 1985.

47. Procianoy RS, Pinheiro CEA: Neonatal hyperinsu-

linism after short-term maternal beta sympathomimetic therapy. J Pediatr 101:612, 1982.

48. Raivio K, Osterlund K: Hypoglycemia and hyperinsulinemia associated with erythroblastosis fetalis. Pediatrics 43:217, 1969.

49. Ramamurthy R, Harris V, Pildes R: Subcutaneous calcium deposition in the neonate associated with intravenous administration of calcium gluconate. Pediatrics 55:802, 1975.

50. Ryan S: Nutritional aspects of metabolic bone disease in the newborn. Arch Dis Child 74:F145, 1996.

51. Sadler TW, Hunter ES III, Wynn RE, et al: Evidence for multifactorial origin of diabetes-induced embryopathies. Diabetes 38:70, 1989.

52. Schwartz R: Hyperinsulinemia and macrosomia. N Engl J Med 323:340, 1990.

53. Seppänen MP, Ojanperä OS, Kääpä PO, et al: Delayed postnatal adaptation of pulmonary hemodynamics in infants of diabetic mothers. J Pediatr 131:545, 1997.

54. Simmons D: Persistently poor pregnancy outcomes in women with insulin dependent diabetes. BMJ 315:263, 1997.

55. Sperling MA, Chernausek SP: Endocrine disorders. In Behrman RE, Kliegman RM, eds: Nelson Essentials of Pediatrics. 15th ed. Philadelphia: WB Saunders, 1996.

56. Swenne I: The fetus of the diabetic mother: Growth and malformations. Arch Dis Child 63:1119, 1988.

57. Tsang R, Chen I, Friedman M, et al: Parathyroid function in infants of diabetic mothers. J Pediatr 86:399, 1975.

58. Tsang R, Oh W: Neonatal hypocalcemia in low-birth-weight infants. Pediatrics 45:773, 1970.

59. Tsang R, Strub R, Brown D, et al: Hypomagnesemia in infants of diabetic mothers: Perinatal studies. J Pediatr 89:115, 1976.

60. Tsang RC, Ballard J, Braun C: The infant of the diabetic mother: Today and tomorrow. Clin Obstet Gynecol 24:125, 1981.

61. Tsang RC: The quandary of vitamin D in the newborn infant. Lancet 1:1370, 1983.

62. Urbach J, Kaplan M, Blondheim O, et al: Neonatal hypoglycemia related to umbilical artery catheter malposition. J Pediatr 106:825, 1985.

63. Venkataraman PS, Blick KE, Dasharathy G, et al: Lowered serum Ca, blood ionized Ca, and unresponsive serum parathyroid hormone with oral glucose ingestion in infants of diabetic mothers. J Pediatr Gastroenterol Nutr 6:931, 1987.

64. Venkataraman PS, Tsang RC, Chen I-W, et al: Pathogenesis of early neonatal hypocalcemia: Studies of serum calcitonin, gastrin, and plasma glucagon. J Pediatr 110:599, 1987.

65. Warram JH, Krolewski AS, Kahn CR: Determinants of IDDM and perinatal mortality in children of diabetic mothers. Diabetes 37:1328, 1988.

66. Weintraub R, Hams G, Merrkin M, et al: High aluminum content of infant milk formulas. Arch Dis Child 61:914, 1986.

67. Weinzimer SA, Stanley CA, Berry GT, et al: A syndrome of congenital hyperinsulinism and hyperammonemia. J Pediatr 130:661, 1997.

68. Wolfsdorf JI: Hyperinsulinemic hypoglycemia of infancy. J Pediatr 132:1, 1998.

69. Zammarchi E, Filippi L, Novembre E, et al: Biochemical evaluation of a patient with a familial form of leucine-sensitive hypoglycemic and concomitant hyperammonemia. Metabolism 45:957, 1996.

Neonatal Hyperbilirubinemia

M. Jeffrey Maisels

Care of the high-risk neonate usually refers to the low-birth-weight infant or the sick term newborn. Whereas hyperbilirubinemia is certainly a matter of concern in these infants, the decisions that must be made regarding jaundice in the high-risk neonate are, in general, less complex than those that must be made for the healthy full-term infant. For the term and near-term infant, shorter hospital stays, the need for outpatient surveillance and management, and the occasional disturbing case of extreme hyperbilirubinemia and even kernicterus raise new issues in the management of neonatal jaundice. Bilirubin has both salutary and toxic effects. At physiologic levels it exerts important antioxidant effects,[107, 113] and, although its toxic effects are well documented, there are also some concerns that aggressive use of phototherapy in very low-birth-weight infants may not be entirely innocuous.[191]

Most neonatal jaundice is the result of a combination of events—an increase in the rate of bilirubin production, reabsorption of bilirubin into the plasma from the gut (the enterohepatic circulation), and inability of the liver to clear sufficient bilirubin from the plasma.

◆ FORMATION STRUCTURE AND PROPERTIES OF BILIRUBIN

Bilirubin is the end product of the catabolism of iron protoporphyrin, or heme, which comes predominantly from circulating hemoglobin (Fig. 12–1). Bilirubin is a tetrapyrrole compound with specific substitutions in the side chains of the four pyrrole rings. The outer pyrrole rings are linked to the inner ones by methene bridges (containing one double bond each), but the two central rings are joined by a methane bridge (no

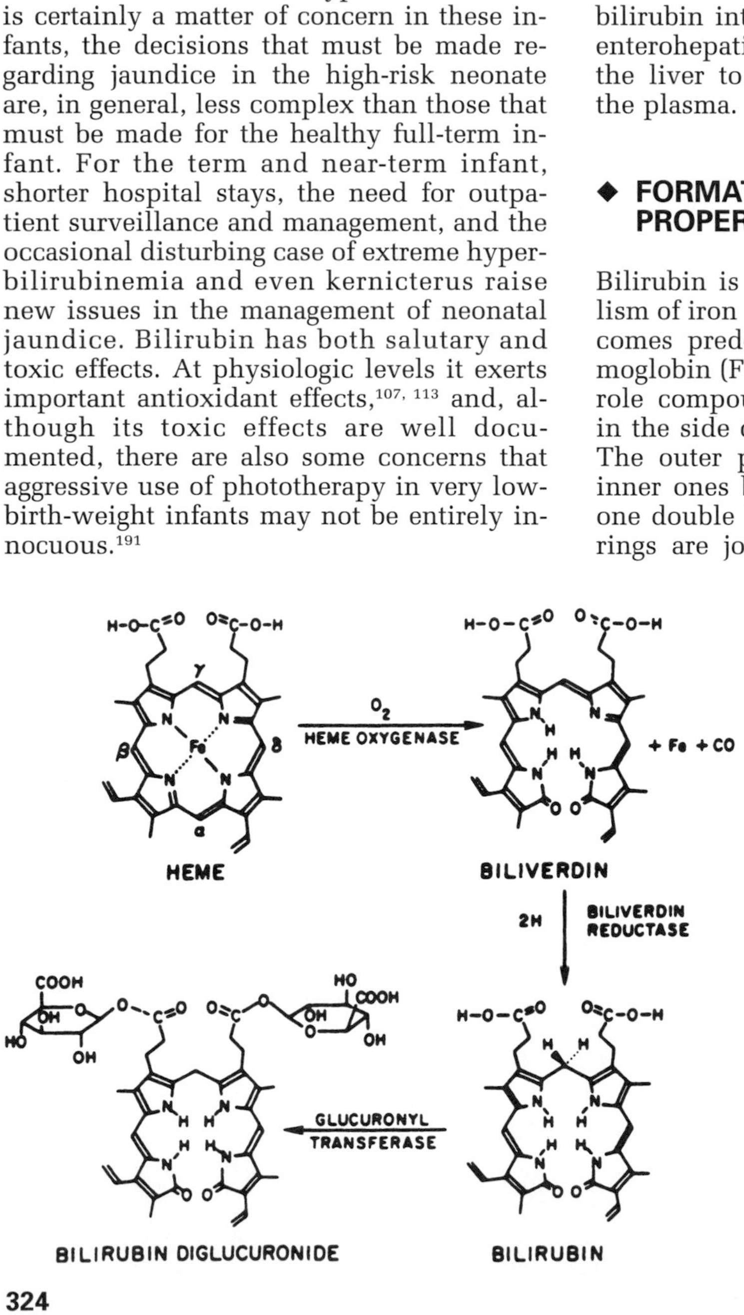

Figure 12–1. Biosynthesis of bilirubin. (From Lightner DA, McDonagh AF: Phototherapy and the photobiology of bilirubin. Semin Liver Dis 8:272–283, 1988.)

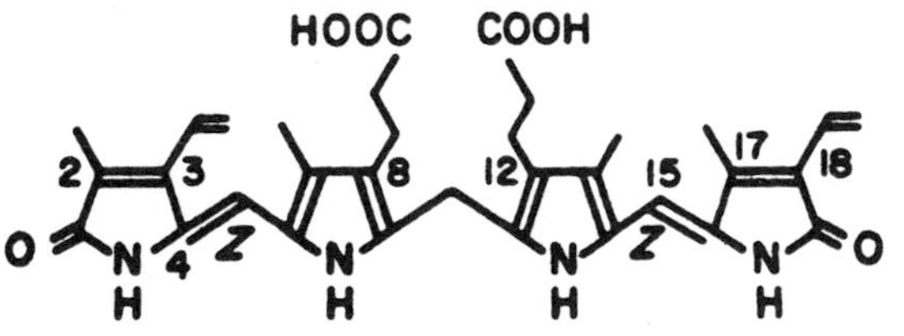

Figure 12–2. The chemical structure of bilirubin. (From McDonagh AF, Lightner DA: "Like a shrivelled blood orange"—bilirubin, jaundice and phototherapy. Pediatrics 75:443–455, 1985.)

double bond). Normally, the methene bridge oxidized in heme is in the α-position, and the resultant isomer is bilirubin IX-α (see Fig. 12–1), the predominant isomer of bilirubin in the body. Although conventionally represented in linear fashion as shown in Figure 12–2, the actual structure of bilirubin revealed by x-ray crystallography is similar to that shown in Figure 12–3, in which the bilirubin molecule is stabilized by the presence of intramolecular hydrogen bonds (stippled lines). In this conformation, the hydrophilic, polar COOH and NH groups are not available for the attachment of water, whereas the hydrophobic hydrocarbon groups are on the perimeter, making the molecule insoluble in water but soluble in nonpolar solvents such as chloroform. The addition of methanol or ethanol interferes with hydrogen bonding and results in an immediate diazo reaction—the basis for measurement of indirect bilirubin by the van den Bergh reaction.

In the jaundiced newborn in whom the primary problem is excessive bilirubin formation or limited uptake and conjugation, unconjugated (i.e., indirect) bilirubin appears in the blood. When bilirubin glucuronide excretion is impaired (i.e., cholestasis), conjugated bilirubin monoglucuronide

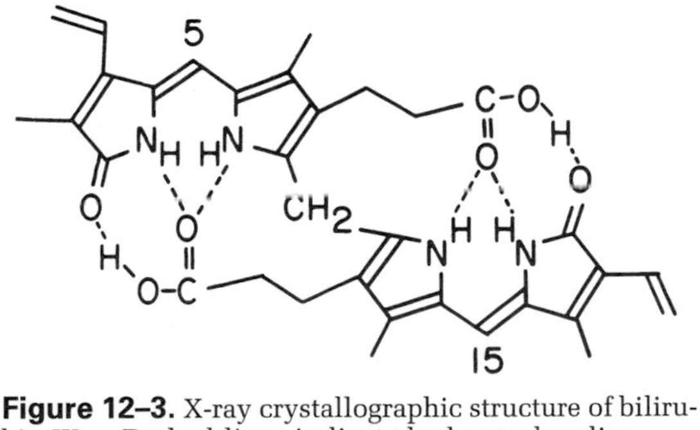

Figure 12–3. X-ray crystallographic structure of bilirubin IX-α. Dashed lines indicate hydrogen bonding.

and diglucuronide (direct reacting bilirubin) accumulate in the plasma and, because of their solubility, also appear in the urine. A fourth bilirubin fraction, known as *delta bilirubin,* is formed nonenzymatically from conjugated bilirubin, is covalently bound to albumin, and reacts directly with the diazo agent.

◆ NEONATAL BILIRUBIN METABOLISM

Heme degradation leads to bilirubin production from two major sources (Fig. 12–4). Approximately 75% of the daily bilirubin production in the newborn comes from senescent erythrocytes (the catabolism of 1 g of hemoglobin yields 35 mg of bilirubin), but 25% is contributed by nonhemoglobin heme contained in the liver (in enzymes such as cytochromes and catalyses and in free heme) and in muscle myoglobin, and from ineffective erythropoiesis in the bone marrow. Once it leaves the reticuloendothelial system, bilirubin is transported in the plasma, bound tightly to albumin so that at physiologic pH the solubility of bilirubin is very low (about 4 nm/L [0.24 mg/dL]).[23] When the bilirubin–albumin complex comes into contact with the hepatocyte, a proportion of the bilirubin, but not albumin, is transported into the cell where it is bound to ligandin and then transported to the smooth endoplasmic reticulum for conjugation. Conversion of unconjugated bilirubin to its water-soluble conjugate must occur before it can be excreted; this is achieved when bilirubin is combined enzymatically with a sugar, glucuronic acid, producing bilirubin monoglucuronide and diglucuronide pigments that are more water soluble and sufficiently polar to be excreted into the bile or filtered through the kidney. The enzyme catalyzing this reaction is uridine diphosphate glucuronosyl transferase (UDPGT), a single form of which (UDPGT1) accounts for almost all of the bilirubin glucuronide in the human liver.[20] The enzyme arises from the UDPGT1 gene complex situated on chromosome 2, at 2q37.[170] Mutations and amino acid substitutions at different loci on this gene are responsible for the inherited unconjugated hyperbilirubinemias: Crigler-Najjar syndrome types I and II and Gilbert disease.

Once conjugated, bilirubin is excreted via

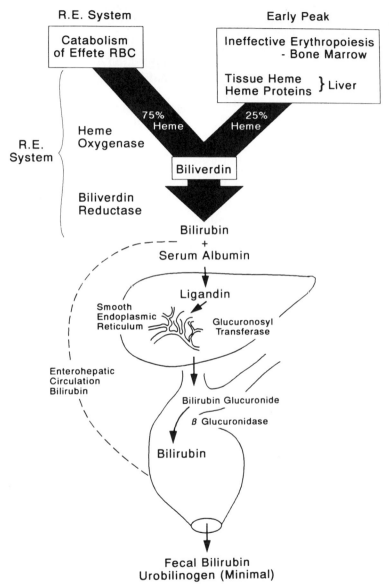

Figure 12–4. Neonatal bile pigment metabolism. RBC, erythrocyte; R.E., reticuloendothelial. (From Maisels MJ: Jaundice. In Avery GB, Fletcher MA, MacDonald MG, eds: Neonatology: Pathophysiology and Management of the Newborn. Philadelphia: JB Lippincott, 1999, pp 765–819.)

the bile canaliculi into the small intestine. A detailed review of the chemistry and metabolism of bilirubin can be found elsewhere.[163]

◆ NORMAL SERUM BILIRUBIN LEVELS AND THE NATURAL HISTORY OF NEONATAL JAUNDICE

Unconjugated bilirubin is transported efficiently via the placenta from fetal blood into the maternal circulation, down a transplacental gradient,[115] and the mean total serum bilirubin (TSB) levels in cord blood range from 1.4 to 1.9 mg/dL (24 to 32 μmol/L),[81, 145] whereas maternal TSB levels are less than 1 mg/dL (17.1 μmol). For years it has been taught that the TSB concentration in normal term infants increases from birth and reaches its apex on about the third day of life, declining to normal levels by 7 to 10 days. Figure 12–5 shows that this is not generally the case. In populations in which 60% to 70% or more of the infants have been fully or partially breast-fed, the TSB levels are substantially higher than in formula-fed infants, do not reach their peak

until the fourth or fifth day, and show no clinically important decline even by the sixth or seventh day. In Figure 12–6, data from eight different studies[17, 31, 46, 95, 118, 145, 184] (Seidman D. Personal Communication, 1998) were used to construct smooth curves that provide a guide to the expected course of bilirubin levels in this type of population. Although these data cannot be applied to all populations, they should be useful for plotting the course of jaundice in term and near-term newborns, and the velocity of the increase in TSB can be used to make decisions about evaluation, follow-up, and potential intervention.

◆ PHYSIOLOGIC JAUNDICE

The normal increase and decrease of TSB levels in the newborn has been termed *physiologic jaundice*, but there is good reason to consider abandoning this term. As shown in Figure 12–5, there are significant differences of TSB levels in different populations, so that what is physiologic for one infant may well be nonphysiologic for another. Particularly in the low-birth-weight infants currently cared for in the neonatal intensive

Total Serum Bilirubin

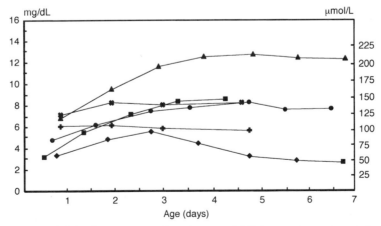

Figure 12–5. Mean total daily bilirubin concentrations in normal full term and near-term infants. (▲) Fifty healthy Japanese newborn infants, 37 to 42 weeks of gestation, all breast-fed, excludes Rh and ABO incompatibility[188]; (✖) 176 term breast-fed Canadian infants, excludes Rh hemolytic disease, includes nine ABO incompatible infants with positive Coombs tests, 17 infants received phototherapy[145]; (✚) 164 Canadian term formula-fed infants, 7 ABO incompatible infants with positive Coombs tests, 3 received phototherapy[145]; (■) 1087 term Israeli infants, 78% fully or partially breast-fed[153]; (●) 56 Nigerian term AGA infants, excludes ABO or Rh incompatibility and G6PD deficiency, infants were "largely breast-fed"[125]; (◆) 29 full-term American infants, all formula fed, about 50% African-American and 50% Caucasian.[47] (From Maisels MJ: Jaundice. In Avery GB, Fletcher MA, MacDonald MG, eds: Neonatology: Pathophysiology and Management of the Newborn. Philadelphia: JB Lippincott, 1999, pp 765–819.)

Total Serum Bilirubin

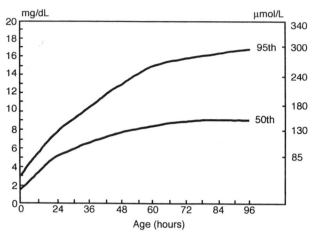

Figure 12–6. Smoothed curves from studies in diverse populations illustrating the expected velocity of total serum bilirubin (TSB) levels and approximate values for the fiftieth and ninety-fifth percentiles. Data for cord blood values come from the studies of Davidson[31] and Saigal,[145] values in the first 12 hours from Frishberg,[46] and subsequent values from Bhutani,[17] Seidman,[153] Maisels,[95] and Wood.[184] Data for the ninety-fifth percentile are primarily obtained from the data of Bhutani,[17] but also from the studies of Newman[118] and Maisels.[95] These data represent values that might be expected in a Western, predominantly breast-fed (60% to 70%) population. In view of the significant variations in different populations (see Fig. 12–5) as well as the variations found in laboratory measurement,[174] the values provided should be used only as rough guidelines. Nevertheless, this graph can be useful in plotting the course of neonatal jaundice because it will demonstrate when the velocity of the TSB increase deviates significantly from the curves shown. *Note that the values must be plotted according to the infant's age in hours, not days.* Infants who have values that exceed the ninety-fifth percentile deserve an evaluation to determine a potential cause for the jaundice and they require careful surveillance and follow-up to prevent the development of extreme hyperbilirubinemia. Infants whose TSB values approach the upper percentiles should also receive closer scrutiny. On the other hand, those whose values fall well below the fiftieth percentile probably require minimal surveillance and follow-up for jaundice.[17] (From Maisels MJ: Jaundice. In Avery GB, Fletcher MA, MacDonald MG, eds: Neonatology: Pathophysiology and Management of the Newborn. Philadelphia: JB Lippincott, 1999, pp 765–819.)

care unit (NICU), the term "physiologic jaundice" has little meaning and is potentially dangerous. If no treatment is given, low-birth-weight infants have prolonged and exaggerated hyperbilirubinemia—the lower the birth weight, the higher the peak bilirubin level. A TSB of 10 mg/dL (171 μmol/L) on day 4 in a 750-g neonate is a normal bilirubin level for that infant and requires no investigation to identify a cause for the jaundice. Nevertheless, most neonatologists would treat this level of TSB in this infant with phototherapy. Thus, TSB levels well within the physiologic range are considered potentially hazardous and are commonly treated with phototherapy. The natural history of hyperbilirubinemia in this population is never observed, and defining these bilirubin levels as physiologic in such infants seems illogical and potentially dangerous. A better term for this phenomenon is *developmental jaundice.*

The jaundice seen in almost every newborn results from a combination of mechanisms:

1. The normal neonate produces about 6 to 8 mg/kg/day of bilirubin, which is about 2.5 times the rate of bilirubin production in the adult.[104]

2. The newborn reabsorbs significant amounts of unconjugated bilirubin from the intestine (the enterohepatic circulation). Unlike the adult, newborns have few bacteria in the small and large bowel and they have greater activity of the deconjugating enzyme β-glucuronidase.[04] As a result, conjugated bilirubin (which cannot be reabsorbed), is not converted to urobilinogen but is hydrolyzed to unconjugated bilirubin. This can be reabsorbed and increases the bilirubin load on the liver.[47, 133]

3. There is a decrease in clearance of bilirubin from the plasma. This is the result of a deficiency in ligandin, the predominant

bilirubin-binding protein in the hepatocyte, and a deficiency of UDPGT, which, at term, has only 1% of the activity found in the adult.[58, 78]

◆ AN APPROACH TO THE JAUNDICED INFANT

The overwhelming majority of both preterm and term infants who are jaundiced are not jaundiced as a result of any pathologic process. Their jaundice is the result of the mechanisms described earlier. A number of epidemiologic factors also exert their influence on one or more of these mechanisms. Those that are most consistently associated with significant nonhemolytic jaundice are listed in Table 12–1.

Who Is Jaundiced?

Jaundice is a clinical sign, and for years clinicians have assessed the intensity of jaundice and used this assessment to decide whether to obtain a serum bilirubin measurement. The American Academy of Pediatrics (AAP) in its algorithm on the management of jaundice recommends measurement of an infant's TSB if the jaundice is "clinically significant by medical judgment."[4] The problem with this recommendation is that the ability of clinicians to diagnose "clinically significant" jaundice varies widely and, in some cases, may be erroneous.[31, 88] In addition, whether the TSB level is "clinically significant" depends both on the actual TSB level as well as the infant's age, in

Table 12–1. Common Obstetric and Neonatal Factors That Significantly Increase the Risk of Nonhemolytic Hyperbilirubinemia in Healthy Term and Near-Term Infants

Previous jaundiced sibling
East Asian race
Oxytocin use in labor
Macrosomic infant of diabetic mother
Bruising cephalhematoma, vacuum extraction
Gestation 35–38 weeks
Male sex
Breast-feeding
Caloric deprivation and larger weight loss
Visible jaundice before discharge
Glucose-6-phosphate dehydrogenase deficiency
Short hospital stay

hours[17] (Figs. 12–6 and 12–7). Nevertheless, newborns whose TSB levels exceed 12 mg/dL (205 μmol/L) are always identified as "jaundiced."[31, 88]

Noninvasive Bilirubin Measurements

The development of noninvasive measurements of bilirubin is an attempt to address the limitations of clinical judgment. The Ingram icterometer (Cascade Healthcare Products, Salem, OR) and the Minolta/Air Shields Jaundice Meter (Air Shields, Hatboro, PA) are useful screening devices, particularly in racially homogenous populations.[100, 152] These devices do not provide a TSB level but they do identify those infants who should have a laboratory measurement of bilirubin.[100, 152] Newer devices such as the TLC-BiliTest (Chromatics Color Sciences International, Inc., New York, NY)[162] and the BiliCheck (Respironics, Pittsburgh, PA)[16] have demonstrated good correlations between the transcutaneous bilirubin and the TSB concentration, even in heterogenous populations. If the data from the initial studies are confirmed, it is possible that the use of these instruments will obviate the need for serum bilirubin determinations in many circumstances.

Laboratory Evaluation—Seeking a Cause for Jaundice

In the NICU, almost all of the neonates are jaundiced simply because they were born too soon and have extremely limited activity of UDPGT (0.1% of adult levels at 30 weeks' gestation).[78] Even in term and near-term infants who are readmitted to hospital in the first 2 weeks of life with TSB levels of 18 to 20 mg/dL (308 to 340 μmol/L), only about 5% have an identifiable pathologic cause for jaundice (Table 12–2).[98]

For years, standard texts have recommended a battery of tests for any infant whose TSB level exceeded 12 to 13 mg/dL (205 to 222 μmol/L) because of the belief that such levels are nonphysiologic and represent potentially "pathologic" jaundice. Not only are there significant differences in TSB levels in different populations (see Fig. 12–5), but recent data show that the 95th percentile for a population of term and near-

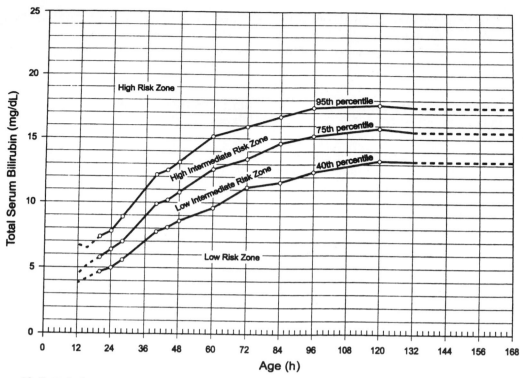

Figure 12–7. Risk designation of term and near-term well newborns based on their hour-specific serum bilirubin values. (Dotted extensions are based on <300 total serum bilirubin values/epoch.) (From Bhutani VK, Johnson L, Sivieri EM: Predictive ability of a predischarge hour-specific serum bilirubin for subsequent significant hyperbilirubinemia in healthy-term and near-term newborns. Pediatrics 103:6–14, 1999.)

term infants is approximately 15 to 17.5 mg/dL (290 to 308 μmol/L).[17, 95, 118] Furthermore, with the exception of blood typing and the Coombs test, the usual laboratory tests performed (complete blood count [CBC], reticulocyte count) are neither specific nor sensi-

Table 12–2. Discharge Diagnosis in 306 Infants Admitted with Severe Hyperbilirubinemia*

Diagnosis	Number	Percentage
Hyperbilirubinemia of unknown cause or breast milk jaundice	290	94.8
Cephalhematoma or bruising	3	1.0
ABO hemolytic disease†	11	3.6
Anti-E hemolytic disease	1	0.3
Galactosemia	1	0.3
Sepsis	0	

*Infants were readmitted after discharge as newborns. Mean age at admission was 5 days (range, 2–17 days), and mean bilirubin level was 18.5 ± 2.8 mg/dL (range 12.7–29.1 mg/dL).

†Mother was type O, infant was type A or B, direct Coombs' test was positive.

From Maisels MJ, Kring E: Risk of sepsis in newborns with severe hyperbilirubinemia. Pediatrics 90:741–743, 1992.

tive.[97, 117] One approach that makes sense is to evaluate the bilirubin level in relationship to the infant's precise age in hours (see Figs. 12–6 and 12–7). Infants whose TSB levels exceed the 95th percentile or in whom the rate of increase appears to be crossing percentiles deserve evaluation and careful follow-up. Tables 12–3 and 12–4 provide an approach to the clinical and laboratory evaluation of the jaundiced newborn, and Table 12–5 lists the causes of indirect hyperbilirubinemia in the newborn.

The timing of the onset of jaundice is very important; jaundice that appears within the first 24 hours or that increases rapidly and crosses percentiles should be considered the result of excessive bilirubin production (hemolysis) until proven otherwise.

◆ PATHOLOGIC JAUNDICE
Hemolytic Disease
Immune-Mediated Hemolytic Disease

The combination of antepartum and postpartum prophylaxis with RhD immunoglob-

Table 12–3. Guidelines for Initial Evaluation and Follow-up of Jaundice in Apparently Healthy Term and Near-Term Infants*

Clinical Observation	Initial Actions	Other Evaluations	Follow-up
Onset of jaundice in first 24 h†	Clinical evaluation‡ Measure TSB and TcB¶	Blood group (ABO, Rh) Direct Coombs' test CBC, smear for red cell morphology, reticulocyte count**	Repeat TSB in 4–24 h§
Onset of jaundice 24–72 h	Clinical evaluation Assess cephalocaudal distribution†† TcB	TSB if indicated by TcB or clinical evaluation	Clinical evaluation and/or TcB or TSB within 24–72 h and repeat as necessary

*These guidelines apply to the evaluation and follow-up of the majority of jaundiced newborns who are cared for in well-baby nurseries and are ≥35 wk of gestation. They cannot take into account all possible situations. The term "apparently healthy" refers to an infant who has no clinical signs suggesting the possibility of other diseases such as respiratory distress, poor feeding, lethargy, temperature instability, and so on.

†Twenty-four hours is a long time in the life of a newborn infant. Jaundice at age 4 h is essentially always due to a hemolytic process, whereas jaundice at age 23 h may be normal.

‡Clinical evaluation refers to a review of the obstetric history, events of labor and delivery, and physical examination of the newborn, which should include an evaluation for cephalhematomas, bruising, and hepatosplenomegaly.

¶In some nurseries, a TcB measurement (using the Minolta/Air Shields Jaundice Meter) is used as a screening device and a decision to measure the TSB is based on the TcB level. If a TSB is done, the simultaneous measurement of a TcB allows subsequent TcB measurements to be used to follow up the baby and to determine the necessity for additional bilirubin measurements. Recently developed TcB devices could largely replace TSB measurements.

§The frequency of obtaining repeated TSB measurements depends on the initial TSB level and the age at which it occurred. A TSB of 5 mg/dL at age 4 h must be repeated within 4 h, whereas the same level at 23 h could be repeated in 12–24 h.

**These investigations lack sensitivity and specificity, but may be helpful in confirming the diagnosis of ABO hemolytic disease or other rarer causes of hemolysis.

††Jaundice is first seen in the face. As the TSB increases, jaundice appears in the trunk, abdomen, and extremities.

TSB, total serum bilirubin; TcB, transcutaneous bilirubin.

Adapted from Maisels J: Epidemiology of neonatal jaundice. In Maisels MJ, Watchko JF, eds: Neonatal Jaundice. London: Harwood Academic, 2000, p 148.

ulin has dramatically reduced the incidence of erythroblastosis fetalis resulting from the RhD antigen, and the incidence of Rh hemolytic disease is estimated to be about 1 in 1000 live births.[26] Approximately half of affected newborns require little or no treatment.[21]

ABO hemolytic disease generally occurs in infants of blood group A or B born to group O mothers. Because approximately

Table 12–4. Additional Laboratory Evaluation of the Jaundiced Term and Near-Term Infant

Indications	Maneuvers
Suspicion of hemolytic disease or anemia (e.g., pallor, early jaundice or TSB >8 mg/dL [137 μmol/L] by 24 h or >13 mg/dL [222 μmol/L] by 48 h of life)	Blood type, group, and Coombs' test, if not obtained with cord blood Complete blood count and smear Reticulocyte count
Either or both parents (or grandparents) of East Asian, Mediterranean, or Nigerian descent with TSB >15 mg/dL (257 μmol/L). Any infant with late-onset jaundice or TSB ≥18 mg/dL (308 μmol/L)	Measure glucose-6-phosphate dehydrogenase
Jaundice beyond 3 wk of age	Direct bilirubin level, urine dipstick for bilirubin, inspect stools for color Check results of newborn thyroid screen, and evaluate infant for signs or symptoms of hypothyroidism
Infant ill	Direct bilirubin level, check urine for reducing substances, check results of newborn screen for galactosemia and other inborn errors, and evaluate for sepsis

From Maisels J: Epidemiology of neonatal jaundice. In Maisels MJ, Watchko JF, eds: Neonatal Jaundice. London: Harwood Academic, 2000, p 149.

TSB, total serum bilirubin concentration.

Table 12–5. Causes of Indirect
Hyperbilirubinemia in Newborn Infants

Increased Bilirubin Production or Load on the Liver

Hemolytic disease
  Immune mediated
    Rh alloimmunization
    ABO and other blood group incompatibilites
  Heritable
    Red cell membrane defects
      Spherocytosis,* elliptocytosis, stomatocytosis,
        pyknocytosis
    Red cell enzyme deficiencies
      Glucose-6-phosphate dehydrogenase
        deficiency,* pyruvate kinase deficiency, and
        other erthyrocyte enzyme deficiencies
    Hemoglobinopathies
      Alpha thalassemia, β-γ-thalassemia
Other causes of increased production
  Sepsis*†
  Disseminated intravascular coagulation
  Extravasation of blood; hematoma; pulmonary,
    cerebral, or other occult hemorrhage
  Polycythemia
  Macrosomic infants of diabetic mothers

Increased Enterohepatic Circulation of Bilirubin

  Breast milk jaundice
  Pyloric stenosis
  Small or large bowel obstruction or ileus

Decreased Clearance

  Prematurity
  Glucose-6-phosphate dehydrogenase deficiency

Metabolic

  Crigler-Najjar syndrome, types I and II; Gilbert
    syndrome
  Tyrosinemia†
  Hypermethioninemia†
  Hypothyroidism
  Hypopituitarism†

---

  *Decreased clearance is also part of pathogenesis of indirect hyperbilirubinemia.
  †Elevation of direct-reading bilirubin also occurs.
  From Watchko JF: Indirect hyperbilirubinemia in the neonate. In Maisels MJ, Watchko JF, eds: Neonatal Jaundice. London: Harwood Academic, 2000, p 52.

45% of Americans of Western European descent have type O blood and a similar percentage are type A, AO incompatibility is the most common form of ABO incompatibility encountered in the United States.[94] Large prospective studies[111, 127] and several smaller studies have found that, although about one of every three group A or B infants born to a group O mother has anti-A or anti-B antibodies attached to their red cells, only one in five of those with a positive direct antibody test (Coombs' test) has a modest to significant degree of hyperbilirubinemia. Thus, although it can, on occasion,

be severe, ABO hemolytic disease is not a common cause of severe hyperbilirubinemia (see Table 12–2).[126, 127] The diagnosis of *ABO hemolytic disease* as opposed to *ABO incompatibility* should generally be reserved for infants who have a positive direct Coombs' test *and* clinical jaundice within the first 12 to 24 hours of life (icterus praecox). Reticulocytosis and the presence of microspherocytes on the smear support the diagnosis. Nevertheless, occasional cases of ABO hemolytic disease have been recorded even in the absence of a positive direct Coombs' test. Such cases may reflect the insensitivity of Coombs' testing or may occur in infants who have a paucity of A and B antigens on their red cells or unusually efficient absorption of serum antibody by A and B antigen epitopes present in body tissues and fluids.[179]

Heritable Causes of Hemolysis

Defects in the red cell membrane include *hereditary spherocytosis, elliptocytosis, stomatocytosis,* and *infantile pyknocytosis.* Although these can occur in the newborn period, newborns frequently exhibit substantial variation in red cell size and shape, and it is not always easy to establish one of these diagnoses.[179] Spherocytes are not usually seen on red cell smears and, when present, suggest the diagnosis of hereditary spherocytosis or ABO hemolytic disease. Because hereditary spherocytosis is inherited autosomal dominantly, a family history can often be elicited. In addition, the presence of severe jaundice in neonates with hereditary spherocytosis is closely related to an interaction with the Gilbert syndrome allele,[63] a phenomenon also observed in infants with glucose-6-phosphate dehydrogenase (G6PD) deficiency.

Red Cell Enzyme Deficiencies

G6PD deficiency is a problem that affects hundreds of millions of people around the world.[74, 165] Nevertheless, most neonatologists in the United States do not (but should) think about this enzyme deficiency as a likely cause for significant hyperbilirubinemia. Although G6PD deficiency occurs in approximately 10% of African-American male neonates, severe hyperbilirubinemia does not develop in most of these newborns. Nevertheless, extreme hyperbilirubinemia and kernicterus have been described in G6PD-deficient infants of African-American descent.[87, 176] G6PD deficiency is an X-linked disorder and hemolysis can occur following exposure to an oxidative challenge. Agents commonly involved include naphthaline (a component of mothballs), dyes, and infection.[165] Interestingly, in most G6PD-deficient infants in whom severe hyperbilirubinemia develops, there are no signs of overt hemolysis (anemia and reticulocytosis). Furthermore, the data of Kaplan and coworkers suggest that significant hyperbilirubinemia associated with G6PD deficiency is primarily the result of abnormal bilirubin clearance rather than hemolysis.[74]

Other researchers disagree with this view and suggest that overt signs of hemolysis are not found because the hemolysis is self-limited and extravascular, and involves an older fraction of the red cell population.[166] The identification of a molecular marker for Gilbert syndrome in the promoter region of the UDPGT1 gene allowed Kaplan and coworkers to demonstrate a remarkable association between hyperbilirubinemia, G6PD deficiency, and Gilbert syndrome. In their study, significant jaundice did not develop in either the neonates with G6PD deficiency alone or in those with only the variant UDPGT1 promoter, whereas TSB levels greater than 15 mg/dL (257 μmol) developed in 50% of those who were homozygous for both abnormalities.[75]

Pyruvate kinase deficiency is an autosomal recessive disorder that is less common than G6PD deficiency but may present with jaundice, anemia, and reticulocytosis.[179]

Other Causes of Increased Bilirubin Production or Load on the Liver

The *hemoglobinopathies* rarely manifest themselves as jaundice in the neonatal period, although such cases have been described occasionally.[179] *Cephalhematomas, intracranial* or *pulmonary hemorrhage*, or any *occult bleeding* may lead to an elevated TSB level from breakdown of the extravascular erythrocytes. In some studies, the presence of periventricular-intraventricular hemorrhage has been associated with an increase in TSB levels in very low-birth-weight infants,[44] but other studies have not reached this conclusion.[3] *Polycythemia* is usually listed as a cause of hyperbilirubi-

nemia because the catabolism of 1 g of hemoglobin produces 35 mg of bilirubin. Nevertheless, mean bilirubin levels and the incidence of hyperbilirubinemia were similar in polycythemic infants randomly assigned to receive either partial exchange transfusion or symptomatic treatment.[18, 48]

Any *small* or *large bowel obstruction, ileus,* or *delayed passage of meconium* exaggerates the enterohepatic circulation of bilirubin (also thought to be the mechanism for hyperbilirubinemia associated with pyloric stenosis). In any of these conditions, correction of the obstruction produces a prompt decline in bilirubin levels. *Macrosomic infants of mothers with insulin dependent diabetes* are at an increased risk of hyperbilirubinemia, probably as a result of increased bilirubin production.[91]

Decreased Bilirubin Clearance

Inherited Unconjugated Hyperbilirubinemia—Inborn Errors of Bilirubin UDPGT Activity

A single form of bilirubin UDPGT (UDPGT1) accounts for almost all of the bilirubin glucuronidation activity in the human liver, and three degrees of inherited UDPGT deficiency are recognized. *Crigler-Najjar syndrome type I* (CN-I) is inherited in an autosomal recessive pattern with marked genetic heterogeneity, and more than 30 different genetic mutations have been identified.[179] Infants with this condition have virtually complete absence of bilirubin UDPGT activity, severe jaundice develops in the first 2 to 3 days of life, and intensive phototherapy and, often, exchange transfusion are required. Unless they receive a liver transplantation, which is curative,[154] these children are committed to lifelong phototherapy, which becomes less and less effective as they get older.

Type II Crigler-Najjar disease (CN-II), also known as Arias syndrome, has a pattern of inheritance that is usually autosomal recessive, but it may also be autosomal dominant. It is characterized by low but detectable activities of bilirubin UDPGT, and the hyperbilirubinemia usually shows some response to phenobarbital therapy. Although jaundice is generally less severe than in the CN-I patients, in some children with CN-II, marked hyperbilirubinemia develops as can kernicterus.

The diagnosis of Gilbert syndrome at one time was never made until adolescence when it manifests as a mild, benign, chronic unconjugated hyperbilirubinemia with no evidence of liver disease or overt hemolysis. Gilbert syndrome affects approximately 6% of the population and both autosomal dominant as well as recessive inheritance patterns have been found. The identification of the genetic basis for this disorder (a variant promoter for the gene encoding UDPGT1) has permitted its identification in the newborn. Newborns who are homozygous for the A(TA)7TAA polymorphism have a greater rate of increase in TSB levels and higher TSB levels in the first days of life than do heterozygous or normal infants.[9, 139] The Gilbert syndrome genotype is also an important contributor to the prolonged indirect hyperbilirubinemia found in some breast-feeding infants. Twenty-seven percent of breast-fed infants who had TSB levels of more than 5.8 mg/dL (100 μmol/L) at age 28 days had the Gilbert syndrome genotype.[114] The association of this genotype with significant jaundice in G6PD-deficient infants and in infants with hereditary spherocytosis is mentioned earlier.

Other Inborn Errors of Metabolism

Jaundiced infants who have vomiting, excessive weight loss, hepatomegaly, and splenomegaly should be suspected of having *galactosemia*. In galactosemia, the hyperbilirubinemia during the first week of life is almost exclusively unconjugated but the conjugated fraction tends to increase during the second week, probably reflecting liver damage. A test of the urine for reducing substances using Clinitest helps to make the diagnosis. Infants with *tyrosinemia* and *hypermethioninemia* are jaundiced primarily as a result of the presence of neonatal liver disease, such that indirect hyperbilirubinemia is generally accompanied by some evidence of cholestasis. Prolonged indirect hyperbilirubinemia is one of the clinical features of *congenital hypothyroidism*, a condition that should be identified by routine metabolic screening programs currently used for the newborn. Other causes of prolonged indirect hyperbilirubinemia are listed in Table 12–6.

Breast-Feeding and Jaundice

A strong association has been found between breast-feeding and an increased inci-

Table 12–6. Causes of Prolonged Indirect Hyperbilirbuinemia

Breast milk jaundice
Hemolytic disease
Hypothyroidism
Extravascular blood
Pyloric stenosis
Crigler-Najjar syndrome
Gilbert syndrome genotype in breast-fed infants

dence of neonatal hyperbilirubinemia,[89, 96, 150] although some studies do not agree.[141] The primary contributors to jaundice associated with breast-feeding are a decreased caloric intake in the first few days of life and an increased enterohepatic circulation.[7, 49] Breast-fed infants usually receive fewer calories in the first days after birth than do those fed formula, and caloric deprivation itself appears to enhance the enterohepatic circulation of bilirubin.[45] Increasing the frequency of breast-feeding significantly reduces the risk of hyperbilirubinemia,[33, 171, 189] providing further support for the important role of caloric deprivation and the enterohepatic circulation in the pathogenesis of breast-feeding jaundice. The stools of breast-fed infants weigh less and their cumulative stool output is lower than that of formula fed infants.[50] In addition, infants fed human milk pass stool significantly less frequently than do formula-fed infants.[50]

Mixed Forms of Jaundice

Sepsis

Jaundice is one sign of bacterial sepsis, but septic infants almost always have other signs and symptoms. Unexplained indirect hyperbilirubinemia as the *only* sign of sepsis is rare (see Table 12–2), and we do not recommend lumbar punctures or blood and urine cultures in jaundiced infants who otherwise appear well.[99] On the other hand, those who appear sick or have direct hyperbilirubinemia or other findings in the physical examination or laboratory evaluation that are out of the ordinary should be evaluated for possible sepsis. Other causes of mixed forms of jaundice include *congenital syphilis*, the *TORCH* (toxoplasmosis, rubella, cytomegalovirus, herpes simplex) *group of intrauterine infections*, and *Coxsackie B virus infection*.[6, 54]

Cholestatic Jaundice

Cholestasis refers to a reduction in bile flow and is the term used to describe a group of disorders associated with conjugated (or direct-reacting) hyperbilirubinemia. Such jaundice indicates inadequate bile secretion or biliary flow. Although frequently transient in the sick low-birth-weight infant, particularly those receiving parenteral nutrition, a pathologic cause must always be ruled out. For a detailed discussion of the causes and management of cholestatic jaundice, refer to recent reviews of this subject.[6, 12, 54]

Conditions associated with conjugated hyperbilirubinemia in the neonatal period are listed in Table 12–7. Cholestasis can be categorized as *hepatocellular* (secondary to immature secretory mechanisms or damage to the hepatocyte canalicular membrane) or *ductal* (an anatomic abnormality of the bile ducts). Approximately 60% to 80% of all cases of conjugated hyperbilirubinemia in early infancy are the result of idiopathic neonatal hepatitis or biliary atresia. *Idiopathic neonatal hepatitis* is characterized by prolonged conjugated hyperbilirubinemia without any obvious evidence of bacterial or viral infection or the other causes listed in Table 12–7. *Extrahepatic biliary atresia* (EHBA) occurs when there is obliteration of the lumen of part of the biliary tract or absence of some or all of the extrahepatic biliary system. EHBA occurs in 1 in 10,000 to 15,000 newborn infants and it is essential to make the diagnosis expeditiously before irreversible sclerosis of the intrahepatic ducts occurs. The identification of cholestatic jaundice and initiation of the necessary diagnostic investigations occur in a timely fashion *if every infant who is clinically jaundiced beyond the age of 3 weeks has a measurement of direct-reacting bilirubin.*[4] Earlier laboratory investigations are mandatory in any jaundiced infant who has pale stools or dark urine (the urine of most newborns is nearly colorless). This simple approach ensures timely evaluation and treatment of infants with EHBA.

Table 12–7. Diseases Associated with Conjugated Hyperbilirubinemia in the Neonatal Period

A. Hepatocellular disturbances in bilirubin excretion
  1. Primary hepatitis
    a. Neonatal idiopathic hepatitis (giant cell hepatitis)
    b. Hepatitis caused by identified infectious agents
      (1) Hepatitis B
      (2) Rubella
      (3) Cytomegalovirus
      (4) *Toxoplasma* organisms
      (5) Coxsackie virus
      (6) Echovirus 14 and 19
      (7) Herpes simplex and varicella zoster
      (8) Syphilis
      (9) *Listeria* organisms
      (10) Tubercle bacillus
  2. "Toxic hepatitis"
    a. Systemic infectious diseases
      (1) *Escherichia coli* (sepsis or urinary tract)
      (2) Pneumococci
      (3) *Proteus* organisms
      (4) *Salmonella* organisms
      (5) Idiopathic diarrhea
    b. Intestinal obstruction
    c. Parental alimentation
    d. Ischemic necrosis
  3. Hematologic disorders
    a. Erythroblastosis fetalis (severe forms)
    b. Congenital erythropoietic porphyria
  4. Metabolic disorders
    a. Alpha$_1$-antitrypsin deficiency
    b. Galactosemia
    c. Tyrosinemia
    d. Fructosemia
    e. Glycogen storage disease type IV
    f. Lipid storage diseases
      (1) Niemann-Pick disease
      (2) Gaucher disease
      (3) Wolman disease
    g. Cerebrohepatorenal syndrome (Zellweger syndrome)
    h. Trisomy 18
    i. Cystic fibrosis
    j. Familial idiopathic cholestasis: Byler disease
    k. Hemochromatosis
    l. Idiopathic hypopituitarism
B. Ductal disturbances in bilirubin excretion
  1. Extrahepatic biliary atresia
    a. Isolated
    b. Trisomy 18
    c. Polysplenia-heterotaxia syndrome
  2. Intrahepatic biliary atresia (nonsyndromatic paucity of bile ducts)
  3. Alagille syndrome (arteriohepatic dysplasia)
  4. Intrahepatic atresia associated with lymphedema
  5. Extrahepatic stenosis and choledochal cyst
  6. Bile plug syndrome
  7. Cystic disease
  8. Tumors of the liver and biliary tract
  9. Periductal lymphadenopathy

From Halamek LP, Stevenson DK: Neonatal jaundice and liver disease. In Fanaroff AA, Martin RJ, eds: Neonatal-Perinatal Medicine. Diseases of the Fetus and Infant. St. Louis: Mosby, 1997, pp 1345–1389.

The initial treatment of EHBA is a portoenterostomy or Kasai procedure in which a loop of small intestine is anastomosed to the porta hepatis following excision of the atretic ducts.[30] About one third of patients who undergo the Kasai procedure survive for more than 10 years without liver transplantation. About one third have adequate bile drainage but complications of cirrhosis develop and liver transplantation is necessary before the age of 10 years. The remaining one third require earlier liver transplantation because bile flow is inadequate following portoenterostomy and progressive fibrosis and cirrhosis develop. Portoenterostomy must be done before there is irreversible sclerosis of the intrahepatic bile ducts[12] and long-term survival following this procedure is best when the procedure is performed before age 60 days. Outcomes are much worse when the operation is performed after 100 days of age.[30]

Perhaps the most common association with cholestasis in the NICU is prolonged use of intravenous alimentation. When total parenteral nutrition (TPN) is used for 2 weeks or longer and, particularly, when such use is exclusive of enteral feedings, cholestatic jaundice may appear. Cholestasis develops in as many as 80% of infants who receive TPN for more than 60 days, and 50% of those with birth weights of less than 1000 g are affected.[13, 158] The pathogenesis of TPN-associated cholestasis is not clear, but it is thought to be related to a combination of factors including immaturity of bile secretion in preterm infants, a decrease in bile flow that occurs with no enteral feeding, and potential toxicity of both trace elements and amino acids.[54, 155]

Jacquemin et al described 92 children who were first seen with cholestasis before the age of 1 month and in whom no etiology for the cholestasis was found.[65] These cases fit the diagnosis of "neonatal hepatitis." The mean duration of jaundice was 3.5 months (range 1.5 to 8 months). Serum conjugated bilirubin concentrations were normal by 6 months in 99% and serum alanine aminotransferase and gamma-glutamyltransferase activities were normal by 1 year. Liver biopsies were performed in 70 of the 92 children and were characterized by the presence of multinucleated giant hepatocytes in 63 (90%). Perinatal events that were commonly associated with this pattern of cholestatic jaundice were prematurity (21%), intrauterine growth retardation (33%), need for assisted ventilation (27%), bacterial infection (22%), and parenteral nutrition (17%). These authors suggest that the term *neonatal hepatitis*, which implies an inflammatory or infectious process, is a misnomer. They prefer the term *transient neonatal cholestasis* because the clinical and biopsy findings are the result of a combination of factors, including (1) immaturity of bile secretion associated with prematurity, (2) chronic or acute ischemia/hypoxia of the liver following intrauterine growth retardation, acute perinatal distress, or lung disease, (3) liver damage caused by perinatal or postnatal sepsis, and (4) decrease in bile flow resulting from delays in enteral feeding.[65]

An approach to the laboratory evaluation of infants with cholestatic jaundice is provided in Table 12–8. Recent descriptions of imaging findings may permit some shortcuts and even avoid the necessity for liver biopsy in some cases. Magnetic resonance cholangiography provides visualization of the extrahepatic bile ducts. Failure to see the bile ducts is highly suggestive of biliary atresia.[53] A Korean study suggests that identification of the "triangular cord" (a triangular or tubular shaped echogenic density just cranial to the portal vein bifurcation on a transverse or longitudinal ultrasound scan) can distinguish infants with EHBA (and the presence of the triangular cord) from those who have other causes of cholestasis. The cord represents the fibrous remnant in the porta hepatis and, when seen, the authors recommend prompt laparotomy without further investigation. When it is absent, hepatic scintigraphy is done.[129]

Treatment of Cholestasis

The treatment of neonatal cholestasis involves treating the cause, although some pharmacologic agents have been used in an attempt to stimulate bile flow. Phenobarbital increases the uptake of bilirubin by the liver, induces conjugation, enhances bile acid synthesis, and increases bile flow. The administration of phenobarbital before performance of hepatic scintigraphy has helped to improve the reliability of this diagnostic test, but the therapeutic use of phenobarbital to improve bile flow and lower serum bilirubin concentrations in conditions such as

Table 12–8. Recommended Laboratory Tests for Evaluation of Neonatal Conjugated Hyperbilirubinemia

A. Liver function tests
  1. Total and direct-reacting serum bilirubin, total serum protein, and serum protein electrophoresis
  2. SGOT (AST), SGPT (ALT), alkaline phosphatase (5'-nucleotidase if alkaline phosphatase [elevated]), and gamma glutamyl transpeptidase (GGTP)
  3. Cholesterol
  4. Serum and urine bile acid concentrations if available
  5. Alpha₁-antitrypsin
  6. Technetium 99m iminodiacetic acid (^{99m}Tc-IDA) scan
  7. Alpha-fetoprotein
B. Hematologic tests
  1. Complete blood count, smear, and reticulocyte count
  2. Direct Coombs' test and erythrocyte glucose-6-phosphate dehydrogenase
  3. Platelet count
  4. Prothrombin time and partial thromboplastin time
C. Tests for infectious disease
  1. Cord blood IgM
  2. VDRL, FTA-ABS, complement fixation titers for rubella, cytomegalovirus, and herpes virus, and Sabin-Feldman dye test titer for toxoplasmosis
  3. HBsAg in both infant and mother
  4. Viral cultures from nose, pharynx, blood, stool, urine, and cerebrospinal fluid
D. Urine test
  1. Routine urinalysis, including protein and reducing substances
  2. Urine culture
  3. Bilirubin and urobilinogen
  4. Amino acid screening
E. Liver biopsy
  1. Light microscopy
  2. Specific enzyme assay (if indicated)
F. Radiologic/ultrasound studies as indicated
G. Additional specific diagnostic studies for metabolic disorders to be performed as indicated or suspected

From Halamek LP, Stevenson DK. Neonatal jaundice and liver disease. In Fanaroff AA, Martin RJ, eds: Neonatal-Perinatal Medicine. Diseases of the Fetus and Infant. St. Louis: Mosby, 1997, pp 1345–1389.

TPN-associated cholestasis has been disappointing.

The use of ursodeoxycholic acid (UDCA) appears to offer more promise. UDCA is a hydrophilic bile acid with a significant choleretic effect. It appears to be a relatively safe agent when used in children who do not have a fixed obstruction to bile flow.[134] It has been used in the treatment of cholestatic jaundice in infants with cystic fibrosis[149] as well as in an infant with erythroblastosis fetalis. In the latter case, a full-term infant with total and direct bilirubin values of 26 mg/dL (445 μmol/L) and 24.5 mg/dL (419 μmol/L), respectively, on the third day of life received UDCA, 25 mg/kg/day divided every 8 hours. Within 2 days, the bilirubin levels had decreased to 8.2 mg/dL (140 μmol/L) and 6.9 mg/dL (18 μmol/L), respectively.[131] UDCA may also be of value in the treatment of extreme hyperbilirubinemia in older children with the Crigler-Najjar syndrome. The mechanism of action of UDCA is not well understood, but it may affect the enterohepatic circulation of endogenous bile salts and increase hepatic bile flow.

◆ BILIRUBIN TOXICITY

The presence of bilirubin pigment at autopsy in the brains of infants who were severely jaundiced was observed more than 100 years ago and the term *kernicterus* was applied to infants who died and demonstrated bilirubin staining of the "kern," or nuclear region of the brain. The regions of the brain most commonly affected are the basal ganglia, particularly the subthalamic nucleus and the globus pallidus (Fig. 12–8); the hippocampus; the geniculate body; various brainstem nuclei, including the inferior colliculus, oculomotor, vestibular, cochlear, and inferior olivary nuclei; and the cerebellum, especially the dentate nucleus and vermis.[2] Neuronal necrosis is the dominant histopathologic feature after 7 to 10 days of postnatal life.

The areas of neuronal injury explain the clinical sequelae of bilirubin encephalopathy. In classic kernicterus, markedly jaundiced infants pass through three clinical phases. Initially, the infant becomes lethargic and hypotonic, and sucks poorly. Subse-

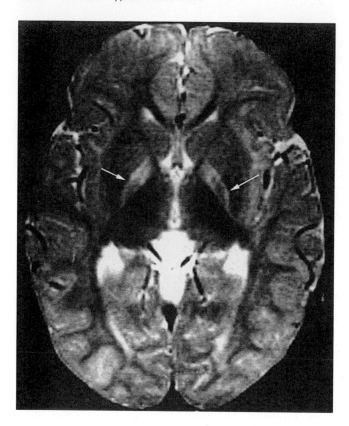

Figure 12–8. Magnetic resonance imaging scan of a 21-month-old male infant who had erythroblastosis fetalis and presented with extreme hyperbilirubinemia and clinical signs of kernicterus at age 54 hours. Note the symmetric, abnormally high-intensity signal from the area of the globus pallidus on both sides *(arrows).* (From Grobler JM, Mercer MJ: Kernicterus associated with elevated predominantly direct-reacting bilirubin. S Afr Med J 87:146, 1997.)

quently, hypertonia, fever, and a high-pitched cry develop. The hypertonia is characterized by backward arching of the neck (retrocollis) and trunk (opisthotonus). After about a week, the hypertonia subsides and is replaced by hypotonia. In those who survive, extrapyramidal disturbances (choreoathetosis), auditory abnormalities (sensorineural hearing loss most severe in the high frequencies), gaze palsies, and dental enamel hypoplasia develop.

The diagnosis of kernicterus can be confirmed by magnetic resonance imaging.[52, 130] The characteristic image is a bilateral, symmetric, high-intensity signal in the globus pallidus seen on both T1- and T2-weighted images (see Fig. 12–8). High signal intensity is also found in the hippocampus and thalamus.[130] Although there is no doubt about the relationship between extremely high bilirubin levels and acute bilirubin encephalopathy, it is possible that this outcome is only the most obvious and extreme manifestation of a spectrum of bilirubin toxicity. At the other end of the spectrum might lie more subtle forms of neurotoxicity that occur at lower bilirubin levels and in the absence of

any obvious clinical findings in the neonatal period.

Hemolytic Disease and Outcome

Initial observations in the late 1940s and early 1950s showed a strong relationship between increasing TSB levels (particularly greater than 20 mg/dL [342 μmol/L]) and the risk of kernicterus in infants with Rh hemolytic disease. Hsia et al[61] reported that the incidence of kernicterus in their erythroblastotic population was 8% for those with TSB levels of 19 to 24 mg/dL (325 to 410 μmol/L), 33% for TSB levels of 25 to 29 mg/dL (428 to 496 μmol/L), and 73% for those with levels greater than 30 mg/dL (513 μmol/L). Subsequent studies, however, found strikingly different outcomes. Of 129 infants born between 1957 and 1958, all of whom had *indirect* bilirubin levels greater than 20 mg/dL (342 μmol/L), neurodevelopmental damage was seen in only 2 of 92 (2%) when they were examined at 5 to 6 years of age with detailed psychometric, neurologic, and audiologic evaluations.[72]

Outcome in Nonhemolyzing Infants

The relationship between hyperbilirubinemia and poor developmental outcome in full-term and near-term infants who do not have hemolytic disease is even less clear. These issues have been addressed in multiple studies and readers are referred to recent extensive reviews that provide details of the individual studies.[69, 70, 119–121, 180] When analyzed as a whole, the data tend to demonstrate that, in otherwise healthy neonates without hemolytic disease, TSB levels that do not exceed approximately 25 mg/dL (428 μmol/L) do not place these infants at risk of adverse neurodevelopmental consequences. In such infants, there has been no convincing demonstration of any adverse affect of these bilirubin levels on IQs, definite neurologic abnormalities, or sensorineural hearing loss. There are no studies, however, specifically looking at infants of 35 to 37 weeks' gestation and the data on infants who have TSB levels of 25 to 30 mg/dL (292 to 513 μmol/L) are insufficient to draw firm conclusions about these TSB levels. In addition, there are limited data on the issue of *length of exposure* to these TSB levels and developmental outcome.[71, 119] Although one might presume that exposure to a TSB level of 23 mg/dL (393 μmol/L) for 48 hours is more hazardous than exposure to that level for 3 hours, this has yet to be demonstrated.

◆ EXTREME HYPERBILIRUBINEMIA AND KERNICTERUS

Several recent reports have identified classical kernicterus occurring in apparently healthy term and near-term newborns who did not have hemolytic disease but in whom extreme hyperbilirubinemia (>30 mg/dL [513 μmol/L]) developed.[24, 103] All of these infants were breast fed, many had excessive weight loss, and almost none were 40 weeks' gestation or older. Of 21 infants reported by Brown and Johnson,[24] all but one remained in hospital for 48 hours or less following birth. There are important lessons to be learned from these case reports and other evidence showing that short hospital stays are associated with a greater risk of severe hyperbilirubinemia.[24, 83, 87, 102, 156] In addition, there is strong and consistent evidence that infants with gestations of 35 to 37 weeks are at much higher risk of development of severe jaundice[102, 156] than those of 40 weeks' gestation or greater. Because these infants are cared for in normal newborn nurseries, it is often forgotten that they are much more likely to have difficulty nursing, to have poor caloric intake, and to experience a greater weight loss than their truly term counterparts. When combined with less effective hepatic clearance because of their prematurity, it is not surprising that they become more jaundiced.

◆ PREMATURE INFANTS

It is generally believed that premature infants are at a greater risk of development of bilirubin encephalopathy than are full-term newborns exposed to similar bilirubin levels, and it has been accepted practice to initiate phototherapy and exchange transfusion for low-birth-weight infants at TSB levels that are much lower than would be used to justify treatment in a full-term newborn (see later). The concern about kernicterus and low TSB levels in low-birth-weight infants arose because of the autopsy finding of kernicterus in infants whose TSB levels never exceeded 10 to 15 mg/dL[181] as well as studies that found impaired psychomotor performance at TSB levels of 10 to 14 mg/dL (171 to 239 μmol/L).[116, 148] Watchko and coworkers[181] have reviewed the history of kernicterus in preterm newborns as well as their experience over a 7-year period at the Magee Women's Hospital in Pittsburgh.[177] In 72 autopsies performed from 1984 through 1991 on newborns of less than 34 weeks' gestation who lived at least 48 hours, only three cases of kernicterus were identified. In the 69 newborns who did not have kernicterus, the peak TSB level ranged from 6.3 to 20.6 mg/dL (108 to 352 μmol/L), and 56% had peak TSB values greater than those suggested for exchange transfusion by the National Institute of Child Health and Human Development (NICHHD) phototherapy study guidelines.[25, 177] Thus, kernicterus in this population is uncommon even when TSB levels are allowed to increase to more than those previously thought to place the premature infant at risk. For reasons that are not clear, the autopsy diagnosis of kernicterus in preterm infants hospitalized in NICUs has decreased dramatically over the past decade or longer.[66, 177] This may be the result of overall improvements in care or the use of prophylactic phototherapy to prevent TSB levels from ever becoming sufficiently great to require exchange transfusion. Phototherapy is capable of controlling bilirubin levels in almost all low-birth-weight infants (see later) and exchange transfusions are rare events in most NICUs.[92]

◆ CELLULAR TOXICITY OF BILIRUBIN

It is not known exactly how bilirubin exerts its toxic effects and no single mechanism of bilirubin intoxication has been demonstrated in all cells. Bilirubin lowers membrane potential, decreases the rate of tyrosine uptake and dopamine synthesis in dopaminergic striatal synaptosomes, and impairs substrate transport, neurotransmitter synthesis, and mitochondrial functions in neurons.[34, 57]

Albumin Binding and the Concept of Free Bilirubin

Bilirubin (B) is transported in the plasma as a dianion bound tightly but reversibly to serum albumin (A):

$$B^{2-} + A \leftrightarrow AB^{2-}$$

The affinity of bilirubin for albumin is high and, as a result, concentrations of unbound (free) bilirubin in plasma are very low. Nevertheless, it is widely accepted that bilirubin toxicity occurs when free bilirubin enters the brain and binds to cell membranes.[182] The presence of albumin mitigates the in vivo and in vitro toxic effects of bilirubin,[182, 183] and drugs that decrease the albumin binding of bilirubin increase the risk of kernicterus.[136] Although there are many techniques available for measuring free or loosely bound bilirubin, none are currently in general use in the clinical management of the jaundiced newborn. Because one molecule of albumin is capable of binding one molecule of bilirubin tightly at the primary binding site, a bilirubin-to-albumin molar ratio of 1 represents about 8.5 mg/g of albumin. Thus, a term infant with a serum albumin concentration of 3 to 3.5 g/dL should be able to bind about 25 to 28 mg/dL of bilirubin (428–479 μmol/L). In sick low-birth-weight infants, the albumin binding capacity is reduced.

In calculating the risks of bilirubin toxicity, factors that affect the binding of bilirubin to albumin should be taken into account. Some of these factors include the concentration of free fatty acids that compete with bilirubin for its binding to albumin, although this does not occur until the molar ratio of free fatty acids to albumin exceeds 4:1.[23] Such ratios are generally not achieved with doses of up to 3 g/kg of intralipid given over 24 hours. The binding of bilirubin to albumin is not affected by changes in serum pH, but a decrease in pH does increase the binding of bilirubin to cells in the central nervous system.

Drugs can affect bilirubin—albumin binding both singly and in combination.[136, 137] Because of their bilirubin displacing capabilities, drugs that should be avoided in the immediate neonatal period, or at least until serum bilirubin levels are less than 5 mg/dL (85 μmol/L), include ethacrynic acid, azlocillin, carbenicillin, cefotetan, ceftriaxone, moxalactam, sulfisoxazole, and ticarcillin.[136]

Entry of Bilirubin Into the Brain

Under normal circumstances, there is a constant influx and efflux of bilirubin in and out of the brain and changes in the brainstem auditory evoked response can be demonstrated at modest elevations of serum bilirubin. These changes reverse as the bilirubin level decreases.[172] Bilirubin also enters the brain when there is a marked increase in the serum level of unbound bilirubin. Even bilirubin bound to albumin can enter the brain when the blood-brain barrier is disrupted,[22] and, in all of these situations, acidosis increases deposition of bilirubin in brain cells.

◆ CLINICAL MANAGEMENT

Has Kernicterus Returned?

There is some evidence that there is a re-emergence of kernicterus, a condition that had almost disappeared from the experience of pediatricians and neonatologists.[24, 36, 87, 103, 176] Contrary to the experience in the 1940s and 1950s, however, these are not infants with Rh hemolytic disease; rather, they are apparently healthy term and near-term newborns who have developed extreme hyperbilirubinemia (TSB >30 mg/dL). Such bilirubin levels occur only in about 1 to 3 in 10,000 infants. Thus, the average practitioner is unlikely to encounter such an infant. Some of the factors that appear to have contributed to this situation include short hospital stays for newborns, increased incidence of neonatal jaundice, less concern by pediatricians regarding jaundice, and failure to apply the meaning of bilirubin levels to the baby's age in hours, not days.

Short Hospital Stays for Newborns

There is evidence that early discharge is associated with an increased risk of significant hyperbilirubinemia[83, 86, 87, 102, 156] and even kernicterus.[24] Recognizing this problem, the AAP has recommended that infants discharged at less than 48 hours be seen within 2 to 3 days of discharge.[4] However, our data and those of Soskolne et al[102, 156] show that the risk of readmission for hyperbilirubinemia is similar whether the infant was discharged at less than 48 hours or between 48 and 72 hours. Reference to Figures 12–6 and 12–7 makes one thing clear: *If newborns leave the hospital before they are 36 hours old, their peak bilirubin level will occur after they are discharged.* Thus, jaundice is primarily an outpatient problem and monitoring and surveillance following discharge are essential if extreme hyperbilirubinemia is to be prevented.

Increased Incidence of Neonatal Jaundice

More significantly jaundiced babies are being seen than were seen in the 1950s and 1960s. The 95th percentile for TSB in the Collaborative Perinatal Project (1959–1966) was a TSB of at least 13 mg/dL (222 μmol/L).[59] In three studies, the 95th percentile was 15.0 to 17.5 mg/dL (265 to 308 μol/L).[17, 95, 118] Factors that may be responsible for this increase in jaundice include an increase in the number of breast-fed infants (30% at discharge in the 1960s; 60% in 1997),[144] an increase in East Asian babies in the United States, and short hospital stays.

Less Concern About Jaundice

Some pediatricians believe that hyperbilirubinemia, no matter how extreme, is harm-less if it occurs in an otherwise healthy breast-fed infant. Reports of kernicterus in such infants indicate that this is not the case.[103]

Failure to Apply Bilirubin Levels to Age in Hours

When erythroblastosis fetalis was prevalent, bilirubin levels in such infants were plotted on charts so that it was immediately obvious when the bilirubin level was increasing beyond the expected rate and could be anticipated to reach a level of 20 mg/dL (340 μmol/L). Exchange transfusions were then performed. Because phototherapy is effective, exchange transfusions may not be needed at these TSB levels, but clinicians still need to be able to identify an infant in whom the velocity of the increase in bilirubin indicates the possibility of an undiagnosed hemolytic process or the likelihood that the bilirubin level might continue to elevate and reach dangerous levels, even though this occurs only in a small percentage of these infants (see later).

Preventing Kernicterus in the Term and Near-Term Newborn

Table 12–1 lists factors that are clinically significant and most consistently associated with an increase in the risk of severe nonhemolytic jaundice. Attention to these risk factors helps identify infants who are at a particular risk of development of significant hyperbilirubinemia. Factors such as breastfeeding and decreasing gestation seem to play a particularly important role in the reported cases of extreme hyperbilirubinemia and kernicterus. Remarkably, essentially every recently described case of kernicterus has occurred in a breast-fed newborn,[24, 87, 103, 130] even when the infant had an underlying hemolytic process.[87, 130] In addition, most cases occurred in infants younger than 40 weeks' gestation.

Universal Newborn Bilirubin Screening

Severe hyperbilirubinemia is more likely to develop subsequently in infants who are clinically jaundiced in the first few days of life.[102] There is also an association between bilirubin levels in cord blood and subsequent bilirubin concentrations.[31, 81] Taking this into account, Bhutani and coworkers have developed a nomogram based on TSB levels obtained in 2840 term and near-term healthy infants.[17] By plotting bilirubin levels against the infant's age in hours, these investigators created percentiles that defined a high-risk (>95th percentile), a low-risk (<40th percentile), and an intermediate risk (40th to 95th percentile) zone (see Fig. 12–7). The results of this study are listed in Table 12–9 and indicate that obtaining a single TSB level on every baby before discharge is a useful way of predicting the risk (or absence of risk) of subsequent significant hyperbilirubinemia. If this is confirmed in other studies, a group of infants could be identified who, *at least as far as hyperbilirubinemia is concerned*, do not require early follow-up—information that could be very useful in populations in which early follow-up is difficult or impossible. Clearly, those infants whose TSB levels fall in the high-risk zone require more careful surveillance and follow-up. In practical terms, the addition of a TSB measurement for every newborn does not require any additional blood sampling in that it can be obtained at the same time as the standard metabolic screen, performed on all infants in the United States.

Measuring Bilirubin Production

When heme is catabolized, carbon monoxide (CO) is produced in equimolar quantities with bilirubin and measurements of end tidal CO, corrected for ambient CO ($ETCO_c$), provide a noninvasive technique for quantifying hemolysis.[157] A measurement of $ETCO_c$ before discharge could identify infants with high rates of bilirubin production and, therefore, in need of more careful follow-up.

◆ PREVENTING EXTREME HYPERBILIRUBINEMIA

If every baby, regardless of risk factors, were seen within 72 to 96 hours of birth, significantly jaundiced infants would be identified and appropriate follow-up and intervention (when necessary) instituted. Such follow-up is not always possible, however, and many infants discharged at less than 48 hours are not being seen earlier than 1 to 2 weeks after discharge.[101] Although the AAP recommends early follow-up only for babies discharged before 48 hours,[4, 5] we and others have shown that infants discharged between 48 and 72 hours are *at as great a risk for readmission with significant jaundice as those discharged before 48 hours.*[102, 156] We, therefore, recommend that any infant discharged before 72 hours of age should be seen by a health care professional within 1 to 2 days of discharge. An approach to the management and follow-up of these infants is summarized in Tables 12–3 and 12–4.

◆ TREATMENT
Term and Near-Term Newborns

Guidelines for the treatment of full-term and near-term infants are provided in Table 12–10. These guidelines, developed by the AAP,[4] refer only to newborns of greater than or equal to 37 weeks' gestation, but there are many infants at 34 to 36 weeks' gestation who are cared for in well-baby nurseries and who are managed no differently. Some clinicians may prefer to use slightly lower TSB levels for intervention with phototherapy or exchange transfusions for infants who are 35 to 36 weeks' gestation. There is little doubt that, if significantly jaundiced infants were identified and these guidelines followed, kernicterus would almost never be seen. Although the treatment levels used are, in my opinion, appropriate, some of the bilirubin levels chosen by the AAP Practice

Table 12–9. Predischarge Bilirubin Levels and Risk of Subsequent Hyperbilirubinemia

TSB Before Discharge		TSB After Discharge
Percentile	n	>95th percentile
>95th	172 (6.1%)	68/172 (39.5%)
76th–95th	356 (12.5%)	46/356 (12.9%)
40th–75th	556 (19.6%)	12/556 (2.15%)
<40th	1756 (61.8%)*	0/1756
Total	2840	126 (4.4%)

*Newborn TSB levels were obtained between 18 and 72 hours of life and 61.8% of all values obtained were below the 40th percentile.
TSB, Total serum bilirubin.
Data from Bhutani VK, Johnson L, Sivieri EM: Predictive ability of a predischarge hour-specific serum bilirubin for subsequent significant hyperbilirubinemia in healthy term and near-term newborns. Pediatrics 103:6–14, 1999.

Table 12–10. Management of Hyperbilirubinemia in the Apparently Healthy Term and Near-Term Newborn

	TSB LEVEL, mg/dL (μmol/L)			
Age (h)	Consider Phototherapy*	Phototherapy	Exchange Transfusion if Intensive Phototherapy Fails†	Exchange Transfusion and Intensive Phototherapy
≤24‡	—	—	—	—
25–48	≥12 (205)	≥15 (260)	≥20 (340)	≥25 (430)
49–72	≥15 (260)	≥18 (310)	≥25 (430)	≥30 (510)
>72	≥17 (290)	≥20 (340)	≥25 (430)	≥30 (510)

*Phototherapy at these TSB levels is a clinical option, meaning that the intervention is available and may be used on the basis of individual clinical judgment.

†Intensive phototherapy should produce a decline of TSB of 1 to 2 mg/dL within 4–6 hours, and the TSB level should continue to decline and remain below the threshold level for exchange transfusion. If this does not occur, it is considered a failure of phototherapy.

‡Term infants who are clinically jaundiced at ≤24 hours old are not considered healthy and require further evaluation.

TSB, total serum bilirubin.

Adapted from American Academy of Pediatrics Provisional Committee for Quality Improvement and Subcommittee on Hyperbilirubinemia: Practice Parameter: Management of hyperbilirubinemia in the healthy term newborn. Pediatrics 96:788–790, 1995.

Parameter for the initiation of phototherapy suggest that the infant may not, in fact, be "healthy." Hence, the title of the table has been modified to read "in the apparently healthy term and near-term newborn." The reason for this somewhat subtle change is that the guidelines recommend phototherapy when the TSB level is greater than or equal to 15 mg/dL (260 μmol/L) in a 25- to 48-hour-old infant (see Table 12–10). But a TSB of greater than or equal to 15 mg/dL (260 μmol/L) at 26 hours is far more than the 95th percentile and is even greater than the 95th percentile for a 48-hour-old infant (see Figs. 12–6 and 12–7).[17, 93] The same applies to a TSB level of 18 mg/dL (310 μmol/L) at 49 to 72 hours and of 20 mg/dL (340 μmol/L) at 72 hours or greater. Infants who develop these TSB levels have either increased bilirubin production or inadequate clearance, or both, and merit investigation for the cause of their hyperbilirubinemia.

Intervention in the Breast-Fed Infant

Of infants with TSB levels high enough to require phototherapy and who do not have evidence of isoimmunization or other obvious hemolytic disease, 80% to 90% are fully or partially breast-fed.[99] It is likely that much of this hyperbilirubinemia is associated with *inadequate* breast-feeding and that increasing the frequency of breast-feeding during the first few days after birth will decrease TSB levels.[33, 171, 189] Supplemental feedings of water or dextrose water should *never* be provided to breast-fed infants because this does not lower their TSB levels.[32, 124] If supplementation is deemed necessary, formula should be provided. It is always undesirable to interrupt nursing and, when the TSB in a breast-fed infant reaches a level at which intervention is being considered, it is our practice to recommend that breast-feeding be continued while the infant undergoes treatment with intensive phototherapy (see Phototherapy).

Low-Birth-Weight Infants

Table 12–11 provides guidelines for the management of hyperbilirubinemia in low-birth-weight infants. Over the past 2 decades, phototherapy has dramatically decreased the necessity for exchange transfusion, a procedure that is currently almost exclusively carried out in the occasional infant who has severe Rh hemolytic disease or extensive bruising. We have not performed a single exchange transfusion in our population of newborns with birth weights less than 1500 g in the past 10 years.[92] As discussed earlier, the criteria previously used for exchange transfusion in the low-birth-weight population have been questioned[177] and the use of more effective phototherapy has obviated the need for exchange transfusion in much of this population. Furthermore, exchange transfusion at very low bili-

Table 12–11. Approaches to the Use of Phototherapy and Exchange Transfusion in Low-Birth-Weight Infants*

Birth Weight (g)	Total Bilirubin Level (mg/dL [μmol/L]†)	
	Phototherapy‡	Exchange Transfusion¶
<1,500	5–8 (85–140)	13–16 (220–275)
1500–1999	8–12 (140–200)	16–18 (275–300)
2000–2499	11–14 (190–240)	18–20 (300–340)

*These guidelines reflect ranges used in neonatal intensive care units. They do not take into account all possible situations. In some units, prophylactic phototherapy is used for all infants who weigh <1500 g. Higher intervention levels may be used for small-for-gestational-age infants, based on gestational age rather than birth weight.

†Consider initiating therapy at these levels. Range allows discretion based on clinical conditions or other circumstances.

‡Used at these levels in therapeutic doses, phototherapy should, with few exceptions, eliminate the need for exchange transfusions.

¶Levels for exchange transfusion assume that bilirubin continues to rise or remains at these levels despite intensive phototherapy.

From Maisels MJ: Jaundice. In Avery GB, Fletcher MA, MacDonald MG, eds: Neonatology: Pathophysiology and Management of the Newborn. Philadelphia: JB Lippincott, 1999, pp 765–819.

rubin levels is inefficient and much less effective than phototherapy in achieving a prolonged reduction of TSB levels in infants with nonhemolytic jaundice.[159] Although there is little evidence to support the practice, it is common to institute phototherapy in low-birth-weight infants according to a sliding scale (see Table 12–11): the lower the birth weight, the lower the TSB level at which phototherapy is instituted. Bilirubin is a powerful antioxidant and some researchers have raised the possibility that maintaining very low TSB levels by the aggressive use of phototherapy might be associated with an increase in severe retinopathy of prematurity (ROP).[191] On the other hand, in a study of 157 surviving infants of 23 to 26 weeks' gestation in our NICU, De-Jonge et al found no association between bilirubin levels, severe ROP, or any stage of ROP.[35]

Elevated Direct-Reacting or Conjugated Bilirubin Levels

There are no good data to guide the clinician in dealing with the occasional infant who has a high TSB as well as a significant elevation of direct-reacting bilirubin. Kernicterus has occurred in infants with TSB levels greater than 20 mg/dL (314 μmol/L) but, because of significant elevations in direct bilirubin levels, the indirect bilirubin levels were well below 20 mg/dL (340 μmol/L). There is evidence that elevated direct bilirubin levels decrease the infant's albumin-binding capacity.[38] The magnetic resonance image shown in Figure 12–8 was obtained from an infant with Rh erythroblastosis fetalis in whom a TSB of 45.2 mg/dL (773 μmol/L) developed, of which 31.6 mg/dL (514 μmol) was direct reacting.[52] It is commonly recommended that the direct bilirubin concentration should not be subtracted from the total bilirubin level unless it exceeds 50% of the TSB concentration. This seems reasonable but would not have benefited the infant with Rh erythroblastosis described previously.[52] One intervention that might be worth trying under these circumstances is the administration of UDCA (see Treatment of Cholestasis).

Hemolytic Disease

Infants with hemolytic disease are generally considered to be at a greater risk for the development of bilirubin encephalopathy than are nonhemolyzing infants with similar bilirubin levels, although the reasons for this are not clear. In Rh hemolytic disease, phototherapy should be used early, as soon as there is evidence for a rapidly increasing bilirubin level. On the other hand, in ABO hemolytic disease, early elevating TSB levels frequently plateau and decline spontaneously and phototherapy is often unnecessary.[126] Nevertheless, if ABO hemolytic disease is suspected, phototherapy is usually instituted at TSB levels 1 to 3 mg/dL (17 to 51 μmol/L) less than those listed in Table 12–10. If, despite intensive phototherapy, TSB levels approach 18 to 20 mg/dL (308–342 μmol/L) in any infant with hemo-

Table 12–12. Radiometric Quantities Used

Quantity	Dimensions	Usual Units of Measure
Irradiance (radiant power incident on a surface per unit area of the surface)	W/m²	W/cm²
Spectral irradiance (irradiance in a certain wavelength band)	W/m² per nm (or W/m²)	μW/cm² per nm
Spectral power (average spectral irradiance across a surface area)	W/m	mW/nm

From Maisels MJ: Why use homeopathic doses of phototherapy? Pediatrics 98:283–287, 1996.

lytic disease, exchange transfusion should be considered. A recent innovation has been the use of intravenous gamma-globulin (IVIG), which, in controlled trials, has been successful in reducing the need for exchange transfusions in both Rh and ABO hemolytic disease.[143, 146] Tin-mesoporphyrin (SnMP) has also decreased TSB levels in infants with Coombs-positive ABO incompatibility and in G6PD deficiency[77, 167] (see Pharmacologic Treatment).

Hydrops Fetalis

The pathogenesis of hydrops fetalis is not fully understood. In the fetal sheep model, acute severe anemia leads to hydrops associated with increased venous pressure and placental edema, whereas the same degree of anemia produced over a longer period does not.[19] Thus, high output failure resulting from anemia is probably not the primary mechanism for hydrops. Profound extramedullary hematopoiesis occurs in the fetus with erythroblastosis fetalis and this leads to both portal hypertension and disruption of normal liver function. It is likely that these are the primary mechanisms responsible for the development of hydrops in isoimmune hemolytic disease.[11, 51, 123] Hydropic infants are commonly hypoxic and severely anemic, and they demand immediate treatment. Exchange transfusion of 50 mL/kg of packed cells soon after birth increases their hematocrits to about 40%. Phlebotomy should not be performed routinely on these infants because they are usually normovolemic and may even be hypovolemic,[11, 122, 132] and their blood volume should not be manipulated without appropriate measurements of central venous and arterial blood pressures. In order to measure central venous pressure (CVP) accurately, the umbilical venous catheter must enter the

inferior vena cava via the ductus venosus. If the catheter is in a portal vein or the umbilical vein, the pressures so measured are meaningless and preclude interpretation of the infant's circulatory status. In addition, before making therapeutic decisions based on measurements of CVP, acidosis, hypercarbia, hypoxia, and anemia (all of which can affect the measured CVP) must be corrected. Serum glucose levels must be monitored carefully because hypoglycemia is common.

◆ PHOTOTHERAPY

Phototherapy is by far the most widely used treatment for hyperbilirubinemia, and it is both safe and effective. Phototherapy works in much the same way as do drugs—the absorption of photons of light by bilirubin molecules in the skin produces a therapeutic effect similar to the binding of drug molecules to a receptor. Whereas drug doses are conveniently measured in units of weight, photon dosages are more difficult to measure and are expressed in less familiar terms. Table 12–12 defines the radiometric quantities used in assessing the dose of phototherapy and Table 12–13 lists the major factors that influence the dose and, therefore, the efficacy of phototherapy.

Light Spectrum

The optical properties of bilirubin and skin determine the light wavelengths that most

Table 12–13. Factors That Determine Dose of Phototherapy

Spectrum of light emitted
Irradiance of light source
Design of phototherapy unit
Surface area of infant exposed to the light
Distance of infant from light source

effectively lower bilirubin; these are wavelengths that are predominately in the blue-green spectrum.[1] *Note that none of the light systems used in phototherapy emit any significant amount of ultraviolet (UV) radiation and ultraviolet light is never used for phototherapy.* A small amount of UV light is emitted by fluorescent tubes, but this UV light is in longer wavelengths (>320 nm) than those that cause erythema and, in any case, almost all UV light produced is absorbed by the glass wall of the fluorescent tube and by the Plexiglas cover of the phototherapy unit.

Irradiance

There is a direct relationship between the efficacy of phototherapy and the *irradiance* used[160] (Fig. 12–9), and irradiance is directly related to the distance between the light and the infant (Fig. 12–10). The irradiance in a certain wavelength band is called the *spectral irradiance* and is expressed as $\mu W/cm^2/nm$. As shown in Figure 12–10, there is strong inverse relationship between the light intensity (measured as spectral irradiance) and the distance from the light source. Thus, the closer the phototherapy lamp is to the infant, the more effective it is. (Certain lamps cannot be put close to the infant because of the risk of a burn; see Halogen Lamps.)

Spectral Power

The *spectral power* is the product of the skin surface irradiance and the spectral irradiance across this surface area. Calculations of spectral power permit comparisons of the dose of phototherapy received by infants under different phototherapy systems. Because infants have a small surface area, fiberoptic systems provide far less spectral power than that obtained from a bank of special blue fluorescent tubes.

Mechanism of Action

It is not known exactly where phototherapy takes place, but a biologic response to light can only occur if the light is absorbed by a photoreceptor molecule.[109] When cultured cells are incubated with bilirubin (allowing the bilirubin to be bound to the cells) and then exposed to visible light, no photoisomers are found, whereas they are found in irradiated samples of bilirubin–albumin mixtures.[27] These data suggest that conversion of bilirubin to photoisomers during phototherapy does not take place in skin cells, but most likely takes place in bilirubin bound to albumin in the blood vessels or in the interstitial space.

Phototherapy detoxifies bilirubin by converting it to photoproducts that are more lipophilic than bilirubin and can bypass the conjugating system of the liver and be excreted without further metabolism.[108] The effectiveness of different light wavelengths is expressed as an *action spectrum,* but when applying the action spectrum to phototherapy, corrections have to be made for the optical properties of skin and the fact that skin blocks shorter wavelengths and visible light more than do longer wavelengths. It

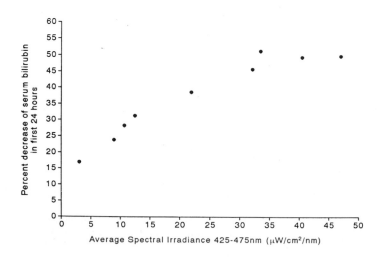

Figure 12–9. Relationship between average spectral irradiance and decrease in serum bilirubin concentration. Full-term infants with nonhemolytic hyperbilirubinemia were exposed to special blue light (Phillips TL52/20W) of different intensities. Spectral irradiance was measured as the average of readings at the head, trunk, and knees. Drawn from the data of Tan.[160] (From Maisels MJ: Why use homeopathic doses of phototherapy? Pediatrics 98:283–287, 1996.)

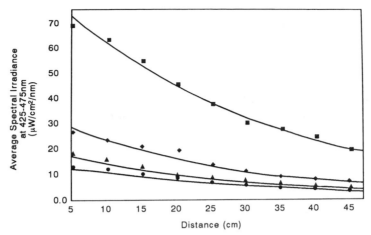

Figure 12–10. Effect of light source and distance from the light source to the infant on average spectral irradiance. Measurements were made across the 425- to 475-nm band using a commercial radiometer (Olympic Bilimeter Mark II). The phototherapy unit was fitted with eight 24-in fluorescent tubes. ■, Special blue, General Electric 20-W F20T12/BB tube; ◆, blue, General Electric 20-w F20T12/B blue tube; ▲, daylight blue, four General Electric 20-W F20T12/D blue tubes and four Sylvania 20-W F20T12/D daylight tubes; ●, daylight, Sylvania 20-W F20T12/D daylight tube. Curves were plotted using linear curve fitting (True Epistat, Epistat Services, Richardson, TX). The best fit is described by the equation $y = Ae^{BX}$. (From Maisels MJ: Why use homeopathic doses of phototherapy? Pediatrics 98:283–287, 1996.)

appears that the most effective light source for phototherapy is one that emits in the blue-green spectral region between 490 and 510 nm.[1]

Bilirubin Photochemistry

During phototherapy, bilirubin absorbs light, and three photochemical reactions have been shown to occur in vivo.[42, 108]

Configurational (Z→E) Isomerization

This process occurs with compounds containing double bonds. The presence of two asymmetrically substituted double bonds in

bilirubin, one at carbon atom C4 and the other at C15 (Fig. 12–11), means that there are four possible configurational isomers of bilirubin (Fig. 12–12). Because of the preference that albumin-bound bilirubin shows for configurational isomerization at the double bond between C15 and C16 rather than C4 and C5, during phototherapy the stable 4Z15Z isomer is converted predominately to the 4Z15E isomer (see Figs. 12–11 and 12–12). Unlike photooxidation or lumirubin formation (see later text), the formation of 4Z15E-bilirubin is spontaneously reversible in the dark, and this reaction occurs rapidly in bile where the 4Z15E bilirubin is converted back to ordinary unconjugated bilirubin.

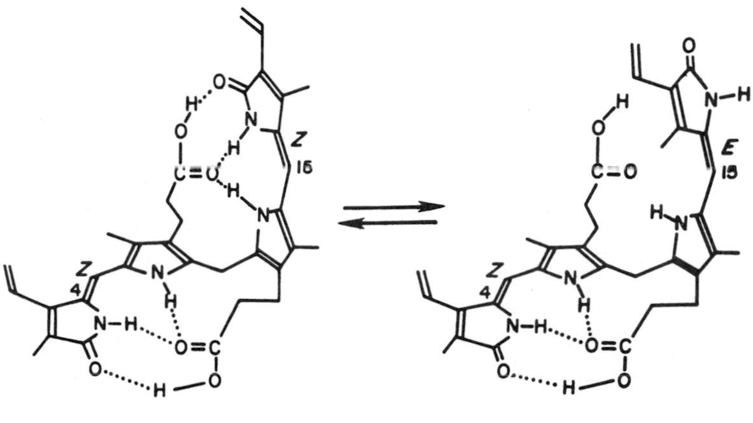

Figure 12–11. Z-E carbon—carbon double bond configurational isomerization of bilirubin in humans. (From McDonagh AF, Lightner DA: "Like a shrivelled blood orange"— Bilirubin, jaundice and phototherapy. Pediatrics 75:443–455, 1985.)

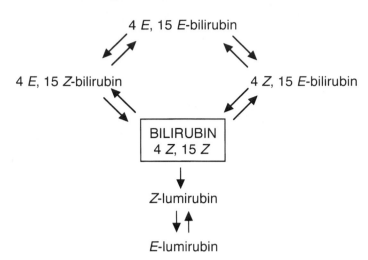

4 E, 15 E-bilirubin

4 E, 15 Z-bilirubin   4 Z, 15 E-bilirubin

BILIRUBIN
4 Z, 15 Z

Z-lumirubin

E-lumirubin

Figure 12–12. Configurational and structural isomers of 4Z, 15Z bilirubin in infants undergoing phototherapy. (From Maisels MJ: Jaundice. In Avery GB, Fletcher MA, MacDonald MG, eds: Neonatology: Pathophysiology and Management of the Newborn. Philadelphia: JB Lippincott, 1999, pp 765–819.)

The whole process of isomerization during phototherapy, the transport of isomers from the skin, and the excretion of isomers in bile is exceptionally efficient. In the Gunn rat, phototherapy produces virtually instantaneous changes in bile composition,[110] but, in infants, *clearance of the light-generated 4Z15E isomer is very slow*[43] and a steady-state concentration of the two isomers is achieved within 3 to 4 hours after initiation of phototherapy. The steady-state amount of the 4Z15E isomer is dependent on the wavelength of the light used, but it is independent of intensity. Thus, although configurational isomerization is rapid and accounts for most of the bilirubin isomerization, it probably plays only a minor role in lowering the serum bilirubin concentration because "although it is formed fastest, it has nowhere to go."[42]

Structural Isomerization

Intramolecular cyclization of bilirubin is an irreversible process that occurs in the presence of light to form a substance known as *lumirubin* (Figs. 12–12 and 12–13). Like the configurational isomer photobilirubin, lumirubin can be excreted in bile (without the need for conjugation) but it is also excreted in urine, although at a much lower rate than in bile.[42] During phototherapy, the configurational isomers formed represent about 20% of the total bilirubin concentration, whereas the concentration of lumirubin is only 2% to 6% of total bilirubin. But lumirubin is cleared from the serum much more rapidly than the 4Z15E isomer, the mean serum half-life of lumirubin being less than 2 hours compared with 15 hours for the 4Z15E isomer.[42] In addition, the formation of lumirubin is not reversible and, once formed, it is excreted unchanged in the bile and the urine. Thus, it is likely that lumirubin formation is mainly responsible for the phototherapy-induced decline in serum bilirubin in the human infant. The general mechanisms of phototherapy are illustrated in Figure 12–14.

It is important to recognize that the proc-

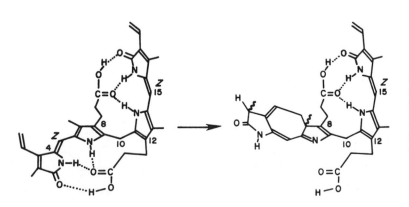

Figure 12–13. Intramolecular cyclization of bilirubin in the presence of light to form lumirubin. (From McDonagh AF, Lightner DA: "Like a shrivelled blood orange"—Bilirubin, jaundice and phototherapy. Pediatrics 75:443–455, 1985.)

Figure 12–14. General mechanisms of phototherapy for neonatal jaundice. Chemical reactions *(solid arrows)* and transport processes *(broken arrows)* are indicated. Pigments may be bound to proteins in compartments other than blood. Some excretion of photoisomers, particularly lumirubin, in urine also occurs. (From McDonagh AF, Lightner DA: "Like a shrivelled blood orange"—Bilirubin, jaundice and phototherapy. Pediatrics 75:443–455, 1985.)

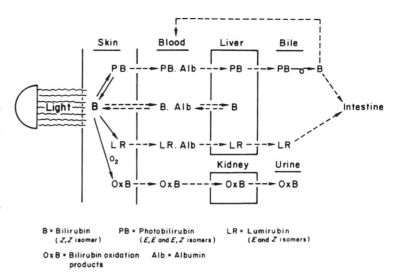

ess of bilirubin detoxification starts as soon as the phototherapy lights are switched on. Because the plasma bilirubin represents only about one third of the bilirubin in the body, a decrease in the serum bilirubin concentration is a secondary effect of phototherapy. Regardless of what happens to the plasma concentration, phototherapy helps to detoxify and eliminate bilirubin.[108]

Photooxidation

Bilirubin gradually disappears from serum samples exposed to sunlight and this bleaching phenomenon is the result of the photooxidation of bilirubin to water-soluble, colorless products that can be excreted in the urine. This process is slow, however, and probably contributes only in a minor way to the elimination of bilirubin during phototherapy.[108]

Clinical Use and Efficacy

Phototherapy is an effective and efficient mechanism for the prevention and treatment of hyperbilirubinemia and dramatically reduces the need for exchange transfusion.[92] There are more than 50 published controlled trials confirming the efficacy of phototherapy.[89] Some idea of the magnitude of the effect of phototherapy can be gauged by the fact that there are many residents in pediatric training programs who, by the end of their 3 years of training, have never seen an exchange transfusion, let alone performed one. The time is not far distant when even those trained in the subspecialty of neonatology might have little exposure to this procedure.[92]

Dose-Response Relationship

Figure 12–9 shows that there is a clear relationship between the dose of phototherapy and the decline in the TSB level and Table 12–13 lists the factors that determine the dose. The initial TSB level is also an important factor that influences the rate of decline of serum bilirubin, the rate being proportional to the initial bilirubin concentration.[68] Because configurational isomers formed during light treatment revert to natural unconjugated bilirubin in the intestine following hepatic excretion, reabsorption of natural bilirubin occurs via the enterohepatic circulation and contributes to the bilirubin load to be cleared by the liver. Both of these phenomena account for why light treatment is most effective during the first 24 hours of therapy, after which the efficacy decreases.

Types of Light

Fluorescent Tubes

Daylight or cool white fluorescent tubes are the most widely used fluorescent light sources. They provide energy in a 300- to 700-nm range with little output in the blue spectrum. They are satisfactory for providing prophylactic phototherapy when the objective is to control a slowly increasing bilirubin level in a preterm or term infant, but they are much less effective than special blue fluorescent tubes, which provide significantly more irradiance in the blue spectrum than any other commercially available tubes (see Fig. 12–10). Special blue tubes are the most effective light source currently available in the United States for phototherapy. They are labeled F20T12/BB (General Electric, Westinghouse) or TL52/20W (Phillips). These are different from regular blue tubes (F20T12/B), which provide only slightly more irradiance than daylight or cool white tubes (see Fig. 12–10).

Halogen Lamps

High-pressure mercury vapor halide lamps provide reasonably good output in the blue range and have the advantage of being much more compact than lamps containing standard fluorescent tubes. An important disadvantage, however, is that, unlike fluorescent lamps they *cannot be brought close to the infant (to increase the irradiance) without incurring the risk of a burn*. Furthermore, the surface area covered by most halogen lamps is small and the spectral power, therefore, is less than that produced by a bank of fluorescent lamps.

Fiberoptic Systems

Fiberoptic phototherapy systems contain a tungsten-halogen bulb that delivers light via a fiberoptic cable to be emitted by the sides and ends of the fibers inside a plastic pad. These systems have the advantage of being less bulky than conventional phototherapy equipment and infants can be held and nursed while they receive phototherapy. In addition, eye patches are unnecessary. They also provide a convenient way of delivering phototherapy above and below the infant simultaneously. The high intensity (irradiance) settings on the fiberoptic pads produce an average spectral irradiance of about 22 to 23 μW/cm^2/nm in the 420- to 480-nm band. Although this output is reasonable (but not nearly as high as that obtained from special blue fluorescent tubes; see Fig. 12–10), fiberoptic pads cover only a small surface area, thus significantly reducing the spectral power achieved. A larger pad would require the light to be distributed over a greater area, thus reducing the irradiance (when compared with a smaller pad with the same light source). To achieve adequate levels of spectral irradiance, the manufacturers have compromised by reducing the size of the pad and, therefore, the overall efficacy of the device.

Light-Emitting Diodes

The use of high-intensity gallium nitride light-emitting diodes (LEDs) permits higher irradiance to be delivered in the spectrum of choice (e.g., blue, blue-green) with minimal heat generation.[153, 175] This is a low-weight, low-voltage, low-power, portable device that could be an effective means of providing intensive phototherapy in the hospital or at home. Only limited clinical trials have been performed.[153]

Using Phototherapy Effectively

In the NICU, phototherapy is used primarily as a prophylactic therapy, to prevent slowly increasing serum bilirubin levels from reaching levels that might require an exchange transfusion. When full-term infants remained in the hospital for 3 to 5 days, phototherapy was also commonly used to treat modestly jaundiced infants. Currently, full-term and near-term infants who need phototherapy are generally those who have left the hospital and are readmitted on days 4 to 7 for treatment of severe hyperbilirubinemia. Such infants need a therapeutic dose of phototherapy (sometimes termed *intensive phototherapy*) in order to diminish the bilirubin as soon as possible.[90] The most effective way of delivering intensive phototherapy is to use special blue fluorescent tubes and to bring them as close as possible to the infant (see Fig. 12–10).[90] To do this, a term or near-term infant *must be in a bassinet, not an incubator* (the top of the incubator prevents the light from being brought sufficiently close to the infant). When needed in low-birth-weight infants or infants in the NICU, the special blue fluorescent lights can be placed between the radiant warmer and the warmer bed. In either case, the light should be no further than 10 cm from the infant. At this distance, special blue fluorescent tubes provide an average spectral irradiance of more than 50 μW/cm^2/nm (see Fig. 12–2). This situation does not produce significant warming of naked full-term infants and, if slight warming does occur, the lamps can be elevated slightly. *Halogen phototherapy lamps cannot be positioned closer to the infant than recommended by the manufacturers without incurring the risk of a burn.*

The use of fiberoptic pads has made it easy to increase the surface area of the infant exposed to phototherapy and this type of "double phototherapy" is approximately twice as effective as single phototherapy in low-birth-weight infants[60, 161] and almost 50% better in full-term infants.[161] The better response of low-birth-weight infants is likely the result of the fact that, at similar levels of irradiance, the fiberoptic pad covers more of a small infant than a large one. Another way of increasing the exposed surface area is to place reflecting material such as aluminum foil around the bassinet or incubator so that light is reflected onto the infant's skin.[40]

Using a combination of special blue tubes and a fiberoptic blanket underneath the infant, we achieve, on average, a decline of 33% in TSB concentrations within 24 hours. Under certain circumstances, even more dramatic declines in the TSB can be achieved.[56] Using two special blue fluorescent units and a fiberoptic pad, Hansen[56] was able to achieve a decline in the TSB of 10 to 11 mg/dL (170 to 185 μmol/L) within 2 to 3 hours in three infants with TSB levels greater than 30 mg/dL (513 μmol/L). Although earlier data suggested that there may be a point beyond which an increase in irradiance produces no added efficacy,[160] it is unknown whether a saturation point exists and, given that the conversion of bilirubin to excretable photoproducts is partly irreversible and follows first order kinetics, there may not be a saturation point. *Certainly with existing equipment there is no such thing as an overdose of phototherapy.*

Intermittent Versus Continuous Therapy

Because light exposure increases bilirubin excretion (compared with darkness), continuous phototherapy should be more efficient than intermittent phototherapy. However, clinical studies comparing these two methods have produced conflicting results.[67] If bilirubin levels are very high, intensive phototherapy should be administered continuously until a satisfactory decline in the TSB level has occurred. On the other hand, in most circumstances, phototherapy does not *need* to be continuous and it should certainly be interrupted during feeding or parental visits when eye patches must be removed to allow appropriate parent-infant contact.

Hydration

Because some of the lumirubin produced during phototherapy is excreted in urine, maintaining adequate hydration and a good urine output does help to improve the efficacy of phototherapy.[185] However, routine supplementation (with dextrose water) of all infants receiving phototherapy is not necessary unless there is evidence that the infant is dehydrated. In such infants it makes more sense to provide both supplemental calories and fluids using a milk-based formula because formula inhibits the enterohepatic circulation of bilirubin and helps to lower the bilirubin level.

Biological Effects and Complications

Even though phototherapy has been used on millions of infants for more than 30 years, reports of significant toxicity are exceptionally rare. Bilirubin is a photosensitizer and, in some circumstances, can act as a photodynamic agent in the presence of light and produce damage. In infants with congenital erythropoietic porphyria,[164] phototherapy produces severe blistering and photosensitivity and congenital porphyria is an absolute contraindication to the use of phototherapy. This proscription has been reinforced recently by reports documenting purpuric or bullous eruptions in infants with hemolytic disease and transient porphyrinemia who received phototherapy.[105, 128] All of these infants had significant direct hyperbilirubinemia and elevated plasma porphyrin levels. Significant accumulation of coproporphyrin has also been described in infants with *the bronze baby syndrome,* which occurs exclusively in phototherapy exposed infants who also have cholestasis. In the bronze baby syndrome, dark, grayish brown discoloration develops in the skin, serum, and urine in infants with cholestatic jaundice who are exposed to phototherapy.[82, 142] The pathogenesis of this syndrome is unknown, but it may be related to an accumulation of porphyrins in the plasma.[73]

A 32-week gestation neonate who received intravenous fluorescein for angiography and subsequently received phototherapy suffered a partial thickness burn, probably related to the phototoxicity from the fluorescein, which has been shown to produce photosensitization by generation of a superoxide anion when exposed to light at a wavelength of 480 nm in the visible light range.[79] Complications of the use of fiberoptic phototherapy blankets have been reported in extremely premature infants (less than or equal to 25 weeks' gestation) and these have included extensive, erythematous denuded areas of skin, resembling a partial thickness burn as well as purplish-red necrotizing lesions.[62, 112] All of these infants had conditions that might reduce skin integrity such as birth trauma, hypotension, poor perfusion of the skin, or bacterial contamination of the incubator or bed. It is important to note that the skin of these extremely premature infants is remarkably fragile.

Although light is toxic to the retina, as long as the infant's eyes are protected with appropriate eye patches, there have been no recorded abnormalities of visual function, electroretinography, or changes in the pattern of visual-evoked potential responses.[15, 37, 140]

Infants receiving phototherapy have an increase in peripheral blood flow and an increase in insensible water loss that, in non–servo-controlled incubators, can be considerable.[186] The use of servo-controlled incubators mitigates these effects.

Phototherapy decreases the expected postprandial increase in blood flow velocity in the superior mesenteric artery[190] and might also increase cerebral blood flow velocity in preterm infants of 32 weeks' gestation or younger.[14] This could be the result of a photochemical reaction to light and might increase the risk of intraventricular hemorrhage. Phototherapy also increases the likelihood of a patent ductus arteriosus in very low-birth-weight infants.[10, 14, 138] In one study, a previously closed ductus arteriosus reopened in 10 of 22 infants receiving phototherapy.[14]

A 6-year follow-up of children in the NICHHD cooperative phototherapy study showed no differences between the phototherapy or control groups in any aspect of growth or developmental outcome.[147]

◆ EXCHANGE TRANSFUSION

Exchange transfusion removes bilirubin-laden blood from the circulation and replaces it with donor blood (usually packed red cells reconstituted with plasma). In addition to removing bilirubin, when used in the treatment of immune-mediated hemolytic disease, it accomplishes the additional goals of:

1. Removal of antibody-coated red blood cells
2. Correction of anemia
3. Removal of maternal antibody
4. Removal of other potential toxic byproducts of the hemolytic process

A double-volume exchange transfusion (approximately 170 mL/kg) removes about 85% of the infant's red blood cells, but because most of the infant's bilirubin is in the extravascular compartment, only 25% of the total body bilirubin is removed.[178] Postexchange bilirubin levels are about 60% of preexchange levels, and the re-equilibration that occurs between the vascular and extravascular bilirubin compartments produces a rapid rebound (within 30 minutes) of serum bilirubin levels to 70% to 80% of preexchange levels. A detailed description of the basic indications for, and contraindications to, performing exchange transfusions has been provided by Edwards and Fletcher.[39] They also provide a detailed description of the necessary equipment, technique, and known complications of this procedure.

As discussed previously, very few exchange transfusions are currently being done. The prevention of Rh hemolytic disease with Rh immunoglobulin and the effective use of phototherapy has led to a dramatic decline in the number of exchange transfusions performed.[92] As fewer of these procedures are done, it is likely that the risks and complications will increase. An overall mortality rate of 0.3 in 100 procedures has been reported, but in term and near-term infants who are relatively well, the risk of death is low.[41, 64, 80] Jackson[64] reported a 15-year experience (1980–1995) of exchange transfusion in 106 infants. Eighty-one were healthy and there were no deaths in these infants, although severe necrotizing enterocolitis requiring surgery did develop in one child. There were 25 sick infants, of whom 3 (12%) had serious complications from the exchange transfusion and 2 (8%) died. There were three additional deaths that were considered "possibly" to be the result of the exchange transfusion. Thus, the total number of deaths in sick infants, possibly as the result of the exchange, was 5 of 25 (20%). Exchange transfusion also carries the usual risk associated with any blood transfusion, although these risks are currently low. The risk estimates (risk per tested unit) for transfusion-transmitted viruses in the United States for the period 1991 to 1993 were as follows: human immunodeficiency virus, 1 in 493,000; human T-cell lymphotropic virus, 1 in 641,000; hepatitis C virus, 1 in 103,000; hepatitis B virus, 1 in 63,000.[151]

◆ PHARMACOLOGIC TREATMENT

Acceleration of Normal Metabolic Pathways for Bilirubin Clearance

Phenobarbital induces conjugation and excretion and increases bile flow and, when given to mothers and infants, can lower TSB levels in the first week of life.[168] But because of concerns about long-term toxicity, it is rarely used.[135, 187]

The *metalloporphyrins* are inhibitors of heme oxygenase, the enzyme necessary for the conversion of heme to biliverdin, one of the first steps in the formation of bilirubin from hemoglobin. In a series of controlled clinical trials, the use of SnMP was shown to be effective in reducing TSB levels and the requirement for phototherapy in full-term and preterm infants as well as infants with G6PD deficiency.[76, 106, 167] The only side effect seen has been a transient, non–dose-dependent erythema that disappeared without sequelae in infants who received phototherapy after SnMP administration.[169] Although there has been no obvious toxicity to date, it is difficult to know how SnMP will be used in the United States. If it is used as a substitute for phototherapy to treat established jaundice, at least 200,000 infants (possibly twice that number) could receive the drug. With these numbers, the possibility of an unanticipated adverse event or complication would certainly increase.

Controlled trials have confirmed that the administration of IVIG to infants with Rh hemolytic disease will significantly reduce the need for exchange transfusion.[29, 143, 173] It is also likely that IVIG will mitigate the course of severe ABO hemolytic disease.[55] The doses usually range from 500 mg/kg given over 2 hours soon after birth to 800 mg/kg given daily for 3 days. The mechanism of action of IVIG is unknown but it is possible that it might alter the course of hemolytic disease by blocking Fc receptors and thus inhibiting hemolysis.

UDCA has been used to treat cholestatic jaundice,[131] and, under some circumstances, could be beneficial in ameliorating indirect hyperbilirubinemia as well (Treatment of Cholestasis).

CASE PROBLEMS

◆

Case One

A 25-year-old G2P1001 mother gave birth to a male infant who weighed 3010 g at 36 weeks' gestation. The baby was born at 11 AM the previous day, is being breast-fed, and you are seeing him for the first time at 8 AM when he is 21 hours old. Discharge is planned for that afternoon, so your admission and discharge examinations are performed at the same time.

◆ **With regard to the risk for hyperbilirubinemia, what would you look for as you examine the baby and review the obstetric and newborn chart?**

What specific questions would you ask the nurses and what questions would you ask the mother when you see her?

◆ *What are the factors that might place this infant at a higher risk for development of significant hyperbilirubinemia?*

Because this infant will be discharged before he is 30 hours old, particular attention should be paid to those factors that might place him at risk for development of significant hyperbilirubinemia. In this infant, these factors are his male sex, gestation of 36 weeks, breast-feeding, and short hospital stay. It is important to ask the mother whether her previous child was significantly jaundiced. A bilirubin level of greater than 15 mg/dL (257 μmol/L) in a previous sibling places the current sibling at a 12-fold greater risk than control infants for development of significant jaundice.[8] Although you do not know the infant's blood group, the fact that the mother is blood group O means that a possibility of OA or OB incompatibility exists. When reviewing the nursing notes, pay particular attention to the notes regarding breast-feeding—how frequently has the infant nursed over the first 21 hours and has the nursing been vigorous or only "fair?" Has the infant voided and stooled?

◆ What physical findings would you pay particular attention to?

Careful examination for clinical jaundice is critical. If jaundice is seen before age 24 hours, a TSB level must be obtained and, if the level is above the 90th to 95th percentile for that age[17] (see Fig. 12–7), an evaluation for the cause of jaundice must be initiated. Look also for cephalhematomas or evidence of bruising, both of which increase the potential for significant hyperbilirubinemia (catabolism of 1 g of hemoglobin produces 35 mg of bilirubin).

◆ When will you schedule a follow-up visit for this baby?

Ideally, this infant should be seen between the age of 48 to 72 hours and no later than 96 hours, perhaps having the mother and infant return to your office within 48 hours (when the infant is about 72 hours old). If significant jaundice had developed, it would be readily identifiable. Occasional cases of kernicterus have occurred in infants first seen between 72 and 96 hours with extremely high TSB levels.[24, 103]

◆ What can be done if the baby is born in the middle of winter and the mother lives 75 miles away and is not willing to drive back to your office over icy roads?

An evaluation can be done before discharge that can help with the decision regarding the need for follow-up. For example, measure a TSB level at the same time that the newborn metabolic screen is performed, before the infant's discharge. Plotting this bilirubin value on the nomogram shown in Figure 12–7 provides guidance regarding the risk for subsequent significant hyperbilirubinemia (see text). If the value is less than the 40th percentile, there is a high degree of reassurance that the TSB level is unlikely ever to exceed the 95th percentile and even less likely to exceed 25 mg/dL (428 μmol/L). On the other hand, if the value is more than the 75th percentile and certainly if it is more than the 95th percentile, the baby could be kept at the hospital for another day so that TSB levels could be measured again, unless the mother can make arrangements to bring the baby back the following day for a TSB level measurement or a visiting nurse can obtain the measurement at the home. Measurement of the $ETCO_c$ concentration provides additional information regarding the infant's rate of bilirubin production.

The baby is nursing well, the mother's previous infant was not jaundiced, and nothing alarming is found on the examination, so you write orders permitting discharge by 5 PM (age 30 hours) and schedule a follow-up visit 2 days after discharge. At 3 PM (when the infant is 28 hours old), you get a call from the nurse saying that she noticed that the baby was slightly jaundiced.

◆ What should be done?

Unless a nurse or physician could evaluate the infant the next day after discharge, a TSB level should be obtained.

◆ The TSB level (returned 1 hour later) is 7.0 mg/dL (120 μmol/L). What should be done next?

This TSB level is between the 75th and 90th percentile for a 28-hour-old infant (see Fig. 12–7). This is not cause for alarm but does require appropriate follow-up. A TSB level should be obtained the next morning, preferably in the laboratory of the hospital of birth or at a conveniently located laboratory. If distance is not a problem, a very useful way to approach this problem is to obtain a transcutaneous bilirubin reading at the same time that the serum bilirubin level is obtained. A repeat transcutaneous measurement can be obtained the following day at home by a visiting nurse or when the mother returns to the hospital. If this value is the same or lower than the value obtained the day before, no further serum bilirubin level need be obtained.

◆ What sort of discharge instructions about jaundice should be given to families before they leave the hospital with their newborn infant?

If the mother is nursing, particular emphasis must be placed on helping the mother to understand how she can tell whether the infant is nursing adequately. The infant must be nursed at least eight times a day and specific instructions must be given regarding the identification of jaundice. For example, demonstrate what jaundice looks like by pressing the baby's nose and showing the mother the yellow color that appears. The mother should be instructed to report if the intensity of the color increases or the jaundice spreads to the chest or abdomen.

Case Two

A 37-week-gestation male infant is born following an uncomplicated pregnancy and delivery. He is breast-fed by his mother and appears to be nursing adequately. He is discharged home at the age of 42 hours with instructions to return to the pediatrician's office 10 days after discharge. Examination at age 40 hours reveals no jaundice. On the morning of the sixth day, he is brought to the office because the mother had noticed that he was increasingly jaundiced over the previous 2 days and had nursed poorly. He had refused the breast completely for the past 12 hours, was lethargic, and had a weight loss of 14% of his birth weight. On closer questioning, the mother acknowledges that he had never nursed very well. Upon examination, the infant appears extremely jaundiced but is otherwise alert and responsive and has no posturing or arching of his back. A stat serum bilirubin level is 29.4 mg/dL (503 μmol/L) and he is admitted to the hospital. The attending pediatrician asks the resident to start phototherapy and requests that a repeat bilirubin level be obtained in 8 hours. The infant is placed under daylight phototherapy lamps that produce an irradiance of 9 μW/cm²/nm in the blue spectrum (420 to 480 nm). The resident asks about sending blood for type and cross-match for a possible exchange transfusion and the attending pediatrician responds "unless we find evidence of hemolytic disease, this sounds like typical breast milk jaundice and these babies never get into trouble. But let's get a type and Coombs' anyway." The resident complies. The baby's blood type is A Rh positive with a weakly positive direct Coombs' test. The mother's blood type was group O Rh positive.

◆ Do you agree with the attending pediatrician's orders?

There are several problems with the way this baby is being managed. The attending pediatrician's assertion that these infants "never get into trouble" is not true. Kernicterus is well described in apparently healthy term and near-term breast-fed newborns. A bilirubin level of 29.4 mg/dL (503 μmol/L) is a medical emergency and demands immediate and intensive phototherapy. Under these circumstances, standard phototherapy lights are inadequate and intensive phototherapy must be used as described above. Special blue fluorescent lamps must be placed 10 to 15 cm above the infant and the infant should lie on at least two fiberoptic pads. The sides of the bassinet should be lined with aluminum foil to increase as far as possible the surface area of the infant exposed to phototherapy. A type and cross-match for blood for exchange transfusion must be obtained immediately because the etiology of this extreme hyperbilirubinemia is unknown and, if a subsequent TSB level remains the same or even increases despite appropriate phototherapy, an immediate exchange transfusion should be performed. Because it is essential to know which way the bilirubin level is moving, a repeat TSB level should be obtained within 2 to 3 hours and certainly no later than 4 hours. In addition, the baby should be given formula in an attempt to reduce the enterohepatic circulation. Because the rate of decline of the TSB under phototherapy is directly related to the initial TSB level (the higher the level, the more rapid the decline), a decrease of at least 2 to 3 mg/dL (and often more) can be expected in the first 4 hours. In addition to limiting the enterohepatic circulation, formula gives needed calories as well as additional fluid. Because the structural isomer lumirubin is excreted in the urine, maintaining a good urine output helps to lower the TSB level more rapidly.

◆ Does this infant have ABO hemolytic disease?

This is unlikely. He was not at all jaundiced at age 40 hours and, although there is AO incompatibility with a positive Coombs' test, four of five such infants do not have TSB levels that exceed 13 mg/dL. If this was truly ABO hemolytic disease, clinical jaundice should have been seen within the first 24 hours and certainly by 36 hours. It is much more likely that this infant has breast-feeding–associated hyperbilirubinemia related to a low caloric intake and exaggeration of the enterohepatic circulation.

A major error in the care of this infant was scheduling a follow-up visit at age 10 days in a newborn discharged at age 42 hours. As emphasized earlier, such infants should always be seen within 48 to 72 hours of discharge, particularly if the baby is breast-fed and younger than 38 weeks' gestation, as was the case here.

◆ What other tests should be ordered for this infant?

In addition to the blood type and Coombs' test, a CBC with smear, reticulocyte count, and G6PD level should be obtained. Measurement of a serum albumin would be helpful. In occasional infants with very low serum albumin levels and, therefore, less ability to bind bilirubin, earlier exchange transfusion might be considered.

◆ *Is it likely that a cause for this hyperbilirubinemia can be specified?*

No, it is not likely. The overwhelming majority of infants readmitted to hospital for hyperbilirubinemia have "breast milk" or "breast-feeding–associated" jaundice with no other identifiable etiology. Nevertheless, it is important to look for specific causes, particularly conditions such as G6PD deficiency, because the risk for kernicterus in such infants appears to be much greater than in other infants with similar TSB levels.

◆ *How could this extreme hyperbilirubinemia have been prevented?*

Follow-up of this infant within 2 days of discharge would have identified an infant who was becoming progressively jaundiced. A TSB level would have been obtained, the mother counseled to improve breast-feeding efforts, and, if necessary, phototherapy would have followed.

◆

Case Three

Hyaline membrane disease develops in a 980-g, 27-week-gestation female infant and she requires assisted ventilation. On the fourth day of life, when she is 80 hours old and being weaned from the ventilator, she is noted to be jaundiced. A TSB level of 14.3 mg/dL (245 μmol/L) is obtained.

◆ *Which of the following should be done?*

1. *Start phototherapy using the standard halogen spot lamp available in the nursery?*
2. *Start intensive phototherapy with special blue lamps and a fiberoptic pad below the baby?*
3. *Perform an exchange transfusion?*
4. *Administer tin-mesoporphyrin (SnMP) 6 μmol/kg?*

The answer is 2. The actual risk to this infant under these circumstances and at this TSB level is ill defined. Nevertheless, the TSB level has reached a point that is of concern and could become a serious problem if, for example, acute hypercapnia develops (as a result of a blocked endotracheal tube or a pneumothorax). Hypercapnia opens the blood–brain barrier. Thus, unlike a similar infant whose bilirubin level was 6 or 7 mg/dL (103 to 120 μmol/L) and who would qualify for "prophylactic" phototherapy using standard phototherapy lights, at this level the use of intensive phototherapy is necessary. In the past, such infants were frequently subjected to exchange transfusion. The data on the outcome of such in-

fants, the efficacy of appropriately used phototherapy, and the potential complications of exchange transfusion make intensive phototherapy a much more rational choice.

◆

Case Four

A healthy full-term female infant is brought to the pediatrician's office at age 2 weeks. The baby is being breast-fed, has had an excellent weight gain, and has a perfectly normal examination except she is slightly jaundiced.

◆ *What questions should be asked of the mother?*

The most important information needed is the color of the baby's stool and urine. If the urine is pale yellow and nearly colorless and the stool is a normal brownish color, the likelihood of cholestatic jaundice is slim. *The mother reports that the baby's stools and urine are normal.*

◆ *What should be done?*

See the baby in a week.

The baby returns in a week (now aged 3 weeks) and is still jaundiced. The mother says that the stools and urine have not changed.

◆ *What should be done?*

Any infant who is jaundiced beyond age 3 weeks *must* have a total and direct bilirubin level measured to rule out cholestatic jaundice and the possibility of EHBA.

◆ *The TSB level is 8.2 mg/dL, the direct bilirubin level 0.5 mg/dL. Do you need to do anything else?*

Although it is overwhelmingly likely that this baby has breast milk jaundice, any baby with prolonged indirect hyperbilirubinemia should have an evaluation of thyroid function because hypothyroidism is one cause of prolonged indirect hyperbilirubinemia. This can easily be done without further testing by referring to the hospital chart (or the state laboratory) and confirming that the metabolic screen was done and that the thyroid function was normal.

The mother comes back when the baby is 10 weeks old and the baby is still jaundiced. TSB level is 7.5 mg/dL (130 μmol/L) and direct bilirubin is 0.4 mg/dL (7 μmol/L).

◆ *What should the mother be told?*

Indirect hyperbilirubinemia up to age 12 weeks is well within the limits of the breast milk jaundice syndrome; reassure the mother that she need not be concerned.

◆ Are there additional questions that should be asked of the mother?

Ask the mother whether there is any history of mild, unconjugated hyperbilirubinemia in her family (Gilbert syndrome). There is a strong association between prolonged hyperbilirubinemia in breast-fed infants and the presence of the abnormal (TA)7 gene promoter of the UGT1A gene. Subjects with Gilbert syndrome are homozygous for this promoter.

Case Five

A 750-g, 26-week-gestation male infant is 24 hours old and receiving assisted ventilation. A TSB level is obtained and is 3.8 mg/dL (65 μmol/L). Cultures from the mother were positive for group B streptococcus. Blood cultures have been obtained and ampicillin and gentamicin administered. Because of this baby's extremely low-birth-weight and need for assisted ventilation, one of the neonatologists would like to start prophylactic phototherapy.

◆ Do you agree with this idea?

Phototherapy probably works on bilirubin that is in the capillaries of the skin and subcutaneous tissues. However, for phototherapy to work, there must be some bilirubin present. At such a low bilirubin level, phototherapy is unlikely to have any impact and any effect would be minimal. Continue to follow the bilirubin level and start standard phototherapy if the bilirubin level exceeds 5 or 6 mg/dL. Note that using aggressive prophylactic phototherapy in such infants deprives them of the potential antioxidant benefits of the bilirubin.

Case Six

A 40-week-gestation male infant is delivered by repeat cesarean section and is being discharged at age 80 hours. He looks jaundiced and a TSB level obtained at 76 hours is 12.8 mg/dL (219 μmol/L). Jaundice is discussed with the mother and she plans to return for a follow-up visit with the infant in 4 or 5 days. The mother asks whether it would be a good idea to place the baby in sunlight.

◆ Is it a good idea to place the baby in sunlight?

Yes. Although there are no appropriate controlled trials of the use of sunlight as a means of providing phototherapy, sunlight and even open shade provide substantial amounts of irradiance in the blue spectrum. It is a good idea to expose infants to the sun, as long as it is done cautiously. Direct sunlight (outside) should be avoided, but having the infant in open shade outside or inside in a sunlit room is a good way to deliver phototherapy. Light in the ultraviolet spectrum is filtered out as the sunlight passes through glass so that the infant does not become tanned. In the original paper describing phototherapy, 13 infants (birth weights 1446 to 3686 g) at the Rochford General Hospital in England were placed naked in direct sunlight for 15 to 20 minutes, alternating with a similar period out of the sun for a total of 2 to 4 hours. This exposure produced a mean decrement in the TSB of 3.9 mg/dL. Only one infant showed no response to sunlight.[28]

REFERENCES

1. Agati G, Fusi F, Donzelli GP, et al: Quantum yield and skin filtering effects on the formation rate of lumirubin. J Photochem Photobiol B 18:197–203, 1993.
2. Ahdab-Barmada M: The neuropathology of kernicterus: Definitions and debate. In Maisels MJ, Watchko JF, eds: Neonatal Jaundice. London: Harwood Academic, 2000, pp 75–88.
3. Amato M, Fouchere JC, von Muralt G: Relationship between peri-intraventricular hemorrhage and neonatal hyperbilirubinemia in very low birth weight infants. Am J Perinatol 4:275–278, 1987.
4. American Academy of Pediatrics Provisional Committee for Quality Improvement and Subcommittee on Hyperbilirubinemia: Practice parameter: Management of hyperbilirubinemia in the healthy term newborn. Pediatrics 94:558–562, 1994.
5. American Academy of Pediatrics: Committee on the Fetus and Newborn Hospital Stay for Healthy Term Newborns. Pediatrics 96:788–790, 1995.
6. Andres JM: Neonatal hepatobiliary disorders. Clin Perinatol 23:352, 1996.
7. Auerbach KG, Gartner LM: Breast feeding and human milk: Their association with jaundice in the neonate. Clin Perinatol 14:89–107, 1987.
8. Bainbridge R, Khoury J, Mimounie F: Jaundice in neonatal sickle cell disease: A case controlled study. Am J Dis Child 148:569, 1988.
9. Bancroft JD, Kreamer B, Gourley GR: Gilbert's syndrome accelerates development of neonatal jaundice. J Pediatr 132:656–660, 1998.
10. Barefield ES, Dwyer MD, Cassady G: Association of patent ductus arteriosus and phototherapy in infants weighing less than 1000 grams. J Perinatol 13:376–380, 1993.
11. Barss VA, Doubilet PM, St. John-Sutton M, et al: Cardiac output in a fetus with erythroblastosis fetalis: Assessment using pulsed Doppler. Obstet Gynecol 70:442–444, 1987.
12. Bates MD, Alsonso MH, Ryckman FC: Biliary atresia: Pathogenesis and treatment. Semin Liver Dis 18:281–293, 1998.

13. Beale EF, Nelson RM, Buccarelli RL, et al: Entero-hepatic cholestasis associated with parenteral nutrition in premature infants. Pediatrics 64:347, 1979.
14. Benders MJNL, van Bel F, van de Bor M: The effect of phototherapy on cerebral blood flow velocity in preterm infants. Acta Paediatr 87:791, 1998.
15. Bhupathy K, Sethupathy R, Pildes RS, et al: Electroretinography in neonates treated with phototherapy. Pediatrics 61:189–189, 1978.
16. Bhutani V, Johnson LH, Gourley G, Adler S: Transcutaneous measurement of total serum bilirubin by multi-wavelength spectral reflectance (Bilicheck): Accuracy and precision in newborn babies. Pediatr Res 45:186A, 1999.
17. Bhutani VK, Johnson L, Sivieri EM: Predictive ability of a predischarge hour-specific serum bilirubin for subsequent significant hyperbilirubinemia in healthy term and near-term newborns. Pediatrics 103:6–14, 1999.
18. Black VD, Lubchenco LO, Koops BL, et al: Neonatal hyperviscosity: Randomized study of effect of partial plasma exchange transfusion on long-term outcome. Pediatrics 75:1048–1053, 1985.
19. Blair DK, Vander Straten MC, Gest AL: Hydrops fetalis in sheep from rapid induction of anemia. Pediatr Res 35:560–564, 1994.
20. Bosma PJ, Seppen J, Goldhoorn B, et al: Bilirubin UDP-glucuronosyl transferase 1 is the only relevant bilirubin glucuronodase isoform in man. J Biol Chem 269:17960–17964, 1994.
21. Bowman JM: The management of alloimmune fetal hemolytic disease. In Maisels MJ, Watcho JF, eds: Neonatal Jaundice. London: Harwood Academic, 2000, pp 23–36.
22. Bratlid D: How bilirubin gets into the brain. Clin Perinatol 17:449, 1990.
23. Brodersen R: Binding of bilirubin to albumin. CRC Crit Rev Clin Lab Sci 11:305–399, 1980.
24. Brown AK, Johnson L: Loss of concern about jaundice and the reemergence of kernicterus in full term infants in the era of managed care. In Yearbook of Neonatal and Perinatal Medicine. St. Louis: Mosby, 1996, pp xvii–xxviii.
25. Brown AK, Kim MH, Wu PYK, et al: Efficacy of phototherapy in prevention and management of neonatal hyperbilirubinemia. Pediatrics 75(Suppl):393–400, 1985.
26. Chavez GF, Mulinare J, Edmonds LD: Epidemiology of Rh hemolytic disease of the newborn in the United States. JAMA 265:3270–3274, 1991.
27. Christensen T, Kinn G: Bilirubin bound to cells does not form photoisomers. Acta Paediatr 82:22–25, 1993.
28. Cremer RJ, Perryman PW, Richards DH: Influence of light on the hyperbilirubinemia of infants. Lancet 1:1094–1097. 1958.
29. Dagoglu T, Ovali F, Samanci N, et al: High-dose intravenous immunoglobulin therapy for haemolytic disease. J Int Med Res 23:264–271, 1995.
30. Davenport M, Kerkar N, Mieli-Vergani G, et al: Biliary atresia: The King's College Hospital experience (1974–1995). J Pediatr Surg 32:479–485, 1997.
31. Davidson LT, Merritt KK, Weech AA: Hyperbilirubinemia in the newborn. Am J Dis Child 61:958–980, 1941.
32. De Carvalho M, Holl M, Harvey D: Effects of water supplementation on physiological jaundice in breast fed babies. Arch Dis Child 56:568–569, 1981.
33. De Carvalho M, Klaus MH, Merkatz RB: Frequency of breastfeeding and serum bilirubin concentration. Am J Dis Child 136:737–738, 1982.
34. De Carvalho M, Robertson S, Klaus M: Fecal bilirubin excretion and serum bilirubin concentration in breast-fed and bottle-fed infants. J Pediatr 107:786–790, 1985.
35. DeJonge MH, Khuntia A, Maisels MJ, Bandagi A: Bilirubin levels and severe retinopathy of prematurity in 23–26 week estimated gestational age infants. J Pediatr 135:102–104, 1999.
36. Department of Clinical Epidemiology and Biostatistics, M.U.H.S.C: How to read clinical journals. III. To learn the clinical course and prognosis of disease. Can Med Assoc J 124:869–872, 1981.
37. Dobson V, Riggs LA, Signeland FR: Electroretinographic determination of dark adaptation functions of children exposed to phototherapy as infants. J Pediatr 85:25, 1974.
38. Ebbesen F: Low reserve albumin for binding of bilirubin in neonates with deficiency of bilirubin excretion and bronze baby syndrome. Acta Paediatr Scand 71:415–410, 1982.
39. Edwards MC, Fletcher MA: Exchange transfusions. In Fletcher MA, MacDonald MG, eds: Atlas of Procedures in Neonatology. Philadelphia: JB Lippincott, 1993, pp 363–372.
40. Eggert P, Stick C, Schroder H: On the distribution of irradiation intensity in phototherapy. Measurements of effective irradiance in an incubator. Eur J Pediatr 142:58–61, 1985.
41. Ellis MI, Hey EN, Walker W: Neonatal death in babies with rhesus isoimmunization. Q J Med 48:211–211, 1979.
42. Ennever JF: Blue light, green light, white light, more light: Treatment of neonatal jaundice. Clin Perinatol 17:467, 1990.
43. Ennever JF, Knox I, Denne SC, Speck WT: Phototherapy for neonatal jaundice, in vivo clearance of bilirubin photoproducts. Pediatr Res 19:205–208, 1985.
44. Epstein MF, Leviton A, Kuban KC, et al: Bilirubin intraventricular hemorrhage and phenobarbital in very low birth weight babies. Pediatrics 82:350, 1988.
45. Fevery J: Fasting hyperbilirubinemia: Unraveling the mechanism involved. Gastroenterology 113:1707–1313, 1997.
46. Frishberg Y, Zelicovic I, Merlob P, Reisner SH: Hyperbilirubinemia and influencing factors in term infants. Isr J Med Sci 25:28–31, 1989.
47. Gartner LM, Lee K-S, Vaisman S, et al: Development of bilirubin transport and metabolism in the newborn rhesus monkey. J Pediatr 90:513–513, 1977.
48. Goldberg K, Wirth FH, Hathaway WE, et al: Neonatal hyperviscosity II. Effect of partial plasma exchange transfusion. Pediatrics 69:419–425, 1982.
49. Gourley GR: Pathophysiology of breast-milk jaundice. In Polin RA, Fox WW, eds: Fetal and Neonatal Physiology. Philadelphia: WB Saunders, 1998, p 1499.
50. Gourley GR, Kreamer B, Arend R: The effect of diet on feces and jaundice during the first three weeks of life. Gastroenterology 103:660, 1992.

51. Grannum PA, Copel JA, Moya FR, et al: The reversal of hydrops fetalis by intravascular intrauterine transfusion in severe isoimmune fetal anemia. Am J Obstet Gynecol 158:914–919, 1988.

52. Grobler JM, Mercer MJ: Kernicterus associated with elevated predominantly direct-reacting bilirubin. S Afr Med J 87:146, 1997.

53. Guibaud L, Lachaud A, Touraine R, et al: MR cholangiography in neonates and infants: Feasibility and preliminary applications. AJR Am J Roentgenol 1:27–31, 1998.

54. Halamek LP, Stevenson DK: Neonatal jaundice and liver disease. In Fanaroff AA, ed: Neonatal-Perinatal Medicine. Diseases of the Fetus and Infant. St. Louis: Mosby, 1997, pp 1345–1389.

55. Hammerman C, Kaplan M, Vreman HJ, Stevenson DK: Intravenous immune globulin in neonatal ABO isoimmunization: Factors associated with clinical efficacy. Biol Neonate 70:69–74, 1996.

56. Hansen TWR: Acute management of extreme neonatal jaundice—The potential benefits of intensified phototherapy and interruption of enterohepatic bilirubin circulation. Acta Paediatr 86:843–846, 1997.

57. Hansen TWR: The pathophysiology of bilirubin toxicity. In Maisels MJ, ed: Neonatal Jaundice. London: Harwood Academic, 1999.

58. Hansen TWR: Fetal and neonatal bilirubin metabolism. In Maisels MJ, Watchko JF, eds: Neonatal Jaundice. London: Harwood Academic, 2000, pp 3–22.

59. Hardy JB, Drage JS, Jackson EC: The First Year of Life: The Collaborative Perinatal Project of the National Institutes of Neurological and Communicative Disorders and Stroke. Baltimore: Johns Hopkins University Press, 1979.

60. Holtrop PC, Ruedisueli K, Maisels MJ: Double versus single phototherapy in low birth weight newborns. Pediatrics 90:674–677, 1992.

61. Hsia DYY, Allen FH, Gellis SS, Diamond LK: Erythroblastosis fetalis. VIII. Studies of serum bilirubin in relation to kernicterus. N Engl J Med 247:668–671, 1952.

62. Hussain K, Sharief N: Dermal injury following the use of fiberoptic phototherapy in an extremely premature infant [see comments]. Clin Pediatr 35:421–422, 1996.

63. Iolascon A, Faienza MF, Moretti A, et al: UGT1 promoter polymorphism accounts for increased neonatal appearance of hereditary spherocytosis. Blood 91:1093, 1998.

64. Jackson JC: Adverse events associated with exchange transfusion in healthy and ill newborns. Pediatrics 99:5, e7, 1997.

65. Jacquemin E, Lykavieris P, Chaoui N: Transient neonatal cholestasis: Origin and outcome. J Pediatr 133:563–567, 1998.

66. Jardine DS, Rogers K: Relationship of benzyl alcohol to kernicterus, intraventricular hemorrhage, and mortality in preterm infants. Pediatrics 83:153–160, 1989.

67. Jährig K, Jährig D, Meisel P, eds: Phototherapy: Treating neonatal jaundice with visible light. München: Quintessenz Verlags-GmbH, 1998.

68. Jährig K, Jährig D, Meisel P: Dependence of the efficiency of phototherapy on plasma bilirubin concentration. Acta Paediatr Scand 71:293–299, 1982.

69. Johnson L: Hyperbilirubinemia in the term infant: When to worry, when to treat. N Y State J Med 91:483–489, 1991.

70. Johnson L, Bhutani VK: Guidelines for management of the jaundiced term and near-term infant. Clin Perinatol 25:555–574, 1998.

71. Johnson L, Boggs TR, Schaffer R, Simopoulous AP: Bilirubin-dependent brain damage: Incidence and indications for treatment. In Odell GB, ed: Phototherapy in the Newborn: An Overview. Washington, DC: National Academy of Sciences, 1974, pp 122–149.

72. Johnston WH, Angara V, Baumal R, et al: Erythroblastosis fetalis and hyperbilirubinemia. A five-year follow-up with neurological, physiological and audiological evaluation. Pediatrics 39:88–92, 1967.

73. Jori G, Reddi E, Rubaltelli FF: Bronze baby syndrome: An animal model. Pediatr Res 27:22–25, 1990.

74. Kaplan M, Hammerman C: Severe neonatal hyperbilirubinemia: A potential complication of glucose-6-phosphate dehydrogenase deficiency. Clin Perinatol 25:575–590, 1998.

75. Kaplan M, Renbaum P, Levi-Lahad E, et al: Gilbert syndrome and glucose-phosphate dehydrogenase deficiency: A dose-dependent genetic interaction crucial to neonatal hyperbilirubinemia. Proc Natl Acad Sci U S A 94:12128–12132, 1997.

76. Kappas A, Drummond G, Henschke C, et al: Direct comparison of Sn-mesoporphyrin, an inhibitor of bilirubin production, and phototherapy in controlling hyperbilirubinemia in term and near-term newborns. Pediatrics 95:468–474, 1995.

77. Kappas A, Drummond GS, Manola T, et al: Sn-protoporphyrin use in the management of hyperbilirubinemia in term newborns with direct Coombs'-positive ABO incompatibility. Pediatrics 81:485–497, 1988.

78. Kawade N, Onishi S: The prenatal and postnatal development of UDP-glucuronyl transferase activity toward bilirubin and the effect of premature birth on this activity in the human liver. Biochem J 196:257–260, 1981.

79. Kearns GL, Williams BJ, Timmons OD: Fluorescein phototoxicity in a premature infant. J Pediatr 107:796–798, 1985.

80. Keenan WJ, Novak KK, Sutherland JM, et al. Morbidity and mortality associated with exchange transfusion. Pediatrics Suppl 75:417–421, 1985.

81. Knudsen A: Prediction of the development of neonatal jaundice by increased umbilical cord blood bilirubin. Acta Pediatr Scand 78:217–221, 1989.

82. Kopelman AE, Brown RS, Odell GB: The "bronze" baby syndrome: A complication of phototherapy. J Pediatr 81:466–466, 1972.

83. Lee K-S, Perlman M, Ballantyne M: Association between duration of neonatal hospital stay and readmission rate. J Pediatr 127:758–766, 1995.

84. Levine RL: Fluorescence quenching studies of the binding of bilirubin to albumin. Clin Chem 23:2292–2292, 1972.

85. Lightner DA, McDonagh AF: Molecular mechanisms of phototherapy for neonatal jaundice. Accts Chem Res 17:417–424, 1984.

86. Liu LL, Clemens CJ, Shay DK, et al: The safety of newborn discharge. The Washington State experience. JAMA 278:293–298, 1997.

87. MacDonald M: Hidden risks: Early discharge and

bilirubin toxicity due to glucose-6-phosphate dehydrogenase deficiency. Pediatrics 96:734–738, 1995.

88. Madlon-Kay DJ: Recognition of the presence and severity of newborn jaundice by parents, nurses, physicians, and icterometer. Pediatrics 100:e3, 1997.

89. Maisels MJ: Neonatal jaundice. In Sinclair JC, Bracken MB, eds: Effective Care of the Newborn Infant. Oxford: Oxford University Press, 1992, pp 507–561.

90. Maisels MJ: Why use homeopathic doses of phototherapy? Pediatrics 98:283–287, 1996.

91. Maisels MJ: Epidemiology of neonatal jaundice. In Maisels MJ, Watchko JF, eds: Neonatal Jaundice. London: Harwood Academic, 2000, pp 37–50.

92. Maisels MJ: Is exchange transfusion for hyperbilirubinemia in danger of becoming extinct? Pediatr Res 45:210A, 1999.

93. Maisels MJ: Jaundice. In Avery GB, Fletcher MA, MacDonald MG, eds: Neonatology: Pathophysiology and Management of the Newborn. Philadelphia: JB Lippincott, 1999, pp 765–819.

94. Maisels MJ: The clinical approach to the jaundiced newborn. In Maisels MJ, Watchko JF, eds: Neonatal Jaundice. London: Harwood Academic, 2000, pp 139–168.

95. Maisels MJ, Fanaroff AA, Stevenson DK, et al: Serum bilirubin levels in an international, multiracial newborn population. Pediatr Res 45:167A, 1000.

96. Maisels MJ, Gifford K, Antle CE, et al: Normal serum bilirubin levels in the newborn and the effect of breast feeding. Pediatrics 78:837–843, 1986.

97. Maisels MJ, Gifford KL, Antle CE, et al: Jaundice in the healthy newborn infant: A new approach to an old problem. Pediatrics 81:505–511, 1988.

98. Maisels MJ, Kring E: Full-term infants with severe hyperbilirubinemia—Do they need a septic workup? Pediatr Res 29:224A, 1991.

99. Maisels MJ, Kring E: Risk of sepsis in newborns with severe hyperbilirubinemia. Pediatrics 90:741–743, 1992.

100. Maisels MJ, Kring E: Transcutaneous bilirubinometry decreases the need for serum bilirubin measurements and saves money. Pediatrics 99:599, 1997.

101. Maisels MJ, Kring EA: Early discharge from the newborn nursery: Effect on scheduling of follow-up visits by pediatricians. Pediatrics 100:72–74, 1997.

102. Maisels MJ, Kring EA: Length of stay, jaundice and hospital readmission. Pediatrics 101:995–998, 1998.

103. Maisels MJ, Newman TB: Kernicterus in otherwise healthy, breast-fed term newborns. Pediatrics 96:730–733, 1995.

104. Maisels MJ, Pathak A, Nelson NM, et al: Endogenous production of carbon monoxide in normal and erythroblastotic newborn infants. J Clin Invest 50:1–9, 1971.

105. Mallon E, Wojnarowska F, Hope P, Elder G: Neonatal bullous eruption as a result of transient porphyrinemia in a premature infant with hemolytic disease of the newborn. J Am Acad Dermatol 33:333–336, 1995.

106. Martinez JC, Garcia HO, Otheguy L, et al: Control of severe hyperbilirubinemia in full-term newborns with the inhibitor of bilirubin production Sn-mesoporphyrin (Sn-MP). Pediatrics 103:1–5, 1999.

107. McDonagh AF: Is bilirubin good for you? Clin Perinatol 17:359–369, 1990.

108. McDonagh AF, Lightner DA: "Like a shrivelled blood orange"—Bilirubin, jaundice and phototherapy. Pediatrics 75:443–455, 1985.

109. McDonagh AF, Lightner DA: Phototherapy and the photobiology of bilirubin. Semin Liver Dis 8:272–283, 1988.

110. McDonagh AF, Ramonas LM: Jaundice phototherapy: Micro flow-cell photometry reveals rapid biliary response of Gunn rats to light. Science 20:829, 1978.

111. Meberg A, Johansen KB: Screening for neonatal hyperbilirubinaemia and ABO alloimmunization at the time of testing for phenylketonuria and congenital hypothyreosis. Acta Paediatr 87:1269–1274, 1998.

112. Medical Device Safety Alert Ohmeda Specialty Products Division of Ohmeda, Inc., Columbia, MD: Medical Device Safety Alert, 1996.

113. Mireles LC, Lum MADPA: Antioxidant and cytotoxic effects of bilirubin on neonatal erythrocytes. Pediatr Res 45:355–362, 1998.

114. Monaghan G, McLellan A, McGeehan A, et al: Gilbert's syndrome is a contributory factor in prolonged unconjugated hyperbilirubinemia of the newborn. J Pediatr 134:441–446, 1999.

115. Monte MJ, Rodriguez-Bravo T, Macias RIR, et al: Relationship between bile acid transport gradients and transport across the fetal-facing plasma membrane of the human trophoblast. Pediatr Res 38:156–163, 1999.

116. Naeye RL: Amniotic fluid infections, neonatal hyperbilirubinemia, and psychomotor impairment. Pediatrics 62:497–503, 1978.

117. Newman TB, Easterling MJ, Goldman ES, Stevenson DK: Laboratory evaluation of jaundiced newborns: Frequency, cost and yield. Am J Dis Child 144:364–368, 1990.

118. Newman TB, Escobar GJ, Branch PT, et al: Incidence of extreme hyperbilirubinemia in a large HMO [abstract]. Amb[ED1] Child Health 3:203, 1997.

119. Newman TB, Klebanoff MA: Neonatal hyperbilirubinemia and long-term outcome: Another look at the collaborative perinatal project. Pediatrics 92:651–657, 1993.

120. Newman TB, Maisels MJ: Does hyperbilirubinemia damage the brain of healthy full-term infants? Clin Perinatol 17:331–358, 1990.

121. Newman TB, Maisels MJ: Evaluation of jaundice in the term newborn: A kinder, gentler approach. Pediatrics 89:809–818, 1992.

122. Nicolaides KH, Clewell WH, Rodeck CH: Measurement of human fetoplacental blood volume in erythroblastosis fetalis. Am J Obstet Gynecol 157:50–53, 1987.

123. Nicolaides KH, Warenski JC, Rodeck CH: The relationship of fetal plasma protein concentration and hemoglobin level to the development of hydrops in rhesus isoimmunization. Am J Obstet Gynecol 152:341–344, 1985.

124. Nicoll A, Ginsburg R, Tripp JH: Supplementary feeding and jaundice in newborns. Acta Pediatr Scand 71:759–761, 1982.

125. Okolo AA, Omene JA, Scott-Emaukpor AB: Physi-

ologic jaundice in the Nigerian neonate. Biol Neonate 53:132–137, 1988.

126. Osborn LM, Lenarsky C, Oakes RC, Reiff MI: Phototherapy in full-term infants with hemolytic disease secondary to ABO incompatibility. Pediatrics 74:371–374, 1984.

127. Ozolek J, Watchko J, Mimouni F: Prevalence and lack of clinical significance of blood group incompatibility in mothers with blood type A or B. J Pediatr 125:87–91, 1994.

128. Paller AS, Eramo LR, Farrell EE, et al: Purpuric phototherapy-induced eruption in transfused neonates: Relation to transient porphyrinemia. Pediatrics 100:360–364, 1997.

129. Park WH, Choi SO, Lee HJ, et al: A new diagnostic approach to biliary atresia with emphasis on the ultrasonographic triangular cord sign: Comparison of ultrasonography, hepatobiliary, scintigraphy, and liver needle biopsy in the evaluation of infantile cholestasis. J Pediatr Surg 11:1555–1559, 1997.

130. Penn AA, Enzman DR, Hahn JS, et al: Kernicterus in a full term infant. Pediatrics 93:1003–1006, 1994.

131. Perez EM, Cooper TR, Moise AA, et al: Treatment of obstructed jaundice in erythroblastosis fetalis with ursodeoxycholic acid (UDCA): A case report. J Perinatol 18:319, 1998.

132. Phibbs RH, Johnson P, Tooley WH: Cardiorespiratory status of erythroblastotic newborn infants. II. Blood volume, hematocrit, and serum albumin concentration in relation to hydrops fetalis. Pediatrics 53:13–23, 1974.

133. Poland RL, Odell GB: Physiologic jaundice: The enterohepatic circulation of bilirubin. N Engl J Med 284:1–6, 1971.

134. Ramirez RO, Sokol RJ: Medical management of cholestasis. In Sushy FJ, ed: Liver Disease in Children. St. Louis: Mosby, 1994, pp 356–388.

135. Reinisch JM, Sander SA, Mortensen EL, et al: In utero exposure to phenobarbital and intelligence deficits in adult men. JAMA 274:1518–1525, 1995.

136. Robertson A, Carp W, Broderson R: Bilirubin displacing effect of drugs used in neonatology. Acta Paediatr Scand 80:1119–1127, 1991.

137. Robertson A, Carp W, Broderson R: Effect of drug combinations on bilirubin-albumin binding. Dev Pharmacol Ther 17:95, 1991.

138. Rosenfeld W, Sadhev S, Brunot V, et al: Phototherapy effect on the incidence of patent ductus arteriosus in premature infants: Prevention with chest shielding. Pediatrics 78:10–14, 1986.

139. Roy-Chowdhury N, Deocharan B, Bejjanki HR, et al: The presence of a Gilbert-type promotor abnormality increases the level of neonatal hyperbilirubinemia. Hepatology 26:370A, 1997.

140. Roy M-S, Caramelli C, Orquin J, et al: Effects of early reduced light exposure on central visual development in preterm infants. Acta Paediatr 88:459–461, 1999.

141. Rubaltelli FF: Unconjugated and conjugated bilirubin pigments during perinatal development. IV. The influence of breast-feeding on neonatal hyperbilirubinemia. Biol Neonate 64:104–109, 1993.

142. Rubaltelli FF, Jori G, Reddi E: Bronze baby syndrome: A new porphyrin-related disorder. Pediatr Res 17:327–330, 1983.

143. Rubo J, Albrecht K, Lasch P, et al: High-dose intravenous immune globulin therapy for hyperbilirubinemia caused by Rh hemolytic disease. J Pediatr 121:93–97, 1992.

144. Ryan AS: The resurgence of breastfeeding in the United States. Pediatrics 99:E12, 1997.

145. Saigal S, Lunyk O, Bennett KJ, Patterson MC: Serum bilirubin levels in breast- and formula-fed infants in the first 5 days of life. Can Med Assoc J 127:985–989, 1982.

146. Sato K, Hara T, Kondo T, et al: High-dose intravenous gammaglobulin therapy for neonatal immune haemolytic jaundice due to blood group incompatibility. Acta Paediatr Scand 80:163–166, 1991.

147. Scheidt PC, Bryla DA, Nelson KB, et al: Phototherapy for neonatal hyperbilirubinemia: Six year follow-up of the NICHD clinical trial. Pediatrics 85:455–463, 1990.

148. Scheidt PC, Mellits ED, Hardy JB, et al: Toxicity to bilirubin in neonates. Infant development during first year in relation to maximum neonatal serum bilirubin concentration. J Pediatr 91:292–297, 1977.

149. Scher H, Bishop WP, McCray PB Jr: Ursodeoxycholic acid improves cholestasis in infants with cystic fibrosis. Ann Pharmacother 9:1003–1005, 1997.

150. Schneider AP: Breast milk jaundice in the newborn. A real entity. JAMA 255:3270–3274, 1986.

151. Schreiber GB, Busch MP, Kleinman SH, Korelitz JJ: The risk of transfusion-transmitted viral infections. N Engl J Med 334:1685–1690, 1996.

152. Schumacher RE: Non-invasive measurements of bilirubin in the newborn. Clin Perinatol 17:417, 1990.

153. Seidman DS, Moise J, Ergaz Z, et al: A new blue light emitting phototherapy device vs conventional phototherapy: A prospective randomized controlled application in term newborns. Pediatr Res 43:193A, 1998.

154. Shevell MI, Bernard B, Adelson JW, et al: Crigler-Najjar syndrome type I: Treatment by home phototherapy followed by orthotopic hepatic transplantation. J Pediatr 110:429, 1987.

155. Sinatra FR: Does total parenteral nutrition produce cholestasis? In Adcock EW III, Lester R, eds. Neonatal Cholestasis: Causes, Syndromes, Therapies. Report of the 87th Ross Conference on Pediatric Research. Columbus, OH: Ross Laboratories, 1984, pp 85–91.

156. Soskolne EL, Schumacher R, Fyock C, et al: The effect of early discharge and other factors on readmission rates of newborns. Arch Pediatr Adolesc Med 150:373–379, 1996.

157. Stevenson DK, Vreman HJ: Carbon monoxide production in neonates. Pediatrics 100:252–254, 1997.

158. Suchy FJ, Mullick FG: Total parenteral nutrition-associated cholestasis. In Balistreri WF, Stocker JT, eds: Pediatric Hepatology. New York: Hemisphere Publishing, 1990, pp 29–40.

159. Tan KL: Comparison of the effectiveness of phototherapy and exchange transfusion in the management of nonhemolytic neonatal hyperbilirubinemia. J Pediatr 87:609–609, 1975.

160. Tan KL: The pattern of bilirubin response to phototherapy for neonatal hyperbilirubinemia. Pediatr Res 16:670–674, 1982.

161. Tan KL: Efficacy of bidirectional fiberoptic phototherapy for neonatal hyperbilirbinemia. Pediatrics 99:e13:5, 1997.

162. Tayaba R, Gribetz D, Gribetz I, Holzman IR: Non-invasive estimation of serum bilirubin. Pediatrics 102:e3, 1998.

163. Tiribelli C, Ostrow JD: New concepts in bilirubin and jaundice: Report of the third international bilirubin workshop, April 6–8, 1995, Trieste, Italy. Hepatology 24:1296–1311, 1996.

164. Tonz O, Vogt J, Filippini L, et al: Severe light dermatosis following phototherapy in a newborn infant with congenital erythropoietic urophyria. Helv Paediatr Acta 30:47–56, 1975.

165. Valaes T: Severe neonatal jaundice associated with glucose-6-phosphate dehydrogenase deficiency: Pathogenesis and global epidemiology. Acta Pediatrica Suppl 394:58–76, 1994.

166. Valaes T: Neonatal jaundice in glucose-6-phosphate dehydrogenase deficiency. In Maisels MJ, Watchko JF, eds: Neonatal Jaundice. London: Harwood Academic, 2000, pp 67–74.

167. Valaes T, Drummond GS, Kappas A: Control of hyperbilirubinemia in glucose-6-phosphate dehydrogenase-deficient newborns using an inhibitor of bilirubin production, Sn-mesoporphyrin. Pediatrics 101;5;e1, 1998.

168. Valaes T, Harvey-Wilkes K: Pharmacologic approaches to the prevention and treatment of neonatal hyperbilirubinemia. Clin Perinatol 17:245–274, 1990.

169. Valaes T, Petmezaki S, Henschke C, et al: Control of jaundice in preterm newborns by an inhibitor of bilirubin production: Studies with tin-mesoporphyrin. Pediatrics 93:1–11, 1994.

170. VanEs HH, Bout A, Liu J, et al: Assignment of the human UDP glucuronosyltransferase gene (UGT1A1) to chromosome region 2Q37. Cytogenet Cell Genet 63:114–116, 1993.

171. Varimo P, Similä S, Wendt L, Kolvisto M: Frequency of breast feeding and hyperbilirubinemia. Clin Pediatr 25:112, 1986.

172. Vohr BR: New approaches to assessing the risks of hyperbilirubinemia. Clin Perinatol 17:293–306, 1990.

173. Voto LS, Sexer H, Ferreiro G, et al: Neonatal administration of high-dose intravenous immunoglobulin and rhesus hemolytic disease. J Perinatol Med 23:443–451, 1995.

174. Vreman HJ, Verter J, Oh W, et al: Interlaboratory variability of bilirubin measurements. Clin Chem 42:869–873, 1996.

175. Vreman HJ, Wong RJ, Stevenson DK: Light-emitting diodes: A novel light source for phototherapy. Pediatr Res 44:804–809, 1998.

176. Washington EC, Ector W, Abboud M, et al: Hemo-lytic jaundice due to G6PD deficiency causing kernicterus in a female newborn. South Med J 88:776–779, 1995.

177. Watchko J, Claassen D: Kernicterus in premature infants: Current prevalence and relationship to NICHD phototherapy study exchange criteria. Pediatrics 93:996–999, 1994.

178. Watchko JF: Exchange transfusion in the management of neonatal hyperbilirubinemia. In Maisels MJ, Watchko JF, eds: Neonatal Jaundice. London: Harwood Academic, 2000, pp 169–176.

179. Watchko JF: Indirect hyperbilirubinemia in the neonate. In Maisels MJ, Watchko JF, eds: Neonatal Jaundice. London: Harwood Academic, 2000, pp 51–66.

180. Watchko JF, Oski FA: Bilirubin 20 mg/dl = vigintiphobia. Pediatrics 71:660–663, 1983.

181. Watchko JF, Oski FA: Kernicterus in preterm newborns: Past, present and future. Pediatrics 90:707, 1992.

182. Wennberg RP, Ahlfors CE, Rasmussen LF: The pathochemistry of kernicterus. Early Hum Dev 31:353, 1979.

183. Wennberg RP, Hance AJ: Experimental encephalopathy: Importance of total bilirubin, protein binding and blood brain barrier. Pediatr Res 20:789, 1986.

184. Wood B, Culley P, Roginski C, et al: Factors affecting neonatal jaundice. Arch Dis Child 54:111–115, 1979.

185. Wu PYK, Hodgman JE, Kirkpatrick BV, et al: Metabolic aspects of phototherapy. Pediatrics 75:427–433, 1985.

186. Wu PYK, Wong WH, Hodgman JE, Levan N: Changes in blood flow in the skin and muscle with phototherapy. Pediatr Res 8:257–257, 1974.

187. Yaffe SJ, Dorn LD: Effects of prenatal treatment with phenobarbital. Dev Pharmacol Ther 15:215, 1990.

188. Yamauchi Y, Yamanouchi I: Transcutaneous bilirubinometry in normal Japanese infants. Acta Paediatr Jpn 31:65–72, 1989.

189. Yamauchi Y, Yamanouchi I: Breast-feeding frequency during the first 24 hours after birth in full-term neonates. Pediatrics 86:171–175, 1990.

190. Yao AC, Martinussen M, Johansen OJ, Brubakk AM: Phototherapy-associated changes in mesenteric blood flow response to feeding in term neonates. J Pediatr 124:309–312, 1994.

191. Yeo KL, Perlman M, Hao Y, Mullaney P: Outcomes of extremely premature infants related to their peak serum bilirubin concentrations and exposure to phototherapy. Pediatrics 102:1426–1431, 1998.

Neonatal Infections

Jill E. Baley
Johanna Goldfarb

The newborn infant is uniquely susceptible to infection, whether it is due to bacterial, viral, or other pathogens. Understanding the anatomic and physiologic basis for this susceptibility can aid in prevention. Bacterial sepsis, when defined as the clinical syndrome resulting from systemic infection and proven by positive blood or other central culture, occurs in approximately one to eight infants per 1000 live births[14, 100] and may be accompanied by meningitis in as many as one fourth of septic infants.[125, 144] The mortality rate ranged from 20% to 30%,[84, 168, 218, 219] but it was as high as 80% to 90% in the presence of bone marrow neutrophil storage pool (NSP) depletion.[40] Clinically, neonatal sepsis has occurred in either of two categories: early onset sepsis, presenting within the first 4 days of life, or late onset sepsis, presenting beyond 4 days of life. As the survival rate of more immature and smaller infants has significantly improved, a third category of disease has become important, that of nosocomial, or nursery-acquired, infection. These nosocomial infections are a subgroup of the late onset category of infections. They predominantly involve the very low birth weight (VLBW) infants. As many as 25% of VLBW infants may have one or more episodes of proven sepsis before discharge.[208] However, these nosocomial infections are also responsible for increasing the morbidity and mortality rates and prolonging the hospital stay. In one study, septic VLBW infants had a 21% mortality rate compared with the nonseptic VLBW infants who had a 9% mortality rate,[65] even though many of the infants did not die during their sepsis episode. In addition, their length of stay (98 days) was significantly longer than in nonseptic VLBW infants (58 days) and they were more likely to suffer severe intraventricular hemorrhage, bronchopulmonary dysplasia, and prolongation of the days spent on a ventilator.

◆ EVOLUTION OF INFECTIONS

The spectrum of etiologic agents and the specific mortality rates for these infections are evolving.[72] In the 1930s, the group A hemolytic streptococci were the most frequent cause of perinatal infections, which came under control with the introduction of penicillin. In the 1940s, the incidence of gram-negative infections, particularly *Escherichia coli*, increased and replaced the streptococci as the most common cause of infection, but by the 1950s, the penicillinase-producing staphylococci (*Staphylococcus aureus*) became predominant. As an understanding of neonatal colonization developed, new cord and skin care practices evolved, which helped to bring staphylococcal infections under control. The gram-negative infections again became prominent in the 1960s, giving way to the group B β-hemolytic streptococci in the 1970s. The evolution of these bacterial epidemics is not completely understood and cannot always be traced to particular changes in the care of the newborn infant. Currently, the group B streptococci (GBS), followed by the enteric microorganisms, remain the most common infecting organisms in the United States in the early postpartum period. At the same time, since the 1980s, nosocomial infections have become predominant in the intensive care nursery. These are more likely to be *Staphylococcus epidermidis* and other gram-positive organisms.[164, 209]

Accompanying this change in infecting organisms, there may be a decrease in actual mortality rate, possibly reflecting the number of infections caused by gram-positive organisms. Overall mortality rate has become as low as 11% to 20%,[20, 218, 219] and, even though meningitis has been previously reported to occur 3 to 17 times more frequently among VLBW infants,[87] the incidence of meningitis among VLBW infants has been reported to be as low as 5%,[89] again possibly reflecting the influence of the gram-positive etiology. Also to be considered are changes in nonbacterial agents. Before the advent of the rubella vaccine, yearly outbreaks of rubella resulted in thousands of congenital infections each year. Following the introduction of the vaccine in 1969, infection rates dropped precipitously.

The current human immunodeficiency virus 1 (HIV-1) epidemic has reached pandemic proportions. In the United States, women and adolescents represent a fast growing group of infected individuals. In parts of sub-Saharan Africa, where HIV is predominantly transmitted heterosexually, pregnant women have rates of infection as high as 20% to 40%, with disastrous effects on their newborns.

◆ TRANSMISSION OF INFECTIONS

Bacteria, viruses, and parasites are transmitted to the fetus and neonate through a variety of routes. Transplacental transmission is responsible for the earliest infections and is well described for the STORCH infections (syphilis, toxoplasmosis, other, rubella, cytomegalovirus [CMV], HSV, and HIV). More commonly, though, infections are transmitted vertically from mother to infant via ascending intraamniotic infection or while the infant is descending through the birth canal. Finally, the infant may be infected after birth. These infections may be transmitted from other infants, hospital staff, or home caretakers, or they may be transmitted from the environment, including from contaminated equipment.

◆ EARLY ONSET INFECTIONS

Most early onset infections present within the first 12 hours of life, although they may develop at any time within the first 4 days. These infections are usually fulminant and multisystemic, with a predilection for pneumonia. The majority of the infants are term, but prematurely born infants are unusually susceptible and have a mortality rate even higher than the 15% to 20% quoted for term infants with early onset disease. Because the organisms are acquired from the mother's birth canal, it is not surprising that there is a very high incidence of obstetric complica-

tions, including premature onset of labor, premature and prolonged rupture of membranes, chorioamnionitis, maternal fever, colonization with GBS, and the need for obstetric intervention. GBS, *E. coli* and other gram-negative bacteria, and enterococcal species were the most common pathogens reported to cause early onset disease at Parkland Memorial Hospital from 1987 through 1994.[98] *Listeria monocytogenes* is also a classic cause.

Among VLBW infants (≤1500 g) from 1991 to 1993, the Neonatal Research Network reported that early onset sepsis was only proven in 1.9% of the infants, although antibiotic therapy was continued beyond 5 days for almost half of the infants, reflecting the uncertainty of diagnosis.[209] The gram-positive organisms (GBS, *Streptococcus viridans*, other streptococci, and coagulase-negative staphylococci) predominated over the gram-negative organisms (e.g., *E. coli, Haemophilus influenzae,* and *Klebsiella).* On a sobering note, early onset sepsis among VLBW infants resulted in significantly higher morbidity, with increased intraventricular hemorrhage, patent ductus arteriosus, and need for prolonged ventilation. Survivors had a prolonged hospital stay (86 days) compared with uninfected infants who stayed a mean of 69 days, even though 26% of the infants with early onset disease died.[208]

◆ LATE ONSET INFECTIONS

Late onset sepsis is more subtle in onset and more likely to result in a focal infection, especially meningitis. Although the etiologic organisms may be acquired from the maternal birth canal, they are more often acquired from the environment. Late onset sepsis is, therefore, more often associated with term infants beyond a week of life and only occasionally related to obstetric complications. In addition, the mortality rate is lower than with early onset disease, approximately 10% to 20%.[119]

◆ NOSOCOMIAL INFECTIONS

Nosocomial infections follow a different pattern. They are inversely related to low-birth-weight and gestational age (Fig. 13–1), and the infected infants were more likely to

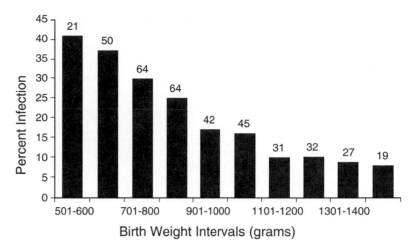

Figure 13–1. Rate of septicemia by 100-g intervals (sample sizes listed above the histogram). (From Fanaroff AA, Korones SB, Wright LL, et al: Incidence, presenting features, risk factors and significance of late onset septicemia in very low birth weight infants. Pediatr Infect Dis J 17:593, 1998.)

suffer complications of prematurity (intubation, catheterization, respiratory distress syndrome, prolonged ventilation, bronchopulmonary dysplasia, patent ductus arteriosus, severe intraventricular hemorrhage, and necrotizing enterocolitis.[65, 208] Freeman and colleagues[73] reported that septic infants were in the hospital an average of 20 days longer than nonseptic infants and that sepsis was 44.5 times more likely to develop in infants weighing less than 750 g at birth than infants with birth weights greater than 2000 g. Among VLBW infants, gram-positive organisms caused 54% of first infections, gram-negative organisms caused 22%, and fungi caused 15%.[65]

◆ RISK FACTORS
Neonatal Factors

The most important risk factor for neonatal sepsis is low birth weight, with the rate of neonatal infection (and mortality) inversely related to birth weight and gestational age.[65, 119, 191, 192, 208] Stoll and colleagues[208] showed that, in as many as 25% of VLBW infants surviving beyond 3 days of life, one or more episodes of blood culture–proven sepsis developed and that these infants were significantly more likely to die (17% mortality rate) than uninfected infants of the same weight (7% mortality rate). Infection with gram-negative organisms or fungi elevated the mortality rate even further, to 40% and 28%, respectively. Likewise, Vesikari and colleagues[219] showed that septic Finnish infants weighing less than 1500 g were twice as likely to die as septic infants weighing

1500 to 2500 g and seven-fold more likely to die than infants weighing greater than 2500 g. Finally, Freeman and colleagues[73] were able to relate birth weight and length of the neonatal intensive care unit (NICU) stay with the risk of developing nosocomial coagulase-negative staphylococcal bacteremia. Many other factors play a role. Sepsis is more likely to develop in male infants than in female infants,[191, 192] particularly with gram-negative organisms, for reasons that are not clear. The first born of twins has an increased rate of infection[191] and low birth weight twins have higher rates of infection than singleton low birth weight infants.[163]

Geographic and ethnic groupings may also influence infections. Mexican women are less likely to be colonized with GBS and their infants to become septic, compared with white and black infants in the same area,[3, 42] also for unclear reasons. In addition, new strains of bacteria, or resistance patterns to antibiotics, may develop in certain regions or nurseries and result in high endemic or epidemic infection rates.

Asphyxia, hypoxemia, and acidosis may impair the immune responses of infants, who already have an immature immune system.[175] Preterm and term neonates need to adapt from an essentially germ-free intrauterine environment to an extrauterine environment of exposure to multiple microorganisms. Yet, compared with adults, neonates have qualitative and quantitative deficiencies of both cellular and humoral immunity. Premature infants, who lack the transplacental transfer of maternal immunoglobulin G (IgG) during the third trimester,[60] have low levels of IgG. These low levels have been associated with increased infection rates among VLBW infants.[65] Both term and preterm infants may lack specific antibody for pathogens, such as the streptococcal carbohydrates or *H. influenzae* b capsular polysaccharide,[60] and they lack IgA in secretions.[175] IgM does not cross the placenta, but synthesis begins by 30 weeks' gestation and it is significantly produced postnatally, becoming the primary immunoglobulin produced by the newborn.[2] Infants have decreased factors of complement, causing delays in activation of both the classic and alternative pathways and thus decreased production of chemotactic factors and opsonization.[175] C3 and factor B are not produced in response to lipopolysaccharide challenge. There are also decreased concentrations of fibronectin. In addition, neonates are unable to localize infections because of alterations in macrophage function. Chemotaxis is decreased. Phagocytosis is decreased without sufficient opsonization and stressed neonates have decreased intracellular bacterial killing.[175] T and B lymphocyte and natural killer (NK) cell function alterations add to the difficulty. Finally, there are reduced bone marrow NSP reserves available to replenish neutrophils during infection.[40]

Of absolute importance to the neonatal host defense is the integrity of the skin and mucosa. Breaks in this integrity may be inherent to the immaturity of the barrier in preterm infants, but they are significantly increased by the invasive procedures and administration of care in the NICU. The tissue of the umbilical cord stump is also a rich source for growth of organisms and subsequent systemic infection.

Infants with galactosemia have a peculiar susceptibility to gram-negative sepsis,[132] which may be related to the altered levels of galactose and glucose, depressing neutrophil function.[198] Likewise, the use of intramuscular iron in neonates has been shown to increase the risk of infection,[15] which may be related to the low levels of iron-binding proteins—lactoferrin and transferrin—in neonates.[224] Exposure of the neonate to other medications, such as steroids,[69] may increase the risk. In contrast, there have been no significant differences shown in the incidence of sepsis among infants with patent ductus arteriosus treated with indomethacin as opposed to surgical ligation.[14]

Maternal Factors

Maternal race, socioeconomic status, and infection also influence the risk of infection in the neonate. Black women are significantly more likely to suffer premature and prolonged rupture of membranes, puerperal infection, and premature birth than white women.[156] Even when controlling for socioeconomic status, young maternal age and premature birth, Schuchat and colleagues[191, 192] attributed 30% of early onset disease and 92% of late onset disease to the black race. Yet, socioeconomic status alone has been related to newborn infection. Poorer women are more likely to deliver premature or low-birth-weight infants, suffer malnutrition, have poor prenatal care, or deliver at a young age, all risk factors by themselves. In addition, infants of alcohol or heroin addicted mothers appear to have an increased risk of infection in the first year of life.[35, 108]

Peripartum fever and focal or systemic infections in the mother carry significant risk for the infant. St. Geme and colleagues[203] showed a four-fold increase in neonatal sepsis with rupture of membranes greater than 24 hours in the presence of maternal chorioamnionitis, yet even rupture of membranes greater than 24 hours alone, without maternal fever or chorioamnionitis, causes the baseline neonatal infection rate to increase to 1.0% from 0.1% to 0.5%.[203] Maternal sepsis, urinary tract infection, cervical infection, or even heavy colonization with a pathogen also carries significant risk for the infant. Finally, any procedure during labor may result in the spread of infection. Fetal scalp monitoring, for example, is associated with a 4.5% incidence of fetal scalp abscesses.

Environmental Factors

In the nursery, crowding, poor hand washing among the staff, and contaminated equipment all add to the risk for the infant. VLBW infants are more likely to experience prolonged endotracheal intubation, which may provide direct access to the tracheal mucosa while bypassing innate cleansing mechanisms, such as the cough and the action of cilia. Contamination of parenteral nutrition solutions and intravenous lipid solutions has also been associated with neonatal infections.[70] The common use of central venous or arterial catheters provides a portal of entry for microorganisms through an intact cutaneous barrier.[70, 153, 204] Probably of no less importance is the use of these catheters to infuse total parenteral nutrition or intravenous lipid emulsions. In one study, the duration of central catheter usage was not longer among infected infants, but the duration of hyperalimentation fluids and fat emulsions was considerably longer.[223] Coagulase-negative staphylococcal infections in preterm infants have been highly correlated with the use of intravenous lipid emulsions alone.[74, 75]

Exposure in the intensive care unit to resistant bacteria and use of antibiotics that alter the indigenous flora of the neonate lead to colonization with more virulent organisms.[46] In contrast, defenses may be improved by the use of human breast milk for feeding. Human milk contains T and B lymphocytes, neutrophils, and macrophages. It is a notable source of secretory IgA, which provides mucosal protection, and bifidus factor, which promotes the growth of *Lactobacillus bifidus*, as opposed to more virulent organisms, in the gut. There are also nonspecific and specific antimicrobial substances and hormones, and epithelial growth factor, which promote the growth of the mucosal epithelium and brush border.

◆ CLINICAL MANIFESTATIONS

Because most episodes of early onset disease begin before birth, the first sign of neonatal sepsis may be that of fetal distress, including fetal tachycardia in the second stage of labor[190] and low 5-minute Apgar scores.[202, 203] Pneumonia has been reported to be present in as many of 40% of the infants when the fetal heart rate is greater than 180 beats per minute (bpm) and in 20% of those with fetal heart rates of 160 to 180 bpm, but it is uncommon with lower fetal heart rates.[190] A septic infant in utero may gasp and be more likely to suffer meconium aspiration. In contrast, an infant younger than 35 weeks' gestation with green amniotic fluid is more likely to have an infection with *Listeria* or other pigment-producing bacteria than meconium staining.

Neonatal bacteremia may occasionally be asymptomatic, although that is rare.[1, 101]

Most frequently, the early signs and symptoms are subtle or minimal, but rapidly progressive. Infants may appear "ill" or feed less vigorously, be less alert, or have lower tone.

Infants may be febrile or hypothermic, have unstable temperature patterns, or have a normal temperature.[145, 225] Weisman and colleagues[225] noted that 85% of infants with early onset GBS disease had normal temperatures on admission to the NICU and that preterm infants were more likely to have hypothermia and less likely to have fever than term infants. However, temperature instability was only found in 11% of VLBW infants with late onset infections.[65] It has also been shown that a difference greater than 3.5°C between the rectal and skin temperature of afebrile term infants with suspected sepsis may be predictive[145] of infection. Upon reviewing the literature, Klein and colleagues[119] found the following:

1. Temperature elevation in full-term infants is uncommon.
2. Temperature elevation is infrequently associated with systemic infection when only a single elevated temperature occurs.
3. Temperature elevation that is sustained for more than an hour is frequently associated with infection.
4. Temperature elevation without other signs of infection is infrequent.

Among febrile infants younger than 2 months of age, Bonadio and colleagues[24] found that alterations in affect, peripheral perfusion, and respiratory efforts were best predictive of infection.

Signs and symptoms of infection in the neonate usually involve multiple organ systems. Respiratory symptoms are prominent. These symptoms include tachypnea, grunting, flaring, retractions and, later, apnea. Respiratory distress syndrome may be indistinguishable from pneumonia clinically or by chest radiograph. Right-sided diaphragmatic hernia or pleural effusion may rarely be seen with GBS sepsis.[95]

Cardiovascular symptoms are of no less importance and include cyanosis, tachycardia, congestive heart failure, and shock, or poor peripheral perfusion. Infants may also develop gastrointestinal symptoms of vomiting and diarrhea, along with the findings of abdominal distention, guaiac-positive stools, ileus, hepatomegaly or, less frequently, splenomegaly. Metabolic derangements, such as hyperglycemia and hypoglycemia and metabolic acidosis, may develop in the sick infant. Hyperbilirubinemia may be found in one third of septic infants and has classically been described as direct, but it may also be indirect.[183] Urosepsis is particularly associated with jaundice.[195] Focal infections may occur as conjunctivitis, otitis, osteomyelitis, and omphalitis before or during the septic episodes. The lower extremity is particularly susceptible to local infection because of the frequent use of umbilical artery catheters in VLBW infants, resulting in seeding with septic emboli. Petechiae may be an early indication of sepsis, whereas purpura, thrombocytopenia, and disseminated intravascular coagulation (DIC) are more likely to occur late. Other skin lesions may include vesicles (especially with herpes simplex virus [HSV]), abscesses, cellulitis, or the granuloma found in listerial infections. Dermal erythropoiesis may be confused with purpura in the "blueberry muffin" baby. These infants are most likely to have nonbacterial infection (STORCH) and often have an associated hepatosplenomegaly and a direct hyperbilirubinemia. They are usually small for gestational age (SGA) as well. Finally, central nervous system findings may be highly variable, ranging from irritability to lethargy, hypertonia or hypotonia, decreased consciousness or

Table 13–2. Presenting Features of First Episode of Septicemia

Clinical Features	% of Total Patients (n = 325)*
Increased apnea/bradycardia	65
Increased oxygen requirement	48
Increased assisted ventilation	38
Gastrointestinal problems†	46
Lethargy/hypotonia	37
Temperature instability	10
Hypotension (systolic/diastolic drop ≥10 mm Hg)	8

*Includes 21 patients with multiple organisms.
†If any of the following: gastric aspirates; feeding intolerance; abdominal distention; blood in stool.
Adapted from Fanaroff AA, et al: Incidence, presenting features, risk factors and significance of late onset septicemia in very low birth weight infants. Pediatr Infect Dis J 17:593, 1998.

coma, and seizures. Only 17% to 18% of infants have a bulging fontanelle, because of the open sutures, and nuchal rigidity is even less common.[215] Klein and Marcy[119] summarized the clinical findings of 455 septic infants at four medical centers (Table 13–1). These findings are similar, but vary in frequency, compared with 325 VLBW infants with sepsis, as described by Fanaroff and colleagues[65] (Table 13–2).

◆ DIAGNOSIS

In order to prove that bacterial sepsis is present, an organism must be isolated in a culture of the blood or other normally sterile body fluid (cerebrospinal fluid [CSF], joint, peritoneal or pleural fluid). A blood culture should be obtained before the initiation of antibiotics and may be effective with as little as 0.2 mL of blood,[53] although ideally there should be two or more cultures sent of 0.5 mL or more in order to optimize the yield.[115] This is often not practical. The incidence of falsely negative cultures is unknown, yet only 82% of infants who died of sepsis, as confirmed by postmortem examination, had a positive blood culture before death in one study.[171] In contrast, samples of blood from capillary sticks or from umbilical catheters that are not just being placed are not acceptable, because there is a high risk of contamination and associated false-positive results. The growth of most organisms is detected within 48 hours using stan-

Table 13–1. Clinical Signs of Bacterial Sepsis in 455 Newborn Infants Studied at Four Medical Centers

Clinical Sign	Infants with Sign (%)
Hyperthermia	51
Hypothermia	15
Respiratory distress	33
Apnea	22
Cyanosis	24
Jaundice	35
Hepatomegaly	33
Lethargy	25
Irritability	16
Anorexia	28
Vomiting	25
Abdominal distention	17
Diarrhea	11

From Klein JO: Bacterial sepsis and meningitis. In Remington JS, Klein JO, eds: Infectious Diseases of the Fetus and Newborn Infant. 5th ed. Philadelphia: WB Saunders, 2001, p 965.

dard techniques,[170] but growth can usually be detected within 24 hours of culture.[186] In addition, a smear of the buffy coat of anticoagulated, centrifuged blood in capillary tubes, stained with either Gram stain and methylene blue or with acridine orange and examined under the microscope, may be used to rapidly identify three fourths of the organisms in neonates with sepsis.[63]

Urine cultures are rarely helpful in early onset disease, but, when needed, these should be obtained by sterile method using suprapubic aspiration or catheterization in the infant older than 3 to 4 days of life.[54, 220] Cultures of tracheal aspirates and Gram stains may be helpful in identifying an organism to guide antibiotic therapy, but they do not discriminate between infection and colonization. Likewise, stool cultures may identify pathogens such as *Salmonella, Shigella, Clostridium difficile,* and *Campylobacter,* but usually they otherwise only identify intestinal colonization. Joint, pleural, peritoneal, and soft tissue aspiration may also be helpful in identifying specific organisms to prove and guide therapy.

Because meningitis may be found in one fourth of infants with bacterial sepsis, all infants with the clinical signs of sepsis should have a lumbar puncture, excluding the very ill infant who may experience cardiac and respiratory compromise during its performance.[80] However, the lumbar puncture has a low yield in the asymptomatic infant receiving treatment primarily because of maternal or obstetric risk factors.[68, 194, 226] In such cases, the use of the lumbar puncture is controversial.

A Gram stain should be examined for all CSF specimens, because detection of organisms may be found in as many as 80% of samples from infants with meningitis.[187] Interpretation of the CSF examination can be challenging. The leukocyte count of neonatal CSF is higher than among children and adults, and it may contain polymorphonuclear leukocytes. The total protein content is also higher than among older children, whereas the CSF glucose is much lower, perhaps as a result of the lower serum glucose levels common among infants. A task force on the diagnosis of meningitis suggested the following values[118]: The white blood cell count (WBC) of the CSF in a healthy newborn ranges from 0 to 32/μL (mean, 8/μL) in the first week, with up to 60% of the cells being polymorphonuclear leukocytes, but

the WBC should be no higher than 10/μL by 1 month of age. The range of protein concentration in the term infant is 20 to 170 mg/dL (mean 90 mg/dL), and in the preterm infant, it is 65 to 150 mg/dL (mean 115 mg/dL). The CSF glucose level varies even more because of the variation in serum glucose in the newborn. If the serum glucose concentration is obtained before the lumbar puncture, the ratio of CSF to blood glucose should average 70:80.

Adding to difficulties in interpretation, the lumbar puncture may be traumatic. Although the resultant red blood cells may be lysed with acetic acid to allow a more accurate count of the leukocytes, there are still the questions of how many leukocytes are present as a result of the contamination of the peripheral blood and how the higher protein level should be interpreted. Many formulas have been proposed, but none are totally reliable. One of the more common estimates allows one leukocyte for every 700 red blood cells[38, 159, 205] or the ratio of the RBC count to the WBC count may be compared in the serum and CSF.

Antigen detection assays may be used to make a more rapid, presumptive diagnosis of certain infections, such as infection with GBS, *E. coli, Neisseria meningitidis,* and *Streptococcus pneumoniae,* or to make a diagnosis when antibiotics are administered before cultures are drawn, making recovery of an organism unlikely. Counter immunoelectrophoresis (CIE) uses type-specific antisera against pathogens in the patient's CSF, serum, or urine. Latex agglutination tests for GBS infection are simple, rapid, and more sensitive than CIE, but not as specific. The sensitivity ranges from 90% to 100%, but specificity may be as low as 81%.[7, 180] False-positive GBS latex agglutination tests are particularly problematic with bagged urine samples, causing many researchers to recommend against their use. Polymerase chain reaction (PCR) involves a newer technology that is currently being explored in diagnosing sepsis.[124]

◆ ADJUNCTIVE TESTS

White Blood Cell Count and Differential

There are many adjunctive tests available to assist the physician in diagnosing neonatal sepsis. The number of tests and their combination into screening batteries indicate their low predictive value and the need for the physician to use clinical judgment.

The most widely used study is the WBC and differential. Manroe et al.[139] have established normal reference values for neutrophilic cells in capillary blood specimens in the first 28 days of life (Fig. 13–2). The lower limit of the total, or absolute, neutrophil count begins at 1750/mm³, peaks at 12 hours of life, at 7200/mm³, and then slowly declines until, at 72 hours of life, the lower limit is again 1750/mm³. The ratio of immature-to-total neutrophils (I:T ratio) remains less than 0.16 to 0.20 in healthy newborns. The timing and source of the blood sampling must be taken into account. Venous and arterial counts are lower than capillary counts.[39] Also, at the start of an infection, a count may still be normal.[41] Neutropenia is more predictive of neonatal sepsis than neutrophilia, but it may also be associated with maternal hypertension, birth asphyxia, and periventricular hemorrhage.[139] Neutropenia in the face of sepsis may be an indicator of bone marrow NSP depletion, which carries a mortality rate of possibly as high as 90%.[40] In another study, the mortality rate associated with neutropenia correlated with the need for assisted ventilation (20%) or an absolute neutrophil count less than 500/mm³ (24%).[12]

Acute Phase Reactants, Cytokines, and Other Screening Methods

The acute phase reactants are proteins made by the liver in response to the inflammation resulting from infection, trauma, or other causes of cellular injury. They are frequently used as adjuncts in the diagnosis of neonatal sepsis, but they do not have sufficient sensitivity and specificity to be of tremendous benefit. The C-reactive protein (CRP) is minimally transferred across the placenta. Concentrations are elevated in 50% to 90% of infants with systemic bacterial infections,[176] but they may also be elevated with meconium aspiration, asphyxia, shock, and prolonged rupture of membranes.

The erythrocyte sedimentation rate (ESR) includes the response of multiple serum acute phase reactant proteins. It also responds to any cause of inflammation and is of limited specificity. Plasma fibronectin[121] is a glycoprotein. It is produced by the liver, but also by endothelial cells, and is important in wound healing and hemostasis and acts as an opsonin. It appears to be decreased early in the presence of infection, but it is also decreased with asphyxia, respiratory distress syndrome, and bronchopulmonary dysplasia, limiting its usefulness.

Cytokines are being studied for their usefulness in diagnosing neonatal sepsis. The two most commonly investigated are tumor

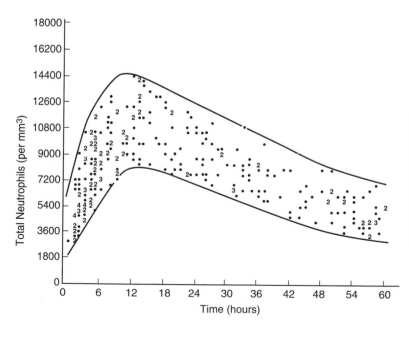

Figure 13–2. The total neutrophil count reference range in the first 60 hours of life. Circles represent single values; numbers represent the number of values at the same point. Heavy lines represent the envelope bounding these data. (From Manroe BL, Weinberg AG, Rosenfeld CR, et al: The neonatal blood count in health and disease. I. Reference values for neutrophilic cells. J Pediatr 95:89, 1979.)

necrosis factor (TNF-α) and interleukin (IL)-6. Both cytokines appear to be elevated in the presence of infection and are less often elevated in its absence. Further study is needed. Measurement of serum fibronectin,[121] soluble CD14,[22] procalcitonin,[37, 151] serial IL-6 levels,[161] and IL-6 in conjunction with CRP, TNF, and IL-8[57, 130, 155] may have some value either in the early diagnosis of neonatal sepsis or in the early discontinuation of antibiotics.

Screening Panels

In an attempt to more accurately identify sepsis before cultures are known or early in the course of the disease, many investigators have combined several tests together. These panels are not very helpful in improving the positive predictive accuracy, but a negative panel does reduce the likelihood of neonatal sepsis by 98% to 100%.[98] Some panels to consider are those by Philip et al,[167, 168] Krediet et al,[123] Tegtmeyer et al,[212] and Gerdes et al.[79]

◆ MANAGEMENT

In any infant suspected of sepsis, antimicrobial therapy should be initiated immediately after completion of the diagnostic evaluation. The progression of the disease is too rapid to await confirmation from blood or other cultures. If the infant is too unstable or in an unfavorable location to perform a lumbar puncture, then antibiotics should be given after obtaining a blood culture and the lumbar puncture should be obtained at a more appropriate time and place. In early onset sepsis, antibiotic coverage is needed for both the gram-positive cocci, most often GBS, and the gram-negative bacilli. In most cases, it is also prudent to cover *L. monocytogenes*, a gram-positive bacillus. These organisms continue to be of concern throughout the newborn period. The GBS remain sensitive to penicillin, ampicillin, and third-generation cephalosporins. *Listeria* is sensitive to ampicillin, but is not well covered by the cephalosporins. The aminoglycosides, including tobramycin, gentamicin, and amikacin, and the cephalosporins, including cefotaxime, ceftazidime, and ceftriaxone, provide reasonable coverage for the gram-negative bacilli. Aminoglycoside se-

rum concentrations are recommended measurements, because ototoxicity and nephrotoxicity can be dose-related complications of aminoglycoside therapy, but fortunately complications are rare in newborns. This toxicity is not a problem with cephalosporins. However, cephalosporin use may facilitate the development of antibiotic resistance among bacteria.[31] Although comparative trials are lacking,[143, 144] the early outcome of neonatal meningitis treated with cephalosporins is apparently comparable to that of neonates given an aminoglycoside, and CSF concentrations of the cephalosporins are high. Thus, initial coverage of neonatal sepsis usually includes ampicillin or penicillin and an aminoglycoside. Which aminoglycoside is chosen should depend on the local sensitivity patterns. This coverage is appropriate for neonatal meningitis, but ampicillin and a cephalosporin, usually cefotaxime, should be considered if gram-negative rods are seen. Neither intraventricular nor intrathecal administration of antibiotics for neonatal meningitis has been beneficial.[143, 144]

In nosocomial sepsis, antibiotics must cover staphylococci and the gram-negative bacilli, including *Pseudomonas*. Sometimes nafcillin or methicillin can be used to cover *S. aureus*. In nurseries where methicillin-resistant strains have emerged or where coagulase-negative staphylococci are frequent pathogens, vancomycin coverage is necessary. There is good *Pseudomonas* coverage with aminoglycosides (except kanamycin) and ceftazidime. All central catheters should be removed immediately. Abscesses, infected joints, or other collections of pus should be drained as well.

It is particularly important to check the susceptibility of microorganisms isolated from culture and to adjust coverage as necessary. Most often, the duration of therapy is at least 10 to 14 days for sepsis, 21 days for meningitis, and longer for osteomyelitis. Persistence of an infiltrate on chest radiograph in the absence of positive cultures may be treated for 7 to 10 days. In the absence of an infiltrate on chest radiograph or positive cultures at 48 to 72 hours, a decision is usually made clinically whether to treat further for neonatal sepsis.

Extracorporeal membrane oxygenation has been successful in recent years in rescuing neonates at high risk of dying of sepsis.[146, 206] Although the trials are conflicting in outcome, there may be some efficacy of granulocyte transfusions in overwhelming neonatal sepsis.[11, 32, 40, 128] However, the value is not proven, and the risks of infection with hepatitis, CMV, and HIV are too significant to justify use of granulocyte transfusions in nonexperimental situations. Successful outcome with IV immunoglobulin (IVIG) therapy has also been reported, but the use of IVIG remains experimental.[99]

EDITORIAL COMMENT: Jenson and Pollock reviewed all published studies of IVIG for the prevention or treatment of neonatal sepsis, which included over 4000 neonates. Using conservative and objective outcome rating criteria, they concluded that "the addition of IVIG to standard therapies is of minimal but demonstrable benefit in preventing sepsis when administered prophylactically to premature low birth weight newborns and of unequivocal benefit in preventing death when administered therapeutically for early-onset neonatal sepsis. The likelihood of newborns with sepsis living past the neonatal period was improved nearly sixfold when IVIG was administered in addition to standard therapies." Lacy and Ohlsson with a similar meta-analysis concurred that the routine administration of IVIG to preterm infants is not recommended. There are efforts to produce designer IG preparations with specific high titers against the common nosocomial infections including coagulase negative staphylococci.

◆———

Jenson HB, Pollock BH: Meta-analyses of the effectiveness of intravenous immune globulin for prevention and treatment of neonatal sepsis. Pediatrics 99:E2, 1997.

Lacy JB, Ohlsson A: Administration of intravenous immunoglobulins for prophylaxis or treatment of infection in preterm infants: Meta-analyses. Arch Dis Child Fetal Neonatal Ed 72:F151–155, 1995.

◆ PROPHYLAXIS

Environmental

The environmental conditions and the invasive procedures to which neonates are exposed are clearly important predisposing factors for sepsis. Those measures that encourage colonization of the newborn with nonpathogenic bacteria while preventing colonization with pathogens are of primary importance. Colonization is initiated on the umbilicus and skin and then spreads to the nasopharynx, eyes, and gastrointestinal tract. The more rapid the rate of colonization, the more likely it is that invasive disease will occur, especially if the infant is colonized with a nursery-acquired, multiply antibiotic-resistant pathogen. Neonates predominantly acquire S. aureus from the hands of nursery personnel. Thus, careful hand washing before and after handling an infant remains crucial to efforts to prevent infection. Careful skin and cord care are also critical. Hexachlorophene has been shown to be effective in controlling S. aureus colonization of the newborn, but the risks of vacuolar neurotoxicity are too significant to risk its routine use in bathing or washing infants.[172] Acceptable agents for cord care include triple dye, silver sulfadiazine, and antibiotic ointments, whereas chlorhexidine and soap baths are being used in skin care. The use of cover gowns is not supported by available data, and their routine use is not required.[14] Cover gowns are still to be used, however, in situations requiring isolation or enteric precautions. Silver nitrate, povidone iodine, or erythromycin eye drops may be used to prevent gonococcal or chlamydial ophthalmic infections.[184]

Judgment must be used in selecting the necessary invasive procedures required in an infant and in limiting the duration of exposure in that infant. Of additional concern is the duration of exposure of an infant to total parenteral nutrition and intravenous fat emulsion via a central catheter.

Although there are few controlled trials supporting its efficacy in prevention of infections, breast milk may provide an advantage over bottle feedings. This is especially true in underdeveloped countries because of unhygienic conditions. Studies have suggested a decrease in gastroenteritis, otitis, respiratory infections, neonatal sepsis, and meningitis.[48, 235]

The use of intravenous immunoglobulin (IVIG) in prophylaxis of infection remains unproven.[7, 65, 99] The use of hyperimmune products may be of more benefit, but needs to be studied.

◆ SPECIFIC NEONATAL INFECTIONS

GBS disease has been intensely studied and massive efforts have been made to eradicate perinatal infection. These efforts and their successes and their failures deserve careful attention.

Group B Streptococcal Disease

In the United States, GBS disease has been a leading cause of bacterial sepsis and death in neonates since the 1970s. GBS disease is also a major cause of urinary tract infection, endometritis, and chorioamnionitis in the pregnant woman.[34] In 1990, it was estimated that 7600 cases of invasive disease and 310 deaths attributed to GBS occurred among infants younger than and up to 90 days of age.[35] Since routine chemoprophylaxis has come into play, GBS infections have been reduced, but still account for 0.5 to 1.0 case per 1000 live births.[131, 152]

Early onset disease (80% of all GBS infections) may occur from birth to 6 days of life, but most cases present by 12 hours of life with an abrupt onset of apnea, respiratory distress, grunting, tachypnea, cyanosis, shock, meningitis, poor feeding, or abdominal distention. The syndrome of sepsis (25% to 40%), pneumonia (35% to 55%), or meningitis (5% to 15%) develops in these infants.[7] The pneumonia may be indistinguishable from respiratory distress syndrome radiographically, but, perhaps in one third, infiltrates will develop and, in others, pleural effusions.[7] Mortality rate remains 10% to 15% and is associated with neutropenia or left shift on complete blood count, shock, apnea, a low 5-minute Apgar score, pleural effusion, prematurity, and delay in treatment.[127, 166] Interestingly, less than one third of infants[191] in the United States with early onset disease were born prematurely,[185] in contrast to 70% of those born in Australia.[78]

Traditionally, late onset disease has presented in infants from 7 days to 3 months of age, but most often at approximately 1 month of age. However, recent reports indicate that 20% of infants are becoming ill beyond 3 months of life.[237] These infants usually have unremarkable neonatal courses. Few of them are premature infants. They have an insidious onset of lethargy, poor feeding, and irritability, but fever, apnea, and sometimes hypotension go on to develop. In 40%, meningitis develops. Fatality rate (2% to 6%)[191, 237] is associated with neutropenia, hypotension, coma, CSF protein greater than 300 mg/dL, and status epilepticus.[6] Hearing loss is a common sequela.

Focal GBS infections may also develop subtly, with decreased to no movement of an extremity at 3 to 4 weeks of life or later, and may involve cellulitis or septic arthritis/osteomyelitis, often at a single site. More than half of the infections are in the hip, followed by the knee and femur. Function, and sometimes growth, may be affected. There is a strong predilection for female infants for arthritis and to a lesser degree for osteomyelitis.[7]

Rarely, there is also recurrence of infection, either during treatment or up to 1½ months later, with the same or different isolates. Inadequate antibiotic dosing may be involved, but persistent mucous membrane colonization has also been implicated.[52, 162]

Three fourths of the infants in whom early onset disease develops can be predicted by three factors: maternal fever greater than 37.5°C, prolonged rupture of membranes greater than 18 hours, and birth at 37 weeks' gestation or less.[7, 26] Infants born to mothers who had a prior infant with GBS disease are at particular risk, as are infants born to mothers with low or absent type-specific antibody.[46] Continued study has yielded other risk factors (Table 13–3).[192] Maternal urinary tract infection may simply

Table 13–3. Multivariate Model: Conditional Logistic Regression of Characteristics Associated With Early Onset Group B Streptococcal Disease

Characteristics	Odds Ratio	95% Confidence Interval	P
Intrapartum fever	11.88	3.83–36.86	0.0001
Rupture of membranes before labor	8.68	3.35–22.51	0.0001
Urinary tract infection during pregnancy	4.33	1.20–15.52	0.02
Labor >12 h	2.23	0.95–5.22	0.06
Maternal age			
<20 y	8.03	0.76–10.5	
20–29 y	2.83	1.47–5.46	0.002
≥30 y	1.00	(reference)	

Adapted from Schuchat A, et al: Multistate case-control study of maternal risk factors for neonatal group B streptococcal disease. Pediatr Infect Dis J 13:623, 1994.

indicate heavier maternal colonization.[192] Indeed, vertical transmission of GBS (colonized mother resulting in colonized infant) occurs with 65% of heavily colonized mothers but only 17% of lightly colonized mothers.[26] Heavy colonization is associated with a 12-fold higher risk of early onset disease and a four-fold risk of late onset disease, compared with light colonization.[55] More recently, GBS disease has been associated with teen mothers (independent of prematurity) and black race (independent of prenatal care)[192] (Fig. 13–3).

Group B streptococci[192] (*Streptococci agalactiae*) colonize the human gastrointestinal and genitourinary tracts in nearly one third of pregnant women and are occasionally found in the pharynx. Vaginal and anorectal cultures placed in selective media should be obtained from the mother at 35 to 37 weeks' gestation to screen for colonization, which is usually constant[34, 45] throughout the pregnancy. Transmission from mother to infant usually occurs in utero or just before delivery and less than 6 hours of incubation is required for early onset disease.[46] Person-to-person and hand-to-person transmission may also occur in the nursery or the community. There are nine serotypes that may cause disease in the infant and mother: Ia, Ib/c, Ia/c, II, III, IV, V, VI, and VII. Serotype III is the predominant cause of infection, especially with meningitis (85%) and late onset disease (89%).[7] However, recent surveys have shown a shift in distribution of serotypes, with serotype V, previously unknown, becoming of increased importance, particularly in the northeastern United States. This creates difficulty in the development of anti-GBS vaccines.[23, 95, 135]

An algorithm for prophylaxis of neonatal GBS infection and empiric therapy of neonates born to mothers who received intrapartum antimicrobial prophylaxis (IAP) has been agreed upon (Figs. 13–4 through 13–6) by the American College of Obstetricians and Gynecologists, the American Association of Pediatricians, and the Centers for Disease Control and Prevention.[34, 45] Two doses of ampicillin need to be administered to the mother (greater than 4 hours of therapy) in order to significantly reduce neonatal transmission.[51]

Treatment for presumptive disease requires penicillin G or ampicillin, plus an aminoglycoside. Penicillin G alone is adequate for GBS when it is positively identified. Duration of therapy should be at least 10 days for bacteremia, 14 to 21 days for meningitis, and greater than 4 weeks for osteomyelitis/arthritis. A repeat lumbar puncture is indicated after 24 hours of treatment in meningitis and may be repeated again if bacteriologic cure is questioned.[46]

There has been considerable concern regarding the emergence of antibiotic resistance as a result of the increased maternal exposure to antibiotics in labor. Penicillin-sensitive mothers are often given erythromycin and clindamycin, but resistance is currently present in 21% and 4% of GBS isolates, respectively.[185] Also, non-GBS bacteria (with ampicillin resistance as high as 87%) may be more commonly causing early

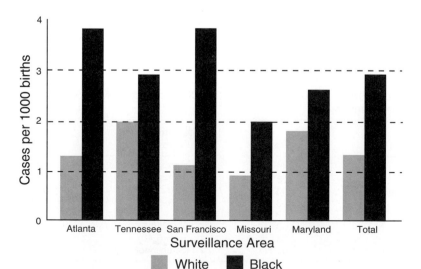

Figure 13–3. Incidence of early onset group B streptococcal disease in cases per 1000 live births by geographic area and race. (From Schuchat A, Deaver-Robinson K, Plikaytis BD, et al: Multistate case-control study of maternal risk factors for neonatal group B streptococcal disease. Pediatr Infect Dis J 13:623, 1994.)

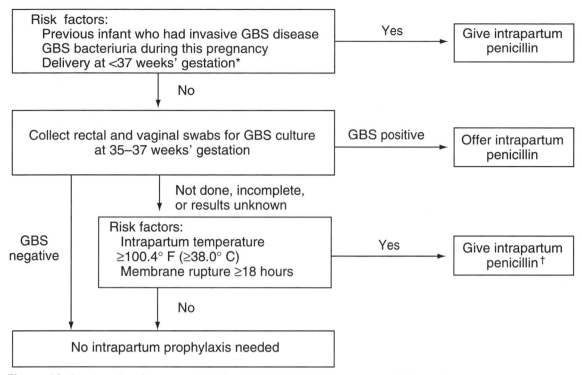

Figure 13–4. Algorithm for prevention of early onset group B streptococcal (GBS) disease in neonates, using prenatal screening at 35 to 37 weeks' gestation.

*If membranes ruptured at <37 weeks' gestation and the mother has not begun labor, collect group B streptococcal culture and either (a) administer antibiotics until cultures are completed and the results are negative or (b) begin antibiotics only when positive cultures are available. No prophylaxis is needed if culture obtained at 35–37 weeks' gestation was negative.

†Broader spectrum antibiotics may be considered at the physician's discretion, based on clinical indications.

(From Centers for Disease Control and Prevention: Prevention of perinatal group B streptococcal disease: A public health perspective. MMWR Morb Mortal Wkly Rep 45:1, 1996.)

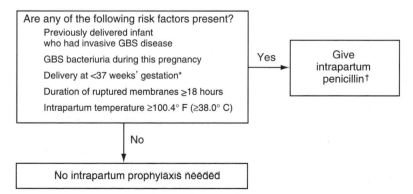

Figure 13–5. Algorithm for prevention of early onset group B streptococcal (GBS) disease in neonates, using risk factors.

*If membranes ruptured at <37 weeks' gestation and the mother has not begun labor, collect group B streptococcal culture and either (a) administer antibiotics until cultures are completed and the results are negative or (b) begin antibiotics only when positive cultures are available.

†Broader spectrum antibiotics may be considered at the physician's discretion, based on clinical indications.

(From Centers for Disease Control and Prevention: Prevention of perinatal group B streptococcal disease: A public health perspective. MMWR Morb Mortal Wkly Rep 45:1, 1996.)

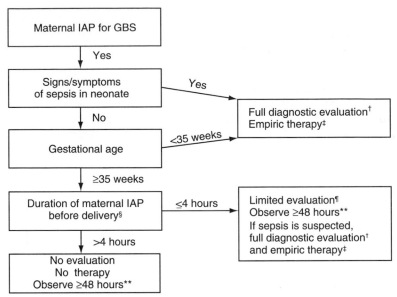

Figure 13–6. Algorithm* for management of a neonate born to a mother who received intrapartum antimicrobial prophylaxis (IAP) for prevention of early onset group B streptococcal (GBS) disease.
*This algorithm is not an exclusive course of management. Variations that incorporate individual circumstances or institutional preferences may be appropriate.
†Includes a complete blood count (CBC) and differential, blood culture, and chest radiograph if neonate has respiratory symptoms. Lumbar puncture is performed at the discretion of the physician.
‡Duration of therapy will vary depending on blood culture and cerebrospinal fluid (CSF) results and the clinical course of the infant. If laboratory results and clinical course are unremarkable, duration of therapy may be as short as 48-72 hours.
§Duration of penicillin or ampicillin chemoprophylaxis.
¶CBC and differential and a blood culture.
**Does not allow early discharge.
(From Centers for Disease Control and Prevention: Prevention of perinatal group B streptococcal disease: A public health perspective. MMWR Morb Mortal Wkly Rep 45:1, 1996.)

onset disease.[214] Similarly, Joseph and colleagues[113] reported that early onset *E. coli* disease was not occurring more frequently, but was more fulminant and more likely to be associated with ampicillin resistance. This needs to be watched carefully.

Staphylococcus epidermidis

Coagulase-negative staphylococci have become the leading cause of nosocomial bacteremia in the nursery, representing as many as 55% of all infections among VLBW infants.[73, 107, 114, 209] Low birth weight, gestational age, and prolonged hospital stay, particularly in an intensive care unit, are major determinants of infection,[65, 73] as well as the multiple complications of prematurity, respiratory distress syndrome, intraventricular hemorrhage, bronchopulmonary dysplasia, necrotizing enterocolitis, and patent ductus arteriosus.[65] These latter factors would ap-

pear to correlate with the need for intensive care. Indeed, prolonged intubation and mechanical ventilation, delayed establishment of enteral feeds, prolonged use of central venous catheters for parenteral nutrition, and the use of steroids are noted to increase the risk.[65, 112, 207] Overcrowding and understaffing in the nursery increases the infection rate,[90] as does lower concentrations of serum IgG among preterm infants.[65] Of particular concern are the studies attributing a large proportion of the risk to intravenous lipid emulsions.[4, 74, 75]

There are multiple strains of coagulase-negative staphylococci, but most infections are caused by *S. epidermidis*. Most species isolated from infections are notable for the production of slime, an extracellular polysaccharide material that aids in bacterial adherence to catheters and other smooth surfaces and probably inhibits chemotaxis and phagocytosis by neutrophils,[59, 92, 103] leading to increased invasiveness. Shunts, catheters, endotracheal tubes, and procedures that lead to breaks in the skin or mucous membranes lead to infection. Using molecular techniques, it has been shown that clones of *S. epidermidis* can be endemic for as long as a decade in the nursery and that nosocomial transmission among infants and staff is of critical importance.[59, 103, 164] Most infecting strains of *S. epidermidis* both produce β-lactamase and are resistant to β-lactamase-resistant penicillins. If the strain is methicillin-sensitive, oxacillin or nafcillin should be used. Otherwise, vancomycin coverage is necessary. Gentamicin and rifampin may add some synergy to vancomycin use. Abscesses need to be drained and foreign materials removed. Contact precautions may interrupt nosocomial spread.

Most episodes of *S. epidermidis* bacteremia are late onset, in that they develop from the strains colonizing the infant. Although the onset may be fulminant, the course is usually more subtle or indolent,[73] with no localized source. Cases present with increasing apnea and bradycardia, respiratory distress and need for support, temperature instability, abdominal distention, gastric aspirates and guaiac-positive stools, lethargy, and poor perfusion.[16, 65, 153, 157] However, metabolic acidosis, a left shift on white blood cell count, thrombocytopenia, and hyperglycemia may be present.[65] Meningitis, omphalitis, cellulitis, and abscesses also can complicate the infection.

Infected infants have longer hospital stays, higher mortality rates, prolonged ventilation, and more severe intraventricular hemorrhage than noninfected infants.[65] There has also been a report of *S. epidermidis* occurring as an early onset sepsis, with severe illness.[65, 207]

Staphylococcus aureus

Large nursery epidemics of *S. aureus*, common in the 1950s and resulting in bacteremias, impetigo, abscesses, and pneumonia, have become less common. Pustules, impetigo, osteomyelitis, arthritis, endocarditis, and conjunctivitis sporadically develop. Scalded skin syndrome or toxic shock syndrome may also develop.[228] Of greater concern is the spread in the nursery of methicillin-resistant *S. aureus*. Molecular epidemiology studies have demonstrated that single or multiple strains may become endemic in the nursery.[137, 157, 201] *S. aureus* commonly colonizes the anterior nares of staff and family members who then can transmit the infection throughout the nursery or in the community, via hands, nasal discharge, or droplets.[56, 197, 210] Antibiotic resistance appears to be increasing over time.[114] Susceptible strains may be treated with oxacillin or methicillin; otherwise, vancomycin is needed. Teicoplanin is being evaluated for use against methicillin-resistant staphylococci.[66] The prevalence of methicillin-resistant *S. aureus* colonization does decrease with time, declining significantly in one study of colonized neonates at 1 year of age to 14%.[148] During a nursery epidemic, mupirocin ointment may be used topically, in the nares, to eliminate nasal carriage.[56]

Systemic Fungal Infections

Systemic candidal infections, once discounted as blood culture contaminants, were recognized in the 1980s as being responsible for 2% to 4% of nosocomial infections among VLBW infants.[9, 110] Currently they are recognized as being responsible for as many as 15% of these infections,[65] and, in some nurseries, are the leading source of nosocomial infections. Previously, 75% of candidal infections were caused by *Candida albicans*,[30] with the remainder caused by non-*albicans* species, such as *Candida tropicalis* (10%), *Candida parapsilosis* (6%), and others. Recently, multiple reports have indicated an increasing frequency of *C. parapsilosis* infections in the nursery.[102, 122, 133, 188, 221] In some nurseries, as many as 50% to 60% of systemic candidal infections may be due to *C. parapsilosis*.

Candida spp. may be transmitted vertically during birth from the mother to the infant. As many as 27% of infants weighing less than 1500 g are colonized with fungi in the NICU.[10] However, there are increasing reports of horizontal transmission within the nursery, particularly in epidemics and particularly with *C. parapsilosis*, as documented by electrophoretic karyotyping, restriction endonuclease analysis of genomic DNA, and other methods.[102, 116, 133, 217, 221]

Candidemia is most common among the VLBW neonates in the NICU. Other risk factors for disease include the use of broad-spectrum antibiotics, which suppress bacterial flora and allow unopposed fungal proliferation,[9, 196, 223] and the use of central venous and arterial catheters, particularly when used for total parenteral nutrition and intravenous lipid.[9, 133, 223] Prolonged endotracheal intubation,[9, 223] the immature skin of preterm infants, and necrotizing enterocolitis also provide access for the fungi.[223] In addition, the immune system of these infants is less effective at inhibiting candidal growth. The use of intravenous hydrocortisone, and possibly other drugs, is a significant risk for disseminated disease.[25] In contrast, most infants weighing greater than 2500 g who have candidiasis have been shown to have congenital anomalies that require prolonged stays in the intensive care unit.[180]

Candida has been cultured from the fetal surface of the placenta in 0.8% of cases of chorioamnionitis[140] and congenital candidiasis may result from ascending infection, across intact fetal membranes. These infants may have a maculopapular rash that desquamates and discrete, yellow plaques or abscesses on the umbilical cord. Systemic treatment may be required if the infant aspirates infected secretions and has respiratory distress[234] or if the infant is VLBW and symptoms present within the first 3 days of life with a severe burnlike dermatitis.[13]

Otherwise, infants are seen at 4 to 6 weeks of age with marked apnea and bradycardia, increasing respiratory distress, generalized erythema, hyperglycemia, temperature instability, and hypotension.[9, 110] Pneumonia may develop and chest film may show generalized haziness or severe bronchopulmonary dysplasia,[9, 165] or the infant may have abdominal distention, feeding intolerance, and guaiac-positive stools, usually without pneumatosis intestinalis[9] or outright necrotizing enterocolitis. A right atrial intracardiac mass may be associated with central venous catheterization, and infected thrombi may be found associated with any central catheter.[110] Meningitis may be found in half the neonates and should be treated aggressively because survival depends on early initiation of therapy.[64] Endophthalmitis appears as a fluffy white mass in a hazy vitreous.[8] Renal involvement is common and may range from pelvic fungal balls causing hydronephrosis to acute renal failure to cortical abscesses.[5, 165] In one report, *Candida* spp. were identified in 42% of hospital acquired urinary tract infections in an intensive care nursery and 52% of infected infants had fungemia, whereas 35%

had renal fungal balls.[169] Involvement may also include osteoarthritis,[174] especially secondary to seeding of lower extremity joints, or cutaneous rashes and abscesses.

Little is known regarding outcome. Reports indicate that mortality rate for candidemia is lower among neonates than adults and lower for *C. parapsilosis* than for *C. albicans*.[122, 238] One report of a case controlled study indicated that infants with candidemia were more likely to die and had a higher grade of intraventricular hemorrhage and that survivors were more likely to be disabled, with a rate as high as 29%. Yet, another study indicated that infants with candidemia had a 95% rate of retinopathy of prematurity, far greater than among uninfected infants (69%), and that they were more likely to reach stage III or more or to require laser surgery.[149]

Diagnosis may be made from sterilely obtained cultures of the blood, CSF, and urine; by skin scrapings; or by ultrasonography and indirect ophthalmoscopy. The therapy of choice remains intravenous amphotericin B, often combined with 5-fluorocytosine in the presence of central nervous system disease.[21] However, many reports are available regarding the use of fluconazole and liposomal amphotericin B, which has fewer side effects, particularly renal side effects, and considerable success, sometimes in infants who had failed amphotericin B therapy.[58, 67, 76, 104, 189, 222, 227]

Another fungal infection, that of *Malassezia furfur*, has occurred in miniepidemics in VLBW infants receiving intravenous lipid emulsions.[181] These infants respond well to discontinuance of the catheter and lipid emulsion.

Listeriosis

L. monocytogenes remains an uncommon, but typical, neonatal pathogen found in some geographic areas more than others. This organism is acquired by ingestion of contaminated foods, most often dairy products.[33] Like GBS disease, both early and late onsets occur. Infection appears to be acquired from an infected mother who, oftentimes, has been ill with nonspecific, flulike symptoms, including fever, chills, and malaise. Headache and muscle pains are often described in the days to weeks before delivery and may be associated with premature delivery and a positive maternal blood culture. Infants with early onset disease may be sick at birth. A transient pustular rash on a red base may be present. Signs of sepsis can be severe and may include a pneumonitis. Infection presenting after the first week of life is often, although not invariably, associated with meningitis. Meningitis is not always immediately suspected, because milder presentations are common, and the diagnosis may not be made until spinal fluid examination is done as part of a fever workup in the young infant. The organism may be seen on Gram stain and the finding of gram-positive rods on CSF examination or in a maternal blood culture should immediately raise the possibility of *Listeria* infection in the infant. Ampicillin remains the antimicrobial of choice, with an aminoglycoside frequently added for initial management. In cases of meningitis, 400 mg/kg of ampicillin should be used and continued for up to 3 weeks. In areas where listeriosis has occurred, pregnant women should avoid potential exposure to the organism by avoiding soft cheeses and unpasteurized milk products, as well as not eating incompletely cooked meat or meat products.[33]

Cytomegalovirus

Congenital infection with CMV is responsible for both symptomatic disease (cytomegalic inclusion disease, or CID), as well as asymptomatic infection in the newborn. It is the most common viral infection transmitted to the newborn. Primary infection during pregnancy is responsible for symptomatic disease, whereas maternal reactivation of latent infection, a common occurrence during pregnancy, is associated with asymptomatic disease in the newborn. Populations with a high baseline rate of infection in women of childbearing age, such as occurs in much of the developing world, have a low incidence of CID because primary infection during pregnancy is unusual. Unlike for most other pathogens, in utero transmission of CMV can occur during reactivation of maternal CMV infection, but this most often results in an asymptomatic infection in the newborn. However, some of these infants will have sequelae, most importantly deafness.[71] Perinatal infection also occurs secondary to viral shedding into the birth canal with infection acquired during labor and delivery, as well

as secondary to viral shedding into breast milk with transmission associated with breast-feeding. Again, when associated with reactivation of infection in the mother, these infections are usually asymptomatic in the infant. Primary maternal infection with transmission during labor and delivery has been associated with severe pneumonitis in the infant.

Transmission related to breast-feeding is almost always asymptomatic and is likely responsible for high infection rates in young children in the developing world. Because the virus is shed into breast milk and is effectively transmitted by breast-feeding, theoretic concerns have been raised about using donor or banked breast milk to feed newborns, especially very premature infants. This is not an issue for the mother's own infant, however, because infection in that setting will likely be asymptomatic, perhaps related to transmission in utero of maternal antibody.

CID should be suspected in the infant born with thrombocytopenia, especially in association with microcephaly, jaundice, and hepatosplenomegaly. Often, but not invariably, infants are premature or small for gestational age. A rash may be present that may be transient and consisting of petechiae alone, although in some cases purpura may also be present. Children with overt signs and symptoms are likely to have permanent sequelae, some of which may evolve over the first months and years of life from continued infection and tissue destruction. Characteristic periventricular intracranial calcifications may help to confirm a suspected clinical diagnosis, but these are only present rarely, even with symptomatic disease.

Children with asymptomatic infection are also at risk for development of sensorineural deafness and, rarely, other neurologic problems. In approximately 7% of asymptomatically infected children, sensorineural hearing loss develops, which may progress over the first months of life.[71] Recognizing this progression raises the possibility that treatment could potentially affect the outcome of infection, but no data yet suggest that either asymptomatic or symptomatic children should be treated with ganciclovir routinely. Studies are ongoing.[231]

Diagnosis, once suspected, can be confirmed by detection of the virus. Serologic techniques are less reliable. The gold standard remains viral culture of urine, blood, or saliva. Rapid tests are increasingly available and include PCR for detection of the virus. Serology can often be used to confirm results and to document primary or secondary infection in the mother by showing significant titer changes, sometimes associated with the presence of a reliable IgM antibody test. The finding of CMV DNA by molecular techniques in the placenta can also be used to confirm the diagnosis of congenital infection in suspected cases.[160]

Acquired Immunodeficiency Syndrome

Women who are infected with HIV may transmit infection during pregnancy and the perinatal period. The risk for transmission appears to depend on factors such as the mother's stage of infection, including the severity of her immune suppression and her viral load, as well as perinatal factors, including the length of rupture of membranes before delivery and delivery via elective cesarean section versus vaginal route.[29, 62, 106, 138] Primary infection during pregnancy appears to carry a risk of 50% for transmission. Rates of transmission during chronic HIV infection have varied, depending on the population studied, but appear to be between 20% and 40%.[126, 141, 154, 173, 182] Clearly, this rate can be significantly decreased if the mother receives antiretroviral therapy during pregnancy, labor, and delivery. The rate is further lowered if the infant continues on therapy for the first weeks after birth. Standard of care is to treat the HIV-infected pregnant woman and newborn with at least zidovudine and possibly with multiple antiretrovirals, depending on the mother's stage of disease. Keeping the mother's viral load as low as possible significantly decreases transmission to the newborn.[77, 150]

The HIV-infected newborn is usually indistinguishable from the uninfected infant. Whereas most children have signs and symptoms in the first years of life, increasingly, older children are being recognized who have congenital infection and who have remained well into childhood. If a pregnant woman is recognized as infected, her newborn should be followed up closely and screened early to make the diagnosis. Most will be on protocols that include zidovudine during the first weeks of life. At about 1 month, trimethoprim/sulfamethoxazole should be added to prevent *Pneumocystis carinii* infection and should be continued until it is clear that the infant is not infected with HIV. Diagnosis can be made by viral culture, PCR, or viral load measurements. It is safest to repeat a positive test, often using a different test, for certainty, before confirming infection. Two negative tests, at least one after 6 months of age, is likely to predict absence of infection, with confirmation by serologic absence of antibody after 15 months of life, when maternal antibody has faded. Babies born to HIV-infected mothers may have more complicated neonatal courses and proportionally more are found in the NICU. This is likely related to the lower socioeconomic class of these mothers and the higher likelihood of poor prenatal care. Breast-feeding is not recommended, unless there is no other safe form of nutrition for the infant, as occurs in underdeveloped countries.

Herpes Simplex Infections

Neonatal herpes simplex infections have also become increasingly common. The herpes viruses are double-stranded DNA viruses. After replication, some viral DNA persists in the dorsal root ganglia for the lifetime of the individual and is responsible for periodic recurrences over the skin and mucosa innervated by that nerve.

Labial and oropharyngeal infections are usually caused by type I (HSV-1) and are transmitted via direct contact or respiratory droplets. HSV-1 infections may cause a gingivostomatitis or mononucleosis-like syndrome.

Transmission of HSV-2 usually occurs during or after adolescence via sexual contact, often with asymptomatic individuals. Pain and burning, followed by paresthesia, then vesicles, which may break down and leave shallow ulcers, may occur on the labia or mucosa, but infections are more likely to be asymptomatic.

A primary infection is one that occurs in a previously uninfected individual, whereas recurrent infections occur with reactivation of the virus. Most infections are recurrent. Recurrence is greater with HSV-2 infection than with HSV-1, in that HSV-2 is more likely to become latent in the inguinal dorsal root ganglia.

There is no history of infection or symptoms or history of intercourse with an infected individual in 70% of women whose infants have HSV infections.[232, 233] Roughly one third of women who asymptomatically shed HSV in labor have been recently infected and their infants are 10 times more likely to be infected than infants born to women with recurrent disease.[27]

Transmission of infection to the neonate occurs by transplacental, intrapartum, and postpartum routes. Congenital infection (transplacental) may represent 5% of all infected infants.[232] These infants may have severe skin scarring, growth retardation, psychomotor retardation, intracranial calcifications, microcephaly, hypertonicity, and seizures. There may also be microphthalmia, cataracts, chorioretinitis, and retinal dysplasia. These infections appear to occur solely with HSV-2, whether primary or recurrent.

Intrapartum transmission is responsible for 85% to 90% of neonatal infection and is more likely with a primary infection, because of the high viral titer, increased likelihood of cervical shedding, and possibly protection from maternal antibody.[229] Half of all neonatal HSV-2 infections occur secondary to recurrent maternal infection, even though only 5% of infants are infected from the mother in this scenario.[179] Neonatal infection occurs, however, in 50% of the infants after a primary third trimester maternal infection.[179] Transmission of the virus is increased with prolonged rupture of membranes (greater than 6 hours) and with the use of fetal scalp monitors, which may breach the intact skin barrier. Antenatal maternal viral cultures are not helpful in predicting which mothers will be shedding virus at delivery.[179]

Lastly, viral transmission (most often of HSV-1) may occur from the environment, postnatally. Spread may occur among babies in a nursery, from either the father or mother, or from hospital personnel. One third of hospital personnel have a history of HSV-1 infections and 1% develop recurrent labial lesions.[97] Individuals with herpetic whitlows should be removed from the nursery. HSV-1 is believed to be responsible for 30% of all neonatal infections.[232]

Two thirds of term newborns with neonatal infection are discharged to home before onset of the infection. These infants may also have a concurrent bacterial infection.

However, half of the infected infants are born prematurely and many of these infants also suffer from respiratory distress syndrome. Asymptomatic neonatal infections almost never occur.

Neonatal infections are clinically classified as (1) disseminated, involving multiple organs, with or without central nervous system involvement, (2) encephalitis, with or without skin, eye, or mouth involvement, and (3) localized infection to the skin, eyes, or mouth.

Disseminated infections predominantly involve the liver, adrenal glands, and lungs, but may involve virtually every organ system. Although there may be earlier, unrecognized symptoms, the usual presentation is at 9 to 11 days of life with signs and symptoms of bacterial sepsis and shock. In one fifth of the infants, skin or mucosal vesicles never develop. Hepatomegaly or hepatitis, with or without jaundice, is usually present. Pneumatosis intestinalis may also be present. DIC is common, resulting in decreased platelets, petechiae, and purpura, and there may be gastrointestinal bleeding. Pneumonia and pleural effusion are associated with a poorer prognosis. Central nervous system involvement may be signaled by irritability, apnea, a bulging fontanelle, seizures, posturing, or coma, but many infants die before these symptoms develop. The virus can be isolated from the CSF in only one third of infants with symptoms, but the CSF may show evidence of hemorrhage.

Encephalitis also presents at 9 to 11 days of life, when brain involvement occurs as a result of viral dissemination or seeding of the brain, but it can also present later, at 16 to 17 days of life, when infection occurs via neuronal transmission, in association with skin, eye, or mouth lesions. Skin vesicles develop in only 60% of these infants. Less than half have virus isolated from the CSF, which usually shows a mild pleocytosis with a predominance of mononuclear cells, an elevated protein concentration, and a normal glucose concentration. Electroencephalograms are usually abnormal, as are brain imaging studies. In these infants, lethargy, poor feeding, irritability, or seizures develop, and nearly half of untreated infants die of neurologic deterioration within 6 months from onset, with virtually all survivors suffering severe sequelae. Blindness, cataracts and microcephaly are common.

Vesicles develop in most infants with

skin, eye, or mouth disease, usually in clusters, and often over the presenting part at birth. Presentation is usually at 10 to 11 days of life. Recurrent skin or oropharyngeal lesions are common. Keratoconjunctivitis, chorioretinitis, microphthalmia, and retinal dysplasia may develop from either HSV-1 or HSV-2 infection. Neurologic symptoms develop later in one third of cases.

Viral isolation (from CSF, stool, urine, conjunctivae, nasopharynx, or skin/mucosal lesions) is diagnostic of infection. Immunofluorescent antibody and enzyme immunoassays have been helpful in earlier recognition, but PCR is of increasing use. Cultures obtained after birth of an infant born to an infected woman can be delayed 24 to 48 hours to help distinguish viral replication from contamination occurring at birth.

Vaginal delivery or cesarean delivery after rupture of membranes in the presence of lesions or positive cultures results in the greatest risk to the newborn. These infants should be isolated and cultured after 24 hours of life. They should be carefully inspected for skin lesions and the complete blood count and liver function tests should be followed. Prophylactic antiviral therapy has not been recommended. The mother should be counseled regarding hand washing, kissing the infant (if there are cold sores), and signs and symptoms of the disease. Ophthalmologic examination may be helpful. The circumcision should be delayed and the mother's breasts should be inspected for herpetic lesions.

Acyclovir is a specific inhibitor for viral DNA polymerase and should be used for a minimum of 14 days. Others advocate longer treatment to prevent recurrences. Survival after acyclovir treatment was 61% for disseminated disease with only 60% of survivors showing normal development at 1 year of life.[229] The relative risk of death was 5.2 for infants in or near coma at onset of treatment, 3.8 for infants with DIC, and 3.7 for premature infants. Pneumonitis, seizures, and infection with HSV-2 also resulted in a higher mortality.[230] Survival rate with encephalitis was 86%, but only 29% of these infants were developing normally at 1 year of life. However, all infants with skin, eye, or mouth disease survived and 98% had normal development at 1 year of life, even though infants with three or more recurrences of vesicles within 6 months were more likely to have sequelae.[229]

Hepatitis

There are at least five specific viruses associated with primary infection of the liver. Congenital infection with the hepatitis viruses occurs regularly with hepatitis B, but only rarely with the other hepatitis viruses.[213] Transmission of hepatitis B vertically to the newborn is a serious worldwide problem, which is avoidable with vaccination. Infants born to mothers who are chronic hepatitis B virus carriers are at significant risk for acquiring infection. If the mother is hepatitis e antigen positive, the risk of transmission can be as high as 90% if no prophylaxis is given.[17] Acute hepatitis B infection during the last trimester of pregnancy is also highly associated with transmission—76% in one study.[193] Transmission of hepatitis B occurs mostly at the time of labor and delivery and is due to exposure of the infant to infected maternal blood. Infection acquired in the neonatal period is usually asymptomatic, but approximately 90% of infected infants become chronic carriers of hepatitis B virus and are at significant risk for chronic liver disease, cirrhosis, liver cancer, and transmission of infection to their children over their lifetimes. Screening all pregnant women for hepatitis B surface antigen allows identification of infants at risk for acquisition of infection. Vaccination of the infant born to a mother who is a hepatitis B carrier (has a positive serology for hepatitis B surface antigen) significantly reduces the chance of infection. The addition of a dose of hepatitis B immunoglobulin given to the baby, ideally in the delivery room or in the hours after delivery, further decreases this risk. With the administration of both vaccine and immunoglobulin, rates of protection are about 95%.[18, 211] A small percentage of children fail this prophylaxis and appear to have had in utero transmission of the infection, a rare but definite occurrence. In endemic areas, neonatal vaccination programs have begun to dramatically decrease perinatal infections. In the United States, a policy of universal hepatitis B vaccination has recently been adopted with initiation of the vaccination series beginning in the neonatal period. This is effective in interrupting perinatal transmission, is less expensive than vaccinating older children or adults (less vaccine required), and gives the best results (highest percent of patients seroconvert to high levels of antibody, well above the apparent protective serum levels). Vaccine schedules vary, and can be the traditional 0-, 1-, and 6-month schedule or a 0-, 1-, and 2-month schedule or, in the child not born to an infected mother, a 2-, 4-, and 6-month schedule has been used. In the child born to an infected mother, the series should begin in the newborn period, as close to delivery as possible, with the rapid schedule offering some theoretic advantages.[83]

The use of interferon-α has been studied in adults and in small numbers of children and is sometimes effective in the treatment of chronic hepatitis B infections. Children with liver disease should be referred to specialists familiar with therapy for evaluation and follow-up for signs of hepatitis and cirrhosis and, as they get older, for liver cancer.

Standard immunoglobulin has not been effective in preventing infection and is not recommended. Breast-feeding is not contraindicated, but the individual mother should be educated about the current understanding of transmission of infection. Children should not be excluded from child care.[50]

The hepatitis viruses transmitted by the fecal-oral route, including hepatitis A and E, are usually not associated with congenital infection.[94] Infection can occur in the neonatal period, but does not appear to be associated with severe or chronic disease. As in the young infant and child, infection is likely to be asymptomatic with hepatitis A. However, infected infants and young children, either in the home or day care settings, are important sources of transmission in the community.

Immunoglobulin used to modify or prevent transmission of hepatitis A must be given within 2 weeks of exposure. Because the period of viral shedding begins 1 to 2 weeks before clinical disease and lasts only briefly after clinical jaundice appears, prophylaxis is difficult to use effectively. Occasionally, a baby is born to a mother with recently diagnosed disease. If this occurs more than 1 to 2 weeks before delivery, it is too late for immunoglobulin to be effective, but administration can be considered when the hepatitis occurs and is recognized within the 2 weeks before delivery. There are effective hepatitis A vaccines available, but they are not for use in newborns.

Hepatitis E (single-stranded RNA virus related to the calcivirus) is one of perhaps several other enterally transmitted viral hepatitides other than A. This infection also is usually asymptomatic in newborns and children, but, unlike the other causes of hepatitis, it is especially dangerous in the pregnant woman during epidemics of infection, as described in Asia, Africa, and Mexico, where the infection is endemic.[117] A fatality rate of up to 20% has been described in pregnant women. Cases in this country are related to travel to endemic areas.

Hepatitis C, like hepatitis B, is transmitted mostly by exposure to blood and blood products and to a much lesser extent by sexual contact. High-risk groups, therefore, include intravenous drug abusers, hemodialysis patients and those who have received multiple blood transfusions or blood products, and women who are partners of hepatitis C-infected individuals. Acute infection is highly associated with persistence and chronic infection, usually with few symptoms. Eventually, most infections result in a chronic hepatitis and cirrhosis develops in approximately 20% of cases. Children, like adults, are usually asymptomatic. Transmission in utero and in the perinatal period is uncommon, but it is estimated to occur in about 5% of pregnancies of infected women and is even higher if the mother is also infected with HIV.[85, 158] There is no proof or evidence of transmission by breast-feeding,[134] but the virus can be detected in colostrum. There is no official contraindication for breast-feeding, but mothers should understand the concerns and be part of the decision to breast-feed or not. Infants born to women with infection should be followed serologically for evidence of infection. Because antibody from the mother is transmitted, antibody titers need to be obtained on newborns or children younger than 2 years of age. Eventually, a universal vaccine recommendation for hepatitis A for children is likely to be adopted in the United States. This will decrease the need for immunoglobulin for prevention and could control the disease completely.

Toxoplasmosis

The risk of congenital toxoplasmosis varies in different populations, with rates in pregnant women reflecting factors such as ingestion of uncooked meat and, more recently, control measures addressed at pregnant women. In the United States, the rate is estimated to be about 1 in 1000, significantly lower than for CMV. Infection acquired early in pregnancy is most likely to result in a severely affected infant, but transmission risk is low during a maternal infection, approximately 10%. In the last trimester, risk of transmission is high, but infection is more likely to be asymptomatic at birth. Only primary infections in the mother are associated with transmission in utero, except for the immunocompromised mother, such as the mother with AIDS, in whom transmission may occur to more than one child. The most severely affected newborns are born with stigmata, including splenomegaly, hepatomegaly, hydrocephalus (or microcephaly), chorioretinitis, CSF pleocytosis, and intracranial calcifications.[142] Nonspecific signs such as fever, jaundice, seizures, and anemia may also be present. These children are at high risk for severe mental retardation. Subclinical infection occurs frequently, especially in later infections. When sought, however, abnormal CSF findings and chorioretinitis may be present.[142] Follow-up is important because other signs may develop over time. It has recently been shown that treatment of children with congenital toxoplasmosis can affect the long-term outcome of infection.[142] Children given sulfadiazine and pyrimethamine and folic acid for the first year of life often had reversal of neurologic findings and many who, without treatment, would likely have been retarded had normal growth and development during early follow-up evaluations. These data stress the importance of early screening for congenital infection to identify infants who can benefit from therapy.[88] Prenatal diagnosis of infection in the pregnant woman can be done using fetal blood sampling. Women who choose to continue the pregnancy can be offered maternal therapy, which can modify the congenital infection.[49]

Gonococcal Infection

Neisseria gonorrhoeae may be responsible for infection in pregnant women who are asymptomatic. Untreated gonorrhea in the mother results in an increased risk for prematurity and perinatal death. Infection of the newborn occurs during birth and occasionally after prolonged rupture of membranes. Infants born to an infected mother may become colonized or infected. About 30% of infants acquire ophthalmic infection after a vaginal delivery.[184] Conjunctivitis is usually severe, with swollen lids and pus exuding from the eyes. Prompt treatment is necessary to avoid spread or local scarring. Diagnosis can be made on Gram stain of the pus and confirmed by culture.

Systemic infection also can occur. Bacteremia in the newborn can present as sepsis, meningitis, endocarditis, or arthritis, often with multiple joints involved. Arthritis alone, presumably after an earlier bacteremia, may occur relatively late, from 1 to 4 weeks after birth. Infection that is not clearly and definitely related to acquisition at birth must be investigated for child abuse.

Prevention is crucial. In the United States, all infants are given eye prophylaxis at birth with 1% silver nitrate, 0.5% erythromycin ophthalmic ointment, or 3.1% tetracycline ophthalmic ointment, in single-use tubes. In infants infected in utero, however, infection may develop despite prophylaxis and needs to be treated. Infants born to women with untreated infection at the time of delivery should also be treated. Women who are found to be infected should also be screened for other sexually transmitted diseases, including syphilis and HIV infection. Newborns should be treated with a third generation cephalosporin, such as ceftriaxone or cefotaxime for a preterm infant, because of the prevalence of penicillin-resistant strains.

Syphilis

The incidence of syphilis is again increasing. Infection is transmitted in utero, with the most significant risk occurring during the last trimester. About 40% of fetal infections result in death either in utero or in the immediate neonatal period. Primary syphilis in the pregnant woman carries the highest risk for the fetus. Chancres are painless ulcers that occur at the site of infection anywhere on the mother's body and are often associated with enlarged regional nodes. Signs of secondary disease may include fever, malaise, a rash, and mucous membrane patches. Untreated syphilis during pregnancy carries the risk of stillbirth, premature delivery, neonatal death, or possible latent infection. Infections have been missed at birth when the mother had a negative serology because not enough incubation time had passed. Therefore, follow-up of newborns with suspicious histories or maternal risk factors must be meticulous. Inadequately documented maternal treatment, treatment in the last trimester of pregnancy, or treatment with an antibiotic other than penicillin is considered inadequate. Signs and symptoms of syphilis in the newborn may include prematurity, a large placenta, unexplained fetal hydrops, symmetric bony lesions involving the metaphyses and diaphyses of the long bones, failure to thrive, rhinitis, intractable diaper rash, jaundice, hepatosplenomegaly, anemia, diffuse pneumonia at birth, chorioretinitis, and aseptic meningitis.

The diagnosis is usually made by serology but can be made by dark field examination for spirochetes from lesions or nasal discharge. Many infected infants are asymptomatic, and the disease is only recognized when the serology is studied. These infants should receive full treatment, especially if adequate follow-up is not guaranteed after discharge. Any child with a positive test, whether treated or not, should be observed for titer change. Titers decline within 6 months if the child has been adequately treated. A positive serology that remains reactive in the first months of life suggests that the infant is infected, and treatment should be repeated. Babies born to women with a reactive rapid plasma reagin test should also have the CSF examined. Presently, regardless of CSF results, it is recommended that treatment be for a minimum of 10 days.

CASE PROBLEMS

Case One

Mrs. A. B. is preparing to take home her 27-weeks' gestational age, 750-g infant girl who is 2 months of postnatal age. Her infant's neonatologist recommends that she take her infant for treatment with palivizumab, beginning in October, to prevent severe infection with respiratory syncytial virus (RSV). It is now July. Mrs. A. B. wants to know about RSV.

◆ *You tell her:*
1. *It is a seasonal virus that peaks in the cold months.*
2. *Infection with RSV confers lifelong immunity to infection.*
3. *RSV is especially likely to progress to lower respiratory tract disease in healthy infants younger than 3 months of age, premature*

infants, those with cyanotic congenital heart disease, or those who are immunosuppressed.
4. *RSV is especially likely to progress to lower respiratory tract disease in infants with bronchopulmonary dysplasia or cystic fibrosis.*

The correct answers are 1, 3, and 4.[81, 82, 91, 136, 200] RSV is a paramyxovirus, which is large and enveloped. It occurs in annual epidemics in winter and spring. Repeated infections are common, even in sequential years. All of the groups noted in answer 3 are at high risk for lower respiratory tract disease.

Mrs. A. B. wants to know how one gets RSV and what her infant might look like if she is infected.

◆ *You tell her:*
1. *Transmission occurs via infected secretions that may be spread as droplets from the respiratory tract.*
2. *Transmission occurs via infected secretions that persist for hours on surfaces in the environment or for at least a half hour on hands.*
3. *Infection initially occurs in the gastrointestinal tract.*
4. *Bronchiolitis, pneumonia, or croup may result from RSV infection.*
5. *Premature infants may require mechanical ventilation for apnea.*

The correct answers are 1, 2, 4, and 5.[93, 120] Humans are the only source for RSV and spread the disease via infected secretions. Initial infection occurs in the nasopharynx and eyes and causes rhinitis, cough, and fever, as well as acute otitis media in one third of infected children. Lower respiratory tract disease may present with respiratory distress, retractions, and difficulty feeding, plus apnea in preterm infants. Lower respiratory tract disease may result in hypoxia, carbon dioxide retention, air trapping, and marked bronchospasm.

Mrs. A. B. also wants to know who should get palivizumab, what the side effects are, and how effective the preparation is.

◆ *You tell her:*
1. *Palivizumab is a humanized monoclonal antibody given intramuscularly during the RSV season.*
2. *Palivizumab resulted in fewer hospital admissions owing to RSV infection and even reduced the number of episodes of acute otitis media.*
3. *Palivizumab is particularly effective in infants with cyanotic congenital heart disease, but also for preterm infants or those with bronchopulmonary dysplasia.*

4. Palivizumab may result in side effects, including hypersensitivity reactions, vomiting, and fever.

The correct answer is 1.[105, 111, 178, 199] Palivizumab, a humanized monoclonal antibody, does decrease the number of hospital admissions due to RSV. It does not, however, decrease otitis media or hospitalizations caused by non-RSV respiratory viruses, although intravenous RSV immunoglobulin does do this. Treatment is contraindicated in infants with cyanotic heart disease, because these infants had a higher incidence of adverse outcomes with heart surgery after intravenous RSV immunoglobulin. Palivizumab is particularly effective in preterm infants and those with bronchopulmonary dysplasia. There is a 3% incidence of reactions at the injection site.

◆ *You also tell Mrs. A. B. that palivizumab is indicated for:*
1. *Infants with bronchopulmonary dysplasia who are less than 2 years of age and have required oxygen therapy within the 6 months before the RSV season.*
2. *Infants of 28 weeks' gestational age or less who are less than 12 months' postnatal age at the beginning of the RSV season.*
3. *Infants of 29 to 32 weeks' gestational age who are less than 6 months' postnatal age at the beginning of the RSV season.*
4. *Infants who are 32 to 35 weeks' gestational age who are in the homes of smokers, are attending day care, or are one of multiple births.*

1 through 4 are all correct answers.[44, 105, 111, 178, 199]

◆

Case Two

Mrs. C. D. comes into the emergency department in active labor and is noted to have active lesions of chickenpox, which developed the day before admission.

◆ *Which of the following are true?*
1. *The infant should be given varicella zoster immune globulin (VZIG) at birth.*
2. *Mother and baby should be isolated.*
3. *The mother and baby should be given acyclovir.*
4. *The baby may remain in the newborn nursery until 7 days of life.*

The correct answers are 1, 2, and 4.[28, 61, 147, 177]

Babies infected in utero are born before the transfer of maternal antibody and are at risk of severe infection, with a mortality rate of 20% to 30%. Therefore, babies born to mothers in whom the rash develops 1 to 5 days before delivery should be given VZIG.

A newborn with a postnatal exposure to varicella zoster whose mother is susceptible should also be considered for VZIG therapy but is at considerably lower risk for severe disease. The incubation period for chickenpox is 10–21 days. An individual is no longer infectious after all lesions have crusted over. Therefore, respiratory isolation is indicated for susceptible individuals for 10 to 21 days after exposure (or 28 days if VZIG is given).

REFERENCES

1. Albers W, Tyler CW, Boxerbaum B: Asymptomatic bacteremia in the newborn infant. J Pediatr 69:193, 1966.
2. Allansmith M, McClennan BH, Butterworth M, et al: The development of immunoglobulin levels in man. J Pediatr 72:276, 1968.
3. Anthony B, Okada DM, Hobel CV: Epidemiology of group B streptococcus: Longitudinal observations during pregnancy. J Infect Dis 137:524, 1978.
4. Avila-Figueroa C, Goldmann DA, Richardson DK, et al: Intravenous lipid emulsions are the major determinant of coagulase-negative staphylococcal bacteremia in very low birth weight newborns. Pediatr Infect Dis J 17:10, 1998.
5. Baetz-Greenwalt B, Debaz B, Kumar ML: Bladder fungus ball: A reversible cause of neonatal obstructive uropathy. Pediatrics 81:826, 1988.
6. Baker C: Nosocomial septicemia and meningitis in neonates. Am J Med 70:698, 1981.
7. Baker C, Edwards MS: Group B streptococcal infections. In Remington JS, Klein JO, eds: Infectious Diseases of the Fetus and Newborn Infant. Philadelphia: Mosby, 1998.
8. Baley J, Annable WL, Kleigman RM: Candida endophthalmitis in the premature infant. J Pediatr 98:458, 1981.
9. Baley J, Kliegman RM, Fanaroff AA: Disseminated fungal infections in very low birth weight infants: Clinical manifestations and epidemiology. Pediatrics 73:144, 1984.
10. Baley J, Kliegman RM, Boxerbaum B, et al: Fungal colonization in the very low birth weight infant. Pediatrics 78:225, 1986.
11. Baley J, Stork EK, Warkentin PI, et al: Buffy coat transfusions in neutropenic neonates with presumed sepsis: A prospective, randomized trial. Pediatrics 80:712, 1987.
12. Baley J, Stork EK, Warkentin PI, et al: Neonatal neutropenia: Clinical manifestations, cause and outcome. Am J Dis Child 142:1161, 1988.
13. Baley J, Silverman RA: Systemic candidiasis: Cutaneous manifestations in low birth weight infants. Pediatrics 82:211, 1988.
14. Baley J, Fanaroff AA: Neonatal infections. I. Infection related to nursery care practices. In Sinclair JC, Bracken M, eds: Effective Care of the Newborn Infant. London: Oxford Press, 1992.
15. Barry D, Reeve AW: Increased incidence of gram-negative neonatal sepsis with intramuscular iron administration. Pediatrics 60:908, 1977.

16. Baumgart S, Hall SE, Campos JM, et al: Sepsis with coagulase-negative staphylococci in critically ill newborns. J Dis Child 137:461, 1983.

17. Beasley RP, Trepo C, Stevens CE, et al: The e antigen and vertical transmission of hepatitis B surface antigen. Am J Epidemiol 105:94, 1977.

18. Beasley R, Hwang LY, Lee GC, et al: Prevention of perinatally transmitted hepatitis B virus infection with hepatitis B immune globulin and hepatitis B vaccine. Lancet 2:1099, 1983.

19. Benirschke K: Routes and types of infection in the fetus and newborn. Am J Dis Child 99:714, 1960.

20. Bennet R, Erikson M, Melen B, et al: Changes in the incidence and spectrum of neonatal septicemia during a fifteen year period. Acta Paediatr Scand 74:687, 1985.

21. Bennett J, Dismukes WE, et al: A comparison of amphotericin B alone and combined with flucytosine in the treatment of cryptococcal meningitis. N Engl J Med 301:126, 1979.

22. Blanco A, Solis G, Arranz E, et al: Serum levels of CD14 in neonatal sepsis by gram-positive and gram-negative bacteria. Acta Paediatr 85:728, 1996.

23. Blumberg H, Stephens DS, Modansky M, et al: Invasive group B streptococcal disease: The emergence of serotype V. J Infect Dis 173:365, 1996.

24. Bonadio W, Hennis H, Smith D, et al: Reliability of observation variables in distinguishing infectious outcome of febrile young infants. Pediatr Infect Dis J 12:111, 1993.

25. Botas C, Kurlat I, Young SM, et al: Disseminated candidal infections and intravenous hyrdo-cortisone in preterm infants. Pediatrics 95:883, 1995.

26. Boyer K, Gadzala CA, Burd LI, et al: Selective intrapartum chemoprophylaxis of neonatal group B streptococcal early onset disease. I. Epidemiologic rationale. J Infect Dis 148:795, 1983.

27. Brown ZA, Benedetti J, Ashley R, et al: Neonatal herpes simplex virus infection in relation to asymptomatic maternal infection at the time of labor. N Engl J Med 324:1247, 1991.

28. Brunell P: Placental transfer of varicella-zoster antibody. Pediatrics 38:1034, 1966.

29. Burns DN, Landesman S, Muenz LR, et al: Cigarette smoking, premature rupture of membranes, and vertical transmission of HIV-1 among women with low CD4+ levels. J Acquir Immune Defic Syndr 7:718,1994.

30. Butler K, Baker CJ: Candida: An increasingly important pathogen in the nursery. Pediatr Clin North Am 35:543, 1988.

31. Byran C, John JF Jr, Pai MS, et al: Gentamicin vs. cefotaxime for therapy of neonatal sepsis. Am J Dis Child 139:1086, 1985.

32. Cairo M, Worcester C, Rucker R, et al: Role of circulating complement and polymorphonuclear leukocyte transfusion in treatment and outcome in critically ill neonates with sepsis. J Pediatr 110:935, 1987.

33. Centers for Disease Control and Prevention: Update: Foodborne listeriosis: US 1988–90. MMWR 41:251, 1992.

34. Centers for Disease Control and Prevention: Prevention of perinatal group B streptococcal disease: A public health perspective. MMWR 45:1, 1996.

35. Centers for Disease Control and Prevention: Decreasing incidence of perinatal group B streptococcal disease. United States 1993–1995. MMWR 46:473, 1997.

36. Chasnoff I: Chemical dependency and pregnancy. Pediatr Res 18:1, 1991.

37. Chiesa C, Panero A, et al: Reliability of procalcitonin concentrations for the diagnosis of sepsis in critically ill neonates. Clin Infect Dis 26:664, 1998.

38. Chow G, Schmidley JW: Lysis of erythrocytes and leukocytes in traumatic lumbar punctures. Arch Neurol 41:1084, 1984.

39. Christensen R, Rothstein G: Pitfalls in the interpretation of leukocyte counts of newborn infants. Am J Clin Pathol 72:608, 1979.

40. Christensen R, Rothstein G, Anstall HB, et al: Granulocyte transfusions in neonates with bacterial infection, neutropenia and depletion of mature marrow neutrophils. Pediatrics 70:1, 1982.

41. Christensen R, Rothstein G, Hill HR, et al: Fatal early onset group B streptococcal sepsis with normal leukocyte counts. Pediatr Infect Dis J 4:242, 1985.

42. Collado M, del Kretschmer RR, Becker I, et al: Colonization of Mexican pregnant women with group B streptococcus. J Infect Dis 143:134, 1981.

43. Committee on Infectious Diseases. American Academy of Pediatrics: Hepatitis C virus infection. Pediatrics 101:481, 1998.

44. Committee on Infectious Disease. American Academy of Pediatrics: Respiratory syncytial virus immune globulin intravenous: Indicators for use. Pediatrics 99:645, 1997.

45. Committee on Infectious Diseases and Committee on Fetus and Newborn: American Academy of Pediatrics: Revised guidelines for prevention of early onset group B streptococcal (GBS) infection. Pediatrics 99:489, 1997.

46. Committee on Infectious Diseases. Group B streptococcal infections. In Peter G, ed: Report on Committee on Infectious Diseases. Elk Grove Village, IL: American Academy of Pediatrics, 1997.

47. Committee on Infectious Diseases, American Academy of Pediatrics: Prevention of hepatitis A infections: Guidelines for use of hepatitis A vaccine and immune globulin. Pediatr 98:1207, 1996.

48. Coppa G, Gabrielli OR, Giorgi P, et al: Preliminary study of breast feeding and bacterial adhesion to uroepithelial cells. Lancet i:569, 1990.

49. Daffos F, Forestier F, MacAleese J, et al: Prenatal management of 746 pregnancies at risk for congenital toxoplasmosis. N Engl J Med 318:271, 1988.

50. Davis L, Weber DJ, Lemon SM: Horizontal transmission of hepatitis B virus. Lancet i:899, 1989.

51. deCueto M, Sanchez MJ, Sampedro A, et al: Timing of intrapartum ampicillin and prevention of vertical transmission of group B streptococcus. Obstet Gynecol 91:112, 1998.

52. Denning D, Bressack M, Troup NS, et al: Infant with two relapses of group B streptococcal sepsis documented by DNA restriction enzyme analysis. Pediatr Infect Dis J 7:729, 1988.

53. Dietzman D, Fischer GW, Schoenknecht FD: Escherichia coli septicemia—Bacterial counts in blood. J Pediatr 85:128, 1974.

54. DiGeronimo R: Lack of efficacy of the urine culture as part of the initial work-up of suspected neonatal sepsis. Pediatr Infect Dis J 9:764, 1992.

55. Dillon H Jr, Khare S, Gray BM: Group B streptococcal carriage and disease: A 6 year prospective study. J Pediatr 110:31, 1987.

56. Doebbling BN: Nasal and hand carriage of *Staphylococcus aureus* in healthcare workers. J Chemother 6(Suppl 2):11, 1994.

57. Doellner H, Arntzen KJ, Haereid PE, et al: Interleukin-6 concentrations in neonates evaluated for sepsis. J Pediatr 132:295, 1998.

58. Driessen M, Ellis JB, Cooper PA, et al: Fluconazole vs. amphotericin B for the treatment of neonatal fungal septicemia: A prospective randomized trial. Pediatr Infect Dis J 15:1107, 1996.

59. Dunne W, Nelson DB, Chusid MJ: Epidemiologic markers of pediatric infections caused by coagulase-negative staphylococci. Pediatr Infect Dis J 6:1031, 1987.

60. Einhorn M, Fanaroff DM, Nohn MH, et al: Concentrations of antibodies in paired maternal and infant sera: Relationship to IgG subclass. J Pediatr 111:783, 1987.

61. Ehrlich R, Turner JA, Clarke M: Neonatal varicella. J Pediatr 53:139, 1958.

62. European Mode of Delivery Collaboration: Elective caesarean section versus vaginal delivery in prevention of vertical HIV-1 transmission: A randomized clinical trial. Lancet i:1035, 1999.

63. Faden H: Early diagnosis of neonatal bacteremia by buffy-coat examination. J Pediatr 99:1032, 1976.

64. Faix R: Systemic candida infections in infants in intensive care nurseries. High incidence of central nervous system involvement. J Pediatr 105:616, 1984.

65. Fanaroff AA, Korones SB, Wright LL, et al: Incidence, presenting features, risk factors and significance of late onset septicemia in very low birth weight infants. Pediatr Inf Dis J 17:593, 1998.

66. Fanos V, Kacet N, Mosconi G, et al: A review of teicoplanin in the treatment of serious neonatal infections. Eur J Pediatr 156:423, 1997.

67. Fasano C, O'Keeffe J, Gibbs D: Fluconazole treatment of neonates and infants with severe fungal infections not treatable with conventional agents. Euro J Clin Microbiol 13:351, 1994.

68. Fielkow S, Reuter S, Gotoff SP: Clinical and laboratory observations. Cerebrospinal fluid examination in symptom free infants with risk factors for infection. Pediatr 119:971, 1991.

69. Fitzhardinge P, Eisen A, Lejtenyi C, et al: Sequelae of early steroid administration to the newborn infant. Pediatrics 53:877, 1974.

70. Fleer A, Senders RC, Visser MR, et al: Septicemia due to coagulase-negative staphylococci in a neonatal intensive care unit: Clinical and bacteriologic features and contaminated parenteral fluids as a source of sepsis. Pediatr Infect Dis 2:426, 1983.

71. Fowler K, McCollister FP, Dahle AJ, et al: Progressive and fluctuating sensorineural hearing loss in children with asymptomatic congenital cytomegalovirus infection. J Pediatr 130:624, 1997.

72. Freedman R, Ingram DL, Gross I, et al: A half century of neonatal sepsis at Yale. Am J Dis Child 135:140, 1981.

73. Freeman J, Platt R, Epstein MF, et al: Birth weight and length of stay as determinants of nosocomial coagulase-negative staphylococcal bacteremia in neonatal intensive care unit populations: Potential for confounding. Am J Epidemiol 132:1130, 1990.

74. Freeman J, Goldmann DA, Smith NE, et al: Association of intravenous lipid emulsions and coagulase-negative staphylococcal bacteremia in neonatal intensive care units. N Engl J Med 323:301, 1990.

75. Freeman J, Goldman DA, et al: Association of intravenous lipid emulsion and coagulase-negative staphylococcal bacteremia in neonatal intensive care units. N Engl J Med 323:301, 1990.

76. Friedlich P, Steinberg I, Fujitani A, et al: Renal tolerance with the use of intralipid-amphotericin B in low-birth-weight neonates. Am J Perinatol 14:1, 1997.

77. Garcia PM, Kalish LA, Pitt J, et al: Maternal levels of plasma human immunodeficiency virus type 1 RNA and the risk of perinatal transmission. N Engl J Med 341:349, 1999.

78. Garland S: Early onset neonatal group B streptococcus infection: Associated obstetric risk factors. Aust N Z J Obstet Gynaecol 31:117, 1991.

79. Gerdes JS, Polin RA: Sepsis screen in neonates with evaluation of plasma fibronectin. Pediatr Infect Dis J 6:443, 1987.

80. Gleason C, Martin FJ, Anderson JV, et al: Optimal position for a spinal tap in preterm infants. Pediatrics 71:31, 1983.

81. Glezen WP, Taber LH, Frank AL, et al: Risk of primary infection and reinfection with respiratory syncytial virus. Am J Dis Child 140:543,1986.

82. Glezen WP, Paredes A, Allision JE, et al: Risk of respiratory syncytial virus infection for infants from low income families in relationship to age, sex, ethnic group, and maternal antibody level. J Pediatr 98:708, 1981.

83. Goldfarb J, Baley J, Medendrop SV, et al: Comparative study of the immunogenicity and safety of two dosing schedules of Engerix B hepatitis B vaccine in neonates. Pediatr Infect Dis J 13:18, 1994.

84. Gotoff S, Behrman R: Neonatal septicemia. J Pediatr 76:142, 1970.

85. Granovsky M, Minkoff HL, et al: Hepatitis C virus infection in the mothers and infants cohort study. Pediatrics 102:355, 1998.

86. Groothuis J, Simoes EAF, Levin MJ, et al: Prophylactic administration of respiratory syncytial virus immune globulin to high risk infants and young children. N Engl J Med 329:1524, 1993.

87. Groover R, Sutherland JM, Landing BH: Purulent meningitis of newborn infants. N Engl J Med 264:1115, 1961.

88. Guerina N, Hsu H, Meissner HC, et al: Neonatal serologic screening and early treatment for congenital *Toxoplasma gondii* infection. N Engl J Med 330:1858, 1994.

89. Hack M, Horbar JD, Malloy MH, et al: Very low birth weight outcomes of the National Institute of Child Health and Human Development Neonatal Network. Pediatrics 87:587, 1991.

90. Haley RW, Bregman DA: The role of understaffing and overcrowding in recurrent outbreaks of staphylococcal infection in a neonatal special care unit. J Infect Dis 145:875, 1982.

91. Hall CB, Powell KR, MacDonald NE, et al: Respiratory syncytial viral infection in children with compromised immune function. N Engl J Med 315:77, 1986.

92. Hall R, Hall SI, Barnes WG, et al: Characteristics of coagulase-negative staphylococci from infants with bacteremia. Pediatr Infect Dis J 6:377, 1987.

93. Hammer J, Numa A, Newth CJ: Acute respiratory distress syndrome caused by respiratory syncytial virus. Pediatr Pulmonol 23:176, 1997.

94. Zhang RJ, Zeng JS, Zhang HZ: Survey of 34 pregnant women with hepatitis A and their neonates. Chin Med J 103:552, 1990.

95. Harris M, Moskowitz WB, Engle WD, et al: Group B streptococcal septicemia and delayed onset diaphragmatic hernia: A new clinical association. Am J Dis Child 135: 723, 1981.

96. Harris L, Elliott JA, Dwyer DM, et al: Serotype distribution of invasive group B streptococcal isolates in Maryland: Implications for vaccine formulation. Maryland Emerging Infections Program. J Infect Dis 177:998, 1998.

97. Hatherly LI, Hayes K, Jack I: Herpes virus in an obstetric hospital. III. Prevalence of antibodies in patients and staff. Med J Aust 2:325, 1980.

98. Hickey SM and McCracken G: Postnatal bacterial infections. In: Fanaroff AA, Martin RJ, eds. Neonatal-Perinatal Medicine: Diseases of the Fetus and Infant. 6th ed. St. Louis: Mosby, 1997.

99. Hill H: Intravenous immunoglobulin use in the neonate: Role in prophylaxis and therapy of infection. Pediatr Infect Dis J 12:549, 1993.

100. Hodgman J: Sepsis in the neonate. Perinatol Neonatol 5:45, 1981.

101. Howard JB, McCracken GJ: The spectrum of group B streptococcal infections in infancy. Am J Dis Child 128:815, 1974.

102. Huang Y, Lin TY, Leu HS, et al: Outbreak of *Candida parapsilosis* fungemia in neonatal intensive care units: Clinical implications and genotyping analysis. Infection 27:97, 1999.

103. Huebner J, Pier GB, Maslow JN, et al: Endemic nosocomial transmission of *Staphylococcus epidermidis* bacteremia isolates in a neonatal intensive care unit over 10 years. J Infect Dis 169:526, 1994.

104. Huttova M, Hartmanova I, Kralinsky K, et al: Candida fungemia in neonates treated with fluconazole: Report of forty cases, including eight with meningitis. Pediatr Infect Dis J 17:1012, 1998.

105. Impact RSV Study Group: Palivizumab, a humanised respiratory syncytial virus monoclonal antibody, reduces hospitalization from respiratory syncytial virus infection in high risk infants. Pediatrics 102:531, 1998.

106. International Perinatal HIV Group: The mode of delivery and the risk of vertical transmission of human immunodeficiency virus type-1: A meta-analysis of 15 prospective cohort studies. N Engl J Med 340:977, 1999.

107. Isaacs D, Barfield C, Clothier T, et al: Late onset infections of infants in neonatal units. J Paediatr Child Health 32:158, 1996.

108. Johnson S, Knight R, Marmer DJ, et al: Immune deficiency in fetal alcohol syndrome. Pediatr Res 15:908, 1981.

109. Johnson DE, Bass JL, Thompson TR, et al: Candida septicemia and right atrial mass secondary to umbilical vein catheterization. Am J Dis Child 135:275, 1981.

110. Johnson DE, Thompson TR, Green TP, et al: Systemic candidiasis in very low birth weight infants (<1500 grams). Pediatrics 73:138, 1984.

111. Johnson S, Oliver C, Prince GA, et al: Development of a humanized monoclonal antibody (MEDI-493) with potent in vitro and in vivo activity against respiratory syncytial virus. J Infect Dis 176:1215, 1997.

112. Johnson-Robbins LA, el-Mohandes AE, Simmens SJ, et al: *Staphylococcus epidermidis* sepsis in the intensive care nursery: A characterization of risk associations in infants <1,000g. Biology Neonate 69:249, 1996.

113. Joseph T, Pyati SP, Jacobs N: Neonatal early onset *Escherichia coli* disease. The effect of intrapartum ampicillin. Arch Pediatr Adolesc Med 15:35, 1998.

114. Kallman J, Kihlstrom E, Sjöberg L, et al: Increase of staphylococci in neonatal septicaemia: A fourteen year study. Acta Paediatr 85:533, 1997.

115. Kennaugh J, Gregory WW, Powell KR, et al: The effect of dilution during culture on detection of low concentrations of bacteria in blood. Pediatr Infect Dis J 3:317, 1984.

116. Khatib R, Thirumoorthis MC, Riederer KM, et al: Clustering of Candida infections in the neonatal intensive care unit: Concurrent emergence of multiple strains simulating intermittent outbreaks. Pediatr Infect Dis J 17:130, 1998.

117. Khuroo M, Teli RM, Skidmore S, et al: Incidence and severity of viral hepatitis in pregnancy. Am J Med 70:252, 1981.

118. Klein J, Feigin RD, McCracken GH Jr: Report of the task force on diagnosis and management of meningitis. Pediatrics 78:959, 1986.

119. Klein J, Marcy SM: Bacterial sepsis and meningitis. In Remington JR, Klein JO, eds: Infectious Disease of the Fetus and Newborn Infant. Philadelphia: Mosby, 1995.

120. Kneyber M, Brandenburg AH, de Groot R, et al: Risk factors for respiratory syncytial virus associated apnea. Eur J Pediatr 157:331, 1998.

121. Kocak U, Ezer V, Vidinlisan S, et al: Serum fibronectin in neonatal sepsis: Is it valuable in early diagnosis and outcome prediction. Acta Paediatr Jpn 39:428, 1997.

122. Kossoff E, Buescher ES, Karlowicz MG: Candidemia in a neonatal intensive care unit: Trends during fifteen years and clinical features of 111 cases. Pediatr Infect Dis J 17:504, 1998.

123. Krediet T, Gerards L, Fleer A, et al: The predictive value of CRP and I:T ratio in neonatal infection. J Perinat Med 20:479, 1992.

124. Laforgia N, Coppola B, Carbone R, et al: Rapid detection of neonatal sepsis using polymerase chain reaction. Acta Paediatr 86:1097, 1997.

125. LaGamma E, Drusin LM, Mackles AW, et al: Neonatal infections: An important determinant of late NICU mortality in infants less than 1,000 g at birth. Am J Dis Child 137:838, 1983.

126. Landesman SH, Kalish LA, Burns DN, et al: Obstetrical factors and the transmission of human immunodeficiency virus type 1 from mother to child. N Engl J Med 334:1617, 1996.

127. Lannering B, Larson LE, Rojas J, et al: Early onset group B streptococcal disease. Seven year experience and clinical scoring system. Acta Paediatr Scand 72:597, 1983.

128. Laurenti F, Ferro R, Isacchi G, et al: Polymorphonuclear leukocyte transfusion for the treatment of sepsis in the newborn infant. J Pediatr 98:118, 1981.

129. Lee B, Cheung PY, Robinson JL, et al: Comparative study of mortality and morbidity in premature infants (birth weight <1250 g) with candidal meningitis. Clin Infect Dis 27:559, 1998.

130. Lehrnbecher T, Schrod L, Rutsch P, et al: Immunologic parameters in cord blood indicating early onset sepsis. Biol Neonate 70:206, 1996.

131. Levine E, Strom CM, Ghai V, et al: Intrapartum management relating to the risk of perinatal transmission of group B streptococcus. Infect Dis Obstet Gynecol 6:25, 1998.

132. Levy H, Sepe SJ, Shih VE, et al: Sepsis due to *Escherichia coli* in neonates with galactosemia. N Engl J Med 297:823, 1997.

133. Levy I, Rubin LG, Vasishtha S, et al: Emergence of *Candida parapsilosis* as the predominant species causing candidemia in children. Clin Infect Dis 26:1086, 1998.

134. Lin HH, Kao JH, Hsu HY, et al: Absence of infection in breast fed infants born to hepatitis C virus-infected mothers. J Pediatr 126:589, 1995.

135. Lin F, Clemens JD, Azimi PH, et al: Capsular polysaccharide types of group B streptococcal isolates from neonates with early onset systemic disease. J Infect Dis 177:790, 1990.

136. MacDonald NE, Hall CB, Suffin SC, et al: Respiratory syncytial viral infection in infants with congenital heart disease. N Engl J Med 307:397, 1982.

137. MacKenzie A, Johnson W, Heyes B, et al: A prolonged outbreak of exfoliative toxin A producing *Staphylococcus aureus* in a newborn nursery. Diagnostic Microbiol Infect Dis 21:69, 1995.

138. Mandelbrot L, LeChenadec J, Berreli A, et al: Perinatal HIV-1 transmission: Interaction between zidovudine prophylaxis and mode of delivery in the French perinatal cohort. JAMA 280:55, 1998.

139. Manroe B, Weinberg AG, Rosenfeld CR, et al: The neonatal blood count in health and disease. I. Reference values for neutrophilic cells. J Pediatr 95:89, 1979.

140. Maudsley RF, Brix GA, Hinton NA, et al: Placental inflammation and infection: A prospective bacteriologic and histologic study. Am J Obstet Gynecol 95:648, 1966.

141. Mayaux MJ, Blanche S, Rouzioux C, et al: Maternal factors associated with perinatal HIV-1 transmission: The French cohort study: 7 years of follow-up observation. J Acquir Immune Defic Syndr Hum Retrovirol 8:188, 1995.

142. McAuley J, Boyer KM, Patel D, et al: Early and longitudinal evaluations of treated infants and children and untreated historical patients with congenital toxoplasmosis: The Chicago Collaborative Treatment Trial. Clin Infect Dis 18:72, 1994.

143. McCracken G Jr, Mize SG: A controlled study of intrathecal antibiotic therapy in gram negative enteric meningitis of infancy: Report of the National Meningitis Cooperative Study Group. J Pediatr 89:66, 1976.

144. McCracken G Jr, Threlkeld N, Mize S, et al: Moxalactam therapy for neonatal meningitis due to gram-negative enteric bacilli: A prospective controlled evaluation. JAMA 252:1427, 1984.

145. Messaritakis J, Anagnostakis D, Kaskari H, et al: Rectal skin temperature difference in septicaemic newborn infants. Arch Dis Child 65:380, 1990.

146. Meyer D, Jessen ME: Results of extracorporeal membrane oxygenation in children with sepsis. The Extracorporeal Life Support Organization. Ann Thorac Surg 63:756, 1997.

147. Meyers J: Congenital varicella in term infants: Risk reconsidered. J Infect Dis 129:215, 1974.

148. Mitsuda T, Arai K, Fujita S, et al: Epidemiological analysis of strains of methicillin-resistant *Staphylococcus aureus* (MRSA) infection in the nursery: Prognosis of MRSA carrier infants. J Hosp Infect 31:123, 1995.

149. Mittal M, Dhanireddy R, Higgins RD: Candida sepsis and association with retinopathy of prematurity. Pediatrics 101:654, 1998.

150. Mofenson LM, Lambert JS, Stiehm ER, et al: Risk factors for perinatal transmission of human immunodeficiency virus type 1 in women treated with zidovudine. N Engl J Med 341:385, 1999.

151. Monneret G, Labaune JM, Isaac C, et al: Procalcitonin and C-reactive protein levels in neonatal infections. Acta Paediatr 86:209, 1997.

152. Moses L, Heath PT, Wilkinson AR, et al: Early onset group B streptococcal neonatal infection in Oxford, 1985–96. Arch Dis Child Fetal Neonatal Ed 79:F148, 1998.

153. Munson D, Thompson TR, Johnson DE, et al: Coagulase-negative staphylococcal septicemia: Experience in a newborn intensive care unit. J Pediatr 101:602 1982.

154. Newell ML, Dunn DT, Peckham CS, et al: Vertical transmission of HIV-1: Maternal immune status and obstetric factors: The European Collaborative Study. AIDS 10:1675, 1996.

155. Ng P, Cheng SH, Chui KM, et al: Diagnosis of late onset neonatal sepsis with cytokines, adhesion molecule, and C-reactive protein in preterm very low birth weight infants. Arch Dis Child Fetal Neonatal Ed 77:F221, 1997.

156. Niswander K., Gordon M: The women and their pregnancies. The Collaborative Perinatal Study of the National Institute of Neurological Diseases and Stroke. U.S. Department of Health, Education and Welfare Publication No. (NIH) 73–379. Washington, DC: U.S. Government Printing Office, 1972.

157. Noel G, Edelson PJ: *Staphylococcus epidermidis* bacteremia in neonates: Further observations and the occurrence of focal infection. Pediatrics 74:832, 1987.

158. Ohto H, Terazawa S, Sasaki N, et al: Transmission of hepatitis C virus from mothers to infants. N Engl J Med 330:744, 1994.

159. Osborne JP, Pizer B: White cell count of contaminating CSF with blood. Arch Dis Child 56:400, 1981.

160. Ozono K, Mushiake S, Takeshima T, et al: Diagnosis of congenital cytomegalovirus infection by examination of placenta: Application of polymerase chain reaction and in situ hybridization. Pediatric Pathol Lab Med 17:249, 1997.

161. Panero A, Pacifico L, Rossi N, et al: Interleukin 6 in neonates with early and late onset infection. Pediatr Infect Dis J 16:370, 1997.

162. Paredes A, Wong P, Yow MD: Failure of penicillin to eradicate the carrier state of group B streptococcus in infants. J Pediatr 89:191, 1976.

163. Pass M, Khare S, Dillon HC Jr: Twin pregnancies: incidence of group B streptococcal colonization and disease. J Pediatr 97:635, 1980.

164. Patrick C, John JF, Levkoff AH, et al: Relatedness of strains of methicillin-resistant coagulase-negative staphylococcus colonizing hospital personnel and producing bacteremias in a neonatal intensive care unit. Pediatr Infect Dis J 11:935, 1992.

165. Patriquin H, Lebowitz R, Perreault G, et al: Neonatal candidiasis: Renal and pulmonary manifestations. Am J Radiol 135:1205, 1980.

166. Payne N, Burke BA, Day DC, et al: Correlation of clinical and pathologic findings in early onset neonatal group B streptococcal infection with disease severity and prediction outcome. Pediatr Infect Dis J 7:836, 1988.

167. Philip A, Hewitt JR: Early diagnosis of neonatal sepsis. Pediatrics 65:1036, 1980.

168. Philip A: Neonatal sepsis: Problems of diagnosis and the need for prevention. In Royal Society of Medicine: Prevention of Infections and the Role of Immunoglobulins in the Neonatal Period. London, 1990.

169. Phillips J, Karlowicz MG: Prevalence of *Candida* species in hospital acquired urinary tract infections in neonatal intensive care units. Pediatr Infect Dis J 16:190, 1997.

170. Pichichero MD, Todd JK: Detection of neonatal bacteremia. J Pediatr 94:958, 1979.

171. Pierce JR, Merenstein GB, Stocker JT: Immediate postmortem cultures in an intensive care nursery. Pediatr Infect Dis 3:510, 1984.

172. Pilapril V: Hexachlorophene toxicity in an infant. Am J Dis Child 111:333, 1966.

173. Pitt J, Brambilla D, Reichelderfer P, et al: Maternal immunologic and virologic risk factors for infant human immunodeficiency virus type 1 infections: Findings from the Women and Infants Transmission Study. J Infect Dis 175:567, 1997.

174. Pittard W III, Thullen JD, Fanaroff AA: Neonatal septic arthritis. J Pediatr 88:621, 1976.

175. Polin RA, St Geme JW 3d: Neonatal sepsis. Adv Pediatr Infect Dis 7:25, 1992.

176. Pourcyrous M, Bada HS, Korones SB, et al: Significance of serial C-reactive protein responses in neonatal infection and other disorders. Pediatrics 92:431, 1993.

177. Preblud S, Bregman DJ, Vernon LL: Deaths from varicella in infants. Pediatr Infect Dis 4:503, 1985.

178. PREVENT Study Group: Reduction of respiratory syncytial virus hospitalization among premature infants and infants with bronchopulmonary dysplasia using respiratory syncytial virus immune globulin prophylaxis. Pediatrics 99:93, 1997.

179. Prober CG, Sullender WM, Yasukawa LL, et al: Low risk herpes simplex virus infections in neonates exposed to the virus at the time of vaginal delivery to mothers with recurrent genital herpes simplex virus infections. N Engl J Med 316:240, 1987.

180. Rabalais G, Samiec TD, Bryant KK, et al: Invasive candidiasis in infants weighing more than 2500 grams at birth admitted to a neonatal intensive care unit. Pediatr Infect Dis J 15:348, 1996.

181. Redline R, Dahms BB: Malasezzia pulmonary vasculitis in an infant on long term intralipid therapy. N Engl J Med 305:1395, 1981.

182. Rodriguez EM, Mofenson LM, Chang BH, et al: Association of maternal drug use during pregnancy with maternal HIV culture positivity and perinatal HIV transmission. AIDS 10:273, 1996.

183. Rooney J, Hills DJ, Danks DM: Jaundice associated with bacterial infection in the newborn. Am J Dis Child 122:39, 1971.

184. Rothenberg R: Ophthalmia neonatorum due to *N. gonorrhoeae*: Prevention and treatment. Sex Transmit Dis 6S2:187, 1979.

185. Rouse D, Andrews WW, Lin FY, et al: Antibiotic susceptibility profile of group B streptococcus acquired vertically. Obstet Gynecol 92:931, 1998.

186. Rowley AH, Wald ER: Incubation period necessary to detect bacteremia in neonates. Pediatr Infect Dis J 5:590, 1986.

187. Sarff L, Platt LH, McCracken GH Jr: Cerebrospinal fluid evaluation in neonates: Comparison of high risk infants with and without meningitis. Pediatrics 88:473, 1976.

188. Saxen H, Virtanen M, Carlson P, et al: Neonatal *Candida parapsilosis* outbreak with a high case fatality rate. Pediatr Infect Dis J 14:776, 1995.

189. Scarcella A, Pasquariello MB, Giugliano B, et al: Liposomal amphotericin B treatment for neonatal fungal infections. Pediatr Infect Dis J 17:146, 1998.

190. Schiano M, Hauth JC, Gilstrap LA: Second stage fetal tachycardia and neonatal infection. Am J Obstet Gynecol 148:79, 1984.

191. Schuchat A, Oxtoby M, Cochi S, et al: Population based risk factors for neonatal group B streptococcal disease: Results of a cohort study in metropolitan Atlanta. J Infect Dis 162:672, 1990.

192. Schuchat A, Deaver-Robinson K, Plikaytis BD, et al: Multistate case-control study of maternal risk factors for neonatal group B streptococcal disease. Pediatr Infect Dis J 13:623, 1994.

193. Schweitzer I, Dunn AE, Peters RL, et al: Viral hepatitis B in neonates and infants. Am J Med 55:762, 1973.

194. Schwersenski J, McIntyre L, Bauer CR: Lumbar puncture frequency and CSF analysis in the neonate. Am J Dis Child 145:54, 1991.

195. Seeler R. Urosepsis with jaundice due to hemolytic *Escherichia coli*. Am J Dis Child 126:414, 1973.

196. Seeling M: The role of antibiotics in the pathogenesis of candida infections. Am J Med 40:887, 1966.

197. Sheretz R, Reagan DR, Hampton KD, et al: A cloud adult: The *Staphylococcus aureus* virus interaction revisited. Ann Int Med 24:539, 1996.

198. Shurin S: *Esherichia coli* septicemia in neonates with galactosemia. N Engl J Med 297:1403, 1977.

199. Simoes E, Sendheimer HM, Top FH Jr, et al: Respiratory syncytial virus immune globulin for prophylaxis against respiratory syncytial virus disease in infants and children with congenital heart disease. J Pediatr 133:492, 1998.

200. Simoes E: Respiratory syncytial virus infection. Lancet ii:847, 1999.

201. Smeltzer M, Pratt FL, Gillaspy AF, et al: Genomic finger printing for epidemiological differentiation of *Staphylococcus aureus* clinical isolettes. J Clin Microbool 34:1364, 1996.

202. Soman M, Green B, Daling J: Risk factors for early neonatal sepsis. Am J Epidemiol 121:712, 1985.

203. St. Geme J Jr, Murray DL, Carter J, et al: Perinatal bacterial infection after prolonged rupture of amniotic membranes: An analysis of risk and management. J Pediatr 104:608, 1984.

204. St. Geme JW III, Bell LM, Baumgart S, et al: Distinguishing sepsis from blood culture contamination in young infants with blood cultures growing coagulase-negative staphylococci. Pediatrics 86:157, 1990.

205. Steele R, Marmer DJ, O'Brien MD, et al: Leukocyte survival in CSF. J Clin Microbiol 23:965, 1986.

206. Stewart DL, Dela-Cruz TV, Ziegler C, et al: The use of extracorporeal membrane oxygenation in patients with gram-negative or viral sepsis. Perfusion 12:3, 1997.

207. Stoll BJ, Fanaroff AA: Early onset coagulase-negative staphylococcal sepsis in preterm neonate. Lancet 345:1236, 1995.

208. Stoll BJ, Gordon T, Korones SB, et al: Late-onset sepsis in very low birth weight neonates: A report from the National Institute of Child Health and Human Development Neonatal Research Network. J Pediatr 129:63, 1996.

209. Stoll BJ, Gordon T, Korones SB, et al: Early onset sepsis in very low birth weight neonates: A report from the National Institute of Child Health and Human Development Neonatal Research Network. J Pediatr 129:72, 1996.

210. Suggs A, Maranan MC, Boyle-Vavra S, et al: Methicillin-resistant and borderline methicillin-resistant asymptomatic *Staphylococcus aureus* colonization in children without identifiable risk factors. Pediatr Infect Dis J 18:410, 1999.

211. Tada H, Yanagida M, Mishina J, et al: Combined passive and active immunization for preventing transmission of hepatitis B virus carrier state. Pediatrics 70:613, 1982.

212. Tegtmeyer FK, Horn C, Richter A, et al: Elastase alpha 1-proteinase inhibitor complex, granulocyte count, ratio of immature to total granulocyte count, and C-reactive protein in neonatal septicaemia. Eur J Pediatr 151:353, 1992.

213. Tong M, Thursby M, Rakela J, et al: Studies on the maternal-infant transmission of the viruses which cause acute hepatitis. Gastroenterology 80:999, 1981.

214. Towers C, Carr MH, Padilla G, et al: Potential consequences of widespread antepartal use of ampicillin. Am J Obstet Gynecol 179:879, 1998.

215. Unhanand J, Mustafa MM, McCracken GH Jr, et al: Gram negative enteric bacillary meningitis: A twenty one year experience. J Pediatr 122:15, 1993

216. U.S. Public Health Service Task Force: Recommendations for the use of antiretroviral drugs in pregnant women infected with HIV-1 for maternal health and for reducing perinatal HIV-1 transmission in the United States. MMWR 47(RR-2):1, 1998.

217. Vazquez J, Boikov D, Boikov SG, et al: Use of electropheretic karyotyping in the evaluation of candida infections in a neonatal intensive care unit. Infect Control Hosp Epidemiol 18:32, 1997.

218. Vesikari T, Janas M, Gronroos P, et al: Neonatal septicaemia. Arch Dis Child 60:542, 1985.

219. Vesikari T, Isolauri E, Tuppurainen N, et al: Neonatal septicemia in Finland 1981–1985: Predominance of group B streptococcal infections with very early onset. Acta Paediatr Scand 78:44, 1989.

220. Visser V, Hall RT: Culture in the evaluation of suspected neonatal sepsis. J Pediatr 94:635, 1979.

221. Waggoner-Fountain L, Walker MW, Hollis RJ, et al: Vertical and horizontal transmission of unique candida species to premature newborns. Clin Infect Dis 22:803, 1996.

222. Walsh T, Seibel NL, Arndt C, et al: Amphotericin B lipid complex in pediatric patients with invasive fungal infections. Pediatr Infect Dis J 18:702, 1999.

223. Weese-Mayer D, Fondriest DW, Brouillette RT, et al: Risk factors associated with candidemia in the neonatal intensive care unit: A case controlled study. Pediatr Infect Dis 6:190, 1987.

224. Weinberg E: Iron and susceptibility to infectious disease. In the resolution of the contest between invader and host iron may be the critical determinant. Science 184:952, 1974.

225. Weisman L, Stoll BJ, Cruess DF, et al: Early onset group B streptococcal sepsis: A current assessment. J Pediatr 121:428, 1992.

226. Weiss M, Ionides SP, Anderson CL: Meningitis in premature infants with respiratory distress: Role of admission lumbar puncture. J Pediatr 119:973, 1991.

227. Weitkamp J, Poets CF, Sievers R, et al: Candida infection in very low birth weight infants: Outcome and nephrotoxicity of treatment with liposomal amphotericin B. Ambisome 26:11, 1998.

228. Whitley CB, Thompson LR, Soteholm MT, et al: Toxic shock syndrome in a newborn infant. Pediatr Res 16:254A, 1982.

229. Whitley RJ, Arvin AM: Herpes simplex virus infections. In Remington JS, Klein JO, eds: Infectious Diseases of the Fetus and Newborn. Philadelphia: WB Saunders, 1995.

230. Whitley RJ, Arvin AM, Prober C, et al: Predictors of morbidity and mortality in neonates with herpes simplex infections. N Engl J Med 324:450, 1991.

231. Whitley RJ, Cloud G, Gruber W, et al: Ganciclovir treatment of symptomatic congenital cytomegalovirus infection: Results of phase II study. J Infect Dis 175:1080, 1997.

232. Whitley RJ, Corey L, Arvin AM, et al: Changing presentation of herpes simplex virus infection in neonates. J Infect Dis 158:109, 1988.

233. Whitley RJ, Nahmias AJ, Visintine AM, et al: The natural history of herpes simplex virus infection of mother and newborn. Pediatrics 66:489, 1980.

234. Whyte R, Hussain Z, deSa D: Antenatal infections with candida species. Arch Dis Child 57:528, 1982.

235. Winberg J, Wessner G: Does breast milk protect against septicaemia in the newborn? Lancet 1:1091, 1971.

236. Word B, Klein JO: Therapy of bacterial sepsis and meningitis in infants and children: A poll of directors of programs in pediatric infectious diseases. Pediatr Infect Dis J 8:635, 1989.

237. Yagupsky P, Menegus MA, Powell KR: The changing spectrum of group B streptococcal disease in infants: An eleven year experience in a tertiary care hospital. Pediatr Infect Dis J 10:801, 1991.

238. Yamamura D, Rothstein C, Nicolle LE, et al: Candidemia at selected Canadian sites: Results from the Fungal Disease Registry, 1992–1994. Fungal Disease Registry of the Canadian Infectious Disease Society. CMAJ 160:493, 1999.

The Heart

Michael M. Brook
Michael A. Heymann
David F. Teitel

Congenital heart disease is one of the most common causes of morbidity and mortality in a pediatric referral hospital. In most children, serious heart disease presents early in the first month of life. Care for these newborns dictates an awareness of the cardiac defects most likely to occur. The data from the New England Regional Infant Cardiac Program concerning the diagnostic distribution of critically ill infants in the first month of life are helpful (Table 14–1), as are the composite autopsy data of Rowe.[91] Together these studies show that 70% of neonates with potentially fatal cardiac malformations have one of the following five types of defects: the hypoplastic left heart syndrome; aortic arch anomalies, including interruption or hypoplasia of the aortic arch and coarctation of the aorta; complete transposition of the great arteries; the hypoplastic right heart syndrome; or severe tetralogy of Fallot.*

EDITORIAL COMMENT: The prevalence of congenital heart disease in Italy during the years 1992 and 1993 varied between 1.8% and 8.1% at 18 regional centers. The average was 4.6%. Isolated ventricular septal defect was the most common lesion (39%), followed by atrial septal defect (7.5%), pulmonary valvar stenosis (7.3%), atrioventricular septal defects (5.4%), patent ductus arteriosus (3.8%), complete transposition (3.7%), tetralogy of Fallot (3.3%), aortic coarctation (2.4%), aortic valvar stenosis (2.2%), and left heart hypoplasia (1.8%). Among the complex cardiovascular anomalies, double inlet ventricle and pulmonary atresia had a proportion of about 2% each; double outlet right ventricle, common arterial trunk, Ebstein's malformation, tricuspid atresia, interrupted aortic arch and total anomalous pulmonary venous connection had a proportion ranging from 0.5% to 0%.

◆

Bosi G, Scorrano M, Tosato G, et al: The Italian Multicentre Study on Epidemiology of Congenital Heart Disease: First Step of The Analysis. Working Party of the Italian Society of Pediatric Cardiology. Cardiol Young 9:291, 1999.

Table 14–1. Diagnostic Distribution of Critically Ill Cardiac Infants 0 to 30 Days of Age, 1968–1971*

Diagnosis (in Rank Order)	No.	%
Transposition of great arteries	81	14
Hypoplastic left ventricle	76	13
Coarctation of aorta (includes simple and complicated)	51	9
Hypoplastic right ventricle (includes pulmonary atresia and tricuspid atresia group)	49	9
Tetralogy of Fallot	44	8
Ventricular septal defect	44	8
Other malpositions	31	5
Single ventricle	21	4
Patent ductus arteriosus	19	3
Atrioventricularis communis	15	3
Pure pulmonary stenosis	14	2
Myocardiopathy	12	2
Total anomalous pulmonary venous return	12	2
Truncus arteriosus	9	2
Others	108	18
TOTAL	586	

*These are babies who were critically ill but did not necessarily die or need surgery to live. The table is also not broken down as to day of onset of illness. Thus, a child with a ventricular septal defect who became ill at 30 days is included and is likely to survive with medical therapy.

Adapted from Fyler D, Buckley L, Hellenbrand W, et al: Report of the New England Regional Infant Cardiac Program. Pediatrics 65(Suppl):375, 1980. Reprinted by permission of Pediatrics. Copyright 1980.

*Classifications of congenital heart disease do not usually include persistent patency of the ductus arteriosus (PDA) in infants born prematurely. A large majority of these infants, particularly very low-birth-weight (<1250 g) pre-term infants, have a PDA of varying hemodynamic severity and therefore require specific care. It is estimated that these infants represent about 1% of all live births, a number approximately equal to that proposed for the incidence of congenital heart disease.

Careful evaluation of the history, physical examination, laboratory data (including the response of upper and lower body blood gases and arterial oxygen saturation in an enriched oxygen environment), x-ray findings, electrocardiogram, echocardiogram, and occasionally cardiac catheterization helps to delineate the specific congenital cardiac defect. In addition, noncardiac disorders such as parenchymal lung disease or disorders associated with persistent pulmonary hypertension may be confused with heart disease. Two-dimensional echocardiography (with Doppler) has eliminated much of the clinical guesswork by providing detailed functional and anatomic data. To make a complete cardiac evaluation, the physician must be familiar with relevant cardiovascular physiology and pathophysiology.

COMMENT: The clinical signs of congenital heart disease may be obscured by the transitional circulation of the neonate. Likewise, the electrocardiogram and chest radiograph are insensitive screening tools at this age. Echocardiography is indicated in a neonate with suspected cardiac disease, but this should be performed by individuals experienced in the diagnosis of congenital heart disease.

Roberta G. Williams

This chapter considers the physiology and pathophysiology of the fetal and neonatal cardiovascular systems, the low-risk newborn with heart disease, and the high-risk newborn with heart disease.

◆ PHYSIOLOGY AND PATHOPHYSIOLOGY

Fetal and Neonatal Circulations

In the adult, the pulmonary and systemic circulations are arranged in series so that oxygenated blood returns from the lungs and is ejected by the left side of the heart to the systemic circulation; in turn, the deoxygenated blood returns from the systemic circulation to the right side of the heart, where it is ejected to the pulmonary circulation. In the fetus, circulation of the blood is more complex (Fig. 14–1). Oxygenated blood returns from the placenta to both the left and the right ventricles. The major portion of the right ventricular output does not perfuse the lungs but bypasses the pulmonary circula-

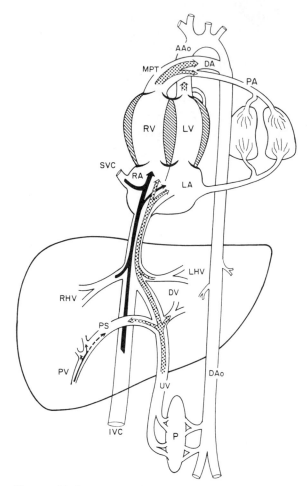

Figure 14–1. Diagrammatic representation of normal fetal circulation. P, placenta; AAo, ascending aorta; DAo, descending aorta; DA, ductus arteriosus; PA, pulmonary artery; MPT, main pulmonary trunk; RHV, right hepatic vein; LHV, left hepatic vein; DV, ductus venosus; UV, umbilical vein; SVC, superior vena cava; IVC, inferior vena cava; RV, right ventricle; LV, left ventricle; RA, right atrium; LA, left atrium; PS, portal system; and PV, portal vein.

tion through the ductus arteriosus and is thereby directed toward the body, returning to the placenta for oxygenation. Because of this parallel circulation, individual organs may receive blood from both ventricles. It has therefore become customary to express the output of the fetal heart as *combined ventricular output* (CVO). In the normal fetus, CVO is approximately 450 mL/kg of fetal body weight/min.*

Approximately 45% (200 mL/kg/min) of this blood perfuses the placenta for oxygen

*In this chapter, all of the data on the fetal circulation are derived from studies on fetal sheep.

uptake and returns via the umbilical veins. Approximately one half of umbilical venous return enters the inferior vena cava directly through the ductus venosus, thereby bypassing the hepatic microcirculation; the remainder passes primarily through the left lobe of the liver and enters the inferior vena cava via the left hepatic vein. Although venous return from the lower body, ductus venosus, and hepatic veins all passes into the thoracic inferior vena cava, these streams do not mix completely, and there is preferential streaming via the inferior vena cava into various cardiac chambers. Blood from the ductus venosus and left hepatic veins tends to stream preferentially across the foramen ovale into the left atrium, providing blood with a higher oxygen content to the left atrium and left ventricle, thereby supplying cerebral and myocardial circulations with blood of a relatively high oxygen content. Venous drainage from the right hepatic veins and the abdominal inferior vena cava tends to stream preferentially to the right atrium and right ventricle. Similarly, desaturated superior vena caval return is preferentially directed to the right ventricle through the tricuspid valve, although some blood may enter the left atrium. The right ventricle ejects much of this relatively undersaturated blood via the ductus arteriosus back to the placenta. Thus, although the circulations are not completely separated, each ventricle primarily performs its postnatal function—the left ventricle delivers blood for oxygen utilization, the right for oxygen uptake.

COMMENT: The streaming of blood from the inferior vena cava to the left heart and from the superior vena cava to the right heart increases the efficiency of oxygen delivery to the most actively metabolizing area of the fetus, the brain, and the delivery of the most oxygen-poor blood to the organ of oxygen supply, the placenta.

Roberta G. Williams

The left and right ventricles do not eject similar volumes in the fetus. The right ventricle is dominant and ejects approximately 65% of the CVO, whereas the left ventricle ejects approximately 35% (the difference is smaller in the human because of the larger brain and greater cerebral blood flow). Of the right ventricular output, only about 12.5% (approximately 30 to 35 mL/kg/min or 8% of CVO) passes to the pulmonary circulation. Left ventricular output is distributed mainly in the upper body, including the brain (approximately 20% of CVO) and the myocardium (3%); the remainder (about 10%) crosses the aortic isthmus to the lower body.

In the fetus, the ductus arteriosus had long been considered a passive conduit that allowed blood to bypass the pulmonary circulation. However, recent studies have shown that vasoactive products of arachidonic acid cause active dilation of the ductus arteriosus during fetal life; prostaglandin E_2 almost certainly is the most important of these substances. The oxygen tension of blood in the fetus (20 to 25 mm Hg) is significantly lower than that in the adult. This lowered oxygen tension may cause the active constriction of the muscular resistance vessels in the lungs which, in turn, permits only a very small flow through the pulmonary circulation. In the presence of the low oxygen environment, other vasoactive substances, which actively constrict the pulmonary circulation, may be released and may also actively control flow through the lungs; products of arachidonic acid metabolism that cause vasoconstriction, such as the leukotrienes, most likely are involved.

COMMENT: The advent of precise measurement of vessel diameter and flow velocity in the human fetus by echocardiography provides insight into the response of the circulation to a variety of physiologic and pathologic circumstances, such as late gestational ductal constriction or redistribution of flow in response to stress.

Roberta G. Williams

Circulatory Changes After Birth

The onset of breathing produces a dramatic increase in pulmonary blood flow (from 30 to 35 mL/kg/min to 350 to 400 mL/kg/min), and a decrease in pulmonary vascular resistance. With the onset of ventilation, air replaces intraalveolar fluid and local oxygen concentration increases markedly, both of which may directly dilate the pulmonary vascular smooth muscle or cause the release of vasodilating substances. Bradykinin, a potent pulmonary vasodilator, is released when the lungs are exposed to oxygen; bradykinin, in turn, stimulates endothelial cell production of nitric oxide (NO), a potent vasodilator. Prostacyclin (prostaglandin I_2), a pulmonary vasodilator derived from the metabolism of arachidonic acid, is released when the lung is mechanically ventilated (not necessarily oxygenated) or exposed to other vasoactive substances, such as bradykinin or angiotensin II; it, too, is produced by pulmonary vascular endothelial cells. Inhibiting prostaglandin production by the administration of a cyclooxygenase inhibitor (such as indomethacin) attenuates the normal ventilation-induced decline in pulmonary vascular resistance, further supporting the role of these vasoactive substances in the establishment of a normal pulmonary circulation after birth.

The initial dramatic decrease in pulmonary vascular resistance is secondary to relaxation of the resistance vessels. There is then a slow, progressive decline over the next 2 to 6 weeks of life as these pulmonary arterioles remodel from their fetal pattern, which has a large amount of smooth muscle in the medial layer, to the adult pattern, with very little muscle in the media. The development of the "physiologic anemia" that normally occurs during this time decreases the viscosity of blood perfusing the lungs and also contributes to the overall decrease in the pulmonary vascular resistance.

COMMENT: Decreasing blood viscosity leads to decreasing shear stress. These mechanical forces may play an active as well as a passive role in the remodeling process.
Roberta G. Williams

COMMENT: The postnatal changes in pulmonary vascular resistance can be divided into those factors that influence the remodeling of the pulmonary vascular bed, which include lung inflation, removal of lung liquids, and maturational changes in the pulmonary resistance vessels, and alterations in blood viscosity. The exact site of the pulmonary resistance vessels is a debatable point and in the fetus and newborn may involve larger vessels than in the adult, where the pulmonary arterioles constitute the major site for resistance changes. The postnatal decrease in viscosity is consequent to the fall in hemoglobin concentration, which takes place over the first 2 to 3 months of life.
Norman Talner

Closure of Foramen Ovale

After the placenta is removed from the circulation, blood flow through the inferior vena cava to both atria decreases dramatically; when breathing begins, blood flow through the pulmonary bed to the left atrium increases. These changes in flow patterns into the heart alter the relationship between left and right atrial pressures: left atrial pressure, which is lower in the fetus than pressure in the right atrium, then exceeds right atrial pressure, thereby causing the valvelike flap of the foramen ovale to close. Although functional closure of the foramen ovale occurs in most infants, anatomic closure is not always complete, and the foramen may remain probe patent for many years, occasionally into adult life.

COMMENT: In the neonate, crying or Valsalva's maneuver can transiently increase right atrial pressure and create a right-to-left shunt across the flap valve of the foramen ovale. Likewise, conditions that create increased left atrial pressure and flow such as PDA may stretch the atrial septum, causing incompetence of the foramen ovale and a left-to-right shunt.
Roberta G. Williams

COMMENT: It is important to point out that any pathologic state that raises pulmonary vascular resistance can permit right-to-left shunting through the foramen ovale as right atrial pressure rises and exceeds left atrial pressure. Under certain circumstances, however, a left-to-right shunt can occur through the foramen ovale as a consequence of an elevation of left atrial pressure and resulting incompetence of the foramen ovale. This has been demonstrated in patients with large-volume left-to-right shunts and obstructive lesions involving the left side of the heart, as well as in any process such as asphyxia or inflammatory disease that could impair myocardial contractility and thereby result in an elevated left atrial pressure.
Norman Talner

Closure of Ductus Arteriosus

Much like the rapid pulmonary vasodilation that occurs after birth, closure of the ductus arteriosus is a complex phenomenon that is not yet fully understood. The fetal ductus arteriosus contains medial smooth muscle that is maintained in a relaxed state, probably by the action of prostaglandins, specifically circulating prostaglandin E_2. Closure after birth reflects removal of the stimuli that maintain relaxation and the addition of factors that produce active constriction. Prostaglandin E_2 is almost completely metabolized as it passes through the pulmonary circulation. Circulating concentrations in the fetus are high because of the very low pulmonary blood flow. After delivery, the placental source of prostaglandin E_2 is removed, and there is a dramatic increase in pulmonary blood flow, which increases the metabolism of any circulating prostaglandin E_2. As a result, serum levels of prostaglandin E_2 decrease, and active constriction of the ductus arteriosus is unopposed. This active constriction is caused by an increase in environmental Po_2 as well as in several vasoactive substances. Bradykinin is released from the lungs with the initial oxygenation and has a constrictor effect on the ductus arteriosus; similarly, other vasoactive substances such as catecholamines and histamine may be involved. The ductus arteriosus constricts rapidly after birth; in mature infants, functional closure generally occurs within the first 12 hours. Permanent closure by intimal cushion formation, intimal proliferation, fibrosis, and thrombosis may take several weeks.

COMMENT: Adverse events such as hypoxia or acidosis in the newborn may encourage persistent ductal patency or stimulate the closed or partially constricted ductus arteriosus to reopen. This is fortuitous in patients with ductal-dependent cardiac lesions, producing a rebound improvement after initial deterioration.
Roberta G. Williams

Persistent patency of the ductus arteriosus occurs relatively frequently in premature infants as compared with full-term infants. The exact mechanisms are not clear. The ductus arteriosus in premature animals is certainly less responsive to the constricting effects of oxygen. The relaxing effects of prostaglandin E_2 and prostacyclin are greater in the immature ductus arteriosus, and the metabolism of prostaglandin E_2 is not efficient. As a result of these phenomena, even small circulating concentrations of prostaglandin E_2 that may be present in the immature infant can cause the ductus arteriosus to remain in a partially relaxed state. Constriction of the ductus arteriosus in premature infants has been achieved by pharmacologic manipulation with inhibitors of prostaglandin synthesis (specifically, indomethacin and ibuprofen).

COMMENT: In the premature infant with pulmonary disease, impaired oxygen exchange in the lung may maintain an elevated pulmonary vascular resistance, masking the presence of PDA. Improvement in the pulmonary disease permits the pulmonary resistance to fall, and signs of a left-to-right ductal shunt to ensue.
Roberta G. Williams

COMMENT: Persistent patency of the ductus arteriosus allowing a left-to-right shunt into the pulmonary circulation constitutes one of the many life-threatening problems facing the preterm infant. The ability to manipulate the ductus arteriosus by pharmacologic means or by surgical ligation, if necessary, permits the clinician to remove the effects of increased pulmonary blood flow on cardiopulmonary function in the premature infant. This allows earlier weaning from ventilatory support and administration of adequate fluids and calories.
Norman Talner

Myocardial Performance and Cardiac Output

Fetal myocardium develops less tension for a given stretch than does adult myocardium. Therefore, ventricular output can be increased only modestly by volume loading and only at relatively low atrial pressures; unlike in the adult, output increases only slightly at levels above 10 mm Hg. Inotropic stimulation of the fetal myocardium also increases cardiac output relatively little. This inability to respond to changes in preload and in the inotropic state is related in part to immaturity of muscle structure. At early gestational ages, there are relatively few contractile elements with immature sarcoplasmic reticulum, and considerable interstitial tissue is present; toward term, more contractile elements are present, and these are more mature and are arranged in a more orderly fashion. Another factor limiting fetal myocardial performance is incomplete sympathetic innervation, which limits response to inotropic stimulation. The fetus is best able to increase ventricular output by increasing its heart rate. There is a linear relationship between ventricular output and heart rate up to about 250 bpm; thereafter, ventricular output reaches a plateau and even starts to decline. As heart rate goes below the normal range, ventricular output decreases dramatically because of the limited ability to increase stroke volume. As a result of all these limitations, the stressed fetus responds by redistributing rather than increasing cardiac output.

COMMENT: It should be emphasized that the neonatal myocardium operates under a high-volume load as compared with the adult myocardium and responds poorly to any increase in ventricular afterload. Although adrenergic support can be supplied either by circulating catecholamines or through neural pathways, the overall quantitative response may be less than in the adult. The control of cardiac rate and the distribution of cardiac output are the major mechanisms for maintenance of circulatory function. In the face of asphyxia with alterations in pH, P_{O_2}, and P_{CO_2}, the net effect is to compromise myocardial performance, and these are factors that must be addressed in an attempt to restore cardiac output and thus improve oxygen transport.

Norman Talner

After birth, left ventricular output increases dramatically, from about 150 mL/kg/min to 350 to 400 mL/kg/min. Right ventricular output does not change significantly. Over the ensuing 6 to 8 weeks, right and left ventricular outputs decrease to less than half this value. Because of the high resting values in the immediate newborn period, ventricular output can be increased only modestly by volume loading or inotropic stimulation; as resting values decrease progressively over the next month, ventricular output can be increased much more. Studies on myocardial contractility have also shown that in the first weeks after birth, resting contractility is high; it decreases progressively over the following month. Thus, isoproterenol produces little change in contractility in the newborn but has a much greater effect in the older infant.

COMMENT: Although this has been observed in the experimental animal when the heart is performing normally, in certain clinical states such as that associated with asphyxia, myocardial contractility may be impaired, whereupon inotropic agents may very well be able to restore contractility toward normal. The newborn heart responds in a positive fashion to inotropic agents such as isoproterenol, dopamine, and dobutamine as well as to the administration of calcium ion.

Norman Talner

Normal Physiologic Data in Newborn

A box diagram is useful in evaluating the hemodynamic data on the heart and great vessels of children with heart defects. Such diagrams are used as illustrations in this chapter.

The normal physiologic values in the

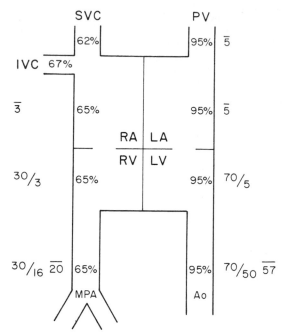

Figure 14–2. Representative blood-oxygen saturation (%) and pressure (mm Hg) in various cardiac chambers and vessels in normal newborn infant. SVC, superior vena cava; IVC, inferior vena cava; PV, pulmonary vein; RA, right atrium; LA, left atrium; RV, right ventricle; LV, left ventricle; MPA, main pulmonary artery; Ao, aorta.

heart and great vessels are shown in Figure 14–2. Pulmonary arterial pressures in the newborn are variable but generally decrease to half of systemic pressure within 8 to 12 hours and to one third of systemic pressure within a day or so. Over the next 4 weeks, there is a further slow, progressive decline to adult levels.

The oxygen saturation on the right side of the heart is approximately 60% to 70%; that on the left side of the heart is 92% to 95%. The oxygen saturations may be used to determine the direction of shunting within the heart or great vessels. For example, an increased saturation in the right atrium suggests a left-to-right shunt at the atrial level; a decreased saturation in the left atrium indicates a right-to-left shunt at the atrial level, if pulmonary venous blood is not desaturated because of pulmonary disease with intrapulmonary right-to-left shunting.

Physical Factors That Control Blood Flow

Flow (Q) through a vascular bed is governed by the resistance to flow (R) and the pressure decrease across the bed (ΔP) (Ohm's law).

$$Q = \frac{\Delta P}{R}$$

Furthermore, by applying Poiseuille's law, resistance to flow is directly related to viscosity of the blood and inversely related to the cross-sectional area of the bed (radius).

An appreciation of the general relationship of pressure, resistance, and flow is important in understanding the pathophysiology and natural history of various congenital heart defects. *Blood flows where resistance is least.*

Vascular resistance is calculated from the formula:

$$Q = \frac{\Delta P}{R}$$

For the systemic circulation, the ΔP (pressure decrease) is systemic arterial pressure (SAP) minus systemic venous pressure (SVP); for the pulmonary circulation, the ΔP is pulmonary arterial pressure (PAP) minus pulmonary venous pressure (PVP).

Pulmonary vascular resistance (PVR) =
$$\frac{PAP - PVP}{Pulmonary\ flow}$$

Systemic vascular resistance (SVR) =
$$\frac{SAP - SVP}{Systemic\ flow}$$

If the pressure decrease is measured in millimeters of mercury and the flow is measured in liters per minute per square meter, then the calculated vascular resistance is considered in *resistance units*. One resistance (or Wood) unit is equal to 80 dynes/cm^2. The maximum normal PVR is 2.5 to 3 units, and the maximum normal SVR is 15 to 20 units.

COMMENT: The calculation of pulmonary and systemic vascular resistances represents an attempt to define alterations from the normal produced by certain disease states. A number of factors influence pulmonary vascular resistance in addition to the pulmonary resistance vessels. These include the height of the pressure on the pulmonary venous side and the volume of blood in the pulmonary vascular bed. Further, changes in blood viscosity may also influence the pulmonary vascular resistance. *It should not be inferred that because there is pulmonary hypertension there is necessarily pulmonary vaso-*

constriction. In certain situations there may be fewer resistance vessels, pulmonary parenchymal alterations (e.g., diaphragmatic hernia), or structural alterations in the pulmonary resistance vessels.

Norman Talner

Peripheral vascular resistance is not the only type of resistance that will affect flow. For example, a narrowed valve provides more resistance to blood flow than does a wide open valve; a small ventricular septal defect provides more resistance to blood flow than does a large ventricular septal defect; and a thick, noncompliant ventricular chamber provides more resistance to blood flow than does a thinner, more compliant ventricular chamber.

If two similar cardiac chambers or arteries (one left sided or systemic and the other right sided or pulmonary) communicate with each other and the opening between them is so large that there is little or no resistance to blood flow, the defect is considered *nonrestrictive*. The pressures on each side of the opening are fully transmitted and approximately equal. If the opening is small *(restrictive)*, there is resistance to blood flow, and the pressures are not fully transmitted. In the presence of a nonrestrictive defect, the resistances to outflow (downstream resistance) from each of the two communicating chambers determine the direction of blood flow. For example, with a large ventricular septal defect (Fig. 14–3) in which ventricular pressures are equal, pulmonary vascular resistance is usually lower than systemic vascular resistance, and pulmonary blood flow is greater than systemic blood flow; that is, a left-to-right shunt is present (see Fig. 14–3*A*). Because the flows and shunting pattern depend on the relationship of the downstream pulmonary and systemic vascular resistances, these are called *dependent shunts*. When the two resistances are equal, no shunt occurs (see Fig. 14–3*B*). When resistance to outflow of the right ventricle exceeds that of the left ventricle (see Fig. 14–3*C*)—as might occur with the development of pulmonary vascular disease or, more commonly, when there is an associated pulmonic stenosis (tetralogy of Fallot)—right-to-left shunting is present. When there is a communication between the two sides of the heart at different anatomic levels (e.g., arteriovenous malformation, left ventricular–right atrial communication), the

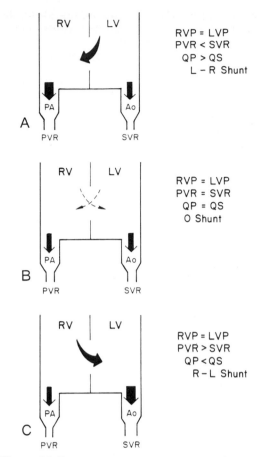

Figure 14–3. Diagrammatic representation of intracardiac shunting patterns as related to outflow resistances of two sides of heart. Q, resistance.

pressure difference between the two chambers or vessels, rather than downstream resistance, dictates the magnitude of the shunt; these are called *obligatory shunts*. For example, in a left ventricular–right atrial shunt, blood shunts continuously through the defect, because the left ventricular pressure is always higher than right atrial pressure, regardless of the distal pulmonary and systemic vascular resistances.

It is customary to relate the cardiac outputs and pressures in each side of the heart. Thus, if there is three times as much flow into the pulmonary artery as into the aorta, there is a 3:1 pulmonary-to-systemic flow ratio. If the pressure in the pulmonary artery is 60 mm Hg and that in the aorta is 90 mm Hg, pulmonary hypertension is at two thirds systemic level.

COMMENT: The pulmonary to systemic blood flow relationship may be somewhat misleading.

For example, if there is severe compromise of systemic perfusion, the pulmonary blood flow may be normal in the face of marked compromise of systemic blood flow. This can result in normalization of arterial oxygen tension, and the development of a metabolic acidemia is the result of the compromise in systemic blood flow.

Norman Talner

◆ THE LOW-RISK NEWBORN

Statistically, the defects encountered most frequently in the newborn are the simple left-to-right shunt lesions. Isolated ventricular septal defect accounts for between 30% and 40% of all congenital heart disease. Atrial septal defect and PDA are less common but important. Occasionally, difficulty occurs late in the neonatal period (3 to 4 weeks of life) from a ventricular septal defect (VSD) or PDA, but this is extremely rare for a simple atrial septal defect.

EDITORIAL COMMENT: An innocent heart murmur in a baby born at term is often related to pulmonary branch stenosis (PBS), particularly if the murmur is still present after 24 hours of age, when most patent ductus arteriosus have closed. In Arlettaz' series, by 6 weeks the murmur had disappeared and the PBS had resolved in 64% of the babies. PBS had resolved in all babies at 6 months.[1] In a study of 7204 consecutive newborn babies, the presence of a murmur prompted echocardiographic examination.[2] A murmur in a neonate was present in less than 1% of the patients and was associated with underlying cardiac malformation in 54% of them. The absence of a murmur in the neonatal period does not rule out congenital heart disease. Indeed, the neonatal examination detected only 44% of cardiac malformations that present during infancy.

◆ ————

1. Arlettaz R, Archer N, Wilkinson AR: Natural history of innocent heart murmurs in newborn babies: controlled echocardiographic study. Arch Dis Child Fetal Neonatal Ed 78:F166, 1998.

2. Ainsworth S, Wyllie JP, Wren C: Prevalence and clinical significance of cardiac murmurs in neonates. Arch Dis Child Fetal Neonatal Ed 80:F43, 1999.

COMMENT: From the standpoint of timing of presentation, the infant with the small ventricular septal defect may be recognized in the immediate newborn period by the presence of the typical murmur in the absence of symptomatology relating to left-to-right shunting into the pulmonary circulation. With the large VSD, however, there is a lag period relating to the delay in the postnatal fall in pulmonary vascular resistance, so that the clinical findings of murmur and the alterations in respiratory function take between 2 and 3 weeks to present themselves. The exception to this situation is encountered in the preterm infant, in whom there may be significant left-to-right shunting via a PDA or ventricular communication within a few days following delivery. Typically, however, the large left-to-right shunt lesion has a lag period before the onset of tachypnea, which represents the change in respiratory pattern attendant on the increase in pulmonary blood flow and alterations in lung compliance.

Norman Talner

Ventricular Septal Defect

In the large, nonrestrictive VSD (see Fig. 14–3), the pressure in the right ventricle and pulmonary artery is at systemic levels. If the thick-walled pulmonary vessels matured normally, the vascular resistance would decrease rapidly, and there would be a large left-to-right shunt with left ventricular failure and pulmonary edema. Such a series of events is unusual. In fact, when a large VSD is present, a heart murmur is not usually heard, even in the newborn period. The left-to-right shunt does not develop rapidly because the pulmonary resistance vessels remain heavily muscular for a longer period than normal and the decrease in pulmonary vascular resistance is delayed. The variation in pulmonary vascular resistance from one child to the next is considerable. Some infants decrease their resistance considerably; others hardly at all. When there is a large defect, the shunt is usually maximal by 2 to 3 weeks of age, so that congestive heart failure, when it occurs, is usually present by 4 weeks of age.

On the other hand, the majority of VSDs are very small and restrictive. In these children, the great resistance to flow between the left and right ventricles allows the pulmonary vessels to mature normally into adult-type vessels. With a rapid decrease in pulmonary vascular resistance, there is a rapid decrease in right ventricular pressure, and a left ventricular–right ventricular pressure gradient will be present. Therefore a left-to-right shunt can develop quickly, so with small defects, the systolic murmur is often present and quite loud (grades 3 to 4/6) even in the newborn period. The murmur may also have a crescendo-decrescendo character typical of a VSD (maladie de

Roger). Despite the low pulmonary vascular resistance, the great resistance to flow at the VSD prevents much left-to-right shunting; therefore, congestive heart failure does not occur frequently. Pulmonary hypertension does not develop readily because the defect is very small. A large percentage of these small defects close spontaneously, and pulmonary hypertension does not develop even in those that remain the same size throughout life.

CASE PROBLEMS

Two cases are illustrated in which there are no symptoms in the newborn period although a heart murmur is heard. The physiologic events during that time are directly related to the eventual course. The preceding discussion of pathophysiology not only helps to answer these questions but also should provide a basis for understanding the very complicated defects to be discussed later.

◆

Case One

At the 2-week checkup, a murmur is heard for the first time in an acyanotic well baby. The diagnosis of VSD with left-to-right shunt is made. The family is very upset with the physician for not having heard the murmur in the newborn period.

◆ *Is the family justified? Why or why not?*

The family is not justified. It is probable, although not definite, that this is a moderately large VSD. If so, then, by definition, the pressure in the right ventricle and pulmonary artery is elevated. The high pulmonary arterial pressure is believed to be one of the factors in delaying maturation of the pulmonary arterioles. The delayed maturation means that pulmonary vascular resistance decreases slowly. Consequently, the left-to-right shunt begins slowly, causing the murmur to develop after the early neonatal period.

COMMENT: The onset of symptomatology in the large left-to-right shunt occurs in a subtle fashion. The earliest finding is that of an increase in respiratory frequency without the presence of respiratory distress. The respiratory rate may be in the range of 60/min without retractions, alar flaring, or wheezing. Tachypnea represents the accumulation of lung water and alterations in lung compliance and is sometimes accompanied by some difficulty in feeding and eventually by failure to thrive. The failure to thrive under these conditions is the result of the increased work of breathing, impaired caloric intake, and probably increased metabolic demands secondary to the release of catecholamines. It should be remembered that although there is a high output state in terms of systemic oxygen transport, there may be significant compromise of oxygen delivery to the tissues.

Norman Talner

◆ *Is it possible that congestive heart failure will develop before the next regularly scheduled visit at 1 month?*
The maximal left-to-right shunt is believed to develop by about 1 month of life, so that when congestive heart failure is recognized, it is usually by then. Occasionally, it is initially diagnosed a little later, but in those patients referred with congestive heart failure at 3 to 4 months, it probably has been present for a while.

◆ *Is pulmonary hypertension likely to be present at this time?*
The larger the defect, the higher the right ventricular pressure. Thus, with large defects and no pulmonary stenosis, high pulmonary arterial pressure must be present no matter what the shunt. With a moderate defect, the pressure is moderately elevated.

◆

Case Two
On the first day of life, the physical examination of a full-term baby is normal, but at 48 hours, the house officer hears a murmur at the lower left sternal border. The child is acyanotic, and the murmur is typical of a VSD with left-to-right shunt.

◆ *Is a VSD possible? Why?*
A VSD is possible. The left ventricular pressure is not transmitted to the right side through the small restrictive VSD. Therefore, nothing impedes the normal decrease in pulmonary vascular resistance. As the pulmonary vascular resistance decreases, the right ventricular pressure decreases as it would normally. Therefore, there is a large pressure gradient between the ventricles, and an early left-to-right shunt is possible.

◆ *Is whatever defect present likely to be small or large?*
The shunt rarely becomes large because of the high resistance to flow through the small defect. The major key to suspecting that the

defect is small is the early onset of the loud, typical murmur.

◆ *Is eventual congestive heart failure likely?*
Heart failure is not likely when the left-to-right shunt is small.

◆ *Is pulmonary hypertension likely?*
When VSDs are small, there is great resistance to flow from one ventricle to the other; thus, there is no transmission of the high left ventricular pressure to the pulmonary arterioles. Consequently, the pulmonary arterioles are not affected by the VSD and mature normally. Pulmonary hypertension is thus unlikely.

One of the house officers argues that the physical examination suggests a large atrial septal defect, which must not be missed. The chief resident, however, counters that unless there is obstruction to flow into the left side of the heart, such as mitral stenosis or atresia, physiologic principles teach that atrial septal defect is not associated with left-to-right shunt in the early newborn period.

◆ *What are the important physiologic principles at work in impedance of left-to-right shunting through an atrial septal defect?*
In the presence of a large atrial septal defect with equalization of right and left atrial pressures, the shunting is determined, at least in part, by the difference in resistance to flow out of the atria. In the newborn period, because the right ventricle is usually thicker than the left, the right ventricular compliance is less (compliance is the inverse of resistance). Because blood flow goes where resistance is least, left atrial blood flows into the left ventricle rather than through the atrial septal defect to the right atrium and then the ventricle.

COMMENT: I would stress that a left-to-right shunt encountered in the immediate newborn period should point to the additional and more important presence of left heart obstructive disease or myocardial dysfunction. In both of these conditions, the foramen ovale may become incompetent with resultant left-to-right shunting.

Norman Talner

◆ *Is it known that the largest simple left-to-right shunt lesions in childhood tend to be atrial septal defects? Are there not dire complications if the defect is not recognized early in life?*
In the first several weeks after the newborn period, because systemic vascular resistance is higher than pulmonary vascular resistance, the left ventricle becomes more mus-

cular and thicker than the right ventricle. Meanwhile, the pulmonary vascular resistance decreases as the fetal vessels mature to adult-type vessels. During infancy, the left-to-right shunt at the atrial level increases gradually. By the time the left-to-right shunt is large, the pulmonary arterioles are mature, thin-walled, and able to dilate maximally. Therefore, the pulmonary arterial pressure is not elevated in childhood.

Consequently, atrial septal defects of the simple type are rarely recognized early in life. Pulmonary hypertension in childhood is virtually unknown, and eventual congestive heart failure in childhood is very uncommon.

Patent Ductus Arteriosus (Fig. 14–4)

The principles discussed for VSD also apply to PDA. However, because there is length to the ductus arteriosus as well as caliber, resistance to flow is greater. A nonrestrictive PDA is less common, so that systemic level pulmonary hypertension is also less common.

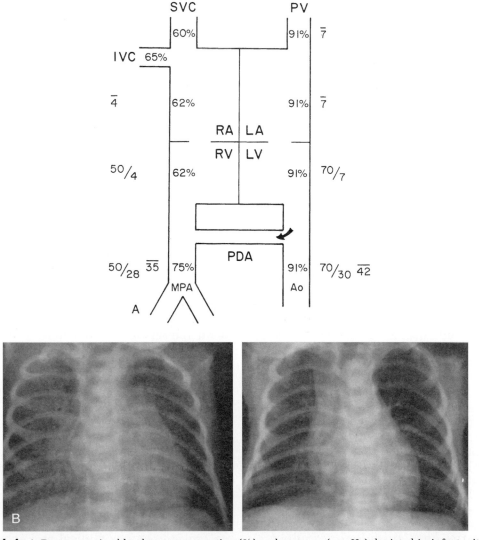

Figure 14–4. *A*, Representative blood-oxygen saturation (%) and pressure (mm Hg) depicted in infant with patent ductus arteriosus (PDA). (See Fig. 14–2 for abbreviations.) *B*, Chest x-ray films of infant with PDA and after pharmacologic closure with indomethacin.

EDITORIAL COMMENT: The exception (see later) is the very low-birth-weight infant with a PDA often complicating respiratory distress syndrome (RDS).

If there is a PDA in the full-term baby, the outcome depends on the size of the channel. With the gradual decrease in postnatal PVR, a left-to-right shunt develops from aorta to pulmonary artery, which produces excessive pulmonary blood flow, increased pulmonary venous return, and left atrial and ventricular dilatation. A small PDA produces only the typical murmur and full pulses. A moderate to large PDA may produce signs of congestive heart failure as well as a typical continuous murmur and wide pulse pressure (bounding pulse), often in the second month of life. Only rarely does failure occur in the newborn period.

PDA in Preterm Infants

As discussed previously, preterm infants and particularly very low-birth-weight infants have a significant incidence of persistent PDA. The PDA of the preterm infant with RDS provides special problems, and in many instances these infants are more high risk in nature, with the PDA seriously complicating management. Although the left ventricle is capable of maintaining near normal systemic blood flow even with a large left-to-right shunt in the premature infant, the increased intravascular blood volume and the associated increase in interstitial fluid aggravate the respiratory distress already present. If left ventricular oxygen demand exceeds supply, the left ventricle may begin to fail, increasing pulmonary venous pressure and further increasing interstitial fluid production. Also, pulmonary arterial pressures may be elevated because of the nonrestrictive PDA itself or because of pulmonary venous hypertension, which may further decrease lung compliance and exacerbate the pulmonary dysfunction. Thus, a PDA in the presence of RDS may seriously affect pulmonary function by a variety of mechanisms.

The diagnosis of a PDA may be difficult in that the typical clinical findings generally are not evident and a continuous murmur is *not* present; an intermittent systolic murmur may be the only auscultatory finding. A wide pulse pressure is often present, as is increased precordial activity. Ventilator therapy and continuous positive airway pressure may mask not only the clinical findings but also the roentgenographic findings of a PDA.

When the roentgenogram shows a large heart and pulmonary venous congestion in the presence of signs of a PDA and a large liver, there is no problem in diagnosis. However, for many reasons, the heart may not be very large, and severe RDS may obscure x-ray findings of cardiomegaly and pulmonary edema. As discussed later, current practice in low-birth-weight preterm infants dictates intervention before this stage so that congestive heart failure should not occur.

In all infants with severe RDS, a PDA must be suspected when the illness is protracted, blood gases suddenly deteriorate and require manipulation of ventilation, or apneic episodes are intensified. Fluid balance must be closely monitored because excess fluid administration may produce a clinically significant PDA and congestive heart failure (see Chapter 6). Infants must be auscultated for murmurs several times each day during the illness and should be briefly removed from the ventilator to permit proper auscultation.

Echocardiography and Doppler mapping have been particularly useful in indicating the presence of a left-to-right shunt through a PDA. Color flow Doppler mapping can detect even a small, hemodynamically insignificant PDA. A large left atrium and left ventricle suggest that the ductus is hemodynamically significant. Other important findings include a hyperdynamic left ventricle, bulging of the atrial septum from left to right indicating increased left atrial pressure, increased pulsations in the descending aorta with retrograde diastolic flow indicating a runoff of blood into the lungs, and reduced diastolic forward flow in branches of the ascending aorta such as the cerebral arteries.

The approach to management of these infants, particularly those of less than 1250 g birth weight, is not clearly established. First, the term *hemodynamic significance* is broadly applied. To some physicians, any change from the standard, expected management of an infant without a PDA constitutes significance; this includes the requirement for fluid and (hence) calorie restriction or the requirement for diuretic administration to prevent obvious clinical and echocardiographic evidence of volume overload. In many institutions, however, the shunt is deemed significant and requires more specific intervention only when severe fluid restriction and diuresis together with aggressive ventilatory management fail. Furthermore, the type and the timing of the intervention are not standard. Whenever feasible, therapy should be aimed at the *cause* of the problem rather than the adverse effects. For PDA, this is possible in most situations; surgical closure can be offered with relatively low risk of morbidity, and, more importantly, pharmacologic closure by inhibition of prostaglandin synthesis with indomethacin has an acceptably low failure rate as well as relatively few adverse effects. A major attempt to control the heart failure would therefore seem unacceptable as a primary approach, especially because digoxin, the drug used in term infants or older children to improve myocardial performance, has little positive effect in premature infants and has a high risk of toxicity. We recommend administering indomethacin on first diagnosis of a PDA (usually by 2 to 3 days after birth) in infants weighing less than 1000 g; in infants of more than 1000 g birth weight, we only administer indomethacin when it is apparent that the PDA is stimulating changes in management or is "hemodynamically significant." Continued deterioration toward true heart failure in any of these situations prompts immediate ligation (for drug therapy of heart disorders see Appendix A–1).

EDITORIAL COMMENT: Permanent closure of the ductus arteriosus requires both effective muscular constriction to block luminal blood flow and anatomic remodeling to prevent later reopening. Narayanan[1] in 257 preterm infants (gestation 24 to 27 weeks) compared prophylactic indomethacin within 15 hours after birth with symptomatic treatment (indomethacin only if clinical symptoms appeared). The prophylactic treatment group had a greater degree of initial ductus constriction, a higher rate of permanent anatomic closure, and a decreased need for surgical ligation than did the symptomatic treatment group. However, even when managed with prophylactic indomethacin, the rate of ductus reopening remained unacceptably high in the most immature infants.

Studies have demonstrated that ibuprofen is equally effective in closing a PDA, but an intravenous preparation is not yet approved for general release in the United States.[2, 3]

◆

1. Narayanan M, Cooper B, Weiss H, Clyman RI: Prophylactic indomethacin: factors determining permanent ductus arteriosus closure. J Pediatr 136:330, 2000.

2. Van Overmeire B, Smets K, Lecoutere D, et al: A comparison of ibuprofen and indomethacin for closure of patent ductus arteriosus. N Engl J Med 343:674, 2000.

3. Clyman RI. Ibuprofen and patent ductus arteriosus. N Engl J Med 343:728, 2000.

Combined or Complicated Shunts

Although an isolated VSD, PDA, or atrial septal defect rarely causes problems in the full-term newborn, combinations of these are more likely to do so. For example, in an infant with the clinical features of VSD, if cardiac failure and respiratory distress develop (see next section) in the first week or two of life, an additional shunt or another cardiac or vascular abnormality might be present. Another situation in which an isolated shunt might produce signs of failure occurs when the lung, particularly the pulmonary vascular bed, is underdeveloped or damaged, such as with diaphragmatic hernia, omphalocele, or chronic lung disease. In these infants, a small shunt seems much larger because of the reduced size of the pulmonary vascular bed.

With an endocardial cushion defect, left ventricular–to–right atrial shunting may occur; this is an *obligatory shunt* not dependent on pulmonary vascular resistance. Thus, this lesion may produce signs of cardiac failure early in life. Mitral or tricuspid insufficiency plus ventricular shunting aggravates the situation.

COMMENT: Endocardial cushion defects are rarely associated with cardiac failure in the newborn, but when this occurs, it is more likely due to associated left heart obstruction or valvular insufficiency than to an obligatory shunt.
Roberta G. Williams

COMMENT: The importance of combined lesions, particularly the association of left heart obstructive disease such as coarctation with a VSD, demands early intervention. It has become apparent that the major problem in most situations relates to the left heart obstructive disease, which must be relieved to maintain systemic perfusion. The removal of the left heart obstruction may then permit the infant to adapt to the shunt lesion, and, in fact, in many instances the shunt lesions may undergo spontaneous closure.
Norman Talner

◆ THE HIGH-RISK NEWBORN

Presentation

Severe forms of congenital heart disease usually present in one of three ways in the immediate newborn period, although there is some overlap. This section discusses these three types of presentation, the most common lesions in each, the diagnostic tests necessary to distinguish among the lesions, subsequent therapy, and the differential diagnosis of noncardiac disease. This section discusses only those lesions with symptoms that require diagnostic and therapeutic interventions. As described in The Low-Risk Newborn, some cases present in the first month of life with murmurs as the only sign of potential heart disease; later, these infants are found to have no heart disease or to have low-risk, isolated lesions. Also, murmurs in the newborn are frequently nonspecific. We believe it is more prudent to reevaluate such infants at several weeks of age: at that time, the physical findings are more specific because adaptation to extrauterine life is complete. Thus, many infants with innocent murmurs or minor lesions would not undergo exhaustive and expensive diagnostic procedures.

During the neonatal period, serious heart disease presents either with persistent cyanosis, respiratory distress, a low systemic output state, or a combination of these. Although complex heart disease usually presents with more than one of these findings, we classify each lesion according to its predominant feature.

COMMENT: Occasionally, neonates with serious forms of heart disease may not exhibit obvious cyanosis, respiratory distress, or low-output state because of persistence of the ductus arteriosus or elevation of pulmonary vascular resistance.

Roberta G. Williams

Generalized Central Cyanosis

Central cyanosis indicates a reduced arterial blood oxygen saturation. The infant with cyanotic heart disease is usually cyanotic in the first few hours of life, although not in respiratory distress. This cyanosis may initially occur with crying or feeding only and then progress as the circulation adapts to postnatal life, particularly as the ductus arteriosus begins to close. The level of sys-temic arterial blood oxygen saturation depends entirely on the effective pulmonary blood flow—that is, the amount of blood oxygenated by the lungs that subsequently passes into the systemic arterial circulation. Pulmonary function is generally normal; therefore, pulmonary venous blood returning to the heart is essentially fully saturated with oxygen. The resultant systemic arterial oxygen saturation depends on the relative O_2 content and amounts of systemic venous and pulmonary venous return and their degree of admixture. There are two major subgroups of lesions that feature cyanosis as the primary finding (Table 14–2): (1) those lesions with decreased pulmonary blood flow, in which the inflow to or outflow from the right ventricle is compromised (e.g., pulmonary atresia; Fig. 14–5), and (2) those lesions with normal or increased pulmonary blood flow but with separation of the pulmonary venous return from the systemic arterial circulation (the transposition complexes; Fig. 14–6). In both subgroups, effective pulmonary blood flow is low.

In practice, the differential diagnosis of these infants is limited to mild pulmonary disease or persistent pulmonary hypertension of the newborn (PPHN). Methemoglobinemia (rarely seen) should always be considered a possible cause. Infants with

Table 14–2. Cardiac Causes of Cyanosis Without Congestive Heart Failure

Decreased Pulmonary Blood Flow

Right ventricular inflow
    Tricuspid atresia with intact ventricular septum or small ventricular septal defect
    Tricuspid stenosis with hypoplastic right side of heart
    Tricuspid insufficiency secondary to myocardial ischemia (often associated with perinatal asphyxia)
    Ebstein anomaly
Right ventricular outflow
    Critical pulmonary stenosis or pulmonary atresia with intact ventricular septum
    Severe pulmonary stenosis with ventricular septal defect (tetralogy of Fallot)
    Pulmonary atresia with ventricular septal defect
    Univentricular heart with severe pulmonary stenosis or atresia

Normal Pulmonary Blood Flow with Poor Mixing

D-Transposition of great vessels
Taussig-Bing anomaly
D-Transposition of great vessels with associated lesions (complex)

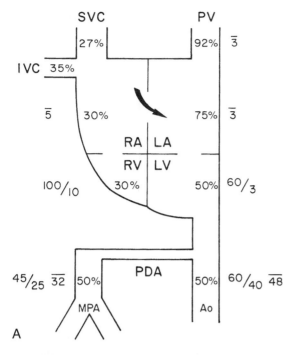

fant with PPHN, however, often has a history of perinatal distress or meconium aspiration. An exception in the cardiac group is tricuspid insufficiency resulting from myocardial ischemia, in which a history of perinatal asphyxia is common. The physical examination rarely distinguishes between the cardiac and noncardiac patients: most are tachypneic but with little or no respiratory distress. (In infants with mild arterial oxygen desaturation, tachypnea can

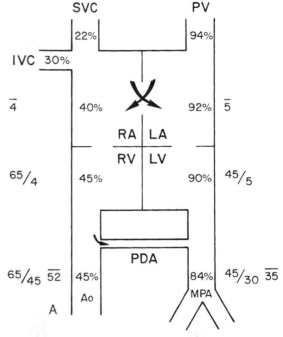

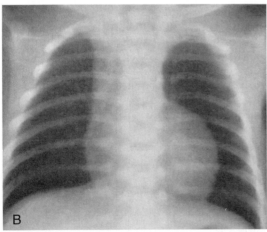

Figure 14–5. *A*, Representative blood-oxygen saturation (%) and pressure (mm Hg) depicted in infant with pulmonary atresia. (See Fig. 14–2 for abbreviations.) *B*, Chest x-ray films of infant with pulmonary atresia.

decreased lung volumes caused by external compression in utero and those with severe parenchymal lung disease presenting with cyanosis invariably show severe respiratory distress; such cases do not enter into the differential diagnosis (they are discussed in the following section).

Initial evaluation usually directs the physician to strongly suspect cardiac disease. The history of the cyanotic infant with heart disease is generally benign, and the pregnancy and delivery are uneventful. The in-

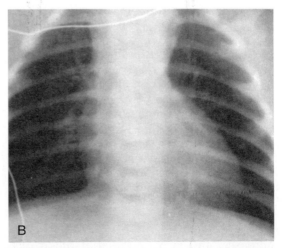

Figure 14–6. *A*, Representative blood-oxygen saturation (%) and pressure (mm Hg) depicted in infant with complete transposition of great arteries. (See Fig. 14–2 for abbreviations.) *B*, Chest x-ray films of infant with complete transposition of great arteries.

develop because of chemoreceptor stimulation.) If the hypoxemia is severe and mild metabolic acidemia develops, respiratory distress may become evident, making it extremely difficult to differentiate from the respiratory distress associated with mild or moderate primary pulmonary disease. Most cyanotic infants have an increased right ventricular impulse resulting from high right ventricular pressure (except in hypoplastic right heart syndrome), and murmurs are frequently present in noncardiac lesions (PPHN with secondary tricuspid insufficiency) or absent in heart disease (transposition with intact ventricular septum and pulmonary atresia with VSD).

Other diagnostic procedures are needed in those infants. It helps to compare arterial blood oxygen saturation or PO_2 (measured directly or transcutaneously) in the right radial artery or upper body (and thus above the ductus arteriosus) with those in the umbilical artery or lower body (below the ductus arteriosus). In most forms of cyanotic heart disease, the two saturations or PO_2s are similar; in PPHN, pulmonary vascular resistance is very high, and the ductus arteriosus, if patent, shows right-to-left ductal shunting with subsequent lowering of the blood oxygen saturation or PO_2 in the descending aorta. If the oxygen saturation in the upper body is lower than that in the lower body, the infant most likely has D-transposition. The "hyperoxia" test, or ventilation with a high inspired oxygen concentration, is frequently considered a valuable diagnostic tool. Although an increase greater than 20 to 30 mm Hg in systemic arterial PO_2 is often seen in primary pulmonary problems (especially because high levels of oxygen tend to dilate the pulmonary arterioles and decrease the pulmonary arterial pressures), the converse, although generally true, is not necessarily so. That is, one may encounter a significant increase in systemic arterial blood oxygen tension or saturation in cyanotic heart disease. As long as effective pulmonary blood flow is reasonable, there is a fair increase in oxygen delivered to the systemic arterial bed. This, in turn, increases the systemic venous blood oxygen saturation as oxygen delivery to the tissues increases, and systemic arterial blood oxygen saturation increases further. If a hyperoxia test is performed, it should be done with transcutaneous saturation or direct oxygen measurements performed simultaneously in the upper and lower body to exaggerate any potential difference and thus help to delineate the presence of a right-to-left ductal shunt. The measurement of upper and lower body saturation during crying can also help to exaggerate potential differences due to ductal shunting.

Chest x-ray films in the first few days of life usually show normal heart size in most lesions. (Exceptions may be those lesions such as Ebstein anomaly in which tricuspid insufficiency is a major problem and marked right atrial enlargement occurs.) Because thymic involution occurs early in cyanotic infants, it is helpful to examine the cardiac contour. Most cyanotic lesions are associated with either a diminutive pulmonary artery (e.g., pulmonary atresia) or one that is transposed to the right; thus, the normal pulmonary artery contour at the upper left region of the cardiac silhouette is absent. The aortic arch should be visualized; the aorta frequently descends to the right of the spine in right-sided obstructive lesions, particularly with an associated VSD (tetralogy of Fallot). Examination of the lung fields may rule out pulmonary abnormalities caused by displacement by abdominal organs. Vascularity may be low, normal, or even increased in cyanotic heart disease. (Consider transposition of the great arteries with VSD in which pulmonary blood flow is high, although effective pulmonary blood flow—that blood then passing to the systemic circulation—may be very low.) Thus, vascularity may not be helpful in diagnosis. When the pulmonary vascularity is low, there is almost always heart disease, but a normal or increased vascularity does not exclude it.

EDITORIAL COMMENT: Assessment of pulmonary vascularity radiographically is dependent on the quality of the film and lung expansion. Overinflated lungs from mechanical ventilation appear to be undervascularized.

An electrocardiogram (ECG) in the first few days of life is often nonspecific because the right ventricle is dominant in the normal fetus and in most forms of cyanotic heart disease. Over the next few weeks, as pulmonary resistance decreases, the T wave normally inverts in the right precordial leads; thus, after this time interval, the T wave in lesions associated with right ventricular hypertrophy can be distinguished. Unfortunately, cyanotic heart disease must be diagnosed much sooner. There are some lesions with specific ECG patterns—right atrial hypertrophy in Ebstein anomaly, left axis deviation and right atrial hypertrophy with decreased right ventricular forces in tricuspid atresia with intact ventricular septum—but these are exceptions.

If the possibility of cyanotic heart disease is entertained after these initial studies, further procedures must be performed. A two-dimensional echocardiogram with color Doppler studies can almost always accurately define the anatomy of the heart.

COMMENT: It may be argued that the chest x-ray film and electrocardiogram are sufficiently nonspecific in the neonate that any evidence for a cardiac lesion should prompt an echocardiographic study as the initial test.

Roberta G. Williams

If the patient is not in a facility where an echocardiogram or cardiac catheterization can be performed, immediate transfer is mandatory. Stabilization before the transport is of utmost importance: metabolic requirements must be reduced to a minimum to provide adequate substrate delivery, and, if oxygen delivery is borderline (measured blood oxygen saturation is less than or equal to 80%, PO_2 is less than or equal to 30 to 35 mm Hg, or the presence of metabolic acidosis), prostaglandin E_1 (Prostin VR) should be infused. Start the infusion at 0.05 μg/kg/min and increase to 0.15 μg/kg/min as needed.

The use of prostaglandin E_1 is based on the physiologic information that prostaglandins dilate the ductus arteriosus. Initially, prostaglandin E_1 was used only in those infants with ductus-dependent lesions, such as hypoplastic right ventricle and pulmonary atresia. In most of these infants, pulmonary blood flow is provided entirely through the ductus arteriosus. When the ductus closes after birth, hypoxemia and acidemia progressively worsen unless a palliative surgical procedure is performed immediately. Prostaglandin E_1 effectively dilates the ductus to provide adequate pulmonary blood flow; the infant's condition can then be stabilized and carefully evaluated. Recently, it became apparent that most infants with complete transposition of the great arteries also have better mixing between the pulmonary and systemic circulations when the

ductus arteriosus is fully dilated with prostaglandin E_1. *It is appropriate, therefore, to infuse prostaglandin E_1 into any infant in whom the diagnosis of cyanotic congenital heart disease is strongly suspected, even before a complete evaluation.* However, prostaglandin E_1 has definite side effects, such as apnea, jitteriness or even frank seizures, hypotension with peripheral vasodilation, and a possible increased risk of infection. Fluid administration is frequently necessary after initiation of prostaglandin E_1 to maintain the arterial blood pressure, because there is significant systemic vasodilation.

In certain patients, cardiac catheterization must be considered. It is necessary to catheterize the newborn when the diagnosis is uncertain, a therapeutic procedure is necessary (e.g., balloon atrial septostomy in transposition of the great arteries), or surgery is imminent and better definition of the anatomy is required (e.g., the right ventricular outflow tract and pulmonary arteries in pulmonary atresia when a pulmonary valvotomy or outflow patch is to be performed). In many infants, because two-dimensional echocardiography can accurately define the anatomy, immediate catheterization is not required and can be delayed beyond the neonatal period, after which time the risks are fewer and the angiographic detail is better.

In summary, an infant with cyanosis and little respiratory distress usually has cardiac disease and requires prompt evaluation and stabilization. When the initial evaluation cannot exclude cardiac disease, it is important to proceed with a complete cardiovascular evaluation. With the dramatic improvements in echocardiography, Doppler technology (including color flow mapping), cardiac catheterization, and neonatal surgery, and the advent of prostaglandin E_1 use to maintain ductal patency, a more normal life can be offered to infants with cyanotic heart disease.

Respiratory Distress

Congenital heart disease that presents with respiratory distress is most difficult to diagnose in infants: their symptoms are usually more insidious and less dramatic than cyanosis, the differential diagnosis is broader, and the yield of heart disease is much less, thus lowering one's index of suspicion. When a physician sees a newborn lying in a crib, blue and comfortable, the diagnosis is almost always cardiac disease; when the infant is acyanotic, tachypneic, and showing retractions, it usually is not.

Infants with respiratory distress usually have modest degrees of systemic blood oxygen desaturation, depending on the type of circulatory derangement and the severity of pulmonary edema. The respiratory distress is related to decreased lung compliance in these patients, and interstitial fluid is usually present. Thus, even with a normal separation of circulations, some degree of hypoxemia is present. A more important source of hypoxemia in many of these infants is the redirection of systemic venous return to the aorta. In fact, infants with respiratory distress on a cardiac basis can be categorized into two major subgroups: (1) those with pure left-to-right shunts, in whom the shunt solely consists of pulmonary venous return being directed back to the pulmonary arterial circulation, so that any arterial desaturation is secondary to alveolar fluid or an intrapulmonary shunt, and (2) those with bidirectional shunts (complete mixing lcsions), in whom there is also systemic venous blood being directed back to the systemic arterial circulation, directly causing some arterial desaturation (Table 14–3). Once again, both groups may have elevated pulmonary venous pressures or pulmonary blood flow that causes interstitial edema,

Table 14–3. Cardiac Causes of Respiratory Distress

Pure Left-to-Right Shunt

Patent ductus arteriosus
Ventricular septal defect (usually with patent ductus arteriosus or atrial septal defect)
Endocardial cushion defect (atrioventricular canal defect)
Aortopulmonary window
Arteriovenous fistula (usually cerebral or hepatic)

Bidirectional Shunt

Total anomalous pulmonary venous connection
Tricuspid atresia with large ventricular septal defect
Univentricular heart or double-outlet right ventricle without severe pulmonic stenosis
Complex D-transposition of great vessels with large ventricular septal defect
Truncus arteriosus
Absent pulmonary valve syndrome

Left Ventricular Inflow Obstruction

Mitral stenosis
Cor Triatriatum

at which point respiratory distress becomes apparent.

In the first subgroup, the blood entering the aorta has the same saturation as that in the pulmonary veins—that is, there is no right-to-left shunt. Atrial septal defect, atrioventricular septal defect (endocardial cushion defect), VSD, aortopulmonary window, PDA, and arteriovenous malformation are examples of left-to-right shunts at each level in the circulation that can produce cardiac failure and thereby respiratory distress. These infants often do not have symptoms in the neonatal period. Exceptions include lesions associated with a large systolic and diastolic shunt (aortopulmonary window or arteriovenous malformation) and prematurity (most typically with a PDA, although we have seen several symptomatic premature infants in heart failure with endocardial cushion defects, atrial septal defects, or VSDs), or in the presence of an associated lesion. The latter is often an obstruction to left ventricular outflow (see the following section), such as coarctation or interruption of the aorta. This is seen most commonly with VSDs or aortopulmonary windows.

The second subgroup of infants represents a wide spectrum of complex congenital heart diseases. Admixture of systemic and pulmonary venous blood may occur at the venous, atrial, ventricular, or arterial level. Admixture at the venous level occurs in total anomalous pulmonary venous connection. There is rarely respiratory distress in this lesion during the neonatal period, unless there is obstruction to pulmonary venous return. This is most commonly seen when the connection is below the diaphragm to the portal venous system. An example of admixture at the atrial level with respiratory distress is tricuspid atresia with a large VSD: because there is no entrance of systemic venous blood to the right ventricle, the blood must cross an interatrial communication into the left atrium and left ventricle. Complete admixture at the ventricular level can be seen in double-outlet right ventricle and in complex univentricular physiology. At the ventriculoarterial level, truncus arteriosus is the classic example. When pulmonary venous obstruction is not present, congestive heart failure usually develops over several weeks as the pulmonary resistance decreases and pulmonary blood flow increases. Even more systemic arterial desaturation occurs in lesions in which there is preferential return of systemic venous blood back to the aorta and pulmonary venous blood back to the pulmonary artery. Increased pulmonary blood flow causes congestive heart failure in the presence of visible cyanosis. This occurs in transposition of the great arteries with a large VSD or occasionally a large PDA and in certain forms of double-outlet right ventricle.

In cases of absent pulmonary valve syndrome, the hemodynamic pattern is similar to that in tetralogy of Fallot, but there often is severe respiratory distress. The massively dilated pulmonary arteries that are present in this syndrome compress the airways and cause ventilatory embarrassment.

Interference with inflow to the left ventricle, as in congenital mitral stenosis or cor triatriatum, may lead to severe pulmonary venous congestion and respiratory distress but may not compromise systemic perfusion to any major degree. Infants with cor triatriatum have been diagnosed as having chronic lung disease and have undergone treatment for many months before a congenital cardiac malformation was suspected.

The differential diagnosis of infants with respiratory distress secondary to heart disease includes parenchymal lung disease and PPHN. The premature infant with resolving RDS who requires increasing respiratory support may have either an increasing ductal shunt or the onset of interstitial lung disease. The full-term infant with total anomalous pulmonary venous connection is often first thought to have PPHN, an aspiration syndrome, or pneumonia. The infant with truncus arteriosus may first appear to have transient tachypnea until it is obviously no longer transient. Thus, it may take several days of careful evaluation before the presence of heart disease is fully appreciated.

The initial evaluation of the infant with respiratory distress rarely points to cardiac problems. The perinatal history is usually benign, but this is also true for infants with early onset pneumonias. The physical examination reveals an infant with tachypnea and retractions, often with no detectable cyanosis, for only when blood oxygen saturations reach quite low levels (about 75%) is cyanosis appreciated in the newborn. Examining the peripheral pulses is helpful when there is a large runoff of blood from the aorta into either the venous system (e.g., arteriovenous malformation) or the low-resistance bed of

the lungs (e.g., PDA and truncus arteriosus). But when the shunt is intracardiac (thus maintaining a normal aortic diastolic pressure) or when there is an associated low-output state, this does not occur. Hepatomegaly is common in both cardiac and lung disease. The assessment of liver size is complicated by the downward displacement of the diaphragm caused by hyperinflation. The precordium is hyperactive because of increased volume load or pulmonary arterial pressures in most shunt lesions as well as occasionally in primary lung disease. The presence of a systolic ejection click suggests lesions in which a large volume of blood is crossing one, usually abnormal, valve, as in truncus arteriosus; this may also be found with the suprasystemic pressures in the pulmonary artery seen in total anomalous venous connection. A single second heart sound may suggest the absence of a pulmonary valve (e.g., truncus arteriosus) or its posterior displacement (e.g., transposition with VSD). Murmurs are more frequent in these lesions than in cyanotic heart disease because there is a large flow of blood across an abnormal connection into the pulmonary artery. A peripheral murmur indicates an arteriovenous malformation (e.g., over the cranium). An important exception is the absence of murmurs in total anomalous pulmonary venous connection.

COMMENT: The presence of tachycardia may obscure auscultatory findings such as an ejection click or splitting of the second heart sound.
Roberta G. Williams

As previously mentioned, values for arterial blood oxygen saturation vary widely depending on the flow patterns and the amount of pulmonary edema. A hyperoxic test is usually unhelpful in infants with respiratory distress caused by congenital heart disease, because a large portion of the desaturation is due to pulmonary edema and thus a significant improvement often occurs when oxygen is administered. The chest x-ray film may show cardiomegaly because of the increased pulmonary blood flow in many of the lesions in this category. Similarly, pulmonary vascularity is often increased, although this may be difficult to interpret when parenchymal disease is present. Passive congestion is seen when the pulmonary venous pressures are markedly elevated. Newborns with pneumonia often have both interstitial pulmonary fluid and cardiomegaly; therefore, these findings are not specific for cardiac disease. The ECG is helpful only when it is specific for particular lesions. For example, in total anomalous pulmonary venous connection, the suprasystemic pressures in the pulmonary artery are often reflected in the ECG by the presence of QR waves in the right precordial leads. However, specific ECG patterns are the exception rather than the rule.

A high index of suspicion is required to consider the presence of heart disease in an infant with respiratory distress. When the course is not classic for pneumonia or another lung disorder, the history does not support lung disease, or there are signs that raise doubts about the diagnosis, it is necessary to consider heart disease. A two-dimensional echocardiogram with Doppler studies and saline contrast injection enables primary lung and cardiac problems to be differentiated. (Shaken saline has "microbubbles" of air out of solution that are highly echoreflectant and thus can be followed as blood travels from the systemic veins throughout the circulation until a capillary bed is reached.) Even in total anomalous pulmonary venous connection, a careful study usually demonstrates the abnormal vessel either above or below the diaphragm. The diagnosis can be confirmed by color Doppler studies showing blood flowing away from the heart in the abnormal vessel or by the absence of contrast (saline) in that vessel alone, because it is the only part of the circulation that is separated from the systemic veins by a capillary bed. It is necessary to consider the possibility of heart disease in any term (and occasionally preterm) infant with respiratory distress.

COMMENT: The pulmonary veins must be identified and traced to the exact point of drainage for the proper echocardiographic diagnosis of anomalous pulmonary venous return. Contrast echocardiography and color Doppler studies may add useful information but should not be the primary evidence for this lesion.
Roberta G. Williams

Children with very severe respiratory distress, who are candidates for extracorporeal support, should all have an echocardiogram before initiation of support. The presentations of severe meconium lung disease and severe obstruction in total anomalous pulmonary venous connection are similar and easily confused. This form of total anomalous pulmonary venous connection remains one of the few cardiac surgical emergencies in the newborn.

Hypoperfusion States

The third common manner of presentation of critical heart disease in the newborn is hypoperfusion. The course may be rapidly progressive over the first few hours of life or insidious in onset over the first few weeks.

COMMENT: Occasionally, low-output state may occur suddenly after several weeks of apparent good health. This may occur with abrupt closure of the ductus arteriosus in a patient with a ductal-dependent systemic circulation.
Roberta G. Williams

The differential diagnosis of noncardiac disease presenting as hypoperfusion covers a wide range of organ systems (Table 14–4). The physician must promptly assess the potential causes of the low-output state and begin treatment before confirmatory studies.

Hypoperfusion is secondary to an inadequate ejection of blood by the left ventricle into the systemic arterial system, with subsequent hypotension and progressive metabolic acidosis. Heart disease that presents in this manner may be divided into two categories: (1) those lesions in which the inflow to or outflow from the left ventricle is obstructed, and (2) those lesions in which flow is unobstructed, but the function of the left ventricle is seriously impaired. Obstructive lesions are far more common, the most common of which are coarctation of the aorta and hypoplastic left heart syndrome (Fig. 14–7). As mentioned previously, hypoperfusion syndromes often have associated findings. Many lesions have some degree of systemic arterial desaturation (e.g., in hypoplastic left heart syndrome, the aorta is perfused by the pulmonary artery via the ductus arteriosus, and thus systemic venous blood returns to the arterial system), and most are associated with respiratory distress in that pulmonary venous pressures are elevated when the left ventricle fails to eject a normal stroke volume. However, infants with the most striking characteristics are lethargic and mottled with pallor and poor pulses.

The differential diagnosis of noncardiac disease is broad: sepsis, adrenal insuffi-

Table 14–4. Causes of Hypoperfusion

Cardiac	Noncardiac
Obstructive Lesions	
Left ventricular inflow obstruction	Adrenal insufficiency
Cor triatriatum	Anemia
Mitral stenosis	Hypovolemia
Supravalvular mitral ring	Inborn errors of metabolism
± Total anomalous pulmonary venous connection	Metabolic (decreased Ca^{2+}, Mg^{2+}, glucose, H^+)
Left ventricular outflow obstruction	Polycythemia
Coarctation of aorta	Sepsis
Hypoplastic left side of heart syndrome	Severe neurologic dysfunction
Interrupted aortic arch	Pneumothorax
Severe aortic stenosis	Interstitial emphysema
	Congenital diaphragmatic hernia
Nonobstructive Lesions	
Arrhythmia	
Complete heart block	
Supraventricular tachycardia	
Intrinsic myocardial abnormality	
Abnormal coronary arteries (arteritis, calcinosis)	
Anomalous left coronary artery	
Endocardial fibroelastosis	
Glycogen storage disease	
Infiltrative disease of myocardium (e.g., congenital leukemia)	
Myocardial ischemia/infarction with normal coronary arteries	
Myocarditis	
Primary cardiomyopathies	
Pericardial disorders	
Cardiac tamponade	
Pneumopericardium	
Hemopericardium	
Hydropericardium (hydrops fetalis)	
Pericarditis	
Diabetic cardiomyopathy	
Asphyxia with myocardial dysfunction	

ciency, anemia, hypovolemia, inborn errors of metabolism, and neurologic instability all may present with hypoperfusion as the major finding. The most frequent misdiagnosis in an infant with heart disease and hypoperfusion is sepsis. Because overwhelming infection is life threatening, it is reasonable to perform a septic workup and even begin specific therapy on any infant with signs of low output, but it is important to consider cardiac disease as well.

The history can help distinguish between cardiac and noncardiac disease and among the specific cardiac lesions. An early presentation within the first few hours to first few days of life is more commonly associated with hypoplastic left heart syndrome in the obstructive group and congenital infection or arrhythmia in the nonobstructive group. Coarctation or interruption of the aorta presents later in the first 1 to 2 weeks of life, as do coronary artery abnormalities. There is sometimes a history of perinatal problems.

A history of recent viral infection in the mother may be elicited in infants with myocarditis. Fetal hydrops occurs in intrauterine supraventricular tachycardia, cardiomyopathy, premature closure of the foramen ovale, and, on rare occasions, hypoplastic left heart syndrome. Maternal diabetes suggests diabetic cardiomyopathy, and a familial history might suggest other forms of cardiomyopathy.

The physical examination uniformly shows a pale, tachypneic, and lethargic infant. The heart rate is markedly elevated (220 to 270 bpm) in supraventricular tachycardia, although it can be greater than 200 bpm in any stressed infant with a sinus tachycardia. Frank cyanosis is most often seen in hypoplastic left heart syndrome, but even then it is uncommon. Peripheral pulses are decreased in low-output states generally, but a differential pulse or blood pressure between the upper and lower extremities can be revealing. In coarctation of the aorta,

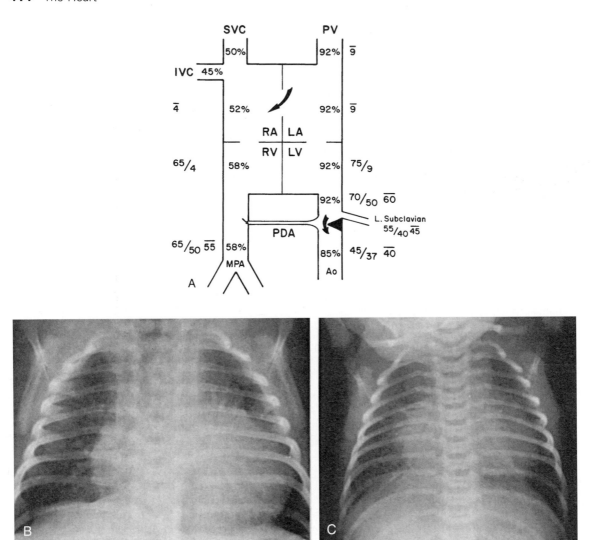

Figure 14–7. *A,* Representative blood-oxygen saturation (%) and pressure (mm Hg) depicted in infant with coarctation of aorta. (See Fig. 14–2 for abbreviations.) *B,* Chest x-ray film of infant with coarctation of aorta. *C,* Chest x-ray film of infant with hypoplastic left side of heart syndrome. Chest x-ray film usually cannot differentiate between left-sided obstructive lesions.

the lower limb pressures may be low (unless the ductus arteriosus is nonrestrictive); in hypoplastic left heart syndrome, the opposite may be true. It is important to realize that the left subclavian artery frequently arises at the origin of the coarctation and thus should not be used to represent ascending aortic pressures in coarctation (see Fig. 14–7*A*). Similarly, the right subclavian artery may arise aberrantly from the descending aorta, making assessment of the ascending aorta difficult. However, a difference in intensity between the carotid pulse and the extremity pulses can be a clue to this diagnosis. The precordial impulse is often nonspecific, usually showing a right

ventricular heave. The second heart sound is single in hypoplastic left heart syndrome but, because of the tachycardia in low-output states, it is often difficult to appreciate a split sound in any of the lesions. Murmurs rarely help the diagnosis in this group: in the presence of severe failure, most lesions are not associated with murmurs or have nonspecific ones. Coarctation of the aorta in which a VSD or subaortic stenosis is present is an exception, but critical aortic stenosis may have little or no murmur when the left ventricular output is low. Rales are heard in most low-output states as a result of elevated pulmonary venous pressures.

Arterial blood gases often show a metabolic acidosis at the time of diagnosis. Differential pulse oximetry measurements between the right hand and foot may be helpful. In coarctation or interruption of the aorta, the saturation in the foot will be lower if the ductus is patent because there will be right-to-left shunting from the pulmonary artery to the descending aorta. Conversely, if the saturation is higher in the descending aorta, transposition with VSD and coarctation should be considered. The chest x-ray study often shows cardiomegaly and interstitial edema in both cardiac and noncardiac lesions once there is severe heart failure and thus is not useful for diagnosis. The ECG is helpful in identifying several lesions. For example, left-sided forces are absent in hypoplastic left heart syndrome; the regular rapid heart rate of supraventricular tachycardia is diagnostic (Fig. 14–8); there are signs of an anterolateral ischemia or infarction in anomalous left coronary artery; endocardial fibroelastosis has prominent Q and R waves in the precordial leads; there usually is marked right ventricular hypertrophy in coarctation of the aorta or critical aortic stenosis; ST-T wave abnormalities are present in myocarditis. The echocardiogram is diagnostic in the obstructive lesions; however, occasionally an isolated aortic coarctation can be masked after the administration of prostaglandin E_1, because the presence of a large PDA decreases the flow through the area. Also, in some patients, ductal tissue wraps around the aorta (so-called ductal sling), causing the obstruction when it contracts and the ductus closes. This area can be dilated by administration of prostaglandin E_1, making diagnosis problematic in its presence. The echocardiogram is also useful in assessing ventricular performance and the response to therapeutic interventions.

An immediate catheterization is best avoided in left-sided obstructive lesions unless absolutely necessary, because infants with such lesions are often barely compensated, and even a small stress could cause rapid metabolic deterioration. Also, these infants do not tolerate large volumes of contrast because of the agent's high osmolarity.

Therapy must be prompt. Once deterioration begins, it is usually rapidly progressive. Initial measures must be directed to the metabolic derangements: partial correction of the metabolic acidosis; maintenance of adequate substrate, hemoglobin, and blood volume; and prompt inotropic support with rapidly acting agents such as isoproterenol or dopamine. Prostaglandin E_1 is of utmost importance when obstructive lesions are considered: by maintaining ductal patency, the lower body may be perfused from the pulmonary artery in interruption or coarctation of the aorta. The entire body can be perfused by this route in critical aortic stenosis and hypoplastic left heart syndrome. Next, a specific diagnosis must be made and appropriate therapy instituted. For example, if the infant has supraventricular tachycardia and is decompensated, cardioversion at 0.25 to 1.0 watt-second should be performed. If the infant is relatively stable after the initial assessment, facial immersion in cold water or pharmacologic cardioversion may be attempted using adenosine. Verapamil is generally contraindicated in the newborn.

In left ventricular obstructive lesions, the infant can be maintained on prostaglandin E_1 before surgery. If the diagnosis is in doubt, antibiotics should be instituted after a sepsis workup, and corticosteroids should be considered if adrenal insufficiency is a possibility.

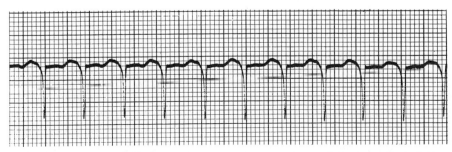

Figure 14–8. Electrocardiogram illustrating paroxysmal atrial tachycardia. Lead II standard electrocardiogram at speed 50. Heart rate = 300 bpm. No P waves are seen.

◆ PRACTICAL HINTS

1. Heart sounds in most newborns with congenital heart disease of a serious nature are usually abnormal. A single second sound after the first 12 hours often indicates heart disease, although with rapid heart rates this can be difficult. A well-split second sound is always abnormal and suggests total anomalous pulmonary venous connection. The presence of a pulmonary systolic ejection click may be normal in the first hours, but after that any systolic ejection click is abnormal, indicating an abnormal pulmonary or aortic valve, an enlarged pulmonary artery or aorta, or truncus arteriosus. If the infant has pulmonary disease without congenital heart disease and has a narrowly split or single second sound, then a high pulmonary vascular resistance is expected.

COMMENT: The clinician should never depend on one finding alone to either rule in or rule out significant cardiac disease. Rather, the various findings should be added to see if they point toward a cardiac etiology. The most important findings relate to the level of arterial oxygen tension, heart size, respiratory pattern, and the adequacy of systemic perfusion.

Norman Talner

2. Visible central cyanosis in the early newborn period usually indicates a very low arterial oxygen tension. Even when the clinical judgment is that of only questionable cyanosis, the arterial Po_2 may be very low.
3. Peripheral cyanosis (acrocyanosis) is normal and must be differentiated from central cyanosis.
4. Systemic arterial blood gases may be helpful in differentiating pulmonary from cardiac cyanosis. A Pao_2 greater than 150 mm Hg in an enriched oxygen environment effectively eliminates severe heart disease with anatomic right-to-left shunt. In questionable cases, hypoxemia without significant hypercapnia (CO_2 retention) tends to suggest primary cardiac disease. However, pulmonary venous congestion, as in the hypoplastic left ventricle syndrome, may result in considerable CO_2 retention. It may also result in a somewhat low Po_2, which increases in a high oxygen environment.

COMMENT: A suspicion of hypoxemia must be verified by arterial blood gas determinations. While peripheral cyanosis may be normal, this is only in the face of adequate systemic perfusion as verified by the volume of the arterial pulsations, skin temperature, and capillary refill. Again, a single finding by itself does not rule in or rule out cardiac disease. It is possible to have a Pao_2 greater than 150 in the face of a lesion such as truncus arteriosus. Further, there may be hypercapnia in the face of pulmonary overcirculation, and, on the other hand, the Pco_2 may be extremely low with impaired systemic perfusion.

Norman Talner

5. Heel-stick blood gases do not provide accurate measures of the arterial Po_2. However, the error is always on the low side, so that, in cyanotic congenital heart disease, a reasonably high heel-stick Po_2 is reassuring.
6. Transcutaneous Po_2 or oximetric measurements are inaccurate at low levels and in the presence of hypoperfusion. They are valuable for monitoring trends or comparing upper and lower body oxygenation.
7. Femoral or pedal pulses must be carefully palpated in all newborn infants. The pulse may be palpable even with significant coarctation of the aorta while the ductus is open, disappearing when the ductus closes.

COMMENT: Occasionally the ductus arteriosus may close and then reopen in the neonate with coarctation so that femoral pulses may be diminished on one examination but restored on subsequent examinations. A colleague's description of diminished femoral pulses should not be dismissed merely because a later examination is unremarkable. Serial assessments are in order.

Roberta G. Williams

8. A high index of suspicion is required to diagnose congenital heart disease early. Careful history taking, physical examination, and laboratory measurements—including chest x-ray studies, ECG, and blood gas or oximetric studies in an enriched oxygen environment—often help to establish the diagnosis. However, two-dimensional echocardiography permits accurate and definitive diagnosis, accomplished without delay.
9. Life-threatening congenital heart disease is sooner or later associated with

respiratory distress or frank cyanosis, or both.

10. The presence of a large liver usually indicates systemic venous congestion, which may not necessarily indicate congestive heart failure. Many conditions in the neonatal period can produce an enlarged liver.

11. When a baby with a congenital heart defect is symptomatic early in the newborn period, death is likely unless a surgical procedure or balloon septostomy can be performed.

12. On occasion, in the presence of RDS and a PDA, congestive heart failure may be diagnosed without cardiomegaly.

13. Although nonspecific systolic murmurs are common (as many as 80% of normal children can have a murmur during the neonatal period), certain murmurs are nearly diagnostic. A to-and-fro (washboard) murmur suggests truncus arteriosus or absent pulmonary valve syndrome. A high-pitched murmur of a small VSD (often with a precordial thrill) in the presence of cyanosis suggests tricuspid atresia with a restrictive VSD. The presence of cyanosis without murmurs, or "silent cyanosis," suggests D-transposition of the great vessels or pulmonary atresia with a VSD (tetralogy of Fallot with pulmonary atresia).

CASE PROBLEMS

One must note the difficulty in recognizing cyanosis caused by right-to-left intracardiac shunting in the first days of life. The degree of desaturation is usually underestimated. It is also important to recognize two major forms of cyanotic congenital heart disease: (1) that associated with insufficient pulmonary blood flow, and (2) that in which there is increased pulmonary blood flow because the oxygenated blood from the pulmonary veins does not reach the systemic circulation.

◆

Case One

A baby girl is considered normal at birth, but at 12 hours of age cyanosis is noted. The heart is quiet. A soft, nonspecific systolic murmur is present, and there is no respiratory distress. On the second day, cyanosis is more obvious, and

the respiratory rate is increased. The child's x-ray film shows a small heart with decreased pulmonary vascularity. The ECG shows right atrial and left ventricular hypertrophy.

◆ *Can a diagnosis be suggested?*

When the heart is quiet and the child is blue, insufficient pulmonary blood flow is suggested. The x-ray finding is consistent. These findings and the ECG indicate that perhaps the right ventricle is hypoplastic.

Two-dimensional echocardiography reveals pulmonary atresia without a VSD and a hypoplastic right ventricle. A cardiac catheterization is performed. The right ventricle is entered with great difficulty.

	Pressure (mm Hg)	Saturation (%)
SVC and RA	m = 10	20
RV	160/10	20
LA	m = 5	50
PV	m = 5	95
LV	80/5	50
Femoral artery	80/50	50

Cineangiograms are done from the right and left ventricles and the aorta.

◆ *Are the physiologic data consistent with the previous diagnosis?*

At catheterization, there is no left-to-right shunt as far as the ventricle, whereas the saturation of 50% in the LA indicates a large right-to-left shunt at the atrial level. The very high RV pressure indicates severe obstruction to outflow, whereas the large difference in pressure between the RV and LV reveals that there must be little or no ventricular communication. Although there is a large right-to-left shunt at the atrial level, the marked difference in pressure between the RA and LA indicates that there is small communication. Thus, the clinical diagnosis fits with the diagnosis of pulmonary atresia with a moderately hypoplastic right ventricle and an intact ventricular septum. Angiography also reveals only small coronary sinusoids from the right ventricular cavity that do not fill the aorta in a retrograde manner.

◆ *How does blood reach the pulmonary circulation?*

All of the systemic venous return flows through the atrial septal defect into the left atrium and then through the left ventricle and aorta. Almost invariably there is a PDA connected to the pulmonary arteries. A moderately hypoplastic main pulmonary artery extends to the atretic pulmonary valve, and the main branch arteries are somewhat small.

◆ *Is there some treatment that can be done before completing the catheterization?*
If not already done, an infusion of prostaglandin E_1 (0.05 µg/kg/min) should be started.

COMMENT: Prostaglandin E_1 infusion should be started when the clinical evidence is that of impaired pulmonary or systemic blood flow so that the infant can be transported in an improved metabolic state consequent to either an increase in systemic perfusion or improved pulmonary blood flow and an increase in PaO_2. In terms of the transport, however, the transport team should be alerted to the possibility of apnea with a PGE_1 infusion and be prepared to ventilate if necessary.

Norman Talner

◆ *Should the surgeon be called?*
Yes, as soon as possible. However, because of the prostaglandin E_1 infusion, surgery can be delayed while the infant is allowed to stabilize.

◆ *How can the surgeon help?*
By making an anastomosis between the aorta and pulmonary artery, thereby increasing pulmonary blood flow (aortopulmonary shunt). The surgeon should also attempt a pulmonary valvotomy and right ventricular outflow patch, if possible, which may help in promoting growth of the right ventricle.

◆ *What is the prognosis?*
The prognosis is not known. Much depends on whether the hypoplastic right ventricle and pulmonary arteries will grow. In general, unless the right ventricle and tricuspid valve are well developed, the outlook is poor.

Case Two

A baby girl is considered normal at birth, but on the second day cyanosis is noted. The heart is quiet. A grade 4/6 holosystolic ejection murmur is heard at the lower left sternal border. There is no respiratory distress.

◆ *At this point, in comparison to Case One, is there any suggestion as to a different diagnosis?*
As in Case One, the heart is quiet, suggesting that cyanosis is associated with decreased pulmonary blood flow. The x-ray study reveals a small heart and decreased pulmonary vascularity. The most important difference is the long, loud murmur.

On the sixth day, cyanosis remains minimal. The chest x-ray study still shows a small heart with questionable decreased pulmonary vascularity. The ECG shows right ventricular hypertrophy.

◆ *Can a diagnosis be suggested?*
The most likely diagnosis is a VSD with pulmonic stenosis and right-to-left shunt (tetralogy of Fallot) or valvular pulmonic stenosis with an atrial right-to-left shunt.

COMMENT: The presence of cyanosis has to be documented by determination of arterial oxygen tension. In the face of pulmonary valve stenosis with a right-to-left atrial shunt, it would seem imperative to perform diagnostic cardiac catheterization to document the severity of the obstruction that is the major hemodynamic problem and that may or may not be accompanied by atrial right-to-left shunting. If there is an atrial right-to-left shunt, this usually accompanies rather severe pulmonary valve obstruction and is of the type that usually requires surgical intervention. With the development of balloon catheter techniques, it may be possible to relieve obstruction in some of these infants and therefore prevent the development of hypoxemia.

Norman Talner

◆ *Should cardiac catheterization be performed?*
Not yet. Eventually catheterization may be required to define the anatomy more clearly, but because the cyanosis is only minimal, an echocardiographic diagnosis is sufficient. The results of the echocardiogram will determine whether catheterization or surgery is required urgently. If no VSD is present, balloon valvoplasty may be indicated.

Case Three

A baby is considered normal at birth, but on the second day of life cyanosis is noted. The heart is hyperdynamic. A grade 2/6 systolic ejection murmur is heard at the upper left sternal border, and there is no respiratory distress. On the third day, the cyanosis is more obvious, and the respiratory rate is increased. The chest x-ray film shows a normal-sized heart. However, there is a suggestion of increased pulmonary vascularity, despite which the pulmonary artery cannot be recognized. The ECG shows the normal right ventricular dominance of a newborn.

◆ *Can a diagnosis be suggested?*
The most striking difference between this case and Cases One and Two is that the heart is hyperdynamic. In addition, pulmo-

nary vascularity is shown by x-ray film to be increased. Thus, the cyanosis is not likely to be caused by decreased pulmonary blood flow but rather by inadequate mixing. The oxygenated pulmonary venous return is not getting to the systemic circulation. This understanding, together with the fact that the pulmonary artery cannot be recognized despite increased pulmonary vascularity, suggests an abnormality of the great arteries.

◆ *What should be done next?*

Because cyanotic congenital heart disease is suspected, prostaglandin E_1 (0.05 μg/kg/min) should be started. The oxygen saturation should be checked in the upper and lower extremities. An upper extremity saturation lower than that in the leg is suggestive of D-transposition. A cardiology consult should be obtained immediately.

Echocardiography shows D-transposition of the great vessels. There is no ventricular septal defect. A small atrial defect is present, and the patent ductus arteriosus is large.

◆ *Is there something that can be done immediately to increase the oxygenation?*

Clearly, more mixing is needed between the two sides. The safest way to accomplish this is to create an atrial septal defect using a balloon catheter. The catheter is placed into the left atrium, blown up with saline, and pulled back hard. This is usually done during cardiac catheterization, but can be done at the bedside using guidance by echocardiography.

A cardiac catheterization is performed.

	Pressure (mm Hg)	Saturation (%)
SVC	m = 5	20
RA	m = 5	40
RV	80/5	40
LA	m = 10	95
PV	m = 10	95
LV	65/10	95
Femoral artery	80/50	40

◆ *What is the likely pulmonary arterial saturation?*

With a femoral arterial saturation of 40%, it is likely that the aorta arises from the right ventricle. The fact that the two ventricles have such different pressures indicates that there is little or no communication between them. The pulmonary artery arises from the left ventricle, and its oxygen saturation will be less than 95%, depending on how much

aorta–to–pulmonary artery shunt there is through a PDA.

◆ *What is the likely pulmonary arterial pressure?*

The pressure in the pulmonary artery can be no more than 65 mm Hg systolic and may be less if there is some mild pulmonic stenosis (pulmonary artery arises from the left ventricle).

◆ *Is surgery resulting in normal systemic saturation possible?*

An arterial switch operation can be performed within the first 2 weeks of life.

◆

Case Four

A full-term baby boy (birth weight 4400 g) was considered to be well at birth, although at examination there was a question of decrease in femoral pulses. The baby was discharged from the hospital at 5 days of age, feeding nicely. The femoral pulses were still difficult to palpate, but this finding was discounted as being common at this age, especially in chubby babies. At 2 weeks of age, the child was admitted to the hospital with respiratory difficulty. He was breathing very rapidly, was sweating profusely, and was moderately cyanotic. The liver was large, femoral pulses were absent, and brachial pulses were weak. Flush pressures were 50 mm Hg in each arm and 40 mm Hg in the legs. A grade 2 short systolic ejection murmur was heard slightly better in the back than at the mid-left sternal border. The x-ray film showed a large heart with pulmonary venous congestion. The ECG showed right ventricular hypertrophy.

◆ *Can a diagnosis be suggested?*

There are strong clues to the diagnosis of coarctation of the aorta despite the lack of blood pressure gradient. The most important clues are that femoral pulses are absent and that the murmur is maximal in the back. (Femoral pulses can appear in the presence of coarctation of the aorta, but they are usually weaker and delayed in relation to the brachial pulses. The murmur may also be louder anteriorly than posteriorly.)

◆ *Explain the lack of blood pressure gradient with the femoral pulse.*

Because of congestive heart failure, the cardiac output may be very low, and there may be insufficient ejectile force to create a high blood pressure even above the coarctation. Thus, there may be little or no systolic gradient across a severe coarctation of the aorta in the presence of congestive heart failure.

◆ *Explain the presence of cyanosis.*

The cyanosis is probably pulmonary, caused by venous congestion resulting from left-sided heart failure and because the low-output state causes stasis.

The patient is intubated and ventilated, the metabolic acidosis is partially corrected, and prostaglandin E_1 is begun. The baby's condition stabilizes over 3 hours, with normal pulses in the arms, slightly reduced pulses in the legs, and normal blood gas values.

◆ *Is cardiac catheterization necessary?*

The diagnosis is evident for simple coarctation of the aorta. Two-dimensional echocardiography and Doppler studies can usually adequately delineate the anatomy. Therefore, except in unusual cases, cardiac catheterization is not necessary. Surgery is often performed without prior catheterization if echocardiography shows an isolated, discrete coarctation.

◆

Case Five

A 4-day-old, full-term baby boy is transferred to the intensive care nursery because of poor feeding for 2 days and recent respiratory difficulties. The child is dusky and sweating profusely and has very poor pulses. The liver is very large. The chest x-ray film shows a large heart with pulmonary venous congestion. The ECG demonstrates no P waves and a ventricular rate of 300 bpm (see Fig. 14–8). The diagnosis of supraventricular tachycardia is made.

◆ *Should a cardiology consultant be called in immediately?*

A cardiology consultant cannot be depended on exclusively for the knowledge necessary to diagnose and treat supraventricular tachycardia (SVT) of infancy. There is not likely to be time for such a luxury. When a child is admitted with congestive heart failure, it usually indicates that the supraventricular tachycardia has been constant for at least 48 hours. Death may be imminent.

◆ *Blood samples are drawn. Which test should be performed and why?*

A radial arterial blood sample was obtained. The child may be quite acidotic. Further, if the Po_2 is low as a result of pulmonary venous congestion, the low Pao_2 and pH may significantly cause an increase in the pulmonary vascular resistance and depress myocardial function. Despite the congestive heart failure, it may be helpful to give sodium bicarbonate as well as oxygen.

◆ *The intern wants to start intramuscular digoxin immediately. Is this correct? If not, what is?*

Because the infant is clearly unstable, the only initial management that should be considered is immediate cardioversion to sinus rhythm. Adenosine (see below) is the first line of therapy. Digoxin, even when administered intravenously, can take 10 to 20 minutes before it has an effect. Digoxin may be appropriate either after conversion to sinus rhythm or if the infant repeatedly relapses into a tachycardia. The intravenous approach is preferred; because of the poor perfusion, intramuscular absorption is unreliable. When digoxin is used, half the total digitalizing dose (30 to 50 µg/kg) is given immediately, with the next quarter dose given 6 to 8 hours later. The second dose can be given in as soon as 1 hour, if needed, for continued stabilization.

◆ *What other pharmacologic or manipulative avenues should be considered?*

When the infant is unstable, no other measures that delay cardioversion should be considered. However, if the child is somewhat more stable or if there is a delay in availability of cardioversion for other reasons, other avenues can be considered. The most appropriate initial management is the administration of adenosine. Adenosine causes complete block at the atrioventricular node. It is administered via a rapid intravenous bolus, followed by immediate flush. This is required because the duration of action is very short, and it is metabolized by the endothelial cells of the blood vessels. The initial dose is 50 µg/kg, up to a dose of 200 µg/kg. A continuous rhythm strip should be recorded during the administration, because the tachycardia may recur after the adenosine is metabolized. The response to the adenosine, even if the tachycardia is not permanently converted, can aid in the exact diagnosis.

Vagal stimulation can convert some patients' tachycardia. Carotid pressure and eyeball massage had been used in the past, but are not indicated. **They do not work and are dangerous.** The placement of ice to the face can stimulate the diving reflex. This requires either placing the infant's face in cold water (holding the nose shut) or applying an ice pack to the entire face for 20 to 30 seconds. An intravenous line and crash cart should be available because there is a risk of ventricular dysrhythmias.

If the baby is hypotensive, a sympathomimetic agent should be used. Isoproterenol, epinephrine, and levarterenol are contraindicated because of the high risk of ventricular fibrillation. Phenylephrine (which causes no cardiac stimulation) is preferable. Even if the baby is not hypotensive and if digitalization has not resulted in sinus rhythm, phenylephrine, to a level that elevates blood pressure above normal, may convert the arrhythmia to sinus rhythm.

The use of other drugs, such as quinidine, procainamide (Pronestyl), or propranolol, is rarely necessary during the acute period. However, a baby occasionally goes in and out of the arrhythmia for many months. In such infants, another maintenance medication, especially propranolol, has been useful in controlling the arrhythmia.

◆ What chance is there that something is structurally wrong with the heart?

The vast majority of the children with supraventricular tachycardia (SVT) have nothing structurally wrong with the heart. One rule of thumb suggesting the prognosis is: when the child is a boy, there will almost invariably be nothing wrong with the heart; if the child is a girl, there is a greater chance of structural abnormality.

◆ Is the patient likely to be prone to supraventricular arrhythmias in the future?

In the few weeks after the first episode of SVT, the rhythm may intermittently revert to abnormal in many children. In most children on medication throughout the first year, another arrhythmia never occurs. In many children with SVT, the tachycardia resolves after 1 year of age. However, in some of those that resolve, the episodes recur later in childhood or during adolescence. In older children and adults, radiofrequency ablation during cardiac catheterization to interrupt the abnormal pathway causing the tachycardia can often be curative.

REFERENCES

1. Adams F, Lind J: Physiologic studies on the cardiovascular status of normal newborn infants with special reference to the ductus arteriosus. Pediatrics 19:431, 1975.
2. Anderson R, Allwork S, Ho S, et al: Surgical anatomy of tetralogy of Fallot. J Thorac Cardiovasc Surg 81:887, 1981.
3. Alverson D, Eldridge M, Dillon T, et al: Non-invasive pulsed Doppler determination of cardiac output in neonates and children. Pediatr 100:46, 1982.
4. Becker A, Becker M, Edwards J: Anomalies associated with coarctation of the aorta: Particular reference to infancy. Circulation 441:1067, 1970.
5. Berman W Jr, Musselman J: Myocardial performance in the newborn lamb. Am J Physiol 237:H66, 1979.
6. Bharati S, McAllister H, Rosenquist G, et al: The surgical anatomy of truncus arteriosus communis. J Thorac Cardiovasc Surg 67:501, 1974.
7. Bharati S, McAllister H, Tatooles C, et al: Anatomic variations in underdeveloped right ventricle related to tricuspid atresia and stenosis. J Thorac Cardiovasc Surg 72:383, 1976.
8. Birk E, Iwamoto HS, Heymann MA: Hormonal effects on circulatory changes during the perinatal period. In Jones CT, ed: Baillière's Clinical Endocrinology and Metabolism. Vol 3, no. 3. Perinatal Endocrinology. London: Baillière Tindall, 1989.
9. Calder L, van Praagh R, van Praagh S, et al: Truncus arteriosus communis: Clinical, angiocardiographic and pathologic findings in 100 patients. Am Heart J 92:23, 1976.
10. Cassady G, Crouse DT, Kirklin JW, et al: A randomized, controlled trial of very early prophylactic ligation of the ductus arteriosus in babies who weighed 1000 grams or less at birth. N Engl J Med 320:1511, 1989.
11. Cassels D: The Ductus Arteriosus. Springfield, IL: Charles C Thomas, Publisher, 1973.
12. Cassin S: Role of prostaglandins and leukotrienes in the control of the pulmonary circulation in the fetus and newborn. Semin Perinatol 11:53, 1986.
13. Castaneda AR, Trusler GA, Paul MH, et al: The early results of treatment of simple transposition in the current era. J Thorac Cardiovasc Surg 95:14, 1988.
14. Casteñeda A, Jonas R, Mayer J, Hanley F: Cardiac Surgery of the Neonate and Infant. Philadelphia: WB Saunders, 1994.
15. Clyman R: Ontogeny of the ductus arteriosus response to prostaglandins and inhibitors of their synthesis. Semin Perinatol 4:115, 1980.
16. Clyman R, Heymann M: Pharmacology of the ductus arteriosus. Pediatr Clin North Am 28:77, 1981.
17. Clyman RI: Ductus arteriosus: Current theories of prenatal and postnatal regulation. Semin Perinatol 11:64, 1987.
18. Cobanoglu A, Metzdorff MT, Pinson CW, et al: Valvotomy for pulmonary atresia with intact ventricular septum: A disciplined approach to achieve a functioning right ventricle. J Thorac Cardiovasc Surg 89:482, 1985.
19. Coceani F, Olley P: Role of prostaglandins, prostacyclin and thromboxanes in the control of prenatal patency and postnatal closure of the ductus arteriosus. Semin Perinatol 4:109, 1980.
20. Cole R, Muster A, Lev M, et al: Pulmonary atresia with intact ventricular septum. Am J Cardiol 21:23, 1968.
21. Crupi G, Macartney F, Anderson R: Persistent truncus arteriosus. Am J Cardiol 40:569, 1977.
22. Danilowicz D, Rudolph A, Hoffman J: Delayed closure of the ductus arteriosus in premature infants. Pediatrics 37:74, 1966.
23. Deeley W: Hypoplastic left heart syndrome: Anatomic, physiologic and therapeutic considerations. Am J Dis Child 121:168, 1971.

24. Ebert PA, Turley K, Stranger P, et al: Surgical treatment of truncus arteriosus in the first 6 months of life. Ann Surg 200:451, 1984.
25. Emery J, Mithal A: Weights of cardiac ventricles at and after birth. Br Heart J 23:313, 1961.
26. Emmanouilides G, Baylen B: Neonatal cardiopulmonary distress without congenital heart disease. Curr Probl Pediatr IX 7:1, 1979.
27. Emmanouilides G, Moss A, Duffie E Jr, et al: Pulmonary arterial pressure changes in human newborn infants from birth to 3 days of age. J Pediatr 65:327, 1964.
28. Foale R, Stefanine L, Rickards A, et al: Left and right ventricular morphology in complex congenital heart disease defined by two-dimensional echocardiography. Am J Cardiol 49:93, 1982.
29. Freed M, Heymann M, Lewis A, et al: Prostaglandin E₁ in infants with ductus arteriosus—dependent congenital heart disease. Circulation 64:899, 1981.
30. Friedman W: The intrinsic physiologic properties of the developing heart. Prog Cardiovasc Dis 15:87, 1972.
31. Fyler D, Buckley L, Hellenbrand W, et al: Report of the New England Regional Infant Cardiac Program. Pediatrics 65(Suppl):375, 1980.
32. Fyler D, Parisi L, Berman L: The regionalization of infant cardiac care in New England. Cardiovasc Clin 4:339, 1972.
33. Gathman G, Nadas A: Total anomalous pulmonary venous connection: Clinical and physiologic observations of 75 pediatric patients. Circulation 42:143, 1970.
34. Gersony W, Bowman F Jr, Steeg C, et al: Management of total anomalous pulmonary venous drainage in early infancy. Circulation 43(Suppl I):19, 1971.
35. Gersony WM, Peckham GJ, Ellison RC, et al: Effects of indomethacin in premature infants with patent ductus arteriosus: Results of a national collaborative study. J Pediatr 102:895, 1983.
36. Goetzman B, Riemenschneider T: Persistence of the fetal circulation. Pediatr Rev 2:37, 1980.
37. Goldberg S, Allen H, Sahn D: Pediatric and Adolescent Echocardiography. Chicago: Year Book Medical Publishers, 1980.
38. Gootman N, Scarpelli E, Rudolph A: Metabolic acidosis in children with severe cyanotic congenital heart disease. Circulation 31:251, 1963.
39. Hastreiter A, Oshima M, Miller R, et al: Congenital aortic stenosis syndrome in infancy. Circulation 28:1084, 1963.
40. Haworth S, Reid L: Persistent fetal circulation: Newly recognized structural features. J Pediatr 88:614, 1976.
41. Haworth S, Sauer U, Buhlmeyer K, et al: Development of the pulmonary circulation in ventricular septal defect: A quantitative study. Am J Cardiol 40:781, 1977.
42. Heymann MA: Fetal cardiovascular physiology. In Creasy RK, Resnik R, eds: Maternal-Fetal Medicine: Principles and Practice. 2nd ed. Philadelphia: WB Saunders, 1989, p 288.
43. Heymann M, Rudolph A: Effects of congenital heart disease on the fetal and neonatal circulations. Prog Cardiovasc Dis 15:115, 1972.
44. Heymann M, Rudolph A, Silverman N: Closure of the ductus arteriosus in premature infants by inhibition of prostaglandin synthesis. N Engl J Med 295:530, 1976.
45. Heymann MA, Soifer SJ: Control of fetal and neonatal pulmonary circulation. In Weir EK, Reeves JT, eds: Pulmonary Vascular Physiology and Pathophysiology. New York: Marcel Dekker, 1989, p 33.
46. Heymann MA, Soifer SJ: Persistent pulmonary hypertension of the newborn. In Fishman AP, ed: The Pulmonary Circulation: Normal and Abnormal. Philadelphia: University of Pennsylvania Press, 1990, p 371.
47. Hirschfeld S, Riggs T: Echocardiographic assessment of normal and abnormal postnatal cardiovascular adaptation. Perinatol Neonatol 1:35, 1977.
48. Hirschklau M, DiSessa T, Higgins C, et al: Echocardiographic diagnosis: Pitfalls in the premature infant with a large patent ductus arteriosus. J Pediatr 92:474, 1978.
49. Hoffmann JIE: Aortic stenosis. In Moller JH, Neall WA, eds: Fetal, Neonatal and Infant Cardiac Disease. East Norwalk, CT: Appleton & Lange, 1990, p 451.
50. Hoffmann JIE: Congenital heart disease: Incidence and inheritance. Pediatr Clin North Am 37:25, 1990.
51. Hoffmann JIE: Ventricular septal defects—Indications for therapy in infants. Pediatr Clin North Am 18:1091, 1971.
52. Hoffmann J, Rudolph A: Natural history of ventricular septal defects in infancy. Am J Cardiol 16:634, 1965.
53. Hoffmann J, Rudolph A, Danilowicz D: Left-to-right shunts in infants. Am J Cardiol 30:868, 1972.
54. Hornberger LK, Sahn DJ, Krabill KA, et al: Elucidation of the natural history of ventricular septal defects by serial Doppler color flow mapping studies. J Am Coll Cardiol 13:1111, 1989.
55. Ikeda M, Hirasawa K: Tetralogy of Fallot. Circulation 38(Suppl 5):21, 1968.
56. Kawabori I, Guntheroth W, Morgan B, et al: Surgical correction in infancy to reduce mortality in transposition of the great arteries. Pediatrics 60:83, 1977.
57. Kersting-Sommerhoff BA, Diethelm L, Stanger P, et al: Evaluation of complex congenital ventricular anomalies with magnetic resonance imaging. Am Heart J 120:133, 1990.
58. Kleinman C, Hobbins J, Jaffe C, et al: Echocardiographic studies of the human fetus: Prenatal diagnosis of congenital heart disease and cardiac dysrhythmias. Pediatrics 65:1059, 1980.
59. Klopfenstein H, Rudolph A: Postnatal changes in the circulation and responses to volume loading in sheep. Circ Res 42:839, 1978.
60. Krovetz L, Goldbloom J: Normal standards for cardiovascular data. II. Pressure and vascular resistances. Johns Hopkins Med J 130:187, 1972.
61. Lakier JB, Lewis AB, Heymann MA, et al: Isolated aortic stenosis in the neonate: Natural history and hemodynamic considerations. Circulation 50:801, 1974.
62. Liebman J, Cullum L, Belloc N: The natural history of transposition of the great arteries. Circulation 40:237, 1969.
63. Lewis A, Freed M, Heymann M, et al: Side effects of therapy of prostaglandin E₁ in infants with critical congenital heart disease. Circulation 64:893, 1981.
64. Levin D, Heymann M, Kitterman J, et al: Persistent pulmonary hypertension of the newborn infant. J Pediatr 89:626, 1976.

65. Levin D, Paul M, Master A, et al: D-transposition of the great vessels in the neonate. Arch Int Med 137:1421, 1977.
66. Luckstead E, Mattioli L, Crosby I, et al: Two-stage palliative surgical approach for pulmonary atresia with intact ventricular septum (Type I). Am J Cardiol 29:490, 1972.
67. Mahony L, Carnero V, Brett C, et al: Prophylactic indomethacin therapy for patent arteriosus in very low-birth-weight infants. N Engl J Med 306:506, 1982.
68. Mahoney LT, Truesdell SC, Krzmarzick TR, et al: Atrial septal defects that present in infancy. Am J Dis Child 140:1115, 1986.
69. Mahony L, Turley K, Ebert P, et al: Long-term results after atrial repair of transposition of the great arteries in early infancy. Circulation 66:253, 1982.
70. Meyer RA: Echocardiography in pediatric patients. Cardiovasc Clin 11:187, 1982.
71. Mirowitz SA, Gutierrez FR, Canter CE, Vannier MW: Tetralogy of Fallot: MR findings. Radiology 171:207, 1989.
72. Mitchell S, Karones S, Berendes H: Congenital heart disease in 56,109 births: Incidence and natural history. Circulation 3:323, 1971.
73. Mody MR: Serial hemodynamic observations in secundum ASD with special reference to spontaneous closure. Am J Cardiol 32:978, 1973.
74. Moller J, Nakib A, Eliot R, et al: Symptomatic congenital aortic stenosis in the first year of life. J Pediatr 69:728, 1968.
75. Moulaert A, Bruins C, Oppenheimer-Dekker A: Anomalies of the aortic arch and ventricular septal defects. Circulation 53:1011, 1976.
76. Murphy J, Rabinovitch M, Goldstein J, Reid L: The structural basis of persistent pulmonary hypertension of the newborn infant. J Pediatr 98:962, 1981.
77. Naeye R: Arterial changes during the perinatal period. Arch Pathol 71:121, 1961.
78. Noonan J: Syndromes associated with cardiac defects. Cardiovasc Clin 11:97, 1980.
79. Noonan J, Nadas A: The hypoplastic left ventricle syndrome: An analysis of 101 cases. Pediatr Clin North Am 5:1029, 1958.
80. Noonan J, Nadas A, Rudolph A, et al: Transposition of the great arteries: A correlation of clinical, physiologic and autopsy data. N Engl J Med 263:592, 1960.
81. Nora J: Etiologic factors in congenital heart disease. Pediatr Clin North Am 18:1050, 1971.
82. Nora J, Nora A: The evolution of specific genetic and environmental counselling in congenital heart disease. Circulation 57:205, 1978.
83. Norwood W Jr: Hypoplastic left heart syndrome. Ann Thorac Surg 52:688–695, 1991.
84. Pigott JD, Murphy JD, Barber G, et al: Palliative reconstructive surgery for hypoplastic left heart syndrome. N Engl J Med 23:308, 1983.
85. Rajasinghe HA, Reddy VM, van Son JA, et al: Coarctation repair using end-to-side anastomosis of descending aorta to proximal aortic arch. Ann Thorac Surg 61:840–844, 1996.
86. Rashkind W, Miller W: Creation of an atrial septal defect without thoracotomy: A palliative approach to complete transposition of the great arteries. JAMA 196:991, 1966.
87. Reid L: The development of the pulmonary circulation. In Peckham G, Heymann M, eds: Cardiovascular Sequelae of Asphyxia in the Newborn. Report of the Eighty-third Ross Conference on Pediatric Research. Columbus, OH: Ross Laboratories, 1982, pp 2–10.
88. Reller MD, Colasurdo MA, Rice MJ, McDonald RW: The timing of spontaneous closure of the ductus arteriosus in infants with respiratory distress syndrome. Am J Cardiol 66:75, 1990.
89. Rice M, Seward J, Hagler D, et al: Impact of two-dimensional echocardiography on the management of distressed newborns in whom cardiac disease is suspected. Am J Cardiol 51:288, 1983.
90. Riggs T, Hirschfeld S, Fanaroff A, et al: Neonatal circulatory changes: An echo study. Pediatrics 59:338, 1977.
91. Rowe R: Severe congenital heart disease in the newborn infant: Diagnosis and management. Pediatr Clin North Am 17:967, 1970.
92. Rudolph A: The changes in the circulation after birth: The importance in congenital heart disease. Circulation 41:343, 1970.
93. Rudolph A, Heymann M, Lewis A: Physiology and pharmacology of the pulmonary circulation in the fetus and newborn. In Hodson W, ed: Lung Biology in Health and Disease. Developmental Biology of the Lung. New York: Marcel Dekker, 1977, pp 497–523.
94. Rudolph A, Heymann M, Spitznas U: Hemodynamic considerations in the development of narrowing of the aorta. Am J Cardiol 30:514, 1972.
95. Saied A, Folger G: Hypoplastic left heart syndrome: Clinicopathologic and hemodynamic correlation. Am J Cardiol 29:190, 1972.
96. Sano S, Brawn WJ, Mee RBB: Total anomalous pulmonary venous drainage. J Thorac Cardiovasc Surg 97:886, 1989.
97. Siassi B, Blanco C, Cabal L, et al: Incidence and clinical features of patent ductus arteriosus in low-birth-weight infants: A prospective analysis of 150 consecutively-born infants. Pediatrics 57:347, 1976.
98. Siassi B, Emmanouilides G, Cleveland R, et al: Patent ductus arteriosus complicating prolonged assisted ventilation in respiratory distress syndrome. J Pediatr 74:11, 1969.
99. Silverman N: Pediatric Echocardiography. Baltimore: Williams & Wilkins, 1993.
100. Sigman J, Perry B, Behrendt D, et al: Ventricular septal defect: Results after repair in infancy. Am J Cardiol 39:66, 1977.
101. Singh A, DeLeval M, Pincott J, et al: Pulmonary artery banding for truncus arteriosus in the first year of life. Circulation 54(Suppl III):17, 1976.
102. Smallhorn JF: Patent ductus arteriosus—Evaluation by echocardiography. Echocardiography 4:101, 1987.
103. Strong W, Liebman J, Perrin E: Hypoplastic left ventricle syndrome: Electrocardiographic evidence of left ventricular hypertrophy. Am J Dis Child 120:511, 1970.
104. Sullivan H, Sulayman R, Replogle R, et al: Surgical correction of truncus arteriosus in infancy. Am J Cardiol 38:113, 1976.
105. Talner N, Berman M: Postnatal development of obstruction in coarctation of the aorta: Role of the ductus arteriosus. Pediatrics 56:562, 1975.
106. Talner N, Ordway N: Acid-base balance in the newborn infant with congestive heart failure. Pediatr Clin North Am 13:983, 1966.

107. Wagenvoort C, Newfeld H, Dushane J, et al: The pulmonary arterial tree in atrial septal defect: A quantitative study of anatomic features in fetuses, infants and children. Circulation 23:733, 1961.

108. Wagenvoort C, Newfeld H, Dushane J, et al: The pulmonary arterial tree in ventricular septal defect: A quantitative study of anatomic features in fetuses, infants and children. Circulation 23:740, 1961.

109. Weidman W, Swan H, Dushane J, et al: A hemodynamic study of atrial septal defect and associated anomalies involving the atrial septum. J Lab Clin Med 50:165, 1957.

110. Wyler F, Rutishauser M: Symptomatic atrial septal defect in the neonate and infant. Helv Paediatr Acta 30:399, 1976.

111. Zackman R, Steinmetz G, Botham R, et al: Incidence and treatment of the patent ductus arteriosus in the ill premature neonate. Am Heart J 87:697, 1974.

112. Zeevi B, Keane JF, Castaneda AR, et al: Neonatal critical valvular aortic stenosis: A comparison of surgical and balloon dilation therapy. Circulation 80:831, 1989.

113. Zuberbuhler J, Allwork S, Anderson R: The spectrum of Ebstein's anomaly of the tricuspid valve. J Thorac Cardiovasc Surg 77:202, 1979.

The Kidney

Beth A. Vogt
Ira D. Davis
Ellis D. Avner

Recent advances in neonatalogy and perinatology have defined new disease processes and raised difficult questions in the field of nephrology. For example, the advent of prenatal ultrasonography has created questions about the prenatal management of urinary tract anomalies. The widespread use of invasive vascular catheters has led to a new set of complications, including renal arterial and aortic thrombosis associated with umbilical artery catheters. The administration of loop diuretics and steroids to infants with bronchopulmonary dysplasia has led to the relatively new complication of neonatal nephrocalcinosis.

This chapter reviews the anatomic and functional development of the kidney, outlines the recommended approach to evaluation of the neonate with suspected renal disease, and comments on the more common nephrologic and urologic problems seen in preterm and term neonates.

◆ ANATOMIC DEVELOPMENT

The definitive mammalian kidney, the metanephros, starts developing at 5 weeks' gestation and begins to produce urine by 12 weeks' gestation. Development of the metanephros occurs through a series of interactions between the metanephric blastema and the ureteric bud. The ureteric bud progressively branches and grows, eventually forming the ureter, renal pelvis, and intrarenal collecting system.

At the same time, mesenchymal cells of the metanephric blastema are induced by the advancing ureteric bud to differentiate into epithelial cells that eventually become the glomeruli and renal tubules. Foci of metanephric blastema cells interact with the surrounding extracellular matrix and condense adjacent to the branching ureteric bud to form comma-shaped bodies, which then elongate to form S-shaped tubular structures (Fig. 15–1). The lower portion of the S-shaped structure becomes associated with a tuft of capillaries and forms the glomerulus; the upper portion forms the tubular elements of the nephron.

The complex process of kidney development appears to be under the control of growth factors, a series of key regulatory genes, and renal innvervation.[57, 64, 88] Recently, a number of genes that control DNA transcription have been identified as crucial in the control of cellular events in renal development.[51, 64] For example, mutation of the transcription factor gene, *Pax 2,* which is normally expressed in developing renal tissue, has been associated with a syndrome characterized by vesicoureteral reflux, hypoplastic kidneys, reduced calyces, and optic nerve colobomas.[30] Mutations in another transcriptional factor gene, *WT-1,* results in renal agenesis, suggesting that this gene product may be crucial for outgrowth of the ureteric bud.[49]

◆ FUNCTIONAL DEVELOPMENT

During intrauterine life, the kidneys play a minor role in regulating fetal salt and water balance in that this function is maintained primarily by the placenta. The primary function of the kidneys prenatally is to elaborate large amounts of hypotonic or isotonic urine to provide adequate amniotic fluid. After birth, a progressive maturation in renal function begins, which appears to parallel the neonate's metabolic needs for growth and development. In general, maturation of most renal functions is complete by 2 years of age (Table 15–1).

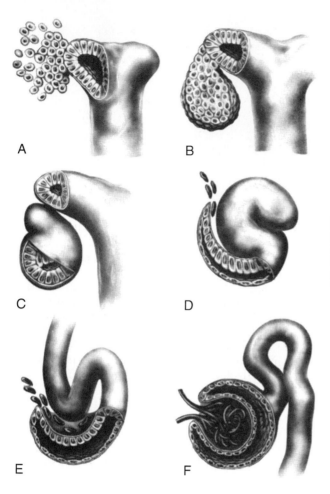

A

B

C

D

E

F

Figure 15–1. Illustration of the early development of the nephron from condensation to the S-shaped body. (From Saxen L: Organogenesis of the kidney. In Barlow PW, Green PB, eds: Developmental and Cell Biology Series. Cambridge: Cambridge University Press, 1987.)

Renal Blood Flow

Both absolute renal blood flow (RBF) and the percentage of cardiac output directed to the kidneys increases steadily with advancing gestational age (see Table 15–1). RBF in the human fetus and term infant are estimated to be as low as 4% and 6% of the cardiac output, respectively. The relatively low RBF of the neonate is related to high renal vascular resistance caused by increased levels of renin, angiotensin, aldosterone, and catecholamines. Postnatally, there is a sharp increase in RBF, which reaches

Table 15–1. Normal Values for Renal Function

Age	Glomerular Filtration Rate (mL/min/1.73 m²)	Renal Blood Flow (mL/min/1.73 m²)	Maximal Urine Osmolality (mOsm/kg)	Serum Creatinine (mg/dL)	Fractional Excretion of Sodium (%)
Newborn					
32–34 wk gestation	14 ± 3	40 ± 6	480	1.3	2–5
Full term	21 ± 4	88 ± 4	800	1.1	<1
1–2 wk	50 ± 10	220 ± 40	900	0.4	<1
6 mo–1 y	77 ± 14	352 ± 73	1200	0.2	<1
1–3 y	96 ± 22	540 ± 118	1400	0.4	<1
Adult	118 ± 18	620 ± 92	1400	0.8–1.5	<1

Adapted from Avner ED, Ellis D, Ichikawa I, et al: Normal neonates and maturational development of homeostatic mechanism. In Ichikawa I, ed. Pediatric Textbook of Fluids and Electrolytes. Baltimore: Williams & Wilkins, 1990.

8% to 10% of cardiac output at 1 week of life and achieves adult values of 20% to 25% of cardiac output at 2 years of age. This dramatic increase in RBF is related to decreasing renal vascular resistance and increasing cardiac output and perfusion pressure.

In addition to the increase in overall RBF, there is a marked change in distribution of blood flow within the neonatal kidney in the postnatal period. Because of a preferential decrease in vascular resistance in the outer cortex, there is a pronounced increase in superficial renal cortical blood flow.

Glomerular Filtration Rate

Glomerular filtration rate (GFR) in the fetal kidney increases with gestational age, and, by 32 to 34 weeks, a GFR of 14 mL/min/1.73 m² is achieved, which further increases to 21 mL/min/1.73 m² at term (see Table 15–1). GFR continues to increase postnatally, achieving adult values of 118 mL/min/1.73 m² by age 2 years. In preterm infants born before 34 weeks' gestation, the GFR remains stable until the conceptual age (gestational age plus postnatal age) exceeds 34 weeks, at which time the GFR begins to increase. Although adult values for GFR are attained by 2 years of life in term infants, achievement of adult GFR is delayed in preterm infants, especially in very low-birth-weight infants and infants with nephrocalcinosis.[24, 99]

Several factors are responsible for the postnatal increase in GFR. Animal studies suggest that the increase in GFR during the initial weeks of postnatal life is primarily due to an increase in glomerular perfusion pressure.[44] Subsequent increases in GFR during the first 2 years of life are primarily due to increases in RBF and maturation of superficial cortical nephrons, which lead to an increase in glomerular filtration surface area.

During the first week of postnatal life, an infant's GFR passes through three distinct phases to maintain fluid and electrolyte homeostasis.[50, 53] The initial 24 hours of life (prediuretic phase) is characterized by a transitory increase in GFR at 2 to 4 hours of life followed by a return to low baseline GFR and minimal urine output regardless of salt and water intake. This phase may extend up to 36 hours of life in the preterm infant, with delay in onset of the transitory increase in GFR. During the second and third days of life (diuretic phase), the GFR increases rapidly and the infant experiences diuresis and natriuresis regardless of salt and water intake. By the fourth to fifth day of life (postdiuretic phase), the GFR decreases slightly, then continues to increase slowly with maturation, with salt and water excretion varying according to intake.

Importantly, the duration and timing of these phases differ among infants, requiring individualization of fluid and electrolyte therapy. If insensible fluid losses are overestimated during the prediuretic phase, excess fluid intake may result in dilutional hyponatremia. On the other hand, a deficiency in fluid intake during this phase may lead to volume contraction and hypernatremia. During the diuretic phase, hypernatremia may develop as a result of excessive urinary fluid losses.

Fluid Compartments

The change in distribution of intracellular fluid (ICF) and extracellular fluid (ECF) in the fetus and newborn infant is summarized in Table 15–2. In the healthy term infant, ECF volume decreases and ICF volume increases in the first few days of life.[19] In the preterm infant, total body water decreases, primarily as the result of ECF losses in the first week of life, a process that is delayed in infants with respiratory distress syndrome.[82] The change in ICF during the first week of life is variable and may be dependent upon total energy intake and corresponding change in body weight during this period. For example, Heimler and colleagues[37] noted a decrease in ECF without an increase in ICF during the first week of life in preterm infants with greater than a 10% loss in body weight compared with a group of infants with minimal weight loss during the same period who displayed an increase in ICF.

Capillary filtration between the intravascular and interstitial fluid compartments is higher in the neonate than it is later in life, leading to a relatively large interstitial fluid compartment. This phenomenon may be due to a number of factors, including increased hydrostatic pressure, decreased intravascular osmotic pressure, and increased levels of atrial natriuretic factor, vasopres-

Table 15–2. Change in Body Water With Maturation

Age	% Body Weight		
	Extracellular Fluid	*Intracellular Fluid*	*Total Body Fluid*
Gestational			
14 weeks	65	27	92
28 weeks	55	25	80
40 weeks	45	30	75
Postnatal			
14 weeks	25	40	65

From Sulyok E: Postnatal adaptation. In Holliday MA, Barratt TM, Avner ED, eds. Pediatric Nephrology. Baltimore: Williams & Wilkins, 1994.

sin, and cortisol.[84] The relatively large interstitial fluid compartment enables the neonate to better tolerate hemorrhage because the large volumes of interstitial fluid can shift into the intravascular space, but it may also lead to reduced ability to excrete a fluid load.

Sodium Handling

Renal sodium losses are inversely proportional to gestational age, and the fractional excretion of sodium (FENa) may be as high as 5% to 6% in infants born at 28 weeks' gestation (Fig. 15–2). As a result, preterm infants younger than 35 weeks' gestation may display negative sodium balance and hyponatremia during the initial 2 to 3 weeks of life as a result of high renal sodium losses and inefficient intestinal sodium absorption.[101] Up to 4 to 5 mEq/kg/day of sodium may be necessary in preterm infants to offset high renal sodium losses during the first few weeks of life.

Healthy term neonates have basal sodium handling similar to that of adults, as demonstrated by a FENa of less than 1.0%, although a transient increase in FENa occurs during the second and third days of life (diuretic phase). Urinary sodium losses may be increased in certain conditions, including hypoxia, respiratory distress, hyperbilirubinemia, acute tubular necrosis, polycythemia, increased fluid and salt intake, and the use of theophylline or diuretics.[44] Pharmacologic agents such as dopamine, labetalol, propranolol, captopril, and enalaprilat that influence adrenergic neural pathways in the kidney and the renin–angiotensin axis may also increase urinary sodium losses in the neonate.

The mechanisms responsible for increased urinary sodium losses in the preterm infant are multifactorial. Glomerulotubular imbalance, which occurs when GFR exceeds the reabsorptive capacity of the renal tubules, occurs because of the preponderance of glomeruli compared with tubular structures, renal tubular immaturity, large extracellular volume, and reduced oxygen availability.[71] Decreased renal nerve activity may also contribute; studies in fetal and newborn sheep demonstrate an inverse relationship between renal nerve stimulation and urine sodium excretion.[71] Finally, fetal and postnatal kidneys exhibit diminished

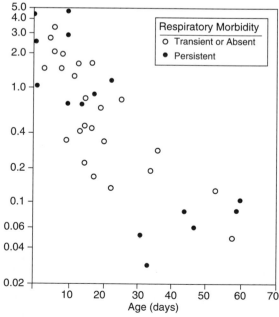

Figure 15–2. Fractional excretion of sodium of neonates at 28 to 33 weeks of gestation during the first 2 months of life. (From Ross B, Cowett RM, Oh W: Renal functions of low birth weight infants during the first two months of life. Pediatr Res 11:1162–1164, 1997.)

responsiveness to aldosterone compared with adult kidneys, resulting in the attenuation of sodium reabsorption.[72]

Urinary Concentration and Dilution

As noted in Table 15–1, renal concentrating capacity is low at birth and progressively increases following delivery from 800 mOsm/kg H_2O in the first 2 weeks of life to greater than 1200 mOsm/kg H_2O at 1 year of age.[8] Maximal urine osmolality reaches adult values of 1400 mOsm/kg H_2O between 1 and 3 years of age. This improvement in ability to excrete a concentrated urine is due to increased urea generation, improved end-organ responsiveness to vasopressin, and anatomic maturation of the renal medulla and its vasculature.

The neonatal kidney's ability to excrete a water load is somewhat limited in comparison to the adult kidney. For example, term and premature newborns can dilute their urine to an osmolality of 50 mOsm/kg and 70 mOsm/kg, respectively, compared with adults, who can dilute their urine to 30 mOsm.[77] This inability to maximally dilute the urine is due to reduced GFR, as well as to decreased activity of transporters in the early distal tubule (diluting segment), which are most prominent in the preterm infant.[84]

Acid–Base Balance

The range of normal serum bicarbonate levels is lower than that of adults, and infants maintain a mild metabolic acidosis (Fig. 15–3). This limitation in acid–base homeostasis seen in neonates, particularly preterm infants, is related to immaturity of both proximal and distal tubular function.

The proximal tubular bicarbonate threshold, defined as the steady-state serum bicarbonate level above which significant amounts of bicarbonate appear in the urine, is much lower in neonates than in adults, leading to incomplete bicarbonate reabsorption. The cause of the low proximal tubular bicarbonate threshold is unknown. Studies in the fetal lamb have demonstrated that renal tubular reabsorption of bicarbonate is inversely proportional to ECF volume.[73] Therefore, expanded ECF compartment characteristic of the preterm and term infant may be related to the low renal bicarbonate

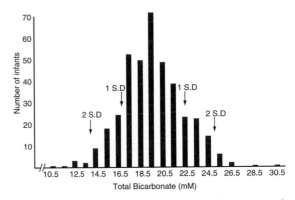

Figure 15–3. Frequency distribution of serum total bicarbonate in low-birth-weight neonates during the first month of life. (From Schwartz GJ, Haycock GB, Chir B, et al: Late metabolic acidosis: A reassessment of the definition. J Pediatr 95:102–107, 1979.)

threshold and low plasma bicarbonate concentration. Limited distal tubular excretion of titratable acid and incomplete development of tubular ammonia production also contribute to the relative metabolic acidosis of the newborn.

Newborn infants may display two forms of acidosis. In the first 24 hours of life, an early type of combined respiratory and metabolic acidosis may develop as a result of stress during birth and disturbances in cardiopulmonary adaptation.[90] Late metabolic acidosis, on the other hand, may develop during the first week of life and is most pronounced in the second and third weeks of life. This type of acidosis is due to an imbalance between net acid input, primarily from dietary protein intake and bone mineralization, and renal capacity for net acid excretion. Late metabolic acidosis may result in poor weight gain or skeletal growth. Late metabolic acidosis usually resolves spontaneously by the end of the first month of life as a result of the rapid postnatal increase in the renal capacity for net acid excretion.

An important consequence of chronic metabolic acidosis in the newborn is enhanced urinary calcium losses, negative calcium balance, and bone demineralization, which may contribute to the phenomenon of osteopenia of prematurity.[50] The mechanism for this process is multifactorial. Acidosis causes release of calcium from bones directly and via parathyroid hormone secretion. Acidosis also inhibits intestinal calcium absorption and impairs 1-alpha-hydroxylation of 25(OH)-vitamin D. Finally, acidosis increases urinary flow rate and urinary calcium excretion.[91] Therefore, persistent metabolic acidosis should be corrected with sodium bicarbonate, with a goal of achieving a serum bicarbonate level of 17 to 18 mEq/L.

Calcium and Phosphorus Balance

Within 24 to 48 hours after birth, the serum calcium concentration decreases, a phenomenon that is most pronounced in preterm infants.[54] Although the exact mechanism of neonatal hypocalcemia is unknown, it appears to be due to suppressed parathyroid hormone secretion and elevated plasma phosphate concentration.[96] In most neonates, the ionized calcium level remains above a physiologically acceptable concentration and the infant experiences no clinical symptoms. Symptomatic hypocalcemia may occur, however, in neonates stressed by illness or in the presence of aggressive fluid administration, diuresis, and sodium supplementation, all of which increase urinary calcium losses.

The normal serum phosphorus level in the newborn ranges from 4.5 to 9.5 mg/dL compared with adult values of 3.0 to 4.5 mg/dL. The higher serum phosphorus level in the newborn is due to enhanced dietary phosphorus intake, particularly in infants fed cow's milk formulas, lower GFR, and higher tubular reabsorption of phosphorus. Tubular reabsorption of phosphorus is lower, however, in preterm infants and increases progressively during gestation as a result of maturation of renal tubular function.[5] Karlen and associates suggested that the enhanced phosphorus excretion seen in premature infants causes a state of relative phosphorus deficiency, which may result in inadequate bone mineralization.[46] Therefore, care must be taken to provide adequate nutritional supplies of phosphorus and calcium in enteral and parenteral formulations for the premature infant.

◆ EVALUATION

The evaluation of an infant with suspected renal disease must be comprehensive and begins with a careful history and thorough physical examination. Selected laboratory studies may be useful in determining the cause and severity of renal dysfunction. Limited radiologic evaluation may be useful in clarifying renal anatomy and detecting complications of vascular catheters.

History

Results of prenatal ultrasonography should be carefully reviewed with particular attention being given to kidney size, echogenicity, malformations, amniotic fluid volume, and bladder size and shape.[69] The presence of small or enlarged kidneys, renal cysts, hydronephrosis, bladder enlargement, or oligohydramnios may suggest significant renal or urologic pathology.

Although most congenital renal disease is unrelated to teratogens, the antenatal history should be reviewed thoroughly, with particular attention being given to medications, toxins, or unusual exposures during the pregnancy. Congenital renal anomalies have been described in infants with antenatal exposure to angiotensin-converting enzyme inhibitors,[10] nonsteroidal anti-inflammatory drugs,[33, 45, 98] gentamicin, corticosteroids,[42] and cocaine.[11, 35] Although older reports have suggested an association between prenatal ethanol exposure and renal anomalies, a recent study showed no increase in incidence of renal anomalies in a group of 84 children with prenatal ethanol exposure.[94]

Finally, review of the family medical history is important, including any prior fetal or neonatal deaths. Although there is no genetic basis for most congenital renal anomalies, there is a clear genetic basis for certain diseases such as polycystic kidney disease.

Physical Examination

Evaluation of blood pressure and volume status is critical in the newborn with suspected renal disease. Hypertension may be present in infants with autosomal recessive polycystic kidney disease, acute renal failure (ARF), or renovascular or aortic thrombosis. Hypotension, on the other hand in addition to cardiovascular disorders, may suggest volume depletion, hemorrhage, or sepsis, all of which may lead to ARF. Edema may be seen in ARF, hydrops fetalis, or with massive urinary protein losses associated with congenital nephrotic syndrome. Ascites may be seen in ARF with volume overload, congenital nephrotic syndrome, or urinary tract obstruction with rupture.

Special attention should be paid to the abdominal examination. In the neonate, the lower pole of both kidneys should be easily palpable because of the neonate's reduced abdominal muscle tone. The presence of an abdominal mass in a newborn should be assumed to involve the urinary tract until proven otherwise, because two thirds of neonatal abdominal masses are genitourinary in origin.[65] The most common renal cause of an abdominal mass is hydronephrosis, followed by multicystic dysplastic kidney. Less common causes of an abdominal mass include polycystic kidney disease, renal vein thrombosis, ectopic or fused kidneys, renal hematoma or abscess, and renal tumors. The newborn bladder should be able to be percussed just above the symphysis pubis and, if enlarged, lower urinary tract obstruction should be suspected. The abdomen should be examined for absence or laxity of the abdominal muscles, which may suggest Eagle-Barrett ("prune-belly") syndrome.

A number of anomalies should alert the physician to the presence of underlying renal defects, including abnormal ears, aniridia, microcephaly, meningomyelocele, pectus excavatum, hemihypertrophy, persistent urachus, bladder or cloacal exstrophy, abnormality of the external genitalia, cryptorchidism, imperforate anus, and limb deformities. A single umbilical artery should raise suspicion of renal disease. In one study, 7% of otherwise normal infants with a single umbilical artery were found to have significant persistent renal anomalies.[16]

A constellation of physical findings called the Potter sequence may be seen in infants with bilateral renal agenesis. Lack of fetal renal function results in severe oligohydramnios, which causes fetal deformation by uterine wall compression. The characteristic facial features include wide-set eyes, depressed nasal bridge, beaked nose, receding chin and posteriorly rotated, low set ears. Other associated anomalies include a small, compressed chest wall and arthrogryposis. The condition is uniformly fatal. "Potter-like" features may be noted in infants with in utero urinary tract obstruction or chronic amniotic fluid leakage. In this group of infants, pulmonary and renal function are generally not as severely impaired and the prognosis is less grim. In infants with significant renal defects, pneumothorax or pneumomediastinum are common clinical associations related to varying degrees of pulmonary hypoplasia.

Urinalysis

Twenty-five percent of male infants and 7% of female infants void at the time of delivery. Although 98% of full-term infants void in the first 30 hours of life,[20, 56] a delay in urination for up to 48 hours should not be a cause for immediate concern in the absence of a palpable bladder, abdominal mass, or other signs or symptoms of renal disease. Failure to void for greater than 48 hours should prompt further investigation, including a kidney and bladder ultrasound to rule out urinary tract anomalies.

Evaluation of the urine should be considered as part of the physical examination in any neonate suspected of having a urinary tract abnormality. Collection of an adequate, uncontaminated specimen is very difficult in the neonate. A specimen collected by cleaning the perineum and applying a sterile adhesive plastic bag may give erroneous results, including a false-positive urine culture. Bladder catheterization is more reliable but may be technically difficult in preterm infants. Suprapubic bladder aspiration is considered the collection method of choice in infants without intra-abdominal pathology or bleeding disorders, and it has been shown to be useful and safe, even in very low-birth-weight infants.[9]

Analysis of the urine should include inspection, measurement of specific gravity, urinary dipstick, and microscopic analysis. The newborn urine is usually clear and nearly colorless. Cloudiness may represent either urinary tract infection or the presence of crystals. A yellow-brown to deep olive-green color may represent increasing amounts of conjugated bilirubin. Porphyrins, certain drugs such as phenytoin, bacteria, and urate crystals may stain the diaper pink and be confused with bleeding. Brown urine suggests bleeding from the upper urinary tract, hemoglobinuria, or myoglobinuria.

Urinary specific gravity may be measured using a clinical refractometer or a urinary dipstick method. The specific gravity of neonatal urine is usually very low (<1.004) but may be factitiously elevated by high-molec-ular-weight solutes such as contrast agents, glucose or other reducing substances, or large amounts of protein. Gouyon showed that dipstick estimation of urinary specific gravity was an unreliable test of urinary concentrating ability in the neonate and suggested that urinary osmolarity is a more reliable measurement of the kidney's concentrating and diluting ability.[34]

Urine dipstick evaluation can detect the presence of heme-containing compounds (red blood cells, myoglobin, and hemoglobin), protein, and glucose. White blood cell products such as leukocyte esterase and nitrite may also be detected on urine dipstick, and should raise suspicion of urinary tract infection, prompting the clinician to obtain a urine culture. Microscopic urinalysis should be obtained in response to an abnormal urinary dipstick and is useful in detecting the presence of red blood cells, casts, white blood cells, bacteria, and crystals.

Laboratory Evaluation

Clinical evaluation of neonatal renal function begins with measurement of serum creatinine level. As discussed previously, normal values for serum creatinine vary with gestational age and postnatal age (see Table 15–1). The serum creatinine level is relatively high at birth, with normal values up to 1.1 mg/dL in term babies and 1.3 mg/dL in preterm infants, but decreases to a mean value of 0.4 mg/dL within the first 2 weeks of life.[8] In general, each doubling of the serum creatinine level represents a 50% reduction in GFR; for example, an increase in creatinine from 0.4 mg/dL to 0.8 mg/dL reflects a 50% reduction in GFR. In addition, the Schwartz formula, which estimates GFR using serum creatinine and body length, has been applied to normal preterm and term infants[17]:

Preterm infants

$$\frac{\text{Estimated GFR}}{(\text{mL/min/1.73 m}^2)} = \frac{0.33 \times \text{height (cm)}}{\text{serum creatinine}}$$

Term infants

$$\frac{\text{Estimated GFR}}{(\text{mL/min/1.73 m}^2)} = \frac{0.45 \times \text{height (cm)}}{\text{serum creatinine}}$$

Radiologic Evaluation

Although intravenous pyelography (IVP) was used in the past to image the urinary tract, renal ultrasound is currently the initial procedure of choice in infants with suspected renal disease.[39] Renal ultrasound offers a noninvasive anatomic evaluation of the urinary tract without the use of contrast agent or radiation exposure. Renal ultrasound can demonstrate kidney size and morphology, presence of nephrocalcinosis or nephrolithiasis, complications of infection (renal abscess, perinephric abscess), obstruction (hydronephrosis, hydroureter), and bladder morphology.

Voiding cystourethrography is the procedure of choice to evaluate the urethra and bladder and to ascertain the presence or absence of vesicoureteral reflux. This study involves urinary catheterization and instillation of radiopaque dye into the infant's bladder. A voiding cystourethrogram should be considered in all infants with urinary tract obstruction, renal dysplasia or anomaly, or documented urinary tract infection.

Other radiologic tests may occasionally be used for diagnostic purposes in the neonate. A MAG-3 (^{99m}Tc mercaptoacetyltriglycine) or DTPA (^{99m}Tc diethylene triamine pentaacetic acid) diuretic renal scan may be helpful in confirming urinary tract obstruction in an infant with hydronephrosis or hydroureter on ultrasonography. DMSA (^{99m}Tc dimercaptosuccinic acid) or ^{99m}Tc glucoheptonate renal scan may help to identify renal scarring related to prior pyelonephritis or umbilical artery catheter-related embolic phenomenon. Computerized tomography may be helpful in evaluating suspected renal abscess, mass, or nephrolithiasis.

◆ SPECIFIC PROBLEMS

HEMATURIA AND PROTEINURIA

Gross hematuria develops at 16 hours of age in a 41-week 4300-g infant born to a mother with gestational diabetes. Physical examination reveals a listless pale infant with a large left flank mass. Urinalysis reveals 1+ protein and 4+ blood with greater than 250 red blood cells/mm³ and no casts. Laboratory evaluation includes hematocrit 36%, platelets 75,000, and serum creatinine 1.0 mg/dL. Renal ultrasound shows the left kidney to be large with a disordered central collection of echoes, consistent with renal venous thrombosis.

The infant undergoes conservative treatment with hydration and careful observation of fluid balance and renal function. Gross hematuria resolves within 24 hours and renal function remains stable. Serial ultrasound examinations show gradual resolution of the thrombosis over the next 7 days, with improvement in renal venous blood flow by Doppler study. On follow-up examination at 6 months of age, serum creatinine is 0.4 mg/dL and renal ultrasound is normal.

Hematuria may be suspected by positive urinary dipstick (microscopic) or visual examination (macroscopic or gross). Confirmation of hematuria requires microscopic examination showing at least five red blood cells per high-power field. A positive urinary dipstick with negative microscopic examination for red blood cells suggests myoglobinuria or hemoglobinuria. Myoglobinuria may be seen in infants with inherited metabolic myopathies, infectious myositis, and rhabdomyolysis related to prolonged seizure activity, corticosteroids, or direct muscle trauma. Hemoglobinuria may be present in erythroblastosis fetalis or other forms of hemolytic disease.

The most frequent cause of hematuria in the neonate is acute tubular necrosis (ATN) following birth asphyxia, nephrotoxic drugs, or sepsis. Another important cause of hematuria is renal venous thrombosis, which must be considered in infants of diabetic mothers, infants with cyanotic congenital heart disease, polycythemia or infants with marked dehydration. Other causes of hematuria include urinary tract infection, blood dyscrasias, bladder hemangioma, renal tumor, nephrolithiasis, congenital urinary tract malformations, and cortical necrosis. Glomerulonephritis, which represents a common cause of hematuria in childhood and adolescence, is extremely uncommon in the neonatal population.

Proteinuria is defined as urinary dipstick greater than or equal to 1 + (30 mg/dL) with specific gravity less than or equal to 1.015, or greater than or equal to 2 + (100 mg/dL) with specific gravity greater than 1.015. False-positive dipsticks for protein may result from very concentrated urine, alkaline urine, infection, and detergents. Average quantitative protein excretion declines with increasing gestational age, from 182 mg/m²/24 hours in premature infants, to 145 mg/m²/24 hours in full-term infants, to 108 mg/m²/24 hours in infants 2 to 12 months of age.[27]

Common causes of neonatal proteinuria include ATN, fever, dehydration, cardiac failure, high-dose penicillin, and contrast agent administration. Persistent massive proteinuria and edema in a neonate should prompt consideration of congenital nephrotic syndrome, an autosomal recessive disorder characterized by proteinuria, failure to thrive, large placenta, and chronic renal dysfunction.

ACUTE RENAL FAILURE

A 2400-g male infant is delivered after a 36-week uncomplicated pregnancy. Thirty minutes before delivery, the fetal heart rate is noted to be 80 beats/minute and a tight nuchal cord is noted at delivery. Apgar scores are 2 at 1 minute and 6 at 5 minutes. Resuscitation measures include positive-pressure ventilation and intravenous sodium bicarbonate. Arterial blood gas at 15 minutes shows pH 7.10, P_{CO_2} 54 mm Hg, and P_{O_2} 93 mm Hg. Initial laboratory work reveals normal electrolytes, blood urea nitrogen (BUN) 7 mg/dL, and creatinine 0.7 mg/dL.

Over the next 72 hours of life, however, the infant becomes oliguric and laboratory work reveals Na 127 mmol/L, K 6.5 mmol/L, Cl 106 mmol/L, HCO_3 15 mmol/L, BUN 18 mg/dL, and creatinine 2.1 mg/dL. Urinalysis shows 2+ blood, 1+ protein, specific gravity 1.015, and pH 6.5. A renal ultrasound study shows no evidence of renal dysplasia or obstruction, but the renal parenchyma appears hyperechoic. With a presumptive diagnosis of ATN, a peritoneal dialysis catheter is placed and dialysis initiated. After 10 days, the infant's urine output improves and, by 14 days, dialysis is discontinued. The infant is discharged to home at 21 days of age with a serum creatinine of 1.0 mg/dL. Follow-up laboratory work 6 weeks later shows the serum creatinine to be normal at 0.3 mg/dL.

ARF is characterized by a sudden impairment in renal function, leading to an inability of the kidneys to excrete nitrogenous wastes. Although the criteria for neonatal ARF have varied between studies, a consensus definition is a serum creatinine level greater than 1.5 mg/dL.[89] Oliguric ARF is characterized by urine flow rate less than 1 mL/kg/min, whereas in nonoliguric ARF, urine flow rate is maintained at greater than this level. Most reports estimate the incidence of ARF in the hospitalized neonatal population to be 6% to 8%,[89] although some estimates reach as high as 23%.[62] The causes of neonatal ARF are multiple and can be divided into prerenal, renal, and postrenal categories (Table 15–3).

Table 15–3. Causes of Acute Renal Failure in the Neonate

Prerenal
    Dehydration
    Hemorrhage
    Sepsis
    Necrotizing enterocolitis
    Congestive heart failure
    Drugs—angiotensin-converting enzyme inhibitors, nonsteroidal anti-inflammatories, amphotericin, tolazoline
Intrinsic
    Acute tubular necrosis
    Renal dysplasia
    Polycystic kidney disease
    Renal venous thrombosis
    Uric acid nephropathy
    Transient acute renal insufficiency of the newborn
Postrenal
    Posterior urethral valves
    Bilateral ureteropelvic junction obstruction
    Bilateral ureterovesical junction obstruction
    Neurogenic bladder
    Obstructive nephrolithiasis

Prerenal ARF

Prerenal (functional) ARF is the most common type of ARF in the neonate and may account for up to 70% of neonatal ARF.[62] Prerenal ARF is characterized by inadequate renal perfusion, which, if promptly treated, is followed by improvement in renal function and urine output. The most common causes of prerenal ARF are dehydration, hemorrhage, septic shock, necrotizing enterocolitis, patent ductus arteriosus, and congestive heart failure as well as medications that reduce RBF, such as indomethacin, tolazoline, and angiotensin-converting enzyme (ACE) inhibitors.

Intrinsic ARF

ATN is one of the most common causes of intrinsic ARF in neonates. Causes of ATN include perinatal asphyxia, sepsis, cardiac surgery, prolonged prerenal state, and nephrotoxic drug administration. The pathophysiology of ATN is complex and appears to involve renal tubular cellular injury, alterations in adhesion molecules, and changes in renal hemodynamics.[95] Cellular injury results from decreased adenosine triphosphate (ATP), increased intracellular calcium influx, and the destructive action of phospholipases, free radicals, and proteases. Alter-ations in cellular adhesion molecules lead to sloughing of injured tubular epithelial cells and subsequent luminal obstruction. Increased endothelin as well as decreased prostaglandins and nitric oxide activity lead to markedly decreased RBF.

Other less common causes of intrinsic ARF in the newborn include renal dysplasia, autosomal recessive polycystic kidney disease, and renal venous thrombosis. Uric acid nephropathy may represent an underestimated cause of ARF in the neonatal population and may occur when uric acid crystals precipitate in the lumen of the nephron following hypoxia, hemolysis, rhabdomyolysis, or cardiac surgery. Finally, transient acute renal insufficiency of the newborn is a poorly understood, rapidly reversible syndrome characterized by oliguric ARF and hyperechogenic renal medullary pyramids on ultrasound.[38, 80] This syndrome has been reported in otherwise healthy full-term infants with sluggish feeding and is thought to be related to deposition of Tamm-Horsfall protein in the renal tubular collecting system.

Postrenal ARF

Postrenal (obstructive) ARF is caused by bilateral obstruction of the urinary tract and can be reversed by relief of the obstruction. Obstructive ARF in the neonate may be related to a variety of congenital urinary tract conditions including posterior urethral valves, bilateral ureteropelvic or ureterovesical junction obstruction, obstructive nephrolithiasis, or neurogenic bladder. Extrinsic compression of the ureters or bladder by a congenital tumor such as a sacrococcygeal teratoma or intrinsic obstruction by renal calculi or fungus balls are rare causes of obstructive ARF.

Evaluation of the Neonate with ARF

Neonates with ARF should have a careful history performed, focusing on prenatal ultrasound abnormalities, perinatal asphyxia, systemic illness, administration of potentially nephrotoxic drugs, and family history of renal disease. Physical examination should focus on the abdomen, genitalia, and a search for other congenital anomalies or signs of Potter sequence. Electrolytes (including acid–base status), BUN, creatinine, calcium, phosphorus, and uric acid should be monitored at least daily and more frequently if significant metabolic abnormalities are present. Urine should be sent for urinalysis, urine culture, and urine sodium and creatinine determination. Calculation of FENa may be helpful in differentiating prerenal ARF from intrinsic ARF.

$$\text{FENa (\%)} = \frac{\text{Urine Na} \times \text{Serum Cr}}{\text{Serum Na} \times \text{Urine Cr}} \times 100\%$$

Neonates with FENa greater than 2.5% to 3.0% generally have intrinsic ARF, whereas those with FENa less than 1.0 have prerenal ARF.[47] Renal ultrasound is helpful in the identification of congenital renal disease and urinary tract obstruction. Voiding cystourethrogram should be performed in neonates with suspected posterior urethral valves, vesicoureteral reflux, or bladder abnormality.

Medical Management

If the neonate is oliguric, a urinary catheter should be placed to rule out lower urinary tract obstruction. If there is no improvement in urine output after bladder drainage is established, a fluid challenge of 10 to 20 mL/ kg should be administered over 1 to 2 hours to rule out prerenal ARF. A lack of improvement in urine output and serum creatinine suggests intrinsic ARF and fluids should be restricted to insensible losses (500 mL/m²), plus urine output and other losses. Daily weights and careful intake and output measurements are optimal to follow volume status.

The goal of medical management of established intrinsic ARF is to provide supportive care until there is spontaneous improvement in the infant's renal function. Nephrotoxic drugs should be discontinued to reduce the risk of additional renal injury. Medications should be adjusted by dose and interval according to the degree of renal dysfunction. Potassium and phosphorus should be restricted in neonates with hyperkalemia or hyperphosphatemia. Metabolic acidosis may require treatment with intravenous or oral sodium bicarbonate. Loop and thiazide diuretics may prove helpful in augmenting urinary flow rate. The role of low-dose dopamine in neonatal ARF management remains unproven.

Renal Replacement Therapy

Renal replacement therapy should be considered if maximal medical management fails to maintain acceptable fluid and electrolyte status. The two purposes of renal replacement therapy are (1) ultrafiltration (removal of water) and (2) dialysis (removal of solutes). Indications for initiation of renal replacement therapy include hyperkalemia, hyponatremia, acidosis, hypocalcemia, hyperphosphatemia, symptomatic volume overload, uremic symptoms, and inability to provide adequate nutrition (Table 15–4).

Peritoneal dialysis is the most commonly employed renal replacement modality in the neonatal population, because it is less technically difficult and does not require vascular access or anticoagulation. In this procedure, hyperosmolar dialysate is repeatedly infused into and drained out of the peritoneal cavity via a catheter, accomplishing both ultrafiltration and dialysis (Fig. 15–4). Cycle length, dwell volume, and the osmolar concentration of the dialysate can be varied to accomplish the goals of therapy. Relative contraindications to peritoneal dialysis include recent abdominal surgery, necrotizing enterocolitis, pleuroperitoneal leak, and ventriculoperitoneal shunt.

Continuous renal replacement therapy (CRRT) is becoming a more frequently employed modality for renal replacement therapy in the unstable neonate.[18, 78] In this procedure, the neonate's blood is continuously circulated through an extracorporeal circuit containing a highly permeable hemofilter. An ultrafiltrate of plasma is removed, a portion of which is returned to the patient in the form of a physiologic replacement fluid. Blood flow can be achieved by using arteriovenous access (continuous arteriovenous he-

Table 15–4. Indications for Dialysis

Hyperkalemia
Hyponatremia
Acidosis
Hypocalcemia
Hyperphosphatemia
Volume overload
Uremic symptoms
Inability to provide adequate nutrition

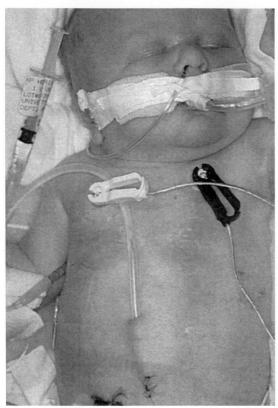

Figure 15–4. Critically ill infant with acute renal failure undergoing treatment with peritoneal dialysis. (Photograph courtesy of Julie H. Corder, PNP, Rainbow Babies and Children's Hospital, Cleveland.)

mofiltration, or CAVH) or by using a pump in conjunction with venovenous access (continuous venovenous hemofiltration, or CVVH). The use of countercurrent dialysate (D) flow can augment solute removal rate (CAVH-D, CVVH-D). The chief advantage of CRRT is the ability to carefully control fluid removal, which makes this modality especially useful in the neonate with hemodynamic instability. The main disadvantages are the need to achieve and maintain central vascular access and the need for continuous anticoagulation.

Acute hemodialysis is a less commonly employed, but technically feasible, mode of renal replacement therapy in the neonatal population.[26] Hemodialysis involves intermittent 3- to 4-hour treatments in which fluids and solutes are rapidly removed from the infant using an extracorporeal dialyzer with rapid countercurrent dialysate flow. The chief advantage of hemodialysis is the ability to rapidly remove solutes or fluid, a characteristic that makes this modality the

therapy of choice in neonatal hyperammonemia,[79] although CRRT has recently been used successfully in the management of inborn errors of metabolism.[29] Critically ill neonates may encounter hemodynamic instability and osmolar shifts with the rapid solute and fluid shifts associated with intermittent hemodialysis.

Prognosis

The prognosis for neonates with ARF is variable. In general, infants with prerenal ARF who receive prompt treatment for renal hypoperfusion have an excellent prognosis. Infants with postrenal ARF related to congenital urinary tract obstruction have a variable outcome that is dependent on the degree of associated renal dysplasia. Infants with intrinsic ARF have the poorest prognosis, with mortality rates as high as 50%.[89]

A study of 23 infants who received peritoneal dialysis in the first month of life showed that, at 1 year, 30% were on dialysis, 9% had chronic renal failure, 26% had made a full renal recovery, and 35% had died in the neonatal period.[15] There was a substantial difference in outcome according to underlying cause of ARF, in that neonates with renal structural anomalies had a 17% mortality rate, whereas those with ATN had a 55% mortality rate.[15] Decreased GFR has been reported in 40% of survivors of neonatal ARF.[4, 21] Other long-term sequelae seen in survivors of neonatal ARF include hypertension, impaired urinary concentrating ability, renal tubular acidosis, and impaired renal growth.

HYPERTENSION

A 4.5-kg male infant is born at 40 weeks' gestation. Initial examination is notable for respiratory distress, a blood pressure of 70/40 mm Hg, and a clinical picture consistent with pulmonary hypertension of the newborn. Mechanical ventilation is initiated and an umbilical artery catheter is placed to the level of T8. On day 7 of life, the blood pressure is 127/80 mm Hg via intraarterial monitoring and the baby's examination suggests congestive heart failure.

Serum electrolytes are notable for sodium 135 mmol/L, potassium 5 mmol/L, chloride 100 mmol/L, bicarbonate 22 mmol/L, BUN 10 mg/dL, and creatinine 0.7 mg/dL. Ultrasonography reveals an irregularly shaped thrombus measur-

ing 2 cm in length in the abdominal aorta, partially occluding the left renal artery. The infant's blood pressure is controlled with sodium nitroprusside and furosemide. The congestive heart failure is treated with dobutamine. Chronic therapy includes captopril and hydrochlorothiazide. At 6 months of age, the child's creatinine is 0.4 mg/dL and a renal ultrasound examination reveals that the left kidney is slightly smaller than the right kidney. By 9 months of age, the infant is able to be successfully tapered off all antihypertensive therapy.

The incidence of neonatal hypertension is reported to be approximately 3%.[2, 85, 87] Determination of the true incidence of neonatal hypertension is problematic because of inconsistencies in the definition of hypertension, variations in blood pressure measurement techniques, normal changes in blood pressure with gestational age and weight, and other factors that affect blood pressure readings.

The definition of neonatal hypertension has not been consistent among various studies. Although some authors have defined hypertension as mean arterial pressure greater than 70 mm Hg,[87] others have defined hypertension as systolic pressures greater than 90 mm Hg in term infants and greater than 80 mm Hg in preterm infants.[2] However, the current gold standard for neonatal hypertension is derived from a large epidemiologic study that defined significant hypertension in term newborn infants as systolic BP blood pressure of at least 96 mm Hg in infants less than 7 days of life and systolic blood pressure of at least 104 mm Hg in infants 8 to 30 days of life.[68] In this same study, significant hypertension in preterm infants was defined as systolic pressure greater than 80 mm Hg and diastolic pressure greater than 50 mm Hg. Although differences exist between measurements taken by aortic blood pressure measurements and to oscillometric measurements using the Dinamap, these are not clinically significant.

In general, normal blood pressure increases with increasing body weight and gestational age. The distribution of normal blood pressures on day 1 of life for newborn infants according to birth weight is presented in Figure 15–5.[103] Furthermore, systolic blood pressure increases by 1 to 2 mm Hg per day between days 3 and 8 of life and increases by 1 mm Hg per week between 5 and 7 weeks of age.[22] Many other factors influence blood pressure measurements in-

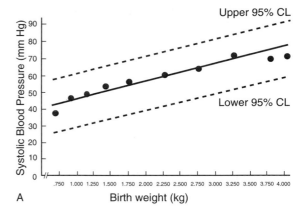

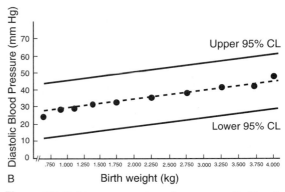

Figure 15–5. Linear regression of mean systolic blood pressure *(A)* and diastolic blood pressure *(B)* on birth weight on day 1 of life. (From Zubrow AB, Hulman S: Determinants of blood pressure in infants admitted to neonatal intensive care units: A prospective multicenter study. Philadelphia Neonatal Blood Pressure Study Group. J Perinatol 15:470–479, 1995.)

cluding anxiety, pain, and level of wakefulness. For example, in term infants, systolic blood pressure is approximately 6 mm Hg higher in awake infants compared with pressures in asleep infants, and may increase by 25% with abdominal palpation, crying, or pain.[22]

Causes of Neonatal Hypertension

The causes of hypertension in the neonate are listed in Table 15–5. Renovascular hypertension is the most frequent cause of neonatal hypertension and accounts for up to 89% of all cases.[2] The most common cause of renovascular hypertension is renal arterial thromboembolism related to umbilical artery catheterization, although congenital renal artery stenosis and renal vein throm-

Table 15–5. Causes of Neonatal Hypertension

Renovascular disease
  Renal arterial thrombosis
  Renal arterial stenosis
Congenital renal malformations
  Polycystic kidney disease
  Hydronephrosis
Renal parenchymal disease
  Acute tubular necrosis
Coarctation of the aorta
Other
  Endocrine disorders
  Bronchopulmonary dysplasia
  Drug exposure—cocaine, methadone,
    corticosteroids, aminophylline
  Abdominal wall closure
  Extracorporeal membrane oxygenation

bosis may also occur. Hypertension may also occur in infants with hypervolemia related to oliguric ARF. A small proportion of neonatal hypertension is related to structural renal disease including autosomal recessive polycystic kidney disease and obstructive uropathy. Other causes of neonatal hypertension include coarctation of the aorta, medications, endocrine disorders, abdominal wall closure, and extracorporeal membrane oxygenation. Finally, in 12% of infants with bronchopulmonary dysplasia, hypertension develops, which is likely multifactorial in origin.[3]

Clinical Presentation

The clinical presentation of hypertension in the neonate is variable. Although some babies may be asymptomatic, nonspecific symptoms such as poor feeding, irritability, and lethargy are common. Significant cardiopulmonary symptoms may be present, including tachypnea, cyanosis, impaired perfusion, vasomotor instability, congestive heart failure, cardiomegaly, or hepatosplenomegaly. Neurologic symptoms such as lethargy, coma, tremors, hypertonicity, hypotonicity, opisthotonos, asymmetric reflexes, hemiparesis, seizures, and apnea may also occur. Hypertensive retinopathy is uncommon in neonates with hypertension and resolves with control of blood pressure.[86] Renal effects of hypertension may include ARF and sodium wasting related to pressure natriuresis.

Evaluation of the Neonate with Hypertension

Evaluation of the hypertensive newborn begins with a careful history and physical examination. Initial laboratory studies should include a urinalysis, serum electrolytes, blood urea nitrogen, serum creatinine, and serum calcium. Although measurement of plasma renin activity is advocated by some authors,[2] the findings are often variable and difficult to interpret. Ultrasonography of the kidneys with Doppler flow study of the aorta and renal arteries should be performed to rule out a renal arterial or aortic thrombus or urinary tract structural anomalies. Echocardiography should be performed to diagnose aortic coarctation and evaluate left ventricular mass. Thyroid function studies and urinary studies for catecholamines, 17-hydroxysteroids, and 17-ketosteroids should be reserved for rare instances when the aforementioned studies are normal.

Management of the Neonate with Hypertension

Neonates with signs and symptoms of a hypertensive emergency such as cardiopulmonary failure, acute neurologic dysfunction, or renal insufficiency require immediate therapy with intravenous medication. The goal of therapy is a prompt decrease in blood pressure to minimize injury to the brain, heart, and kidneys. Blood pressures should not be lowered below the 95th percentile until 24 to 48 hours of therapy in order to avoid cerebral and optic disc ischemia.

Antihypertensive medications used in the neonate are summarized in Table 15–6. Sodium nitroprusside is the most common intravenous medication used for treating hypertensive emergencies in neonates. The safety and efficacy of this drug at doses of 0.5 to 8.0 µg/kg/min is well described, and adverse effects such as tachyphylaxis and metabolic acidosis are uncommon.[12] Occasionally, tachycardia is treated with intravenous labetalol at doses of 1 to 2 mg/kg/h. Infants with renovascular disease respond very well to angiotensin-converting enzyme inhibitors such as captopril[14] or enalaprilat[100] and to β-blockers such as propranolol. Careful attention to urine output, serum potassium, and serum creatinine is recom-

Table 15–6. Antihypertensive Medications

Drug	Dose	Route	Dosing Interval	Action	Comment
Sodium nitroprusside	0.5–8.0 μg/kg/min	IV	Continuous	Vasodilator	Drug of choice
Labetalol	0.25–3 mg/kg/h 0.20–1.0 mg/kg	IV IV	Continuous Bolus q 6 h	Alpha, beta blockade	Drug of choice
Diazoxide	2–5 mg/kg (bolus)	IV	q 12 h	Vasodilator	Second line drug
Hydralazine	0.1–0.4 mg/kg/ dose	IV	bolus q 4 h	Vasodilator	Second line drug
Enalaprilat	5–30 μg/kg/d	IV	q 6–24 h	ACE inhibitor	Second line drug
Captopril	0.03–2.0 mg/kg/d	p.o.	q 6–12 h	ACE inhibitor	
Nifedipine	0.2–0.3 mg/kg	p.o./SL	q 30 min–4 h	Ca channel antagonist	Oral/sublingual administration
Propranolol	0.5–4.0 mg/kg/d	p.o.	q 6–12 h	Beta blockade	Contraindicated in heart block and heart failure
Furosemide	1–10 mg/kg/d	p.o./IV/ continuous drip	q 8–24 h	Loop diuretic	
Chlorothiazide	20–40 mg/kg/d	p.o./IV	q 12 h	Distal tubule diuretic	Give 30 minutes before furosemide

q, every; IV, intravenous; p.o., oral; SL, sublingual; ACE, angiotensin-converting enzyme.

mended when initiating treatment with these agents because neonates may be extremely sensitive to the reduction in renal blood flow associated with administration of these agents. Patients with hypervolemia resulting from oliguric acute renal failure frequently benefit from hydralazine, nifedipine, or furosemide.

The long-term prognosis for children with neonatal hypertension is excellent. Among 17 children reported by Friedman and Hustead with hypertension diagnosed either in the nursery or at follow-up by 18 weeks of age, no children were receiving antihypertensive medication at 24 months of age.[31]

Renal Arterial Thrombosis

In the neonatal population, renal arterial thrombosis is most commonly associated with an indwelling umbilical arterial catheter. The incidence of thrombus formation in the aorta in the presence of umbilical artery catheters ranges from 26% using ultrasonography[81] to 95% as determined by aortography.[61] Risk factors for complications from umbilical artery catheters include maternal diabetes, sepsis, dehydration, birth trauma, perinatal asphyxia, patent ductus arteriosus, and cocaine exposure. Although 30% to 40% of infants with arterial thrombosis may be asymptomatic, hypertension occurs in

approximately 25% of patients and may be associated with hematuria, oliguria, renal failure, congestive heart failure, or lower extremity ischemia.

Ultrasonography of the kidneys with Doppler flow study of the aorta and renal arteries is the diagnostic study of choice when renal arterial thromboembolism is suspected. Patients with suspected renal arterial thromboembolism with a normal renal ultrasound and Doppler study may require confirmation with renal radionuclide imaging using either MAG-3 or DTPA. Aortography may be necessary even in the presence of a normal ultrasound in a sick child with lower extremity vascular insufficiency, congestive heart failure, or acute renal failure.

The primary treatment for hypertension associated with arterial thromboembolism is removal of the umbilical artery catheter and institution of antihypertensive therapy with an angiotensin-converting enzyme inhibitor or a β-blocker. Heparinization and fibrinolytic therapy are reserved for patients at high risk for complete occlusion or those with either oliguric ARF, congestive heart failure, or severe lower extremity ischemia. In this situation, successful use of systemic or intrathrombic urokinase or streptokinase has been reported.[55, 70] Aortic thrombectomy must be considered in patients resistant to anticoagulants and fibrinolytic agents.[97]

However, spontaneous recanalization of an aortic clot with development of collateral circulation of permanently occluded renal arteries has been described.[58]

Although children with renovascular hypertension secondary to renal arterial thromboembolism from umbilical artery catheters do not typically require antihypertensive medications beyond 12 months of age, several long-term issues exist. In a report of 12 children studied at a mean follow-up of almost 6 years, Adelman noted that 5 of 11 patients displayed unilateral renal atrophy on ultrasound or intravenous pyelography despite having normal creatinine clearances.[1] Furthermore, follow-up radionuclide scans remained abnormal in all patients studied, even in patients without renal atrophy on ultrasound. The long-term significance of these findings regarding the likelihood of chronic hypertension or renal insufficiency with prolonged follow-up is unknown.

NEPHROCALCINOSIS

A 4-month-old former 24-week premature infant with bronchopulmonary dysplasia, periventricular leukomalacia, and retinopathy of prematurity was incidentally noted to have medullary nephrocalcinosis while undergoing an abdominal ultrasound study for unrelated reasons. She had required chronic corticosteroid and loop diuretic administration to manage her lung disease. Urinalysis revealed 1+ blood, negative protein, specific gravity 1.020, and pH 5.5. Urine culture was sterile and urine calcium-to-creatinine ratio was 1.65.

Loop diuretics were discontinued and chlorothiazide initiated to reduce urinary calcium excretion. She was able to be tapered off of corticosteroids over the next 2 months as her lung disease improved. Urine calcium-to-creatinine ratio decreased to 0.8 and serial ultrasound examinations showed gradual resolution of nephrocalcinosis. At 8 months of age, chlorothiazide was discontinued and a follow-up renal ultrasound study at 1 year of age was normal.

Renal medullary calcifications were first described in the premature infant in 1982 by Hufnagle.[41] Since then, nephrocalcinosis has become a well-known complication in the neonatal population, occurring in 27% to 65% of hospitalized premature infants.[43, 74, 83] Nephrocalcinosis in infants may present with microscopic or gross hematuria, granular material in the diaper, ARF related to ureteral obstruction, or urinary tract infection. Nephrocalcinosis may also be discovered incidentally on abdominal ultrasound examination.

The majority of infants with nephrocalcinosis have had exposure to loop diuretics for management of bronchopulmonary dysplasia. However, nephrocalcinosis has been reported in infants with no prior exposure to loop diuretics. Furosemide and other loop diuretics enhance urinary calcium excretion, predisposing to deposition of calcium oxalate crystals in the renal interstitium. Other factors that may contribute to the development of neonatal nephrocalcinosis include fluid restriction, the hypercalciuric effect of corticosteroids or xanthine derivatives, decreased urinary concentration of stone inhibitors such as citrate and magnesium, hyperuricosuria,[13] increased oxalate excretion related to parenteral hyperalimentation,[40] and familial history of nephrolithiasis.[48]

In infants with nephrocalcinosis or nephrolithiasis, use of agents that increase urinary calcium excretion, such as loop diuretics and corticosteroids, should be minimized or discontinued if possible. A high urinary flow rate should be maintained to reduce the probability of urinary crystallization. Oral calcium supplements should be discontinued and metabolic acidosis, if present, should be treated with bicarbonate because chronic acidosis enhances urinary calcium excretion. Thiazide diuretics such as chlorothiazide may be effective in reducing urinary calcium excretion,[41, 74] although serum calcium should be monitored closely to avoid hypercalcemia.

The long-term consequences of neonatal nephrocalcinosis are not clearly defined. In approximately 50% of affected infants, nephrocalcinosis spontaneously resolves within 5 to 6 months of discontinuation of diuretic with no known adverse consequences.[23, 66] However, other studies suggest that persistent nephrocalcinosis can lead to diminished renal growth and deterioration of renal function.[24, 25, 28]

CONGENITAL RENAL DISEASE

A 2200-g female infant was delivered at 33 weeks by cesarean section. Oligohydramnios had been noted in the third trimester by ultrasound. Apgar score was 8 at 1 minute and 9 at

5 minutes. Physical examination was normal, including the absence of abdominal masses. She fed poorly and became listless. Laboratory evaluation revealed a persistent metabolic acidosis and a progressively increasing serum creatinine, which reached 4.5 mg/dL on day 5 of life. Renal ultrasound revealed absence of a kidney in the right renal fossa and a small, hyperechoic left kidney.

The infant was diagnosed with chronic renal failure related to left renal dysplasia and right renal agenesis. With parental consent, a peritoneal dialysis catheter was placed and dialysis initiated. The infant's parents were trained by the nephrology team to perform home dialysis, supplemental nasogastric feedings, and administer multiple medications for renal failure management. She continued on home dialysis until 3 years of age when she received a living related renal transplant from her father.

Renal Agenesis

Unilateral renal agenesis or congenital absence of the kidney occurs in 1 in 500 to 1 in 3200 individuals, whereas bilateral renal agenesis occurs in 1 in 4000 to 1 in 10,000 live births.[75] Renal agenesis occurs when the ureteric bud fails to induce proper differentiation of the metanephric blastema, an event that may be related to both a genetic predisposition and environmental factors.

Renal agenesis may be seen in infants with VACTERL (vertebral defects, imperforate anus, cardiac defects, tracheoesophageal fistula, radial and renal anomalies, limb anomalies) association, caudal regression syndrome, branchio-oto-renal syndrome, and multiple chromosomal defects,[75] but it may also be seen in otherwise healthy infants. Because contralateral urinary tract abnormalities, including vesicoureteral reflux, ureteropelvic junction obstruction, renal dysplasia, and ureterocele, occur in up to 90% of individuals with unilateral renal agenesis,[7] a thorough evaluation of the urinary tract including a voiding cystourethrogram is warranted in all patients.

Renal Dysplasia

Renal dysplasia is characterized by abnormal fetal renal development, leading to replacement of the renal parenchyma by cartilage and disorganized epithelial structures. The pathogenesis of renal dysplasia may involve mutations in developmental genes,[51]

altered interaction of the ureteric bud with extracellular matrix, abnormalities of renal growth factors, and urinary tract obstruction.[102]

Renal dysplasia is frequently present in infants with obstructive uropathy, and a variety of congenital disorders including Eagle-Barrett syndrome (prune-belly syndrome), VACTERL association, branchio-oto-renal syndrome, CHARGE (coloboma of iris, choroid, or retina, heart defects, atresia choanae, retarded growth and development, genital anomalies or hypogonadism, ear anomalies or deafness) syndrome, trisomy 13, 18, and 21, and Jeune syndrome. The function of dysplastic kidneys is variable and infants with bilateral dysplasia may exhibit signs of renal insufficiency as early as the first few days of life. Concentrating and acidification defects may also be present, whereas hematuria, proteinuria, and hypertension are unusual findings. Progressive renal insufficiency generally develops in children with bilateral renal dysplasia during childhood and adolescence.

Multicystic Dysplastic Kidney

A multicystic dysplastic kidney represents the most severe form of renal dysplasia, and is defined as a nonfunctional, dysplastic kidney with multiple large cysts and ureteral atresia. Multicystic dysplastic kidney represents the most common unilateral abdominal mass in the neonatal period and its incidence is estimated at 1 in 4300 live births.[76] Multicystic dysplastic kidney usually occurs as a sporadic event, although it may be associated with VACTERL association, branchio-oto-renal syndrome, Williams syndrome, Beckwith-Wiedemann syndrome, trisomy 18 syndrome, and 49,XXXXX syndrome. Because contralateral urinary tract abnormalities are present in up to 50% of patients with unilateral multicystic dysplastic kidney,[76] a careful evaluation of the urinary tract including a voiding cystourethrogram is warranted in all patients.

The majority of unilateral multicystic dysplastic kidneys undergo spontaneous involution while the contralateral kidney, if unaffected by other urologic malformations, grows larger than expected as a result of compensatory hypertrophy. In view of the small but real risk of hypertension[92] and malignancy,[63, 67] some clinicians advocate surgical removal of the unilateral multicystic dysplastic kidney in infancy.

Polycystic Kidney Disease

Both autosomal dominant polycystic kidney disease (ADPKD) and autosomal recessive polycystic kidney disease (ARPKD) may present in the neonatal period. ADPKD has an incidence of 1 in 200 to 1 in 1000 and represents the most common inherited renal disease.[32] The PKD1 and PDK2 genes have been identified, and mutations in these genes may alter a multimeric protein complex, which has an important regulatory role in kidney development to trigger ADPKD.[59] Clinical presentation of ADPKD in the neonatal period may vary from a severe form with significant renal failure to asymptomatic renal cysts found on ultrasound.

ARPKD is a much less common disorder, with an incidence of 1 in 6000 to 1 in 40,000, but the majority of cases present in infancy. Prenatal ultrasound may show oligohydramnios and bilaterally large, hyperechoic kidneys. Characteristic neonatal findings include palpable abdominal masses, severe hypertension, pulmonary hypoplasia, congenital hepatic fibrosis, and renal insufficiency. Primary management concerns include control of hypertension, management of renal insufficiency, and ventilatory support.

HYDRONEPHROSIS

At 18 weeks' gestation, a screening ultrasound reveals moderate bilateral fetal hydronephrosis. Serial ultrasounds show persistence of the hydronephrosis, development of hydroureters, and a large bladder with a thickened wall. The infant is delivered at 36 weeks' gestation. A bladder catheter is placed immediately to secure adequate bladder drainage. A renal ultrasound shows moderate bilateral hydronephrosis and hydroureter, a trabeculated bladder, and a dilated proximal urethra. A voiding cystourethrogram confirms the diagnosis of posterior urethral valves as well as the presence of bilateral grade III vesicoureteral reflux.

The infant undergoes primary valve ablation to relieve the urinary tract obstruction. Antibiotic prophylaxis is administered daily to reduce the possibility of urinary tract infection. Serum creatinine at hospital discharge is 1.3 mg/dL and 0.8 mg/dL at 6 months of age, suggesting mild chronic renal insufficiency.

In the past, hydronephrosis or dilation of the proximal collecting system was most commonly discovered on postnatal ultrasound study performed to evaluate an abdominal mass or urinary tract infection. However, the advent of antenatal ultrasonography has led to increasingly common prenatal detection of hydronephrosis. Although the ability to predict long-term renal function by prenatal ultrasonography remains limited,[69] prenatal diagnosis may allow parents to adjust to the diagnosis of a congenital anomaly, may maximize coordination of surgical and medical intervention, and may prevent symptomatic illness such as urinary tract infection or fluid and electrolyte imbalance. In one study, children with prenatal diagnosis of hydronephrosis had better growth and a lower incidence of reduced renal function than did those with postnatal diagnosis.[60]

Neonates with moderate to severe hydronephrosis on prenatal ultrasonography should have a repeat ultrasound performed within the first 2 days of life. Because the degree of hydronephrosis may be significantly underestimated as a result of the low GFR of the newborn, a repeat ultrasound is mandatory within several weeks. Infants with only mild hydronephrosis on prenatal ultrasonography should have their initial postnatal ultrasound performed at 2 weeks of age. Further evaluation, including voiding cystourethrogram and radionuclide renal scans, should be coordinated by a pediatric nephrologist or urologist.

Ureteropelvic Junction Obstruction

Ureteropelvic junction (UPJ) obstruction is the most common cause of congenital hydronephrosis and may be the result of incomplete recanalization of the proximal ureter, abnormal development of ureteral musculature, abnormal peristalsis, ureteral valves, or polyps. UPJ obstruction is more common in male infants and may be associated with other congenital anomalies, syndromes, or other genitourinary malformations. Diagnosis is confirmed by an obstructive pattern on diuretic-enhanced radionuclide scan. Many clinicians advocate antibiotic prophylaxis to prevent urinary tract infection, although this practice remains somewhat controversial in cases of

UPJ obstruction without reflux. Definitive treatment involves surgical repair.

Ureterovesical Junction Obstruction

Ureterovesical junction (UVJ) obstruction is the second-most common cause of congenital hydronephrosis and is characterized by hydronephrosis with associated ureteral dilatation. This disorder may be related to underdevelopment of the distal ureter or the presence of a ureterocele. Diagnosis is confirmed by radionuclide scan and voiding cystourethrogram. UVJ obstruction is usually unassociated with other congenital malformations. Many clinicians advocate antibiotic prophylaxis to prevent urinary tract infection, although this practice remains somewhat controversial in cases of UVJ obstruction without associated reflux. Definitive treatment involves surgical repair.

Posterior Urethral Valves

Posterior urethral valves are the most common cause of infravesicular urinary tract obstruction, with an incidence of 1 in 5000 to 1 in 8000 males. Prenatal ultrasound may show hydronephrosis, dilated ureters, thickened trabeculated bladder, a dilated proximal urethra, and oligohydramnios. Antenatal presentation may include a palpable, distended bladder, poor urinary stream, and signs and symptoms of renal and pulmonary insufficiency. Voiding cystourethrogram is diagnostic for posterior urethral valves and may reveal associated vesicoureteral reflux in 30% of patients.

Treatment is centered on securing adequate drainage of the urinary tract, initially by placement of a urinary catheter and later by primary ablation of the valves, vesicostomy, or upper tract diversion. The long-term outcome of infants with posterior urethral valves is dependent on the degree of associated renal dysplasia. As many as 30% of boys with posterior urethral valves whose symptoms present in infancy are at risk for progressive renal insufficiency in childhood or adolescence.

Eagle-Barrett Syndrome

Eagle-Barrett syndrome (EBS), also formerly known as prune-belly syndrome, is characterized by deficiency of abdominal wall musculature, a dilated nonobstructed urinary tract, and bilateral cryptorchidism. The estimated incidence is 1 in 35,000 to 50,000 live births, with more than 95% of cases occurring in males. Two current theories of pathogenesis include in utero urinary tract obstruction and a specific mesodermal injury between the 4th and 10th weeks of gestation.[93]

The most common urinary tract abnormalities in infants with EBS are renal dysplasia or agenesis, vesicoureteral reflux, and a large-capacity, poorly contractile bladder. Cardiac, pulmonary, gastrointestinal, and orthopedic anomalies occur in a large percentage of EBS patients. Treatment in the neonatal period involves optimization of urinary tract drainage, management of renal insufficiency, and antibiotic prophylaxis if vesicoureteral reflux is present. Management later in childhood may include surgical repair of reflux, orchiopexy, reconstruction of the abdominal wall, and renal transplantation.

Vesicoureteral Reflux

Vesicoureteral reflux is defined as retrograde propulsion of urine into the upper urinary tract during bladder contraction. The underlying cause of vesicoureteral reflux is believed to be ectopic insertion of the ureter into the bladder wall, resulting in a shorter intravesicular ureter, which acts as an incompetent valve during urination. Vesicoureteral reflux appears to have a genetic component, in that the incidence of reflux is at least 30% in first-degree relatives.[36] In infants and children evaluated for their first urinary tract infection, at least one third have vesicoureteral reflux on voiding cystourethrogram.[36]

Primary vesicoureteral reflux tends to resolve over time as the intravesical segment of the ureter elongates with growth, with the greatest rate of spontaneous resolution in the lowest grades of reflux. Daily oral antibiotic prophylaxis is important in the prevention of urinary tract infection. Surgical repair is considered in children with breakthrough urinary tract infections or high-grade reflux. Long-term complications of vesicoureteral reflux include hypertension, renal scarring, and chronic renal failure.[6]

REFERENCES

1. Adelman R: Long-term follow-up of neonatal reno-vascular hypertension. Pediatr Nephrol 1:35–41, 1987.
2. Adelman RD: Neonatal hypertension. Pediatr Clin North Am 25:99–110, 1978.
3. Alagappan A, Malloy MH: Systemic hypertension in very low-birth weight infants with bronchopulmonary dysplasia: Incidence and risk factors. Am J Perinatol 15:3–8, 1998.
4. Anand SK, Northway JD, Crussi FG: Acute renal failure in newborn infants. J Pediatr 92:985–988, 1978.
5. Arant BS: Developmental patterns of renal functional maturation compared in the human neonate. J Pediatr 92:705–712, 1978.
6. Arant BS: Vesicoureteral reflux and renal injury. Am J Kidney Dis 5:491–511, 1991.
7. Atiyeh B, Husmann D, Baum M: Contralateral renal abnormalities in patients with renal agenesis and noncystic renal dysplasia. Pediatrics 91:812–815, 1993.
8. Avner ED, Ellis D, Ichikawa I, et al: Normal neonates and maturational development of homeostatic mechanisms. In Ichikawa I, ed: Pediatric Textbook of Fluids and Electrolytes. Baltimore: Williams & Wilkins, 1990, pp 107–118.
9. Barkemeyer BM: Suprapubic aspiration of urine in very low birth weight infants. Pediatrics 92:457–459, 1993.
10. Barr M: Teratogen update: Angiotensin-converting enzyme inhibitors. Teratology 50:399–409, 1994.
11. Battin M, Albersheim S, Newman D: Congenital genitourinary tract abnormalities following cocaine exposure in utero. Am J Perinatol 12:425–428, 1995.
12. Benitz WE, Malachowski N, Cohen RS, et al: Use of sodium nitroprusside in neonates: Efficacy and safety. J Pediatr 106:102–110, 1985.
13. Berard E, Dageville C, Bekri S, et al: Nephrocalcinosis and prematurity: Importance of urate and oxalate excretion. Nephron 69:237–241, 1995.
14. Bifano E, Post EM, Springer J, et al: Treatment of neonatal hypertension with captopril. J Pediatr 100:143–146, 1982.
15. Blowey DL, McFarland K, Alon U, et al: Peritoneal dialysis in the neonatal period: Outcome data. J Perinatol 13:59–64, 1993.
16. Bourke WG, Clarke TA, Mathews TG, et al: Isolated single umbilical artery—The case for routine renal screening. Arch Dis Child 68:600–601, 1993.
17. Brion LP, Fleischman AR, McCarton C, et al: A simple estimate of glomerular filtration rate in low birthweight infants during the first year of life: Noninvasive assessment of body composition and growth. J Pediatr 109:698–707, 1986.
18. Bunchman TE, Donckerwolcke RA: Continuous arterial-venous diahemofiltration and continuous veno-venous diahemofiltration in infants and children. Pediatr Nephrol 8:96–102, 1994.
19. Cheek DB, Wishart J, MacLennan A, et al: Cell hydration in the normally grown, the premature and the low weight for gestational age infant. Early Hum Dev 10:75–84, 1984.
20. Clark DA: Time of first void and stool in 500 newborns. Pediatrics 60:457–459, 1977.
21. Dauber IM, Krauss AN, Symchych PS, et al: Renal failure following perinatal anoxia. J Pediatr 88:851–855, 1976.
22. de Swiet M, Fayers P, Shinebourne EA: Systolic blood pressure in a population of infants in the first year of life: The Brompton study. Pediatrics 65:1028–1035, 1980.
23. Downing GJ, Egelhoff JC, Daily DK, et al: Furosemide-related renal calcifications in the premature infant. Pediatr Radiol 21:563–565, 1991.
24. Downing GJ, Engelhoff JC, Daily DK, et al: Kidney function in very low birth weight infants with furosemide-related renal calcifications at ages 1 to 2 years. J Pediatr 120:599–604, 1992.
25. Downing GJ, Thomas MK, Daily DK: Nephrocalcinosis (NC) associated renal function (RF) impairment in furosemide (F) treated VLBW infants at 1 year of age. Pediatr Res 29:1252, 1991.
26. Donckerwolcke RA, Bunchman TE: Hemodialysis in infants and small children. Pediatr Nephrol 8:103–106, 1994.
27. Ettenger RB: The evaluation of the child with proteinuria. Pediatr Ann 23:486–494, 1994.
28. Ezzedeen F, Adelman RD, Ahlfors CE: Renal calcification in preterm infants: Pathophysiology and long-term sequelae. J Pediatr 113:532–539, 1988.
29. Falk MC, Knight JF, Roy LP, et al: Continuous venovenous haemofiltration in the acute treatment of inborn errors of metabolism. Pediatr Nephrol 8:330–333, 1994.
30. Favor J, Sandulache R, Neuhauser-Klaus, et al: The mouse Pax2^{1Neu} mutation is identical to a human PPAX2 mutation in a family with renal-coloboma syndrome and results in developmental defects of the brain, ear, eye, and kidney. Proc Natl Acad Sci U S A 93:13870–13875, 1996.
31. Friedman AL, Hustead VA: Hypertension in babies following discharge from a neonatal intensive care unit. A 3-year follow-up. Pediatr Nephrol 1:30–34, 1987.
32. Gabow PA: Autosomal dominant polycystic kidney disease. N Engl J Med 329:332–341, 1993.
33. Gloor JM, Muchant DG, Norling LL: Prenatal maternal indomethacin use resulting in prolonged neonatal renal insufficiency. J Perinatol 13:425–427, 1993.
34. Gouyon JB, Houchan N: Assessment of urine specific gravity by reagent strip test in newborn infants. Pediatr Nephrol 7:77–78, 1993.
35. Greenfield SP, Rutigliano E, Steinhardt G, et al: Genitourinary tract malformations and maternal cocaine abuse. Urology 37:455–459, 1991.
36. Greenfield SP, Wan J: Vesicoureteral reflux: Practical aspects of evaluation and management. Pediatr Nephrol 10:789–794, 1996.
37. Heimler R, Doumas BT, Jendrzejczak B, et al: Relationship between nutrition, weight change and fluid compartments in preterm infants during the first week of life. J Pediatr 122:110–114, 1993.
38. Hijazi Z, Keller MS, Gaudio KM, et al: Transient renal dysfunction of the neonate. Pediatrics 82:929–930, 1988.
39. Hilton SVW, Kaplan GW: Imaging of common problems in pediatric urology. Urol Clin North Am 22:1–20, 1995.
40. Hoppe B, Hesse A, Neuhaus T, et al: Urinary saturation and nephrocalcinosis in preterm infants: Effect of parenteral nutrition. Arch Dis Child 69:299–303, 1993.
41. Hufnagle KG, Khan SN, Penn D, et al: Renal calci-

fications: A complication of long-term furosemide therapy in pre-term infants. Pediatrics 70:360–363, 1982.

42. Hulton SA, Kaplan BS: Renal dysplasia associated with in utero exposure to gentamicin and corticosteroids. Am J Med Genet 58:91–93, 1995.

43. Jacinto JS, Modanlou HD, Crade M, et al: Renal calcification: Incidence in very low birth weight infants. Pediatrics 81:31–35, 1988.

44. Jose PA: Neonatal renal function and physiology. Curr Opin Pediatr 6:172–177, 1994.

45. Kaplan BS, Restaino I, Raval DS, et al: Renal failure in the neonate associated with in utero exposure to non-steroidal anti-inflammatory agents. Pediatr Nephrol 8:700–794, 1994.

46. Karlen J, Aperia A, Zetterstrom R: Renal excretion of calcium and phosphate in preterm and term infants. J Pediatr 106:814–819, 1985.

47. Karlowicz MG, Adelman RD: Acute renal failure in the neonate. Clin Perinatol 19:139–158, 1992.

48. Karlowicz MG, Katz ME, Adelman RD, et al: Nephrocalcinosis in very low birth weight neonates: Family history of kidney stones and ethnicity as independent risk factors. J Pediatr 122:635–638, 1993.

49. Kreidberg JA, Sariola H, Loring JM, et al: WT-1 is required for early kidney development. Cell 74:679–691, 1993.

50. Lemann J, Litzow JR, Lennon EJ: The effects of chronic acid loads in normal man: Further evidence for the participation of bone mineral in defence against chronic metabolic acidosis. J Clin Invest 45:1608–1614, 1966.

51. Lipschultz JH: Molecular development of the kidney: A review of the results of gene disruption studies. Am J Kidney Dis 31:383–397, 1998.

52. Lorenz JM, Kleinman LI: Ontogeny of the kidney. In Tsang R, Nichols B, eds: Nutrition During Infancy. Philadelphia, Hanley and Belfus, 1988, pp 58–85.

53. Lorenz JM, Kleinman LI, Ahmed G, et al: Phases of fluid and electrolyte homeostasis in the extremely low birth weight infant. Pediatrics 96:484–489, 1995.

54. Loughead JL, Mimouni F, Tsang RC: Serum ionized calcium concentrations in normal neonates. Am J Dis Child 142:516–518, 1988.

55. Moltèni KH, George J, Messersmith R, et al: Intrathrombic urokinase reverses neonatal renal artery thrombosis. Pediatr Nephrol 7:413–415, 1993.

56. Moore ES, Galvez MB: Delayed micturition in the newborn period. J Pediatr 80:867–873, 1972.

57. Mugrauer G, Ekblom P: Contrasting expression patterns of three members of the myc family of protooncogenes in the developing and adult mouse kidney. J Cell Biol 112:13–25, 1991.

58. Munoz-Arizpe R, Walsh RF, Edge W: Obstructive aortic renal thrombosis in the newborn—Spontaneous recovery. Pediatr Nephrol 6:190–191, 1992.

59. Murcia N, Avner ED: The molecular pathophysiology of polycystic kidney disease. Pediatr Nephrol 12:721–726, 1998.

60. Murphy JI, Kaplan GW, Packer MG, et al: Prenatal diagnosis of severe urinary tract anomalies improves renal function and growth. Child Nephrol Urol 9:290–294, 1988.

61. Neal WA, Reynolds JW, Jarvis CW, et al: Umbilical artery catheterization: Demonstration of arterial thrombosis by aortography. Pediatrics 50:6–13, 1972.

62. Norman ME, Assadi FK: A prospective study of acute renal failure in the newborn infant. Pediatrics 63:475–479, 1979.

63. Oddone M, Marino C, Sergi C, et al: Wilms' tumor arising in a multicystic kidney. Pediatr Radiol 24:236–238, 1994.

64. Orellana SA, Avner ED: Cell and molecular biology of kidney development. Semin Nephrol 18:233–243, 1998.

65. Pinto E, Guignard J-P: Renal masses in the neonate. Biol Neonate 68:175–184, 1995.

66. Pope JC, Trusler LA, Klein AM, et al: The natural history of nephrocalcinosis in premature infants treated with loop diuretics. J Urol 156:709–712, 1996.

67. Rackley RR, Angermeier KW, Levin H, et al: Renal cell carcinoma arising in a regressed multicystic dysplastic kidney. J Urol 152:1543–1545, 1994.

68. Report of the Second Task Force on Blood Pressure Control in Children—1987. Pediatrics 79:1–25, 1987.

69. Reznik VM, Budorick NE: Prenatal detection of congenital renal disease. Urol Clin North Am 22:21–30, 1995.

70. Reznik VM, Anderson J, Griswold WR, et al: Successful fibrinolytic treatment of arterial thrombosis and hypertension in a cocaine-exposed neonate. Pediatrics 84:735–738, 1989.

71. Robillard JE, Segar JL, Smith FG, et al: Regulation of sodium metabolism and extracellular fluid volume during development. Clin Perinatol 19:15–31, 1992.

72. Robillard J, Smith F, Guillery E, et al: Mechanisms regulating renal sodium excretion during development. Pediatr Nephrol 6:205–213, 1992.

73. Robillard JE, Sessions C, Burmeister L, et al: Influence of fetal extracellular volume contraction on renal reabsorption of bicarbonate in the lamb fetus. Pediatr Res 11:649–655, 1977.

74. Robinson CM, Cox MA: The incidence of renal calcifications in low birth weight (LBW) infants on Lasix for bronchopulmonary dysplasia (BPD). Pediatr Res 20:359A, 1986.

75. Robson WL, Leung AKC, Rogers RC: Unilateral renal agenesis. Adv Pediatr 42:575–592, 1995.

76. Robson WL, Leung AKC, Thomason MA: Multicystic dysplasia of the kidney. Clin Pediatr 34:32–40, 1995.

77. Rodriguez-Soriano J, Vallo A, Castillo G, Oliveros R: Renal handling of water and sodium in infancy and childhood: A study using clearance methods during saline diuresis. Kidney Int 20:700–704, 1981.

78. Ronco C, Parenzan L: Acute renal failure in infancy: Treatment by continuous renal replacement therapy. Intens Care Med 21:490–499, 1995.

79. Rutledge SL, Havens PL, Haymond MW, et al: Neonatal hemodialysis: Effective therapy for the encephalopathy of inborn errors of metabolism. J Pediatr 116:125–128, 1990.

80. Salisz JA, Kass EJ, Cacciarelli AA: Transient acute renal failure in the neonate. Urology 41:137–140, 1993.

81. Seibert JJ, Taylor BJ, Williamson SL, et al: Sonographic detection of neonatal umbilical artery thrombosis: Clinical correlation. Am J Radiol 148:965–968, 1987.

82. Shaffer SG, Bradt S, Hall R: Postnatal changes in total body water and extracellular volume in preterm infant with respiratory distress syndrome. J Pediatr 109:509–514, 1986.

83. Short A, Cooke RW: The incidence of renal calcification in preterm infants. Arch Dis Child 66:412–417, 1991.

84. Simpson J, Stephenson T: Regulation of extracellular volume in neonates. Early Hum Dev 34:179–190, 1993.

85. Singh HP, Hurley RM, Myers TF: Neonatal hypertension. Incidence and risk factors. Am J Hypertens 5:51–55, 1992.

86. Skalina MEL, Annable WL, Kliegman RM, et al: Hypertensive retinopathy in the newborn infant. J Pediatr 103:781–786, 1983.

87. Skalina MEL, Kliegman RM, Fanaroff AA: Epidemiology and management of severe symptomatic neonatal hypertension. Am J Perinatol 3:235–239, 1986.

88. Slotkin TA, Lau C, Kavlock RJ, et al: Role of sympathetic neurons in biochemical and functional development of the kidney: Neonatal sympathectomy with 6-hydroxydopamine. J Pharmacol Exp Ther 246:427–433, 1988.

89. Stapleton FB, Jones DP, Green RS: Acute renal failure in neonates: Incidence, etiology and outcome. Pediatr Nephrol 1:314–320, 1987.

90. Sulyok E: Postnatal adaptation. In Holliday M, Barratt T, Avner E, eds: Pediatric Nephrology. Baltimore: Williams & Wilkins, 1994, pp 267–286.

91. Sulyok E, Guignard J-P: Effect of ammonium chloride–induced metabolic acidosis on renal electrolyte handling in human neonates. Pediatr Nephrol 4:415–420, 1990.

92. Susskind MR, Kim KS, King LR: Hypertension and multicystic kidney. Urology 34:362–366, 1989.

93. Sutherland RS, Mevorach RA, Kogan BA: The prune-belly syndrome: Current insights. Pediatr Nephrol 9:770–778, 1995.

94. Taylor CL, Jones KL, Jones MC, et al: Incidence of renal anomalies in children prenatally exposed to ethanol. Pediatrics 94:209–212, 1994.

95. Thadhani R, Pascual M, Bonventre JV: Acute renal failure. N Engl J Med 334:1448–1460, 1996.

96. Tsang RC, Chen IW, Friedman MA, et al: Neonatal parathyroid function: Role of gestational and postnatal age. J Pediatr 83:728–738, 1973.

97. Vailas GN, Brouillette RT, Scott JP, et al: Neonatal aortic thrombosis: Recent experience. J Pediatr 109:101–108, 1986.

98. Vander Heijden BJ, Carlus C, Narcy F, et al: Persistent anuria, neonatal death, and renal microcystic lesions after prenatal exposure to indomethacin. Am J Obstet Gynecol 171:617–623, 1994.

99. Vanpee M, Blennow M, Linne T, et al: Renal function in very low birth weight infants: Normal maturity reached during early childhood. J Pediatr 121:784–788, 1992.

100. Wells TG, Bunchman TE, Kearns GL: Treatment of neonatal hypertension with enalaprilat. J Pediatr 117:664–667, 1990.

101. Wilkins B: Renal function in sick very low birthweight infants. Sodium, potassium, and water excretion. Arch Dis Child 67:1154–1161, 1992.

102. Woolf AS: Clinical and biological basis of renal malformations. Semin Nephrol 15:361–372, 1995.

103. Zubrow AB, Hulman S, Kushner H, et al: Determinants of blood pressure in infants admitted to neonatal intensive care units: A prospective multicenter study. Philadelphia Neonatal Blood Pressure Study Group. J Perinatol 15:470–479, 1995.

Hematologic Problems

D. Wade Clapp
Kevin M. Shannon
Roderic H. Phibbs

Clinically important problems of hemostasis and blood cell production and function frequently develop in both premature and term neonates. The approach to all of the commonly encountered hematologic problems seen in the high-risk newborn includes (1) obtaining family, obstetric, and perinatal histories; (2) physical examination of the infant with particular attention paid to assessment of skin, mucous membranes, skeleton, liver, and spleen; and (3) selective use of laboratory tests to define the severity of a particular hematologic problem and to establish the cause. Simple procedures that require little blood from the infant, such as hematologic studies of the parents (especially of the mother) and examination of the blood smear, often yield a correct diagnosis rapidly. During infancy, the normal values for many laboratory studies differ markedly from those in healthy older children. This chapter selectively reviews basic physiologic principles of neonatal hemostasis and hematopoiesis as a way of providing a rational basis for approaching hematologic problems in the high-risk infant. Diagnosis and initial management of the more common disorders are also discussed. The work of Oski and Naiman[73] is recommended for a more detailed discussion of the problems described in this chapter.

◆ COAGULATION IN THE NEWBORN

The coagulation system is often taught (and therefore learned) as consisting of discrete fluid-phase (circulating proteins), cellular (platelet), and vascular (vessel wall) compartments. Even though this approach is useful in classifying specific disorders, the component parts of the hemostatic system are functionally and biochemically interrelated. Clot formation is best viewed as a precisely regulated local event, which occurs as a result of molecular interactions between the endothelial surface of an injured blood vessel, the circulating coagulation proteins, and the platelets. Although most pediatricians are familiar with the procoagulant factors and how they function, proteins that limit the extent and location of clot formation by promoting the degradation of activated thrombin and factor X are equally essential. These molecules include antithrombin III, protein C, and protein S. Certain tests provide valuable information about the functional status of the coagulation system in newborns; however, these assays are more useful for defining the causes of hemorrhage than for evaluating infants with unexplained thrombosis. In addition, the living vascular surface cannot be duplicated in the clinical laboratory. For this reason, most laboratory studies should be viewed as measures of global hemostatic function and may not provide useful information about the process of local thrombus formation.

Initial Laboratory Evaluation

Specific issues related to the laboratory evaluation of infants with hemorrhage or thrombosis have been reviewed in detail.[59] Studies that should be obtained to evaluate neonatal hemorrhage include the prothrombin time (PT) and partial thromboplastin time (PTT), a complete blood count with differential and platelet count, and examination of the blood smear. The PT and PTT measure the overall function of the proteins involved in the coagulation cascade. These factors are shown in Figure 16–1 and are classified as compo-

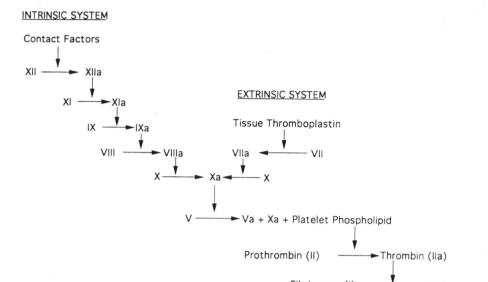

INTRINSIC SYSTEM

Contact Factors

EXTRINSIC SYSTEM

Tissue Thromboplastin

Figure 16–1. Overview of the coagulant proteins of the intrinsic system (upper left) and extrinsic system (upper right), which both feed into the common pathway (bottom).

nents of extrinsic, intrinsic, or common pathways. Coagulation factor VII, the only factor unique to the extrinsic pathway, is activated by tissue factor and directly induces the conversion of factor X to its active form (Xa) at the start of the common pathway (see Fig. 16–1). The PT (Quick test) measures factor VII activity as well as the integrity of the "downstream" factors of the common pathway (factors X, V, II [thrombin], and I [fibrinogen]).

The intrinsic arm of the cascade is initiated by the activities of contact factor on factor XII (Hageman factor) and includes factors XI, IX, and VIII. Factor VIIIa forms a phospholipid complex with factor X, thereby triggering activation of the common pathway. The PTT measures the activities of factors XII, XI, IX, and VIII in the intrinsic

pathway, as well as testing the integrity of the common pathway.

There are a number of pitfalls in performing and interpreting the PT and PTT in neonates. First, the upper limits of normal for both tests are much longer in newborns than in adults (Table 16–1). Normal ranges for PT and PTT vary somewhat between laboratories. Second, the PTT is exquisitely sensitive to heparin. In our opinion, coagulation times should never be obtained from indwelling catheters that are being flushed with solutions containing heparin. If heparin contamination is suspected as the cause of a prolonged PTT, the plasma can be mixed 1 to 1 with normal plasma and the test repeated. If the PTT normalizes, the cause is not heparin. Protamine sulfate and the thrombin time can also be used to estab-

Table 16–1. Normal Values for Coagulation Screening Tests

Test	Older Child	Full-Term Newborn	Healthy Growing Premature Infant
Platelets (per mm³)	150,000–400,000	150,000–400,000	150,000–400,000
Prothrombin time (s)	10–14	11–15	11–16
Partial thromboplastin time (s)	25–35	30–40	35–80
Fibrinogen (mg/dL)	175–400	165–400	150–325
Fibrin degradation products (μg/mL)	<10	<10	<10

From Buchanan GR: Neonatal hemorrhagic diseases. In Nathan DG, Oski FA: Hematology of Infancy and Childhood. 3rd ed. Philadelphia: WB Saunders, 1987.

lish whether a prolonged PTT is due to the presence of heparin in the specimen. Third, it is critical that the blood sample be added to the tube before any clotting has occurred and that the tube be allowed to fill completely. Samples are collected into tubes containing sodium citrate, an anticoagulant that acts by binding free calcium. Because the PT and PTT measurements are performed by adding a known amount of calcium back to the decalcified plasma, it is essential that the anticoagulant in the collecting tube be diluted with the proper amount of blood.

The platelet count should be measured routinely as part of the initial evaluation of the bleeding neonate. The range of normal platelet counts is the same in newborns as in older patients (see Table 16–1). Fictitious thrombocytopenia is a common problem in the nursery, particularly in capillary blood specimens. The blood smear should always be examined in infants with thrombocytopenia to exclude clumping, to assess whether the platelets are morphologically normal, to determine whether giant platelets (suggestive of early release of young platelets) are present, and to search for abnormalities of white and red blood cells.

Other tests of coagulation include the bleeding, thrombin, and whole blood clotting times, platelet aggregometry, measurement of the level of fibrinogen and of other coagulation factors, and urea clot solubility.

We do not believe that any of these studies are useful as screening tests in the bleeding neonate unless there is strong historical or clinical evidence to support a specific diagnosis. The indications for each of these tests are incorporated into the discussion of individual disorders.

◆ THROMBOCYTOPENIC BLEEDING

It is useful in clinical practice to approach the bleeding neonate by first asking whether thrombocytopenia is present. Serious hemorrhage is usually not due to thrombocytopenia alone if the platelet count is greater than 50,000 per mm³. It has been suggested that some infants with thrombocytopenic bleeding "look sick" whereas others "look well" and that clinical appearance provides an important clue as to the correct diagnosis.[10] In general, babies with thrombocytopenia resulting from disseminated intravascular coagulation (DIC), intrauterine infection, or congenital leukemia are quite ill, whereas those with decreased platelet counts resulting from immunologic destruction or impaired marrow production are frequently asymptomatic except for mild clinical bleeding. Table 16–2 summarizes salient clinical and laboratory features of the thrombocytopenic bleeding syndromes discussed below.

Table 16–2. Conditions Associated With Bleeding and Thrombocytopenia

Diagnosis	Appearance	Prothrombin Time	Partial Thromboplastin Time	Other Useful Tests
Disseminated intravascular coagulation	Sick	↑	↑	Fibrinogen; fibrin degradation products
TORCH (toxoplasmosis, rubella, cytomegalovirus, herpes simplex)	Sick	Normal or ↑	Normal or ↑	Liver function tests; fibrinogen; fibrin degradation products
Leukemia	Sick	Normal	Normal	Bone marrow
Maternal immune thrombocytopenic purpura	Well	Normal	Normal	Maternal platelet count
Alloimmune thrombocytopenia	Well	Normal	Normal	Maternal platelet count and platelet antigen typing (PAI-1)
Giant hemangioma	Well	Normal or ↑	Normal or ↑	Fibrinogen; fibrin degradation products
Defective platelet production	Well	Normal	Normal	Bone marrow examination

Disseminated Intravascular Coagulation

Whereas normal hemostasis is a tightly regulated process localized to injured endothelial surfaces, DIC involves diffuse, inappropriate activation of the clotting system throughout the vascular space. Bleeding primarily results from depletion of clotting proteins and platelets. There is a wide range of clinical severity associated with DIC. Whereas DIC is acute and fulminant in some infants with diffuse hemorrhage and ongoing consumption, other babies may have a milder picture with only mild depression of clotting factor levels. Septicemia (including viremia) is the most common cause of severe DIC in neonates; other causes are included in Table 16–3. Infants with severe DIC are typically very sick with multiorgan failure. Bruising, petechiae, bleeding from puncture sites, and pulmonary hemorrhage are common. Screening laboratory evaluation reveals thrombocytopenia and marked prolongation of the PT and PTT. The blood smear often shows red cell fragments and giant platelets. Neutropenia is common in preterm babies with sepsis, and the granulocytes may be vacuolated or contain toxic granulations. Although no single laboratory test unequivocally establishes the presence of DIC, the fibrinogen level is typically depressed and fibrin degradation products are increased as a result of excessive fibrinogen consumption and fibrin turnover. Many clinical laboratories no longer measure total fibrin degradation products in patients suspected of having fibrinolysis. Instead, plasma D-dimer assays have been adopted; these are more specific and are less prone to technical problems.

The first principle in managing DIC is to identify and treat the underlying cause in order to eliminate the stimulus that has dysregulated the normal hemostatic mechanism. Immediate replacement of platelets and clotting factors is essential when DIC is associated with hemorrhage. Even mild bleeding should be treated aggressively in infants with laboratory evidence of significant DIC because the coagulopathy is frequently progressive. Controlling acute bleeding requires replenishing the coagulation factors, particularly fibrinogen. For this reason, cryoprecipitate should be given in addition to fresh frozen plasma and platelet concentrates. Table 16–4 summarizes the blood components available in most blood banks, what factors they contain, and common indications for their use. Fibrinogen is concentrated in cryoprecipitate so that large amounts can be transfused in small volumes. For the infant who does not require rapid infusions to immediately control life-threatening bleeding, double volume exchange transfusion with fresh whole blood is an excellent strategy. If fresh whole blood is not available, the exchange can be performed with packed red blood cells diluted in fresh frozen plasma with concurrent administration of cryoprecipitate and platelets to maintain the fibrinogen at greater than 100 mg/dL. A stable or increasing fibrinogen is often the first sign that severe DIC is resolving. The platelet count, PT, and PTT should be measured every 4 to 6 hours to determine the need for transfusions of platelets and plasma. There are no convincing data that heparin is useful in neonatal DIC, and regulating the heparin dose is problematic in sick infants.[66] Anticoagulant therapy should be considered only in refractory cases of DIC and should be initiated only after consulting a hematologist with expertise in managing coagulopathies in neonates.

Table 16–3. Etiologic Factors in Newborn Disseminated Intravascular Coagulation

---

Septicemia
  Bacterial
  Viral
  Parasitic
  Rickettsial
  Mycotic
Tissue release
  Antigen-antibody complexes
  Abruptio placentae
  Intravascular hemolysis
  Malignancy
  Cardiopulmonary failure, asphyxia, hypoxia, shock
  Burns
Giant hemangioma (platelet trapping)
Purpura fulminans
Hepatitis and cirrhosis

TORCH Infections

Thrombocytopenia is a common finding in congenital viral infections caused by the TORCH (toxoplasmosis, rubella, cytomegalovirus, and herpes simplex) agents (see Chapter 13). Infants with full-blown TORCH

Table 16–4. Products Used in Treatment of Neonatal Coagulopathies

Product	Contents	Usual Dose	Indications
Fresh frozen plasma	All factors	10–20 mL/kg	Disseminated intravascular coagulation (DIC); liver disease; protein C deficiency
Exchange transfusion*	All factors; platelets	Double volume	Severe DIC; liver failure
Cryoprecipitate	Factors VIII and XIII; VWF; fibrinogen	1 bag†	DIC; liver disease; factor VIII or XIII deficiency; von Willebrand disease
Factor IX concentrates	Factor IX	50–100 U/kg	Factor IX deficiency
Factor VIII concentrates	Factor VIII	25–50 U/kg	Factor VIII deficiency
Vitamin K		1–2 mg	Suspected vitamin K deficiency
Platelet concentrates	Platelets	1–2 units/5 kg‡	Bleeding caused by thrombocytopenia
Intravenous gamma globulin	IgG	1–2 g/kg	Severe sepsis; thrombocytopenia caused by transplacental antibodies

*If fresh whole blood is used for exchange.
†One bag of cryoprecipitate contains approximately 250 mg of fibrinogen and 80 to 120 units of factor VIII.
‡Response to platelets can vary markedly, depending on underlying condition (see text for details).

infection generally appear ill with microcephaly, chorioretinitis, hepatosplenomegaly, pallor, and purpura. Multiple factors contribute to the bleeding diathesis seen in infants with congenital TORCH infections. Impaired marrow platelet production, increased peripheral destruction caused by coexisting DIC, and sequestration in the enlarged spleen are thought to be important mechanisms. In addition to revealing thrombocytopenia, screening laboratory studies may reveal prolongation of the PT, PTT (caused by either DIC or impaired production of clotting factors as a result of hepatitis), and anemia. The anemia is associated with reticulocytosis and increased numbers of nucleated red cells on the blood smear. Once the extent and nature of the coagulopathy is established by measuring levels of fibrinogen and fibrin split products as well as the PT, PTT, and platelet count, significant hemorrhage is treated by replacing deficiencies.

Maternal Thrombocytopenia

Obtaining a maternal medical history and platelet count is mandatory in evaluating neonatal thrombocytopenia. This is especially true in the baby who "looks well," has an unremarkable physical examination except for signs of bleeding, and has a normal white blood cell count, hemoglobin, PT,

and PTT. Maternal immune thrombocytopenic purpura (ITP) and systemic lupus erythematosus (SLE) are common conditions associated with transplacental passage of IgG antiplatelet antibodies, which bind to the infant's platelets and induce premature destruction. The same mechanisms are operative in the mother, resulting in the important diagnostic clue of maternal thrombocytopenia. The blood smear often contains giant platelets, which are released prematurely from the marrow to compensate for rapid platelet destruction. Maternal platelet count is often a poor predictor of the degree of neonatal thrombocytopenia; however, the level of maternal plasma antiplatelet antibody may be predictive.[22] There is considerable debate among perinatologists regarding indications for cesarean section, the utility of fetal blood sampling to measure the platelet count, and the value of maternal pretreatment with corticosteroids or intravenous gamma globulin. Severe hemorrhage is uncommon in the infants of women with ITP.[11] Management of these newborns depends on the severity of the bleeding diathesis. Many infants either are asymptomatic or have only a mild petechial rash and require no specific therapy. Intracranial hemorrhage is a feared complication and is usually seen in infants with profound thrombocytopenia who are delivered vaginally. We believe that severe bleeding should be treated with intravenous gamma globulin (1 to 2 g/kg) and platelet concentrates. Combination therapy is recommended because gamma globulin can increase the survival of antibody-coated platelets by inducing a temporary blockade of the reticuloendothelial system.[34] Infants who do not initially show severe thrombocytopenia require careful observation because the platelet count may decrease after birth. Thrombocytopenia resolves after 1 to 3 months as the level of maternal IgG declines. In addition to maternal ITP and SLE, antibody-mediated thrombocytopenia may occur in mothers and infants in association with maternal use of certain drugs (e.g., sulfonamides and quinines).

Neonatal Alloimmune Thrombocytopenia

The pathogenesis of this condition is analogous to that of hemolytic anemia resulting from Rh incompatibility. In alloimmune thrombocytopenia, the infant's platelets carry a surface antigen inherited from the father, which is recognized as foreign by the maternal immune system. Transplacental passage of antibodies produced against this antigen causes destruction of the baby's platelets by immunologic mechanisms similar to those in maternal ITP. However, an important distinction between the two conditions is that the mothers of infants with alloimmune thrombocytopenia have normal platelet counts because the antiplatelet antibody is specific for the baby's platelets. Although many infants with alloimmune thrombocytopenia appear well, the risk of severe bleeding is considerably higher than in maternal ITP. Alloimmune thrombocytopenia should be suspected in a phenotypically normal newborn in whom the only hematologic abnormality is a low platelet count. The presence of giant platelets on the smear suggests that thrombocytopenia is due to an increased rate of platelet destruction. Antibodies against an antigen associated with the platelet glycoprotein (GP) IIb/IIIa complex called PAI-1 account for more than 90% of all cases of alloimmune thrombocytopenia.[95] Because more than 95% of the population express PAI-1, the finding that the mother is PAI-1 negative supports the diagnosis. In infants with alloimmune thrombocytopenia who require transfusions for significant hemorrhage, infusing the mother's platelets can be diagnostic as well

as therapeutic. Because most people express PAI-1 on their platelets, transfusions of random-donor platelets usually does not result in a significant increase in the platelet count. In contrast, because the mother's platelets do not express the target antigen, they survive normally in the infant's circulation and produce a sustained increase in the platelet count. It is important to establish the diagnosis of alloimmune thrombocytopenia because subsequent pregnancies are at high risk of severe hemorrhage. Bussel and associates[12] have shown that maternal treatment with intravenous gamma globulin markedly improves the infant's platelet count. We recommend gamma globulin and random-donor platelet concentrates for cases of severe bleeding in which maternal platelets are not available. Because alloimmune thrombocytopenia is associated with a considerable risk of severe perinatal hemorrhage, close fetal monitoring, intrauterine platelet transductions, and elective caesarean delivery are indicated in certain infants.

Giant Hemangioma (Kasabach-Merritt Syndrome)

Neonatal thrombocytopenia may be caused by platelet consumption within congenital hemangiomas. Large hemangiomas may occur anywhere in the body and are typically associated with either thrombocytopenia (low flow rate hemangiomas) or arteriovenous shunting and congestive heart failure (high flow rate hemangiomas). An important consideration is that hemangiomas frequently enlarge during the first few months of life. Sluggish blood flow through hemangiomas is thought to predispose to activation of the coagulation system with consumption of platelets and fibrinogen. Infants with hemangiomas may appear well until the sudden onset of local hemorrhage. Bleeding is frequently accompanied by acute enlargement of the hemangioma and by petechiae around the lesion and elsewhere on the body. Laboratory evaluation reveals an acute decrease in the platelet count and may show prolongation of the PT and PTT, hypofibrinogenemia, and an increase in the level of fibrin degradation products (including D-dimers). Giant platelets and red blood cell fragments are common on the blood smear. Treatment must be individualized. In general, a trial of corticosteroids is reasonable in symptomatic babies in that it is rarely associated with significant morbidity. Radiation should be used only as a last resort.

Thrombocytopenia Resulting From Impaired Platelet Production

Neonatal thrombocytopenia is occasionally due to a primary disorder of marrow platelet production. These problems are rare and are discussed briefly as a group. Parental consanguinity should be excluded, and specific history should be sought regarding first-degree relatives with congenital anomalies, childhood bleeding disorders, bone marrow failure, or leukemia. Anomalies of the radii are frequently associated with primary megakaryocytic hypoplasia in babies with the syndrome of thrombocytopenia and absence of the radii (TAR), trisomy 18, and Fanconi anemia. These infants may be small for gestational age and have associated anomalies. The Wiskott-Aldrich syndrome is an X-linked disorder characterized by eczema, immunodeficiency, and thrombocytopenia with small platelets. Affected boys may first come to medical attention because of neonatal hemorrhage. Laboratory evaluation of infants with primary defects of platelet production reveals a normal PT and PTT. Bone marrow examination shows rare megakaryocytes, which may appear dysplastic. Other diagnostic studies (e.g., cytogenetic analysis, immunologic evaluation, chromosomal breakage testing) are useful in selected cases. Platelet transfusions should be reserved for severe bleeding or surgical procedures because frequent exposures cause alloantibody formation.

Other Causes of Thrombocytopenia

Thrombocytopenia is common in high-risk infants. Prospective studies have shown that the incidence of thrombocytopenia is 30% to 40% in intensive care nurseries, with rates of more than 70% in babies who were clinically sick. Thrombocytopenia is an early sign of a number of nonhematologic conditions including sepsis, necrotizing enterocolitis, hyperviscosity, and renal vein thrombosis. Exchange transfusion with platelet-deficient blood, particularly packed red blood cells reconstituted in fresh frozen plasma, washes out the infant's platelets and

often causes thrombocytopenia. The likelihood of determining a specific hematologic cause increases as the platelet count decreases (Fig. 16–2). In light of these data, we first search for nonhematologic explanations for thrombocytopenia when the platelet count is greater than 50,000 per mm³ and then perform a limited number of laboratory tests. In infants who are otherwise well, the platelet count can be followed daily with an extensive workup reserved for infants with profound thrombocytopenia and for babies whose counts do not increase spontaneously. Finally, thrombocytopenia is common in infants with moderate and severe hemolysis caused by Rh incompatibility. This problem is discussed later in the chapter.

Platelet Transfusions

There are a number of special considerations involved in administering platelet transfusions in neonates. Matching donor

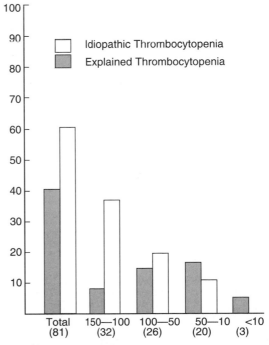

Figure 16–2. Numbers of neonates with thrombocytopenia (vertical axis) grouped by platelet counts (horizontal axis). The percentage of infants with an identifiable cause of thrombocytopenia increases as the platelet count decreases. (From Oski FA, Naiman JL, eds: Hematologic Problems in the Newborn. 3rd ed. Philadelphia: WB Saunders, 1982. Originally from Hathaway WE, Bonnar J: Perinatal Coagulation. New York: Grune and Stratton, 1978.)

and recipient for HLA, ABO, and Rh types is indicated in only a few circumstances. First, female Rh-negative infants should be transfused with Rh-negative platelets or should be given intramuscular Rh immunoglobulin (Rhogam) around the time of transfusion to prevent sensitization. Second, babies with disorders characterized by megakaryocytic hypoplasia should receive HLA-matched platelets whenever possible to reduce alloantibody formation. Third, although the risks of transfusion-transmitted graft versus host disease are not well defined,[2] we routinely irradiate all transfusions in infants who are younger than 32 weeks' gestation. In general, transfusing 1 unit of platelets elevates the platelet count by 50,000 per mm³ per 5 kg of body weight in conditions not associated with accelerated peripheral destruction.

when both genes are inactivated, these disorders are rare in nonconsanguineous families. In contrast, because the genes encoding factors VIII and IX are located on the X chromosome, a single mutation causes the common inherited bleeding disorders hemophilia A and hemophilia B in affected male infants. Although most cases of hemophilia and of the autosomal dominant bleeding disorder von Willebrand disease (VWD) are diagnosed later in life, they may present in the neonatal period. We use the PT and PTT to screen infants with suspected bleeding, and we reserve the bleeding time and other studies for selected patients. In our experience, template bleeding times are difficult to perform and interpret in neonates. The common entities are discussed in the following paragraphs, and salient clinical and laboratory findings are summarized in Table 16–5.

◆ BLEEDING IN INFANTS WITH NORMAL PLATELET COUNTS

The differential diagnosis of nonthrombocytopenic bleeding includes a number of acquired and inherited conditions. All of the coagulation proteins of the intrinsic, extrinsic, and common cascades except factors VIII and IX are encoded by autosomal genes. Mutant alleles are uncommon in the general population. Because clinically significant neonatal hemorrhagic disease results only

Hemorrhagic Disease of the Newborn (Vitamin K Deficiency)

Vitamin K acts on the precursors of factors II (thrombin), VII, IX, and X to generate active procoagulants. Its biochemical function involves creating calcium-binding sites in these proteins by carboxylating specific glutamic acid residues. The anticoagulant protein C is also a vitamin K–dependent factor. Neonates normally have low levels of the precursor proteins at birth. In addition, pro-

Table 16–5. Conditions Associated With Bleeding and Normal Platelet Count

Diagnosis	Appearance	PT	PTT	Other Useful Tests
Hemorrhagic disease of newborn	Well	↑	↑	Fibrinogen; fibrin degradation products
Hepatic disease	Sick	↑	↑	Albumin; fibrinogen; fibrin degradation products; liver function tests
von Willebrand disease*	Well	Normal	Normal or ↑	Bleeding time (see text)
Hemophilia	Well	Normal	↑	Mixing tests; factor VIII and IX assays
Factor XIII deficiency	Well	Normal	Normal	Urea clot solubility
Afibrinogenemia	Well	↑	↑	Fibrinogen, fibrin degradation products; thrombin time
Disorders of platelet function*	Well	Normal	Normal	Bleeding time, platelet aggregometry

*Some patients with these disorders show mild to moderate thrombocytopenia (see text for details).
PT, prothrombin time; PTT, partial thromboplastin time.

gressive prolongation of the PT and PTT develop during the first week of life if the infants are not given vitamin K. Because it is common practice to routinely administer parenteral vitamin K after birth, hemorrhagic disease of the newborn is a rare condition. It classically presents between the second and fifth day of life with oozing from the umbilicus, bleeding from circumcision and puncture sites, and gastrointestinal hemorrhage. Intracranial hemorrhage may also occur. Screening laboratory tests reveal a normal platelet count and an abnormal PT and PTT. The PT is often markedly prolonged compared with the PTT. Levels of fibrinogen and fibrin degradation products, and the thrombin time are all normal. For hemorrhages that are not life threatening, parenteral vitamin K can be used to rapidly correct the bleeding diathesis. Vitamin K works within a few hours because it generates active procoagulants from the precursors with no requirement for new protein synthesis. Fresh frozen plasma should be given to stop severe bleeding. A number of special considerations apply to the high-risk newborn. Infants born to mothers who are receiving hydantoin anticonvulsants are also at increased risk for hemorrhage and may benefit from additional doses of vitamin K. Vitamin K production by bacteria in the gut is reduced by illnesses that require enteral feedings be delayed or interrupted. Treatment with broad-spectrum antibiotics also decreases vitamin K synthesis. For these reasons, we routinely administer weekly vitamin K to babies who are not being fed and to those who are being treated with parenteral antibiotics. Infants with cystic fibrosis, biliary atresia, and other diseases characterized by gastrointestinal malabsorption are at risk of development of "late" vitamin K deficiency weeks to months after receiving parenteral vitamin K at birth. Intracranial hemorrhage associated with vitamin K deficiency has also been described in 2- to 3-month-old Asian infants who are exclusively breast-fed.[16] For a succinct discussion of the clinical and biochemical features of neonatal vitamin K deficiency, refer to the review of Lane and Hathaway.[54]

Liver Disease

Intrinsic or acquired liver disease may be associated with bleeding that results from impaired production of coagulation proteins. Screening laboratory tests reveal a normal platelet count with a prolonged PT and PTT. In contrast to vitamin K deficiency, the fibrinogen is reduced because of a generalized impairment of hepatic protein synthesis. The diagnosis is also supported by a low serum albumin and by abnormal liver function studies. Severe bleeding is best treated with fresh frozen plasma. Cryoprecipitate is indicated for patients with severely reduced fibrinogen levels. Because the hemostatic disorder is a result of global hepatic dysfunction, the overall aim is to identify and reverse the underlying condition.

The Hemophilias

Hemophilia A and hemophilia B are X-linked bleeding disorders caused by congenital deficiencies of proteins in the intrinsic coagulation cascade. Hemophilia A (or classic hemophilia) is due to a deficiency of factor VIII and accounts for 85% of cases. Hemophilia B (Christmas disease) results from absence or decrease of factor IX activity and is responsible for the remaining 15%. Hemophilia A and hemophilia B are clinically indistinguishable. The percentage of factor VIII or IX coagulant activity is used to classify the hemophilias as severe (<2%), moderate (2% to 5%), or mild (5% to 15%). Even though a positive family history is helpful in making the diagnosis, new mutations account for about one third of all cases of factor VIII deficiency. The bleeding symptoms in infants with hemophilia range between mild and catastrophic. Approximately 50% of patients with severe hemophilia bleed excessively following circumcisions. Other cases present with severe visceral (particularly intracranial) hemorrhage after difficult vaginal deliveries. These infants may be acutely ill from hypovolemia or local hemorrhage into vital organs. Laboratory evaluation reveals a normal platelet count and PT with marked prolongation of the PTT (to greater than 100 seconds in severe cases). Specific assays for factors VIII and IX quickly confirm the diagnosis, but these are not available in all laboratories. When hemophilia is suspected in a male infant with a prolonged PTT and factor assays are not immediately available, other studies are helpful. The PTT should be repeated using a 50:50 mix of patient and normal plasma. In hemophilia, the PTT corrects to normal. Even small clinical laboratories often have a stock of factor VIII–deficient plasma. If the PTT corrects with normal plasma, the mixing study is repeated with this factor VIII–deficient plasma. If the PTT corrects to normal, hemophilia A is excluded and hemophilia B is the likely diagnosis. If the PTT does not correct to normal, factor VIII deficiency is the presumptive diagnosis.

Lyophilized concentrates of factor VIII or factor IX have been the mainstay for treating bleeding in patients with hemophilia. In the early 1980s, use of these concentrates was associated with a high incidence of transfusion-transmitted human immunodeficiency virus (HIV) infection. Routine heating of factor concentrates in the manufacturing process has apparently eliminated this problem. Factor VIII and IX peptides with procoagulant activity have been produced in vitro using recombinant DNA technology. These recombinant products are the treatment of choice for neonates with hemophilia who require therapy. The dose of factor VIII or IX used to treat hemorrhagic complications depends on the severity of the bleeding. Life-threatening hemorrhages in infants with hemophilia A should be treated with an initial dose of factor VIII concentrate of 50 U/kg followed either by a continuous infusion of 8 to 10 U/h or by boluses of 50 U/kg every 8 hours. Babies with hemophilia B who have severe bleeding are given a bolus of 75 to 100 U of factor IX concentrate followed either by a continuous infusion starting at 5 U/kg/h or by bolus doses given every 12 hours. Lower doses are recommended for less severe bleeding.[57] Inhibitors are rare in neonates. The duration of replacement therapy is based on the location and extent of the bleeding, and on the clinical response of the patient. Less severe hemorrhages (such as those that typically follow circumcision) often resolve after application of pressure to the wound or may require a single bolus doses of 10 to 25 U/kg factor VIII concentrate or 15 to 30 U/kg of factor IX concentrate. Replacement therapy is not indicated for infants with hemophilia who are not bleeding unless they require surgery. Cryoprecipitate contains factor VIII but not factor IX and can, therefore, be used to treat bleeding complications in hemophilia A. One unit of cryoprecipitate per 5 kg of body weight increases the factor VIII level by about 40%. Recommended doses of factor

concentrates and cryoprecipitate are summarized in Table 16–4.

von Willebrand Disease

Although VWD is probably the most common inherited bleeding disorder, it is rarely diagnosed in the nursery. The von Willebrand factor (VWF) is the product of an autosomal gene, and the common form of VWD is transmitted as a dominant condition. VWF plays a central role in hemostasis by promoting platelet adherence to the vascular endothelium, a reaction mediated through a specific receptor on the platelet called GP Ib. VWF is stored in platelet granules and is also released from the endothelial cell lining of the injured vessel. VWF circulates as high-, intermediate-, and low-molecular-weight complexes called multimers. In addition to its role in platelet adherence, VWF associates with and stabilizes factor VIII. This, in turn, delivers factor VIII to sites of vascular injury. Whereas there is extraordinary clinical heterogeneity in the common, autosomal dominant type of VWD, hemorrhage typically occurs in the skin and mucosal surfaces. Screening tests usually reveal a normal PT and platelet count, although some patients have mild thrombocytopenia. The PTT is either normal or mildly prolonged. Laboratory investigation of affected adults in the family is a good initial step in evaluating infants suspected of having VWD. The results may be used to determine the best test (or tests) for the baby. However, even this approach has pitfalls, particularly because pregnancy markedly alters VWF levels, rendering evaluation of the mother unreliable. Some plasma-derived factor VIII concentrates are manufactured so that they also contain VWF. These products are an excellent treatment for bleeding complications in neonates with VWD. Cryoprecipitate is another effective therapy for treating hemorrhage in infants with a family history of VWD. Most lyophilized factor VIII concentrates do not contain significant amounts of VWF and are ineffective. Circumcision should not be performed if a parent has VWD. In the absence of significant bleeding, we routinely defer the laboratory workup of infants with a family history of VWD until after 6 months of age.

The autosomal recessive form of VWD is a much rarer condition. Affected infants have a severe bleeding disorder caused by a combination of profoundly abnormal platelet function and low factor VIII levels, and they require regular treatment with cryoprecipitate or with an appropriate concentrate.

Disorders of Platelet Function

Inherited disorders of platelet function are rare. In general, they present with petechiae, purpura, and bleeding from puncture sites, circumcisions, and umbilical cord. Because these disorders are uncommon and are often inherited as autosomal recessive conditions, a history of consanguinity is especially important. The PT and PTT are normal. In some disorders (e.g., the gray platelet syndrome, Bernard-Soulier syndrome), there is mild thrombocytopenia and the platelets are morphologically abnormal. Careful examination of the blood smear is therefore mandatory whenever an inherited disorder of platelet function is suspected. In certain diseases (e.g., Glanzmann thrombasthenia), both the platelet count and platelet appearance are normal. A hallmark of inherited disorders of platelet function is marked prolongation of the bleeding time. Studies of platelet aggregation in response to various stimuli, antibody staining for antigens expressed on the surface of the platelets, electron microscopy, and molecular analysis are all useful in selected cases. Transfusions of platelet concentrates are given for severe bleeding.

◆ THROMBOSIS

Despite prolongation of the PT and PTT well beyond the normal adult range, many experts in neonatal hematology believe that neonates should be viewed more as "hypercoagulable."[10] Indeed, thrombotic complications are more common in the neonatal period than at any other time during the first two decades of life and are receiving increased attention as more high-risk patients survive with invasive medical interventions. Why newborns suffer from a relatively high incidence of thrombosis is unknown; however, increased blood viscosity resulting from a high hematocrit at birth may play an important role. Polycythemia may partially account for why infants of diabetic mothers are at high risk of thrombosis. In addition,

the levels of protein C, a vitamin K–dependent serine protease, are low at birth.

Although thrombosis is a serious complication in high-risk infants, this problem has received relatively limited attention until recently. Investigators at McMaster University estimated that there was an incidence of clinically apparent thrombotic episodes of 2.4 per 1000 admissions to the neonatal intensive care unit on the basis of a multicenter survey of 97 cases.[83] Ninety percent of cases in their series were associated with indwelling catheters and included 21 infants with renal vein thrombosis, 39 with right atrial thrombosis or other major venous thromboses, and 33 with arterial thrombosis. Because severe thrombosis is relatively uncommon in neonates, there are almost no controlled data addressing the efficacy of thrombolytic or anticoagulant therapies.

Thrombosis Associated With Indwelling Catheters

Thromboembolic complications are clearly an important risk associated with the use of venous and arterial catheters. Although significant thrombosis has been reported in 1% of all infants who undergo umbilical artery catheterization, severe vascular obstruction by thrombus is rare, in our experience, as long as good technique is used in managing the catheter. However, the incidence of asymptomatic clot formation in the aorta is high. In one study, continuous infusion of heparin at a dose of 0.5 to 3.5 U/kg/h improved catheter patency, reduced the rate of thrombus formation, and decreased the incidence of hypertension.[43] It is uncertain whether higher doses of heparin provide any additional benefit or whether the incidence of intraventricular hemorrhage is higher with heparin administration.[43, 85] Damping of the arterial pressure wave tracing is a frequent early sign of catheter thrombosis. Blanching or cyanosis of a "downstream" anatomic area suggests obstruction. Ultrasonography is a useful, noninvasive initial test,[85, 94] and may be followed by arteriography in severe cases. The involved segment may include only the tip of a toe, or it may encompass an entire extremity or even half of the body. Hypertension is common because there is reduced renal blood flow. Umbilical venous catheters may lead to thrombi in the portal circulation or in the inferior vena cava, depending on the location of the catheter (Appendix I–2). Portal hypertension is a late complication of thrombosis in the portal system. Management of severe thrombosis should be individualized. Systemic heparinization, treatment with fibrinolytic agents, and thrombectomy have all been used.[43, 83, 85] In infants without evidence of major vessel obstruction, removing the catheter is often followed by resolution of symptoms.

Protein C Deficiency

Severe protein C deficiency is a recessive disorder associated with catastrophic thrombosis and necrosis of dependent tissues, consumption of coagulation factors, and DIC.[27, 63] A history of consanguinity or of thrombotic disease in multiple adult relatives may be elicited. Infants with severe protein C deficiency are severely ill with "purpura fulminans"—diffuse tissue infarction with secondary hemorrhage particularly in the skin. The PT and PTT are prolonged, the platelet count and fibrinogen are reduced, and there is an elevated level of fibrin degradation products. An important diagnostic clue that helps distinguish protein C deficiency from DIC is its propensity to be associated with prominent areas of segmental tissue infarction. Even though the diagnosis is strongly supported by demonstrating profoundly reduced levels of protein C, Manco-Johnson and coworkers[60] observed transient reductions in some infants, which later improved. Their data emphasize the importance of parental blood studies and of serial testing to confirm the diagnosis. Treatment may initially include exchange transfusions, infusions of fresh frozen plasma at a dose of 10 to 15 mL/kg every 12 hours to raise the protein C level and replenish consumed coagulation factors, and heparinization.[63] Warfarin is preferred for long-term management.[63]

Factor V Leiden

A missense mutation in the factor V gene was first associated with resistance to the action of activated protein C in adults with venous thrombosis. This allele encodes a molecule called factor V Leiden, which is relatively insensitive to inactivation by pro-

tein C and is most prevalent in Northern European populations. Individuals who are heterozygous for the factor V Leiden mutation show a 5- to 10-fold increase in the incidence of venous thrombosis as young adults, and homozygotes are at very high risk. Recent studies addressing the role of factor V Leiden in pediatric patients with thrombosis have shown a higher-than-expected incidence of the mutant allele in affected patients.[39, 71] In one study, the strongest association was seen in infants with arterial thrombotic events involving the central nervous system.[39]

Evaluation of Infants With Thrombosis

In general, thrombosis appears to be both underdiagnosed and undertreated in neonates. Symptoms and signs are highly variable and depend on the location and severity of the thrombotic process. In addition to the high percentage of patients with indwelling catheters, thrombosis often occurs in the context of systemic infection. A constellation of hematuria, abdominal mass, and thrombocytopenia is observed in many infants with renal vein thrombosis. Although the PT, PTT, and platelet count should all be measured, these are frequently unremarkable in infants with thrombosis. The mother should be screened for the presence of antiphospholipid antibodies (lupus anticoagulant) because these may be associated with neonatal thrombosis. In addition, studies should be performed to exclude hereditary conditions including the factor V Leiden mutation and deficiencies of antithrombin III, protein C, and protein S. With the exception of DNA analysis for the factor V Leiden mutation, all of these tests may be unreliable in the setting of acute thrombosis. For this reason, we suggest that parents be screened initially with follow-up testing performed on the infant as indicated. Even though contrast angiography is the most definitive modality for demonstrating thrombi, Doppler ultrasonography is preferred by most clinicians because it can be performed at the bedside.[83] Prospective studies have not been reported comparing the sensitivity of contrast angiography and Doppler ultrasonography in infants with thrombosis. We believe that it is imperative to use imaging studies to evaluate clinically significant thrombotic events because this assists in therapeutic decision making and provides a baseline for clinical follow-up. Infants should not be exposed to the risks of systemic anticoagulant therapy unless thrombosis is well documented.

Anticoagulant and Fibrinolytic Therapy

The paucity of controlled data and the clinical heterogeneity seen in newborns with thrombosis preclude definitive recommendations regarding which infants are likely to benefit from treatment and which agents, doses, and schedule should be used. The following discussion describes the guidelines and therapeutic agents for such therapy. The Children's Thrombophilia Network (1-800-NO-CLOTS) offers telephone advice on managing infants and children with thrombosis. Even though it is very useful, we believe that the optimal use of this service is in combination with on-site pediatric hematology consultation. In order to exclude intracranial hemorrhage or hemorrhagic infarction, it is essential that central nervous system imaging be performed before administering systemic anticoagulant or thrombolytic therapy in the neonatal intensive care unit.

Heparin is the mainstay of anticoagulant therapy for infants with acute thrombosis. McDonald and Hathaway[66] studied continuous heparin infusions in 15 infants with significant thrombosis. They achieved plasma heparin levels in the therapeutic range at doses from 16 to 27 U/kg/h and found that infants who had large thrombi showed the most rapid clearance. Because of the very wide range of normal PTT values, the authors followed micro whole blood clotting times to monitor heparin effect. We recommend that initial heparin therapy consist of a loading dose of 50 U/kg followed by a continuous infusion at 20 U/kg/h. Heparin should be continued for at least 7 days in infants with significant thrombosis.

Low-molecular-weight heparin (LMWH) products have been thoroughly tested in adults with a variety of thrombotic disorders.[42] Advantages of these agents include having a longer plasma half-life than standard heparin, which permits subcutaneous dosing, and having less variability in anticoagulant effects between individual patients. Given the difficulties of administering and

monitoring heparin in neonates, these drugs appear to offer considerable theoretic advantages over standard heparin in managing thrombosis in the neonatal intensive care unit. There are important differences in the biochemical mechanisms of action of heparin and LMWH. In particular, while heparin markedly accelerates the rate of thrombin inactivation through its ability to form a stable ternary complex that includes antithrombin III and thrombin, the major anticoagulant effect of LMWH is mediated through antithrombin III–mediated destruction of activated factor X. The PTT is therefore not a useful test for measuring the anticoagulant effects of LMWH, which can be monitored by following anti–factor Xa levels. Studies have begun to elucidate optimal dosing for neonates. In a series that included 7 infants and 18 older children, Massicotte and colleagues[64] found that infants required higher doses of enoxaparin per kilogram to achieve therapeutic anti–factor Xa levels than older children. In a much larger study examining 147 courses of enoxaparin in pediatric patients, the same group reported clinical resolution of thromboembolic events in 84% of patients.[31] Randomized controlled trials comparing standard heparin with LMWH in pediatric patients are planned.

Warfarin is a competitive inhibitor of vitamin K and therefore depresses the levels of active procoagulant factors II, VII, IX, and X and of the anticoagulant proteins C and S.[96] Warfarin is not an appropriate treatment for acute thrombosis, but it may be instituted later and be used as long-term therapy in some infants with ongoing hypercoagulable disorders. There is little published experience using warfarin in neonates, and dosing is problematic given the rapid rate in growth and dietary changes that occur during the first few months of life.

The fibrinolytic agents urokinase, streptolysin, and tissue plasminogen activator are used in the acute management of certain types of vascular occlusion in adults.[62] Although these compounds might also prove beneficial for neonatal vascular occlusion, experience is limited. Clot formation in indwelling lines that are essential for patient care and thrombotic occlusions involving an extremity are potential indications in high-risk infants. An initial urokinase dose of 4400 U/kg over 20 minutes followed by a continuous infusion at a rate of 4400 U/kg/h has been suggested.[84] Laboratory responses include a decrease in the fibrinogen level and an increase in D-dimers. A hematologist with experience in managing neonatal thrombosis should be consulted when fibrinolytic treatment is considered.

◆ WHITE BLOOD CELLS

The blood leukocytes include myeloid and lymphoid cells. Because they are derived from distinct populations of immature hematopoietic progenitors, differ in their morphology and function, and respond to different endogenous and exogenous stimuli, it is logical to discuss them separately. However, nonlymphoid and lymphoid cells cooperate in generating many types of immunologic responses. For example, intracellular processing and presentation of specific antigens by monocytes is essential before lymphocytes are able to recognize and respond to many infections. High-risk newborns, especially those born prematurely, are immunologically immature. Defects exist in both lymphocyte and phagocyte function. Granulocyte production in response to severe bacterial infections and the generation of specific antibodies by lymphocytes are impaired. For this reason, infants are highly susceptible to severe viral and bacterial infections and may not manifest clinical signs of infection typical of older patients. An important aspect of neonatal leukocyte counts is that some normal values differ markedly from those in older children and adults, and they change dramatically over time. This is particularly true of neutrophil counts during the first few days of life. Appendices C–6 and C–7[61] depict the normal ranges of total and immature (band forms) neutrophil counts as a function of time after birth. These data emphasize that knowing the age of the infant at the time a white blood cell count is obtained is essential in interpreting the results.

Blood Cell Production

The amount of time blood cells remain in the circulation ranges from a few hours for granulocytes to about 10 days for platelets to years for some types of lymphocytes. As a result of this "planned obsolescence," hematopoietic tissues must continuously produce new blood cells to maintain stable circulating numbers. Experience in patients undergoing bone marrow transplantation has conclusively established that all of the mature blood elements are derived from hematopoietic stem cells capable of amplification, differentiation, and self-renewal. The most immature stem cells become lymphoid or myeloid progenitors in response to signals, which remain poorly defined. Hematopoietic progenitors are identified by their ability to form distinctive in vitro colonies in specialized culture systems.[33, 38] The most immature nonlymphoid progenitor is the colony-forming unit (CFU)–granulocyte, erythroid, megakaryocyte, monocyte (GEMM). As its name indicates, CFU-GEMM gives rise to colonies that contain a mixture of four cell types. Progenitors become more restricted as they mature in the bone marrow. In the myeloid series, the CFU–granulocyte, monocyte (CFU-GM) differentiates into progenitors committed to become either monocytes or macrophages (CFU-M) or granulocytes (CFU-G). Late progenitors of the myeloid, erythroid, and megakaryocytic lineages mature into identifiable precursors in the bone marrow. These cells undergo terminal differentiation within the marrow and are ultimately released into the circulation. Developmental pathways for lymphoid progenitors are not restricted to the bone marrow. For example, the thymus plays a crucial role in the functional maturation of cellular immune responses mediated by T lymphocytes. Figure 16–3 presents a simplified overview of hematopoietic cell development beginning with the earliest stem cell and proceeding forward to the progenitor, precursor, and mature effector cell compartments.

Recombinant Hematopoietic Growth Factors

The development of culture systems supporting the growth of colonies derived from different classes of hematopoietic progenitors has facilitated the isolation, characterization, and molecular cloning of a number of proteins essential for the growth of certain types of colonies.[38] Complementary DNA molecules encoding some of these hematopoietic growth factors have been inserted into expression vectors to facilitate large-scale production in mammalian cell lines. Therapeutic quantities of many hematopoietic growth factors are available for

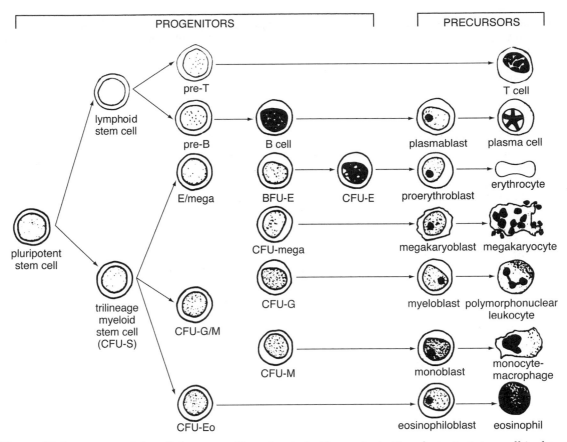

Figure 16–3. Overview of the cellular stages of hematopoiesis. The most primitive pluripotent stem cell is shown at the far left. As they differentiate, hematopoietic progenitor cells become committed to a single lineage. This diagram does not emphasize the large increase in the number of cells (amplification) which occurs in the progenitor and precursor compartments. (From Lipton JW, Nathan DG: The anatomy and physiology of hematopoiesis. In Nathan DG, Oski FA, eds: Hematology of Infancy and Childhood. 3rd ed. Philadelphia: WB Saunders, 1987.)

clinical trials. These growth factors include proteins that predominantly act on cells committed to a single lineage (e.g., monocyte-CSF [M-CSF], granulocyte-CSF [G-CSF], erythropoietin, and thrombopoietin) as well as on those that act on more immature progenitors (e.g., granulocyte, monocyte-CSF [GM-CSF], interleukin-3 [IL-3], and interleukin-11 (IL-11). Hematopoietic growth factors are important to clinicians because of their potential therapeutic application in a number of disorders.[38] Premature and other high-risk infants are a particularly interesting patient population in that functional immaturity of the cells that normally release hematopoietic growth factors may be important in the pathogenesis of many hematologic problems encountered in the neonatal period. The role of impaired erythropoietin production in the anemia of prematurity (see Red Blood Cells) illustrates this concept. In addition, several small pilot studies have been conducted to evaluate the safety and potential efficacy of recombinant G-CSF and GM-CSF for treatment of neonatal sepsis. These studies are discussed later as acquired causes of neutropenia.

Low Neutrophil Counts (Neutropenia)

Neutropenia may result from impaired bone marrow production of granulocytes, from increased peripheral destruction of mature cells, or from an abnormal distribution of neutrophils resulting from excessive margination or an increase in the size of the storage pool. Impaired production is a major factor in most cases of neutropenia encountered in high-risk neonates. Infants with inadequate neutrophil production either have intrinsic abnormalities of their progenitors or of the marrow microenvironment (primary neutropenias) or are neutropenic in response to exogenous stress. Although neutropenia is relatively common in high-risk newborns,[3, 61] the primary neutropenias are rare. Certain physiologic features of myelopoiesis suggest why neonates might develop neutropenia in a variety of clinical settings. Neutrophil counts increase during the third trimester. This increase necessitates vigorous myelopoiesis because it is accomplished while the body weight (and blood volume) is expanding rapidly. It is not surprising then that a high proportion of CFU-GM are actively synthesizing DNA.[19] One potentially deleterious consequence of this high proliferative rate is a reduction in the number of quiescent myeloid progenitors available to respond to infection or other stress. Even though this aspect of neonatal myelopoiesis might partially explain the propensity for neonates to become neutropenic, there is no direct evidence that the number of CFU-GM is limiting. Furthermore, several studies both in humans and animal models have indicated that neonatal progenitors are equally responsive to cytokines.[41, 82, 87, 99] However, immature immune responses that result in either reduced growth factor production of cytokines that enhance granulocyte production[56, 82] or increased production of proinflammatory cytokines observed in patients in septic shock may be important in the acquired neutropenia observed in septic newborns.[55, 100]

Conditions associated with acquired neutropenia in the high-risk newborn are listed in Table 16–6. Neutropenia is common in neonatal infection.[3] In a prospective study of 119 infants with neutropenia, 73 (40%) had infections. Neutropenia was particularly likely in infants with necrotizing enterocolitis.[81] The finding that more than 20% of the neutrophils are immature forms (bands and myelocytes) is especially suggestive of severe infection in neutropenic infants. In severe infection, the total neutrophil count is frequently depressed for about

Table 16–6. Conditions Associated With Acquired Neonatal Neutropenia

Infection
Intrauterine growth retardation caused by severe preeclampsia
Hemolysis caused by Rh incompatibility
Neonatal alloimmune neutropenia

Table 16–7. Primary Causes of Neonatal Neutropenia

Severe congenital neutropenia (Kostmann agranulocytosis)
Familial benign neutropenia
Cyclic neutropenia
Cartilage/hair hypoplasia
Reticular dysgenesis
Congenital neutropenia with humoral immunodeficiency

24 hours, and then it increases rapidly. The onset of neutrophilia may be a helpful confirmatory finding in infants suspected of infection. As discussed in Chapter 13, neonatal bacterial infections are associated with substantial morbidity and mortality and therefore require aggressive treatment. Maternal hypertension and preeclampsia are also important causes of neutropenia. Neutropenia in the infants of hypertensive mothers is due to decreased production and is more severe in infants delivered prematurely and in those with intrauterine growth retardation.[52] Immune-mediated neutropenia is rare but should be considered if both mother and infant have low granulocyte counts.

Neonatal neutropenia may also be caused by intrinsic diseases of the bone marrow. These primary neutropenias are listed in Table 16–7. All are rare; refer to detailed information and literature citations for further information.[24, 46] When the known causes of acquired neutropenia are excluded or considered unlikely, evaluation should include a family history, physical examination, and diagnostic studies on the baby and parents. A history of parental consanguinity suggests the possibility of severe congenital neutropenia (Kostmann agranulocytosis). Detecting neutropenia in either parent may indicate familial benign neutropenia or cyclic neutropenia. The baby should be examined for evidence of cartilage or hair hypoplasia and other abnormalities. Bone marrow examination is an essential part of the workup and should ideally include assessment of in vitro CFU-GM colony formation in cultures stimulated with G-CSF, GM-CSF, and other hematopoietic growth factors. Bone marrow smears generally have normal cellularity with a characteristic arrest at the promyelocyte-myelocyte stage of differentiation. Until recently, the diagnosis of Kostmann agranulocytosis carried a dismal prognosis without bone marrow transplantation. However, patients may respond dramatically to treatment with G-CSF.[7] Similarly, early results suggest that G-CSF therapy is highly effective in children with cyclic neutropenia who suffer from recurrent infections. Recent data indicate that mutations in the ELA2 gene cause most cases of severe congenital neutropenia and cyclic neutropenia.[44] Because the clinical experience with G-CSF and other recombinant growth factors is limited and because these patients may be predisposed to the acquisition of myelodysplasia or leukemia, a hematologist familiar with their use should be consulted before initiating treatment.

Treatment of Acquired Neutropenia

Any discussion of treatment for acquired neutropenia must distinguish two groups of patients: those who are infected and those who are not. A number of clinical trials in the 1980s examined the efficacy of leukocyte transfusions in neutropenic neonates with evidence of bacterial sepsis. The rationale for granulocyte transfusions is based on the historically high mortality rate in such patients and on evidence that neutrophil storage pools may be exhausted.[18] Cairo[14] reviewed the results of clinical trials that administered granulocyte transfusions to neonates with suspected sepsis. The data are inconsistent, with three of five trials showing improved outcomes among babies who were transfused, and two others demonstrating no benefit. These five studies differ in some important respects, including inclusion criteria and the method used to collect leukocytes for transfusion. Granulocyte transfusions may transmit cytomegalovirus or other pathogens. Furthermore, most studies that examined the efficacy of granulocytes were conducted before the availability of recombinant cytokines.

The recombinant growth factors G-CSF and GM-CSF represent potential new therapies for newborns with sepsis and neutropenia. Several small clinical trials to evaluate the pharmacokinetics and safety of administration of these molecules have been conducted.[15, 36, 53, 81] It is intriguing that some septic neonates show a sustained elevation in the neutrophil count after a single granulocyte transfusion. This is in contrast to cancer patients with chemotherapy-induced myelosuppression who never demonstrate a significant increase in peripheral blood neutrophil counts after leukocyte transfusions and suggests that many newborns with sepsis retain myeloid progenitors that might respond to growth factors. In the limited number of patients that have been studied, no serious side effects have been observed. However, no study conducted to date has had sufficient power to ascertain whether these drugs will reduce the mortality rate associated with sepsis.

The risk of acquired infection in healthy neutropenic neonates is unknown. In their study of 119 consecutive babies with neutropenia, Baley et al[3] found increased short-term mortality rates only among infants with absolute neutrophil counts of less than 500/mm³. Many of these babies were not known to have neutropenia before signs of infection developed. Koenig and Christensen[52] observed a 23% risk of nosocomial infection, but no deaths, among 35 infants whose neutropenia was associated with maternal hypertension. Two subsequent studies have confirmed these observations.[13, 32] The neutropenia is associated with a decreased production of leukocytes based on the reduction in the absolute number of progenitors isolated and the number of progenitors that are proliferating. The etiology for the reduced production is not clear. However, these studies emphasize the importance of diagnosis and prompt treatment of neutropenic infants in whom signs suggestive of infection develop. Whether prophylactic treatment with G-CSF or GM-CSF might decrease infections in healthy neonates with neutropenia is unknown; multicenter trials using either GM-CSF or G-CSF are in progress.

Elevated Neutrophil Counts

Like neutropenia, neonatal granulocytosis is rarely due to intrinsic disorders of the marrow. As noted in the section on thrombocytopenia, neonatal leukemia and the transient myeloproliferative disorder seen in infants with trisomy 21 are usually associated with large numbers of circulating immature myeloid cells and with hepatosplenomegaly. The diagnosis is established by bone marrow examination, which should include cytogenetic analysis of unstimulated marrow. The most common identifiable cause of neonatal neutrophilia is infection. Birth asphyxia and other causes of acute or chronic hypoxia can induce the marrow to prematurely release immature myeloid and erythroid cells into the circulation. Nucleated erythrocytes are "seen" by electronic cell counters as leukocytes, so it is important to correct for the presence of nucleated red blood cells when interpreting the white blood cell count.

Disorders of Neutrophil Function

These uncommon disorders rarely present in the newborn period unless there is a strong family history of the disease or morphologic abnormalities of the neutrophils. Because the neonatal immune system is functionally immature, organisms that are generally not pathogenic after the neonatal period cause infections in normal newborns. In addition, the invasive nature of modern neonatal intensive care compromises the integrity of mucosal and dermal barriers. Finally, immunologically normal infants who receive multiple courses of broad-spectrum antibiotics are at risk for invasive infections with opportunistic pathogens. For all of these reasons, it is difficult to identify the rare infant in whom infection is due to an inherited defect in neutrophil function. Chronic granulomatous disease (CGD) is the most common inherited disorder of leukocyte function. Most cases are X-linked; the remaining are autosomal recessive. The "oxidative burst" is defective in the leukocytes

of patients with CGD.[69] This results in impaired hydrogen peroxide production and in inefficient intracellular killing of phagocytized organisms. CGD neutrophils are unable to reduce the dye nitroblue tetrazolium. The genes responsible for CGD have been cloned so the precise molecular lesion can be determined in many families. Many patients improve clinically when treated with recombinant gamma interferon.[46] The other disorders of neutrophil function are rare.

Disorders of Lymphocytes

Lymphoid immune responses are poorly developed at term and are severely impaired in premature babies. Immaturity of cellular immune responses mediated by T lymphocytes renders neonates susceptible to certain invasive viral infections, particularly those caused by herpes viruses. B lymphocytes are functionally immature, and infants rely on transplacental transfer of maternal IgG for protection against many pathogens. Because little IgG crosses the placenta until the third trimester, small premature infants have low levels of antibody. These low levels of antibody led to the hypothesis that intravenous gamma globulin might play a role in the prevention and treatment of neonatal infection.[51] Two large multicenter trials were conducted to determine whether administration of intravenous immunoglobulin would reduce the frequency of nosocomial sepsis in premature infants. The results of one trial suggested that the administration of the drug

Table 16–8. Features of Selected Congenital Immunodeficiency Disorders

Disorder	Type of Deficiency	Inheritance	Clinical Features
X-linked agammaglobulinemia (Bruton disease)	B cell	X linked	Recurrent bacterial sinopulmonary infections, diarrhea, otitis media
Wiskott-Aldrich syndrome	T cell	X linked	Severe eczema, thrombocytopenia with small platelets, recurrent infection with encapsulated bacteria
Ataxia-telangiectasia	T cell	Autosomal recessive	Telangiectasia, ataxia, recurrent sinopulmonary infection, malignancy
DiGeorge anomaly	T cell	Sporadic	Characteristic facial features include hypertelorism and ear anomalies; abnormalities of aortic arch and neonatal hypocalcemia common
Severe combined immunodeficiency	T and B cell	Autosomal recessive or X linked	Recurrent or chronic bacterial, viral, fungal, and protozoal infections; 30% of patients have adenosine deaminase deficiency

Adapted from Ammann AJ, Shannon KM: Pediatr Rev 7:101, 1985. Reproduced by permission of Pediatrics. Copyright 1985.

was efficacious, whereas the other trial did not. One potential limitation to the therapy may be the lot-to-lot variability of the drug.

Inherited deficiencies of lymphoid immunity that may present during the neonatal period are listed in Table 16–8. Circulating lymphopenia and the absence of a normal thymic shadow on chest radiographs are commonly seen in these disorders. Babies with abnormalities limited to B lymphocytes are usually protected from infections by maternal IgG until beyond the immediate neonatal period. In contrast, life-threatening infections can develop in infants with defects of T lymphocyte function, often within a few weeks of birth. Some inherited immunodeficiencies are diagnosed in the nursery because of associated nonimmunologic problems such as thrombocytopenia in boys with Wiskott-Aldrich syndrome or hypocalcemia and cardiac disease in the DiGeorge syndrome. The number of infants with congenital immunologic disorders is miniscule compared with the incidence of pediatric acquired immunodeficiency syndrome (AIDS). Pediatric AIDS is discussed in Chapter 13. Consultation with a pediatric immunologist should be obtained to order and interpret the results of functional and phenotypic studies of lymphoid immunity in babies suspected of immunodeficiency. In immunodeficient infants, graft versus host reactions can develop from small numbers of viable lymphocytes in transfused blood products. It is essential that infants suspected of immunodeficiency be recognized early in life so that they receive only irradiated blood products.

◆ RED BLOOD CELLS

Fetal Erythropoiesis

The fetus must sustain a high rate of red blood cell production to keep pace with rapid growth. Blood volume expands in proportion to weight gain, and the fetal intravascular space is much larger than that of the newborn infant because it includes the fetal placental circulation. This combined blood volume averages 115 mL/kg of fetal body weight at term and is even larger in the preterm fetus. At the same time that the blood volume is increasing, the hematocrit is increasing: from a mean of 40% at 28 weeks of gestation to 50% at term. This

places additional demands on fetal erythropoietic tissues. Elevated reticulocyte counts and the presence of circulating nucleated red blood cells at birth reflect active intra-uterine erythropoiesis. (See Appendices C–4 and C–5 for normal hematologic values in term and premature newborns.) At term, red blood cell production has largely shifted from the liver to the bone marrow.

Distribution of Blood at Birth and the Placental Transfusion

At the moment of birth, the partition of blood volume between the infant's body and the fetal placental vasculature is almost 2:1 (75 mL/kg body weight in the infant and 40 mL/kg body weight in the placenta). Unless the umbilical cord is clamped immediately, circulation continues through the umbilical arteries and vein, resulting in a net shift of blood from placenta to infant. This is called the placental transfusion and has a major effect on the blood volume, hematocrit, and hemoglobin concentration in the first days of life. In the first 30 seconds after birth, the infant gains about 14 mL/kg of blood, resulting in a blood volume of 89 mL/kg. Over the next several hours, the blood volume decreases to 83 mL/kg as a result of a decrease in plasma volume and the hematocrit increases proportionately. Infants who receive an excessive placental transfusion have a greater elevation in hematocrit. In contrast, in babies who receive little or no

Table 16–9. Processes Affecting Volume of Placenta-to-Infant Transfusion at Birth

Increase	Decrease
Late cord clamping	Early cord clamping
Baby >20 cm below mother before clamping	Baby >20 cm above mother before clamping
Forceful uterine contractions before clamping (spontaneous or secondary to oxytocin treatment)	Maternal hypotension
	Cesarean delivery
Prolonged asphyxia before delivery	Asphyxia within a few minutes before delivery
	Umbilical cord compression that occludes vein but not arteries

placental transfusion, plasma volume increases, raising total blood volume toward 83 mL/kg, and hematocrit decreases after birth. Table 16–9 lists factors that increase or decrease the placental transfusion. Postnatal adjustments of blood volume and hematocrit begin within 15 minutes after birth and, although largely complete within 2 hours, may continue for as long as 6 hours. Capillary hematocrits are consistently higher than simultaneous venous hematocrits; however, the correlation between the two is poor in sick infants.

Changes in Erythropoiesis After Birth

Erythropoietin levels decline rapidly and erythropoiesis almost ceases by the end of the first week of life (Fig. 16–4). This is accompanied by the expected changes in the bone marrow and peripheral blood. In the presence of a pathologic process, which re-

sults in a high level of fetal erythroid activity (such as intrauterine hemolytic anemia), the postnatal decline in erythropoiesis takes somewhat longer but proceeds even in the face of continued anemia. This low level of erythroid activity persists for more than a month and hematocrit gradually declines. When it approaches 30% late in the second or third month of life, the serum erythropoietin level increases and erythropoiesis resumes.

Thereafter, the red cell mass increases. However, because total blood volume increases in proportion to weight gain, the hematocrit does not increase a great deal. This process follows a different schedule in the preterm infant.

Data from animal species and humans indicate that fetal erythropoiesis is regulated by endogenous erythropoietin, which is produced in the liver.[86] Anephric fetuses have normal levels of erythropoietin in their plasma at birth.[97] When erythropoiesis recommences in infancy, the erythropoietin

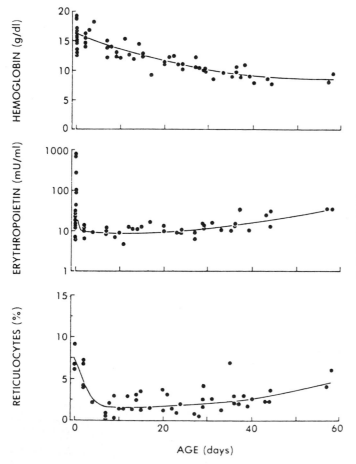

Figure 16–4. Developmental changes in hemoglobin, erythropoietin, and reticulocyte count in untransfused preterm infants from birth to 60 days of age. (From Brown MS, Phibbs RH, Garcia JF, et al: Postnatal changes in erythropoietin levels in untransfused premature infants. J Pediatr 103:612, 1983.)

comes mainly, if not exclusively, from the kidneys. There is a single erythropoietin gene in humans, and the nucleotide sequences of complementary DNA molecules isolated from fetal liver and adult kidney are identical.[33, 47]

Fetal and Adult Hemoglobin

At birth, more than 80% of the hemoglobin in the circulation is fetal hemoglobin, which is composed of two alpha and two gamma globin chains ($\alpha_2\gamma_2$). Adult hemoglobin is composed of two alpha and two beta globin chains ($\alpha_2\beta_2$). The switch from synthesis of mainly γ chains to mainly β chains and, therefore, from hemoglobin F to A begins around 34 weeks' gestation and continues into early infancy. When erythroid activity resumes in the second and third months of life, most of the new hemoglobin is A. There are some exceptions to this. For example, when the very preterm infant recovers from anemia of prematurity with the return of erythropoiesis, there is a transient period during which hemoglobin F is the predominant hemoglobin synthesized.

The most important functional difference between hemoglobins F and A is their different oxygen binding properties as shown in their respective oxygen dissociation curves (see Fig. 9–1). The higher oxygen affinity of hemoglobin F is advantageous in the fetus because oxygen uptake occurs in the placenta, producing an umbilical venous Po_2 of just 35 to 40 torr, which is the highest Po_2 in the fetal circulation. This left-shifted oxygen dissociation curve achieves a higher O_2 content in this situation, but it is no longer an advantage after birth because of the relatively high oxygen tension (usually >75 torr) in the pulmonary capillaries. Relatively high PaO_2 values can usually be maintained, even in the presence of severe lung disease, by oxygen and ventilator therapy. The disadvantage of the high oxygen affinity of hemoglobin F is that the Po_2 in the capillary blood must decrease to lower level before an equivalent amount of oxygen is released by hemoglobin F for tissue metabolism. These differences in oxygen affinity imply that a newborn suffering from cardiopulmonary disease might be better off with hemoglobin A than with F, and clinical studies tend to support this concept. Exchange transfusions that did not raise hematocrit but did replace hemoglobin F with hemoglobin A produced a substantial improvement in survival in extremely premature babies during the first days of life.[30, 37] Frequent phlebotomies for laboratory studies plus multiple small transfusions of packed red blood cells eventually have the same effect on the type of hemoglobin in the circulation of very low-birth-weight infants.

◆ ANEMIA

Hemorrhagic Anemias

The fetus may lose blood through a variety of routes. Hemorrhage commonly occurs through the placenta into the mother's circulation and may be detected by performing a Kleihauer-Betke test on the mother's blood. In monozygotic twin gestations, one fetus may hemorrhage through placental vascular anastomosis into the other (see Twin-to-Twin Transfusion Syndrome). The fetus may also bleed through the placenta into the birth canal. In many cases of placental abruption, the vaginal blood contains a mixture of fetal and maternal blood. The fetus may lose a large volume of blood into the fetal placental circulation at the time of birth by processes noted in Table 16–9. This has the same effect as hemorrhage. Some of these mechanisms of blood loss such as placental abruption and trapping of blood in the placenta by cord compression also produce asphyxia, and the coexistence of asphyxia with hypovolemia complicates both the assessment and the management of the infant. Even though most asphyxiated babies are not hypovolemic, there is a subset of infants who have lost blood volume around the time of delivery and most also suffered asphyxia.

Internal (particularly intracranial) hemorrhage may occur before delivery. The true incidence of antenatal intracranial bleeding is not known but the increased use of ultrasonography for fetal surveillance suggests that it is more common than had previously been appreciated. Internal hemorrhage can also occur around the time of delivery from birth trauma. Important locations include subgaleal hematomas, hepatic subcapsular hematomas, mediastinal hematomas, intracerebral and cerebellar hemorrhage, and hematomas in fractured limbs. Hemorrhages caused by trauma generally occur during difficult term deliveries, particularly in large for gestational age infants. Splenic rupture is uncommon but may lead to catastrophic intraabdominal hemorrhages in infants with hemophilia and in babies in whom intrauterine splenomegaly develops as a result of erythroblastosis or other causes. Extensive trauma to the perineum in breech deliveries can also produce hypovolemia and anemia, particularly in preterm infants.

The severity of anemia at birth depends on the interval between the hemorrhage and delivery. Because there is insufficient time for hemodilution, infants who suffer hemorrhages shortly before birth may not be anemic initially. These babies show clinical signs referable to hypovolemia and hematocrit decreases during the first hour after birth. An elevated reticulocyte count in response to anemia is seen only when the anemia has been present for days. However, hypoxia without anemia causes the release of erythropoietin and subsequent increase in nucleated red blood cells and reticulocyte counts in the peripheral blood.

Treatment of hemorrhagic anemias largely depends on the cardiorespiratory effects of the blood loss. The fetus has a virtually limitless reservoir of saline for volume replacement by way of the rapid transport of fluid across the placenta. If fetal blood loss occurs long enough before delivery to allow for this fluid replacement, the only concern becomes the reduced oxygen-carrying capacity from the anemia. This becomes important during labor because the anemic fetus may not tolerate the intermittent hypoxemia associated with uterine contractions. When infants with anemia are asphyxiated, partial correction of the anemia is an essential part of resuscitation. If the blood volume is judged to be low, a transfusion of 5 to 10 mL/kg of packed red blood cells can be given over 5 to 10 minutes and the response observed. This may need to be repeated several times. Elevating the hematocrit to the range of 30% to 40% provides adequate oxygen-carrying capacity. If there is concern that simple transfusions will induce volume overload, partial exchange transfusion with packed red blood cells can be performed to elevate the hematocrit without increasing blood volume. Depending on the severity of the anemia, the baby's blood volume and the hematocrit of the packed red blood cells used, an exchange of between 30 and 50 mL/kg body weight may be needed to elevate the hematocrit to the desired level.

More often, hemorrhage occurs acutely during delivery and the hematocrit does not fully reflect the degree of blood loss because there has been little hemodilution. Management in this situation requires aggressive treatment of shock with careful attention to cardiorespiratory parameters (arterial and central venous pressures, capillary filling time, and metabolic acidosis). As noted earlier, most babies with acute hypovolemic shock at birth have suffered intrapartum asphyxia and the findings of asphyxia can confound the assessment of shock. In this circumstance, the circulation must be reassessed and shock must be treated after asphyxia has been at least partially corrected. Immediate volume replacement with blood has been shown to be more effective than administration of crystalloid followed in a few hours with packed red blood cells.[74] Many cases can be anticipated by the presence of maternal vaginal bleeding, and type O, Rh-negative whole blood or packed cells cross-matched against the mother's should be available in the delivery room. Shock is treated with a series of infusions of 5 mL/kg of blood, each given over about 5 minutes. This treatment is repeated until signs of adequate circulation return. Severe cases require cumulative replacement in the range of 40 mL/kg.

Twin-to-Twin Transfusion Syndrome

The twin-to-twin transfusion syndrome can produce one polycythemic and one anemic twin. This occurs in monochorionic placenta twins in whom there may be vascular anastomosis between the circulations of the twins. These anastomoses may be arterial to arterial, venous to venous, or arterial to venous; the latter is thought to be responsible for most of the clinical cases.

Both the degree of transfusion from one into the other and the time course can be highly variable. Bleeding may have been relatively recent before delivery or it may begin in the second trimester and have been longstanding by the time the twins are delivered. Depending on the severity and time course, the clinical findings at birth are quite different. The donor twin becomes anemic and has increased erythropoiesis in response to blood loss. In some cases, there is even a dermal erythropoiesis. The recipient fetus becomes polycythemic. With ongoing significant bleeding, the recipient twin grows normally while the donor becomes progressively smaller for gestational age. As the process becomes more severe, polyhydramnios and ultimately, possibly, hydrops fetalis develops in the recipient. Oligohydramnios develops in the donor fetus. Myocardiopathy with poor ventricular function may develop in either twin. Hydrops may also occur in the donor fetus, but this is unusual. In severe cases, the growth-retarded twin may die and intravascular coagulation in the dead twin may lead to embolization through the vascular anastomoses into the surviving fetus. When embolization occurs, it commonly involves the brain and may also involve the kidneys and gastrointestinal tract. Recent embolization of the gastrointestinal tract may present as perforation, whereas old embolization may present as an atretic area of the bowel. When twins suffering from this syndrome are delivered, management during resuscitation may be extremely complicated. The pediatrician taking care of such babies is usually forewarned, however. Findings in the mother usually lead to close ultrasonic surveillance and prenatal recognition of twin-to-twin transfusion syndrome. The polycythemic baby needs the hematocrit reduced (see Polycythemia). Management of the anemic donor is less straightforward. For relatively recent blood loss, the management is the same as for any other type of hypovolemic anemia. However, *if* myocardiopathy has developed, the infant may not tolerate blood volume expansion. In this case, the proper therapy is partial exchange transfusion with packed cells to elevate the hematocrit to a normal level. One should be prepared to monitor both arterial and central venous pressures beginning immediately after birth in order to make the correct adjustments in both hematocrit and intravascular volume. Most often, these babies are born prematurely. When they are born relatively late in gestation and the anemia is not too severe, the anemic twin generally has fewer cardiopulmonary complications than the polycythemic twin.

In some monochorionic twin sets, there may be vascular anastomosis in the placenta and discordant intrauterine growth with oligohydramnios in the small-for-gestational-age infant and polyhydramnios in the appropriate-for-gestational-age infant, yet the hematocrits are near normal and similar in both twins, emphasizing the point that the pathophysiology of the twin-to-twin vascular anastomosis syndrome is not well understood.

Nonhemorrhagic Anemias

In comparison with older children, hyperbilirubinemia is far more common and more severe in neonates with hemolytic anemia. The bilirubin may increase rapidly in the first hours after birth. For this reason, diagnosing and treating the underlying cause is especially important. A family history of anemia or neonatal jaundice should be obtained, and both the baby and the blood smear should be examined. Because transplacental passage of maternal IgG alloantibodies against a paternal antigen expressed on the infant's erythrocytes accounts for most cases of hemolytic anemia, the direct antiglobulin (Coombs') test should first be checked. Other diagnostic tests are often suggested by morphologic abnormalities on the blood smear. We reserve extensive laboratory investigation for infants with a negative Coombs' test who show marked or persistent hyperbilirubinemia, a declining hematocrit, and reticulocytosis. Bone marrow examination is almost never indicated in infants with evidence of hemolysis, but it is essential in the rare baby in whom a primary disorder of erythropoiesis is suspected.

Hemolysis Caused by Maternal Antibodies

Alloimmune disease accounts for most cases of hemolytic anemia in newborn infants. Of these, Rh disease, although preventable, remains the most common cause of severe anemia. At birth, the direct antiglobulin (Coombs') test is strongly positive and reticulocytes are elevated in all but the mildest cases. Anemia varies from mild to severe. The most important aspect of good management is antenatal assessment. This includes maternal screening and, in sensitized pregnancies, frequent surveillance of fetal well-being to establish when to intervene with premature delivery or intrauterine transfusions. Hyperbilirubinemia (see Chapter 12) is a problem in almost all cases; some affected infants cannot be managed with phototherapy alone and require exchange transfusions. More severe cases require correction of anemia at birth. Many of these infants are born prematurely; some have intrapartum asphyxia and subsequent cardiorespiratory distress. Correction of anemia to increase oxygen-carrying capacity is a crucial component of resuscitation in this group of patients. Hydrops in utero develops in the most severe cases, further complicating resuscitation. (See reference 75 for review of alloimmune hemolytic disease and differential diagnosis of hydrops.)

Infants who have undergone treatment with intrauterine transfusions are different. These babies often have mild to moderate anemia with all of their circulating red cells derived from intrauterine transfusions. The direct antiglobulin test may be negative, but the indirect antiglobulin test is strongly positive. In many, there is no reticulocytosis despite moderate anemia and, because all of the donor-derived blood is Rh negative, no hemolysis. Such infants require very close observation during the first several months after birth when the donor erythrocytes die off. Often, late anemia develops, resulting from a combination of decreased marrow stimulation because of low erythropoietin levels and an increased rate of hemolysis. As these babies begin to synthesize their own Rh-positive cells, they are then attacked by residual maternal antibodies.[68, 75] In severe cases, the direct antiglobulin test may persist at +2 positive as late as 6 months after birth and the infants become severely anemic. These infants need supplemental folic acid to meet the demands of increased erythropoiesis.[75]

Alloimmune disease may also occur as a result of other blood group incompatibilities (anti-c, anti-e, and anti-C in the Rh system and anti-Kell are the most common). The course is similar to that with anti-D Rh disease, and these causes of alloimmune disease are not preventable by anti-D immunoglobulin treatment of mothers to prevent sensitization.

The third form of alloimmune disease is due to ABO incompatibility. This is a frequent cause of hyperbilirubinemia but rarely results in significant anemia. The direct antiglobulin test may be only weakly positive. The diagnosis can be made by examination of the peripheral blood smear, which shows microspherocytes. In virtually all cases, the mother is group O, whereas the baby is either A or B. Clinical disease rarely occurs in group A mothers with B babies or group B mothers with A babies.

Congenital Infections

Congenital infections may be associated with hemolytic anemia. This may occur in any of the TORCH infections (see Chapter 13), but it is most common in cytomegalovirus infection. Hemolytic anemia may also be accompanied by a coexisting DIC. The mechanism of hemolytic anemia in these infections is not known. Fetal infection with the B-19 strain of parvovirus presents a special case. This virus is tropic for erythroid progenitors and produces severe erythroid hypoplasia. The anemia may be severe and, as in anti-D Rh alloimmune disease, the worst cases may progress to hydrops fetalis.[77]

Hemoglobinopathies and Thalassemias

Because the fetus has mainly hemoglobin F, the common hemoglobinopathies resulting from mutations in β-globin (e.g., sickle cell anemia) are clinically silent at birth and appear later as the baby switches from γ to β chain synthesis. The same applies to mutations that reduce β-globin chain production (the thalassemias). β-thalassemia resulting from large structural deletions of the β-globin cluster (thalassemia) is a rare familial cause of neonatal microcytic anemia and hyperbilirubinemia. Although infants with sickle cell disease and severe β-thalassemia have normal red blood cell counts at birth, these disorders can be detected in term and near-term infants by demonstrating an absence of hemoglobin A on electrophoresis. In many states, umbilical cord blood is routinely screened to identify infants with sickle cell disease or thalassemia before they become symptomatic. This is done because overwhelming infection may be the first sign of sickle cell disease in infants and young children, and penicillin prophylaxis is effective in reducing the risk of sepsis.[35]

The situation is different in the α-thalassemias. Humans have two pairs of α-globin genes located on chromosome 16. The genes are required for normal intrauterine hemoglobin production.[23] In the fetus, a complete deficiency of chain synthesis results in an absence of hemoglobin F and in the production of Bart's hemoglobin, which is composed of tetrads of γ-chains (γ_4). This hemoglobin has profoundly abnormal oxygen dissociation characteristics, which severely impedes off-loading oxygen to tissues. Although the anemia in these cases is usually mild (hematocrit in the low 30s), fetal tissue oxygen delivery is severely compromised and leads to hydrops fetalis and death. Infants who have one or two functional α-globin genes have microcytosis at birth (mean corpuscular volume is less than 95) and an elevated percentage of Bart's hemoglobin on electrophoresis.

Glucose-6-Phosphate Dehydrogenase Deficiency

Glucose-6-phosphate dehydrogenase (G6PD) is the rate-limiting enzyme in the hexose monophosphatase shunt pathway of glycolysis. The purpose of this system is to generate reduced glutathione, which, in turn, protects the red blood cell membrane from oxidant damage. G6PD deficiency is common worldwide and certain molecular variants are associated with neonatal hemolysis and hyperbilirubinemia. The G6PD gene is on the X chromosome, so significant deficiency occurs almost exclusively in males. The most common G6PD mutation in the North American population is the A− variant present in 10% of African Americans. Term infants are rarely symptomatic; however, this type of G6PD deficiency is associated with neonatal jaundice in preterm babies. Jaundice may occur in the absence of known oxidant exposure. In contrast to G6PD A−, G6PD Canton, a variant common in South China, is commonly associated with significant neonatal jaundice, even though most nurseries carefully avoid using medications that cause hemolysis. There is

increasing evidence that most cases of jaundice in G6PD-deficient neonates is due to diminished bilirubin conjugation by the liver rather than hemolysis.[5, 49] However, sometimes a fetus or newborn infant is exposed to an oxidant, resulting in hemolysis and severe jaundice. For example, severe hemolysis has occurred in fetuses from mothers eating fava beans and in newborn infants exposed to baby clothes stored in naphtha. The diagnosis of G6PD-deficient hemolytic anemia should be suspected in male infants with evidence of acute hemolytic anemia and a negative Coombs' test. The reticulocytes of G6PD-deficient individuals contain relatively high levels of G6PD, and the oldest cells with the lowest levels of G6PD are the first to be hemolyzed, so screening tests of G6PD are less reliable immediately after an episode of hemolysis when there is a brisk reticulocytosis. Heinz bodies are clumps of oxidatively denatured hemoglobin that may be detected in the red cells of G6PD-deficient individuals with active hemolysis after staining with 1% methyl violet. Family studies and measurements of G6PD activity 2 to 3 months after an acute hemolytic episode may be required to establish the diagnosis.

Other Congenital Anemias

Red cell enzymopathies other than G6PD deficiency are rare. Pyruvate kinase deficiency is the most common defect, frequently presenting as neonatal anemia and hyperbilirubinemia. Inherited abnormalities of one of the proteins that form the red cell skeleton may be associated with neonatal hemolysis and jaundice. Hereditary spherocytosis, which is transmitted as an autosomal dominant condition, is the most common of these disorders. Most cases of spherocytosis result from decreased production of spectrin. A negative family history does not exclude the diagnosis because new mutations are common. Examination of the blood smear is particularly helpful in infants suspected of hemolysis caused by abnormalities of the red cell skeleton.

Anemias resulting from inadequate red blood cell production are extremely rare in neonates. Blackfan-Diamond syndrome (also called congenital hypoplastic anemia) is the most common. Infants are often small for gestational age and may have other malformations (especially renal anomalies). Both familial and sporadic cases have been reported. Affected babies show variable degrees of anemia during the newborn period with normal white blood cell and platelet counts. Fanconi anemia is often diagnosed in the nursery because of the associated malformations of the radial ray, but neonatal anemia is rare. Other congenital aplastic anemias are extremely rare.

Anemia of Prematurity

There are three separate mechanisms operating in this condition. The first mechanism is phlebotomy required for laboratory studies. Even with micromethods and the conservative use of laboratory studies, the small, sick preterm infant on assisted ventilation loses more than 5 mL of blood per day for laboratory studies. At this rate, an 800-g infant would lose his or her entire blood volume for laboratory studies in approximately 13 days. This is less of a problem in bigger infants because their blood volumes are much larger.

The second process involved in anemia of prematurity is somatic growth. The very low-birth-weight infant will more than double his or her body weight and blood volume by the time of discharge from the nursery. The third process is the prolonged cessation of erythropoietin release. This system becomes inactive as it does in term infants in the first week after birth. However, reactivation of the erythropoietin system appears to follow a biologic clock in the prematurely born infant. There is no response even to severe anemia until the infant reaches a corrected gestational age of about 34 to 36 weeks. After that, the system responds when the hematocrit declines into the range of 25% to 30% and the reticulocyte count increases rise about 1 week after the increase in erythropoietin.[9, 91, 92] Transfusion with packed red blood cells during this critical period suppresses the release of endogenous erythropoietin and delays the recovery from anemia of prematurity.[8] Some seriously ill infants may not respond until even a later corrected gestational age.[20] Because of the improved oxygen delivery of hemoglobin A,

an infant who has received many transfusions will have to become more anemic than an infant who has not received transfusions in order to achieve a low enough tissue oxygen tension to stimulate erythropoietin release.

Once premature infants mount an erythroid response, they require supplemental iron. Term infants are born with large iron stores, which are mainly acquired during the last month of intrauterine life. Preterm infants not only lack these stores but also have a more rapid rate of growth (and therefore expansion of the blood volume) during the first 6 months of life.

Multiple randomized, controlled trials have shown that treatment of extremely preterm infants with recombinant human erythropoietin (r-HuEPO) during the period when their endogenous erythropoietin system is inactive will stimulate erythropoiesis, maintain a higher hematocrit, and reduce the need for transfusions. Reticulocytosis appears about 1 week after the start of treatment.[58, 67, 72, 88] The main target population is considered to be infants born before 30 completed weeks of gestation.

The smaller and less mature in this group are likely to have the greatest benefit. Treatment is usually started after the infant has tolerated the introduction of enteral feedings. Treatment prevents the later transfusions but does not prevent those given in the first week of life.

The r-HuEPO should be given subcutaneously. Doses of 100 U/kg body weight given 5 days a week or 250 U/kg given three times a week are equally effective and there is no evidence that larger doses are more effective. We use the 3 day per week schedule because it is usually less expensive. All suitable infants undergo treatment on Mondays, Wednesdays, and Fridays and a single 2000-U bottle of r-HuEPO usually is sufficient to treat all of the qualifying infants in a relatively large neonatal intensive care unit.*

Usually treatment can be discontinued as the infant approaches 34 to 35 weeks cor-

---

*Clinicians choosing to use r-HuEPO should follow the other components of therapy used in the trials. The infants received multivitamins, including a total intake of vitamin E of 15 U/day. Also, they were started on enteral iron at or soon after the start of r-HuEPO. The iron should be increased as tolerated to total enteral dose of 6 mg/kg/day.

Table 16–10. Indications for Packed
Erythrocyte Transfusions

Transfuse infants at hematocrit ≤20%
  If symptomatic with reticulocytes <100,000/μL
Transfuse infants at hematocrit ≤30%
  If receiving <35% supplemental hood oxygen
  If on CPAP or mechanical ventilation with mean
    airway pressure <6 cm H_2O
  If significant apnea and bradycardia are noted (>9
    episodes in 12 h or two episodes in 24 h
    requiring bag-and-mask ventilation) while
    receiving therapeutic doses of methylxanthines
  If heart rate >180 beats/min or respiratory rate
    >80 breaths/min persist for 24 h
  If weight gain <10 g/d is observed over 4 d while
    receiving ≥100 kcal/kg/d
  If undergoing surgery
Transfuse for hematocrit ≤35%
  If receiving >35% supplemental hood oxygen
  If intubated on CPAP or mechanical ventilation
    with mean airway pressure ≥6–8 cm H_2O
Do not transfuse
  To replace blood removed for laboratory tests
    alone
  For low hematocrit alone

CPAP, continuous positive airway pressure by nasal or
endotracheal route.
From Shannon KM, Keith JF, Mentzer WC, et al: Recombinant human erythropoietin stimulates erythropoiesis and reduces erythrocyte transfusions in very low birth weight infants. Pediatrics 95:1, 1995.

rected gestational age. The r-HuEPO will continue to have an effect on the reticulocyte count and hematocrit for 2 weeks beyond the end of treatment.[89] If the hematocrit is between 30% and 35%, which is usual, it will take 2 weeks for it to decline sufficiently to stimulate the release of endogenous erythropoietin.

Erythrocyte Transfusion

Infants who have significant cardiopulmonary disease are transfused when they become anemic, because it is thought that a higher oxygen-carrying capacity improves their tolerance of cardiorespiratory distress. Extremely low-birth-weight infants are the most heavily transfused. Indications for red blood cell transfusion are an area of controversy and there has been a recent trend toward the more conservative use of transfusions.[48, 50, 88, 93, 98] There is wide variation in transfusion practices between neonatal intensive care units without apparent adverse effects in the units using more conservative practices.[78] Table 16–10 shows the relatively

conservative guidelines that were used in a multicenter, randomized, controlled trial of r-HuEPO for anemia of prematurity.* The table is based on the paradigm that there is no single critical hematocrit that always requires transfusion in sick neonates. Rather, it assumes that there is a range of critical hematocrits, most of which will apply to the same individual at different times during the course of neonatal illness. In general, the sicker the infant, the higher the critical hematocrit. There are only a few clinical studies that are beginning to define the critical hematocrits for some parts of the whole range of pathophysiologic states.[1, 4, 6, 70, 79, 90]

There is also considerable variation in the volume of packed red blood cells transfused to correct anemia. It is popular to give 10 mL/kg over 1 to 3 hours. However, this is often too little to have a significant effect on hematocrit; volumes of 15 or 20 mL/kg are needed in many cases.[45] Most infants tolerate 15 mL/kg, and the 20 mL/kg can be given as two transfusions of 10 mL/kg with a pause of a few hours between the two. A single dose of furosemide can be given if there is particular concern about temporary volume overload, for example, in infants with serious chronic lung disease. To accurately measure the effect of a transfusion, hematocrit should be measured more than an hour after the end of the transfusion when post-transfusion adjustments in blood volume have occurred.

◆ POLYCYTHEMIA

Conditions that lead to intrauterine polycythemia are summarized in Table 16–11. Most infants who develop polycythemia severe enough to be of clinical significance have both a relatively high hematocrit in utero from one of the causes listed in Table 16–11 and receive a normal to excessive placental transfusion at delivery (see Table 16–9). Small placental transfusions can offset the effect of intrauterine polycythemia. For example, the infant of a poorly controlled diabetic mother who is then delivered by

*These guidelines are for use in preterm infants without congenital anomalies. Infants with some congenital heart lesions benefit from higher hematocrits than would be achieved by these guidelines (see Chapter 14).

Table 16–11. Conditions Associated With Polycythemia in Utero

---

Chronic hypoxia from maternal toxemia and
    placental insufficiency
Placental insufficiency with postmaturity syndrome
Pregnancy at high altitudes
Diabetic pregnancy
Trisomy, particularly trisomy 21

---

cesarean section with early cord clamping is likely to end up with a normal hematocrit.

As hematocrit increases, it reaches a point where viscosity is so high that it interferes with circulation into a variety of tissues and organs. Those most commonly involved include the following:

1. Skin: delayed capillary filling time and plethora.
2. Kidneys: hematuria and proteinuria, or, in severe cases, a syndrome indistinguishable from renal vein thrombosis.
3. GI tract: necrotizing enterocolitis if there is associated early feeding.
4. Pulmonary: reversal of the pulmonary to systemic vascular resistance and a form of pulmonary hypertension.
5. Central nervous system: irritability, abnormal cry, poor feeding in mild cases, apnea in moderate cases, seizures, and cerebral infarction in severe cases.
6. Hematologic: thrombocytopenia and jaundice.

Diagnosis and Treatment

There is no precise hematocrit at which symptoms appear in all infants, in part because viscosity is affected by factors other than hematocrit and measurement of blood viscosity is not available at most hospitals. Symptoms are common when the venous hematocrit exceeds 66%, but serious signs of organ dysfunction develop in some infants with lower hematocrits. Because capillary blood hematocrits are generally higher than central venous values but may correlate poorly with them, it is essential that the presence of polycythemia be confirmed by measuring venous blood hematocrit.

The treatment for infants with symptomatic polycythemia is partial exchange transfusion replacing blood with a plasma substitute. Isotonic saline has been shown to be as effective as plasma or a mixture of saline and albumin. The equation for the volume to be exchanged is as follows:

$$V = (Hct_I - Hct_D \times Body\ weight\ (kg) \\ \times 90\ mL)/Hct_I$$

Where V = the exchange volume, Hct_I is the infant's hematocrit and Hct_D is the desired hematocrit. Hct_D should be 50%. Commonly, after this procedure, there is further hemoconcentration and the hematocrit increases again. If the hematocrit is only lowered to 55%, it often increases again to a dangerous range.

Asymptomatic babies with high hematocrits pose a therapeutic dilemma. One option is to observe and only treat those with symptoms. However, if the first symptoms are neurologic, one may have waited too long. Even though there is an increased incidence of neurologic handicaps in children who had untreated neonatal polycythemia,[29] the definitive controlled trial to examine the risks and benefits of prophylactic partial exchange in asymptomatic polycythemic infants is yet to be done. We routinely perform partial exchange transfusions in asymptomatic infants who have venous hematocrits greater than 66% on the first day of life.

CASE PROBLEMS

◆

Case One

You are called to evaluate a 12-hour-old infant who was noted to have a petechial rash soon after delivery. The nurse obtains a complete blood count, which reveals a platelet count of 11,000.

◆ *What is your initial approach?*

The baby should be examined. The first goal is to determine whether there is clinical evidence of severe pathology (i.e., does the baby look "sick"). Thrombocytopenic bleeding may be the first sign of sepsis or necrotizing enterocolitis. Maternal fever, prolonged rupture of the placental membranes, and premature birth all predispose to invasive infection. If the baby appears ill, a sepsis workup should be performed and parenteral antibiotics should be initiated. Physical examination may disclose other abnormalities, suggesting the correct diagnosis. Babies with thrombocytopenia from congenital viral infections often show microcephaly and hepatosplenomegaly. Radial and thenar aplasia or hypoplasia suggest a primary defect in platelet production (e.g., Fanconi anemia or the syndrome of thrombocytopenia with absence of the radii).

The baby weighs 3450 g and vaginal delivery is uncomplicated. She appears well except for scattered petechiae and bruising from heel-stick and venipuncture sites. The remainder of the complete blood count is unremarkable (white blood cell count—10,000/mm³ with a normal differential and hemoglobin—17.2 g/dL).

◆ **What should be done next?**

Factitious thrombocytopenia should always be considered but is unlikely in this case because of the presence of clinical signs. The blood smear should be examined for normal-appearing red and white blood cells and for giant platelets, which, if present, suggest an increased rate of peripheral platelet destruction with the marrow attempting to compensate by releasing young platelets into the circulation. The mother's platelet count should be checked and she should be questioned regarding medication use and to determine whether she has a history of ITP, lupus, or other collagen-vacuolar disorder. Maternal thrombocytopenia is an important clue that suggests transplacental transmission of maternal antiplatelet IgG autoantibodies. This is a common cause of neonatal thrombocytopenia in babies who "look well."

The baby's blood smear reveals giant platelets and marked thrombocytopenia but is otherwise normal. The mother's platelet count is normal and there is no history suggesting maternal autoimmune disease.

◆ **What is the most likely diagnosis and what should be done?**

The most likely diagnosis is alloimmune thrombocytopenia from transplacental passage of a maternal antibody that specifically recognizes an antigen that the infant inherited from her father. The PAI-1 antigen accounts for the vast majority of cases. The mother's platelets should be typed for PAI-1. If she is negative, a presumptive diagnosis can be made. The baby's platelet count should be measured at least daily for the first few days of life, and she should be observed for signs of active hemorrhage.

While discussing the probable diagnosis with the parents, you are called urgently to the nursery because the baby has developed worsening petechiae and has gross hematuria. Her vital signs are stable.

◆ **What should be done?**

The baby now has evidence of significant active hemorrhage and should receive a platelet transfusion. However, 97% of Caucasians express the PAI-1 antigen on the surface of their platelets. PAI-1–positive platelets will be destroyed rapidly in the infant's circulation. An excellent solution to this problem is to use the mother as a pheresis donor for platelets. Her PAI-1–negative platelets will not be recognized by circulating alloantibody and will survive normally in the baby. Alternatively, the blood bank may be able to provide PAI-1–negative platelets from an unrelated donor.

The mother is PAI-1–negative. The baby's platelet count increases and she stops bleeding after she is transfused with maternal platelets. The parents are interested in having other children and are concerned about the recurrence risk.

◆ **What do you tell them?**

Subsequent pregnancies are at high risk of severe neonatal hemorrhage. The mother should be followed up as a "high-risk" patient. Recent data indicate that the administration of intravenous gamma globulin to the mother before delivery decreases the incidence of neonatal thrombocytopenia.

◆─────────────────────────────

Case Two

A baby girl is born at 38.5 weeks' gestation and weighs 3 kg. The mother is a 26-year-old who was G2 P1 AB1 at the start of the pregnancy. Her first child was born at term and had no neonatal problems. At her first prenatal visit, the mother is found to be group O Rh-negative and an antibody screen is negative. Other routine perinatal screening tests are negative. The mother has continuing prenatal care until 22 weeks but then misses further care. She does not receive hyperimmune anti–Rh-globulin. She goes into labor at 38.5 weeks' gestation. There is rapid progression of labor and rapid delivery vaginally without complications. The baby is vigorous at birth and has Apgar scores of 7 and 9 but is noted shortly after birth to be pale. Heart rate, blood pressure, and respiratory rate are normal. On physical examination, the liver is of normal size and the spleen is not enlarged. There is no cardiorespiratory distress.

At 30 minutes of age, hematocrit measured from capillary blood sample from the heel shows 37%. At 45 minutes, a venous blood he-

matocrit is 32%. Further laboratory work shows the baby is group O, Rh(D)-positive. The direct antiglobulin (Coombs') test is negative. Reticulocyte count is 150,000 (5%), platelet count is 270,000, and the white blood cell count is normal with a normal differential.

◆ *What diagnostic studies should be done and in what order? What specific instructions should you give to the mother's obstetrician?*

This is not Rh disease. The direct antiglobulin test is invariably strongly positive when the disease is severe enough to produce this amount of anemia, and the reticulocyte count would be elevated. The spleen and liver would probably be enlarged with this degree of anemia. It is not ABO disease because mother and baby are group O and other isoimmune disease is extremely unlikely in the absence of a positive direct antiglobulin test. The baby is the wrong sex for G6PD deficiency. The lack of an elevated reticulocyte count suggests that the anemia is of very recent onset, most likely the result of blood loss. The greatest concern is that the blood loss is transplacental. If this is true, the standard dose of hyperimmune anti–Rh globulin may not be sufficient to prevent this mother from becoming sensitized to the Rh(D) antigen. Because mother and baby are both group O, the mother is at even greater risk of becoming sensitized to the D antigen. The obstetrician should be told to perform a Kleihauer-Betke test on the mother's blood immediately to look for fetal cells. If there are increased numbers of fetal cells, a larger dose of hyperimmunoglobulin must be given to the mother to prevent sensitization. The size of the fetomaternal bleed can be calculated from the baby's estimated blood loss (based on hematocrit and blood volume).

REFERENCES

1. Alverson DC, Isken VH, Cohen RS: Effect of booster blood transfusion on oxygen utilization in infants with bronchopulmonary dysplasia. J Pediatr 113:722, 1988.
2. Anderson KC, Weinstein HJ: Transfusion-associated graft versus host disease. N Engl J Med 323:315, 1990.
3. Baley JE, Stork EK, Warkentin PI, et al: Neonatal neutropenia: Clinical manifestations, cause, and outcome. Am J Dis Child 142:1161, 1988.
4. Bard H, Fouron J-C, Chessex P, et al: Myocardial, erythropoietic, and metabolic adaptations to anemia of prematurity in infants with bronchopulmonary dysplasia. J Pediatr 132:630, 1998.
5. Beulter E: Glucose-6-phosphate dehydrogenase deficiency. N Engl J Med 324:169, 1991.
6. Bifano EM, Smith F, Borer J: Relationship between determinants of oxygen delivery and respiratory abnormalities in preterm infants with anemia. J Pediatr 120: 292, 1992.
7. Bonilla MA, Gillio AP, Ruggerio M, et al: Effects of recombinant human granulocyte colony-stimulating factor on neutropenia in patients with congenital agranulocytosis. N Engl J Med 320:1564, 1989.
8. Brown M, Berman E, Luckey D: Prediction of the need for transfusion during anemia of prematurity. J Pediatr 116:773, 1990.
9. Brown MS, Phibbs RH, Garcia JF, et al: Decreased response of plasma immunoreactive erythropoietin to "available oxygen" in anemia of prematurity. J Pediatr 105:793, 1984.
10. Buchanan GR: Neonatal hemorrhagic diseases. In Nathan DG, Oski FA, eds: Hematology of Infancy and Childhood. 3rd ed. Philadelphia: WB Saunders, 1987.
11. Burrows RF, Kelton JG: Low risk in pregnancies associated with idiopathic thrombocytopenic purpura. Am J Obstet Gynecol 163:1147, 1990.
12. Bussel JB, Berkowitz RL, McFarland JG, et al: Antenatal treatment of neonatal alloimmune thrombocytopenia. N Engl J Med 319:1974, 1988.
13. Cadnapaphornchai M, Faix RG: Increased nosocomial infection in neutropenic low birth weight (2000 grams or less) infants of hypertensive mothers. J Pediatr 121:956, 1992.
14. Cairo MS: Neonatal neutrophil host defense. Am J Dis Child 143:40, 1989.
15. Cairo M, VandeVan C, Toy C, et al: Lymphokines: Enhancement by granulocyte-macrophage and granulocyte colony-stimulating factors of neonatal myeloid kinetics and functional activation of polymorphonuclear leukocytes. Rev Infect Dis 12:492, 1990.
16. Chaou WT, Chou ML, Eitzman DV: Intracranial hemorrhage and vitamin K deficiency in early infancy. J Pediatr 105:880, 1984.
17. Chirico G, Rondini G, Plebani A, et al: Intravenous immunoglobulin therapy for prophylaxis of infections in high risk neonates. J Pediatr 110:437, 1987.
18. Christensen R, Rothstein G, Anstall H, et al: Granulocyte transfusions in neonates with bacterial infection, neutropenia, and depletion of mature marrow neutrophils. Pediatrics 70:1, 1982.
19. Christensen RD, Harper TE, Rothstein G: Granulocyte-macrophage progenitor cells (CFU-GM) in term and preterm neonates. J Pediatr 109:1047, 1986.
20. Christensen RD, Hunter DD, Godell H, et al: Evaluation of the mechanism causing anemia in infants with bronchopulmonary dysplasia. J Pediatr 120:593, 1992.
21. Christensen RD, Rothstein G: Exhaustion of mature marrow neutrophils in neonates with sepsis. J Pediatr 96:316, 1980.
22. Cines DB, Dusak B, Tomaksi A, et al: Immune thrombocytopenic purpura and pregnancy. N Engl J Med 306:826, 1982.
23. Clapp D, Shannon K: Embryonic and fetal erythropoiesis. In Feig S, Freedman M, eds: Clinical Disorders and Experimental Models of Erythropoietic Failure. Boca Raton: CRC Press, 1993, pp 1–38.

24. Clapp D: Bone marrow failure syndromes in the neonate and infant. In Christensen R, ed: Hematologic Problems of the Neonate. Philadelphia: W.B. Saunders, 1999, pp 79–89.

25. Clapp DW, Kliegman RM, Baley JE, et al: Use of intravenously administered immune globulin to prevent nosocomial sepsis in low birth weight infants: Report of a pilot study. J Pediatr 115:324, 1989.

26. Clark SC, Kamen R: The human hematopoietic colony stimulating factors. Science 236:1229, 1987.

27. Clouse LH, Comp PC: The regulation of hemostasis: The protein C system. N Engl J Med 314:1298, 1986.

28. Curnutte JT, Boxer LA: Disorders of granulopoiesis and granulocyte function. In Nathan DG, Oski FA, eds: Hematology of Infancy and Childhood. 3rd ed. Philadelphia: WB Saunders, 1987.

29. Delaney-Black V, Camp BW, Lubchenco LO, et al: Neonatal hypoviscosity association with lower achievement and IQ scores at school age. Pediatrics 83:662, 1989.

30. Delivoria-Papadopoulos M, Miller LD, Forster RE II, et al: The role of exchange transfusions in the management of low-birth-weight infants with and without severe respiratory distress syndrome I. J Pediatr 89:273, 1976.

31. Dix D, Andrew M, Marzinotto V, et al: The use of low molecular weight heparin in pediatric patients: A prospective cohort study [see comments]. J Pediatr 136:439, 2000.

32. Doron MW, Makhlouf RA, Katz VL, et al: Increased incidence of sepsis at birth in neutropenic infants of mothers with preeclampsia. J Pediatr 125:452, 1994.

33. Egrie JC, Browne J, Lai P, et al: Characterization of recombinant monkey and human erythropoietin. Prog Clin Biol Res 191:339, 1985.

34. Fehr J, Hoffman V, Kappeler U: Transient reversal of thrombocytopenia in idiopathic thrombocytopenic purpura by high-dose intravenous gamma globulin. N Engl J Med 306:1254, 1982.

35. Gaston M: Why we should screen newborns for sickle cell disease. Contemp Pediatr 1:175, 1989.

36. Gillan ER, Christensen RD, Suen Y, et al: A randomized, placebo-controlled trial of recombinant human granulocyte colony-stimulating factor administration in newborn infants with presumed sepsis: Significant induction of peripheral and bone marrow neutrophilia. Blood 84:1427, 1994.

37. Gottuso MA, Williams ML, Oski FA: The role of exchange transfusions in the management of low-birth weight infants with and without severe respiratory distress syndrome II. J Pediatr 89:279, 1976.

38. Groopman JE, Molina JM, Scadden DT: Hematopoietic growth factors. Biology and clinical applications. N Engl J Med 321:1449, 1989.

39. Hagstrom JN, Walter J, Bluebond-Langner R, et al: Prevalence of the factor V leiden mutation in children and neonates with thromboembolic disease. J Pediatr 133:777, 1998.

40. Hammond WP, Price TH, Souza LM, et al: Treatment of cyclic neutropenia with granulocyte-colony stimulating factor. N Engl J Med 320:1306, 1989.

41. Haneline LS, Marshall KP, Clapp DW: The highest concentration of primitive hematopoietic progenitor cells in cord blood is found in extremely premature infants. Pediatr Res 39:820, 1996.

42. Hirsh J, Levine MN: Low molecular weight heparin. Blood 79:1, 1992.

43. Horgan MJ, Bartoletti A, Polansky S, et al: Effect of heparin infusates in umbilical artery catheters on frequency of thrombotic complications. J Pediatr 111:774, 1987.

44. Horwitz M, Benson KF, Person RE, et al: Mutations in ELA2, encoding neutrophil elastase, define a 21-day biological clock in cyclic haematopoiesis. Nat Genet 23:433, 1999.

45. Hudson I, Cooke A, Holland B, et al: Red cell volume and cardiac output in anaemic preterm infants. Arch Dis Child 65:672, 1990.

46. International Chronic Granulomatous Disease Study Group: A controlled trial of interferon gamma to prevent infections in chronic granulomatous disease. N Engl J Med 324:509, 1991.

47. Jacobs K, Shoemaker C, Rudersdorf R, et al: Isolation and characterization of genomic and cDNA clones of human erythropoietin. Nature 313:806, 1985.

48. Joshi A, Gerhardt T, Shandloff P, et al: Blood transfusion effect on the respiratory pattern of premature infants. Pediatrics 80:79, 1987.

49. Kaplan M, Rubatelli FF, Hammerman C, et al: Conjugated bilirubin in neonates with glucose-6-phosphate dehydrogenase deficiency. J Pediatr 128:695, 1996.

50. Keyes WG, Donohue PK, Turner MC, et al: Assessing the need for transfusion of premature infants and the role of hematocrit, clinical signs and erythropoietin level. Pediatrics 84:412, 1989.

51. Kliegman R, Clapp D, Berger M: Targeted immunoglobulin therapy for the prevention of neonatal infections. Rev Infect Dis 12:443, 1990.

52. Koenig JM, Christensen RD: Incidence, neutrophil kinetics, and natural history of neonatal neutropenia associated with maternal hypertension. N Engl J Med 321:557, 1989.

53. La Gamma EF, Alpan O, Kocherlakota P: Effect of granulocyte colony-stimulating factor on preeclampsia-associated neonatal neutropenia. J Pediatr 126:457, 1995.

54. Lane PA, Hathaway WE: Vitamin K in infancy. J Pediatr 106:351, 1985.

55. Lauterbach R, Pawlik D, Kowalczyk D, et al: Effect of the immunomodulating agent, pentoxifylline, in the treatment of sepsis in prematurely delivered infants: A placebo-controlled, double-blind trial. Crit Care Med 27:807, 1999.

56. Lieschke GJ, Grail D, Hodgson G, et al: Mice lacking granulocyte colony-stimulating factor have chronic neutropenia, granulocyte and macrophage progenitor cell deficiency, and impaired neutrophil mobilization. Blood 84:1737, 1994.

57. Lusher JM, Warrier I: Hemophilia. Pediatr Rev 12:275, 1991.

58. Maier RF, Obladen M, Scigalla P, et al: The effects of epoetin beta (recombinant human erythropoietin) on need for transfusion in very-low-birth weight infants. N Engl J Med 330:1173, 1994.

59. Male C, Johnston M, Sparling C, et al: The influence of developmental haemostasis on the laboratory diagnosis and management of haemostatic disorders during infancy and childhood. Clin Lab Med 19:39, 1999.

60. Manco-Johnson MJ, Marlar RA, Jacobson LJ, et al: Severe protein C deficiency in newborn infants. J Pediatr 113:359, 1988.
61. Manroe BL, Weinberg AG, Rosenfeld CR, et al: The neonatal blood count in health and disease. Reference values for neutrophilic cells. J Pediatr 95:89, 1979.
62. Marder VJ, Sherry S: Thrombolytic therapy: Current status. N Engl J Med 318:1512, 1988 (part 1); 318:1585, 1988 (part 2).
63. Marlar RA, Montomery RR, Broekmans AW, et al: Diagnosis and treatment of homozygous protein C deficiency. Report of the Working Party on Homozygous Protein C Deficiency of the Subcommittee on Protein C and Protein S, International Committee on Thrombosis and Haemostasis. J Pediatr 114:528, 1989.
64. Massicotte P, Adams M, Marzinotto V, et al: Low-molecular-weight heparin in pediatric patients with thrombotic disease: A dose finding study. J Pediatr 128:313, 1996.
65. Mayer P, Geissler K, Ward M, et al: Recombinant human leukemia inhibitory factor induces acute phase proteins and raises the blood platelet counts in nonhuman primates. Blood 81:3226, 1993.
66. McDonald MM, Hathaway WE: Anticoagulant therapy by continuous heparinization in newborn and older infants. J Pediatr 101:451, 1982.
67. Meyer MP, Commerford A, et al: Recombinant human erythropoietin for the treatment of the anemia of prematurity. Pediatrics 93:918, 1994.
68. Millard DD, Gidding SS, Socol ML, et al: Effects of intravascular, intrauterine transfusion on prenatal and postnatal hemolysis and erythropoiesis in severe fetal isoimmunization. J Pediatr 117:447, 1990.
69. Morgenstern DE, Gifford MAC, Li LL, et al: Absence of respiratory burst in X-linked chronic granulomatous disease mice leads to abnormalities in both host defense and inflammatory response to *Aspergillus fumigatus.* J Exp Med 185:1, 1997.
70. Nelle M, Hocker C, Zilow EP, et al: Effects of red cell transfusion on cardiac output and blood flow velocities in cerebral and gastrointestinal arteries in preterm infants. Arch Dis Child 71:F45, 1994.
71. Nowak-Gottl U, Debus O, Findeisen M, et al: Lipoprotein (a): Its role in childhood thromboembolism. Pediatrics 99:E11, 1997.
72. Ohls RK, Osborne KA, Christensen RD: Efficacy and cost analysis of treating very low birth weight infants with erythropoietin during their first two weeks of life: A randomized placebo-controlled trial. J Pediatr 126:421, 1995.
73. Oski FA, Naiman JL: Hematologic Problems in the Newborn. 3rd ed. Philadelphia: WB Saunders, 1982.
74. Paxson C, Heaton G, Adcock E, et al: Treatment of early postnatal cardiovascular shock with autologus fetal blood transfusions. Pediatr Res 10:430, 1976.
75. Phibbs RH, Naiman JL: Erythroblastosis fetalis. In Mentzer WC, ed. Congenital hemolytic anemias. Basil: Karger, 1989, pp 324–329.
76. Quisenberry P, Levitt L: Hematopoietic stem cells. N Engl J Med 301:755 (part 1); 819 (part 2); 868 (part 3), 1979.
77. Rodis JF, Hovick TJ, Quinn DL, et al: Human parvovirus infection in pregnancy. Obstet Gynecol 72:733, 1988.
78. Ringer SA, Richardson DK, Sacher RA, et al: Variations in transfusion practice in neonatal intensive care. N Engl J Med 101:194, 1998.
79. Ross MP, Christensen RD, Rothstein G, et al: A randomized trial to develop criteria for administering erythrocyte transfusions to anemic preterm infants 1 to 3 months of age. J Perinatol 9:246, 1990.
80. Sachs L: The molecular control of blood cell development. Science 238:1374, 1987.
81. Schibler KR, Osborne KA, Leung LY, et al: A randomized, placebo-controlled trial of granulocyte colony-stimulating factor administration to newborn infants with neutropenia and clinical signs of early-onset sepsis. Pediatrics 102:6, 1998.
82. Schibler KR, Liechty KW, White WL, et al: Production of granulocyte colony-stimulating factor in vitro by monocytes from preterm and term neonates. Blood 82:2478, 1993.
83. Schmidt B, Andrew M: Neonatal thrombosis: report of a prospective Canadian and international registry. Pediatrics 96:939, 1995.
84. Schmidt B, Andrew M: Report of Scientific and Standardization Subcommittee on Neonatal Hemostasis Diagnosis and Treatment of Neonatal Thrombosis. Thromb Haemost 67:381, 1992.
85. Schmidt B, Andrew M: Neonatal thrombotic disease: Prevention, diagnosis, and treatment. J Pediatr 113:407, 1988.
86. Shannon K: Anemia of prematurity: Progress and prospects. Am J Pediatr Hematol Oncol 12:14, 1990.
87. Shannon K, Naylor GS, Torkildson JC, et al: Circulating erythroid progenitors in the anemia of prematurity. N Engl J Med 317:728, 1987.
88. Shannon KM, Keith JF, Mentzer WC, et al: Recombinant human erythropoietin stimulates erythropoiesis and reduces erythrocyte transfusions in very low birth weight infants. Pediatrics 95:1, 1995.
89. Soubasi V, Kremenopaulos G, Diamanti E, et al: Follow-up of very low birth weight infants after erythropoietin treatment to prevent anemia of prematurity. J Pediatr 127:291, 1995.
90. Stockman JA III, Clark DA: Weight gain: A response to transfusions in selected preterm infants. Am J Dis Child 138:828, 1984.
91. Stockman JA III, Garcia JF, Oski FA: The anemia of prematurity: Factors governing the erythropoietin response. N Engl J Med 296:647, 1977.
92. Stockman JA III, Graeber JE, Clark DA, et al: Anemia of prematurity, determinants of erythropoietin response. J Pediatr 105:786, 1984.
93. Strauss RG: Transfusion therapy in neonates. Am J Dis Child 145:904, 1991.
94. Vailas GN, Brouillette RT, Scott JP, et al: Neonatal aortic thrombosis: Recent experience. J Pediatr 109:101, 1986.
95. von der Borne AEGK, van Leeuwen EF, von Riesz LE, et al: Neonatal alloimmune thrombocytopenia: Detection and characterization of the responsible antibodies by the platelet immunofluorescence test. Blood 57:649, 1981.
96. Wessler S, Gitel SN: Warfarin. N Engl J Med 311:645, 1984.

97. Widness JA, Philips AF, Clemons GK: Erythropoietin levels and erythropoiesis at birth in infants
with Potter syndrome. J Pediatr 117:155, 1990.

98. Widness JA, Seward VJ, Kromer IJ, et al: Changing
patterns of red blood cell transfusion in very low
birth weight infants. J Pediatr 129:680, 1996.

99. Yoder MC, Hiatt K, Dutt P, et al: Characterization
of definitive lymphohematopoietic stem cells in
the day 9 murine yolk sac. Immunity 7:335, 1997.

100. Zimmerman JJ: Appraising the potential of pentoxifylline in septic premies. Crit Care Med
27:695, 1999.

Brain Disorders of the Fetus and Neonate

Mark S. Scher

A physician's knowledge of prenatal cerebral and noncerebral development greatly enhances the neurologic assessment of the newborn.[2, 78, 165] Pathologic processes may occur during prenatal life that subsequently modify expected neonatal brain functions. Any discussion of the neurologic evaluation of the newborn, therefore, must take into account historical and physical examination components that synthesize intrauterine and extrauterine time periods, during which congenital or acquired events may have occurred. Specifically, the evaluation of the neonate must take into account familial, maternal, fetal, environmental, and placental factors in order to better determine the developmental niche of the fetus or neonate when stress or disease occurred.

This chapter contains three sections, each highlighting a different perspective on accurate neurologic diagnosis: consideration of fetal development and disease, serial and systematic bedside examinations, and laboratory investigations of the newborn, emphasizing classic components of neurologic assessment and, finally, selected neurologic conditions that underscore the importance of integrating historical and examination findings in the evaluation of brain disorders of the fetus and neonate.

◆ STAGES OF PRENATAL BRAIN DEVELOPMENT

Maturation of the brain is defined through descriptions of sequential and overlapping developmental processes, during which the following anatomic, biochemical, and physiologic processes occur: neural induction followed by neuronogenesis, programmed cell death and neuroblast migration, formation of axons and dendrites, continuous energy generation to provide membrane excitability, synaptogenesis, neurotransmitter biosynthesis, and myelination of axons. At least

in part, these represent prenatal time periods of brain development. Regional differences in the rate of maturation of the nervous system also must be recognized. Different brain structures do not express equivalent function at specific times during the development of the fetus, prenate, or full-term neonate. Table 17–1 lists the major prenatal developmental sequences in brain maturation within the cerebrum and cerebellum, listing representative disorders at each stage. Both volume and gyral-sulcal complexity increase during prenatal development, with prominent changes in the last 3 months of gestation[35] (Fig. 17–1), reflecting major molecular and histologic maturational changes during the formation of maturing cortical-subcortical cellular connections.

◆ TOOLS FOR FETAL NEUROLOGIC DIAGNOSIS

Diagnostic techniques of the fetus have improved over the past several decades, providing morphologic, biochemical, and physiologic diagnoses. Many medical conditions can be better documented during the prenatal period:

Indications for the use of these tests are enumerated in both obstetric and pediatric guidelines[36] (Table 17–2). Most of the following investigative tools are invasive, with specific indications:

1. Amniocentesis is usually performed at 16 weeks' gestational age or earlier if necessary.[27] Fluid can be evaluated for karyotyping as well as a variety of biochemical investigations. The most commonly used tests are alpha-fetoprotein and screening studies for specific chromosomopathies or neural tube defects.[59] (See Chapter 1.)
2. Chorionic villous sampling can be undertaken from 8 weeks' gestation or beyond to be used for chromosomal studies by

Table 17-1. Major Stages of Central Nervous System Development

Stage	Peak Time of Occurrence	Major Morphologic Events in Cerebrum	Major Morphologic Events in Cerebellum	Main Corresponding Disorders*
Uterine implantation	1 wk			
Separation of 3 layers	2 wk	Neural plate		Enterogenous cysts and fistulae
Dorsal induction Neurulation	3–4 wk	Neural tube, neural crest, and derivatives Closure of anterior (d24) and posterior (d29) neuropores	Paired alar plates	Anencephaly, encephalocele, craniorachischisis, spina bifida, meningoceles
Caudal neural tube formation	4–7 wk	Canalization and regressive differentiation of cord	Rhombic lips (d35), cerebellar plates	Diastematomyelia, Dandy-Walker syndrome, cerebellar hypoplasia
Ventral induction	5–6 wk	Forebrain and face (cranial neural crest) Cleavage of prosencephalon into cerebral vesicles (d33). Optic placodes (d26), olfactory placodes Diencephalon	Fusion of cerebellar plates	Holoprosencephaly, median cleft face syndrome
Neuronal and glial proliferation	8–16 wk	Cellular proliferation in ventricular and subventricular zone (interkinetic migration) Early differentiation of neuroblasts and glioblasts	Migration of Purkinje cells (9–10 wk) Migration of external granular layer (10–11 wk)	Microcephaly, megalencephaly
Migration	12–20 wk	Radial migration and accessory pathways (e.g., corpus gangliothalamicum). Formation of corpus callosum	Dendritic tree of Purkinje cells (16–25 wk)	Lissencephaly-pachygyria (types I and II), Zellweger syndrome, glial heterotopia, microgyria (some forms), agenesis of corpus callosum
Organization†	24 wk to postnatal	Late migration (to 5 months) Alignment, orientation, and layering of cortical neurons Synaptogenesis Glial proliferation/differentiation well into postnatal life	Monolayer of Purkinje cells (16–28 wk) Migration of granules to form internal granular layer (to postnatal life)	Minor cortical dysplasias, dendritic/synaptic abnormalities, microgyria (some forms)
Myelination	24 wk to 2 y postnatally			Dysmyelination, clastic insults

*Disorders do not necessarily correspond to abnormal development. They may also result from secondary destruction/disorganization.

†Programmed cellular death takes place throughout the second half of pregnancy and the first year of extrauterine life.

Adapted from Aicardi J, Bax M, Gillberg C, Ogier H: Diseases of the Nervous System in Childhood. Clinics in Developmental Medicine. 2nd ed. New York: MacKeith Press, 1998.

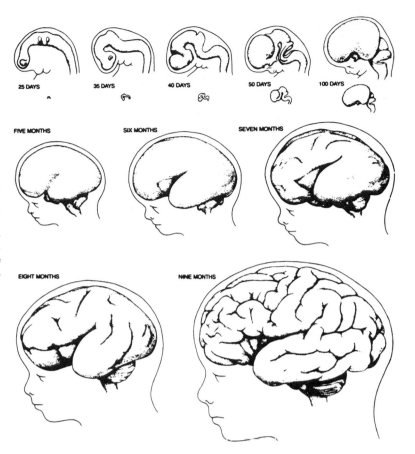

Figure 17–1. Schematic diagram of gyral development in the human brain from 25 days to 9 months. Note the prominent increase in volume and gyral complexity in the last 3 months of gestation. (From Cowan WM: The development of the brain. Sci Am 241:113, 1997.)

direct examination or culture as well as for biochemical analysis.[36]

3. Fetal blood sampling guided under ultrasound examination from 18 weeks' gestation onward can clarify ambiguous amniocentesis or chorionic villous sampling results and diagnose fetal infections, isoimmunization, or other hematologic problems.

4. Ultrasound examination with transvaginal probes can detect structural abnormalities as early as the embryonic period, but abdominal probes are used at 15 to 20 weeks' gestation and the examination can be repeated as required. Evaluation of fetal maturity and the assessment of intrauterine growth are powerful measures for the antenatal diagnosis of many neurologic and nonneurologic fetal conditions.[27, 46, 161, 171] Table 17–3 lists selected brain malformations that can be diagnosed antenatally by sonography. Whereas abnormal fetal sonographic findings might be discovered fortuitously, previous pregnancy complica-

tions or current medical difficulties during early pregnancy usually prompt the proactive use of one or more studies. In routine practice, the sensitivity of sonography is not uniformly satisfactory,[2] but improved reliability has been reported[130] (Fig. 17–2).

5. Biochemical, cytogenetic, and molecular biologic techniques can assess for specific enzyme assays or other biochemical products that have a relationship to specific genetic conditions.[173] Techniques of DNA analysis make possible prenatal diagnosis of specific inherited biochemical abnormalities, detection of mutant genes, and linkage studies with fragment length polymorphisms or other DNA markers for a specific familial condition.[3]

6. Techniques for physiologic fetal well-being versus distress. In utero surveillance of physiologic functions of the fetus can also be achieved using fetal sonography. Specific fetal activities include gross body movements,[123] eye movements,[18] sucking movements, heart rate patterns,[16]

Table 17–2. Indications for Prenatal Diagnostic Techniques

General risk factors*
  Maternal age 35 years or older at time of expected delivery†
Specific risk factors
  Previous child with malformation or chromosomal abnormality
  Previous history of stillbirth or neonatal death
  Structural abnormality in mother or father (e.g., neural tube defect)
  Balanced chromosomal translocation in one parent
  Family history of inherited disease in first-degree relatives
  Maternal diabetes mellitus, phenylketonuria, exposure to teratogens or some infectious disease
Risk factors peculiar to certain ethnic groups
  Tay-Sachs disease (screening in Ashkenazi Jews of Eastern European origin)
  Sickle cell disease (screening in African and Afro-American blacks)
  Thalassemia (screening in some Mediterranean and some Asian populations)

*Mostly for chromosomal anomalies.
†Risk of Down syndrome increases significantly after 35 years. Other chromosomal abnormalities are also increasingly common and double or treble the overall risk.
  Modified from D'Alton ME, DeCherney AH: Prenatal diagnosis. N Engl J Med 328:114–120, 1993, with permission.

respiratory patterns, and quantitative determination of amniotic fluid volume.[25] Components can be cumulatively calculated as a fetal biophysical score, which may reflect fetal physiologic well-being.[64] Early or midgestation assessments are controversial; during the last trimester, studies of fetal behaviors may help document altered functional brain maturation by defining dysfunctional fetal state organization of different behaviors[118] (Table 17–4).

7. Intrauterine fetal therapies involve direct intervention of the fetus by a variety of techniques to treat specific conditions.[45] For instance, fetal exchange transfusion is used to treat the anemia and secondary consequences of hematologic disorders. Withdrawal of fluid from body cavities (e.g., pleural, peritoneal), catheterization of the bladder, and, in rare situations, fetal surgery for hydrocephalus can be considered.[3]

◆ RELATIONSHIPS BETWEEN SYSTEMIC AND NEUROLOGIC FETAL DISORDERS

Table 17–5 lists a number of nonneurologic abnormalities that might be associated with neurologic conditions on a genetic or acquired basis. Fetal consultations with a pediatric neurologist may help generate a list of diagnostic possibilities for a variety of medical conditions that share systemic nonneurologic disorders with brain disorders. Some conditions are genetic, syndromic, or acquired. Figure 17–3 illustrates two examples of nonneurologic structural abnormalities that may indicate brain disorders.

◆ SPECIFIC MEDICAL CONDITIONS TO BE CONSIDERED IN THE GENESIS OF FETAL BRAIN DISORDERS

Following is a brief synopsis of selected fetal disease conditions, in which brain disorders play a major or supportive role.

Table 17–3. Major Malformations That Can Be Diagnosed Antenatally by Sonography

Condition Diagnosed	Dates When Diagnosis Is Possible* (weeks' gestational age)	Percentage at 20–24 wk†
Anencephaly	12–16	100
Encephalocele	12–20	75–100
Meningomyelocele	14–32	60–95
Hydrocephalus	20–36	25
Microcephaly‡	18–36	25
Callosal agenesis	>20	Probably high
Lissencephaly	>20	Occasional reports

*Associated malformations are often the most capacious and can lead to discovery of central nervous system abnormalities.
†Frequency estimates using best technique available in 1990.
‡This group includes cases of lissencephaly, true genetic microcephaly, and microcephaly caused by early destructive lesions.
Adapted from Aicardi J, Bax M, Gillberg C, Ogier H: Diseases of the Nervous System in Childhood. Clinics in Developmental Medicine. 2nd ed. New York: MacKeith Press, 1998, with permission.

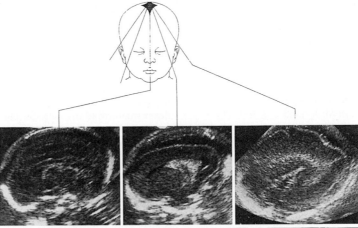

Figure 17–2. List of brain structures imaged on three separate views using fetal sonography—median and two oblique views. (From Timor-Tritsch IE, Monteagudo A, Cohen HL: Ultrasonography of the Prenatal and Neonatal Brain. Stamford, CT: Appleton & Lange; 1996, p 45.)

MEDIAN	OBLIQUE-1	OBLIQUE-2
Corpus callosum	Lateral ventricle	Insula
Cavum septi pellucidi	Anterior horn	Parietal operculum
Caudate nucleus	Posterior horn	Temporal operculum
Thalamus	Atrium	Lateral sulcus
Tela choroidea	Choroid plexus	
Tectum	Thalami	
Corpora quadrigemina		
Vermis		
4th ventricle		
Cisterna magna		

Infectious Diseases

Both the embryo (i.e., less than 8 weeks' gestation) and fetus (i.e., greater than 8 weeks' gestation) are vulnerable to a number of infectious agents. Infections during the first and early second trimesters usually result in congenital malformations, more commonly than destructive lesions. Later infections during the third trimester generally result in destructive changes of the brain. The inflammatory response by infectious agents results in glial scarring of the brain, usually after 26 to 28 weeks' gestation.[10, 12]

The brain may appear markedly atrophic, with calcification of neurotic areas, documented by computed tomography (CT) scan of the head after birth. Major destructive lesions may also have been noted on fetal sonography or neonatal neuroimaging (Fig. 17–4). The most frequent infections that can affect fetal brain integrity and development include those caused by cytomegalovirus (CMV), rubella virus, herpes simplex virus, *Toxoplasma gondii*, *Treponema pallidum*, and human immunodeficiency virus (HIV).

Clinical neonatal manifestations for fetal infectious disease may include organo-

Table 17–4. Major Features of Neonatal Behavioral States in Term Infants*

	Eyes Open	Respiration Regular	Gross Movements	Vocalization
State 1	−	+	−	−
State 2	−	−	±	−
State 3	+	+	−	−
State 4	+	−	+	−
State 5	±	−	+	+

*Data from Ref. 121.
−, absent; +, present; ±, present or absent.
Adapted from Volpe JJ: Neurology of the Newborn. 3rd ed. Philadelphia: WB Saunders, 1995, with permission.

Table 17–5. Nonneurologic Findings Associated With Neurologic Diagnoses

Nonneurologic Finding	Neurologic Diagnosis
Cardiac rhabdomyoma	Tuberous sclerosis
Hypoplastic left heart syndrome	Brain malformations (e.g., microgyria, agenesis of corpus callosum)
Multicystic dysplastic kidney	Brain malformations with specific genetic syndromes vs. destructive brain lesions
Diaphragmatic hernia	Brain malformations (e.g., cerebellar hypoplasia)
Polyhydramnios	Brain malformations with genetic syndromes or destructive brain lesions
Hydrops fetalis	Congenital syndromes (e.g., Turner syndrome) or destructive brain lesions, usually of vascular or infectious origin (e.g., asphyxia, parvovirus, metabolic disorders)
Cleft lip and palate	Midline brain malformations (e.g., holoprosencephaly)
Arthrogryposis	Neuromuscular disease or destructive brain lesions (e.g., congenital muscular dystrophies)
Multiple gestation pregnancy	Destructive brain lesions of white or gray matter (e.g., periventricular leukomalacia)
Omphalocele/gastroschisis	Neural tube defects

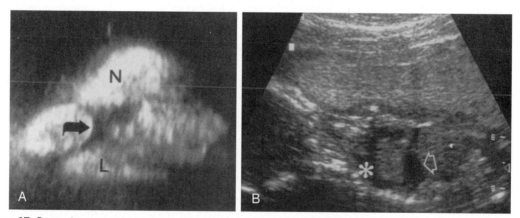

Figure 17–3. Fetal sonography views of nonneurologic findings that may suggest brain disease. *A,* Unilateral cleft lip *(arrow)* end; N, nose; L, lip. *B,* Sagittal view of fetal trunk. Pleural effusion (*) surrounds the fetal lung. Fetal ascites is present *(arrow).* (From Sanders RC: Structural Fetal Abnormalities. St. Louis: Mosby, 1996.)

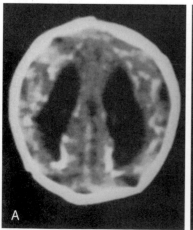
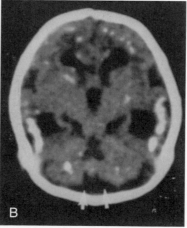

Figure 17–4. Congenital cytomegalovirus infection seen on two computed tomography scans on a 5-day-old newborn. *A,* Periventricular and diffuse cerebral calcifications, and ventriculomegaly. *B,* Cerebellar hypoplasia and large cisterna magna *(arrows).* (From Volpe J: Neurology of the Newborn. 3rd ed. Philadelphia: WB Saunders, 1995, p 680.)

megaly, intrauterine growth retardation (IUGR), jaundice, microcephaly, intracranial calcification, osseous lesions, encephalitis, and chorioretinitis, particularly with CMV infection.[154] Specifically for rubella, any combination of brain, eye, heart, or ear involvement is possible, and some children may have irritability, lethargy, and hypotonia at birth, whereas others only suffer hearing loss, depending on when the fetus was infected.[88] Children with herpes simplex infections are either acutely ill during the immediate postdelivery period or may become symptomatic over the first several weeks of life.[155] Intractable seizures and coma may also highlight their neonatal clinical course. Congenital toxoplasmosis involves a severe neonatal form, which includes hepatosplenomegaly, fever, and purpura. Ventricular dilatation may exist in utero, as documented by fetal sonography, and chorioretinitis is a common feature seen on retinal examination in the newborn period. Clinical presentation of a child with congenital syphilis also involves hepatosplenomegaly, retinitis, and osteochondritis, but these may appear only after several months of life with irritability, vomiting, cranial nerve deficits, and chronic hydrocephalus.[43] HIV infection can be transmitted as early as 15 weeks' gestation; most neonates are asymptomatic with positive serology for up to several years.[1] Diagnosis in the neonatal period is generally difficult. However, some infants receive a large viral load in utero and may be born prematurely with microcephaly and calcification of the basal ganglia.

Less common viruses that also affect the brain but have no consistent pattern of fetal injury include influenza, measles, hepatitis, variola, and enteroviruses and adenoviruses. One viral infection, parvovirus B19,[22] has been associated with nonimmune hydrops fetalis, which may indirectly affect fetal brain integrity by uteroplacental insufficiency, leading to vasculopathies.

Fetal Circulatory and Vascular Disorders

Both ischemic and hemorrhagic cerebrovascular lesions can result from circulatory disorders of the mother, fetus, or placenta.[76]

Consequences of intrauterine circulatory and vascular disorders may only present after birth in the immediate neonatal period

as a result of systemic diseases of the mother, including maternal anemia, hypertensive disorders of pregnancy, or uncontrolled maternal seizures leading to severe hypoxia. Direct trauma to the mother's abdomen, indirect consequences from maternal accidents, and gas intoxication by carbon monoxide or butane poisoning are other examples of maternal pathologic conditions that promote vascular brain injury. Vascular lesions related to fetal conditions include multiple gestation births, particularly when one macerated twin is present (Fig. 17–5), prenatal arterial occlusions from altered angiogenesis, blood dyscrasias from hemolytic disease or thrombocytopenia, and hydrops fetalis from hematologic, infectious, or other congenital causes. Finally, placental or cord anomalies, including fetal-maternal hemorrhage, chronic placental insufficiency with fetal distress, abruptio placenta, true cord knots, and long or short cords may contribute to vascular compromise to the fetus, either in the antepartum or intrapartum periods (Table 17–6).

Circulatory disturbances affect fetal brain differently, depending on the stage of brain development.[2] Brain injuries before the 70th day in utero result in abnormal migratory patterns of neuronal groups within the white matter or neocortex without major cavitation, whereas later injuries result in destructive (encephaloclastic) lesions on an ischemic or hemorrhagic basis. For example, schizencephaly may be the result of faulty vascular supply to the developing neocortex

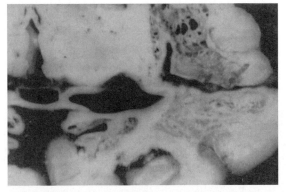

Figure 17–5. Multicystic encephalomalacia in the brain of a monozygotic twin whose stillborn co-twin was macerated. Note honeycomb appearance of subcortical white matter on postmortem examination. (From Aicardi J, Bax M, Gillberg C, Ogier H: Diseases of the Nervous System in Childhood. 2nd ed. New York: MacKeith Press, 1998, p 15.)

Table 17–6. Main Causes of Fetal Encephalopathies of Circulatory Origin

Lesions Related to Maternal Pathologic Conditions

Systemic diseases
  Maternal anemia
  Toxemia with chronic hypertension
  Renal diseases
  Repeated seizures during second trimester of
    pregnancy
  Severe hypoxia
Maternal trauma
  Direct trauma to abdomen
  Maternal accidents
Gas intoxication
  Carbon monoxide
  Butane

Lesions Related to Fetal Conditions

Twinning (especially with one macerated twin)
Prenatal arterial occlusions
Blood dyscrasias
  Hemolytic disease with or without incompatibility
  Thrombocytopenia (genetic, isoimmune, or of
    infective origin)
Nonimmune hydrops fetalis

Lesions Related to Placental or Cord Abnormalities

Fetomaternal hemorrhage
Chronic placental insufficiency with fetal distress
Abruptio placentae
Cord knotting

Adapted from Larroche J-C: Fetal encephalopathies of circulatory origin. Biol Neonate 50:61–74, 1986.

before the 70th day of gestation, resulting in a "true porencephaly," with an ependymal lined cleft or tract between the intraventricular and subarachnoid spaces. In contrast, bilateral carotid artery ligations in fetal monkeys between 70 and 100 days of gestation result in hydranencephaly from destructive ischemic lesions.[93]

In general, the migratory process of neocortical cells, angiogenesis of the blood vessels, and gliogenesis of supportive cellular elements occur in an overlapping manner. Therefore, it may be difficult to precisely predict the specific brain injury because of the unknown timing of the insult or insults that precede or follow critical stages of brain maturation. Circulatory disturbances generally damage the periventricular white matter of the preterm infant. Ischemic or hemorrhagic injuries in the preterm brain tend to occur between 26 and 34 weeks' gestation, whether occurring prenatally in the fetal brain or postnatally in the preterm infant's brain. Alternatively, cortical, subcortical, and basal ganglia regions are more suscepti-

ble to injury after 34 weeks' gestation in either the near-term or term infant, because of the more advanced maturation of brain vasculature. These vascular lesions may also be produced before or after birth, depending on the timing of the insult after 36 weeks' gestation. This topic is discussed in greater detail under the section concerning asphyxia.

Clinical manifestations of fetal circulatory and vascular disorders may be difficult to ascertain, either before or after birth. Unexpected alterations in fetal movements may be helpful, as perceived by the mother, or with abdominal sonography, but they are perceived largely through serendipity; fetal growth restriction, hydrops fetalis, or hydramnios are other examples of more obvious suspicious features. Multiple gestation pregnancies or maternal trauma can also be associated with circulatory abnormalities within the fetal brain. Conversely, vascular lesions may result even with the lack of documentation of maternal, fetal, or placental disorders.

Following birth, specific clinical and laboratory findings may suggest in utero brain injury on a circulatory basis; marked neonatal anemia, microcephaly at birth, marked rigidity or spasticity, or isolated seizures in the absence of post–hypoxic-ischemic brain disorder raise suspicions of antepartum disorders. Early neuroimaging (CT or magnetic resonance imaging [MRI]) within 48 hours after birth should distinguish an acute from a chronic brain lesion. Specific CT or MRI images[71] (i.e., inversion-recovery sequences or diffusion-weighted views) may distinguish acute stages of cellular edema with transmembrane diffusion of intercellular and intracellular fluid contents, whatever the etiology but presumably after a recently occurring pathogenetic process (e.g., asphyxia, infection, trauma), from gliotic scarring, irregular ventricular borders, ventriculomegaly, or brain maldevelopment, alternatively implying a remote brain injury.

Inherited Metabolic and Neurodegenerative Diseases of Fetal Onset

Although it may be difficult to definitively identify children with metabolic or neurodegenerative disorders during fetal life, specific clues can raise concerns before or after birth.[13] Specific disease entities may present in the neonatal period with hypotonia, decreased levels of arousal, or intractable neonatal seizures inappropriate to events around birth. Decreased arousal or coma after formula feedings may suggest a biochemical disorder involving carbohydrate, protein, or fat metabolism. A constellation of minor brain or somatic anomalies may heighten one's clinical suspicions. Limb contractures, an underdeveloped thorax, or decreased muscle mass, for instance, may suggest congenital neuromuscular diseases. Careful ophthalmologic evaluation of the anterior chamber of the eye may document an anterior chamber (i.e., embryotoxon) anomaly associated with peroxisomal diseases, or colobomata of the iris or retina, which represent a nonspecific arrest in ocular development from either metabolic and genetic or developmental disorders. Association with nonimmune hydrops or IUGR may also be clues to the diagnosis. Careful inspection of placental specimens may document destructive lesions, congenital anomalies, or storage material that reflects timing or etiology of disease states (Fig. 17–6).

Exogenous and Endogenous Toxic Disorders

Even though the placenta is usually an effective barrier between maternal and fetal circulations, specific exogenous or endogenous toxins may nonetheless reach the fetus to produce malformations or destructive disturbances, depending on the timing of the toxin exposure[2]: examples of exogenous agents include therapeutic agents, industrial pollutants, and recreational substances. These are listed in Table 17–7, which also lists the various patterns of damage that may occur. An example of endogenous toxicity involves maternal diabetes mellitus. All forms of diabetes may produce problems for the fetus and neonate. Careful control of diabetes can prevent most major congenital malformations to brain and spinal cord, yet developmental and destructive insults can result during fetal life, parturition, or after birth, including immaturity of brain development, sacral agenesis, intracranial venous thromboses from hyperviscosity-polycythemia syndrome, or peripheral nerve injury from shoulder dystocia after impaction of a hypotonic-macrosomic fetus against the pelvic inlet during delivery. Postnatal polycythemia, hypoglycemia, and hypocalcemia may all result in neonatal seizures or coma, or both.

Immunologic and Blood Disorders in the Fetus

Blood type incompatibility has classically been associated with erythroblastosis fetalis and can be prevented by isoimmunization and the administration of globulins. Blood dyscrasias can also contribute to hydrops fetalis on either an immune or nonimmune basis; association with cerebrovascular lesions in the fetus is described earlier. Nonimmune hydrops fetalis, for instance, may occur after infection with parvovirus B19[22] or as the result of different inherited metabolic disorders, cardiac diseases, or chromosomal diseases, such as Turner syndrome. Fetal-maternal and twin-to-twin transfusion syndromes are also frequently implicated in fetal brain disease, usually resulting from ischemic or hemorrhagic injuries because of venous stasis (i.e., hyperviscosity-polycythemia syndrome) or arterial ischemia (i.e., anemia). Intrauterine thrombocytopenia, either the result of isoimmunization against fetal platelets or idiopathic causes, may produce fetal brain damage.[94] Recent research inquiries concerning the inflammatory process have implicated specific components within the cascade of chemical reactions of inflammation as contributory to fetal brain damage in the child with cerebral palsy.[96]

Intrauterine Growth Restriction

Fetal growth restriction may be associated with children at higher risk for neurologic

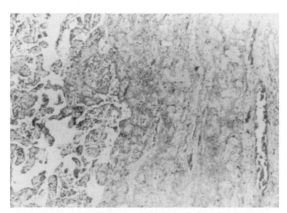

Figure 17–6. Chronic placental infarction superimposed on a more recent retroplacental hemorrhage.

Table 17–7. Main Substances That Can Be Transmitted From Mother to Fetus and Produce Neurologic Damage

Category	Pattern of Damage
Therapeutic Agents	
Antiepileptic drugs (phenytoin, barbiturates, carbamazepine, diones, sodium valproate)	Fetal growth retardation, small head, dysmorphism of face and fingers, clefts, congenital heart disease, and other defects
Benzodiazepines	Poorly defined
Warfarin and other coumarin derivatives	Punctate chondrodystrophy, deafness
Vitamin A	Hydrocephalus, ear, and heart anomalies (uncertain)
Retinoic acid, isotretinoin	Central nervous system (CNS) migration disorder
Industrial Pollutants	
Methylmercury	Abnormal neuronal migration, deranged cortical organization
Polychlorinated biphenyls (PCBs)	Microcephaly, large fontanelles, behavioral disturbances
Carbon monoxide	Hypoxic-ischemic lesions
Recreational Substances	
Alcohol	Fetal growth retardation, facial dysmorphism, brain malformations with excess neuronal migration, and other CNS defects
Narcotics (heroin, codeine, methadone)	Virtually all such substances may produce fetal growth retardation, and narcotics may produce withdrawal symptoms in neonates. In addition, cocaine can induce abruptio placentae and fetal death and may be responsible for skull and brain malformations and vascular damage with infarcts or hemorrhage
Other "street drugs" (amphetamines, pyrobenzamine, phencyclidine)	
Cocaine	
Toluene and other inhalants	Microcephaly, minor craniofacial anomalies, limb anomalies
Tobacco	Growth retardation, possible effects on cognitive development

Adapted from Aicardi J, Bax M, Gillberg C, Ogier H: Diseases of the Nervous System in Childhood. Clinics in Developmental Medicine. 2nd ed. New York: MacKeith Press, 1998.

problems. IUGR is variably defined, usually as somatic growth less than the second percentile, or at least 2 standard deviations less than the mean for the gestational age.[28] Symmetric versus asymmetric growth restriction implies a different time course for a disease state.[75] A child with early gestational disorders from chromosomal or syndromic disorders is more likely to demonstrate balanced growth retardation (i.e., both head and somatic growth compromised). Asymmetric growth retardation occurs during the last trimester from acquired deficits, which tend to spare head growth. Children who are small for gestational age as a compensatory response to in utero stress may escape subsequent neurologic sequelae, whereas other children with IUGR suffer brain injury. The fetus with IUGR exhibits malformations or dysmorphic syndromes at a much higher rate than the general population (5% to 15%).[2] Therefore, the possible association of intrauterine growth restriction and brain injury should be taken in the context of other historical and physical examination factors.

◆ APPROACH TO NEUROLOGIC EXAMINATION OF THE NEWBORN

Even though the nervous system of the newborn is structurally and functionally immature, general strategies for the performance of a neurologic examination should parallel the bedside approach used with the older infant and child.[165] Neuronal networks in the neonatal brain with limited dendritic and synaptic interconnections, as well as immature myelination patterns, contribute to the expression of immature neurologic function. Therefore, clinical neurologic signs reflect, to a larger extent, subcortical structures and, to a more limited extent, cortical function. Therefore, judicious coordination of careful neurologic clinical examination with neurobehavioral state assessment, with electroencephalographic (EEG) and polygraphic analyses, can better assess brain function.

To reinforce the discussion in the previous section concerning fetal brain development and its unique susceptibilities to maldevelopment or injury, the present discussion of the clinical evaluation of the newborn explores how the newborn's clinical repertoire reflects prenatal, peripartum, and postnatal disease processes.

Systematic neonatal examination techniques must be followed in a sequential and repetitive fashion, emphasizing specific levels of the neuraxis (Table 17–8). The preterm infant has a more limited clinical repertoire because of greater immaturity; yet, serial examination findings can optimize the validity of normal or suspicious findings. Knowledge of the evolution of signs and symptoms over the early postnatal period can contribute to the clinician's diagnostic and prognostic abilities. Abnormalities found on neurologic examination reflect moment-to-moment functional integrity of the child and may have little bearing on the location or extent of brain damage that occurred during fetal or neonatal life; it only becomes more demonstrable at older ages.

Estimation of Gestational Age

Estimation of the maturity of a child is crucial to understanding the neurodevelopmental niche into which a child is situated when an examination is performed. Responses to the neonatal neurologic examination change with the child's maturational level. Also, disease entities are expressed in unique characteristics of newborns who are born appropriate for gestational age compared with those who are small for gestational age. Finally, specific types of insults to the brain have varying impact on different parts of the nervous system, depending on a child's gestational maturity.[165]

The most useful historical data for estimating gestational age, especially in preterm infants, is the date of the mother's last menstrual period.[133] Techniques for estimating gestational maturity by clinical examination include careful anthropometric measurements such as body weight, length, and head circumference, as well as descriptions of external characteristics such as body hair, skin texture, skin creases, and areola size.[8, 50] Laboratory evaluations also provide estimates of maturity; these include radiographic study of bone growth, neurophysiological measures of EEG or nerve conduction velocities,[145] and neuroimaging descriptions of sulcal, gyral, and myelination features.[67]

Characteristics of the Head

Examination of the head comprises four areas: skin characteristics, head circumference, shape of the head, and rate of head growth.

The skin should be carefully inspected for the presence of (1) dimples or tracts, which are associated with brain malformations; (2) subcutaneous masses that reflect trauma, tumors, or encephaloceles; and (3) cutaneous lesions, which may be associated with specific congenital vascular abnormalities or neurocutaneous syndromes, such as Sturge-Weber syndrome, linear sebaceous nevus syndrome, or incontinentia pigmenti. Description of skin lesions may help diagnose a medical condition with important manifestations to brain. For instance, the port wine stain of Sturge-Weber syndrome can be associated with abnormalities in choroidal vessels in the eye and meninges, which may result in glaucoma and cortical lesions, respectively. Skin lesions may evolve with maturation. For example, pale macular lesions with Sturge-Weber syndrome become more deeply stained red or purple with age[158] (Fig. 17–7).

Head circumference should be consid-

Table 17–8. Neonatal Neurologic Examination—Basic Elements

Level of alertness
Cranial nerves
  Olfaction (I)
  Vision (II)
  Optic fundi (II)
  Pupils (III)
  Extraocular movements (III, IV, VI)
  Facial sensation and masticatory power (V)
  Facial motility (VII)
  Audition (VIII)
  Sucking and swallowing (V, VII, IX, X, XII)
  Sternocleidomastoid function (XI)
  Tongue function (XII)
  Taste (VII, IX)
Motor examination
  Tone and posture
  Motility and power
  Tendon reflexes and plantar response
Primary neonatal reflexes
  Moro reflex
  Palmar grasp
  Tonic neck response
Sensory examination

Adapted from Volpe JJ: Neurology of the Newborn. 3rd ed. Philadelphia: WB Saunders, 1995, p. 95.

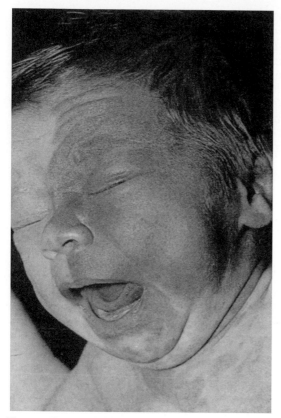

Figure 17–7. Angiomata in a newborn characteristic of Sturge-Weber syndrome.

be associated with craniosynostosis, ranging from Treacher-Collins syndrome to congenital hypothyroidism.

Finally, the rate of head growth is extremely important to note on serial examinations. Appropriate postnatal growth rates are difficult to define, but certain generalities should be considered: modest head shrinkage, reflected by overriding sutures, can be seen during the first several days in the near-term or term infant.[172] For the premature infant, increases in head growth by a mean of approximately 0.5 cm in the second week and 0.75 in the third week, as well as 1 cm on a weekly basis thereafter, should be expected for a healthy premature infant.[56, 148] The clinician must recognize that the sick preterm infant with systemic disease may require initial time for "catch-up head growth," which may exceed the expected rate. However, extremes in growth arrest or excessive growth must be considered as part of a pathologic process (e.g., continued nutritional deprivation, genetic influences, or progressive hydrocephalus).[149] A pathologic condition should be considered in all infants with changes in head growth that are more than 2 standard deviations above or below the mean for all infants at that corrected age.

Levels of Alertness

As with a patient at any older age, the formal neurologic examination of the newborn should include an assessment of the level of alertness. Terms such as *state* or *vigilance*

ered as a surrogate measurement of brain and cerebrospinal fluid (CSF) volumes. Generalized or localized scalp edema affects the accuracy of the head circumference measurement. True macrocephaly or microcephaly can be estimated based on whether the child's head size is greater than or less than the 2nd or 98th percentiles, respectively.

The shape of the head also requires careful inspection. Skull deformities may be a result from acquired or congenital processes. Molding of the skull may result from a difficult vaginal descent and extraction. Scalp edema, cephalohematomas, or subgaleal hematomas may have occurred. Knowledge of all cranial sutures is necessary (Fig. 17–8). Craniosynostosis (i.e., premature closure of a cranial suture) may be a congenital cause of a malformed shape. Sagittal synostosis is the most common type, resulting in an elongated shape with a high forehead. Different head shapes result from closure of coronal, metopic, or lambdoidal sutures; several sutures may also be fused. Genetic disorders or endocrinologic syndromes can

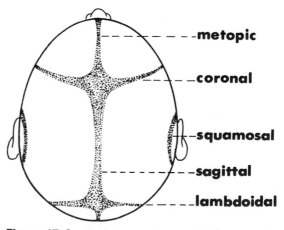

Figure 17–8. Diagram depicting cranial sutures in the skull of the newborn.

have been ascribed to these criteria, and they usually imply a description of the two initial states of quiet (state 1) and active (state 2) sleep, respectively, followed by progressively increased levels of arousal from an awake-sleep transition (state 3) through quiet wakefulness (state 4) and vigorous crying with wakefulness (state 5).[20, 119] The infant varies in levels of alertness relative to feeding or environmental stimuli, as well as disease states. Behavioral or polygraphic criteria help define these state transitions (see Table 17–4).[121] Recent events in the nursery, such as painful procedures, bathing, feeding, or medications also affect the child's state of alertness.

Abnormalities in levels of alertness are one of the more common neurologic deficits noted in the newborn period. Detection of such abnormalities may be subtle and require consideration of environmental influences as well as the maturity of the child. General categories for decreased levels of arousal include lethargy, stupor, and coma. The appearance of the infant in a resting state, his or her arousal response, and the quality and quantity of motor responses allow the examiner to approximate whether the child should be considered stuporous rather than asleep; diminished or absent arousal responses and reduced motor responses are noted in the child who is abnormally lethargic.[60, 150] The distinction between stupor and coma is also based on the quality and quantity of motor responses relative to the gestational maturity. After 28 weeks of gestational age, stimulation consistently results in the infant's waking for several minutes. By 32 weeks of gestational age, no stimulation is needed for arousal. After 36 weeks of gestational age, increased alertness is readily observed, with well-formed sleep-wake cycles by term age.[109, 121] In general, the examiner should assume bilateral cortical dysfunction or disturbance of the reticular activating system within the gray matter of the diencephalon, midbrain, and upper pons if wakefulness cannot be achieved, even with vigorous stimulation.[117]

Cranial Nerves

There are 12 pairs of cranial nerves that are identified by specific functions within the cortex and brainstem. Cranial nerve functions and abnormalities referable to a partic-ular region of the brain are elaborated in the following text.

Olfaction (I)

Olfaction is often ignored in the neurologic evaluation of the neonate, but it may be associated with various disease conditions. A sensory stimulus such as a cotton pledget soaked with peppermint extract elicits a consistent response in a child of 30 to 32 weeks of gestational age, with a sucking arousal or withdrawal response; more immature infants may normally lack this response.[135] Olfactory discrimination has been demonstrated for the newborn, who prefer odors from the mother, with rapid associative learning within 48 hours.[86, 157] An absent response should be considered in infants in whom the olfactory bulbs and tracts may not have developed, sometimes noted with disturbances of midline brain development such as holoprosencephaly.[135] This could be present in infants of diabetic mothers who have a higher risk for this type of brain anomaly.[38]

Vision (II)

Specific visual responses are subserved by the second cranial nerves. Blinking to light begins by approximately 25 to 26 weeks of gestational age[131]; by 32 weeks, infants sustain prolonged eye closure as long as the light source remains present.[111] By 34 weeks of gestational age, infants can track a large red object, and by 37 weeks, they can follow ambient light. Optokinetic nystagmus elicited by a rotating drum or striped cloth may be seen after 36 weeks of gestational age. Anatomic localization for visual fixation and following responses does not require the occipital cortex and may be subserved by subcortical structures such as the superior colliculus of the midbrain and the pulvinar, which link with the retina and optic nerves.[68]

It is far more difficult to study the visual abilities of acuity, color perception, contrast sensitivity, and visual discrimination in the newborn. Estimations of these responses can be ascertained by careful observation of functional abilities using age-specific visual fixation devices.[19] By 35 weeks of gestational age, newborns prefer complex patterns with curved contours over straight lines. However, acuity, binocular visual acuity, and appreciation of depth perception vary widely in the newborn, and these only rapidly improve during the first 3 to 4 postnatal months.[6] Therefore, the evaluation of visual function may be hampered by one's ability to assess these visual functions at the bedside. Nonetheless, infants with periventricular leukomalacia (PVL) involving parieto-occipital regions exhibit delayed visual acuity when studied later in infancy.[44]

The funduscopic examination of cranial nerve II is an extremely valuable aspect of neurologic assessment of the newborn. Optic discs may reflect significant disease processes if alterations in color, depth of cup, and circumference are noted. Careful inspection of the anterior chamber, retinal grounds, and external eye structures by a pediatric ophthalmologist is essential. Evidence of corneal clouding, glaucoma, cataracts, colobomata, or chorioretinitis are examples of ophthalmologic findings that have clinical importance for both acquired and genetic fetal disorders. Indirect ophthalmologic evaluation by this specialist more fully examines the fundus, particularly the posterior pole of the retinal surface. Major abnormalities of the optic fundus during the newborn period include colobomata, optic disc hypoplasia or atrophy (Fig. 17–9), retinal and preretinal hemorrhages, chorioretinitis, retinopathy of prematurity, and retinoblastoma. Congenital malformations associated with optic disc hypoplasia usually occur early during the first trimester of pregnancy (e.g., septooptic dysplasia, agenesis of the corpus callosum). As many as 50% of affected children subsequently exhibit other neurologic disorders.[124] Atrophy suggests an acquired injury or ongoing metabolic or degenerative process. Retinal hemorrhages may suggest increased ocular venous pressure, blood dyscrasias, or asphyxia, but they can also be present in 20% to 40% of all newborns.[15] Chorioretinitis may suggest a congenital infection, and retinopathy of prematurity implies dilatation[54] and tortuosity of vessels as a result of a variety of etiologies in premature infants. The uncommon presentation of retinoblastoma or an embryotoxon would be helpful in the diagnosis of a neoplasm or a genetic or metabolic disease, respectively. Retinoblastoma in neonates usually presents with a white pupil and strabismus. Embryotoxon signifies an arrest in development within the anterior chamber, requiring documentation with an indirect ophthalmoscope.

Pupils (II and III)

Pupillary function is associated with both the second and third cranial nerves and appears by 30 weeks of gestational age, with consistent responses occurring between 30 and 32 weeks of gestational age.[125] Abnormalities in function of the pupillary pathways are reflected by the overall size and symmetry of the pupils; bilateral cortical disease such as asphyxia or medication effects must be considered. Unilateral changes may imply autonomic dysfunction to central

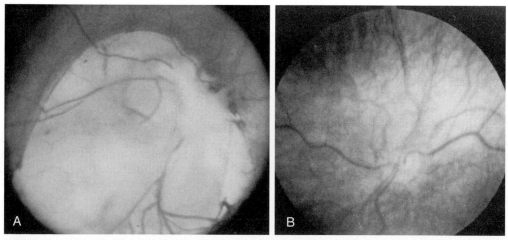

Figure 17–9. *A,* Coloboma of optic nerve, retina, and choroid. Yellow-white sclera is visible and retinal vessels can be seen coursing through the coloboma. There is malformation resulting from faulty closure of the fetal fissure within the first month of gestation. *B,* Hypoplasia of the optic disc half the normal size.

or peripheral nervous portions of the pupillary pathways. These can be associated with brachial plexus injuries, with herniation effects involving unilateral mass lesions (e.g., from infarction or intracranial hemorrhage), and with the mass effect of supratentorial brain structures along the course of the third cranial nerve in which the parasympathetic fibers are encased.[165]

Extraocular Movements (III, IV, and VI)

Attention must be directed to the infant's eye position, spontaneous eye movements, and movements elicited by oculovestibular (i.e., doll's eyes response) or oculocaloric (i.e., cold or warm water response) maneuvers. Three cranial nerves interconnect within the brainstem to subserve these functions, and doll's eyes can be observed in the infant as early as 25 weeks of gestational age. The eyes normally move conjugately in the direction opposite head movement, given the child's degree of prematurity.[168] Caloric stimulation can be performed after 30 weeks, and spontaneous roving eye movements are expected after 32 weeks.[42]

Abnormalities in extraocular movements include dysconjugate gaze, skew or downward deviation, and opsoclonus; these can be seen in healthy neonates.[66] These disorders of ocular motility usually resolve over the first 6 months of life, but they may indicate persistent gaze palsies related to ocular strabismus or intracranial diseases within the brainstem or cortical visual pathways. Intermittent abnormal eye movements may also be associated with seizure abnormalities. Some nonseizure pathologic processes include hydrocephalus, mass lesions, and genetic and metabolic diseases.[23, 164]

Facial Sensation and Masticatory Power (V)

The trigeminal nerve has both sensory and motor components. Facial sensation is best assessed by facial grimaces to noxious stimuli. The three divisions of the trigeminal nerve must be distinguished from the first and second cervical root sensory distributions over the posterior scalp and neck, respectively. Masseter and pterygoid muscle strength also reflect fifth nerve motor function and may be affected if the neonate exhibits suck and swallow abnormalities. Corneal reflexes are also subserved by the autonomic pathway within the fifth cranial nerve, which becomes functional by the 25th to 26th week of gestation.

Facial Motility (VII)

Facial nerve function involves amplitude and symmetry of both spontaneous and sensory-elicited facial movements. Major causes of facial weakness in the neonatal period occur throughout all levels of the neuraxis (i.e., cerebral, nuclear, peripheral nerve, neuromuscular junction, or muscle).[164] For example, the presence of a bilateral facial weakness may be secondary to severe hypoxic-ischemic encephalopathy, but bilateral or unilateral facial weakness may also be associated with brainstem hypoplasia or aplasia of the motor nuclear groups known as Möbius syndrome. Injury to the facial nerve may also occur during labor or delivery as a result of compression of the face against the maternal sacrum or by forceps compression. Finally, weakness at either neuromuscular junction or the muscle may be associated with congenital myasthenia, myopathies, or mitochondrial disorders. Asymmetry of the child's face while crying may be associated with hypoplasia or absence of a specific muscle, the depressor anguralis oris, on the side that the face does not depress.

Audition (VIII)

The child of 28 weeks of gestational age startles or blinks to loud sudden noise. The lemniscal or auditory pathway that subserves this sensory function is functionally active early in the third trimester of development.[131] Auditory acuity, localization, and discrimination are present in the neonate.[152] Detection of significant hearing deficits may be quite important in the examination of the neonate. Four categories of eighth nerve disturbances include familial forms of deafness, bilirubin-induced injury to the auditory pathway, congenital infections, and congenital defects of the head and neck. Premature infants have a distinctly increased incidence of significant hearing loss.[165] The term infant may suffer hearing loss from asphyxial causes that occur any time throughout the perinatal period; for example, one specific pulmonary problem called persistent pulmonary hypertension of the newborn (PPHN) may result in peripheral injury to the eighth nerve.[62] Use of the brainstem auditory evoked response may more precisely localize the site of the deficit to the peripheral nerve or auditory pathway.[32]

Sucking and Swallowing (V, VII, IX, X, and XII)

Sucking involves coordinated action of breathing, sucking, and swallowing with two coordinated phases that are linked in a synchronous action. The swallow response has a voluntary followed by involuntary phase, both of which physiologically improve with maturity. Whereas rooting appears as early as 28 weeks of gestational age, the synchronous action of swallowing does not appear until 30 to 34 and is not coordinated with breathing until 37 weeks. Gag responses subserved by cranial nerves IX and X are essential for the response of the posterior pharyngeal muscles, particularly to close the larynx and prevent aspiration; the gag reflex appears in the child of 28 weeks of gestational age.[24] Disturbances in suck and swallow functions may originate throughout the neuraxis, ranging from the cerebral cortex through the brainstem nuclear groups to peripheral nerve, neuromuscular junction, and muscle levels.[165]

Sternocleidomastoid Function (XI)

The function of the sternocleidomastoid muscle is mediated by the cranial nerve XI, which allows the child to flex and rotate the neck and head. Disorders in this function are usually related to a contracture or weakness of the muscle, such as from fetal positioning or trauma to the muscle. There are also children with congenital torticollis that reflect congenital, musculoskeletal, and brain abnormalities referable to the cervicomedullary junction. Malformations during the embryonic or fetal periods can result in anomalies such as Klippel-Feil syndrome, syringobulbia, or basilar impression.

Tongue Function (XII)

Tongue movements are usually best assessed spontaneously or by observing the child's suck on the examiner's fingertip. Abnormalities in tongue function usually involve neurons of the hypoglossal nerve or muscle. Atrophy or fasciculations may suggest a pathologic condition to the brainstem nu-

clear group subserving tongue movement, ranging from congenital (e.g., progressive spinal muscular atrophy) to destructive processes (e.g., brainstem infarction). The size of the tongue may imply syndromic or metabolic disorders (e.g., macroglossia with hypothyroidism, Beckwith-Wiedemann syndrome, or specific storage diseases). The clinician should also consider that a tongue may appear enlarged because the oral cavity is reduced in size (e.g., in Pierre-Robin syndrome).

◆ MOTOR EXAMINATION

Major features of the motor examination of the newborn involve descriptions of muscle tone, posture of limbs, motility, muscular power, deep tendon reflexes, and plantar responses. As with all aspects of the neurologic examination, observations of motor function rely on gestational maturity, levels of alertness, and serial examinations. Knowledge of medications, feeding, disease states, and noxious stimuli must also be considered because they affect the neonate's motor responses.

Tone and Posture

Tone is best assessed by passively manipulating the limbs with the head in the midline. It is important to avoid head turning, which elicits a tonic neck reflex, leading to a false sense of asymmetry in tone. Eighty percent of infants spontaneously prefer right-sided head turning. Developmental aspects of tone have been carefully documented by earlier researchers; in general, a caudal to rostral progression in tone development occurs with increasing gestational maturity. Minimal resistance is present at 28 weeks of gestational age. By 32 weeks, distinct flexor tone begins in the lower extremities. By 36 weeks, flexor tone is prominent in the lower extremities and palpable in the upper extremities. When assessing a child's level of maturity, observations of tone and posture imply measurement or observation of the angle of a limb around a joint, at rest or with gentle traction.[4, 120]

The quantity, quality, and symmetry of motility and muscular power are also important aspects of the motor examination. The initial myoclonic movements of the preterm infant evolve into larger amplitude, slower movements in the near-term and term infant. Also, as the child matures, alternating rather than symmetric movements begin to be observed. By term, an awake infant has the ability to momentarily lift the head off his or her chest and remain upright for several seconds while being supported in a vertical position.[131]

Deep Tendon Reflexes and Plantar Responses

Deep tendon reflexes are initially elicited in the preterm infant after 32 to 34 weeks of gestational age. Pectoralis, biceps, brachioradialis, knee, and ankle reflexes should be assessed. Symmetric ankle clonus of 5 to 10 beats may be an acceptable finding in a healthy full-term newborn. The plantar response is usually extensor in the newborn; therefore, its pathologic significance is assigned only if asymmetry is noted.

In general, abnormalities found on motor examination include altered muscle tone with or without weakness, abnormalities in deep tendon reflexes and plantar responses, and abnormal spontaneous movements. A brief description of these abnormalities follows:

One must always consider normal maturational changes in motility, tone, and reflexes before ascribing pathologic significance. Therefore, the presence of low tone or hypotonia—the most common motor abnormality in neonates—must be considered with respect to possible patterns of muscle weakness that usually are present with low tone. Levels of the neuraxis that may be involved with hypotonia include focal or bilateral cerebral, brainstem, spinal cord, low motor neuron, nerve root, peripheral nerve, neuromuscular junction, and muscle involvement[165] (Table 17–9). Focal injury to the cerebrum results in contralateral hemiparesis. Parasagittal cerebral injury, usually from asphyxia, affects the border zone vascular regions over the cerebral convexities, resulting in increased weakness of the upper extremities more than lower extremities. Periventricular injury, primarily situated in deep white matter structures, largely affect tone and strength in the lower extremities. Spinal cord involvement usually spares the face and other functions of cranial nerves while involving sphincteric as well as motor

and sensory functions below the site of the spinal lesion. Other lower motor neuron sites include primarily focal weakness situated in nerve roots or, more commonly, generalized weakness localized to the peripheral nerve, neuromuscular junction, or muscular levels.

Hypertonia is a less common feature of neonatal neurologic disease, but it is one that may have important significance. Increased tone in the newborn period is commonly noted with mild acute postasphyxial dysfunction, meningitis, or subarachnoid hemorrhage, or as a result of severe intrauterine injury from asphyxia or malformation earlier in gestation as a fetus. The chronic phase of bilirubin encephalopathy, prenatal substance exposure (e.g., cocaine and amphetamines), and continuous muscle fiber activity (Isaac syndrome) are rare clinical conditions in the newborn that are also associated with hypertonicity. An unusual genetic or familial syndrome known as hyperexplexia may also be expressed in a child with increased muscle tone, usually accentuated by sensory stimuli.

Abnormalities in deep tendon reflexes and plantar responses also follow the general rule of localization at the site of neurologic injury above or below the motor neuron level. Preserved reflexes are seen with pathologic processes above the lower motor neuron unit, that is, lesions of the cerebrum down to the anterior horn cell of the spinal cord. Disease entities in the lower motor neuron unit, below the anterior horn cell on the peripheral nerve, neuromuscular junction, or muscle levels, result in absent or diminished responses. Unlike in the child older than 1 year, plantar responses (i.e., the Babinski sign), in general, are extensor, and, therefore, are only clinically helpful if they are asymmetric.

Spontaneous Abnormal Movements

There are a variety of movements that may suggest neurologic abnormalities: tremulousness, excessive startles, fasciculations, complex movements, and myotonia can all occur in the neonate. Tremulousness is a common feature noted in children with neuronal hyperirritability after asphyxial stress, metabolic disturbances such as hypocalcemia and hypoglycemia, or drug withdrawal. Fasciculations are associated with

Table 17–9. Main Causes of Generalized Hypotonia in the Newborn Infant

Site of Major Pathology	Disorder
Anterior horn cell	Spinal muscular atrophy
	Other anterior horn cell disease (in association with cerebellar atrophy)
Peripheral nerves or roots	Congenital polyneuropathies (several types)
Muscle	Congenital muscular dystrophy (several types including Fukuyama type and "occidental" types with and without merosine deficiency)
	Congenital myotonic dystrophy
	Congenital myopathies
	Central core disease
	Centronuclear myopathy
	Nemaline myopathy
	Congenital fiber type disproportion
	Other structural myopathies
	Glycogen storage diseases types II and III
	Mitochondrial myopathies (deficit in cytochrome *c* oxidase)
	Severe type
	Transient type
Neuromuscular junction	Neonatal myasthenia (infants of myasthenic mothers)
	Congenital myasthenia and myasthenic syndromes (several types)
	Infantile botulism
Central nervous system	Hypoxic-ischemic encephalopathy
	Brain malformations (including trisomy 21)
	Hemorrhagic and other brain damage
	Drug intoxication
Mixed origin (mainly central nervous system)	Zellweger syndrome and related peroxisomal disorders
	Prader-Willi syndrome
	Hypothyroidism
Connective tissue abnormality	Marfan syndrome
	Ehlers-Danlos syndrome

Adapted from Aicardi J, Bax M, Gillberg C, Ogier H: Diseases of the Nervous System in Childhood. Clinics in Developmental Medicine. 2nd ed. New York: MacKeith Press, 1998.

low motor neuron disease, particularly within the anterior horn cells of the spinal cord. Excessive startles are noted with metabolic, genetic, or familial disturbances, and myotonia can be seen with specific forms of congenital muscular dystrophy, such as myotonic dystrophy. One striking movement disorder has been described in preterm infants following severe bronchopulmonary dysplasia at near-term or term corrected ages, as well as after bilirubin encephalopathy. Athetotic, choreiform, and dystonic movements have been described, reflecting neuronal injury within the basal ganglia or extrapyramidal pathways connected to these midline gray matter structures.[115]

Primitive Fetal and Neonatal Reflexes

There are many primitive reflexes that should be part of the neonatal neurologic examination. Five major responses to be elicited include the Moro reflex, palmar and plantar grasp, tonic neck responses, placing, and stepping reflexes.[131]

The Moro reflex has an onset between 28 to 32 weeks of gestational age and is well established by 37 weeks; it is no longer active after 4 months of corrected age. The palmar grasp also appears at 28 weeks of gestational age, becomes well established by 32 weeks, and disappears by 2 months of age. The tonic neck reflex does not appear until 35 weeks of gestational age and is well established at 1 month, but disappears by 5 to 7 months. Placing and stepping reflexes are usually elicited by 37 weeks of gestational age and later become integrated with supporting reflexes after 2 months of age.

Abnormalities in primitive reflex testing usually involve reproducible asymmetry or the incomplete or exaggerated response of a reflex. Any of the reflexes, when asymmetric, may reflect either a cortical, brainstem, plexus, or peripheral nerve disease. The complete repertoire of reflex testing should be performed to ascertain whether dysfunction of the upper or lower motor unit exists.

◆ SENSORY EXAMINATION

Even though sensory examination is an extremely important part of the newborn neurologic examination, alerting and withdrawal responses are the most practical expressions of either cortical or peripheral sensory abilities. A serial response to pinprick over the medial aspect of the extremity should result in a response that can be described by latency, limb movement, facial reaction, localization, and habituation.[165] A lower level of response as well as an exaggerated response should be noted. Some major generalizations serve as caveats for abnormalities of the sensory examination. Most illustrative is the sensory deficit in infants with brachial plexus injuries that are seen in a segmental manner, depending on what portion of the plexus has been injured. A spinal cord injury should be considered if a sensory level can be appreciated over the thorax, trunk, and legs. Genetic syndromes involving the sensory system rarely present in the newborn period. One example of a genetic disorder that encompasses peripheral sensory and autonomic nervous systems as well as higher cortical structures is Riley-Day syndrome, or familial dysautonomia. These infants characteristically display irritability, lack the ability to express tears, fail to maintain temperature, demonstrate areflexia on tendon reflex testing, and lack fungiform papillae on the posterior part of the tongue.

Importance of Serial Neonatal Neurologic Examinations

Although more limited in the newborn infant, the neurologic examination remains an essential aspect of neurologic diagnosis in the newborn, from which formulations of diagnostic and therapeutic strategies are based. Even though the examination permits evaluation of functions that may be subcortical in location, the constellation of persistently abnormal neurologic findings over time are strong predictors of neurologic deficits at older ages.[21, 162] Specific clinical abnormalities may predict static motor encephalopathies, collectively referred to as cerebral palsy. Various abnormalities of limb, neck, or trunk tone (Fig. 17–10); diminished cry; weak or absent suck and swallow; the need for gavage or tube feeding; and diminished levels of activity or arousal carry substantially increased risks.[97] Consideration of both clinical and laboratory findings provide the clinician with compelling bedside evidence of possible neurologic abnormalities.

◆ LABORATORY EVALUATIONS OF THE NEWBORN INFANT

After obtaining maternal, fetal, and neonatal histories, and after performing a careful bedside examination, neonatal neurologic assessment must then include judicious use of specialized studies that assess the structural

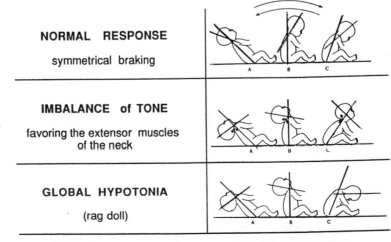

Figure 17–10. Abnormalities of active tone in the neonate at term.

NORMAL RESPONSE
symmetrical braking

IMBALANCE of TONE
favoring the extensor muscles of the neck

GLOBAL HYPOTONIA
(rag doll)

RAISE TO SIT MANEUVER and RETURN BACKWARD

and functional integrity of the child's nervous system. Two diagnostic modalities include tests of structure versus function. Several highlights should be kept in mind. The early and repetitive use of specialized studies may not only shed light on the severity of the encephalopathic state of the child but also elucidate aspects of etiology and timing during fetal life. Structural and functional studies are complementary and are therefore useful when combined with historical and clinical data. Furthermore, serial laboratory studies may provide insight into the persistence or resolution of a pathologic process to the brain as a function of the child's gestational age and adaptation of brain function to either stress or injury.

Cerebrospinal Fluid Examination

Examination of the CSF is one important aspect of neurologic evaluation of the newborn. The principal components of this specific fluid examination include measurements of intracranial pressure, assessment of color of the spinal fluid (i.e., bloody or xanthochromia), turbidity of spinal fluid (i.e., purulence), the red and white blood cell counts, the neutrophil differential count, concentrations of protein and glucose, and the detection of microorganisms as well as specific metabolites. Normal values for preterm and full-term neonates have been studied[126, 134] and are summarized elsewhere in the text, with the following highlights to be kept in mind. The clinical suspicion of meningitis should always be a part of the general concern for clinical sepsis. CSF might be infected despite the absence of infection in the peripheral blood. Values for blood cell, protein, and glucose concentrations in the CSF may be difficult to interpret, and clinical considerations may need to be preferentially considered. Careful examination of the supernate after centrifugation, documenting xanthochromia, particularly with elevated CSF protein, strongly suggests the possibility of an intracranial hemorrhage. The presence of nucleated red blood cells in the spinal fluid as well as the peripheral blood may point to an intrauterine pathologic process of longer duration than the peripartum period. See Appendix F.

Diagnostic Imaging of the Neonatal Brain

Important tools have been developed to assist in the structural assessment of the immature brain: cranial ultrasonography, computerized tomography (CT), magnetic resonance imaging (MRI), spectroscopy (MRS), and positron emission tomography (PET). During the neonatal period, the clinical usefulness of PET is limited.

Cranial Ultrasonography

Ultrasonography is a rapid, noninvasive cribside imaging technique that has been the method of choice for detecting and following the evolution of specific brain lesions. Excellent reviews are available for consultation.[47, 57, 79, 161] Clinicians should be aware of the limits of visibility and accuracy of images, which are confined primarily to the periventricular regions and ventricular space within the brain. Identification of normal features should be initially mastered (Fig. 17–11A), including the ventricular outline, choroid plexus, and thalami. Visualization of the germinal matrix, intraventricular hemorrhage (see Fig. 17–11B), periventricular echodensities (see Fig. 17–11C) in the white matter, and intraparenchymal echodensities are the principal abnormalities. Normal ultrasound examination results do not rule out the presence of cortical injury or malformation. Intraparenchymal or meningeal locations of brain lesions are not readily detected. Furthermore, visualization of posterior fossa structures is limited.

Computed Tomography Scans

CT scanning of the neonatal brain continues to have important applications to neonatal neurologic assessment, despite the more recent availability of MRI studies. Two situations—acute hemorrhage and intracerebral calcifications—may be better visualized by CT than MRI during the neonatal period (see Fig. 17–4). It is also relatively easier to obtain a CT scan than an MRI scan; however, the limited resolution of CT clearly is a factor. Early ischemic injuries and more subtle malformations are generally not as well localized using CT.

Magnetic Resonance Imaging

Even though the indications for an MRI scan are essentially the same as for a CT scan of the newborn, the higher contrast resolution of MRI permits more sensitive assessment of white and gray matter structures; specific

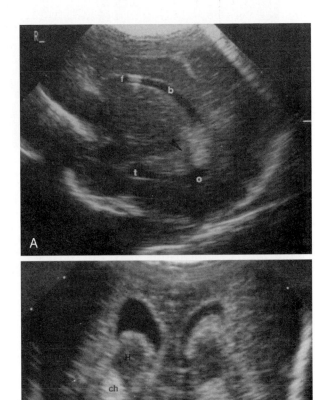

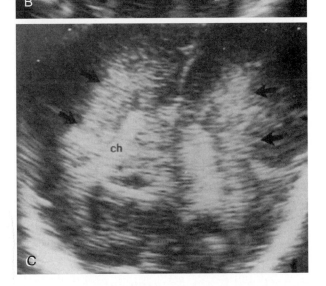

Figure 17–11. *A,* Normal lateral ventricle in the right paramedian plane on cranial sonography of the newborn. Arrowhead points to the choroid plexus in the atrium of the lateral ventricle; f, frontal horn; b, body; o, proximal portion of the occipital horn; t, temporal horn of the lateral ventricle. *B,* Grade III IVH (coronal plane). H signifies large clot in the left dilated anterior horn in a 7-day-old 29-week GA newborn. Arrowhead indicates small amount of blood in the third ventricle. *C,* Periventricular leukomalacia in the first day of life for a preterm infant. Symmetric echogenic regions noted *(arrows),* to be distinguished from the choroid plexus, labeled as ch. (From Timor-Tritsch IE, Monteagudo A, Cohen HL: Ultrasonography of the Prenatal and Neonatal Brain. Stamford, CT: Appleton & Lange, 1996, p 229.)

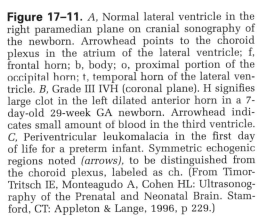

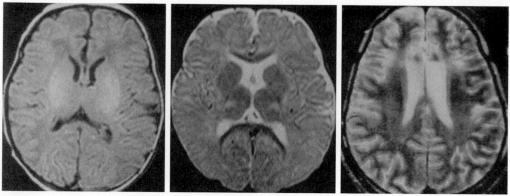

Figure 17–12. Hypoxic-ischemic encephalopathy in term infant: MRI scans. *Left,* Intense T2-weighted signal from basal ganglia on axial cuts. *Center,* Extensive low T1-weighted signal from basal ganglia and thalami. *Right,* Multifocal corticosubcortical damage in another infant. (From Aicardi J, Bax M, Gillberg C, Ogier H: Diseases of the Nervous System in Childhood. 2nd ed. New York: MacKeith Press, 1998.)

radiologic features such as acute hemorrhage and calcifications may not be as readily discernible as with the CT scan. Newer signal processing techniques using MRI can better discern regional developmental changes within white and gray matter structures, localization of pathologic processes to specific regions such as the basal ganglia, and early cytotoxic changes with diffusion of water into the extracellular space (Fig. 17–12). Identification of normal age-specific aspects of brain development must first be mastered,[11, 29] particularly the process of myelination.[17] T1- and T2-weighted images (for increased and decreased white matter signals, respectively), as well as diffusion-weighted images,[71] are currently recommended. Morphometric measurements provide quantitative estimates of either developmental or destructive changes.[49]

Magnetic Resonance Spectroscopy

MRS is a new method for the measurement of energy metabolism; it can be sensitive in situations in which impaired energy metabolism is suspected (Fig. 17–13). This technique may be particularly useful for more pervasive, less severe lesions that are more localized and not identified by ultrasound or conventional MRI.[71, 99]

Functional Brain Assessments

Electroencephalography

EEG is an extremely sensitive technique during the neonatal period to confirm the clinical suspicion of neonatal seizures, as well as provide accurate information regarding maturation of regional and hemispheric brain function.[145] Combined EEG/polysomnographic recordings can better assess sleep state transitions and brain organization, which has an important bearing on predicting brain integrity. Serial measurements of EEG/sleep studies document important maturational changes (Fig. 17–14), which can be visually analyzed by expert decision making or digitally by computerized systems that quantitate and correlate multiple neuronal systems, such as EEG power, car-

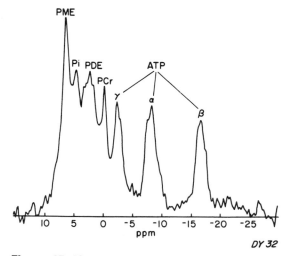

Figure 17–13. Nuclear magnetic resonance ³¹P spectrum of a normal infant showing individual peaks. PME, phosphomonoesterase; Pi, inorganic phosphates; PDE, phosphodiesterase; PCr phosphocreatine; ATP, adenosine triphosphate. (From Volpe J: Neurology of the Newborn. 3rd ed. Philadelphia: WB Saunders, 1995.)

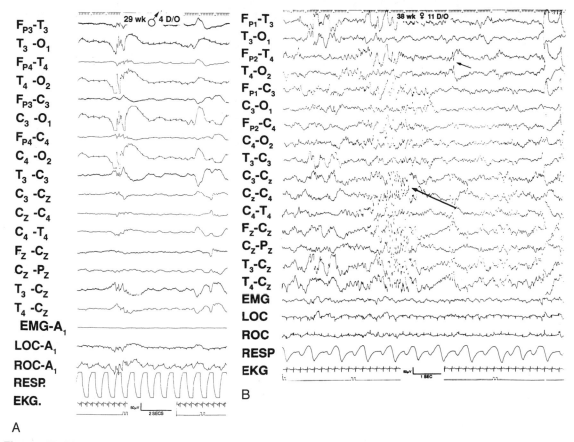

Figure 17–14. *A,* Segment of an electroencephalogram (EEG) of a healthy preterm infant of 29 weeks' gestational age and 4 days old, demonstrating discontinuous background with discrete regional patterns characteristic of this postconceptional age. *B,* Segment of an EEG for a 38-week, 11-day-old female, demonstrating normal patterns, including prominent rhythmic theta alpha activity at the midline *(long arrow)* and isolated sharp waves in the right temporal region *(small arrow).*

diorespiratory regularity, eye movements, and motility.[146]

Evoked Potentials

Three types of short-latency sensory evoked potentials can be useful for evaluation of the newborn. Brainstem auditory evoked responses can objectively assess the function of the auditory pathways of children suspected of abnormalities within the eighth cranial nerve or brainstem.[132, 156] Visual evoked responses are useful to screen for major visual pathway disturbances.[159] Somatosensory evoked potentials can preferentially monitor the motor pathways that may be involved with specific disease states.[32]

Electromyography and Nerve Conduction Velocities

On rare occasions, electromyelographic (EMG) and nerve conduction velocity stud-

ies may be helpful in the newborn nursery.[73] This is particularly applicable to children with suspected myopathic or motor neuron diseases before considering a muscle or nerve biopsy. For instance, with the simultaneous administration of neostigmine or edrophonium, an EMG may be used to diagnose connatal and neonatal forms of myasthenia gravis. Assessment of peripheral nerve or nerve root function using nerve conduction velocities can grade the severity of a neurologic lesion at facial nerve, brachial plexus, or other peripheral nerve location.

Placental Examination

Incorporating information regarding the gross and microscopic examinations of placental and cord specimens can be extremely helpful in the assessment of the etiology and timing of the disease state of the newborn.[81] The placental weight may not correlate with the weight of the infant; placental weights greater than or less than the 10th percentile for the gestational maturity and infant weight, respectively, may suggest placental insufficiency. Cord length as well as anomalies of the cord such as true knots and anomalous development of the cord may also have important bearing on fetal and neonatal neurologic diseases.

Microscopic evaluation of the placenta may reveal acute hemorrhage, villous edema, or the presence of purulent material, possibly suggesting acute or subacute pathologic processes. Conversely, the presence of altered size or development of the placental cotyledons, more longstanding vascular changes with or without infarction of the placenta, and deeply stained layers of the amnion and chorion with meconium within macrophages may be relevant to the fetal or maternal disease processes. These pathologic descriptions have relevance to both the pathogenesis and chronicity that ultimately may affect fetal brain (see Fig. 17–6).

◆ REPRESENTATIVE FETAL AND NEONATAL NEUROLOGIC DISEASES

This discussion of several disease processes of the fetus and neonate reinforces the previous sections pertaining to history taking, neurologic examination, and laboratory assessment. Four topics exemplify the overlapping nature of neonatal clinical signs and symptoms that reflect the etiology and timing of neurologic disease in the newborn. Hypoxic-ischemic–induced brain dysfunction or injury, cerebrovascular lesions, and neonatal seizures are commonly overlapping clinicopathologic entities in the newborn period (Table 17–10). The final topic is hypotonia, which is another major clinical sign with an extensive differential diagnosis and which extends beyond consideration of only children who suffered asphyxia.

Hypoxic-Ischemic Encephalopathy

Hypoxic-ischemic encephalopathy (HIE) occurs in 1.5 per 1000 live births and is the single most important fetal or neonatal dis-

ease state.[165] Yet, the definition of HIE is difficult to address with respect to the role of events during the intrauterine or peripartum periods that result in neurologic dysfunction and in relation to either the presence or timing of brain injury. Fetal brain disorders that occur before labor and delivery may contribute to the condition of the infant who is seen with postasphyxial encephalopathy syndrome after birth. The clinician must also recognize that HIE reflects a neurologic condition of dysfunction with or without coincident or subsequent damage.[14, 112]

The definition of asphyxia implies two overlapping mechanisms: (1) hypoxia, or reduced supply of oxygen in the blood, and (2) ischemia, or reduced perfusion of blood flow. The conventional standard of measurement concerning an asphyxial state involves the ascertainment of a blood gas determination, which documents metabolic acidosis; specific values for the P_{CO_2}, P_{O_2}, bicarbonate, and base excess must also be considered. A greater degree of acidosis may imply an increased production of lactate from an incomplete catabolism of glucose (i.e., metabolic acidosis), although hypercarbia from respiratory insufficiency may also explain an acidotic state (i.e., respiratory acidosis), which is associated with less morbidity. Metabolic acidosis eventually depletes high energy stores of phosphate, which ultimately results in cellular dysfunction because of inadequate energy production. The initial stage of HIE is one of cellular dysfunction. Two successive stages in the pathophysiologic process of HIE occur over several hours, during which time excessive membrane depolarization and release of excitatory amino acid neurotransmitters (e.g., glutamate) lead to calcium influx mediated by N-methyl D-aspartate and alpha-amino-3-hydroxy-5 methyl-4-isoxazole propionic acid (NMDA and AMPA) membrane receptors.[82] With an accumulation of cytosolic calcium, intracellular activation of lipases, proteases, and nucleases results in further injury to essential cellular proteins. Free radicals are also generated as a direct or indirect result of increased cytosolic calcium and nitric oxide.[37, 87] This entire cascade ultimately produces membrane injury, cytocellular disruption, and, finally, cell disintegration. Several therapeutic options are being considered that might abort this cytotoxic cascade, including use of calcium channel blockers,[105] excitatory amino acid antagonists,[61] (e.g., magnesium),[95] inhibitors of nitric oxide synthesis,[37] free radical scavengers,[105] and agents that inhibit free radical formation such as allopurinol.[104] Moderate hypothermia by either total body cooling or direct brain cooling is being evaluated in asphyxiated infants.[166]

Neuropathology

Brain damage from HIE has been described in experimental animal models in two general forms.[93] The acute total asphyxial model usually leads to death because of circulatory collapse or the pattern of brain injury; these immature animals are usually stillborn or die shortly after birth. A small number may survive and have evidence of predominant brainstem and diencephalic damage. Symmetric lesions within the brainstem, basal ganglia, and spinal cord structures are noted on postmortem examination.[77] Recent studies using MRI have also documented this pattern of injury in surviving neonates after HIE who die or suffer severe sequelae[127] (see Fig. 17–12).

The partial prolonged model of HIE-induced brain damage has also been described.[93] In this model, brain lesions are more diffuse within the cortex, subcortical white matter, and basal ganglia. Clinical scenarios in which these two hypothetic asphyxial situations occur include antepartum, intrapartum, and neonatal periods.

The following is a brief discussion of the common brain lesions associated with asphyxia.

Periventricular Leukomalacia

The most commonly occurring lesion of HIE in the preterm infant is PVL. These are symmetric bilateral lesions that result from coagulation necrosis. They are located adjacent to the external angles of the lateral ventricle, with or without cavitation. Extensive lesions produce multicystic encephalomalacia.[40] The occurrence of PVL is directly related to the immaturity of the vascular supply to the central white matter of the preterm brain. Arterial end zones lack adequate collateral blood flow to the deep white matter.[39] PVL is often associated with periventricular-intraventricular hemorrhage (PIVH).[163] Many pathophysiologic condi-

tions may contribute to this cerebrovascular white matter stroke, but usually it results from decreases in systemic blood pressure. This systemic hypotension immediately results in a decrease in cerebral blood flow, because the immature cerebral vasculature reactivity in the premature brain causes a pressure-passive state of brain hemodynamics.[122] This physiologic immaturity in the preterm infant brain is contrasted by the mature cerebral blood flow response of the term infant who can better maintain adequate cerebral perfusion over a wider range of systemic blood pressure values. PVL may also result after the elaboration of vasoactive cellular byproducts (i.e., cytokines, cytokenes) in response to infection or inflammation.[114] Such endotoxic agents contribute to cerebrovascular occlusion and consequential ischemic-induced injury in combination with asphyxia.[80]

Selective Neuronal Necrosis

In near-term and term infants after HIE, cortical and basal ganglia injury can occur, including subcortical white matter lesions with selective or extensive gyral involvement. Neuronal necrosis may be localized, multifocal, or diffuse and is preferably noted in the left greater than right hemisphere.[165] Cellular necrosis occurs with reactive astrocytic gliosis and resultant laminar injury to the cortical mantle, resulting in alterations in gyral thickness after destruction of layers of gray matter (i.e., ulegyria)[110] End zone perfusion between territories of major intracerebral arteries are also more likely to be compromised in the brain of the term newborn, with injuries resulting in these specific vascular regions within the cortex.

Parasagittal Pattern of Injury

A parasagittal pattern can result after HIE, contributing to a specific pattern of motor deficits in the proximal upper extremities, referable to the motor strip in each cerebral hemisphere. Although uncommon, these lesions have been demonstrable on neuroimaging studies.[74]

Lesions of the Basal Ganglia

Lesions within the basal ganglia are other important sites of brain injury that can re-

Table 17–10. Clinical Features and Ultimate Outcome in Four Types of Perinatal Brain Damage

Gestational Age	Timing	Risk Situations	Anatomic Findings	Acute Clinical Features	Confirmed by	Late Outcome
Hypoxic-Ischemic Encephalopathy (Severe)						
Full term or after term	Intrapartum or immediate postnatal	Acute birth asphyxia (abruptio placentae, hemorrhage, cord compression, mechanical injury) Prolonged subacute asphyxia (prenatal or intrapartum) Inadequate resuscitation	Brain edema, massive cellular necrosis (cortex, basal ganglia, brain stem), ± hemorrhage (intraventricular, subdural, or intracerebral)	Major CNS depression, repeated seizures (often subtle in comatose child), ± brainstem signs (no spontaneous respiration, no suck) Usually systemic signs of acute hypoxia-ischemia (e.g., acute renal tubular necrosis, paralytic ileus)	EEG findings Critical and severe interictal abnormalities Ultrasound and CT scan findings Edema ± hemorrhage within first wk Cerebral necrosis of various degrees and localization, but imaging often normal acutely	Severe sequelae in 50% of survivors, with microcephaly, multiple handicaps, ± epilepsy Motor handicap always more severe than cognitive Less severe degree of neuromotor, sensorial, intellectual, or behavioral deficit in others Normal or subnormal outcome possible
Hypoxic-Ischemic Encephalopathy (Moderate or Mild)						
Same as above	Same as above	Same circumstances as above but less severe and for shorter duration	Brain edema ± cellular damage ± subarachnoid hemorrhage	In moderate cases, CNS depression ± isolated seizures In "mild" cases, hyperexcitability and tone abnormalities (no depression, no seizures)	EEG moderate or no abnormalities Ultrasound usually normal Purely clinical diagnosis based on signs within first wk of life	Any type of permanent deficit including cerebral palsy in about 20% of moderate cases Normalization fast and complete in most mild cases and about 50% of "moderate" cases MBD at school age in about 30% of moderate cases
Periventricular Leukomalacia						
Any age	Any time (prenatal or postnatal)	Chronic fetal distress (± intrauterine growth retardation) Low CBF Acute hypotension (may be associated with apneic spell and bradycardia, cardiac arrest, or hemorrhagic shock) Chorioamnionitis	Ischemic necrosis of periventricular white matter (centrum semiovale, corona radiata, occipital and temporal zones) Coagulation necrosis in acute stage ± hemorrhage Cavitation and gliosis later Distribution often asymmetric	CNS depression within first wk Poor visual pursuit and poor axial tone at 40 wk corrected age	Ultrasound findings Periventricular leukomalacia including echogenicity Organization within 1 mo: porencephalic cysts ± ventricular enlargement caused by cerebral atrophy	Persisting neurologic findings (including typical spastic diplegia) ± sensorial and intellectual deficit of various degrees

Intraventricular Hemorrhage

Prematurity (below 34 wk)	Postnatal (first wk of life)	Immaturity + RDS leading to hypoxia, hypercarbia, unstable CBF Pneumothorax	Hemorrhage in germinal matrix (grade I) Intraventricular hemorrhage without ventriculomegaly (grade II) Intraventricular hemorrhage with ventriculomegaly (grade III) Hemorrhagic venous infarction (grade IV)	Major CNS depression ± seizure, onset at birth or later Nonspecific and unexplained deterioration Often silent	Ultrasound findings Resorption of blood in about 10 d Normalization in grades I and II Organization of periventricular leukomalacia often associated with grade III within 1 mo (see above)	Usually excellent in grades I and II Poor or very poor in grade III, especially when associated with extensive periventricular leukomalacia Possible hydrocephalus (10%–30% risk)

Cerebral Infarction (arterial territory)

Any age (frequently full term)	Mainly prenatal; can occur intrapartum or first 24 h	Embolization in twin-to-twin transfusion, placental abnormality Thrombophilia Thrombosis in DIC, sepsis, maternal cocaine Often no predisposing factors Low risk full term	Infarction of both white matter and cortex in arterial distribution Contraction of affected area, multiple cystic degeneration Middle cerebral artery most common (2 times more than other arteries) Left hemisphere mainly (3 times more than right)	Repeated focal seizures within first 3 d No major depression Asymmetric findings in case of middle cerebral artery	CT scan within 48 h of birth: wedge-shaped area of low attenuation with irregular margins; may be normal if scan too soon after actual infarction Rescanning a few mo later to evaluate loss of tissue EEG findings: focal seizures	Improvement of neuromotor function within first year, with mild residual hemiparesis (usually walk alone) Mild mental deficit or none No speech disorder, usually Epilepsy uncommon

RDS, respiratory distress syndrome; CBF, cerebral blood flow; DIC, disseminated intravascular coagulation; CNS, central nervous system; EEG, electroencephalogram; CT, computed tomography; MBD, minimal brain dysfunction.

sult after HIE in the near-term or term infant brain. Status marmoratus (i.e., the marbleized appearance of injury caused by the increased myelinated patterns in caudate, putamen, and thalamus) has been classically described by neuropathologists.[52] These deep gray matter structures possess a high concentration of excitatory neurotransmitters[69]; consequently, these brain regions are vulnerable to the cytotoxic cascade that results after release of the neurotransmitters into the extracellular space, leading to further neuronal injury and death.

Focal Cerebral Lesions

Focal lesions in the brain may be due to arterial infarction, usually within border zone territories between major cerebral arteries.[53] Thrombotic or embolic infarctions may occur,[33] which can convert from ischemic to hemorrhagic lesions.[26]

Clinical and Neuroimaging Correlates of HIE

As described in the earlier section of fetal neurologic disease, it is difficult for the clinician to distinguish fetal distress that occurs because of events during labor and delivery from an antepartum versus intrapartum occurrence of brain injury. In some neonates who exhibit classic signs of intrauterine fetal distress, neither neurologic symptoms nor brain injury develop subsequently. More commonly, asymptomatic infants at birth have already sustained brain injury before parturition. Even though fetal surveillance techniques detect the presence of fetal distress (as documented by electronic fetal monitoring of the heart and fetal scalp pH monitoring) and, after birth, neonatal clinical signs of depressed arousal and muscle tone reflect an encephalopathy, these expressions of dysfunction may not be responsible for brain injury that preceded the time when fetal distress was first noted.[9, 85]

Symptoms and signs of HIE are also different between preterm and term infants. For the near-term or term infant, three general grades of encephalopathy have been described.[136] Stage I HIE syndrome is a mild form during which the child is hyperalert and tremulous during the first 24 hours, with excessive responsiveness to external stimulation. Muscle tone is generally increased and tendon reflexes are hyperactive.

Stage II, or moderate, HIE syndrome is characterized by stupor or lethargy lasting at least 24 to 48 hours. While the child can be aroused followed by tremulousness, muscle tone is generally decreased after birth, although hypertonus may be seen with tactile stimulation. Weakness is noted in the shoulder and proximal arm muscles. The clinical condition of the child may worsen or improve within 48 to 72 hours, with or without seizures. Stage III, or severe, HIE usually results in a stuporous or comatose child with seizures that develop within the first 24 to 48 hours of life. Seizures are difficult to distinguish from nonepileptic seizure-like events, as discussed under the section on neonatal seizures. In children who are profoundly hypotonic, unresponsive, and ventilatory dependent, cranial nerve abnormalities and other focal motor abnormalities may be present with a full, bulging fontanelle, suggesting increased intracranial pressure. Such children have the highest likelihood for neurologic sequelae or death.[63]

Conversely, in the preterm child, the neonate with HIE may exhibit fewer clinical signs. The preterm child may appear ill based on respiratory distress, sepsis, or other organ system problems, but the neurologic manifestations of HIE are more difficult to ascertain because of the immaturity in the clinical expression of the neurologic function. The two lesser degrees of HIE are much less well defined.

Neurophysiologic and Neuroimaging Correlates of HIE

EEG can be useful in determining the progression of HIE and may have strong prognostic significance. For moderate-to-severe HIE, the EEG background abnormalities include suppression of electric activities (i.e., frequencies and amplitude of wave forms) or may consist of a suppression burst pattern. The expression of continuous EEG rhythms with age-appropriate rhythms that spontaneously change between active and quiet sleep states carries a more favorable outcome. Immature patterns on the EEG without amplitude/frequency suppression or burst suppression patterns on the EEG may suggest a more chronic in utero occurrence of an HIE process.[145]

Neuroimaging techniques can document the structural injury associated with HIE as well as suggest timing of the injury. The ultrasonographic appearance of PVL in preterm infants has been extensively studied.[57] Well-defined areas of echodensity along the lateral ventricle appear between 7 and 14 days after a presumed asphyxial insult.[114] These echodensities generally disappear or are replaced by small cysts over subsequent weeks. More sophisticated neuroimaging techniques (i.e., CT and MRI) document more details of neuroanatomy and pathology.[51, 128] Cortical enhancement, particularly in the depths of the sulci and of lesions within the basal ganglia, shows brain lesions associated with HIE in the near-term and term infant. Chronic changes include calcifications. Other abnormalities such as focal ischemic lesions in the border zone between major cerebral arteries are more readily documented by either CT or MRI scans.[10] Certain features on neuroimaging may suggest a more remote occurrence of a brain injury caused by an asphyxial insult during the antepartum rather than peripartum period. Cerebral atrophy or well-formed cystic cavitation at the time of birth as seen on ultrasound, CT, or MRI scan signifies the process of liquefaction necrosis, which requires 2 to 6 weeks during intrauterine life to appear.[52] Irregularity of the ventricular borders, white matter multicystic lesions, and the appearance of basal ganglia calcification or overall brain atrophy also suggest more chronic injuries. Therefore, despite the clinical expression of HIE, brain injury may have already resulted from clinical silent events before the onset of fetal distress. This generalization has obvious ramifications concerning the evaluation of therapeutic interventions to treat HIE. The use of glutamate antagonists, for instance, may not be recommended in a child who has already suffered remote intrauterine asphyxia. Conversely, those children with well-documented intrapartum or postnatal disease conditions may suffer hypoxic-ischemic–induced brain injury, which may respond to therapeutic strategies of brain resuscitation.[98]

Cerebrovascular Lesions of the Neonate

Cerebrovascular lesions occur in both the preterm and full-term brain, either as a result of varying pathologic processes (e.g., asphyxia), infection, or blood disorders.[33]

Two manifestations of cerebrovascular disease processes may occur: intracranial hemorrhage (ICH) and intracranial ischemic lesions.

The demographics of ICH have changed considerably over the past several decades. Two specific forms of ICH have decreased in occurrence: subdural hemorrhage in term infants and IVH in preterm infants. In general, however, cerebrovascular-related brain injuries remain important structural correlates to neurologic sequelae.

Periventricular-Intraventricular Hemorrhage

PIVH is the most frequent type of intracranial hemorrhage in the neonate, overwhelmingly noted in the preterm infant (60% of infants weighing less than 1000 g compared with 20% in larger infants).[113] PIVH in preterm infants originates primarily in the subependymal germinal matrix, a highly vascular area that gives rise to neurons and glia during brain maturation.[165] The germinal matrix eventually is resorbed into the head of the caudate. Hemorrhages within the subependymal region may be clinically silent, even if ventricular dilatation occurs. Intraventricular hemorrhage results when venous stasis causes the ependymal lining to rupture, with extravasation of blood into the extravascular space, which may extend into the ventricular space. Severity of PIVH is graded based on the coincident presence of ventriculomegaly and the occurrence of intraventricular blood[108] (see Fig. 17–11B) (Table 17–11). Whereas PIVH is a hemorrhagic event caused by rupture of blood through thin endothelial lining of vessels within the germinal matrix, the hemorrhage originates because of venous stasis. More severe venous stasis affects blood drainage more proximally within the terminal vein or the medullary veins of the deep white matter below the developing neocortex. A hemorrhagic infarction may then result and is graded as the most severe form of IVH, documented as a parenchymal hemorrhage within a region of ischemia on neuroimaging or postmortem examination.[58] Unlike the symmetric ischemic pattern of injury noted with PVL, which is in an arterial distribution, the venous infarction associated with PIVH is asymmetric and may be extensive with accompanying ventriculomegaly.

PIVH may subsequently cause hydro-

Table 17–11. Severity of Periventricular-Intraventricular Hemorrhage

Severity	Staging of Papile et al. (1978)[108]	Staging of Volpe (1995)[165]
Grade I	Subependymal bleeding only	*Idem*, or <10% of ventricular area filled with blood.
Grade II	<50% of ventricular area filled with blood. No ventricular dilation.	10–50% of ventricular area filled with blood.
Grade III	>50% of ventricular area filled with blood. Blood in the white matter of centrum semiovale.	>50% of ventricular area filled with blood.

cephalus as a result of posthemorrhagic adhesive arachnoiditis. Whereas compensatory ventriculomegaly during the first several weeks after hemorrhage is expected, the time course after which progressive hydrocephalus is established is unknown. Both the initial hemorrhagic venous infarction and progressive hydrocephalus contribute to long-term neurologic sequelae.

Periventricular Leukomalacia

This arterial stroke of the preterm brain is described previously in the section on asphyxia. The tissue destruction that follows after an ischemic event results in gliosis and cavitation, usually limited to the white matter region within the trigone of the white matter, above the occipital horns, along the optic radiations, or more anteriorly along the body and frontal horns of the lateral ventricles. Twenty-five percent of children with PVL may also suffer PIVH; extensive forms of PVL produce multicystic encephalomalacia. Unlike the asymmetric presentation with PIVH, PVL lesions are largely symmetric (see Fig. 17–11C).

Other Intracranial Hemorrhages of the Neonate

Other hemorrhagic events within the brain occur less commonly. Subdural hemorrhage results from tentorial tears after rupture of the straight sinus, vein of Galen, or small afferent veins. Subdural hemorrhages are mainly of traumatic origin in term infants at higher birth weight. Posterior fossae subdural hemorrhage may also occur as a result of excessive head molding in the vertex presentation or after excessive traction on the skull of a child in a breech presentation.[55, 165]

A third form of hemorrhage occurs within the cerebellar tissue within the posterior fossae, either after asphyxia or as the result of mechanical trauma from occipital osteodiastasis or traumatic cerebellar injury.[169] Other intraparenchymal hemorrhage within the cortex can occur in either term or preterm infants, usually associated with children with subarachnoid hemorrhage.[116]

Thalamic hemorrhage is an uncommon but potentially devastating form of intraparenchymal hemorrhage, more commonly noted in the term infant.[41]

Primary subarachnoid hemorrhage (SAH) is perhaps the most common form of intracranial hemorrhage and occurs in children even after seemingly nontraumatic deliveries.[55] The true incidence of SAH remains elusive because many children remain asymptomatic, with generally a low incidence of neurologic sequelae. Clinical features and outcome for the different forms of cerebrovascular disease with or without asphyxia are summarized in Chapter 2.

◆ NEONATAL SEIZURES

Even though neonatal seizures remain one of the few neurologic emergencies, this condition may indicate significant dysfunction or damage to the immature nervous system both on a remote and on an acute basis.[140] Advances in neurophysiologic monitoring of the high-risk infant have spurred the development of an integrated classification of both clinical and electrographic criteria for seizures diagnosis.[90] Synchronized video EEG/polygraphic techniques as well as computer-assisted analyses allow the clinician to better characterize suspicious clinical behaviors that may or may not be associated with coincident surface-generated electrographic seizures (Fig. 17–15). Nonetheless, with a reliance on detecting suspicious clinical behaviors, recognition of neonatal seizures is still hampered by both overestimation and underestimation. Clinical criteria for suspected seizures may not easily distinguish seizure activity either from normal or

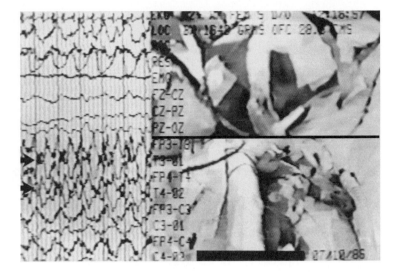

Figure 17-15. Segment of a video electroencephalogram for a 32-week gestational age, 5-day-old female with electroclinical seizures characterized by bitemporal electrographic discharges coincident with tonic posturing to the left.

pathologic nonepileptic behavior; coincident EEG is needed to best define the diagnosis. Subclinical EEG seizures may also occur, which escape detection by clinical observation alone. Conversely, EEG criteria may not adequately monitor ictal patterns that originate from subcortical brain regions, but no universal classification based on clinical criteria can distinguish subcortical seizures from nonepileptic paroxysmal activity, although recent speculation regarding electroclinical disassociation has been suggested. Certain clinical seizures originate within subcortical structures and only intermittently propagate to the cortical surface where EEG recordings can readily record electrographic seizures.[167] One pragmatic approach to the diagnosis and management of neonatal seizures is, therefore, based on the documentation of seizures by surface-recorded EEG studies. A therapeutic end point for the use of antiepileptic medications can be more practically achieved using EEG documentation, in that clinical signs may be absent, minimal, or nonepileptic in origin.

Seizure Detection: Clinical Versus EEG Criteria

Neonates are unable to sustain generalized tonic followed by clonic seizures as noted in older patients, although separately occurring generalized tonic and clonic events do appear, even in the same neonate. Most seizures are brief and subtle, and consequently are expressed as clinical behaviors

that are unusual to recognize. Five clinical categories of neonatal seizures have been described.[165] Several caveats should be considered before reviewing these five clinical criteria.[140] First, the clinician should be suspicious of any abnormal repetitive stereotypic behavior that could represent a possible seizure. Second, certain behaviors such as orbital and buccolingual movements, tonic posturing, and myoclonus can be associated either with normal neonatal sleep behaviors or nonepileptic pathologic behaviors. Third, clinical events may have only an inconsistent relationship with coincident electrographic seizures.

Subtle or Fragmentary Seizures

Subtle or fragmentary seizures constitute the most frequently observed clinical group of seizure-like phenomena, including repetitive facial activity, unusual bicycling or pedaling movements, momentary fixation of gaze, or autonomic dysfunction. Specific autonomic signs such as apnea rarely occur in isolation but usually occur in the context of other seizure phenomena in the same neonate.[48] Even though these clinical expressions appear unimpressive, they may reflect significant brain dysfunction or injury. An inconsistent relationship between specific subtle behaviors and EEG seizures has been documented using synchronized video EEG/polygraphic recordings, emphasizing the need for further classification.[89] The temporal relationship between suspicious clinical behaviors and EEG seizure patterns is generally considered standard practice.

Clonic Seizures

Clonic seizures consist of rhythmic movements of muscle groups in a focal or multifocal distribution. Rapid followed by slow movement phases distinguish clonic movements from the symmetric to-and-fro movements of nonepileptic tremulousness or jitteriness.[34, 151] Whereas gentle flexion of the extremity can suppress tremors, this is not possible with clonic seizure activity. The clonic event may involve any muscle group of the face, limbs, or torso. Focal clonic seizures may be associated with localized brain injury, but they can also accompany generalized cerebral disturbances.[30, 144] Following seizures, newborns may also have a transient period of paresis or paralysis, called *Todd's phenomenon.*

Tonic Seizures

Tonic seizures are characterized by sustained flexion or extension of either axial or appendicular muscle groups, such as decerebration or dystonic posturing (see Fig. 17–15). Focal head/eye turning or tonic flexion or extension of an extremity exemplifies tonic seizures. Even though some tonic behaviors are coincident with EEG seizures, there is a high false-positive correlation with tonic behavior in the absence of coincident electric seizure activity.[72]

Myoclonic Seizures

Myoclonic movements are rapid, isolated jerks involving the midline musculature or a single extremity either in a generalized or multifocal fashion. Unlike the fast or slow phase seen in clonic seizures, myoclonic movements lack this two-phase movement. Healthy preterm and term infants may demonstrate abundant myoclonic movements, either during sleep or wakefulness.[34, 151] However, sick neonates may also exhibit myoclonus, which is verified as either seizures on the EEG or as a manifestation of nonepileptic abnormal motor activity.[137]

EEG Seizure Criteria

EEG remains an invaluable tool for the assessment of both ictal and interictal cerebral activities, as expressed on surface recordings. Even though an EEG finding is rarely pathognomonic for a particular disease, important information about the presence and severity of a brain disorder with or without seizures can result from careful visual interpretation.[145] Major EEG background rhythm disturbances in the absence of seizures carry major prognostic implications for compromised outcome. Specific interictal EEG abnormalities on serial EEG recordings offer invaluable information to the clinician on the presence, severity, and persistence of an encephalopathic state of the neonate.

Interictal EEG

Background EEG abnormalities have prognostic significance for both preterm and full-term infants.[92, 160] Such patterns include suppression burst, electrocerebral inactivity, low voltage invariant, and persistent multifocal sharp wave abnormalities (Fig. 17–16). Other interictal EEG abnormalities, such as dysmaturity between EEG and polygraphic activities, also carry prognostic importance but require greater skills of visual analysis to describe.[145]

Ictal EEG patterns

Ictal EEG patterns of the newborn are composed of repetitive waveforms of sufficient duration and similar morphology that evolve in response to frequency, amplitude, and electric field. The electroencephalographer readily can identify seizures that are at least 10 seconds in duration.[143] Four categories of ictal patterns have traditionally been described: focal ictal patterns with normal background, focal ictal patterns with abnormal background, focal monorhythmic periodic patterns of various frequencies, and multifocal ictal patterns.[83]

Neonatal encephalopathies should be characterized in functional terms based on both interictal and ictal abnormalities as well as on severity and persistence over time.[138] The persistence of abnormal patterns on serial studies is more significantly correlated with neurologic sequelae, even though EEG patterns rarely specify a particular disease state. Brain lesions documented on neuroimaging or postmortem examination may have had an electrographic signature on EEG studies, either on an acute, subacute, or chronic basis. Therefore, EEG patterns must be analyzed in the context

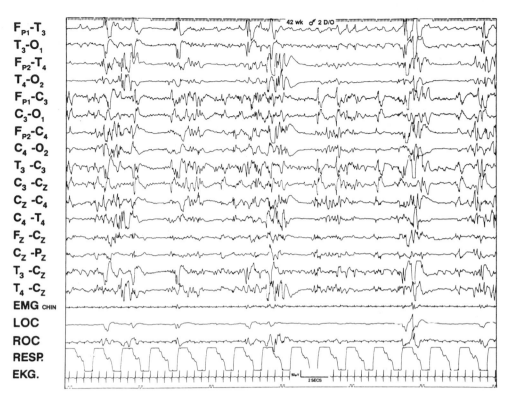

Figure 17–16. Segment of an electroencephalogram record for a 42-week gestational age, 2-day-old male, demonstrating a burst suppression pattern with multifocal sharp waves and attenuation of activity in the right temporal and midline (T_4 and C_z) region.

of history, clinical findings, and laboratory information, including neuroimaging.

Clinical Correlation of Neonatal Seizures

Neonatal seizures are not disease specific and may be caused by a combination of medical conditions. Establishing a specific reason for seizures in any infant is essential both for treatment as well as for prediction of neurologic outcome. Neonates with an encephalopathy or brain disorder may or may not have seizures and they commonly come to attention for a variety of disturbances.[145]

Asphyxia

Postasphyxial encephalopathy, the principal disorder during which neonatal seizures may occur, can also be accompanied by hypoglycemia, hypocalcemia, cerebrovascular accidents, or intraparenchymal hemorrhage.

Each individually or in combination can contribute to seizures.

Most neonates suffer asphyxia either before or during parturition. In only 10% of affected neonates does asphyxia result from postnatal causes. Intrauterine factors leading to asphyxia before or during labor and delivery compromise gas exchange or glucose movement across the placenta. These factors may be maternal (e.g., toxemia) or uteroplacental (e.g., abruptio placentae or cord compression) in origin. However, other maternal conditions such as antepartum trauma or infection, as detected by fetal sonography or cranial imaging of the infant immediately after birth, are not only associated with acquired brain insults from asphyxia but also may contribute to the formation of congenital malformations during early pregnancy. Respiratory distress syndrome, pulmonary hypertension of the newborn, and severe right-to-left cardiac shunts in children with congenital heart disease are other major causes of postnatal asphyxia in a newborn who may also suffer with seizures. Therefore, the events that lead to asphyxia must be taken in the context of the maternal, placental, and neonatal examinations, as well as the corroborative laboratory findings. Adverse events during labor and delivery may reflect longer standing maternal placental or cord diseases that contribute to postnatal seizures, hypotonia, or coma. HIE, including neonatal seizures, develops in only 45% of infants who suffer asphyxia at the time of birth.[114] Similarly, meconium staining of skin, placental tissue, or cord tissue can occur in association with asymptomatic infants with or without intrauterine insults. Meconium-laden macrophages distributed throughout the placental amnion generally indicate fetal distress in the antepartum period.[7] Placental weights less than the 10th or greater than the 90th percentiles, altered placental villous morphology, lymphocytic infiltration, and erythroblastic proliferation in the villi implicate more chronic stress to the fetus, whether or not seizures occur during the immediate neonatal period in a child who is neurologically depressed. Recently, neonates with electrically confirmed seizures during the first 2 days of life were found to have been associated with longer standing placental lesions; over a 15-week interval, the odds that chronic placental lesions were associated with a group of neonates with EEG-confirmed seizures increased by a factor of 12.[147] Other findings on neurologic examination, such as hypertonia, joint contractures without profoundly depressed consciousness, seizures within the first hours after delivery, growth restriction, and neuroimaging evidence of encephalomalacia, separately or collectively point to the antepartum time period when brain injury occurred.

Hypoglycemia

Low blood sugar can result in seizures either associated with asphyxia or as a separate metabolic consequence. Infants of diabetic or toxemic mothers, those born as one of multiple gestation siblings, and, rarely, those with metabolic diseases may also have hypoglycemia. (See Chapter 11.)

Hypocalcemia

Whereas hypoglycemia can be associated with children with neonatal seizures with asphyxia, hypocalcemia may be seen in the context of trauma, hemolytic disease, or metabolic disease. Hypomagnesemia may also occur in the child with hypocalcemia. Rarely, a form of hypocalcemia may be due to congenital hypoparathyroidism or with delayed onset occurrence in a child who received a high-phosphate infant formula. Congenital cardiac lesions may be associated with the child with either hypocalcemia or hypomagnesemia.[84] (See Chapter 11.)

Cerebrovascular Lesions

Intracranial hemorrhage as well as ischemic cerebrovascular lesions can occur as a result of asphyxia, trauma, or infection, or from developmental or congenital lesions. PIVH in the preterm infant who also has seizures has already been discussed.[141] However, full-term infants with seizures may also have intraventricular hemorrhage, usually arising within the choroid plexus or thalamus. Other sites of intracranial hemorrhage (e.g., subdural space, subarachnoid space, or into the parenchyma) can also be associated with seizures with or independent of postasphyxial encephalopathy.

Arterial and venous infarctions have been noted in neonates with seizures.[30, 144] Cerebral infarctions can occur during the antepartum, intrapartum, or neonatal periods, depending on diverse etiologies such as persistent pulmonary hypertension, polycythemia, and hypertensive encephalopathy. Neonates with isolated seizures without an accompanying encephalopathy have etiologies timed to the antepartum period.[142]

Infection

Central nervous system infection acquired in utero or postnatally may give rise to neonatal seizures.[70] Congenital infections that are usually associated with a severe encephalitis also include seizures and major interictal EEG background disturbances. For instance, neonatal herpes encephalitis is associated with severe ictal and interictal EEG pattern abnormalities, consisting of multifocal seizures as well as multifocal periodic discharges.[91] Acquired in utero or postnatal bacterial infections from *Escherichia coli* or Group B streptococcal infections may result in neonatal seizures. *Listeria monocytogenes* and mycoplasma infections can also produce areas of lymphocytic infiltration and resultant encephalomalacia.

Central Nervous System Malformations

Brain lesions that result from either genetic or acquired defects during early fetal brain development also contribute to neonatal seizures (Fig. 17–17). Such lesions include microgyria, heterotopia, and lissencephaly. Other dysgenic central nervous system conditions such as holoprosencephaly, schizencephaly, and congenital hydrocephalus may also be associated with neonatal seizures.[106]

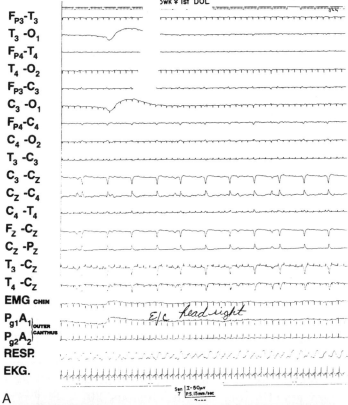

Figure 17–17. *A,* Segment of an electroencephalogram (EEG) for a 35-week gestational age, 1-day-old female with periodic discharges at the midline (C_z). *B,* A computed tomography scan documenting a lobar holoprosencephaly. EEG is depicted in A.

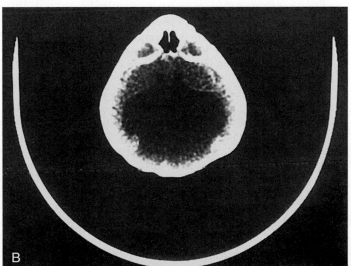

Inborn Errors of Metabolism

Inherited biochemical defects are rare causes of neonatal seizures.[139] Peculiar body odors, intractable seizures that occur later in the newborn period, or persistently elevated lactate, pyruvate, ammonia, or amino acid values in the blood may reflect inherited biochemical disorders rather than transient postasphyxial insults. Neonates with metabolic disease may also have otherwise normal prenatal and delivery histories. The emergence of food intolerance, increasing lethargy, and late onset of seizures may be the only indication of an inborn error of metabolism. Certain conditions are responsive to supplements; for example, vitamin B_6 dependency is a rare form of metabolic disturbance that can lead to intractable seizures that are unresponsive to conventional antiepileptic medication.[31]

Neonatal Epileptic Syndromes

Few clinical situations regarding neonatal seizures represent a chronic epilepsy syndrome. Most newborns with seizures reflect transient disturbances that resolve over days (e.g., asphyxia, metabolic-toxic conditions, infections). Rarely, a newborn has an ongoing epileptic condition that is independent of, but perhaps is triggered by, adverse events during fetal or neonatal life. A rare form of familial neonatal seizures has been described as an autosomal dominant condition.[129] The diagnosis requires careful exclusion of acquired causes. Two pedigrees were assigned the genetic defect for this condition to two genetic loci on chromosome 20. Whereas most newborns respond promptly to antiepileptic drug treatment and develop age appropriately, some children are delayed at older ages. A defect in potassium-dependent channel kinetics has been described.

Other rare epileptic states include progressive syndromes associated with severe myoclonic seizures and progressive developmental delay. These children have been described as an early infantile epileptic encephalopathy (i.e., Ohtahara syndrome) and usually have severe brain dysgenesis.[100]

Treatment of Neonatal Seizures

Before antiepileptic medications are administered, an acute rapid infusion of glucose or other electrolytes such as calcium or magnesium should be considered. Determination of low magnesium or altered sodium metabolism is a less common reason for neonatal seizures that do not require antiepileptic medications.[139]

Questions persist with respect to when, how, and for how long to treat neonates with antiepileptic medications who suffer neonatal seizures. Some believe that neonates should undergo treatment only when the clinical seizures are recognized and that brief electrographic seizures need not be treated. Others argue that this practice may be potentially harmful, in that undetected repetitive or continuous electrographic seizures may adversely affect immature brain metabolism and cellular integrity. Consensus is lacking with respect to the necessity for treatment of minimal or absent clinical seizure phenomena.[140]

Major antiepileptic drug choices have been used to treat neonatal seizures: phenobarbital is the most commonly used antiepileptic medication, with a recommended loading dose of 20 mg/kg and a maintenance dose of 3 to 5 mg/kg/d. Half-life of the drug is long, 45 to 173 hours, and there is no consensus on how long to maintain phenobarbital levels after seizures have been controlled.[102]

Phenytoin is the second-most commonly used medication for the treatment of seizures. A loading dose of phenytoin is 15 to 20 mg/kg, but it is necessary to maintain an intravenous administration because the drug rapidly redistributes to body tissues when given orally.[102]

Some clinicians prefer using benzodiazepines for the acute treatment of seizures, particularly when phenobarbital or phenytoin are no longer effective. Depending on the type of benzodiazepine, the half-life may vary; furthermore, these drugs have not been studied as well in the neonatal population. Diazepam is one choice in this class of medication, and the recommended intravenous dose is 0.5 mg/kg.[153] However, other forms of benzodiazepines such as Ativan, lorazepam, or midazolam have also been used (Table 17–12).

Free or unbound drug fractions have recently been suggested to assess the efficacy and potential toxicity of antiepileptic drugs in pediatric populations, including the neonatal population.[101] Binding of drugs in neonates with seizures has only recently been

Table 17-12. Treatment of Neonatal Seizures with Antiepileptic Medications

	Phenobarbital	Phenytoin	Diazepam	Lorazepam
Delivery route	IV, IM, p.o.	IV	IV	IV
Initial loading dose	20 mg/kg	20 mg/kg	0.25 mg/kg	0.05 to 0.1 mg/kg
Rate of administration	Give IV dose over 20 min	Give IV dose no faster than 1 mg/kg/min with ECG monitoring	Give IV dose over 2 min	Give IV dose over 2 min
Maintenance dosage	3–4 mg/kg/d divided every 12 h	3–4 mg/kg/d divided every 12 h	0.25 mg/kg every 15–30 min after load p.r.n.	0.05 to 0.1 mg/kg p.r.n. (after loading dose)
Timing of first maintenance dose	12–24 h after loading	12–24 h after loading	15–30 min after loading	Up to 12 h
Therapeutic level	20–40 μg/mL	10–20 μg/mL	—	—
Serum half-life	Varies from 40 to 100 h depending on age and duration of drug usage	Newborn: approximately 104 h; by 1 mo, 2–7 h	31–75 h but seizure control may be much shorter	12 h
Possible adverse effects	Respiratory depression, hypotension, lethargy—if given in excess or too rapidly	Heart block, hypotension if given too rapidly	Respiratory depression; hypotension	Respiratory depression; hypotension; dystonic movements

IV, intravenous; IM, intramuscular; p.o., by mouth; ECG, electrocardiographic; p.r.n., as needed.

reported; such binding can be altered significantly in the sick neonate with metabolic dysfunction. Biochemical alterations may cause toxic side effects by increasing the free fraction of the drug, which readily affects cardiovascular or respiratory function. Serial drug determinations and computerized EEG analysis based on seizure cessation before toxic side effects ensue may improve the optimal titration of antiepileptic drugs.[103]

The decision to maintain or discontinue antiepileptic drug treatment is fraught with uncertainty.[139] Discontinuation of drugs before discharge from the neonatal intensive care unit should be attempted, specifically for the infant who shows no demonstrable brain lesions on cranial imaging, who exhibits age-appropriate findings on neurologic examination, and who expresses normal interictal EEG background patterns.[165] Prompt cessation of antiepileptic pharmacotherapy may be justified even in patients who are at higher risk for seizures beyond the neonatal period because there is a "honeymoon" period that lasts months to years before seizures may recur. Because there is the potential for damage of the developing nervous system by antiepileptic medications, prompt discontinuation in the late neonatal or early infancy period is recommended.

Despite the urgency to establish a cause of the seizure, several unique aspects of neonatal seizures impede prompt diagnosis and treatment. As discussed previously, there are a number of etiologic possibilities associated with seizures, and the efficacy of conventional antiepileptic drugs to control seizures remains controversial. Neonatal seizures can reflect either acute or remote etiologies or represent a series of insults that began in the antepartum period, with extension to include events during the intrapartum or postnatal periods.

◆ HYPOTONIA

Evaluation of tone in the neonate requires considerable experience and perseverance by the clinician. The section on clinical examination technique discusses evaluation of the motor system and the evaluation of the child with altered tone, principally hypotonia and, less commonly, hypertonia (Fig. 17–18). Clearly, the approach to the diagno-

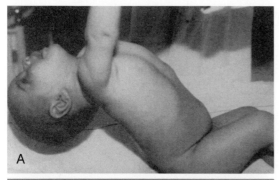

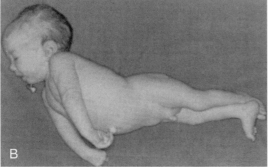

Figure 17–18. *A,* A 3-month-old with marked hypotonia resulting from neuromuscular disease. *B,* Decerebrate posturing after severe asphyxia in a term infant.

sis of hypotonia requires an understanding of the neuroanatomic location within the neuraxis that may be responsible for producing low tone in the neonate. Such locations include the cerebrum, spinal cord, peripheral nerve, and neuromuscular junction or muscle (Table 17–9). The clinical approach to the hypotonic neonate is summarized in Table 17–13. Most hypotonic neonates have disorders of the cerebrum. In these situations, hypotonia is usually not accompanied by profound weakness, and other signs of brain dysfunction such as lethargy, swallowing difficulties, and abnormal primitive reflexes are present. Hypotonia can be one prominent clinical manifestation of HIE (as discussed previously) or of other acute forms of neonatal disease derived from metabolic or infectious causes. Other cerebral causes of hypotonia include congenital infections and genetic diseases, including inherited disorders of metabolism involving glucose, amino acids, fatty acids, or peroxisomal pathways.

Peripheral causes of neonatal hypotonia also usually result in greater degrees of weakness, often including respiratory and swallowing difficulties. With situations of hypotonia associated with anterior horn cell disease (i.e., progressive spinal muscular atrophy), infants are alert and their behavior is otherwise normal. In other clinical situations, such as neonatal myotonic dystrophy or Prader-Willi syndrome, there may be a mixture of central and peripheral involvement to motor pathways, causing hypotonia as well as other disorders of cerebral or systemic function.[163, 170]

Neonatal myasthenia gravis in offspring of myasthenic mothers should be considered in neonates with hypotonia located at the neuromuscular junction. These infants exhibit cranial nerve deficits such as facial diparesis, ptosis, and ophthalmoplegia, as well as respiratory depression.[107] Exogenous causes of hypotonia include the administration of drugs to the mother, such as inappropriate systemic or local injections of local anesthetics, introduced to the infant through placental circulation or directly into the baby's scalp at the time of paracervical or pudendal blocks.[65] These medications may cause a characteristic syndrome of hypotonia, respiratory depression, and seizures during the first day of life. Magnesium and aminoglycoside administration each may result in transient neuromuscular dysfunction, resulting in profound weakness and hypotonia.

Connective tissue abnormalities also may be associated with low tone, particularly involving mesochymal tissue, such as Marfan syndrome or Ehlers-Danlos syndrome.

Myopathies either associated with specific muscular dystrophies or congenital myopathies can present with neonatal hypotonia and are generally associated with some degree of weakness or decrease in muscle bulk. A mixture of lower and upper motor neuron diseases is noted with certain congenital muscular dystrophies as well as mitochondrial myopathies.

◆ QUESTIONS

True or False

◆ *A newborn who is neurologically depressed at the time of birth with evidence of fetal acidosis, low Apgar scores, and neonatal seizures is always associated with asphyxia that occurred during the intrapartum period.*

The presence of asphyxia as documented by clinical and laboratory examination can be seen in children with antepartum as well

Table 17–13. Approach to Diagnosis of Hypotonia

Anatomic Site	Pathogenesis	Clinical Features							Laboratory Aids			
		Alertness	Cry	Eye Movements	Tongue Fasciculation	Deep Tendon Reflexes	Muscle Bulk	Electro-myography	Muscle Biopsy	Muscle Enzyme (CPK)*	Prostigmine
Cerebral	Malformation Hemorrhage Hypoxia-ischemia Metabolic Infection Drugs	Poor	Poor	Occasionally abnormal	No	Normal or increased	Normal	Normal	Normal	Normal	Negative
Spinal cord	Injury	Good	Normal	Normal	No	Decreased or increased	Normal	Normal	Normal	Normal	Negative
Anterior horn cell	Spinal muscular atrophy† (Werdnig-Hoffmann)	Good	Normal/weak	Normal	Yes	Absent	Decreased	Neurogenic pattern	Neurogenic group	Normal	Negative
Neuromuscular junction	Neonatal myasthenia gravis	Good	Weak	Abnormal	No	Normal	Normal	±Normal	Normal	Normal	Negative
Muscle	Congenital myopathy Myotonic dystrophy‡ Glycogen storage disease	Good	Good	Normal	No	Decreased or normal	Decreased	Myopathic pattern	Myopathic change	Normal or elevated	Negative

*CPK, creatine phosphokinase. CPK is grossly elevated in Duchenne dystrophy, which does not usually manifest as hypotonia in neonates.
†Molecular diagnosis identifies survival motor neuron (SMN) gene deletions or mutations from blood, amniotic fluid, or tissue.
‡Molecular diagnosis of myotonic dystrophy = CTG triplet repeat expansion.

as intrapartum etiologies for asphyxia. Even though children may become symptomatic during a problematic labor and delivery that leads to asphyxia, the intrapartum period may not be the time course during which brain damage occurred. Therefore, the statement is false.

◆ *The elongated head shape of a preterm infant who is a corrected age of 44 weeks suggests craniosynostosis, and an immediate neurosurgical referral should be made.*

Even though craniosynostosis must be suspected in a child with an abnormal head shape, premature infants commonly have inhibition of lateral head growth because the head is turned to either side in contact with the mattress. In most of these children, no premature closure of the sagittal suture can be documented. Therefore, the statement is false.

◆ *A 37-week gestational age female neonate has spontaneous appearance of lateral eye movements, buccolingual and orbital twitching, irregular respirations, and low tone. This constellation of signs occurred intermittently over a 15- to 20-minute period followed by cessation of these movements, regular cardiorespiratory rates, and increased muscle tone. A coincident EEG would most likely document neonatal seizures during the first of the two observation intervals.*

This is a description of appropriate clinical phenomena associated with active followed by quiet sleep in a near-term child. The movements during rapid eye movement sleep superficially may resemble seizures but have no EEG correlate; therefore, the statement is false.

◆ *A cranial ultrasound documents a bilateral echodensity surrounding the ventricular outline. In addition, there is extension of the echodensity into the left brain substance with high density signal within the ventricular space. The neuroimaging report concludes that both IVH and PVL occurred in this preterm infant.*

This is a true statement. These two forms of cerebrovascular lesions can occur in the same preterm infant.

◆ *A full-term newborn whose mother had premature rupture of membranes and a fever to 39° C has bulging fontanelle, seizures, and irritability. Spinal fluid shows evidence of 100 white blood cells and elevation in the CSF protein to 200 µg/dL. The clinician makes the diagnosis of bacterial meningitis.*

This is a true statement. The child has an increased risk because of premature rupture of membranes in a mother with probable maternal chorioamnionitis. Careful examination of placenta reveals lymphocytic infiltration, villous edema, and intravascular thrombin deposition.

◆ *A growth-restricted newborn of 37 weeks' gestation has irritability, hypotonia, hepatosplenomegaly, and chorioretinitis. Congenital infection is suspected, and the attending neonatologist should obtain a CT scan rather than an MRI scan.*

This choice of neuroimaging technique is reasonable because a CT scan better documents calcifications associated with congenital infection. An MRI study would otherwise be preferred for a child suspected to have brain lesions that require higher resolution to document structural anomalies or injury.

◆ *A full-term infant who is clearly awake does not move below the neck except for fine myoclonic movements of the fingers and toes and fasciculations of the tongue. The neonatologist should request a specific serum blood study to diagnose progressive spinal muscular atrophy.*

This is a true statement. Anterior horn cell disease (i.e., spinal muscular atrophy, historically termed Werdnig-Hoffmann disease) can be expeditiously diagnosed by genetic analysis using a serum sample to document a deletional defect on chromosome 7. This genetics study has largely replaced the more laborious and indirect diagnostic investigations including EMG and muscle biopsy, which nonetheless still lack genetic specificity.

CASE PROBLEMS

◆ ───────────────────────────

Case One

M. C. is a 2400-g female infant, born at term to a 30-year-old mother with known epilepsy who has undergone treatment throughout pregnancy with phenobarbital, 120 mg a day. During the initial day of life, the child appears neurologically normal but subsequently lethargy, hypotonia, depressed Moro reflex, and a weak cry develop. The deep tendon reflexes are normal, and the tongue does not have fasciculations. The child's anterior fontanelle is full and bulging, and the neck is supple. Head circumference is 33 cm. Funduscopic examination is normal. The child's temperature is 35.2° C.

◆ *Did the mother's antiepileptic medications contribute to the child's hypotonia and other neurologic findings?*

One does not anticipate cerebral depression in an infant whose mother was prescribed the appropriate doses of an antiepileptic medication. A withdrawal syndrome may be associated with barbiturate use, and the newborn may show poor sleep, agitation, and crying rather than hypotonia and a weak, incomplete Moro reflex. Other medications do not cause this specific withdrawal syndrome. Although antiepileptic medications may result in coagulation defects of the neonate that lead to intracranial hemorrhage, this possibility was anticipated and the child's anticoagulation studies were all within normal limits. It is also unlikely that the drugs taken by the mother would cause depression and hypotonia after a day of life because these drugs would have caused problems immediately after birth rather than after a delay of a day.

◆ *What diagnostic steps are indicated?*
In a child with hypotonia, lethargy, and a poor cry with normal deep tendon reflexes, one must consider an "upper motor neuron" explanation for the child's hypotonia rather than a low motor neuron disease. Given the rapid onset of symptoms and the lack of history of intrapartum asphyxia, trauma, or malformation, an intracranial infection or metabolic derangement would more likely cause cerebral depression and low tone. A complete blood count; spinal tap; blood, urine, skin, and throat cultures; blood sugar, calcium, potassium, and sodium concentrations; and blood gas determination should be performed. An x-ray study of the chest and urinalysis should also be included.

Results of these evaluations show a hematocrit of 58 and white blood cell count of 14,000 with 80% segmented polymorphonuclear cells. Urinalysis is normal. Blood sugar is 38 mg/dL, calcium is 6.3 mg/dL, sodium is 132 mmol/L, potassium is 4.9 mmol/L, pH is 7.37, P_{CO_2} is 38 mm Hg, and P_{O_2} is 95 mm Hg. Chest x-ray results are negative. Spinal fluid is xanthochromic with 102 white blood cells, 60% polymorphs, a CSF glucose measurement of 10 mg/dL, and a CSF protein of 300 mg/dL. The Gram stain of the spinal fluid is negative for organisms.

◆ *Despite the negative Gram stain of the CSF, should this child be treated presumptively for meningitis?*
Definitely. The child should be treated for bacterial meningitis given the clinical picture described. The absence of a stiff neck should not deceive the physician that the child has meningitis, particularly when the fontanelle is full. In addition, cultures of the blood and CSF did grow out *E. coli* after 48

hours of culture. For at least one third of cases with neonatal septicemia, meningitis will also occur.

Subsequently, the mother reported having had a urinary tract infection with *E. coli.* Given the early signs of infection in the mother, chorioamnionitis of placental tissues or blood-borne infection of the fetus before delivery resulted in the newborn's infectious illness.

◆

Case Two
A. P. is delivered at 36 weeks' gestation by cesarean section to a 32-year-old Gravida 4, Para 0 mother. His birth weight is 1490 g, length is 40 cm, and head circumference is 27 cm. The mother had severe preeclampsia and had a coagulopathy of the blood, which was treated with large molecular weight heparin. She maintained a hypertensive state from the 15th week of gestation and required methyldopa to maintain her blood pressure. A fetal ultrasound at 27 weeks' gestation documented asymmetry of the lateral ventricles with an irregular border on the right. Fetal heart monitoring was obtained with the onset of premature labor at 30 weeks' gestation, which showed poor variability. Mother also noted decreased fetal movements. The child is born with Apgar scores of 1 at 1 minute and 7 at 5 minutes. He requires intubation and resuscitation. Initial arterial blood gas is pH of 7.26, P_{CO_2} of 19, and a base excess of -13 mEq/L. The child's initial blood pressure is 48/32 mm Hg in the first hour of life. Respiratory distress syndrome develops and is treated with continuous positive pressure ventilation, surfactant administration, and oxygen for 3 days. Hyperbilirubinemia develops with a maximum peak bilirubin of 9 mg/dL and is treated with phototherapy. Feedings are begun on the sixth day of life.

Neurologically, the child appears appropriate for gestational maturity of 30 weeks. No suspicious movements suggesting seizures are noted. A lumbar puncture is obtained on day 3, and results are normal. Cranial ultrasound on day 2 of life is obtained, and results are normal. An EEG documents positive rolandic sharp waves at 5 days of age on the left greater than right.

By 3 weeks of age, at 33 weeks of postconceptional age, the head circumference has grown to 29 cm, and the sutures and fontanelle are normal. The child's neurologic examination remains normal but low tone is noted in the legs. Repeat ultrasound documents irregularity of the ventricular outline, greater on the right. MRI scan documents porencephaly with hemosiderin noted in the right ventricle.

The child is discharged at 36 weeks' corrected age. The parents do not return for follow-up until the child is 6 1/2 months old, at which time he recently acquired head control but his legs were quite stiff. His social ability is poor and he cries excessively. His head circumference is 2 standard deviations greater than the mean. He is unable to sit. An MRI scan indicates ventriculomegaly, and he is referred to a neurosurgeon who places an intraventricular shunt device.

Subsequently, he is followed up for developmental milestones. He begins walking at 22 months, but he has poor fine motor function and increased tone in the lower extremities, left greater than right. At 2 years of age, his developmental quotient is 74. Repeat MRI scan documents a right porencephaly with bilateral high signal lesions seen in the central white matter, right greater than left, on the T2-weighted signal.

◆ When did the lesions occur?

There are two cerebrovascular lesions described over the course of this child's evaluation. One lesion was hemorrhagic and the other lesion was ischemic in nature. These are the two principal cerebrovascular lesions noted in preterm infants. Given the mother's severe toxemia of pregnancy and the presence of disseminated intravascular coagulation, this raises the possibility of a blood dyscrasia in the fetus, which may have resulted in IVH, as suggested on fetal sonography. The positive rolandic sharp waves noted on the EEG after birth suggest IVH or PVL; each can be associated with this particular EEG abnormality. The irregular ventricular border on the second cranial ultrasound together with the MRI finding suggest that coincident PVL may have occurred in association with IVH.

◆ Why was the initial ultrasound normal at 3 days of age?

Clearly, the cystic lesions that chronically appear with PVL eventually collapse, resulting in an irregularity of the ventricular border; this may not have been noted shortly after birth before sufficient atrophy of brain subsequently was visually evident. Follow-up ultrasounds later documented the emerging brain atrophy.

◆ Could the cerebrovascular lesions have occurred during the intrapartum period rather than during the antepartum period?

Although the child was depressed during the fetal and immediate neonatal periods, there is EEG and neuroimaging evidence to suggest an event preexisting the labor and delivery. This must be taken in the context of the mother's significant medical history during the antepartum period, which consisted of toxemia complicated by disseminated intravascular coagulation.

◆ Why did the child appear normal at birth in the newborn period only to show developmental delay at a later time?

The immaturity of the brain during the early months of life does not allow clinical expression of children with static motor encephalopathies (i.e., cerebral palsy). If the family had attended an earlier follow-up appointment, documentation of abnormalities at an earlier stage than 6 months may have been detected.

◆ Can the cerebrovascular deficits described be prevented?

Even if fetal surveillance is aggressive with serial prenatal studies, these cerebral lesions could not have been avoided. One could attempt to treat the mother's medical condition in the hopes of avoiding brain injury in the infant. It is unclear, however, whether the child would have survived or had greater deficits if no treatment had been offered to the mother during her pregnancy.

◆ Could earlier intervention have made a difference before 6 months of age when the child returned for his first follow-up visit?

Early intervention programs provide additional stimulation and prevent contractures from abnormal hypertonicity of the legs. Developmental monitoring may also provide an incentive for parents to supplement stimulation at both an earlier time and on a more frequent basis. Even though other comorbid conditions cannot be avoided in children with cerebrovascular accidents (e.g., learning disabilities and behavioral problems), it is still unclear whether earlier aggressive interventional strategies result in a greater degree of brain plasticity and ultimately improved developmental outcome in an already damaged child.

REFERENCES

1. Abrams EJ, Matheson PB, Thomas PA, et al: Neonatal predictors of infection status and early death among 332 infants at risk of HIV-1 infection monitored prospectively from birth. Pediatrics 97:451–458, 1996.
2. Aicardi J, Bax M, Gillberg C, Ogier H: Diseases of the Nervous System in Childhood. Clinics in Developmental Medicine. 2nd ed. New York: MacKeith Press, 1998.
3. American Academy of Pediatrics Committee on

Genetics: Prenatal genetic diagnosis for pediatricians. Pediatrics 93:1010–1015, 1994.

4. Amiel-Tison C: Neurological evaluation of the maturity of newborn infants. Arch Dis Child 43:89–93, 1968.

5. Amiel-Tison C, Korobkin R: Neurologic problems. In Klaus MH, Fanaroff AA: Care of the High-Risk Neonate, 4th ed. Philadelphia: WB Saunders, 1993.

6. Atkinson J: Human visual development over the first 6 months of life. A review and a hypothesis. Hum Neurobiol 3:61–74, 1984.

7. Aultschuler G, Herman AA: The medical-legal imperative: Placental pathology as epidemiology. In Stevenson D, Sunshine P, eds: Fetal and Neonatal Brain Injuries. New York: BC Decker, 1989, pp 250–263.

8. Ballard JL, Khoury JC, Wedig K, et al: New Ballard score, expanded to include extremely premature infants. J Pediatr 119:417–423, 1991.

9. Barabas RE, Barmada MA, Scher MS: Timing of brain insults in severe neonatal encephalopathies with isoelectric EEG. Pediatr Neurol 9:39–44, 1993.

10. Barkovich AJ: MR and CT evaluation of profound neonatal and infantile asphyxia. AJNR Am J Neuroradiol 13:959–972, 1992.

11. Barkovich AJ, Kjos BO, Jackson DE, et al: Normal maturation of the neonatal and infant brain: MRI imaging at 1.5 T1. Radiology 166:173–180, 1988.

12. Barkovich AJ, Lindan CE: Congenital cytomegalovirus infection of the brain: Imaging analysis and embryologic considerations. AJNR Am J Neuroradiol 15:703–715, 1994.

13. Barth PG, Fukuyama Y, Suzuki Y, et al: Inherited progressive disorders of the fetal brain: A field in need of recognition. In Fukuyama Y, Suzuki Y, Kamoshita S, Caesar P, eds: Fetal and Perinatal Neurology. Basel: S Karger AG, 1992, pp 299–313.

14. Bax M, Nelson KB: Birth asphyxia: A statement. Dev Med Child Neurol 35:1022–1024, 1993.

15. Besio R, Caballero C, Meerhoff E, et al: Neonatal retinal hemorrhages and influence of perinatal factors. Am J Ophthalmol 87:74–76, 1979.

16. Biale Y, Brawer-Ostrovsky J, Insler V: Fetal heart rate tracings in fetuses with congenital malformations. J Reprod Med 30:43–47, 1985.

17. Bird CR, Hedberg M, Drayer BP, et al: MR assessment of myelination in infants and children: Usefulness of marker sites. AJNR Am J Neuroradiol 10:731–740, 1989.

18. Birnholz JC: Ultrasonic fetal neuro-ophthalmology. In Hill A, Volpe JJ, eds: Fetal Neurology. New York: Raven Press 1989, pp 41–56.

19. Boothe RG, Dobson V, Teller DY: Postnatal development of vision in human and nonhuman primates. Annu Rev Neurosci 8:495–545, 1985.

20. Brazelton TB: Neonatal Behavioral Assessment Scale. Philadelphia: JB Lippincott 1973.

21. Brown JK, Purvis RJ, Forfar JO, et al: Neurological aspects of perinatal asphyxia. Dev Med Child Neurol 16:567–580, 1974.

22. Brown KE: What threat is human parvovirus B19 to the fetus? A review. Br J Obstet Gynaecol 96:764–767, 1989.

23. Buckley EG: The clinical approach to the pediatric patient with nystagmus. Int Pediatr 5:225–248, 1990.

24. Bu'Lock F, Woolridge MW, Baum JD: Develop-ment of coordination of sucking, swallowing and breathing: Ultrasound study of term and preterm infants. Dev Med Child Neurol 32:669–678, 1990.

25. Chamberlain PF, Manning FA, Morrison L, et al: Ultrasound evaluation of amniotic fluid volume. 1: The relationship of marginal and decreased amniotic fluid volumes to perinatal outcome. Am J Obstet Gynecol 150:245–249, 1984.

26. Chaplin ER, Goldstein GW, Norman D: Neonatal seizures, intracerebral hematoma and subarachnoid hemorrhage in full-term infants. Pediatrics 63:812–815, 1979.

27. Chard T, Macintosh M: Antenatal diagnosis of congenital abnormalities. In Chard T, Richards MPM, eds: Obstetrics in the 1990s: Current Controversies. Clinics in Developmental Medicine. New York: MacKeith Press, 1992.

28. Chiswick ML: Intrauterine growth retardation. BMJ 291:845–848, 1985.

29. Christmann D, Haddad J: Magnetic resonance imaging: Application to the neonatal period. In Haddad J, Christmann D, Messer J, eds: Imaging Techniques of the CNS of the Neonates. New York: Springer-Verlag, 1991.

30. Clancy R, Malin S, Larague D, et al: Focal motor seizures heralding a stroke in full-term neonates. Am J Dis Child 139:601–606, 1985.

31. Clarke TA, Saunders BS, Feldman B: Pyridoxine-dependent seizures requiring high doses of pyridoxine for control. Am J Dis Child 133:963–965, 1979.

32. Cooke RWI: Somatosensory evoked potentials. In Eyre JA, ed: The Neurophysiological Examination of the Newborn Infant. New York: MacKeith Press, 1992.

33. Coker SB, Beltran RS, Myers TF, IImura L: Neonatal stroke: Description of patients and investigation into pathogenesis. Pediatr Neurol 4:219–223, 1988.

34. Coulter DL, Allen RJ: Benign neonatal sleep myoclonus. Arch Neurol 39:191–192, 1982.

35. Cowan WM: The development of the brain. Sci Am 241:113–120, 1979.

36. D'Alton ME, DeCherney AH: Prenatal diagnosis. N Engl J Med 328:114–120, 1993.

37. Dawson TM, Dawson VL, Snyder SH: A novel neuronal messenger molecule in brain: The free radical, nitric oxide. Ann Neurol 32:297–311, 1992.

38. Dekaban AS, Magee KR: Occurrence of neurologic abnormalities in infants of diabetic mothers. Neurology 8:193, 1958.

39. De Reuck J, Chattha AS, Richardson EP: Pathogenesis and evolution of periventricular leukomalacia. Arch Neurol 27:229–231, 1972.

40. DeVries LS, Connell JA, Dubowitz LMS, et al: Neurological, electrophysiological and MRI abnormalities in infants with extensive cystic leukomalacia. Neuropediatrics 18:61–66, 1987.

41. DeVries LS, Smer M, Goemans N, et al: Unilateral thalamic haemorrhage in the pre-term and full-term newborn. Neuropediatrics 23:153–156, 1992.

42. Donat JF, Donat JR, Lay KS: Changing response to caloric stimulation with gestational age in infants. Neurology 30:776–778, 1980.

43. Dorfman DH, Glaser JH: Congenital syphilis presenting in infants after the newborn period. N Engl J Med 323:1299–1302, 1990.

44. Eken P, van Nieuwenhuizen O, van der Graaf Y, et

al: Relation between neonatal cranial ultrasound abnormalities and cerebral visual impairment in infancy. Dev Med Child Neurol 36:3–15, 1994.

45. Evans MI, Schulman JD: Medical fetal therapy. In Evans MI, Fletcher JC, Dixler AO, Schulman JD, eds: Fetal Diagnosis and Therapy: Science, Ethics and the Law. Philadelphia: Lippincott, 1989, pp 403–412.

46. Ewigman BG, Crane JP, Frigoletto FD, et al: Effects of prenatal ultrasound screening on perinatal outcome. RADIUS Study Group. N Engl J Med 329:821–827, 1993.

47. Fawer CL, Calame A: Ultrasound. In Haddad J, Christmann D, Messer J, eds: Imaging Techniques of the CNS of the Neonate. New York: Springer-Verlag, 1991.

48. Fenichel GM, Olson BJ, Fitzpatrick JE: Heart rate changes in convulsive and nonconvulsive apnea. Ann Neurol 7:577–582, 1979.

49. Filipek PA, Kennedy DN, Caviness VS: Volumetric analyses of central nervous system neoplasm based on MRI. Pediatr Neurol 7:347–351, 1991.

50. Finnstrom O: Studies on maturity in newborn infants. II. External characteristics. Acta Paediatr Scand 61:24–32, 1972.

51. Fitzhardinge PM, Flodmark O, Fitz CR, Ashby S: The prognostic value of computed tomography of the brain in asphyxiated premature infants. J Pediatr 100:476–481, 1982.

52. Friede RL: Developmental Neuropathology. New York: Springer-Verlag, 1989.

53. Fujimoto S, Yokochi K, Togari H, et al: Neonatal cerebral infarction: Symptoms, CT findings and prognosis. Brain Dev 14:48–52, 1992.

54. Gobel W, Richard G: Retinopathy of prematurity—Current diagnosis and management. Eur J Pediatr 152:286–290, 1993.

55. Govaert P: Cranial Haemorrhage in the Term Newborn Infant. Clinics in Developmental Medicine No. 109. London: MacKeith Press, 1993.

56. Gross SJ, Eckerman CO: Normative early head growth in very low birthweight infants. J Pediatr 107:946–949, 1983.

57. Govaert P, DeVries LS: An Atlas of Neonatal Brain Sonography. Clinics in Developmental Medicine No. 141/142. London: MacKeith Press, 1997.

58. Guzzetta F, Shackelford GD, Volpe S, et al: Periventricular intraparenchymal echodensities in the premature newborn: Critical determinant of neurologic outcome. Pediatrics 78:995–1006, 1986.

59. Haddow JE, Palomaki GE, Knight GJ, et al: Prenatal screening for Down's syndrome with use of maternal serum markers. N Engl J Med 327:588–593, 1992.

60. Hall WG, Oppenheim RW: Developmental psychobiology: Prenatal, perinatal, and early postnatal aspects of behavioral development. Annu Rev Psychol 38:91–128, 1987.

61. Hattori H, Morin AM, Schwartz PH, et al: Posthypoxic treatment with MK-801 reduces hypoxic-ischemic damage in the neonatal rat. Neurology 39:713–718, 1989.

62. Hendricks-Munoz KD, Walton JP: Hearing loss in infants with persistent fetal circulation. Pediatrics 81:650–656, 1988.

63. Hill A: Perinatal asphyxia: Clinical aspects. Clin Perinatol 16:435–457, 1989.

64. Hill A, Volpe JJ: Fetal Neurology. New York: Raven Press, 1989.

65. Hillman LS, Hillman RE, Dodson WE: Diagnosis, treatment, and follow-up of neonatal mepivacaine intoxication secondary to paracervical and pudendal blocks during labor. J Pediatr 94:472–477, 1979.

66. Hoyt CS, Mousel DK, Weber AA: Transient supranuclear disturbances of gaze in healthy neonates. Am J Ophthalmol 89:708–713, 1980.

67. Huppi PS, Warfield S, Kikincs R, et al: Quantitative magnetic resonance imaging of brain development in premature and mature newborns. Ann Neurol 43:224–235, 1998.

68. Jan JE, Wong PK, Groenveld M, et al: Travel vision: Collicular visual system? Pediatr Neurol 2:359–362, 1986.

69. Johnston MV: Neurotransmitter alterations in a model of perinatal hypoxic-ischemic brain injury. Ann Neurol 13:511–518, 1983.

70. Kairam R, DeVivo DC: Neurologic manifestations of congenital infection. Clin Perinatol 8:455–465, 1981.

71. Kauppinen RA, Williams SR, Busza AL, et al: Applications of magnetic resonance spectroscopy and diffusion-weighted imaging to the study of brain biochemistry and pathology. Trends Neurosci 16:88–95, 1993.

72. Kellaway P, Hrachovy RA: Status epilepticus in newborns: A perspective on neonatal seizures. In Delgado-Escueta AV, Wasterlain CG, Treiman DM, et al, eds: Status Epilepticus: Mechanisms of Brain Damage and Treatment. New York: Raven Press 1983, pp 93–99.

73. Khater-Boidin J, Duron B: Nerve conduction. In Eyre JA, ed: The Neurophysiological Examination of the Newborn Infant. New York: MacKeith Press, 1992.

74. Kragelon-Mann I, Petersen D, Magberg G, et al: Bilateral spastic cerebral palsy. MRI pathology and origin. Analysis from a representative series of 56 cases. Dev Med Child Neurol 37:379–397, 1995.

75. Kramer MS, Olivier M, McLean FH, et al: Impact of intrauterine growth retardation and body proportionality on fetal and neonatal outcome. Pediatrics 85:707–713, 1990.

76. Larroche J-C: Fetal encephalopathies of circulatory origin. Biol Neonate 50:61–74, 1986.

77. Leech RW, Brumback RA: Massive brain stem necrosis in the human neonate: Presentation of three cases with review of the literature. J Child Neurol 3:258–262, 1988.

78. Levene MI, Lilford RJ, eds: Fetal and Neonatal Neurology and Neurosurgery. 2nd ed. London: Blackwell Scientific, 1995.

79. Levene MI, Williams JL, Fawer CL: Ultrasound of the Infant Brain. London: Blackwell Scientific, 1985.

80. Leviton A, Gilles FH: Acquired perinatal leukoencephalopathy. Ann Neurol 16:1–8, 1984.

81. Lewis SH, Gilbert-Barness E: The placenta and its significance in neonatal outcome. Adv Pediatr 45:223–266, 1998.

82. Lipton SA, Rosenberg PA: Excitatory aminoacids as a final common pathway for neurologic disorders. N Engl J Med 330:613–622, 1994.

83. Lombroso CT: Neonatal polygraphy in full-term and pre-term infants: A review of normal and abnormal findings. J Clin Neurophysiol 2:105–115, 1985.

84. Lynch BJ, Rust RS: Natural history and outcome of neonatal hypocalcemic and hypomagnesemic seizures. Pediatr Neurol 11:23–27, 1994.

85. MacDonald HM, Mulligan JC, Allen AC, Taylor PM: Neonatal asphyxia I: Relationship of obstetric and neonatal complications to neonatal mortality in 38,405 consecutive deliveries. J Pediatr 96:898–903, 1980.

86. MacFarlane A: Olfaction in the development of social preferences in the human neonate. Parent-Infant Interaction: CIBA Foundation Symposium, Washington, DC, 33, 1975.

87. McCord JM: Oxygen-derived free radicals in post-ischemic tissue injury. N Engl J Med 312:159–163, 1985.

88. Miller E, Cradock-Watson JE, Pollock TM: Consequences of confirmed maternal rubella at successive stages of pregnancy. Lancet 2:781–784, 1982.

89. Mizrahi EM, Kellaway P: Characterization and classification of neonatal seizures. Neurology 37:1837–1844, 1987.

90. Mizrahi EM, Kellaway P: Diagnosis and Management of Neonatal Seizures. Philadelphia: Lippincott-Raven, 1998.

91. Mizrahi EM, Tharp BR: Characteristic EEG pattern in neonatal herpes simplex encephalitis. Neurology 32:1215–1220, 1982.

92. Monod N, Pajot N, Guidasci S: The neonatal EEG: Statistical studies and prognostic value in full-term and pre-term babies. Electroencephalogr Clin Neurophysiol 32:529–544, 1972.

93. Myers RE: Two patterns of brain damage and their conditions of occurrence. Am J Obstet Gynecol 112:246–276, 1972.

94. Naidu S, Messmore H, Caserta V: CNS lesions in neonatal iso-immune thrombocytopenia. Arch Neurol 40:552–554, 1983.

95. Nelson KB: Magnesium sulfate and risk of cerebral palsy in very low birth-weight infants. JAMA 276:1843–1844, 1996.

96. Nelson KB, Danbrook JM, Grether JK, et al: Neonatal cytokines and coagulation factors in children with cerebral palsy. Ann Neurol 44:665–675, 1998.

97. Nelson KB, Ellenberg JH: Neonatal signs as predictors of cerebral palsy. Pediatrics 64:225–232, 1979.

98. Nelson KB, Grether JK: Selection of neonates for neuroprotective therapies. Arch Pediatr Adolesc Med 153:393–398, 1999.

99. Novotny E, Ashwal S, Shevell M: Proton magnetic resonance spectroscopy: An emerging technology in pediatric neurology research. Pediatr Res 44:1–10, 1998.

100. Ohtahara S: Clinico-electrical delineation of epileptic encephalopathies in childhood. Asian Med J 21:7–17, 1978.

101. Painter MJ, Minnigh B, Mollica L, et al: Binding profiles of anticonvulsants in neonates with seizures. Ann Neurol 22:413–420, 1987.

102. Painter MJ, Pippenger C, Wasterlain C, et al: Phenobarbital and phenytoin in neonatal seizures, metabolism, and tissue distribution. Neurology 31:1107–1112, 1981.

103. Painter MJ, Scher MS, Stein AD, et al: Phenobarbital compared with phenytoin for the treatment of neonatal seizures. N Engl J Med 341:485–489, 1999.

104. Palmer C, Smith MB: Assessing the risk of kernic-terus using nuclear magnetic resonance. Clin Perinatol 17:307–329, 1990.

105. Palmer C, Vannucci RC: Potential new therapies for perinatal cerebral hypoxia-ischemia. Clin Perinatol 20:411–432, 1993.

106. Palmini A, Andermann E, Andermann F: Prenatal events and genetic factors in epileptic patients with neuronal migration disorders. Epilepsia 35:965–973, 1994.

107. Papazian O: Transient neonatal myasthenia gravis. J Child Neurol 7:135–141 and erratum p 325, 1992.

108. Papile LA, Burstein J, Burstein R, Koffler H: Incidence and evolution of subependymal and intraventricular hemorrhage: A study of infants with birthweights less than 1,500 gm. J Pediatr 92:529–534, 1978.

109. Parmelee AH, Schultz HR, Disbrow MA: Sleep patterns of the newborn. J Pediatr 58:241, 1961.

110. Pasternak JF: Parasagittal infarction in neonatal asphyxia. Ann Neurol 21:202–204, 1987.

111. Peiper A: Cerebral Function in Infancy and Childhood. New York: Consultants Bureau, 1963.

112. Perlman JM, Risser R: Severe fetal acidemia: Neonatal neurological features and short-term outcome. Pediatr Neurol 9:277–282, 1992.

113. Perlman JM, Volpe JJ: Intraventricular hemorrhage in extremely small premature infants. Am J Dis Child 140:1122–1124, 1986.

114. Perlman JM, Risser R, Broyles RS: Bilateral cystic periventricular leukomalacia in the premature infant: Associated risk factors. Pediatrics 97:822–827, 1996.

115. Perlman JM, Volpe JJ: Movement disorder of premature infants with severe bronchopulmonary dysplasia: A new syndrome. Pediatrics 84:215–218, 1989.

116. Pierre-Kahn A, Renier D, Sainte-Rose C, Hirsch JF: Acute intracranial hematomas in term neonates. Childs Nerv Syst 2:191–194, 1986.

117. Plum F, Posner JB: The Diagnosis of Stupor and Coma. Philadelphia: FA Davis, 1966.

118. Prechtl HFR: Fetal behavior. In Hill A, Volpe JJ, eds: Fetal Neurology. New York: Raven Press, 1989, pp 1–16.

119. Prechtl HFR, Beintema D: The Neurological Examination of the Full Term Newborn Infant. London: William Heinemann, 1964.

120. Prechtl HF, Fargel JW, Weinmann HM, et al: Postures, motility and respiration of low-risk preterm infants. Dev Med Child Neurol 21:3–27, 1979.

121. Prechtl HFR, O'Brien MJ: Behavioural states of the full-term newborn. The emergence of a concept. In Stratton P, ed: Psychobiology of the Human Newborn. New York: John Wiley & Sons, 1982.

122. Pryds O, Greiser G, Lou H, et al: Heterogeneity of cerebral reactivity in preterm infants supported by mechanical ventilation. J Pediatr 115:638–645, 1989.

123. Rayburn WF: Antepartum fetal monitoring fetal movements. In Hill A, Volpe JJ, eds: Fetal Neurology. New York: Raven Press 1989, pp 17–36.

124. Roberts-Harry J, Green SH, Willshaw HE: Optic nerve hypoplasia: Associations and management. Arch Dis Child 65:103–106, 1990.

125. Robinson J, Fielder AR: Pupillary diameter and reaction to light in preterm neonates. Arch Dis Child 65:35–38, 1990.

126. Rodriguez AF, Kaplan SL, Mason EO Jr: Cerebrospinal fluid values in the very low birth weight infant. J Pediatr 116:971–974, 1990.

127. Roland EH, Poskitt K, Rodriguez E, et al: Perinatal hypoxic-ischemic thalamic injury: Clinical features and neuroimaging. Ann Neurol 44:161–166, 1998.

128. Rutherford MA, Schwieso J, et al: Hypoxic-ischemic encephalopathy: Early and late magnetic resonance imaging findings in relation to outcome. Arch Dis Child 75:F145–F151, 1996.

129. Ryan SG, Wiznitzer M, Hollman C, et al: Benign familial neonatal convulsions: Evidence for clinical and genetic heterogeneity. Ann Neurol 33:696–705, 1976.

130. Saari-Kemppainen A, Karjalainen O, Ylostalo P, Heinon OP: Ultrasound screening and perinatal mortality: Controlled trial of systematic one-stage screening in pregnancy. The Helsinki Ultrasound Trial. Lancet 336:387–391, 1990.

131. Saint-Anne Dargassies S: Neurological Development in the Full-Term and Premature Neonate. New York: Excerpta Medica, 1977.

132. Salamy A, Mendelson T, Tooley WH: Developmental profiles for the brainstem auditory evoked potential. Early Hum Dev 6:331–339, 1982.

133. Sanders M, Allen M, Alexander GR, et al: Gestational age assessment in preterm neonates weighing less than 1500 grams. Pediatrics 88:542–546, 1991.

134. Sarff LD, Platt LH, McCracken GH Jr: Cerebrospinal fluid evaluation in neonates: Comparison of high-risk infants with and without meningitis. J Pediatr 1976;88:473–477, 1976.

135. Sarnat HB: Olfactory reflexes in the newborn infant. J Pediatr 92:624–626, 1978.

136. Sarnat HB, Sarnat MS: Neonatal encephalopathy following fetal distress: A clinical and electroencephalographic study. Arch Neurol 33:696–705, 1976.

137. Scher MS: Pathological myoclonus of the newborn: Electrographic and clinical correlations. Pediatr Neurol 1:342–348, 1985.

138. Scher MS: Neonatal encephalopathies as classified by EEG-sleep criteria: Severity and timing based on clinical/pathologic correlations. Pediatr Neurol 11:189–200, 1994.

139. Scher MS: Neonatal seizures. Seizures in special clinical settings. In Wyllie E, ed: The Treatment of Epilepsy, Principles & Practice. 3rd ed. Baltimore: Williams & Wilkins. (In press.)

140. Scher MS: Seizures in the newborn infant. Diagnosis, treatment and outcome. Clin Perinatol 24:735–772, 1997.

141. Scher MS, Aso K, Beggarly ME, et al: Electrographic seizures in preterm and full-term neonates: Clinical correlates, associated brain lesions, and risk for neurological sequelae. Pediatrics 91:128–134, 1993.

142. Scher MS, Belfar H, Martin J, et al: Destructive brain lesions of presumed fetal onset: Antepartum causes of cerebral palsy. Pediatrics 88:898–906, 1991.

143. Scher MS, Hamid MY, Steppe DA, et al: Ictal and interictal durations in preterm and term neonates. Epilepsia 34:284–288, 1993.

144. Scher MS, Klesh KW, Murphy TF, et al: Seizures and infarction in neonates with persistent pulmonary hypertension. Pediatr Neurol 2:332–339, 1986.

145. Scher MS: Neonatal EEG-sleep, normal and abnormal features. In Neidermeyer E, da Silva L, eds: Electroencephalography. 4th ed. Baltimore: Williams & Wilkins, 1999.

146. Scher MS, Sun M, Hatzilabrou GM, et al: Computer analyses of EEG-sleep in the neonate: Methodological considerations. J Clin Neurophysiol 7:417–441, 1990.

147. Scher MS, Trucco J, Beggarly ME, et al: Neonates with electrically-confirmed seizures and possible placental associations. Pediatr Neurol 19:37–41, 1998.

148. Sher PK, Brown SB: A longitudinal study of head growth in preterm infants I: Normal rates of head growth. Dev Med Child Neurol 17:705–710, 1975.

149. Sher PK, Brown SB: A longitudinal study of head growth in preterm infants II: Differentiation between "catch-up" head growth and early infantile hydrocephalus. Dev Med Child Neurol 17:711–718, 1975.

150. Shimada M, Segawa M, Higurashi M, et al: Development of the sleep and wakefulness rhythm in preterm infants discharged from a neonatal care unit. Pediatr Res 33:159–163, 1993.

151. Shuper A, Zalzberg J, Weitz R, et al: Jitteriness beyond the neonatal period: A benign pattern of movement in infancy. J Child Neurol 6:243–245, 1991.

152. Simmer ML: Newborn's response to the cry of another infant. Dev Psychobiol 5:136, 1971.

153. Smith BI, Misoh RE: Intravenous diazepam in the treatment of prolonged seizure activity in neonates and infants. Dev Med Child Neurol 13:030–634, 1971.

154. Stagno S: Cytomegalovirus. In Remington JS, Klein OJ, eds: Infectious Disease of the Fetus and Newborn Infant. 3rd ed. Philadelphia: WB Saunders, 1990, pp 241–281.

155. Stagno S: Herpesvirus infections of pregnancy. Part II: Herpes simplex virus and varicella-zoster virus infections. N Engl J Med 313:1327–1330, 1985.

156. Stapells DR, Kurtzberg D: Evoked potential assessment of auditory system integrity in infants. Clin Perinatol 18:497–518, 1991.

157. Sullivan RM, Taborsky-Barba S, Mendoza R, et al: Olfactory classical conditioning in neonates. Pediatrics 87:511–518, 1991.

158. Tallman B, Tan OT, Morell JG, et al: Location of port-wine stains and the likelihood of ophthalmic and/or central nervous system complications. Pediatrics 87:323–327, 1991.

159. Taylor MJ: Visual evoked potentials. In Eyre JA, ed: The Neurophysiological Examination of the Newborn Infant. New York: MacKeith Press, 1992.

160. Tharp BR, Cukier F, Monod N: The prognostic value of the electroencephalogram in premature infants. Electroencephalogr Clin Neurophysiol 51:205–208, 1981.

161. Timor-Tritsch IE, Monteagudo A, Cohen HL: Ultrasonography of the Prenatal and Neonatal Brain. Stamford, CT: Appleton and Lange, 1996.

162. Touwen BC, Lok-Meijer TY, Huisjes HJ, et al: The recovery rate of neurologically deviant newborns. Early Hum Dev 7:131–148, 1982.

163. Trounce JQ, Fagan D, Levene MI: Intraventricular haemorrhage and periventricular leucomalacia: Ultrasound and autopsy correlation. Arch Dis Child 61:1203–1207, 1986.

164. Tychsen L, Lisberger SG: Maldevelopment of visual motion processing in humans who had strabismus with onset in infancy. J Neurosci 6:2495–2508, 1986.

165. Volpe JJ: Neurology of the Newborn, 3rd ed. Philadelphia: WB Saunders, 1995.

166. Wagner CL, Eichen NJ, Katikaneni D, et al: The use of hypothermia: A role in the treatment of neonatal asphyxia? Pediatr Neurol 21:429–443, 1999.

167. Weiner SP, Painter MJ, Scher MS: Neonatal seizures: Electroclinical disassociation. Pediatr Neurol 7:363–368, 1991.

168. Weisman BM, DiScenna AO, Leigh RJ: Maturation of the vestibulo-ocular reflex in normal infants during the first 2 months of life. Neurology 39:534–538, 1989.

169. Welch K, Strand R: Traumatic parturitional intracranial haemorrhage. Dev Med Child Neurol 28:156–164, 1986.

170. Wharton R, Bresnan MJ: Neonatal respiratory depression and delay in diagnosis in Prader-Willi syndrome. Dev Med Child Neurol 31:231–236, 1989.

171. Whittle MJ: Routine fetal anomaly screening. In Drife JO, Donnai D, eds: Antenatal Diagnosis of Fetal Abnormalities. Berlin: Springer 1991, pp 35–43.

172. Williams J, Hirsch NJ, Corbet AJ, et al: Postnatal head shrinkage in small infants. Pediatrics 59:619–622, 1977.

173. Winchester B: Prenatal diagnosis of enzyme defects. Arch Dis Child 65:59–67, 1990.

The Outcome of Neonatal Intensive Care

Maureen Hack

Technical advances and improvements in obstetric and neonatal care have been mainly responsible for the improved survival of high-risk neonates (Fig. 18–1). A major concern persists, however, that neonatal intensive care results in an increase in the number of permanently handicapped children.

The initial follow-up studies of preterm infants in the early 1970s described a decrease in unfavorable neurodevelopmental sequelae as compared with the era before neonatal intensive care. However, despite the continued decrease in mortality rates, the incidence of neurosensory and developmental handicaps remained constant in the 1980s.[9, 10] The absolute number of both healthy and neurologically impaired children in the population has thus increased. Furthermore, the increased survival of extremely low-birth-weight infants (<1 kg), and infants of extremely low gestation (<26 weeks), many of whom were previously considered nonviable, resulted in a high handicap rate (30% to 40%) in the subpopulation of infants born weighing less than 750 g or

at less than 26 weeks. The increased survival rate of smaller and sicker babies requiring neonatal intensive care also resulted in an extended morbidity of various medical complications, including chronic pulmonary disease, increased susceptibility to infection, sequelae of necrotizing enterocolitis, multiple rehospitalizations, and poor physical growth.[4, 18]

The introduction of surfactant therapy to prevent or treat respiratory distress syndrome (RDS) improved the survival rate of infants with RDS born since 1990 but has not decreased the rate of periventricular hemorrhage, ischemic encephalopathy, infections, or necrotizing enterocolitis.[14]

EDITORIAL COMMENT: When evaluating outcome results there is a considerable difference in the actual figures quoted in different reports. One reason for this variation is the fact that selection of patients by birth weight by no means guarantees a homogeneous group, and such populations studied in one center may differ considerably from those studied in another center. There are several reasons for these differences. One of the most important factors is

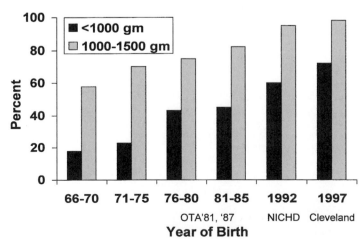

Figure 18–1. Improvement in survival. Data from 1966–1985, publications of U.S. Office of Technology Assessment[21]; 1992, National Institute of Child Health and Human Development[18]; 1997, Rainbow Babies & Children's Hospital, Cleveland, unpublished data.

the pattern of referral to the neonatal intensive care unit (ICU). An "inborn" unit, which limits admissions to babies born in an adjoining obstetric unit, has a population sample most closely approximating a normal sample. On the other hand, units that receive admissions from numerous outlying hospitals have a selected population that may contain a disproportionate number of the sickest babies or may contain only those infants deemed well enough to transport. In addition, patients treated in the inborn unit have the advantage of consistent and, presumably, good obstetric care coupled with the opportunity for immediate postnatal resuscitation and management. Inadequate resuscitation at birth and prolonged hypoxia and acidemia, together with the cold stress of transport that is seen so frequently in the referred patient, influence not only the immediate neonatal period but also the type and frequency of developmental sequelae. Other factors that may influence the outcome of weight-selected samples are (1) the socioeconomic profile of the parents; (2) the proportion of infants with intrauterine growth retardation; (3) the incidence of extreme prematurity, i.e., 28 weeks or less; (4) a selective admission policy; (5) a selective treatment policy; and (6) changes in therapy during the selection period.

P. Fitzhardinge

Measures of the outcomes of neonatal care include mortality rate before and after discharge from the neonatal intensive care nursery, sequelae related to health problems including rates of rehospitalization, and chronic illness such as asthma and growth attainment. Neurodevelopmental sequelae include subnormal and borderline cognitive (mental) function and neurosensory sequelae. These outcomes have traditionally been used as outcome measures.[6] More recently other outcomes are being considered. These include functional measures and the child's ability to perform activities of daily living.[11, 15] Other measures include special health care needs such as technologic aids, excessive physician visits and medications for chronic conditions, occupational and physical therapy, and the need for special education and counseling.

Additional measures have included impact on the family,[16] quality of life,[13] and cost of care.[17] This chapter pertains specifically to the clinical, medical, and developmental type of follow-up programs provided by neonatal intensive care nurseries.

Regional outcome results reflect a more accurate picture of outcome because they include all infants born in an area. These studies have rarely been undertaken in the United States, although they have been done in Canada, the United Kingdom, and Australia. Results have recently been obtained from multicenter studies or randomized controlled trials for various therapies (Table 18–1).[2, 12, 22]

A higher risk for neurodevelopmental problems exists as birth weight and gestational age decrease. Additional risk factors include the occurrence of neonatal seizures, severe periventricular hemorrhage,[12, 19] periventricular leucomalacia,[3] an oxygen requirement at 36 weeks' postconceptional age, and severe intrauterine or neonatal growth failure with a microcephalic (≤ 2 standard deviations [SD]) head circumference at discharge. Children born to mothers of low educational and socioeconomic status or in poverty demonstrate the additional detrimental effects of the environment. Among term-born children, risk factors for later neurologic sequelae in addition to the above include perinatal asphyxia, neonatal seizures, an abnormal neurologic finding at discharge, and persistent fetal circulation requiring prolonged ventilator treatment or extracorporeal membrane oxygenation (ECMO).[23] Children born with multiple major malformations also constitute a group that generally has a poor developmental outcome (Table 18–2).

Table 18–1. Measures of Very Low-Birth-Weight Outcome

Survival
  To discharge
  After discharge
Medical morbidity
  Rehospitalization
  Chronic lung disease
  Growth failure
Neurodevelopmental outcome
  Motor dysfunction (cerebral palsy)
  Mental retardation
  Seizures
  Vision problems
  Hearing disorder
  Behavior
  School age outcomes
Functional outcomes
  Health or illness
  Activity and skills of daily living
  Ambulation
  Need for technologic aids (gastric tube, oxygen)
  Need for special services
Quality of life
Impact on family
Cost of care

Table 18–2. Factors Affecting Outcomes of the Very Low-Birth-Weight Child

Birth weight <750 g, or <26 weeks' gestation
Periventricular hemorrhage (grade III, IV)
Periventricular leucomalacia
Persistent ventricular dilatation
Neonatal seizures
Chronic lung disease
Neonatal meningitis
Subnormal head circumference
Poverty or parental deprivation

◆ IMPORTANCE OF FOLLOW-UP FOR HIGH-RISK INFANTS

Follow-up clinics should be an integral part of every neonatal ICU. Specialized care of problems of growth, chronic disease, and adaptation is best provided within the setting of such a neonatal follow-up program. This care should initially be provided by the neonatologists themselves and then gradually transferred to a developmental specialist. This initial continuity of care is important to the family, who will find reassurance in the fact that the same people who were responsible for the life-saving decisions are continuing to assume responsibility for the child's adaptation into home life. There is also a moral obligation to maintain this contact. Furthermore, even if the neonatologist does not continue the follow-up for a long period, he or she will benefit greatly by maintaining contact with the nursery graduates and recognizing the sequelae of the early neonatal interventions.

Minor Transient Problems

The first few months after discharge can be considered a period of convalescence for the infant and the parents as well. Many infants have minor problems specifically related to being born preterm, but these may seem major problems to their parents. They include anemia of prematurity, umbilical and inguinal hernias (inguinal hernia is present in 26% of very low-birth-weight males [<1.5 kg]), relatively large dolichocephalic "preemie shaped" heads, and subtle behavioral differences. Most healthy preterm infants are discharged home at 36 to 37 weeks' gestation (or when they weigh 1.9 kg). At this age they tend still to sleep most of the day, waking only for feedings; to feed slowly and not always demonstrate hunger; to be jittery sometimes; and to have "preemie" vocalizations, which include grunts and a relatively high-pitched cry.

Transient Neurologic Abnormality

There is a very high incidence of transient neurologic abnormalities (ranging from 40% to 80%) in preterm infants. These include abnormalities of muscle tone such as hypotonia or hypertonia. They present as poor head control at 40 weeks' corrected age (the expected term date), poor back support at 4 to 8 months, and sometimes a slight increase in tone of the upper extremities. Because there is normally some degree of physiologic hypertonia during the first 3 months, it is difficult to diagnose the early developing spasticity related to cerebral palsy. Initially, children in whom cerebral palsy later develops present with hypotonia (poor head control and back support) and only later with spasticity of the extremities combined with truncal hypotonia. Spasticity during the first 3 to 4 months is a poor indicator of prognosis. Mild hypertonia or hypotonia persisting at 8 months usually resolves by the second year. Persistence of primitive reflexes might be a sign of early cerebral palsy. Major neurologic handicap appears obvious during the first 6 to 8 months after term in about 10% of newborns in the most high-risk categories; however, 90% of high-risk newborns will be or become normal neurologically during the first year.

Neurologic Sequelae

Major neurologic handicap can usually be defined during the latter part of the first year of life or even earlier if severe. Major neurologic handicap is usually classified as cerebral palsy (spastic diplegia, spastic quadriplegia, or spastic hemiplegia or paresis); hydrocephalus (with or without accompanying cerebral palsy or sensory deficits); blindness (usually caused by retinopathy of prematurity); or deafness. The developmental/intellectual outcomes of these children differ according to the neurologic diagnosis. For example, children with spastic quadriplegia usually have severe mental retardation, whereas children with spastic diplegia or hemiplegia may have relatively intact mental functioning. Furthermore, this is not always measurable until after 2 to 3 years of age.

Physical Sequelae and Chronic Disease

Chronic diseases of prematurity, mainly chronic lung disease (bronchopulmonary dysplasia), gradually resolve during infancy. Scars from various neonatal surgery procedures (tracheotomy, thoracocentesis, Broviac lines, shunt procedures) tend also to fade gradually and appear less significant as the children grow. There is, however, a high rate of rehospitalization, especially for those children of extremely low-birth-weight with chronic lung diseases or neurologic sequelae. Fifty percent of children who have chronic lung disease will be hospitalized in the first year after discharge. Many hospitalizations in winter have been associated with respiratory syncytial virus (RSV) infections. Children with neurologic sequelae such as cerebral palsy or hydrocephalus have a higher rate of rehospitalization for shunt complications, orthopedic correction of spasticity, and eye surgery for strabismus.

Physical Growth

Intrauterine and/or neonatal growth retardation is present in up to 50% of very low-birth-weight neonates who receive intensive care and require prolonged hospitalizations. For children born appropriate for gestational age (AGA), poor neonatal growth is related to inadequate nutrition during the acute phase of neonatal disease, to increased caloric requirements related to breathing in chronic lung disease, to poor feeding in neurologically impaired children, and to the lack of parental care or an optimal environment for growth in the nursery. As these conditions gradually resolve and when an optimal home environment is provided, catch-up of body growth may occur during the first 2 to 3 years of life. However, up to 20% of these infants still remain subnormal in weight and height by their third year.

The prognosis for catch-up growth is not as good in children born small for gestational age (SGA). This is because their initial period of growth failure occurred earlier in gestation and extended for a longer time during the critical perinatal period of growth.

Growth attainment after discharge is a very good measure of physical, neurologic, and environmental well-being. To promote optimal catch-up growth of high-risk infants, neonatal nutrition needs to be maximized and sufficient calories provided during the recovery phase. This is especially important because catch-up of head circumference in both AGA and SGA children occurs only during the first 6 to 12 months postterm.

Predictors of poor catch-up growth include severe intrauterine growth failure, severe neonatal complications including chronic lung disease with prolonged ventilator and oxygen dependence, and neurologic impairment such as cerebral palsy. Neurologically impaired children might also fall off in growth after discharge as a result of failure to thrive. The genetic potential as measured by parental height also determines eventual catch-up growth.[5]

The increased calorie formulas providing 22 calories per ounce might enhance growth during the first few months after discharge home; however, there are no reported studies of their longer term effects on growth.

EDITORIAL COMMENT: There is a rapid spurt in growth when a healthy premature infant is discharged home. Daily weight gain may jump from 20 to 30 g in the hospital to as much as 60 to 90 g. A check-up at 7 to 14 days after discharge with measurement of weight gain is useful in the early detection of environmental (nonorganic failure to thrive) or physical problems.

Extremely low-birth-weight children with chronic lung disease who can feed orally are usually discharged home on oxygen when they reach the expected date of delivery or even earlier. These children need close follow-up by pediatric pulmonary specialists or neonatologists with expertise and interest in follow-up care. As the children are gradually weaned from oxygen, close attention needs to be paid to optimizing growth with the use of increased calorie formulas and to gradual weaning of any medications the child might be receiving such as diuretics or antireflux medication. Such children also require RSV immunization in winter.

Most neurologic or physical problems either resolve or become permanent during the first year of life. Clinical follow-up is essential for all high-risk infants during this period. After the first year, new problems that become evident are usually subtle motor, visuomotor, and behavioral difficulties, which are best diagnosed and treated in an educational rather than a medical setting. Furthermore, during the second year of life, the environmental effects of parental education and social class begin to influence the outcome measures.

◆ FOLLOW-UP—WHO, WHAT, HOW, AND WHEN

Infants at highest risk should be observed. These include children who had severe asphyxia complicated by seizures or signs of brain edema, intraventricular or other intracranial hemorrhage, meningitis, or multisystem congenital malformations; those who required assisted ventilation; and those born with very low-birth-weights (especially those weighing <1 kg).

Growth (weight, height, and head circumference), neurologic development, psychomotor development, ophthalmologic status, vision, and hearing should all be examined on a regular basis.

Timing of Follow-up Visit

The initial follow-up visit should be 7 to 10 days after discharge. This is essential to evaluate how the child is adapting to the home environment. This visit usually occurs around the time of the expected date of delivery.

A clinic visit at 4 months' corrected age is important to document problems of inadequate catch-up growth and severe neurologic abnormality that might require intervention or physical therapy.

Eight months' corrected age is a good time to confirm the presence of developing cerebral palsy or other neurologic abnormality. It is also an excellent time for the first developmental assessment (preferably the Bayley Scales of Infant Development) to be performed because the children show very little outward or combative stranger anxiety at this age and are most cooperative. (Some physicians, however, prefer 12 months of age for the first developmental assessment.)

By 18 to 24 months of age, most transient neurologic findings have resolved, and the neurologically abnormal child shows some adaptation to neurologic sequelae. Furthermore, most of the potential catch-up growth has been achieved, and some prediction can be made of the child's ultimate growth attainment. The mental scale of the Bayley Scales provides at this age some assessment of the child's ultimate mental performance. Before 1 year of age, this is not easily measured, in that most of the test is based on motor function.

The Bayley score attained at 8 to 12 months' corrected age tends to decrease by the second year (partly a function of the test and partly because of the increased effect of the environment) and is not of great prognostic significance. However, low scores (<80) are predictive of poor later functioning.

When a child is 3 years of age, a Stanford-Binet IQ test can be performed. This test further validates the child's mental abilities. Language is easily measurable at this age.

From 4 years of age, more subtle neurologic, visuomotor, and behavioral difficulties are measurable. These difficulties affect school performance even in those children who have normal intelligence.[8, 20]

◆ NEUROSENSORY AND DEVELOPMENTAL ASSESSMENT

Neurodevelopmental handicap is usually defined in children suffering from a neurologic abnormality or a developmental quotient or IQ of less than 80. However, some researchers include only a subnormal IQ (<70), whereas others include all children with IQ less than 1 SD from the norm (IQ <84). Neurologic abnormality is usually classified by neurologic diagnosis, which can include hypotonia or hypertonia, cerebral palsy (spastic diplegia or quadriplegia), hydrocephalus, blindness, or deafness.

The neurologic examination during infancy is best based on changes in muscle tone that occur during the first year of life. We use the scale developed by Amiel-Tison.[1] This measures the progressive increase in active muscle tone (head control, back support, sitting, standing, and walking) together with the concomitant decrease in passive muscle tone. Furthermore, it documents visual and auditory responses and some primitive reflexes. This method gives a qualitative assessment of neurologic integrity, which is defined as normal, suspect, or abnormal during the first year. The Amiel-Tison method of evaluation extends into early childhood.[1]

Psychomotor Developmental Tests

Bayley Scales of Infant Development

The Bayley Scales of Infant Development are the recognized standard for measuring infant development and may be used between early infancy and 42 months of age. Separate motor and mental scales each yield a developmental index with a mean of 100. The scales were revised and restandardized in 1993. In the first year, motor skills are weighted heavily, even in the mental scale, but by the second year, cognitive functions, including speech, may be more reliably measured.

In the preschool years and into adolescence, the following tests are often used clinically and for research:

The Stanford-Binet Intelligence Scale is used from age two years into the elementary school years. It provides a measure of intelligence that is highly correlated with school performance.

The Wechsler Scales (WPPSI-R for preschoolers and the WISC-III for ages 6 to 16 years) yield verbal, performance, and full scale scores with means of 100.

The Kaufman Assessment Battery for Children is used between the ages of 3 and 10 years. Like the Stanford-Binet and Wechsler tests, it has a number of subscales to assess various components of intelligence.

The McCarthy Scales of Child Development provide measures of cognitive, perceptual performance, and quantitative abilities in children between ages 2 1/2 and 8 years as well as a composite score (comparable to an IQ) and measures of motor and memory functions. However, this test has not been restandardized since 1972, and it is likely that the norms are outdated.

The Denver Developmental Screening Test is used as a clinical screening tool in the first 6 years. It is not highly sensitive and fails to identify a significant number of at-risk children. Because it is not a quantitative assessment, it cannot be used to document outcome in specific high-risk populations.

Visual Testing

An ophthalmologic examination should be performed on all high-risk children before discharge. Infants younger than 30 to 32 weeks' gestation should have been followed serially in the nursery for signs of developing retinopathy of prematurity. Those who have residual findings at discharge or who have undergone laser or cryotherapy should be followed up with an ophthalmologist until the abnormal findings resolve. All children should have a repeat eye examination between 12 and 24 months of age. Infants of extremely low-birth-weight or gestational age who have had severe retinopathy of prematurity might require correction with glasses during infancy or early childhood.

Hearing

Hearing should be screened before discharge from the neonatal intensive care nursery. Most nurseries use base of brain evoked responses or otoacoustic emissions. Hearing should be reexamined between 12 and 24 months because the most common cause of hearing loss is related to middle ear infections, which occur after the neonatal period and during the first 2 years of life.

◆ EARLY INTERVENTION

Early environmental enrichment with close attention to the family's needs may improve the developmental outcome of normal birth-weight and low-birth-weight infants, especially that of children of deprived homes.[7] Studies of early intervention have shown a decrease in beneficial effects after discontinuation of the intervention. Initial home visits during early childhood by experienced nurses are important for surveillance of the child's growth and medical needs, for education concerning preterm behavior and development, and for support of the mother. Such home visits can gradually be phased out as the mother becomes more confident and, when needed, the child becomes enrolled in an educational enrichment program.

◆ POINTS TO REMEMBER

1. Correct for gestational age (preterm birth) until at least 3 years of age.

Table 18–3. Outcome Variables

	Birthweight (g) 501–800	Gestational Age (Weeks)		
		23	*24*	*25*
Total followed (N)	1000	77	323	554
Severe disability	9–37%	34%	22–45%	12–35%
Cerebral palsy	5–37%		11–15%	3–20%
Subnormal cognitive (MDI <70)	13–47%		14–39%	10–30%
Blindness	2–25%		0–9%	3–10%
Deafness	0–7%			

Adapted from Hack M, Fanaroff AA: Outcomes of children of extremely low birthweight and gestational age in the 1990s. Semin Neonatol 5:89–106, 2000.

2. Do not emphasize to the parents the many abnormalities observed during the 3-month postdischarge period of convalescence because most are transient and have little prognostic significance.

3. Be available, be honest, be optimistic. After the initial abnormal diagnosis is made, most children show improvement, restitution, and growth.

4. The majority of high-risk children do well.

5. In some cases, the diagnosis of cerebral palsy, hydrocephalus, blindness, or cortical atrophy has to be accepted during the first year of life. Early intervention with the child and supportive psychological help that can be facilitated by the follow-up clinic are crucial.

6. Except when a severe neurologic or sensory disorder persists, ultimate development depends on parental education, social class, and environment.

7. The functional capacity attained is more important than the medical diagnosis of abnormality.

EDITORIAL COMMENT: Outcome data for infants surviving at the cusp of viability are very sparse. A summary of some outcome variables is included in Table 18–3. We emphasize the importance of early identification of developmental deficits in order to plan and establish early appropriate interventions. Developmental outcomes of children are influenced by many risk factors including social, genetic, and biologic ones. For children of extremely low birthweight, the neonatal risk factors tend to predominate.[24]

REFERENCES

1. Amiel-Tison C, Grenier A: Neurologic Examination of the Infant and Newborn. New York: Masson Publishers, 1983.
2. Bregman J, Kimberlin LVS: Developmental outcome in extremely premature infants. Impact of surfactant. Pediatr Clin N Am 40:937–953, 1993.
3. Fazzi E, Lanzi G, Gerardo A, et al: Neurodevelopmental outcome in very-low-birth-weight infants with or without periventricular haemorrhage and/or leucomalacia. Acta Pædiatr 81:808–811, 1992.
4. Hack M, Fanaroff AA: Outcomes of children of extremely low birthweight and gestational age in the 1990s. Early Hum Dev 53:193–218, 1999.
5. Hack M, Weissman B, Breslau N, et al: Health of very low birth weight children during their first eight years. J Pediatr 122:887–892, 1993.
6. Hack M, Klein NK, Taylor HG: Long-term developmental outcomes of low birth weight infants. The Future of Children 5:176–196, 1995 [Packard Foundation publication].
7. The Infant Health and Development Program: Enhancing the outcomes of low-birth-weight, premature infants: A multi-site, randomized, trial. JAMA 263:3035, 1990.
8. Klein NK, Hack M, Breslau N, Fanaroff A: Children who were very low birthweight: Development and academic achievement at nine years of age. Dev Behav Pediatr 10:32, 1989.
9. Lee K-S, Kim BI, Khoshnood B, et al: Outcome of very low birth weight infants in industrialized countries: 1947–1987. Am J Epidemiol 141:1188–1193, 1995.
10. Lorenz JM, Wooliever DE, Jetton JR, Paneth N: A quantitative review of mortality and developmental disability in extremely premature newborns. Arch Pediatr Adolesc Med 152:425–435, 1998.
11. McCormick MC, Brooks-Gunn J, Workman-Daniels K, et al: The health and developmental status of very low-birth-weight children at school age. JAMA 267:2204–2208, 1992.
12. Ment LR, Vohr B, Oh W, et al: Neurodevelopmental outcome at 36 months' corrected age of preterm infants in the multicenter indomethacin intraventricular hemorrhage prevention trial. Pediatrics 98:714–718, 1996.
13. Saigal S, Feeny D, Rosenbaum P, et al: Self-perceived health status and health-related quality of life of extremely low-birth-weight infants at adolescence. JAMA 276:453–459, 1996.
14. Soll RF, McQueen MC: Respiratory distress syndrome. In Sinclair JC, Bracken MB, eds: Effective Care of the Newborn Infant. Oxford: Oxford University Press, 1992.
15. Stein REK, Jones JD: Functional status II [R]: A measure of child health status. Med Care 28:1041–1055, 1990.

16. Stein REK, Riessman CK: The development of an Impact-on-Family Scale: Preliminary findings. Med Care 18:465–472, 1980.
17. Stevenson RC, Pharoah POD, Cooke RWI, Sandhu B: Predicting costs and outcomes of neonatal intensive care for very low birthweight infants. Publ Health 105:121–126, 1991.
18. Stevenson DK, Wright LL, Lemons JA, et al: Very low birth weight outcomes of the National Institute of Child Health and Human Development Neonatal Research Network, January 1993 through December 1994. Am J Obstet Gynecol 179:1632–1639, 1998.
19. Stewart A, Kirkbride V: Very preterm infants at fourteen years: Relationship with neonatal ultrasound brain scans and neurodevelopmental status at one year. Acta Paediatr Suppl 416:44–47, 1996.
20. Taylor HG, Hack M, Klein N, Schatschneider C: Achievements in <750 gm birthweight children with normal cognitive abilities: Evidence for specific learning disabilities. J Pediatr Psychol 20:703–719, 1995.
21. US Congress, Office Technology Assessment: Neonatal intensive care for low-birthweight infants: Cost and effectiveness. Health Technology Case Study 38. Washington, DC, US Congress, 1987.
22. Vohr BR, Dusick A, Steichen JJ, et al: Neurodevelopmental and functional outcome of extremely low birth weight [ELBW] infants in the National Institute of Child Health and Human Development Neonatal Research Network, 1993–1994. Pediatrics 105:1216–1226, 2000.
23. Walsh-Sukys MC, Bauer R, Cornell DJ, et al: Severe respiratory failure in neonates: Mortality, morbidity and neurodevelopmental outcome. J Pediatr 125:104, 1994.
24. Hack M, Wilson-Costello D, Friedman H, et al: Neurodevelopment and predictors of <1000 gram birth weight children born 1992–1995. Arch Pediatr Adolesc Med 154:725–731, 2000.

Ethical Issues in the Perinatal Period

Lawrence J. Nelson

Despite great advances in perinatal medicine, not all newborns born alive can stay alive or survive without suffering from severe—perhaps even devastating—physical and mental problems. This is particularly true for extremely low-birth-weight infants (ELBW). In one study, for example, 47% of ELBW infants survived to discharge.[21] Thus, many ELBW infants can and do survive despite being born much too soon, although they not infrequently suffer from significant chronic lung disease,[37] neurologic and cognitive abnormalities such as mental retardation and subnormal intelligence,[27, 28, 37] and secondary morbidities such as necrotizing enterocolitis, poor growth, blindness, and chronic illness.[10, 27]

In at least some of these cases, physicians, nurses, or parents raise questions about whether initial or continued aggressive treatment is ethically correct, who should make these decisions, and what criteria they should use. These questions have been publicly asked and answered in a variety of ways since 1973 when Duff and Campbell acknowledged that they, their neonatal intensive care unit (NICU) staff, and the involved parents allowed some infants to die because of their poor chances of survival or of having a reasonable quality of life.[9] No single "standard of care" exists in this area. One study has shown what clinical experience and common sense posit: physicians' practices regarding the use or withholding of resuscitative therapy in the NICU is not consistent.[20]

This chapter explores some answers to these enduring and fundamental questions by presenting and commenting upon a recent case. In doing so, I consider the most pressing questions and dominant myths about forgoing treatment of newborns and briefly explain why the myths should be discarded by ethical and humane practitioners of neonatal medicine. These myths deserve attention because they are both widely held and dangerous to the interests of infants, parents, and medicine. Unnecessary legalism, improper disenfranchisement of parents, simplistic reliance on a single popular standard of questionable meaning, and rejection of quality of life considerations are still the deepest and most insidious traps into which physicians and nurses caring for newborns fall.

◆ THE CASE*

Mark and Karla Miller filed a negligence lawsuit against a hospital, Women's Hospital of Texas, and the company that owns the hospital, Columbia/HCA Healthcare Corporation, following the premature birth of their daughter, Sydney. She was born at 22 weeks' gestation and weighed 1.5 pounds. The parents claimed that the hospital had "callously ignored the couple's request not to artificially prolong the child's life at birth" and that resuscitating such an underdeveloped baby amounted to "medical experimentation on humans." They also accused the hospital of being motivated to impose treatment in order to collect the large revenues that would thereby be generated.

Mrs. Miller had developed an infection "of the sac holding her fetus," which had spread, and she was hospitalized. "With her own life in potential danger, she and her husband agreed with the doctor to induce

---

*This case report is based entirely upon four articles published in the *Houston Chronicle*, on January 6, 1998 (Section A, page 9), January 17, 1998 (Section A, page 1), January 31, 1998 (Section A, page 29), and April 18, 1998 (Section A, page 36). All direct quotes are taken from these articles. The accuracy and comprehensiveness of this information has to be considered in this context. None of the articles discussed why the attending physicians were not named as defendants in the suit.

labor." They were notified about the "uncertain odds of survival in such a young pregnancy" and the "baby's unlikely prospects for survival so early in pregnancy." After "much agonizing," they decided to have the baby delivered [following induction] but "to let nature take its course." According to the parents' lawyer, they saw it as "God's will" if the newborn had "not developed to the extent that it could survive without artificial means"; they wanted no "special heroics" performed. The parents claimed they had repeatedly requested that doctors not resuscitate the newborn if she had not developed adequately to sustain life on her own.

The hospital administrator of the NICU allegedly told the father that "it was against hospital policy to refuse resuscitation efforts no matter what," but could not produce a written policy to this effect. She also allegedly informed the father that "his only option would be to take his wife to another hospital, which he could not risk because of her condition." When the father said he would be in the delivery room and would stop physicians from performing resuscitation, this administrator said police would be called to remove him from the premises.

The hospital disputed the parents' version of the facts and claimed it had an ethical and legal obligation to keep the baby alive. It denied that treatment decisions were related to financial considerations, that its administrator had made any threats or statement to the father as he had alleged, and that it had any responsibility for medical decisions that were made by the physicians and family involved. It claimed that the attending physicians had drafted a "birth plan" with the parents' full consent and produced several consent forms signed by the father for medical services.

Furthermore, the father allegedly never questioned the physician's actions to keep the child alive either in the delivery room or later. The hospital also asserted that the physicians honored the parents' decision not to restart the child's heart if she went into arrest. However, she had a heartbeat when born, although her "lungs and other vital organs" were not working at birth, and received vigorous treatment.

Sydney was born with her eyes fused shut and is legally blind at age 7. She remained hospitalized for nearly a year at a cost of about $1 million. She is severely brain damaged and requires extensive care, because

she is almost totally incapacitated. Her mother ended her career as an equities fund broker to care for her daughter full-time because the family could not afford the $200,000 annual cost of professional care.

Eleven days after the start of the trial and after 2 days of deliberations, the jury returned $42.9 million verdict against the hospital and Columbia/HCA by a vote of 10 to 2: $29.4 million for the costs of the child's past and future medical care and $13.5 million in punitive damages. Pretrial interest of $22.4 million on the damages awarded made the total verdict worth $65.3 million. The parents' lawyer stated that the key issue was "who will make the basic medical decisions—families or medical specialists who do not have to live with the consequences." One juror reported that he and other jurors believed the Millers rather than the hospital and that there was evidence that indicated "arrogance" on the part of the hospital and Columbia/HCA.

Defense witnesses had testified that the care delivered to both the mother and infant met the applicable standard of care and that the "newborn's condition was adequate enough to require them to try to sustain life." These witnesses also stated that denying "proper care could subject the doctors to penalties and sanctions, or even suit alleging negligence."

The trial court judge approved the verdict in its entirety, and the hospital and Columbia/HCA are appealing. The defendants will be liable for the standard 10% interest on the judgment while the case is being appealed.

Several months later, the trial court denied three motions to alter the verdict: one was to reverse the verdict in its entirety, the second was to lower the amount of money damages, and the third was to grant a new trial. The defendants' lawyer argued that allowing the verdict to stand would "condone discrimination against handicapped children by giving judicial approval of withholding treatment." The parents' lawyer argued that legal precedent allows "doctors and hospitals to be sued for care of handicapped children if the parents were misled before birth."

◆ **Is there a legal and ethical obligation to resuscitate all newborns and continue providing treatment until a child is imminently dying?**

Some, perhaps many, physicians and nurses believe that no choice exists but to resuscitate every newborn infant in the delivery room, no matter how small, and continue aggressive medical treatment in the NICU until he or she is headed inevitably and imminently toward death. Once the infant has "declared herself" to be close to death despite aggressive medical management, then and only then can physicians and parents choose to withhold or withdraw life-sustaining treatment.

First, it is incorrect to claim either that all infants are in fact resuscitated at birth or that the standard of care requires that they be resuscitated. In one study of delivery room resuscitation decisions and mortality for infants born at 23 to 26 weeks, 32% were not resuscitated with intubation or cardiopulmonary resuscitation (CPR) at delivery.[7] Other articles in the medical literature support the position that resuscitation in the delivery room is not professionally and ethically required in all cases.[4, 15]

Second, it is false to claim on the merits that a strict ethical and legal obligation exists to resuscitate each and every newborn regardless of his or her condition, prognosis, or parental desires about resuscitation. For example, if prenatal testing and ultrasound had unambiguously detected anencephaly, the parents had given their informed consent to nontreatment, and this condition was clearly present at birth, no obligation to resuscitate such an infant would exist because of his or her permanent unconsciousness, the nature of the anomaly as incompatible with biological and biographical life, and the reasonableness of the parents' desire to avoid prolonging the dying of an unconscious and doomed child.

In other words, there may be cases in which enough can be known about a child's diagnosis and prognosis before birth that a parental decision to refuse resuscitation is morally justified and within the bounds of parental discretion. Such cases are likely to involve an infant with one of the following three diagnoses: severe congenital anomalies, ELBW, and severe perinatal asphyxia.[15]

On the other hand, an extremely premature child can be born alive with no prenatal indication of any specific anomaly or disease, and his or her medical condition and prognosis might be so uncertain that the attending physicians cannot honestly assess the particular child's prospects for survival and outcome at birth. In this situation or a similar one, the physicians and nurses could

legitimately conclude that they were under an ethical obligation to resuscitate the child initially because of legitimate uncertainty about his or her true diagnosis and prognosis. If this is the case, however, they would also be obligated promptly to ascertain more accurately the particular child's medical condition and the prospects for a life not characterized by excessive pain, burdensome interventions, or inability to consciously interact with others.

From this point of view, the absence of reasonably accurate medical information at birth needed to ground the value judgment that must inevitably be made about forgoing treatment renders a parental decision against initial resuscitation uninformed, poorly (if at all) justified, and not prima facie morally binding on the health care providers. Even assuming the validity of this rationale, it still remains true that after more clinical information has been gathered and more deliberation has occurred, the physicians, nurses, and hospital should then respect parental decisions to forgo further treatment in appropriate cases.

The facts of the Miller case as presented herein make it very difficult to determine precisely what the parents were told about their child's likely condition and prospects if born at 22 weeks' gestation and weighing 1.5 lb. The case report makes reference to a "birth plan" agreed to by parents and providers alike, but both its management content and medical and ethical rationale are unknown. Moreover, the parents' informed consent to this "birth plan" is suspect in light of their claim that they were "misled before birth" by the physicians or hospital about their child's situation.

The case report also makes no mention whatsoever of what the attending physicians and nurses (or, for that matter, the hospital representative) told the Millers about their ethical position on the propriety of not resuscitating in the delivery room or on stopping treatment at some point after resuscitation. The health care providers should have disclosed their interpretation of the medical facts known about this individual child's condition and prospects, as well as the values or principles that would govern their decision whether to honor a parental refusal of treatment.

To be sure, a child born at 22 weeks and at an estimated weight of 1.5 lb. would generally be expected to have "uncertain" or "unlikely" odds of survival. Nevertheless, a substantial ethical argument exists that the child's best interests are best advanced by making an irrevocable decision not to treat and maintain the child's life *only after* both a careful and honest medical assessment is made of the particular child's postbirth condition and after time for careful reflection and moral deliberation by everyone involved has passed—time for parents, physicians, nurses, and hospital alike. Human moral responsibility for respecting the life of every person is generally incompatible with precipitously made decisions that use incomplete or inaccurate facts, or ill-founded medical generalizations. With one study showing that 80% of ELBW infant deaths occur within the first 3 days of life and that the survival rate of those who live until day 4 is 81%, waiting a few days to reflect on forgoing treatment may generate more clinical information and greater predictability about the child's diagnosis and prognosis.[21]

Whatever the merits of this brief moral analysis, it is a myth that the *law* requires all infants to receive aggressive resuscitation and treatment until they are imminently dying. The ultimate source of this myth is the so-called "Baby Doe" law, the Child Abuse Amendments of 1984.[35] These amendments to the Child Abuse Prevention and Treatment Act and the implementing regulations issued by the Department of Health and Human Services (DHHS)[6] constitute the Baby Doe law that is in effect in the United States. This law requires a state to establish certain procedures for reporting alleged instances of "medical neglect," including the withholding of "medically indicated treatment," to local child protective services authorities and for the investigation of such reports—*if* the state wishes to receive federal child abuse prevention grants. On their face, the DHHS regulations permit treatment to be forgone only in very limited circumstances.

Many physicians are under the impression that the Baby Doe law directly imposes on them certain duties to care for newborns and that they will suffer federal penalties if they fail to do so. However, this impression is *mistaken*. The Baby Doe law does *not* apply directly to physicians or parents of critically ill newborns; it only requires states receiving federal funds to do certain things. In particular, this law does *not* create federally mandated standards of medical care for newborns, nor does it directly limit the discretion that parents would otherwise have under state law when deciding about treatment of their child.[25]

Contrary to some claims,[22] the Baby Doe law *does not authorize* any civil or criminal penalties against physicians, hospitals, or parents who are involved in forgoing treatment of a severely ill newborn. Such penalties could be imposed under state law, but there is not a single reported appellate court case in any state upholding any penalty against a physician or nurse for withholding or withdrawing treatment from a newborn with parental consent. If the Baby Doe law strictly forbade forgoing treatment and was being enforced vigorously, surely there would be some reported examples of its enforcement since the law has been in effect—but none exist. Interestingly, defense witnesses in the Miller case claimed that the physicians would have been subject to legal penalties and sanctions if they denied the child "proper care." But this claim, of course, begs the ethical and legal question: Was the care they allegedly imposed on this child and her parents ethically and legally mandatory regardless of the parents' wishes?

The obligation of individual medical professionals to report instances of child abuse or neglect, including medical neglect, arises out of the law of an individual state, not the federal Baby Doe law.[31] The substantive legal standards applicable to a determination of whether a particular decision by a physician and parents to forgo life-sustaining treatment of a newborn is unacceptable are established by state law, not the Baby Doe law.[25, 32]

State law typically does not contain explicit or detailed standards for determining when treatment is being improperly withheld or withdrawn from a child. California, for example, requires physicians and other licensed providers to report as child neglect parental refusals of "adequate medical care," but not when the parents have made an "informed and appropriate medical decision" after consulting with a physician who has actually examined the child.[3] Because there is no statutory definition of "informed and appropriate medical decision," the practical meaning of the term is left to clinicians who must decide whether an "inappropriate" medical decision has been made and consequently whether they are going to make a report to child protective services.

It is wrong to claim that the Baby Doe law or most state laws expressly require very aggressive treatment of all newborns until death is close at hand. Many commentators have concluded that the law regarding the treatment of newborns is fundamentally the same currently as it was before the Baby Doe law was enacted.[11, 16, 23] Weil[38] rightly points out that the Baby Doe law "does not mandate that every disabled infant be treated. It does not prescribe how any child should be treated. It does not place government persons in the role of medical decision makers. It does not allow physicians to treat infants without the consent of parents." He argues that if physicians opt for the "safe" response to the Baby Doe law and treat every infant aggressively, then "that is a course of their own choosing and not one imposed upon them by the government."

Perhaps more important, evidence exists that the Baby Doe law as understood by many physicians is generating significant harm as a result of overtreatment of children whose chances of survival and even minimal human interaction are dismal. One influential study has shown that between 23% and 33% of the pediatricians surveyed agreed that they practiced differently as a result of the Baby Doe law and that many of them agreed that infants with very poor chances for survival were being overtreated in neonatal intensive care units.[17] This response appears to be consistent across the nation and even in states where the Baby Doe law is not in operation. Reports issued by the Inspector General of the DHHS suggest that the law has exerted pressure toward overly aggressive treatment.[18, 19]

One veteran clinician believes that the Baby Doe law "is usually taken as a mandate to rescue many infants by the application of available technology, even though families and their health and other advisors often hold that quality of life and other considerations, including staggering costs and low benefits, clearly support a different choice." He accuses an influential portion of the medical profession of helping the federal government to create "a law, which, chiefly on ideological or biological grounds, often mandates treatment that careful reflection by those most intimately involved finds is inappropriate."[8]

It is possible that the Millers wanted no "special heroics" (a vague and ambiguous phrase that always needs specific interpretation and explanation) even at birth because they were afraid that once the physicians started to treat, they would refuse to stop until the child was literally a few minutes or hours from death. This fear is not unwarranted in light of the myth of the legal requirement for treatment and the failure of physicians and hospitals to honestly disclose their policies about stopping treatment. The Miller case demonstrates a lack of clarity, or perhaps outright dishonesty, on this point of institutional and medical policy. Other cases demonstrate it as well.[24]

Consequently, the most invidious effect of the mandatory treatment myth surrounding the Baby Doe law appears to be how it has replaced careful attention to the humane and compassionate treatment of disabled and severely ill newborns with preoccupation about abstract legal formulas and fears of remote possibilities of legal liability. Insofar as their misinterpretation of the Baby Doe law has led physicians to overtreat infants with very poor prognoses and thereby cause them (and others) suffering with no corresponding benefit, or to disenfranchise parents from giving informed consent to the treatment of their infants because "the law" has made the decision for them, we all have been done a profound disservice, most especially the infants who are supposed to be the ones served by the physicians who care for them.

◆ Should physicians or hospitals, rather than parents, make decisions to forgo resuscitation or treatment of an extremely low-birth-weight newborn?

In my clinical experience, parents of severely ill newborns are frequently disenfranchised, in whole or in part, from participating in the decisions pertaining to their child's medical treatment. There are a number of reasons for this phenomenon. First, as discussed earlier, physicians are intimidated by what they often misunderstand to be the legal restrictions on forgoing treatment of a newborn. In fairness, they also are probably genuinely puzzled about the ethics of the matter. As a result, though, they have serious trouble identifying the legal and ethical boundaries of medical and parental discretion in deciding to let a newborn die by forgoing life-sustaining treatment.[24] Peremptorily ignoring parental requests to consider forgoing treatment or adopting a policy of never forgoing treatment before a child's death is inevitable and imminent eliminates the need to confront and practically resolve the underlying ethical issue.[34]

Second, at least some physicians simply consider themselves to be best qualified and solely responsible for determining the medical fate of their infant patients.

Third, many physicians and nurses assume that parents of severely ill newborns are so influenced by anxiety, grief, and guilt that they could not possibly make good decisions about their child's fate. They may even distrust the motives and character of any parent who wants anything other than full, aggressive treatment. Finally, physicians and nurses commonly experience serious difficulty both coping with the inherent uncertainty of their diagnoses and prognoses and trying to explain this to parents.

Whatever its causes, routine disqualification of parents from participating in the medical treatment plans for their newborns is wrong. Parents have rather broad legal and moral authority to give or withhold their consent to treatment of their children, although this authority is certainly *not* unlimited. The President's Commission for the Study of Ethical Problems in Medicine rightly notes that there is a "presumption, strong but rebuttable, that parents are the appropriate decision-makers for their infants. Traditional law concerning the family, buttressed by the emerging constitutional right of privacy, protects a substantial range of discretion for parents."[29] The US Supreme Court has approved of the statement that the "decision to provide or withhold medically indicated treatment is, except in highly unusual circumstances, made by the parents or legal guardian."[36]

Parents have unique natural bonds of love for and loyalty to a child. The child is their flesh and blood and exists in a family they have created. Of course, not all parents treat their children properly, and they can make unacceptably bad decisions about treatment in some cases. Nevertheless, in the absence of strong evidence to the contrary, we must assume that the parents are the proper decision makers. Furthermore, there is no assurance that strangers—be they physicians, nurses, judges, or lawyers—who have no bonds of love or loyalty to a child will make a better decision about treatment than the parents.[24]

Assuming it is true that the Millers had repeatedly requested that physicians not resuscitate their child if she had not developed adequately to sustain her own life and that the hospital (and presumably the attending physicians and nurses as well) "callously disregarded the couple's request," then the health care providers improperly ignored the parents' presumptive moral and legal authority to make medical decisions for their child. Even if the providers conscientiously disagreed with the parents, they have the obligation to express the factual and moral grounds for their disagreement clearly and plainly. More important, they are obliged to disclose whether and under what circumstances they will honor parental decisions to refuse treatment. The jury's verdict in the Miller case (whether upheld on appeal or not) should serve as a stern warning to physicians, nurses, and hospitals that ignoring parental wishes, particularly in an arrogant and peremptory manner, does not sit well with the public and may carry serious legal consequences.

None of this is to imply that physicians, nurses, and other clinicians have no role in determining the course of medical treatment for a newborn. To the contrary, the attending clinicians must be involved: they, together with the child's parents, should be deciding how best to care for a severely ill newborn. Clinicians are not just the tools of the parents' wishes; they are moral agents who bear responsibility for the child as well. Clinicians should provide parents with honest and accurate disclosure of both the child's medical diagnosis and prognosis (with any attendant uncertainty) and their own carefully thought out recommendation for a plan of action in light of relevant ethical, medical, and legal considerations. But they may not simply ignore the parents. The jury's verdict in the Miller case shows that members of the public will not automatically defer to the clinicians or hospital and permit them to act arrogantly toward parents who do, quite literally, have to live with the consequences of all the medical decisions that are made on behalf of their children.

Assuming, then, that decisions to forgo treatment of severely ill newborns ought to be in the hands of the attending clinicians *and* of the child's parents—and *not* the law except in very rare cases—there remains the question of what standards should be used to make such decisions.

◆ *Is the "best interests of the child" the only standard that should be used in making decisions to forgo treatment or newborns, and does it have a clear and generally accepted meaning?*

The "best interests of the child" constitutes the single most popular principle brought to bear on the controversial subject of forgoing life-sustaining treatment of a child. Many commentators agree that the infant's best interests is the *sole* ethical criterion upon which to base an ethically defensible decision, although these same people disagree on unavoidably related subjects such as which infants should be treated, which conditions count as exceptions to the general duty to preserve life, and whether parents, physicians, and/or ethics committees ought to have a major role in the decision.[13, 29, 39]

While noting how this standard possesses a "remarkable vogue in medical ethics," Brody[2] has seriously questioned its coherence and adequacy as a substantive ethical principle. He perceives the best interests standard as trying not only to make a very complex matter simple, but also magically to avoid abuse of parental discretion in deciding against treatment (as occurred in the original Baby Doe of Bloomington case). Brody sees decisions to forgo treatment of newborns as inherently complex in light of (1) the near impossibility of having a reliable prognosis, (2) the medical and social differences between newborns and adults, (3) the difficulty predicting which medical interventions will help and which will hurt the child, and (4) the vast differences among families in adapting to the substantial changes that must occur in the life of a family with a severely ill newborn. His insightful analysis of the best interests standard deserves careful consideration.

Among other things, Brody's criticism of the best interests standard rests upon the following factors: (1) an infant's interests are unknowable, (2) the best interests standard can yield results that seem inhumane, and (3) the interests of persons other than the infant deserve consideration at least in certain circumstances.

With respect to the first factor, Brody argues that once we move beyond basic needs such as food and shelter, we cannot really know what is in someone's interests without knowing a good deal about that person's individual plans and desires about life. But a newborn has no such plans or desires. He offers the example of two neonatologists arguing over how aggressively to treat an infant born with a high meningomyelocele and hydrocephalus. One argues the infant's best interests are served by early surgical intervention, noting the high probability of death or life with worse retardation without surgery. She cites the occasional success story of another infant with an equally severe defect who turned out to have only mild retardation and physical impairment. The other argues that an early death is in the infant's best interests and points to the very high odds of major mental and physical handicap, plus the need for repeated, painful surgeries to treat the condition and its sequelae. Brody correctly points out that what these physicians are really arguing about is what *they* think ought to be done. The phrase "the infant's best interests" is a rhetorical flourish that does no useful work in the discussion.

Second, the best interests standard can yield inhumane or unjust results because it implies that whenever the benefits of treatment outweigh burdens even to a slight degree, that fact alone fixes an obligation to treat—even if the burdens are minuscule or the burdens horrendous. He cites the case of children so severely retarded as to be unable to recognize other people or form any human relationship, who can perceive only primitive sensations such as light and color, but show no sign of suffering. Because such children get some primitive pleasure out of living and suffer little, a best interests analysis would require that any newborn with such a future should have its life prolonged, even by invasive or aggressive means.[1] Brody[2] claims that to save a child in order to let it live such a life "may well do nothing of real, substantial benefit for the child; and to use expensive resources to save it may well [unjustly] squander those resources."

Finally, Brody agrees with Strong[33] that the refusal to consider any interests other than the infant's own is an arbitrary rather than a principled ethical choice, although this refusal is required by the best interests standard. In the many cases in which treatment will result in clear and substantial benefits to the infant, then its interests override those of others. However, in other cases in which the benefit to the infant is lesser or more questionable, then the interests of the family ought to be factored into the decision. Similarly, given the increasing scarcity of health care resources and the requirements of justice to others, it may be that the interest of an individual child may have to give way to the interests of society and its members. For example, although some individual newborns might benefit somewhat from it, society may be justified in refusing to reimburse hospitals for the use of a new, high-tech machine for maintaining extreme premature infants because it benefits too few while costing society too much.

In summary, despite its popularity and frequent invocation, the best interests standard as traditionally understood is not necessarily either the best or the most intelligible one to use in making decisions to forgo treatment of newborns. Physicians, other clinicians, and parents should be using a complex set of factors when making decisions about newborns, and should be careful in concluding just what the "best interests of the infant" may mean in any given case. One provocative and useful set of such factors is mentioned here. Rhoden[30] posits that aggressive treatment is not mandatory if an infant (1) is in the process of dying, (2) will never be conscious, (3) will suffer unremitting pain, (4) can live only with major, highly restrictive technology that is intended to be temporary (e.g., mechanical ventilation), (5) cannot live past infancy, or (6) lacks potential for human interaction as a result of profound retardation.

◆ Is the present and future quality of an infant's life relevant to a decision to forgo resuscitation or life-sustaining treatment of a premature or seriously ill newborn?

It is a myth that an infant's quality of life is utterly irrelevant to a decision to forgo treatment, although this claim is false only in its extreme form. The appeal to quality of life can be both false and pernicious when it is made in a manner that sanctions nontreatment of children who are only mildly physically or intellectually impaired, or when it is taken to mean that the simple presence of physical disability or mental retardation is a sufficient reason to deny treatment. Denying medically needed treatment to a child *simply* because he has Down syndrome or some form of spina bifida *is* a misuse of quality of life as an ethically proper consideration in forgoing treatment.

The alleged complete irrelevance of quality of life considerations is false, and more-over potentially inhumane, when it is taken to mean that the life expectancy of a child, his or her level of physical and intellectual functioning, and the relative burdens and benefits of treatment make no difference whatsoever when parents and clinicians decide to intervene medically. The irrelevance of quality of life is typically embedded in the application of a "medical benefit" standard, which holds that medical intervention must occur when it is likely, in the exercise of reasonable medical judgment, to bring about its intended medical result. The use of such a medical benefit standard not only blindly falls into the trap of the technologic imperative (whatever can be done, should be done), but also denies that medicine is an enterprise devoted to being of benefit to an individual person whose life in the world cannot be reduced to the technical "success" of an operation, a medicine, or a machine. "To adequately assess benefit, the nature of the life being preserved cannot be ignored."[30] Put differently, people are not meant to be the passive objects of medical technology.

Consider the generally accepted view that newborns with anencephaly should not receive any life-prolonging treatment other than basic supportive care. This view is usually justified on the basis that children lacking a cerebral cortex are irretrievably dying and should not have their agony prolonged. However, on closer analysis, this justification is flawed in several ways. First, while it is true that such infants cannot live indefinitely, it is not true that their deaths are necessarily imminent. Most anencephalics die *quickly* precisely because they do not receive any treatment, which is a human choice rather than a fact of nature. In fact, at least one anencephalic has lived for 4.5 years.[12, 14] Thus, if we choose to, we could keep at least some of these infants alive for quite some time.

Second, because anencephalics are permanently unconscious, they experience neither agony nor pain nor anything else during their lives.[5] Deciding not to treat them aggressively does not truly spare them any unpleasantness (although it may spare parents, nurses, and physicians terrible pain and frustration). More honestly put, it is ethically proper not to resuscitate and treat such newborns aggressively precisely because they have no ability to survive indefinitely and no capability of experiencing even primitive human interaction. In other words, they have an unacceptably poor quality of life.

Paradoxically, the Baby Doe law and its implementing regulations contain an *express* condemnation of quality of life considerations and yet also contain two exceptions to the general duty to preserve an infant's life, which rest upon quality of life. The first exception approves of forgoing treatment when the infant is "chronically and irreversibly comatose." Because some of these infants could live indefinitely and the exception does not depend upon their imminent demise, the only justification left for not treating them is their poor quality of life: unconscious infants have no potential for human life as we understand it, and thus there is no ethical obligation to prolong their lives. "With no cognitive capacity, these infants are alive in only the most minimal sense possible: they have nothing more than cardiac, respiratory, and excretory functions."[30]

The second exception encompasses treatment that would be "virtually futile in terms of the survival of the infant and the treatment itself under such circumstances would be inhumane." Thus, treatment can be withheld because the infant's quality of life would be seriously compromised by the pain and burden of intervention and the lack of compensating benefit. At bottom, medical procedures are "inhumane" and contraindicated only because of certain features pertaining directly to the infant's quality of life.

In summary, quality of life should be a factor in decisions to forgo treatment fundamentally because the very purpose of medicine is to benefit persons. Benefit to persons "must be defined in terms of the whole person, and not merely in terms of isolated organ systems or purely biological responses."[30] Virtually all medical interventions have some risk attached: pain, side effects, complications, even death. The first principle of medical ethics—above all, be useful, or at least do no harm—requires that the potential harm of an intervention be prudently balanced by a countervailing benefit.[26] Perhaps most important, to be the possible subject of benefit, a patient must have the potential for partaking in human relationships. While life must hold at least some potential for interaction with others for it to be truly human, this potential does not have

to be that for normal or near normal intelligence.

We need to recognize that we should neither avoid quality of life judgments nor act as if medicine can always preserve a life worth living. Quality of life is not an inherently dirty or discriminatory concept, although it does contain potential danger. But this is true of medicine itself: it can do great good, but it can also cause bitter suffering and loss. We should not abandon medicine because its results are not always happy. We should not abandon the search for figuring out what quality of life means in the life of a newborn because this meaning is often elusive.

REFERENCES

1. Arras JD: Toward an ethic of ambiguity. Hastings Cent Rep 14:25–33, 1984.
2. Brody H: In the best interests of.... Hastings Cent Rep 18:37–39, 1988.
3. California Penal Code §11165.2(a) and (b) (Supp 1991).
4. Campbell AG, McHaffie HE: Prolonging life and allowing death: Infants. J Med Ethics 22:339–344, 1995.
5. Cranford R: The persistent vegetative state. Hastings Cent Rep 18:27–32, 1988.
6. Department of Health and Human Services: Child abuse and neglect prevention and treatment program. Fed Reg 50:14878–14901, 1985.
7. Doran MW, et al: Delivery room resuscitation decisions for extremely premature infants. Pediatrics 102(3 Pt 1):574–582, 1998.
8. Duff RS: "Close-up" versus "distant" ethics: deciding the care of infants with poor prognosis. Semin Perinatol 11:244–253, 1987.
9. Duff RS, Campbell AGM: Moral and ethical dilemmas in the special care nursery. N Engl J Med 289:890–894, 1973.
10. Dusick A, et al: Factors affecting growth outcome at 18 months in extremely low birth weight infants. Ped Res 43:213A, 1998.
11. Elias S, Annas GJ: Reproductive Genetics and the Law. Chicago: Year Book, 1987.
12. Flannery EJ: One advocate's viewpoint: Conflicts and tensions in the baby K case. J Law Med Ethics 23:7–12, 1995.
13. Fost N: Counseling families who have a child with a severe congenital anomaly. Pediatrics 67:321–324, 1981.
14. Glover JJ, Rushton CH: From baby Doe to baby K: Evolving challenges in pediatric ethics. J Law Med Ethics 23:5–6, 1995.
15. Goldsmith JP, et al: Ethical decision in the delivery room. Clin Perinatol 23:529–550, 1996.
16. Gustaitis R: Right to refuse life-sustaining treatment. Pediatrics 81:317–321, 1988.
17. Kopelman LM, Irons TG, Kopelman AE: Neonatologists judge the "baby Doe" regulations. N Engl J Med 318:677–683, 1988.
18. Kusserow RP: Infant Care Review Committees Un-

der the Baby Doe Program, US Department of Health and Human Services publication no. OAI-03-87-0042. Washington, DC: Government Printing Office, September 1987.

19. Kusserow RP: Survey of State Baby Doe Programs, US Department of Health and Human Services publication no. OAI-03-87-0018. Washington, DC: Government Printing Office, September 1987.

20. Lantos JD, et al: Providing and forgoing resuscitative therapy for babies of very low birth weight. J Clin Ethics 3:283–287, 1992.

21. Meadow W, et al: Birth weight-specific mortality for extremely low birth weight infants vanishes by four days of life. Pediatrics 97:636–643, 1996.

22. Moskop JC, Saldanha RL: The baby Doe rule: Still a threat. Hastings Cent Rep 16:8–14, 1986.

23. Murray TH: The final, anticlimactic rule of baby Doe. Hastings Cent Rep 15:5–9, 1985.

24. Nelson LJ: And the truth shall set you free: The case of baby boy Cory. In Culver C, ed: Ethics at the Bedside 40–70. Hanover, NH: University Press of New England, 1990.

25. Nelson LJ: Perinatology/neonatology and the law: Looking beyond baby Doe. In Klaus M, Fanaroff A, eds: 1988 Year Book of Perinatal/Neonatal Medicine 5–10. Chicago: Year Book, 1988.

26. Nelson LJ: Primum utilis esse: The primacy of usefulness on medicine. Yale J Biol Med 51:322–29, 1978.

27. Pena IC, et al: The neurodevelopmental outcome of the extremely low birth weight infant remains precarious in the 1990s. Pediatr Res 34:275A, 1996.

28. Piecuch RE, et al: Outcome of infants born at 24–26 weeks' gestation: II. Neurodevelopmental outcome. Obstet Gynecol 90:809–814, 1997.

29. President's Commission for the Study of Ethical Problems in Medicine and Biomedical and Behavioral Research: Deciding to Forgo Life-Sustaining Treatment. Washington, DC: US Government Printing Office, 1983.

30. Rhoden NK: Treatment dilemmas for imperiled newborns: Why quality of life counts. South Cal Law Rev 58:1283–1347, 1985.

31. Smith SR: Disabled newborns and the federal child abuse amendments: Tenuous protection. Hastings Law J 37:765–825, 1986.

32. Illinois Statutes §325–513 (2000).

33. Strong C: Defective infants and their impact on families: Ethical and legal considerations. Law Med Health Care 11:168–181, 1983.

34. Torasse U: Keeping extremely early newborns alive tests emotions, ethics. San Francisco Examiner 2:A1, 1999.

35. US Child Abuse Prevention and Treatment Amendments of 1984, Public Law 98–457.

36. United States Supreme Court. Bowen v. American Hospital Association, 106 S.Ct. 2101, 1986.

37. Vohr BR, et al: Survival and outcome characteristics of VLBW infants <750 g born in the 1990s. Pediatr Res 41:213A, 1997.

38. Weil WB: The baby Doe regulations: Another view of change. Hastings Cent Rep 16:12–13, 1986.

39. Weir RF: Selective Nontreatment of Handicapped Newborns. New York: Oxford University Press, 1984.

Appendices

Drugs Used for Emergency and Cardiac Indications in Newborns

Ricardo J. Rodriguez

Agent	Dosage	Comments
Adenosine (Adenocard)	IV (rapid push) starting dose 50 µg/kg. Increase every 2 minutes if no response; max dose 250 µg/kg.	Facial flushing and irritability may occur. Apnea in a premature baby has been reported. Preferably use 12-lead ECG monitoring during administration.
Atropine	IV (rapid push) or SC: 0.01–0.03 mg/kg; max 0.04 mg/kg. May be given via endotracheal tube.	Low doses may result in paradoxical bradycardia.
Calcium chloride 10% (27 mg Ca²⁺/mL)	IV (over 10 minutes): 0.15–0.3 mL/kg up to 1 mL/kg.	Dilute 1:1 with normal saline to reduce osmolality. Monitor HR during administration. Extravasation may lead to tissue necrosis.
Calcium gluconate 10% (9 mg Ca²⁺/mL)	Emergency dose IV (over 10 min): 1–4 mL/kg/dose; up to 5 mL in premature infants and 10 mL in term babies. Maintenance PO or IV fluids: 30–80 mg/kg/d of elemental calcium (3.3–9 mL/kg/d), diluted and divided q 4 h.	
Digoxin	Total digitalizing dose (TDD): divided into three doses, given q 8 h or q 6 h IV (over 15 minutes): Premature infants (1000–1499 g): 15–23 µg/kg. Premature infants (1500–2500 g): 23–30 µg/kg. Term newborns: 45 µg/kg Term infants (older than 1 month): 60 µg/kg. PO or IM: TDD is increased by one third. Daily maintenance dose: PO, IM, or IV: one fourth of TDD divided q 12 h.	Serum levels by radioimmunoassay are not useful in neonates (interference by endogenous digoxin-like substances). Avoid hypokalemia, hypocalcemia.
Dobutamine	IV (continuous infusion): 2–50 µg/kg/min.	Tachycardia may occur.
Dopamine	IV constant infusion: 2–20 µg/kg/min. "Renal dose": 0.5–3.0 µg/kg/min. Cardiotonic: 3–8 µg/kg/min. Vasopressor: >8 µg/kg/min.	Pharmacologic effect is dose dependent. Extravasation may lead to necrosis; phentolamine (Regitine) infiltration is an antidote.
Epinephrine	IV or ET: 0.1–0.3 mL/kg (0.01–0.03 mg/kg) or 1:10,000 solution. IV (continuous infusion): 0.05–1 µg/kg/min.	Follow ET dose with 1 mL of NS.
Hydralazine (Apresoline)	IV or IM: 0.15 mg/kg every 6 h; increase by 0.1 mg/kg every 6 h prn. Dose not to exceed 2 mg/kg/dose. PO: 0.7 mg/kg/d in divided doses of twice the effective IV dose.	May cause lupus-like syndrome.

Agent	Dosage	Comments
Indomethacin	PDA: IV q 8–12 h. Total of 3 doses: <48 h of life: 0.2/0.1/0.1 mg/kg 2–7 days of life: 0.2/0.2/0.2 mg/kg >7 days of life: 0.2/0.25/0.25 mg/kg Prolonged treatment: After standard regimen give 0.2 mg/kg/dose per day for 5 days. For IVH prophylaxis, give 0.1 mg/kg/24 h for 3 days starting between 6 and 12 h of life.	Monitor urine output, electrolytes, BUN, creatinine, and platelet count.
Isoproterenol (Isuprel)	IV (constant infusion): 0.05–1.5 μg/kg/min.	Increases myocardial oxygen consumption.
Lidocaine	IV (over 5–10 min): 1–2 mg/kg/dose given as 1% injection. May repeat in 10 min. Maximum dose: 5 mg/kg. IV (constant infusion): 10–50 μg/kg/min.	May cause seizures, apnea, asystole. Decrease dose with hepatic dysfunction, congestive heart failure, and cyanosis.
Milrinone (Primacor)	Bolus dose: 10–50 μg/kg, followed by continuous infusion of 0.25–0.75 μg/kg/min.	Afterload reducing agent.
Naloxone (Narcan)	IV, IM, or SC: 0.1 mg/kg/dose (equals 0.25 mL/kg/dose of solution 0.4 mg/mL). Repeat prn for the treatment of respiratory depression secondary to prenatal opiates administered to the mother.	Caution: may trigger acute withdrawal syndrome in babies born to opiate addicted mothers.
Neostigmine (Prostigmine)	Myasthenia gravis: 0.1 mg IM (30 min prior to feedings). IM: 0.04 mg/kg. IV: 0.025 mg/kg after atropine 0.02 mg/kg to reverse neuromuscular blockade.	
Nitroprusside, sodium (Nipride)	IV (constant infusion): 0.3–10 μg/kg/min; titrate to therapeutic response.	Must have continuous intraarterial blood pressure monitoring. May produce severe hypotension and thiocyanate intoxication. Protect from light. Should be used with anticholinergic agents (atropine).
Procainamide (Pronestyl)	IV over 10–30 minutes: 2–6 mg/kg. IV (constant infusion): 20–80 μg/kg/min. PO: 40–60 mg/kg/d divided q 6 h.	Therapeutic serum level 4–10 μg/mL (10–30 μg/mL if combined with NAPA [N-acetyl-procainamide]).
Propranolol (Inderal)	0.01–0.15 mg/kg/dose slow IV push; then 0.5–1.0 mg/kg/d divided q 6 h PO. For hypertension: 1 mg/kg/d divided q 6 h PO. For tetralogy of Fallot spells 0.15–0.25 mg/kg/dose IV.	
Prostaglandin E$_1$ (alprostadil)	IV: Begin infusion at 0.1 μg/kg/min. Once response is established, decrease infusion to lowest therapeutic dose. Usual dose range: 0.01–0.2 μg/kg/min.	May cause apnea; be prepared to perform endotracheal intubation and mechanical ventilation.
Quinidine	IM: 2–10 mg/kg q 2–6 h. Total dosage: 10–30 mg/kg/d. 5–15 mg/kg q 6 h PO. Maintain therapeutic serum levels between 2 and 5 μg/mL.	Increases digoxin levels; need to decrease digoxin dose.
Sodium bicarbonate	IV: 1–3 mEq/kg/dose (equals 2–6 mL/kg/dose 0.5 mEq/mL NaCO$_3$).	Adequate ventilation is necessary to avoid worsening respiratory acidosis.
Tolazoline (Priscoline)	IV (over 10 minutes): 1–2 mg/kg followed by continous infusion of 0.25–2 mg/kg/h.	Monitor blood pressure. Side effects include hypotension and gastrointestinal and pulmonary hemorrhage.

IV, intravenous; max, maximum; ECG, electrocardiogram; SC, subcutaneous; PO, by mouth; q, every; HR, heart rate; prn, as needed; BUN, blood urea nitrogen; IM, intramuscular; ET, endotracheal tube; IVH, intraventricular hemorrhage; PDA: patent ductus arteriosus.

A–2

Drug Dosing Table

Andrew P. Ten Eick
Ricardo J. Rodriguez
Michael D. Reed

Medication (Trade Name) Route of Administration	Mechanism of Action/Dosing	Important Adverse Events	Special Considerations
Acetaminophen (Tylenol) PO/PR	Inhibits prostaglandins in the central nervous system. Inhibition of the hypothalamic thermal regulating center. PO: 10–15 mg/kg q 6–8 h PR: 20–25 mg/kg q 6–8 h	Liver toxicity in overdose (acute or chronic)	Avoid aspartame-containing products (e.g., chewable tablets) in patients with phenylketonuria.
Acetazolamide (Diamox) IV	Competitively inhibits carbonic anhydrase IV: 5 mg/kg/dose q 6 h, increasing to 100 mg/kg/d	Drowsiness, fever, metabolic acidosis, seizures, renal calculi, polyuria, hyperpnea	Monitor electrolytes. Avoid if patient has sulfa hypersensitivity. IM administration is extremely painful.
Acyclovir (Zovirax) PO/IV	Inhibits viral phosphorylation of adenosine monophosphate (AMP) PO: 20 mg/kg/d divided q 12 h for HSV in premature neonates. 1500 mg/m²/d divided q 8 h or 30–45 mg/kg/d divided q 8 h for HSV in term neonates.	Renal dysfunction	Maintain proper hydration, monitor renal function. Administer small and frequent doses orally to enhance amount absorbed.
Adenosine (Adenocard) IV	Slows AV conduction, thereby interrupting reentry pathway. IV: 0.05 mg/kg/dose q 2 min for a total of 0.25 mg/kg or maximum of 12 mg.	Momentary complete heart block after administration Bronchoconstriction in patients with reactive airways disease	Administer rapidly and as close to IV insertion site as possible. Not effective in atrial flutter, atrial fibrillation, or ventricular tachycardia. Do administer to patients with second or third degree heart block. Methylxanthines antagonize adenosine pharmacodynamic effect and therefore larger dose may be needed.
Albuterol (Proventil, Ventolin) PO/Neb/MDI	β₂-agonist Nebulized 0.1–0.5 mg/kg dose q 2–6 h PO: 0.1–0.3 mg/kg/dose q 6–8 h	Tachycardia, hypokalemia with continuous administration, increased blood pressure	Oral administration may be associated with more systemic adverse events.
Alprostadil (Prostaglandin E₁, Caverject, Edex) IV	Prostaglandin E₁ analog that produces direct vasodilatation. 0.05–0.1 µg/kg/min via continuous IV infusion	Hypotension, flushing, bradycardia, tachycardia, hypoglycemia, inhibition of platelet aggregation, diarrhea, gastric outlet obstruction (≥5 d of use), cortical hyperostosis (with long-term administration >6 mo)	Apnea occurs in ~10%–12% of neonates within the first hour of infusion.

Table continued on following page

Medication (Trade Name) Route of Administration	Mechanism of Action/Dosing	Important Adverse Events	Special Considerations
Amikacin (Amikin) IM/IV	Inhibits bacterial protein synthesis by inhibiting the 50s ribosomal subunit. Postnatal age 0–4 wk: <1200 g: 7.5 mg/kg/dose q 18–24 h Postnatal age ≤7 d: 1200–2000 g: 7.5–10 mg/kg/dose q 12–18 h >2000 g: 10 mg/kg/dose q 12 h Postnatal age >7 days: 1200–2000 g: 7.5–10 mg/kg/dose q 8–12 h >2000 g: 10 mg/kg/dose q 8 h	Nephrotoxic, additive neuromuscular blockade with neuromuscular blocking agents (e.g., vecuronium and pancuronium)	Monitor serum concentrations. Therapeutic peak serum concentration 25 to 40 µg/mL. Therapeutic trough serum concentration <10 µg/mL. Should not be concurrently administered in same IV line with extended spectrum penicillins (possible inactivation). Synergist antibacterial actions with penicillins and other antibiotics.
Aminophylline (Aminophyllin, Phyllocontin) PO/IV	Competitively inhibits adenosine receptor. Loading dose: 4–6 mg/kg IV or PO Maintenance dose: 1.5–3 mg/kg/dose q 8–12 h	Gastroesophageal reflux, diarrhea, tachycardia, ventricular dysrhythmias, feeding intolerance	80% theophylline by weight. Monitor theophylline and caffeine serum concentrations. Therapeutic serum concentrations 6–15 µg/mL (theophylline + caffeine). Theophylline clearance may be modified by disease state and many drugs. Phenobarbital and rifampin may decrease theophylline serum concentrations. Cimetidine and macrolides (e.g., erythromycin) may increase theophylline serum concentrations.
Amphotericin B (Fungizone)	Binds to fungal ergosterol, compromising fungal cell wall integrity. Amphotericin B: 0.25–1 mg/kg/d over 4–6 h	Infusion-related adverse events: hypotension, phlebitis, fever, rigors, chills, nephrotoxicity, hypokalemia, hypomagnesemia	Monitor renal function. May consider premedication with acetaminophen, steroids, meperidine, and heparin. Less renal toxicity with lipid-based formulations.
Lipid amphotericin B (Abelcet, AmBisome) IV	Liposomal amphotericin B: 1–5 mg/kg/d over 1–2 h		

Drug (Route)	Action/Dosage	Adverse Effects	Comments
Ampicillin (Omnipen, Polycillin, Principen) IM/IV	Inhibits bacterial cell wall synthesis by binding to specific penicillin-binding proteins. Postnatal age ≤7 days: ≤2000 g: 50–100 mg/kg/d divided q 12 h >2000 g: 75–150 mg/kg/d divided q 8 h Postnatal age >7 days: <1200 g: 50–100 mg/kg/d divided q 12 h 1200–2000 g: 75–100 mg/kg/d divided q 8 h >2000 g: 100–200 mg/kg/d divided q 6 h	Few adverse events; similar to penicillins	Poor oral absorption—use amoxicillin. Administer higher doses for meningitis.
Atropine PO/IV/ET	Competitively inhibits actions of acetylcholine by binding to postsynaptic acetylcholine receptors. Oral: <5 kg: 0.02 mg/kg/dose >5 kg: 0.01–0.02 mg/kg/dose (maximum 0.4 mg/dose) Bradycardia 0.01–0.03 mg/kg/dose, may repeat every 10–15 min (maximum dose 0.04 mg/kg) ET: administer 2–3 times the IV dose	Tachycardia, urinary retention, decreased GI motility	Administer rapidly and undiluted. Slow administration may result in paradoxical bradycardia.
Aztreonam (Azactam) IM/IV	Inhibits bacterial cell wall synthesis by binding to penicillin-binding proteins. Postnatal ≤7 d: ≤2000 g: 60 mg/kg/d divided q 12 h >2000 g: 90 mg/kg/d divided q 8 h Postnatal >7 days: <1200 g: 60 mg/kg/d divided q 12 h 1200–2000 g: 90 mg/kg/d divided q 8 h >2000 g: 120 mg/kg/d divided q 6–8 h	Rash, thrombophlebitis	Rare cross hypersensitivity reactions with penicillins and cephalosporins.
Beractant (Survanta) IT	Modified bovine pulmonary surfactant analog. 4 mL/kg/dose divided into 4 aliquots administered as soon as possible. Up to 3 doses, if necessary, should be administered within 48 h.	Reflux of surfactant up ET, decreased oxygenation, bradycardia	For intratracheal administration only. Suspension should be at room temperature before administering. Do not artificially warm. Swirl the suspension; do not shake or filter suspension. Administer via ET using a shortened 5-French end-hole catheter. Instill one fourth of dose then gently rotate the infant's head and torso to a different position. Continue to administer one fourth of the dose and rotate baby. Remove catheter and ventilate baby for 30 sec between each administration. *Table continued on following page*

Medication (Trade Name) Route of Administration	Mechanism of Action/Dosing	Important Adverse Events	Special Considerations
Bumetanide (Bumex) PO/IV	Reversibly binds to Na/K/Cl ion pump and inhibits chloride reabsorption in the ascending loop of Henle. 0.01–0.05 mg/kg/dose q 6–48 h Continuous IV: 0.007 mg/kg/h	Metabolic alkalosis, fluid and electrolyte abnormalities (potassium, chloride, magnesium, bicarbonate)	Possible cross hypersensitivity in sulfa-allergic patients. Monitor urinary output.

Caffeine, citrate PO/IV	Competitively inhibits phosphodiesterase, increasing intracellular cyclic AMP concentrations.
	Loading dose:
	  20–40 mg/kg
	Maintenance:
	  5–8 mg/kg/d divided q 12–24 h
		Tachycardia, cardiac dysrhythmias, insomnia, GI disturbances, gastroesophageal reflux	Therapeutic serum concentration range 8–20 µg/mL; toxicity associated with serum concentrations >50 mg/mL. Active metabolite of theophylline. Sodium benzoate displaces bilirubin from binding; therefore, avoid in neonates with hyperbilirubinemia.

Calcitriol (Calcijex, Rocaltrol) PO/IV	Vitamin D analog. Promotes calcium absorption in the intestines and inhibits calcium renal excretion. IV: 0.05 mg/kg/d PO: 1 µg/d	Polyuria	May be administered intranasally. Monitor total and ionized serum calcium concentrations.
Captopril (Capoten) PO/IV	Competitively inhibits angiotensin-converting enzyme. Premature neonate: 0.01 mg/kg/dose q 8–12 h Neonate: 0.05 mg–0.1 mg/kg/dose q 8–24 h Maximum dose: 0.5 mg/kg/dose q 6–24 h	Reflex tachycardia, angioedema, renal dysfunction, hypotension	Monitor renal function. Dose based upon individual response.

Cefazolin (Ancef, Kefzol) PO/IM/IV	Inhibits bacterial cell wall synthesis by binding to penicillin-binding proteins.
	Postnatal age ≤7 d:
	  40 mg/kg/d divided q 12 h
	Postnatal age >7 d:
	  ≤2000 g: 40 mg/kg/d divided q 12 h
	  >2000 g: 60 mg/kg/d divided q 8 h
		Similar to penicillins	Rare hypersensitivity reactions Possible cross reactivity in penicillin-allergic neonates. Poor CNS penetration.

Cefotaxime (Claforan) IM/IV	Inhibits bacterial cell wall synthesis by binding to penicillin-binding proteins.
	Neonates 0–4 wk:
	  <1200 g: 100 mg/kg/d divided q 12 h
	Postnatal age ≤7 d:
	  1200–2000 g: 100 mg/kg/d divided q 12 h
	  >2000 g: 100–150 mg/kg/d divided q 8–12 h
	Postnatal age >7 d:
	  1200–2000 g: 150 mg/kg/d divided q 8 h
	  >2000 g: 150–200 mg/kg/d divided q 6–8 h
		Similar to penicillins	Rare hypersensitivity reactions. Possible cross reactivity in penicillin-allergic neonates. Metabolized to an active metabolite.

Drug (route)	Action/Dose	Side effects/toxicity	Comments
Ceftazidime (Ceptaz, Fortaz) IM/IV	Inhibits bacterial cell wall synthesis by binding to penicillin-binding proteins. Neonate 0–4 wk: <1200 g: 100 mg/kg/d divided q 12 h. Postnatal age ≤7 d: 1200–2000 g: 100 mg/kg/d divided q 12 h; >2000 g: 100–150 mg/kg/d divided q 8–12 h. Postnatal age >7 d: ≥1200 g: 150 mg/kg/d divided q 8 h	Similar to penicillins	Rare hypersensitivity reactions. Possible cross reactivity in penicillin-allergic neonates.
Ceftriaxone (Rocephin) IM/IV	Inhibits bacterial cell wall synthesis by binding to penicillin-binding proteins. Postnatal age ≤7 d: 50 mg/kg/d divided q 24 h. Postnatal age >7 d: ≤2000 g: 50 mg/kg/d divided q 24 h; >2000 g: 50–75 mg/kg/d divided q 24 h	Similar to penicillins	Rare hypersensitivity reactions. Possible cross reactivity reaction in penicillin-allergic neonates.
Chloral hydrate (Aquachloral Supprettes, Noctec) PO/PR	CNS depressant. Infrequently used as a sedative. Oral/PR: 25–75 mg/kg/dose	Prolonged sedation, respiratory depression	Dependence may occur with long-term administration. Active metabolite, trichloroethanol, may accumulate with repeated dosing.
Chloramphenicol (Chloromycetin) IV	Inhibits bacterial protein synthesis by binding to the 50s ribosomal subunit. Loading dose: 20 mg/kg followed 12 h later by maintenance dose: Postnatal age: ≤7 d: 25 mg/kg/d q 24 h; >7 d and ≤2000 g: 25 mg/kg/d q 24 h; >7 d and >2000 g: 50 mg/kg/d q 12 h. Monitor serum concentrations to adjust dose and avoid toxicity.	Cardiotoxicity, left ventricular dysfunction, gray baby syndrome, bone marrow suppression, aplastic anemia, optic neuritis, peripheral neuropathy	Hemolysis may occur in patients with G-6-PD deficiency. Bone marrow suppression may be associated with serum concentrations >25 µg/mL and is reversible with discontinuation of medication. Gray baby syndrome may be associated with persistent serum concentrations ≥50 µg/mL. Aplastic anemia is an idiosyncratic reaction and not dose related, occurring in approximately 1 in 40,000 cases.
Chlorothiazide PO/IV	Inhibition of Na reabsorption in the proximal and distal renal tubules. Oral: 20–40 mg/kg/d divided q 12 h. IV: 2–8 mg/kg/d divided q 12 h	Hypochloremic alkalosis; fluid and electrolyte disorders	Synergistic effect with loop diuretics (e.g., furosemide). Possible hypersensitivity reaction in neonates allergic to sulfa.
Cimetidine (Tagamet) PO/IV/IM	Competitively antagonizes H$_2$ receptors decreasing gastric acid secretion. 5–10 mg/kg/d divided q 8–12 h	Possible endocrine side effects with long-term dosing	Inhibits cytochrome P450 3A4; many possible drug-drug interactions (i.e., cisapride, erythromycin, phenytoin, metronidazole, propranolol, theophylline, and warfarin).

Table continued on following page

Medication (Trade Name) Route of Administration	Mechanism of Action/Dosing	Important Adverse Events	Special Considerations

Clindamycin (Cleocin) PO/IM/IV	Inhibits bacterial protein synthesis by reversibly binding to the 50s ribosome subunit.
	Postnatal age ≦7 d:
	  ≤2000 g: 10 mg/kg/d divided q 12 h
	  >2000 g: 15 mg/kg/d divided q 8 h
	Postnatal age >7 d:
	  <1200 g: 10 mg/kg/d divided q 12 h
	  1200–2000 g: 15 mg/kg/d divided q 8 h
	  >2000 g: 20 mg/kg/d divided q 6–8 h
		Clostridium difficile associated diarrhea, pseudomembranous colitis, phlebitis at the site of injection	Adjust dosage according to patient's renal and/or liver function. Slowly administer intravenously (~ 30–60 min).

Dexamethasone (Dalalone, Decadron) PO/IV/IM	Potent corticosteroid, inhibits and promotes synthesis of proinflammatory and anti-inflammatory mediators, respectively. 0.25–0.6 mg/kg/d divided q 4–12 h	May aggravate fluid retention, pituitary-adrenal axis suppression, possible GI disturbances	Taper dexamethasone therapy after 7–10 d of continuous administration. Approximately 6–7 times more potent than prednisone.

Diazepam (Valium) PO/IV/IM/PR	Sedative, antianxiolytic reversibly binds to central GABA receptors, enhancing GABA effects, the major inhibitory neural transmitter in the CNS.
	Status epilepticus:
	  IV: 0.05–0.3 mg/kg/dose over 2–3 min and may repeat every 3 min.
	  Rectal: 0.5 mg/kg then 0.25 mg/kg in 10 min.
	Sedation:
	  Oral: 0.2–0.3 mg/kg (maximum dose 10 mg)
	  IM/IV: 0.04–0.3 mg/kg (maximum dose 0.6 mg/kg/d q 8 h)
		Hypotension, cardiac dysrhythmias, cardiac arrest, phlebitis (adverse event probably associated with the propylene glycol dilulent)	Respiratory depression may occur when administered with other respiratory and CNS depressants (e.g., opioids, chloral hydrate). IM administration is extremely painful. Increased pharmacodynamic effects when administered with P450 inhibitors (e.g., erythromycin, cimetidine). Injectables contain benzyl alcohol and propylene glycol.

Diazoxide (Hyperstat) IV	Potent antihypertensive given IV and inhibits insulin release from the pancreas. 8–15 mg/kg/d divided q 8–12 h	Hypotension, tachycardia, seizures, hypoglycemia	Oral administration for hyperinsulin conditions.

Digoxin (Lanoxin) PO/IV	Reversibly binds to the Na/K/Ca pump and increases calcium influx within myocardial cells.
	Loading dose:
	  Preterm: IV: 15–25 μg/kg
	    PO: 20–30 μg/kg
	  Term: IV: 20–30 μg/kg
	    PO: 25–35 μg/kg
	Maintenance dose:
	  Preterm IV: 4–6 μg/kg/d
	    PO: 5–7.5 μg/kg/d
	  Term: IV: 5–8 μg/kg/d
	    PO: 6–10 μg/kg/d
		Atrial and ventricular dysrhythmias; first, second, and third degree AV block; feeding intolerance	Many possible drug interactions (i.e., amphotericin B, erythromycin, cyclosporine, itraconazole, phenobarbital, phenytoin, and quinine sulfate). Monitor serum concentrations. Digoxin toxicity associated with serum concentrations >2 ng/mL. Contraindicated in patients with AV block, idiopathic hypertrophic subaortic stenosis, constrictive pericarditis.

Drug	Mechanism/Dose	Adverse effects	Comments
Dobutamine (Dobutrex) IV	Reversibly binds to and stimulates the β_1-adrenergic receptor. 2–25 µg/kg/min continuous IV infusion: titrate to blood pressure or mean arterial pressure	Hypertension, tachycardia, phlebitis	Do not concurrently administer with β_1- or α_1-adrenergic antagonists
Dopamine IV	Stimulates α-, β-adrenergic and dopaminergic receptors. 1–20 µg/kg/min continuous IV infusion	Hypertension, tachycardia, phlebitis	Low dose 1–5 µg/kg/min stimulates dopaminergic receptors. Moderate dose 5–10 µg/kg/min mainly stimulates β-adrenergic receptors. High dose >10 µg/kg/min α-adrenergic stimulation predominates. Contains sulfites.
Enalapril (Vasotec) PO/IV	Blood pressure and cardiac effects resulting from competitive inhibition of angiotensin-converting enzyme. PO: 0.04–0.1 mg/kg/dose q 12–24 h IV: 0.005–0.01 mg/kg/dose q 8–24 h	Reflex tachycardia, angioedema, renal dysfunction	Monitor renal function. Individualize dose based on patient's response.
Epinephrine (Adrenalin) IV/IM/SQ/IO/ET	Stimulates α-, β-adrenergic and dopaminergic receptors. IV: 0.01–0.03 mg/kg/dose q 3–5 min ET: Administer 2–3 times the IV dose Use 1:10,000 concentration	Hypertension, tachycardia, phlebitis	Intratracheal administration.
Epoetin alfa (Epogen, Procrit) IV/SQ	Synthetic analog of erythropoietin-stimulating erythrocyte production. 5–500 U/kg/dose 3 times per week	Hypertension, edema	Monitor hematocrit, which should not exceed 36% (temporarily discontinue if hematocrit >40 mg/dL). Consider repleting iron stores. Do not shake bottle.
Erythromycin (E-mycin, E.E.S.) PO/IV	Inhibits bacterial protein synthesis by reversibly binding to the 50s ribosome subunit. Postnatal age ≤7 d: 20 mg/kg/d divided q 12 h Postnatal age >7 d: <1200 g: 20 mg/kg/d divided q 12 h ≥1200 g: 30 mg/kg/d divided q 8 h	Ventricular dysrhythmias with rapid intravenous administration, GI disturbances, cholestatic hepatitis, jaundice, thrombophlebitis	Sodium content: intravenous erythromycin should be administered over 60 min. Inhibits P450 3A4 isozyme. Many possible drug-drug interactions (i.e., theophylline, digoxin, and cyclosporine).
Fentanyl (Duragesic, Sublimaze) IV/IM	Potent opioid analgesic/sedative. 1–4 µg/kg/dose every 2–4 h Continuous IV: 0.5–5 µg/kg/h	Respiratory depression, rigid chest syndrome, GI disturbances	Dependence may occur with long-term administration. Closely monitor respiratory rate, blood pressure, heart rate, oxygen saturation, and bowel sounds. Effects reversed by naloxone. 5–10 times more potent than morphine.
Ferrous salts PO/IV	See iron.		

Table continued on following page

557

Medication (Trade Name) Route of Administration	Mechanism of Action/Dosing	Important Adverse Events	Special Considerations
Fluconazole (Diflucan) PO/IV	Reversibly binds to fungal CYP P450, inhibiting sterol C-14 α-demethylation and decreasing ergosterol synthesis. ≤29 wk gestational age and postnatal age: 0–14 d: 5–6 mg/kg/dose q 72 h >14 d: 5–6 mg/kg/dose q 48 h 30–36 wk gestational age and postnatal age: 0–14 d: 3–12 mg/kg/dose q 48 h >14 d: 3–12 mg/kg/dose q 24 h	Increased liver function tests	Fluconazole is a weak inhibitor of CYP 450 3A4 isozyme. Increased serum concentrations of warfarin, cyclosporine, and phenytoin. May inhibit metabolism of cisapride, rifampin, and zidovudine.
Flucytosine (Ancobon) PO	Converted within fungal cells to fluorouracil, which competitively competes with the incorporation of uracil in fungal RNA. 50–150 mg/kg/d divided q 6 h	GI disturbances, bone marrow suppression, increased liver function, renal dysfunction	Increase dosing interval in patients with decreased glomerular filtration rate. Monitor serum concentrations. Adult therapeutic serum concentration 25–100 µg/mL. Increased toxicity observed with serum concentrations >100 µg/mL.
Fosphenytoin (Cerebyx) IV/IM	Phenytoin prodrug. Inhibits sodium ion influx and stabilizes neuronal membranes. See phenytoin. Loading dose: 10–20 mg/kg of phenytoin equivalent	See phenytoin	May administer IM. May administer much more rapidly than phenytoin (100–150 mg/min). Maximal pharmacodynamic effect observed approximately 20–30 min after administration. Does not contain propylene glycol.
Furosemide (Lasix) PO/IV	Reversibly binds to Na/K/Cl ion pump and inhibits chloride reabsorption in the ascending loop of Henle. IV: 0.5–2 mg/kg/dose q 12–24 h PO: 1–6 mg/kg/dose q 12–24 h	Hypochloremic alkalosis, renal calculi, rare hearing deficit	Synergistic effect with proximal and distal tubule inhibitors (e.g., thiazides). Possible hypersensitivity reaction in neonates allergic to sulfa.
Gentamicin (Garamycin) IV/IM	Inhibits bacterial protein synthesis by inhibiting the 50s ribosomal subunit. Neonates 0–4 wk: <1200 g: 2.5 mg/kg/dose q 18–24 h Postnatal age ≤7 d: 1200–2000 g: 2.5 mg/kg/dose q 12–18 h >2000 g: 2.5 mg/kg/dose q 12 h Postnatal age >7 d: 1200–2000 g: 2.5 mg/kg/dose q 8–12 h >2000 g: 2.5 mg/kg/dose q 8 h	Nephrotoxic, additive neuromuscular blockade with neuromuscular blocking agents (e.g., vecuronium and pancuronium)	Administer IV over 30–60 min. Peak serum concentration should be obtained 30 min after end of infusion. Monitor serum concentrations. Therapeutic peak serum concentration 6–12 µg/mL. Therapeutic trough serum concentration <1 µg/mL. Should not be concurrently administered in same IV line with extended spectrum penicillin. Synergistic antibacterial actions with penicillin. Consider less frequent dosing.

Drug (Route)	Action/Dosage	Adverse Effects	Comments
Glucagon IV/IM/SQ	Increases hepatic glycogenolysis and gluconeogenesis. 0.3 mg/kg/dose Maximum 1 mg/dose	Hypotension, GI disturbances	
Heparin (Hep-Lock, Liquaemin) IV/IM	Potentiates the action of antithrombin III, inactivates thrombin, inhibits the conversion of fibrinogen to fibrin. Loading dose: 50 U/kg Maintenance dose: 15–25 mg/kg/h Reverse heparin effects with protamine (1 mg protamine will neutralize approximately 90 U of heparin).	Hemorrhage, thrombocytopenia	Use caution when administering with drugs with anticoagulant effect (warfarin) or affect platelet function (NSAIDs). Monitor aPTT. Therapeutic anticoagulation aPTT/INR = 1.5–2.5 times normal/INR 2–3.
Hydralazine (Apresoline) PO/IV	Peripheral α_2 agonist; potent vasodilator. PO: 0.25–1 mg/kg/dose divided q 6–12 h IV: 0.1–0.5 mg/kg/dose 6–8 h	Hypotension, tachycardia, flushing, GI disturbances	Positive ANA, lupus-like syndrome has been observed.
Hydrochlorothiazide (HydroDIURIL) PO	Inhibition of Na reabsorption in the proximal and distal renal tubules. 2–4 mg/kg/d divided q 12 h	Hypochloremic alkalosis; fluid and electrolyte abnormalities	Synergistic effect with loop diuretics (e.g., furosemide). Possible hypersensitivity reaction in neonates allergic to sulfa.
Hydrocortisone (A-Hydrocort) PO/IV	Corticosteroid that inhibits and promotes synthesis of pro-inflammatory and anti-inflammatory mediators, respectively. Adrenal insufficiency: 1–2 mg/kg/d then 25–150 mg/d divided q 6 h	May aggravate fluid retention, pituitary-adrenal axis suppression, possible GI disturbances	Taper hydrocortisone therapy after 7–10 d of continuous administration. Physiologic replacement is approximately 6–8 mg/m²/d.
Imipenem/cilastatin (Primaxin) IV/IM	Inhibits bacterial cell wall synthesis by binding to penicillin-binding proteins. Neonates 0–4 wk: <1200 g: 20 mg/kg/d divided q 18–24 h Postnatal age ≤7 d: ≥1200 g: 40 mg/kg/d divided q 12 h Postnatal age >7 days: 1200–2000 g: 40 mg/kg/d divided q 12 h >2000 g: 60 mg/kg/d divided q 8 h	GI disturbances, rash, and possible seizures with high doses in patients with poor renal function; possible bacterial or fungal overgrowth	Rare hypersensitivity reactions. Possible (rare) cross reactivity in penicillin-allergic neonates. Cilastatin possesses no antibacterial; prevents metabolism of imipenem by inhibiting dehydropeptidase I in proximal tubule.
Indomethacin (Indocin) PO/IV	Competitively inhibits cyclooxygenase and decreases the formation of prostaglandins. Initial: 0.2 mg/kg, then: Postnatal age <48 h: 0.1 mg/kg q 12 h for 2 doses Postnatal age 2–7 d: 0.2 mg/kg q 12 h for 2 doses Postnatal age >7 d: 0.25 mg/kg q 12 h for 2 doses	Hypertension, edema, GI disturbances, increased bleeding time, renal toxicity	May decrease diuretic efficacy; diuretics may decrease indomethacin effect. Monitor urine output; adjust interval appropriately. Therapeutic serum concentration 1–3 µg/mL.
Insulin (Humulin) IV/SQ	Increases glucose intracellular transport. SQ: 0.5–1 U/kg/d divided q 6–12 h Continuous IV: 0.01–0.1 U/kg/h	Hypoglycemia and associated signs and symptoms	
Ipratropium (Atrovent) Neb, MDI	Bronchodilator that reversibly antagonizes postsynaptic acetylcholine receptors. 25–100 µg/kg/dose 6–8 h	Constipation, palpitations, tachycardia, hypotension, xerostomia, dry secretions	

Table continued on following page

Medication (Trade Name) Route of Administration	Mechanism of Action/Dosing	Important Adverse Events	Special Considerations
Iron PO/IV/IM	Routine supplemental doses: PO: 2–4 mg/kg/d divided in 3–4 doses IV: 1–4 mg of elemental iron/kg/d divided q 12–24 h Patients receiving erythropoietin: 6 mg/kg/d divided q 12–24 h	GI disturbances, discolored stool; IM dose painful and may stain skin	Oral absorption is dependent on an acid environment. Iron dextran for IV results in rare hypersensitivity reactions. Dextran-allergic patients use iron gluconate in sucrose.
Isoproterenol (Isuprel) Neb/IV	Nonselective β_1- and β_2-adrenergic agonist. Nebulized: 0.1–0.5 µg/kg/dose 2–6 h IV: 0.05–0.5 µg/kg/min (maximum dose 2 µg/kg/min)	Tachycardia, hypokalemia with continuous administration, increased blood pressure	
Levothyroxine (Synthroid) PO/IV	Triiodotyrosine is peripherally converted to thyroxine as thyroid replacement therapy. PO: 8–14 µg/kg/d IV: 5–8 µg/kg/d	Tachycardia, cardiac dysrhythmias, tremors, GI disturbances, diaphoresis	
Lidocaine (Dilocaine, Xylocaine) IV/ET	Class IB antiarrhythmic 0.5–1 mg/kg/dose, which may be repeated 5–10 min to maximum of 3 mg/kg. Continuous IV: 20–50 µg/kg/min ET: Administer 2–3 times IV dose	Bradycardia, hypotension, heart block, lethargy, coma	Monitor serum concentrations. Therapeutic serum concentrations 1–5 µg/mL. Toxicity often associated with serum concentrations >6 µg/mL.
Lorazepam (Ativan) PO/IV/IM	Reversibly binds to GABA receptors, enhancing GABA effects, the major inhibitory neural transmitter. Status epilepticus: 0.05–0.2 mg/kg/dose over 2 min; may repeat q 10–15 min Sedation: 0.1–0.4 mg/kg/dose q 4–6 h	Hypotension, cardiac dysrhythmias, phlebitis (adverse event probably associated with diluent)	Do not exceed 2 mg/min or 0.05 mg/kg over 2–5 min. Respiratory depression may occur when administered with other respiratory and CNS depressants (e.g., opioids). Increased pharmacodynamic effects when administered with P450 inhibitors. (e.g., erythromycin, cimetidine). Injectables contain benzyl alcohol, polyethylene glycol, and propylene glycol.
Meperidine PO/IV	Opioid analgesic/sedative. 1 mg/kg/dose q 4 h	Hypotension, vasodilation, flushing, pruritus, respiratory depression, rigid chest syndrome, GI disturbances, seizures	Nor-meperidine (seizuregenic metabolite of meperidine) may accumulate in neonate with poor renal function and possibly lower seizure threshold.
Meropenem (Merrem) IV/IM	Carbapenem inhibits bacterial cell wall synthesis by binding to penicillin-binding proteins. Serious infections: 40 mg/kg/d divided q 12 h Meningitis: 120 mg/kg/d divided q 8 h	GI disturbances, rash, and possible bacterial or fungal overgrowth	Rare hypersensitivity reactions. Possible (rare) cross reactivity in penicillin-allergic neonates.

Drug	Action/Dosage	Adverse Effects	Comments
Methylprednisolone (Adlone, Depo-Medrol) PO/IV/IM	Potent corticosteroid, which inhibits and promotes synthesis of proinflammatory and anti-inflammatory mediators, respectively. 0.5–30 mg/kg/dose q 6–24 h	May aggravate fluid retention, pituitary-adrenal axis suppression, possible GI disturbances	Only sodium succinate salt may be administered intravenously. Taper therapy after 7–10 d of continuous administration.
Metoclopramide (Clopra, Reglan) PO/IV	Gastroprokinetic that reversibly antagonizes dopamine-1 and enhances acetylcholine receptor stimulation. 0.1–0.3 mg/kg/d divided q 6–8 h	Extrapyramidal reactions, oculogyric reaction, SVT, bradycardia, diarrhea	Increased motility may decrease absorption of some oral medications.

Metronidazole (Flagyl, Metro) PO/IV/IM	Breaks helical structure of DNA, resulting in strand breaking in anaerobes (including *C. difficile*)/trichomonas.
	Neonates 0–4 wk:
	  <1200 g: 7.5 mg/kg/dose q 48 h
	Postnatal age ≤7 d:
	  1200–2000 g: 7.5 mg/kg/d q 24 h
	  ≥2000 g: 15 mg/kg/d divided q 12 h
	Postnatal age >7 d:
	  1200–2000 g: 15 mg/kg/d divided q 12 h
	  ≥2000 g: 30 mg/kg/d divided q 12 h
		Seizures, insomnia, GI disturbances, hairy tongue, darkening of urine, thrombophlebitis	100 mg = 2.8 mEq of sodium.
			Phenobarbital may increase metabolism of metronidazole.

Midazolam (Versed) PO/IV/IM/IN	Reversibly binds to GABA receptors, enhancing GABA effects, the major inhibitory neural transmitter. Intermittent IV: 0.05–0.15 mg/kg/dose q 2–4 h Continuous IV infusion: <32 wk: 0.01 mg/kg/h >32 wk: 0.06 mg/kg/h Intranasal/sublingual: 0.2–0.3 mg/kg/dose q 2–4 h PO: 0.3–0.5 mg/kg/dose q 2–4 h	Hypotension, cardiac dysrhythmias, phlebitis	May be administered by the intranasal route. Administer intravenous infusions slowly. Titrate dose to individual response Respiratory depression may occur when administered with other respiratory and CNS depressants (e.g., opioids). Increased pharmacodynamic effects when administered with P450 inhibitors (e.g., erythromycin and cimetidine). Injectable does not contain benzyl alcohol, polyethylene glycol, or propylene glycol.
Morphine (Astramorph, Duramorph) PO/IV/IM/SQ	Opioid analgesic/sedative. 0.05–0.2 mg/kg/dose q 2–4 h Continuous IV infusion: 0.025–0.05 mg/kg/h	Hypotension, vasodilation, flushing, pruritus, respiratory depression, rigid chest syndrome, GI disturbances	Dependence may occur with long-term administration. Closely monitor respiratory rate, blood pressure, heart rate, oxygen saturation, and bowel sounds. Metabolized to an active metabolite. Effects reversed by naloxone.

Table continued on following page

Medication (Trade Name) Route of Administration	Mechanism of Action/Dosing	Important Adverse Events	Special Considerations
Nafcillin (Nafcil, Nallpen, Unipen) IV/IM	Inhibits bacterial cell wall synthesis by binding to penicillin-binding proteins. Neonates 0–4 wk: <1200 g: 50 mg/kg/d divided q 12 h Postnatal age ≦7 d: 1200–2000 g: 50 mg/kg/d divided q 12 h >2000 g: 75 mg/kg/d divided q 8 h Postnatal age >7 d: 1200–2000 g: 75 mg/kg/d divided q 8 h >2000 g: 100 mg/kg/d divided q 6–8 h Administer 200 mg/kg/d q 6 h for meningitis.	Skin rash, GI disturbances, increased liver function tests, acute interstitial nephritis, thrombophlebitis	Rare hypersensitivity reactions. Dose adjustment necessary in patients with both renal and liver dysfunction.
Naloxone IV	Opioid analog/Mμ receptor antagonist. 0.01–0.1 mg/kg dose; may be repeated q 2–3 min	Possible signs and symptoms of opioid withdrawal	Reverses the effects of morphine and other opioids. Half-life of naloxone may be shorter than opioids; therefore, repeated doses or a constant infusion of naloxone may be necessary. May precipitate withdrawal symptoms in neonates receiving long-term opioid administration.
Nitroprusside (Nitropress) IV	Potent peripheral arterial and venous vasodilator. 0.3–0.5 μg/kg/min continuous IV infusion Metabolized to cyanide/thiocyanate. Administer 1:10 mixture of nitroprusside:thiosulfate.	Hypotension, thyroid suppression, very rare cyanide intoxication (metabolic acidosis, tachycardia, methemoglobinemia)	Dilute with only D$_5$W. Protect from light. Coadministration with thiosulfate prevents cyanide toxicity. Titrate to individual response.
Nystatin (Mycostatin, Milstat) PO, topical	Binds to sterols in fungal cell membranes and increases permeability. 100,000 U 4 times per day	GI disturbances	Very poor systemic absorption.
Oxacillin (Bactocill) PO/IV/IM	Inhibits bacterial cell wall synthesis by binding to penicillin-binding proteins. Postnatal age ≦7 d: ≦2000 g: 50 mg/kg/d divided q 12 h >2000 g: 75 mg/kg/d divided q 8 h Postnatal age >7 d: ≦1200 g: 50 mg/kg/d divided q 12 h 1200–2000 g: 75 mg/kg/d divided q 8 h >2000 g: 100 mg/kg/d divided q 6 h	Skin rash, GI disturbances, increased liver function tests, acute interstitial nephritis, thrombophlebitis (less than nafcillin)	Rare hypersensitivity reactions.

Drug	Mechanism/Dosage	Adverse Effects	Comments
Pancuronium (Pavulon) IV	Reversibly binds to postsynaptic cholinergic receptor antagonizing acetylcholine. Intermittent IV: 0.04–0.15 mg/kg q 60–120 min Continuous IV infusion: 0.1 mg/kg/h	Tachycardia, hypertension	Possible increased neuromuscular blockade when concurrently administered with aminoglycosides, clindamycin, and erythromycin.
Penicillin G (Pfizerpen) IV/IM	Inhibits bacterial cell wall synthesis by binding to penicillin-binding proteins. Postnatal age ≤7 d: ≤2000 g: 50,000 U/kg/d divided q 12 h; for meningitis, 100,000 U/kg/d divided q 12 h >2000 g: 75,000 U/kg/d divided q 8 h; for meningitis 150,000 U/kg/d divided q 8 h Postnatal age >7 d: ≤1200 g: 50,000 U/kg/d divided q 12 h; for meningitis, 100,000 U/kg/d divided q 12 h >1200–2000 g: 75,000 U/kg/d divided q 8 h; for meningitis 150,000 U/kg/d divided q 8 h >2000 g: 100,000 U/kg/d divided q 6 h; for meningitis, 200,000 U/kg/d divided q 6 h	Skin rash, GI disturbances, seizures, thrombophlebitis (less than nafcillin)	Rare hypersensitivity reactions. Contains 1.7 mEq of potassium and 0.3 mEq of sodium per 1 million U of penicillin G.
Pentobarbital PO/IV/IM/PR	Reversibly binds to the GABA receptor and enhances the pharmacodynamic activity of GABA. 2–6 mg/kg/24 h	Hypotension, dysrhythmias, laryngospasms	Intravenous preparation contains propylene glycol. Pentobarbital may increase metabolism of many drugs (see phenobarbital). May be administered as a continuous IV to induce a pentobarbital coma.
Phenobarbital (Barbita, Luminal) PO/IV/IM	Reversibly binds to the GABA receptor and enhances the pharmacodynamic activity of GABA. Loading dose: 15–20 mg/kg, then 3–5 mg/kg/d q 24 h	Hypotension, skin eruptions, megaloblastic anemia, hepatitis, respiratory depression	Long-term use stimulates CYP 450 isozyme activity, leading to decreased serum concentrations of ritonavir, saquinavir, delavirdine, warfarin, chloramphenicol, β-blockers, theophylline, and corticosteroid. Chloramphenicol may inhibit the metabolism of phenobarbital. Monitor serum concentrations. Therapeutic concentrations 15–40 µg/mL. Increased toxicity associated with acute serum concentrations >40 µg/mL.

Table continued on following page

Medication (Trade Name) Route of Administration	Mechanism of Action/Dosing	Important Adverse Events	Special Considerations
Phenytoin (Dilantin) PO/IV/IM	Antiseizure/antiarrhythmic agent, which inhibits sodium ion influx and stabilizes neuronal/cardiac cell membranes. Loading dose: 15–20 mg/kg, then 4–8 mg/kg/d divided q 8–24 h. Better oral absorption with chewable tablets vs suspension (consider crushing chewable tablets into slurry)	Lethargy, nystagmus, hypotension, bradycardia, dysrhythmias, hirsutism, Stevens-Johnson syndrome, gingival hyperplasia, blood dyscrasias, hepatitis, thrombophlebitis, lupus-like syndrome	Slowly infuse. Do not exceed 0.5 mg/kg/min. IM administration is extremely painful. Monitor free and bound (total) serum concentrations. Therapeutic free concentration: 0.8–1.5 μg/mL. Therapeutic bound concentrations: 8–15 μg/mL. Phenytoin may decrease serum concentrations of ritonavir, saquinavir, delavirdine, warfarin, corticosteroids, cyclosporine, theophylline, chloramphenicol, rifampin, and nondepolarizing skeletal muscle relaxants. Concurrent administration of phenytoin with nasogastric feeding may decrease phenytoin oral absorption. Injectables contain approximately 40% propylene glycol.
Piperacillin / tazobactam (Zosyn) IV/IM	Inhibits bacterial cell wall synthesis by binding to penicillin-binding proteins. Tazobactam irreversibly binds to β-lactamase. 150–300 mg of piperacillin/kg/d divided q 6–8 h	Hypertension, edema, rare hypokalemia, skin rash, GI disturbances, increased liver function tests, thrombophlebitis	Rare hypersensitivity reactions. IM administration is extremely painful.
Propranolol (Betachron, Inderal) PO/IV	Nonspecific antagonist of β_1- and β_2-adrenergic receptors. Oral: 0.25 mg/kg/dose q 6–8 h (maximum 3.5 mg/kg/dose q 6 h) IV: 0.01–0.15 mg/kg/dose q 6–8 h Thyrotoxicosis: 2 mg/kg/d divided q 6–8 h	Hypotension, bradycardia, hypoglycemia, hyperglycemia, GI disturbances, bronchospasms	Cimetidine may increase propranolol serum concentration; phenobarbital and rifampin may decrease propranolol serum concentrations. Administer slowly over 10 to 20 min.
Ranitidine (Zantac) PO/IV	Competitively antagonizes H_2 receptors, inhibiting gastric acid secretion. 1.5–2 mg/kg/dose q 6–12 h Continuous infusion: 0.04 mg/kg/h (maximum 1 mg/kg/q 24 h)		May decrease absorption of drug requiring an acid gastric environment (e.g., ketoconazole). Monitor gastric pH and dose appropriately.

Drug	Action/Dose	Adverse Effects	Comments
Rifampin (Rifadin, Rimactane) PO/IV	Inhibits bacterial RNA synthesis by reversibly binding to the β subunit of DNA-dependent RNA polymerase, thereby inhibiting RNA transcription. PO: 10–20 mg/kg/d q 24 h IV: 5–10 mg/kg/d q 24 h	Lethargy, rash, cholestatic jaundice, hepatitis, reddish color to bodily fluids (e.g., urine, tears), influenza-like syndrome.	Rifampin induces CYP 450 isozymes. Rifampin may decrease serum concentrations of digoxin, cyclosporine, corticosteroids, warfarin, theophylline, barbiturates, chloramphenicol, opiates, azoles, and ketoconazole.
Secobarbital (Seconal) IV/IM/PO/PR	Barbiturate that reversibly binds to the GABA receptor and enhances the pharmacodynamic activity of GABA. Hypnotic IM: 3–5 mg/kg IV: 1–3 mg/kg Sedation PO: 2–6 mg/kg Rectal: 4–6 mg/kg Usual maximum dose: 50–100 mg	Hypotension, cardiac dysrhythmias, megaloblastic anemia, hepatitis, respiratory depression, thrombophlebitis	Secobarbital may decrease serum concentrations of ritonavir, saquinavir, delavirdine, warfarin, chloramphenicol, β-blockers, theophylline, and corticosteroids. Chloramphenicol may inhibit the metabolism of secobarbital.
Sotalol PO	Class III antiarrhythmic 1–4 mg/kg/dose q 12 h (maximum dose 4 mg/kg/dose q 12 h)	Bradycardia, decreased peripheral perfusion, constipation, diarrhea	Administer cautiously to neonates with reactive airway disease or second or third degree AV block.
Spironolactone (Aldactone) PO/IV	Competitive aldosterone antagonist increasing potassium reabsorption. 1–3 mg/kg/d q 12–24 h	Hyperkalemia, gynecomastia	Suspension may be made by crushing tablets in water and glycerin. Titrate dose to decrease in urinary K^+ excretion.
Streptokinase (Kabikinase, Streptase) IV	Fibrinolytic that promotes conversion of plasminogen to plasmin. Clotted catheter: 10,000–25,000 U in normal saline; instill into catheter for approximately 1 h	Hemorrhage, allergic reactions, bronchospasms	Allergic reaction has been observed with repeated doses. Allergic reaction may occur if administered after a recent streptococcal infection.
Tobramcyin (Nebcin) IV	Inhibits bacterial protein synthesis by reversibly binding to 50s ribosomal subunits. Neonates 0–4 wk: <1200 g: 2.5 mg/kg/dose q 18–24 h Postnatal age ≤7 d: 1200–2000 g: 2.5 mg/kg/dose q 12–18 h >2000 g: 2.5 mg/kg/dose q 12 h Postnatal age >7 d: 1200–2000 g: 2.5 mg/kg/dose q 8–12 h >2000 g: 2.5 mg/kg/dose q 8 h	Nephrotoxic, additive neuromuscular blockade with neuromuscular blocking agents (e.g., vecuronium and pancuronium)	Administer IV over 30–60 min. Peak serum concentration should be obtained 30 min after end of infusion. Monitor serum concentrations. Therapeutic peak serum concentration 6–12 µg/mL. Therapeutic trough serum concentration <1 µg/mL. Should not be concurrently administered in same IV line with extended spectrum penicillin. Synergistic antibacterial actions with penicillin. Consider less frequent dosing.
Tolazoline (Priscoline) IV	Vasodilator competitively antagonizes α-adrenergic receptors. 1–2 mg/kg, then 1–2 mg/kg/h	Hypotension, tachycardia, dysrhythmias, GI disturbances, oliguria	Monitor preductal and postductal oxygen saturation, arterial blood gases.

Table continued on following page

Medication (Trade Name) Route of Administration	Mechanism of Action/Dosing	Important Adverse Events	Special Considerations
Urokinase IV	Fibrinolytic which promotes conversion of plasminogen to plasmin. Clotted catheter: 5000 U and instill into catheter for 1–4 h	Hemorrhage, allergic reactions, bronchospasms	Efficacy unaffected by recent streptococcal infection. If not available may use TPA 1 mg/mL of normal saline; fill catheter and wait 1 hour.
Vancomycin (Lyphocin, Vancocin) PO/IV	Inhibits glycopeptide polymerization by competitively binding to D-anyl-D-alanine. Postnatal age ≤7 d: <1200 g: 15 mg/kg/dose q 24 h 1200–2000 g: 5–7.5 mg/kg/dose q 12–18 h >2000 g: 10–15 mg/kg/dose q 8–12 h Postnatal age >7 d: <1200 g: 15 mg/kg/dose q 24 h 1200–2000 g: 5–7.5 mg/kg/dose q 8–12 h >2000 g: 15–20 mg/kg/dose q 8 h	Red-man syndrome, fever, chills, phlebitis, ototoxicity, nephrotoxicity	Infuse slowly for 45–60 min. Obtain peak serum concentration 1 hour after completion of a 1-hour infusion. Therapeutic peak serum concentration 25–40 µg/mL. Therapeutic trough serum concentrations 5–10 µg/mL. Reduce infusion rate if the patient experiences "red-neck syndrome"; may respond to antihistamine premedication. Oral vancomycin is not to be administered for systemic infections.
Vecuronium (Norcuron) IV	Competitively antagonizes postsynaptic acetylcholine receptors 0.1 mg/kg/dose, then 0.03–0.15 mg/kg/dose q 1–2 h as needed	Bradycardia, tachycardia, hypotension, muscle weakness	Muscle weakness is associated with concurrent administration of corticosteroids and extended infusions of vecuronium. Titrate dose to patient's response. Increase neuromuscular blockade when coadministered with aminoglycosides, erythromycin, and clindamycin.
Vitamin K-phytonadione (AquaMEPHYTON, Konakion)	Cofactor for liver synthesis of clotting factors (II, VII, IX, X) Prophylaxis: 0.5–1 mg within 1 h of birth; may repeat 6–8 h later Treatment: 1–2 mg/dose/d	Flushing, hypotension, anaphylactoid reactions	Antagonizes warfarin anticoagulant effects. Anaphylactoid reactions have occurred immediately after IV administration in children and adults. Infuse slowly.
Zidovudine (Retrovir)	Phosphorylated intracellularly and is incorporated within viral RNA, interrupting HIV replication. Premature neonates: PO: 1.5–2 mg/kg/dose q 8–12 h Neonates: PO: 2 mg/kg/dose q 6 h IV: 1.5 mg/kg/dose q 6 h		

aPTT, activated partial thromboplastin time; AV, atrioventricular; CNS, central nervous system; ET, endotracheal tube; GI, gastrointestinal; G6PD, glucose-6-phosphate dehydrogenase; HIV, human immunodeficiency virus; HSV, herpes simplex virus; IM, intramuscular; IN, intranasal; IO, intraosseous; IT, intrathecally; IV, intravenous; MDI, metered dose inhaler; Neb, nebulizer; NSAIDs, nonsteroidal anti-inflammatory drugs; PO, by mouth; PR, per rectum; q, every; SQ, subcutaneous; SVT, supraventricular tachycardia; TPA, tissue plasminogen activator.

Drug Compatibility

Leta Houston Hickey

Name	Concentration*	Dosage	Indications	Side Effects†	Compatibility‡	Considerations	Mathematics*
Epinephrine	1:1000 = 1 mg/mL	0.05–1.0 μg/kg/min	Asystole Severe bradycardia	Tachycardia, hypertension, arrhythmias, tremors, decreased renal and splanchnic blood flow Ischemia and necrosis of tissue if IV infiltration occurs	D_5W, $D_{10}W$, NS, TPN, KCl, and heparin, with Y-site administration, amikacin, dopamine, dobutamine, isoproterenol. *Never give with bicarbonate. Incompatible* with intralipid, phenobarbital, pentobarbital, aminophylline, and hyaluronidase.	Never give through UAC or other artery. Do not retrograde anything into epinephrine line. Discard if brown or pink color observed. Attempt to correct any acidosis before infusion begins. Protect from light.	Multiply wt in kg ___ × 0.6 = mg/100 mL ___ mg ÷ 1 mg/mL = ___ ml/100 mL = 0.1 μg/kg/min @ 1 mL/hr
Lidocaine	2% = 20 mg/mL	*Initial bolus:* 0.5–1 mg/kg over 5 min *Continuous infusion:* 10–50 μg/kg/min	Ventricular tachycardia Ventricular arrhythmias	Hypotension, bradycardia, CNS effects (drowsiness, agitation, seizures), respiratory depression/arrest, arrhythmias, heart block, asystole	D_5W, $D_{10}W$, NS, TPN. Terminal injection site: KCl, aminophylline, heparin, calcium salts, digoxin, dobutamine, $NaHCO_3$. *Incompatible* with phenytoin.	Reconstitute with D_5W. Therapeutic serum levels are 1–5 μg/mL.	Multiply wt in kg ___ × 60 = mg/100 mL ___ ÷ 20 mg/mL = ___ ml/100 mL D_5W = 10 μg/kg/hr @ 1 mL/hr
Nitroglycerin	50 mg/10 mL = 5 mg/mL	0.2–6.0 μg/kg/min up to 10 μg/kg/min	Hypertension Congestive heart failure	Hypotension, bradycardia, tachycardia, restlessness	Furosemide, heparin, lidocaine, aminophylline. May be piggybacked with dopamine or dobutamine. *Incompatible* with phenytoin and hydralazine.	Mix with D_5W, or NS. Adsorbed onto plastic, therefore mix small amounts of q4h in a syringe. Do not use filters. Concentration should not exceed 0.4 mg/mL. Little information available on neonates.	Multiply wt in kg ___ × 6 = mg/100 mL ___ mg ÷ 5 mg/mL = ___ ml/100 mL = 1 μg/kg/min @ 1 mL/hr
Prostaglandin E₁ (alprostadil) (Prostin VR)	500 μg/mL = 0.5 mg/mL	0.05–0.1 μg/kg/min	Maintain patency of ductus arteriosus	Apnea, hypotension, hyperthermia, seizures, diarrhea, inhibition of platelet aggregation, flushing, bradycardia	D_5W, NS. Terminal injection site: aminophylline, gentamicin, dopamine, furosemide, KCl, and heparin.	Give through UAC only if absolutely necessary and if flow is not interrupted by obtaining lab specimens. Requires constant, patent IV access.	Multiply wt in kg ___ × 0.6 = mg/100 mL ___ mg ÷ 0.5 mg/mL = ___ mL/100 mL = 0.1 μg/kg/min @ 1 mL/hr

Drug	Concentration*	Dose	Indication	Side effects/toxicity†	Compatible solutions/incompatibilities‡	Comments	Calculation
Sodium bicarbonate (NaHCO₃)	4.2% = 0.5 mEq/mL	1–2 mEq/kg/hr	Metabolic acidosis	Local tissue necrosis, hypocalcemia, hypernatremia, IVH with rapid infusion	D₅W, D₁₀W, NS. *Precipitates* with calcium or phosphate; *Inactivates* epinephrine, norepinephrine, dobutamine, and dopamine.	If administered via UVC make sure of placement. Needs to be in right atrium or IVC.	Multiply wt in kg × $\dfrac{2}{1}$ = ___ mL/hr mEq/kg/hr
Sodium nitroprusside (Nipride)	50 mg/2 mL = 25 mg/mL	*Initial dose:* 0.25–0.5 μg/kg/min Usual maintenance dose: 3 μg/kg/min	Hypertension	Hypotension, decreased thyroid function, possible thiocyanate toxicity	Reconstitute with *D₅W or NS only.* Terminal injection site: aminophylline, dopamine, dobutamine, heparin, insulin, lidocaine, MSO₄, nitroglycerin, KCl, and pancuronium.	Monitor BP and HR continuously. Follow thiocyanate levels in patients with impaired renal function or who are on drug for >48 hr. Level should be <50 μg/mL. Administer via peripheral IV or central venous catheter. Always cover bag. Discard tubing after 24 hr.	Multiply wt in kg × ___ 60 = mg/100 mL D₅W ___ mg ÷ 25 mg/mL = ___ ml/100 mL = 10 μg/kg/min @ 1 mL/hr
Tolazoline (Priscoline)	100 mg/4 mL = 25 mg/mL	*Initial bolus:* 1–2 mg/kg over 10–20 min *Continuous infusion:* 0.5–2 mg/kg/hr	Persistent pulmonary hypertension	Severe hypotension, GI hemorrhage, oliguria, hematuria, tachycardia, flushing, pulmonary hemorrhage, diarrhea, vomiting, nausea, TCP	D₅W, D₁₀W, NS. Terminal injection site: dopamine, dobutamine, aminophylline, TPN, calcium gluconate, gentamicin, NaHCO₃, and vancomycin.	(CAUTION: decrease dose with oliguria)	Multiply wt in kg × ___ 100 = mg/100 mL ___ mg ÷ 25 mg/mL = ___ ml/100 mL = 1 mg/kg/hr @ 1 mL/hr

*Note concentration on vial. If different, the amount of mL of medication placed into the diluent will be different.
†Most common; not a complete list.
‡Not a complete list. Please consult a pharmacology text for more information.
BP, blood pressure; D₅W, 5% dextrose in water; D₁₀W, 10% dextrose in water; GI, gastrointestinal; HR, heart rate; IV, intravenous; IVC, inferior vena cava; IVH, intraventricular hemorrhage; KCl, potassium chloride; NS, normal saline; TCP, thrombocytopenia; TPN, total parenteral nutrition; UAC, umbilical artery catheter; UVC, umbilical vein catheter.

Blood Chemistry Values in Premature Infants During the First 7 Weeks of Life* (Birth Weight 1500–1750 g)

Constituent	Age 1 Week			Age 3 Weeks			Age 5 Weeks			Age 7 Weeks		
	Mean	SD	Range	Mean	SD	Range	Mean	SD	Range	Mean	SD	Range
Na (mEq/L)	139.6	±3.2	133–146	136.3	±2.9	129–142	136.8	±2.5	133–148	137.2	±1.8	133–142
K (mEq/L)	5.6	±0.5	4.6–6.7	5.8	±0.6	4.5–7.1	5.5	±0.6	4.5–6.6	5.7	±0.5	4.6–7.1
Cl (mEq/L)	108.2	±3.7	100–117	108.3	±3.9	102–116	107.0	±3.5	100–115	107.0	±3.3	101–115
CO_2 (mM/L)	20.3	±2.8	13.8–27.1	18.4	±3.5	12.4–26.2	20.4	±3.4	12.5–26.1	20.6	±3.1	13.7–26.9
Ca (mg/dL)	9.2	±1.1	6.1–11.6	9.6	±0.5	8.1–11.0	9.4	±0.5	8.6–10.5	9.5	±0.7	8.6–10.8
P (mg/dL)	7.6	±1.1	5.4–10.9	7.5	±0.7	6.2–8.7	7.0	±0.6	5.6–7.9	6.8	±0.8	4.2–8.2
BUN (mg/dL)	9.3	±5.2	3.1–25.5	13.3	±7.8	2.1–31.4	13.3	±7.1	2.0–26.5	13.4	±6.7	2.5–30.5
Total protein (g/dL)	5.49	±0.42	4.40–6.26	5.38	±0.48	4.28–6.70	4.98	±0.50	4.14–6.90	4.93	±0.61	4.02–5.86
Albumin (g/dL)	3.85	±0.30	3.28–4.50	3.92	±0.42	3.16–5.26	3.73	±0.34	3.20–4.34	3.89	±0.53	3.40–4.60
Globulin (g/dL)	1.58	±0.33	0.88–2.20	1.44	±0.63	0.62–2.90	1.17	±0.49	0.48–1.48	1.12	±0.33	0.5–2.60
Hb (g/dL)	17.8	±2.7	11.4–24.8	14.7	±2.1	9.0–19.4	11.5	±2.0	7.2–18.6	10.0	±1.3	7.5–13.9

*Adapted from Thomas J, Reichelderfer T: Premature infants: Analysis of serum during the first seven weeks. Clin Chem 14:272, 1968.

Other Serum Values

Ammonia (ng/dL)	Newborn	90–150
	0–2 wk	70–129
Cholesterol (ng/dL)	Full term	50–120
	1–2 y	70–190
Fatty acids, "free" (mEq/L)	Newborn	0–1845
Phenylalanine (ng/dL)	Newborn	Up to 4
Serum Enzymes		
Creatine phosphokinase (CPK) (U/L)	Premature	37.0–106.9
	3–12 wk	30.1–70.2
Lactate hydrogenase (U/L)	Birth	290–501
	1 d–1 mo	185–404
Aspartate aminotransferase (SGOT) (U/L)	Birth–10 d	6–25

Adapted from Meites S, ed: Pediatric Clinical Chemistry: A Survey of Normals, Methods and Instruments. Washington, DC: American Association for Clinical Chemistry, 1977.

Plasma-Serum Amino Acids in Premature and Term Newborns (μmol/L)

Amino Acid	Premature (First Day)	Newborn (Before First Feeding)	16 d–4 mo
Taurine	105–255	101–181	
OH-proline	0–80	0	
Aspartic acid	0–20	4–12	17–21
Threonine	155–275	196–238	141–213
Serine	195–345	129–197	104–158
Asp + Glut	655–1155	623–895	
Proline	155–305	155–305	141–245
Glutamic acid	30–100	27–77	
Glycine	185–735	274–412	178–248
Alanine	325–425	274–384	239–345
Valine	80–180	97–175	123–199
Cystine	55–75	49–75	33–51
Methionine	30–40	21–37	15–21
Isoleucine	20–60	31–47	31–47
Leucine	45–95	55–89	56–98
Tyrosine	20–220	53–85	33–75
Phenylalanine	70–110	64–92	45–65
Ornithine	70–110	66–116	37–61
Lysine	130–250	154–246	117–163
Histidine	30–70	61–93	64–92
Arginine	30–70	37–71	53–71
Tryptophan	15–45	15–45	
Citrulline	8.5–23.7	10.8–21.1	
Ethanolamine	13.4–10.5	32.7–72	
α-Amino-*n*-butyric acid	0–29	8.7–20.4	
Methylhistidine			

Data from Dickinson JC, Rosenblum H, Hamilton PB: Ion exchange chromatography of the free amino acids in the plasma of the newborn infant. Pediatrics 36:2, 1965, and Dickinson JC, Rosenblum H, Hamilton PB: Ion exchange chromotography of the free amino acids in the plasma of infants under 2,500 gm at birth. Pediatrics 45:606, 1970.

Source: Behrman RE: Neonatal-Perinatal Medicine: Diseases of the Fetus and Infant. 2nd ed. Table 20, Appendix. St. Louis: CV Mosby, 1977.

Reference Serum Amino Acid Concentrations That Have Been Proposed as Standards for Neonates (μmol/L)

Amino Acids	Term Infant Fed Human Milk	Cord Blood
Isoleucine	26–93	21–76
Leucine	53–169	47–120
Lysine	80–231	181–456
Methionine	22–50	8–42
Phenylalanine	22–71	24–87
Threonine	34–168	108–327
Tryptophan	18–101	19–98
Valine	88–222	98–276
Alanine	125–647	186–494
Arginine	42–148	28–162
Aspartic A	5–51	18 ± 17
Glutamic A	24–243	92 ± 57
Glycine	77–376	123–312
Histidine	34–119	42–136
Proline	82–319	72–278
Serine	0–326	57–174
Taurine	1–167	41–461
Tyrosine	38 119	34–83
Cystine	35–132	4–37

Modified from Hanning RM, Zlotkin SH: Amino acid and protein needs of the neonate: Effects of excess and deficiency. Semin Perinatol 13:131, 1989. See also Moro G, et al: Postprandial plasma amino acids in preterm infants: Influence of the protein source. Acta Paediatr 88:885–889, 1999.

Normal Hematologic Values

Value	Gestational Age (wk)		Full-Term Cord Blood	Day 1	Day 3	Day 7	Day 14
	28	*34*					
Hb (g/dL)	14.5	15.0	16.8	18.4	17.8	17.0	16.8
Hematocrit (%)	45	47	53	58	55	54	52
Red cells (mm³)	4.0	4.4	5.25	5.8	5.6	5.2	5.1
MCV (μ³)	120	118	107	108	99	98	96
MCH (pg)	40	38	34	35	33	32.5	31.5
MCHC (%)	31	32	31.7	32.5	33	33	33
Reticulocytes (%)	5–10	3–10	3–7	3–7	1–3	0–1	0–1
Platelets (1000s/mm³)			290	192	213	248	252

MCV, mean corpuscular volume; MCH, mean corpuscular hemoglobin; MCHC, mean corpuscular hemoglobin concentration.

Hematologic Values in the First Weeks of Life Related to Gestational Maturity

◆ MEAN CORPUSCULAR HEMOGLOBIN CONCENTRATION (PERCENT)*

Weeks	3 Days	1	2	3	4	6	8	10
<1500 g								
28–32 wk	32	32	32	33	33	33	33	32
1500–2000 g								
32–36 wk	32	32	32	33	33	33	33	32
2000–2500 g								
36–40 wk	32	32	33	33	33	33	33	33
>2500 g								
Term	32	33	33	33	33	33	33	33

*MCV and MCH, the mean corpuscular volume and mean corpuscular hemoglobin in μ^3 and pg, respectively, depend upon red cell counts that are not generally reliable.

◆ HEMOGLOBIN (g/dL)—MEAN ± [1 SD]

Weeks	3 Days	1	2	3	4	6	8	10
<1500 g	17.5	15.5	13.5	11.5	10.0	8.5	8.5	9.0
28–32 wk	[1.5]	[1.5]	[1.1]	[1.0]	[0.9]	[0.5]	[0.5]	[0.5]
1500–2000 g	19.0	16.5	14.5	13.0	12.0	9.5	9.5	9.5
32–36 wk	[2.0]	[1.5]	[1.1]	[1.1]	[1.0]	[0.8]	[0.5]	[0.5]
2000–2500 g	19.0	16.5	15.0	14.0	12.5	10.5	10.5	11.0
36–40 wk	[2.0]	[1.5]	[1.5]	[1.1]	[1.0]	[0.9]	[0.9]	[1.0]
>2500 g	19.0	17.0	15.5	14.0	12.5	11.0	11.5	12.0
Term	[2.0]	[1.5]	[1.5]	[1.1]	[1.0]	[1.0]	[1.0]	[1.0]

◆ HEMATOCRIT (PERCENT)—MEAN ± [1 SD]

Weeks	3 Days	1	2	3	4	6	8	10
<1500 g	54	48	42	35	30	25	25	28
28–32 wk	[5]	[5]	[4]	[4]	[3]	[2]	[2]	[3]
1500–2000 g	59	51	44	39	36	28	28	29
32–36 wk	[6]	[5]	[5]	[4]	[4]	[3]	[3]	[3]
2000–2500 g	59	51	45	43	37	31	31	33
36–40 wk	[6]	[5]	[5]	[4]	[4]	[3]	[3]	[3]
>2500 g	59	51	46	43	37	33	34	36
Term	[6]	[5]	[5]	[4]	[4]	[3]	[3]	[3]

◆ RETICULOCYTE COUNT (PERCENT)—MEAN ± [1 SD]

Weeks	3 Days	1	2	4	6	8	10
<1500 g	8.0	3.0	3.0	6.0	11.0	8.5	7.0
28–32 wk	[3.5]	[1.0]	[1.0]	[2.0]	[3.5]	[3.5]	[3.0]
1500–2000 g	6.0	3.0	2.5	3.0	6.0	5.0	4.5
32–36 wk	[2.0]	[1.0]	[1.0]	[1.0]	[2.0]	[1.5]	[1.5]
2000–2500 g	4.0	3.0	2.5	2.0	3.0	3.0	3.0
36–40 wk	[1.0]	[1.0]	[1.0]	[1.0]	[1.0]	[1.0]	[1.0]
>2500 g	4.0	3.0	2.0	2.0	2.0	2.0	2.0
Term	[1.5]	[1.0]	[1.0]	[1.0]	[0.5]	[0.5]	[0.5]

White Cell and Differential Counts in Premature Infants

Birth Weight	<1500 g			1500–2500 g		
Age in Weeks	1	2	4	1	2	4
Total count (× 10³/mm³)						
Mean	16.8	15.4	12.1	13.0	10.0	8.4
Range	6.1–32.8	10.4–21.3	8.7–17.2	6.7–14.7	7.0–14.1	5.8–12.4
Percent of Total						
Polymorphs						
Segmented	54	45	40	55	43	41
Unsegmented	7	6	5	8	8	6
Eosinophils	2	3	3	2	3	3
Basophils	1	1	1	1	1	1
Monocytes	6	10	10	5	9	11
Lymphocytes	30	35	41	9	36	38

Leukocyte Values and Neutrophil Counts in Term and Premature Infants

◆ LEUKOCYTE VALUES IN TERM AND PREMATURE INFANTS (10³ cells/μL)

Age (h)	Total White Cell Count	Neutrophils	Bands/Metas	Lymphocytes	Monocytes	Eosinophils
Term Infants						
0	10.0–26.0	5.0–13.0	0.4–1.8	3.5–8.5	0.7–1.5	0.2–2.0
12	13.5–31.0	9.0–18.0	0.4–2.0	3.0–7.0	1.0–2.0	0.2–2.0
72	5.0–14.5	2.0–7.0	0.2–0.4	2.0–5.0	0.5–1.0	0.2–1.0
144	6.0–14.5	2.0–6.0	0.2–0.5	3.0–6.0	0.7–1.2	0.2–0.8
Premature Infants						
0	5.0–19.0	2.0–9.0	0.2–2.4	2.5–6.0	0.3–1.0	0.1–0.7
12	5.0–21.0	3.0–11.0	0.2–2.4	1.5–5.0	0.3–1.3	0.1–1.1
72	5.0–14.0	3.0–7.0	0.2–0.6	1.5–4.0	0.3–1.2	0.2–1.1
144	5.5–17.5	2.0–7.0	0.2–0.5	2.5–7.5	0.5–1.5	0.3–1.2

From Oski F, Naiman J: Hematologic Problems in the Newborn. Philadelphia: WB Saunders, 1982.

◆ TOTAL NEUTROPHIL COUNT REFERENCE RANGE IN THE FIRST 60 HOURS OF LIFE*

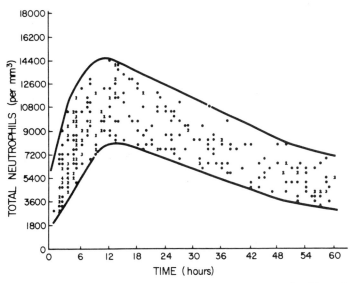

*Manroe BL, Weinberg AG, Rosenfeld CR, et al: The neonatal blood count in health and disease. I. Reference values for neutrophilic cells. J Pediatr 95:91, 1979.

Urine Amino Acids in Normal Newborns (μmol/d)

Amino Acid	μmol/d
Cysteic acid	Tr–3.32
Phosphoethanolamine	Tr–8.86
Taurine	7.59–7.72
OH-proline	0–9.81
Aspartic acid	Tr
Threonine	0.176–7.99
Serine	Tr–20.7
Glutamic acid	0–1.78
Proline	0–5.17
Glycine	0.176–65.3
Alanine	Tr–8.03
α-Aminoadipic acid	
α-Amino-*n*-butyric acid	0–0.47
Valine	0–7.76
Cystine	0–7.96
Methionine	Tᵣ–0.892
Isoleucine	0–6.11
Tyrosine	0–1.11
Phenylalanine	0–1.66
β-Aminoisobutyric acid	0.264–7.34
Ethanolamine	Tr–79.9
Ornithine	Tr–0.554
Lysine	0.33–9.79
1-Methylhistidine	Tr–8.64
3-Methylhistidine	0.11–3.32
Carnosine	0.044–4.01
β-Aminobutyric acid	
Cystathionine	
Homocitrulline	
Arginine	0.088–0.918
Histidine	Tr–7.04
Sarcosine	
Leucine	Tr–0.918

Adapted from Meites S, ed: Pediatric Clinical Chemistry: A Survey of Normals, Methods and Instruments. Washington, DC: American Association for Clinical Chemistry, 1997.

Source: Fanaroff AA, Martin RJ, eds: Neonatal-Perinatal Medicine, Diseases of the Fetus and Infant. 6th ed. Table B-13. St. Louis: CV Mosby, 1997.

Siggaard-Anderson Alignment Nomogram

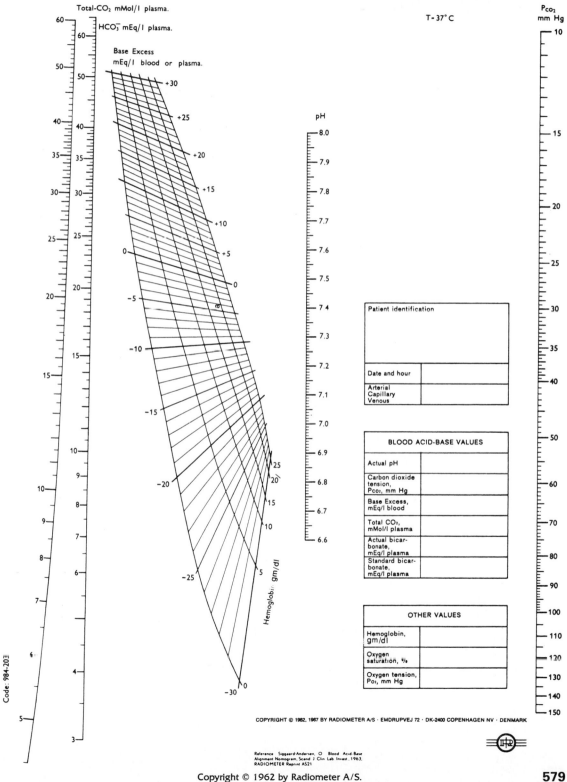

T-37°C

Total-CO₂ mMol/l plasma.

HCO₃⁻ mEq/l plasma.

Base Excess
mEq/l blood or plasma.

pH

Hemoglobin gm/dl

Pco₂
mm Hg

Patient identification

Date and hour	
Arterial Capillary Venous	

BLOOD ACID-BASE VALUES	
Actual pH	
Carbon dioxide tension, Pco₂, mm Hg	
Base Excess, mEq/l blood	
Total CO₂, mMol/l plasma	
Actual bicarbonate, mEq/l plasma	
Standard bicarbonate, mEq/l plasma	

OTHER VALUES	
Hemoglobin, gm/dl	
Oxygen saturation, %	
Oxygen tension, Po₂, mm Hg	

Code: 984-203

Reference: Siggaard-Andersen, O. Blood Acid-Base
Alignment Nomogram, Scand J Clin Lab Invest, 1963.
RADIOMETER Reprint AS21

579

Cerebrospinal Fluid Findings in Term and Premature Infants

◆ CEREBROSPINAL FLUID EXAMINATION IN HIGH-RISK NEONATES WITHOUT MENINGITIS

	Term	Preterm
WBC count (cells/mm³)		
No. of Infants	87	30
Mean	8.2	9.0
Median	5	6
SD	7.1	8.2
Range	0–32	0–29
± 2 SD	0–22.4	0–25.4
Percentage PMN	61.3%	57.2%
Protein (mg/dL)		
No. of Infants	35	17
Mean	90	115
Range	20–170	65–150
Glucose (mg/dL)		
No. of infants	51	23
Mean	52	50
Range	34–119	24–63
CSF/blood glucose (%)		
No. of infants	51	23
Mean	81	74
Range	44–248	55–105

PMN, polymorphonuclear cells; CSF, cerebrospinal fluid.
Adapted from Sarff L, Platt L, McCracken G: Cerebrospinal fluid evaluation in neonates: Comparison of high risk infants with and without meningitis. J Pediatr 88:473, 1976.

◆ CEREBROSPINAL FLUID FINDINGS IN FIRST 24 HOURS OF LIFE IN 135 FULL-TERM INFANTS

	Range	Mean	2 SD
Red blood cells	0–1070	9	0–884
Polymorphs	0–70	3	0–27
Lymphocytes	0–20	2	0–24
Protein	32–240	63	27–144
Sugar	32–78	51	35–64
Chloride	680–760	720	660–780

From Naidoo T: The cerebrospinal fluid in the healthy newborn infant. South Afr Med J 42:933, 1968.

◆ CEREBROSPINAL FLUID FINDINGS ON FIRST AND SEVENTH DAYS IN FULL-TERM INFANTS

	Day 1 (n = 135)		Day 7 (n = 20)	
	Range	*Mean*	*Range*	*Mean*
Red blood cells	0–620	23	0–48	3
Polymorphs	0–26	7	0–5	2
Lymphocytes	0–16	5	0–4	1
Protein	40–148	73	27–65	47
Sugar	38–64	48	48–62	55
Chloride	680–760	720	720–760	720

From Naidoo T: The cerebrospinal fluid in the healthy newborn infant. South Afr Med J 42:933, 1968.

◆ CEREBROSPINAL FLUID VALUES OF HEALTHY TERM NEWBORNS

	Age			
	0–24 Hours	*1 Day*	*7 Days*	*>7 Days*
Color	Clear or xanthochromic	Clear or xanthochromic	Clear or xanthochromic	
Red blood cells/mm³	9 (0–1070)	23 (6–630)	3 (0–48)	
Polymorphonuclear leukocytes/mm³	3 (0–70)	7 (0–26)	2 (0–5)	
Lymphocytes/mm³	2 (0–20)	5 (0–16)	1 (0–4)	
Protein (mg/dL)	63 (32–240)	73 (40–148)	47 (27–65)	
Glucose (mg/dL)	51 (32–78)	48 (38–64)	55 (48–62)	
Lactate dehydrogenase (IU/L)	22–73	22–73	22–73	0–40

Modified from Naidoo BT: The cerebrospinal fluid in the healthy newborn infant. S Afr Med J 42:933, 1968, and Neches W, Platt M: Cerebrospinal fluid LDH in 287 chilidren, including 53 cases of meningitis of bacterial and nonbacterial etiology. Pediatrics 41:1097, 1968.

◆ CEREBROSPINAL FLUID VALUES IN VERY LOW-BIRTH-WEIGHT INFANTS ON BASIS OF BIRTH WEIGHT

	≤1000 g		1001–1500 g	
	Mean ± SD	*Range*	*Mean ± SD*	*Range*
Birth weight (g)	763 ± 115	550–980	1278 ± 152	1020–1500
Gestational age (wk)	26 ± 1.3	24–28	29 ± 1.4	27–33
Leukocytes/mm³	4 ± 3	0–14	6 ± 9	0–44
Erythrocytes/mm³	1027 ± 3270	0–19,050	786 ± 1879	0–9750
PMN leukocytes (%)	6 ± 15	0–66	9 ± 17	0–60
MN leukocytes (%)	86 ± 30	34–100	85 ± 28	13–100
Glucose (mg/dL)	61 ± 34	29–217	59 ± 21	31–109
Protein (mg/dL)	150 ± 56	95–370	132 ± 43	45–227

PMN, polymorphonuclear; MN, mononuclear.
Modified from Rodriguez AF, Kaplan SL, Mason EO: Cerebrospinal fluid values in the very low birth weight infant. J Pediatr 116:971, 1990.

Comparison of WBC Counts in Neonates With and Without Meningitis

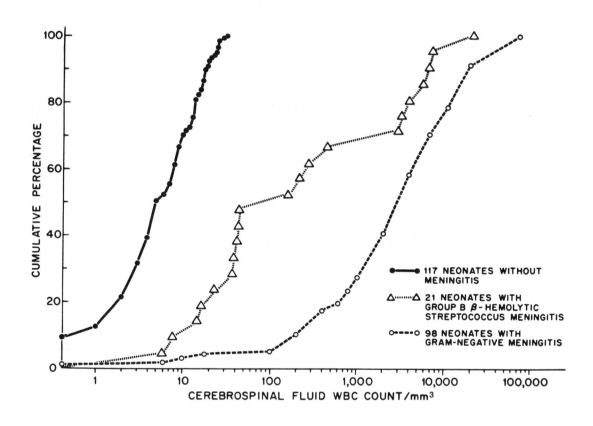

Fetal Growth Curves for Trimmed and Raw Data

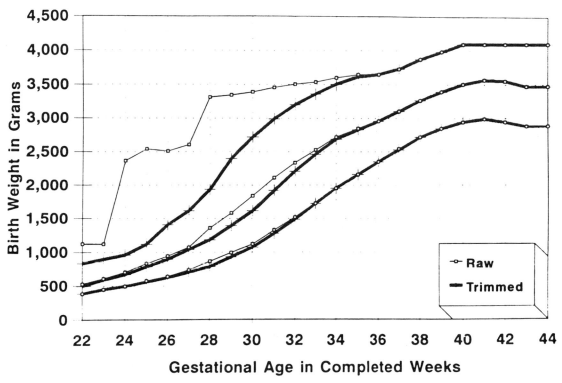

From Alexander GR, et al: A United States reference for fetal growth. Obstet Gynecol 87:163, 1996.

Fetal Growth by Selected References

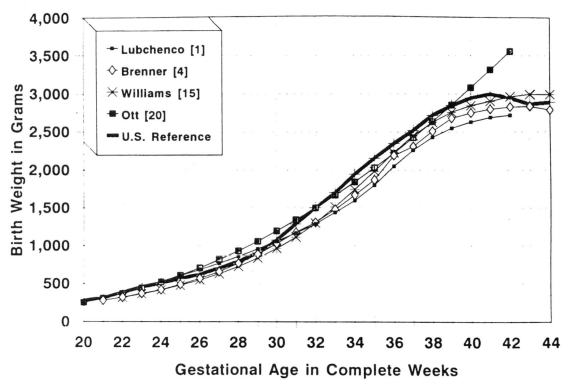

From Alexander GR, et al: A United States reference for fetal growth. Obstet Gynecol 87:163, 1996.

Smoothed Percentiles of Birth Weight (g) for Gestational Age: US 1991 Single Live Births to Resident Mothers

Gestational age (wk)	Percentile				
	5th	*10th*	*50th*	*90th*	*95th*
20	249	275	412	772	912
21	280	314	433	790	957
22	330	376	496	826	1023
23	385	440	582	882	1107
24	435	498	674	977	1223
25	480	558	779	1138	1397
26	529	625	899	1362	1640
27	591	702	1035	1635	1927
28	670	798	1196	1977	2237
29	772	925	1394	2361	2553
30	910	1085	1637	2710	2847
31	1088	1278	1918	2986	3108
32	1294	1495	2203	3200	3338
33	1513	1725	2458	3370	3536
34	1735	1950	2667	3502	3697
35	1950	2159	2831	3596	3812
36	2156	2354	2974	3668	3888
37	2357	2541	3117	3755	3956
38	2543	2714	3263	3867	4027
39	2685	2852	3400	3980	4107
40	2761	2929	3495	4060	4185
41	2777	2948	3527	4094	4217
42	2764	2935	3522	4098	4213
43	2741	2907	3505	4096	4178
44	2724	2885	3491	4096	4122

From Alexander GR, et al: A United States reference for fetal growth. Obstet Gynecol 87:163, 1996.

Growth Record for Infants

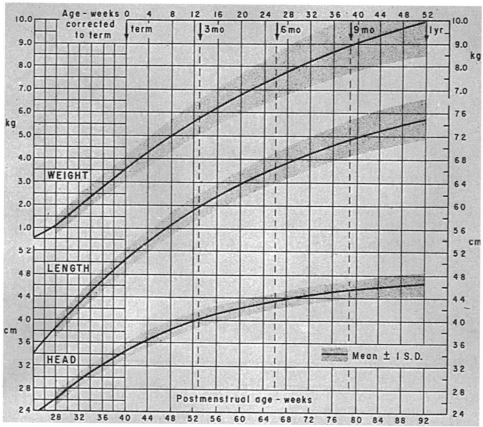

Growth record for infants in relation to gestational age and fetal and infant norms (combined sexes), University of Oregon. (From Babson S: Growth of low-birthweight infants. J Pediatr 77:11, 1970.)

Head Circumference

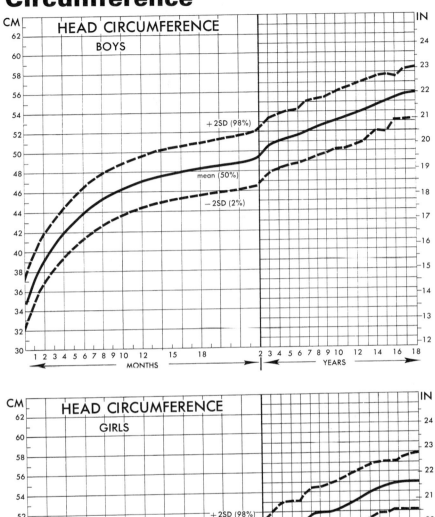

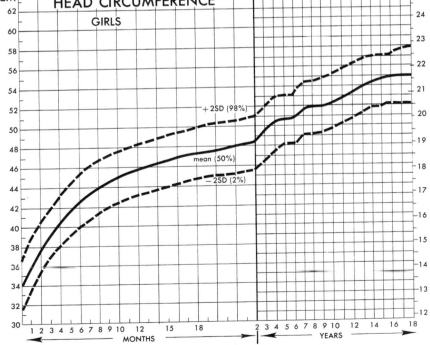

From Nellhaus G: Composite international and interracial graphs. Pediatrics 41:106, 1968. Reproduced by permission of Pediatrics.

Intrauterine Growth Curves

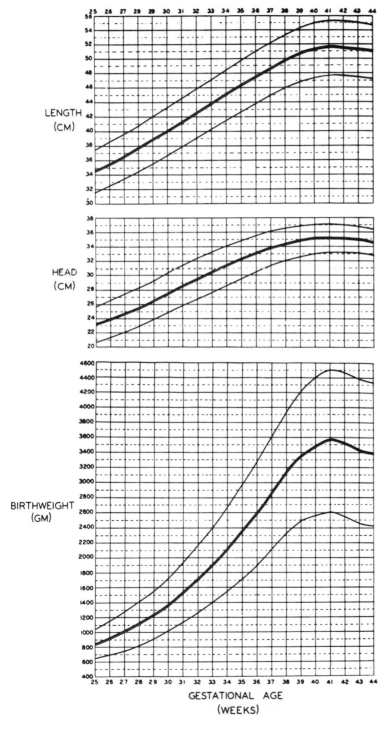

Intrauterine growth curves for length, head circumference, and weight for singleton white infants born at sea level (mean ± 2 standard deviations). (Composite of graphs from Usher R, McLean F: Intrauterine growth of liveborn Caucasian infants at sea level: Standard obtained in 7 dimensions of infants born between 25 and 44 weeks of gestation. J Pediatr 74:901, 1969.)

Low-Birth-Weight Infants Daily Growth—Weight

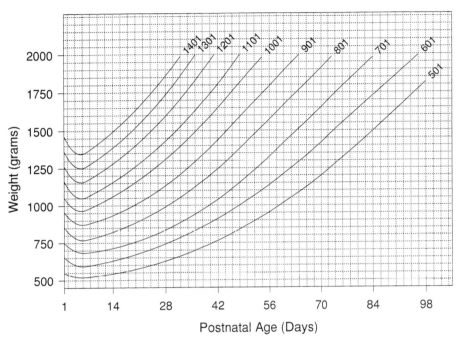

Average daily body weight versus postnatal age in days for infants stratified by 100-g birth weight intervals. (From Ehrenkranze RA, et al: Longitudinal growth of hospitalized very low birth weight infants. Pediatrics 104:280, 1999.)

Low-Birth-Weight Infants Weekly Growth—Head Circumference

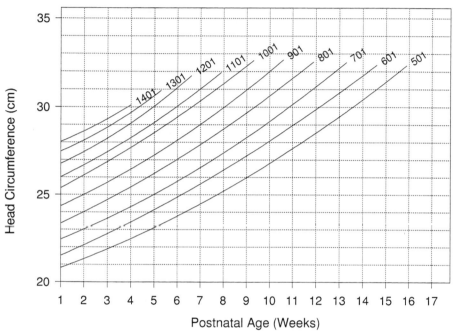

Average weekly head circumference versus postnatal age in weeks for infants stratified by 100-g birth weight intervals. (From Ehrenkranze RA, et al: Longitudinal growth of hospitalized very low birth weight infants. Pediatrics 104:280, 1999.)

Low-Birth-Weight Infants Growth Curves, With and Without Major Morbidities

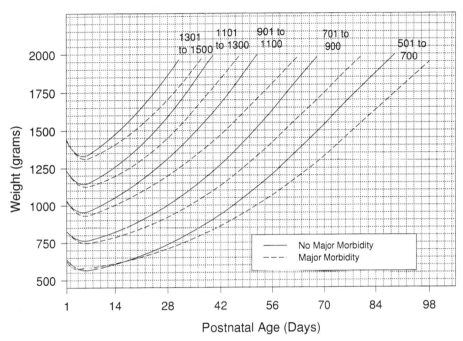

Growth curves of infants with major morbidities *(dashed lines)* and of reference infants without major morbidities *(solid line)* plotted by postnatal age in days. The infants are stratified by 200-g birth weight intervals. Reference infants without major morbidities were appropriate for gestational age and survived to discharge without development of chronic lung disease, severe intraventricular hemorrhage, necrotizing enterocolitis, or late onset sepsis. (From Ehrenkranze RA, et al: Longitudinal growth of hospitalized very low birth weight infants. Pediatrics 104:280, 1999.)

Time of First Void and Stool

Time of 1st Voiding by 920 Full-Term Infants			
Time	No.	Percent	Cumulative %
Delivery room	139	15.1	15.1
Hours			
1–24	743	80.8	95.9
24–48	35	3.8	99.7
>48	3	0.3	100.0

Time of Passage of 1st Stool by 920 Full-Term Infants			
Time	No.	Percent	Cumulative %
Delivery room	210	22.8	22.8
Hours			
1–24	674	73.3	96.1
24–48	35	3.8	99.9
>48	1	0.1	100.0

Time of Passage of 1st Urine by 280 Premature Infants			
Time	No.	Percent	Cumulative %
Delivery room	62	22.1	22.1
Hours			
1–24	201	71.8	93.9
24–48	17	6.1	100.0
>48			

Time of Passage of 1st Stool by 280 Premature Infants			
Time	No.	Percent	Cumulative %
Delivery room	30	10.7	10.7
Hours			
1–24	191	68.2	78.9
24–48	46	16.4	95.3
>48	13	4.7	100.0

Adapted from Sherry S, Kramer I: The time of passage of the first stool and first urine by the newborn infant. J Pediatr 46:158, 1955; Kramer I, Sherry S: The time of passage of the first stool and urine by the premature infant. J Pediatr 51:353, 1957; and Clark D: Times of first void and stool in 500 newborns. Pediatrics 60:457, 1977. Reproduced by permission of Pediatrics.

Mean Arterial Blood Pressure by Birth Weight

◆ **OSCILLOMETRIC MEASUREMENTS: Mean Arterial Blood Pressure**

Birth Weight	Mean MAP ± SD		
	Day 3	Day 17	Day 31
501–750 g	38 ± 8	44 ± 8	46 ± 11
751–1000 g	43 ± 9	45 ± 7	47 ± 9
1001–1250 g	43 ± 8	46 ± 9	48 ± 8
1251–1500 g	45 ± 8	47 ± 8	47 ± 9

From Fanaroff AA, Wright E for the NICHD Neonatal Research Network, Bethesda, MD: Profiles of mean arterial blood pressure (MAP) for infants weighing 50–1500 grams. Pediatr Res 27:205A, 1990.

Blood Pressure by Age and Gestational Age

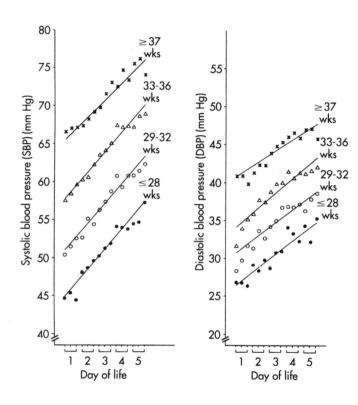

Systolic blood pressure and diastolic blood pressure are plotted for first 5 days of life, with each day subdivided into 8-hour periods. Infants are categorized by gestational age into four groups: ≤28 weeks (n = 33), 29 to 32 weeks (n = 73), 33 to 36 weeks (n = 100), and ≥37 weeks (n = 110). (From Zubrow AB, Hulman S, Kushner H, Falkner B: Determinants of blood pressure in infants admitted to neonatal intensive care units: A prospective multicenter study. Philadelphia Neonatal Blood Pressure Study Group. J Perinatol 15:470, 1995.)

Blood Pressure by Age

Blood pressure ranges in premature infants over first week of life. (From Hegyi T, Anwar M, Carbone MT, et al: Blood pressure ranges in premature infants: II. The first week of life. Pediatrics 97:336, 1996.)

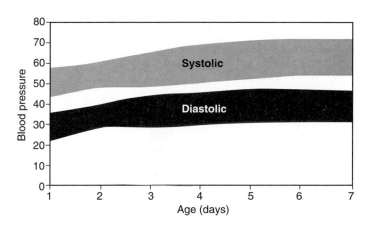

Percent Mortality and Major Morbidity by Birth Weight

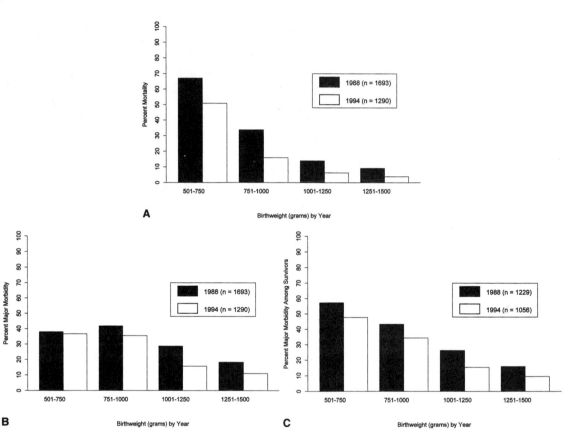

A, Mortality rate for very low-birth-weight infants cared for in National Institute of Child Health and Human Development Neonatal Research Network Centers (n = 5) in 1988 and 1994 by 250-g birth weight intervals. *B,* Major morbidity for all very low-birth-weight infants cared for in National Institute of Child Health and Human Development Neonatal Research Network Centers (n = 5) in 1988 and 1994 by 250-g birth weight intervals, including severe intracranial hemorrhage, chronic lung disease, and confirmed necrotizing enterocolitis. *C,* Major morbidity among very low-birth-weight infant survivors cared for in the National Institute of Child Health and Human Development Neonatal Research Network (n = 5) in 1988 and 1994 by 250-g birth weight intervals, including severe intracranial hemorrhage, chronic lung disease, and confirmed necrotizing enterocolitis. (From Stevenson DK, Wright LL, Lemons JA, et al: Very low birthweight outcomes of the National Institute of Child Health and Human Development Neonatal Research Network, January 1993 through December 1994. Am J Obstet Gynecol 179:1632–1639, 1998.)

Mortality Risk by Birth Weight and Gestational Age

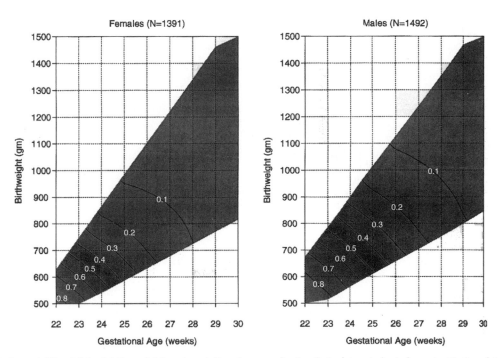

Estimated mortality risk by birth weight and gestational age on basis of singleton infants born in National Institute of Child Health and Human Development Neonatal Research Network Centers between January 1, 1993, and December 31, 1994. (From Stevenson DK, Wright LL, Lemons JA, et al: Very low birthweight outcomes of the National Institute of Child Health and Human Development Neonatal Research Network, January 1993 through December 1994. Am J Obstet Gynecol 179:1632–1639, 1998.)

Equipment Found on the Umbilical Catheterization Tray, University Hospitals, Cleveland, Ohio

2 2-mL Luer-Lok syringes
1 Small needle holder
2 Curved mosquito hemostats
1 Straight iris scissors
2 Straight mosquito hemostats
1 Straight suture scissors
1 Smooth straight iris forceps
2 Smooth deep-curved iris forceps
1 Medium glass
2 Cord ties (10 in long)
2 3-way stopcocks
4 3 × 3 inch gauze sponges
1 Size 5–0 silk suture set with needle (#682)
1 Eye treatment sheet
2 Needle caps

Umbilical Vessel Catheterization

Ricardo J. Rodriguez

Use of central catheters requires careful consideration of the risks involved. The relatively easy accessibility to the umbilical vessels makes these vessels a very good option for central access in emergency situations. A central catheter inserted into the aorta via an umbilical artery may be required in the management of the sick neonate for monitoring of blood pressure, intermittent blood sampling to monitor acid-base status, and, while in place, infusion of parenteral fluids and medications.

Umbilical artery catheters must be precisely located. A major objective is to avoid the origin of the renal arteries, because a catheter may occlude a renal artery and catheters in the area may produce thrombosis.[4] Both situations can result in renal infarction. Our preference is to position the catheter in the midthoracic aorta (high); others prefer the location of the catheter tip between L3 and L4 (low). Thrombotic complications are reported with both high and low placement.[9] Resolution of the thrombus or development of collateral circulation generally occurs, even when extensive thrombosis (aorta distal to renal arteries, common iliac) has been documented.[3, 4] Occasionally a neonatal death is considered a direct consequence of complications related to umbilical vessel catheterization.[8] Hypertension in the neonate following use of high umbilical artery catheters has been described. However, in a prospective study, the incidence of hypertension was similar with low and high catheters.[6]

Hemorrhage, as a result of loose connections or careless use of the stopcocks, or occurring at the time of removal, is a major complication of arterial catheters. Another major complication is thrombus formation with release of microemboli to the systemic circulation. It is speculated that the catheter tip can traumatize the vessel wall, which may release tissue thromboplastin and activate intravascular coagulation. Alternatively, the presence of the catheter itself may produce clot formation. More rare complications include intimal flap formation and aneurysmatic dilatation of the abdominal artery. Ultrasonographic examination of the abdominal aorta and its branches is indicated when any of these complications is suspected.

Arterial blood samples may be obtained by multiple arterial punctures (i.e., radial artery) or an indwelling radial artery cannula as the method of choice or when umbilical artery catheterization is unsuccessful.[1, 7]

In general, umbilical vein catheterization is technically easier. However, it should be avoided except when immediate access to a vein is needed for an unexpected emergency (delivery room resuscitation), because complications may be serious and difficult to avoid. An umbilical vein catheter tip may locate in a branch of the portal vein and lead to areas of liver necrosis without perforation of the vein wall following infusions of hypertonic solutions, such as sodium bicarbonate and hypertonic glucose. Portal vein thrombosis and aseptic abscess formation have also occurred with and without infection. In addition, spontaneous perforation of the colon following exchange transfusion via an umbilical vein catheter has been reported. X-ray verification of catheter tip location was not done in any of these cases; most likely, the catheter tip was in the portal vein, and the cause of perforation was local necrosis of bowel wall following hemorrhagic infarction as a result of retrograde microemboli or obstructive hemodynamic changes. A more rare complication, air embolism in the portal system, has also been observed.

In the first hour or so of life in a normal term infant, or for many hours and occasionally for many days in a sick or preterm infant, an umbilical venous catheter may be passed through the ductus venosus into the inferior vena cava.

Depending on the circumstances and preference of the physician, exchange transfusions can be done using either vessel or both, but not infusing into the artery.

The umbilical vessel catheter should be removed as soon as possible and a peripheral intravenous line substituted, if necessary. In the undistressed newborn infant requiring parenteral fluids, under no circumstances should an umbilical vessel catheter be used when a peripheral intravenous line could be started via a scalp vein or an extremity vein. In the extremely low-birth-weight group, in whom parenteral nutrition is essential until enteral feeds are established, we routinely place percutaneous indwelling central catheters and remove umbilical lines as soon as possible.

◆ TECHNIQUE OF CATHETERIZATION

In the small premature infant, the entire procedure should be done as an operating room procedure in an incubator or under a radiant warmer to prevent hypothermia. In the delivery room, a radiant heater should be used.

When not precluded by an emergency (e.g., acute asphyxia), the following protocol should be followed. The operator carefully scrubs hands and arms to the elbows and puts on sterile gloves. A 3.5–4 (for infants weighing less than 1500 g) or a 5 French catheter with rounded tip, which has a radiopaque line and end hole (Argyle umbilical artery catheter) is attached to a syringe by a three-way stopcock. The system is filled with heparinized saline solution (1 unit heparin/mL of normal or ½ normal saline). (Appendix I–1 lists the equipment found on the catheterization tray.) Before the procedure is begun, the length of the catheter to be inserted should be marked according to the location desired (Figs. I–1 and I–2). After the umbilical stump and surrounding abdominal wall are carefully prepared with an antiseptic solution, sterile towels are placed around the stump and a circumcision drape is placed with the hole over the stump. The base of the cord is then loosely tied with umbilical tape taking care to avoid the skin. The cord stump is then grasped and cut perpendicular to its axis to within about 1.5 cm of the abdominal wall with a surgical blade. The exposed vessels are identified—a thin-walled oval vein and two smaller thick-walled round arteries with tightly constricted lumens. Occasionally, only one artery may be present. The cord is stabilized by grasping the Wharton's jelly with one or two Kelly clamps.

The lumen of the vessel to be used is gently dilated with a curved iris dressing forceps or small obturator (Fig. I–3A and B). The catheter is then inserted and gently advanced. Obstruction at the level of the abdominal wall may be relieved by gentle traction on the umbilical cord stump accompanied by steady but gentle pressure for about 30 seconds. During umbilical artery catheterization, obstruction may also occur at the level of the bladder. It may be overcome by gentle, steady pressure for 30 seconds. Alternatively, marked resistance could be found where the umbilical artery meets the internal iliac artery (usually at 5 cm). The operator should avoid applying undue pressure to overcome this point of resistance because of the possibility of perforation of the vessel and severe hemorrhage. If continued resistance is met, the other artery should be used. If at any point during or after the line placement persistent blanching or cyanosis of the ipsi- or contralateral extremity is observed, the catheter should be promptly removed. Cyanosis involving toes or part of the foot on the side of the catheter may be relieved by warming the contralateral foot; when this is not successful, the catheter should be removed. Both lower extremities and buttocks should be carefully watched for alterations in blood supply when an umibical artery catheter is in place.

If an umbilical vein catheterization is performed, the next site of obstruction after the abdominal wall is the portal system. (The catheter meets resistance several centimeters before the distance marked on the catheter is reached.) The catheter should be withdrawn several centimeters, gently rotated, and reinserted in an attempt to get the tip through the ductus venosus into the inferior vena cava. Gentle application of caudal traction of the umbilical cord stump sometimes facilitates the introduction of an umbilical venous line. Occasionally it is not possible to get the catheter into the inferior vena cava for anatomic reasons, and vigorous attempts to advance the catheter are to be avoided.

An umbilical vessel catheter should be

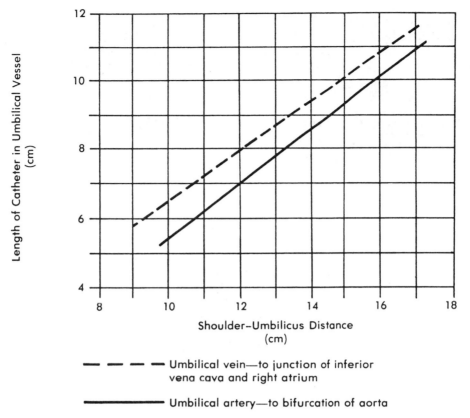

Figure I–1. Determination of length of catheter to be inserted for appropriate arterial or venous placement. The length of the catheter read from the diagram is to the umbilical ring; the length of the umbilical cord stump present must be added. The shoulder-umbilicus distance is the perpendicular distance between parallel lines at the level of the umbilicus and through the distal ends of the clavicles. (Adapted from data of Dunn P: Localization of the umbilical catheter by post-mortem measurement. Arch Dis Child 41:69, 1966.)

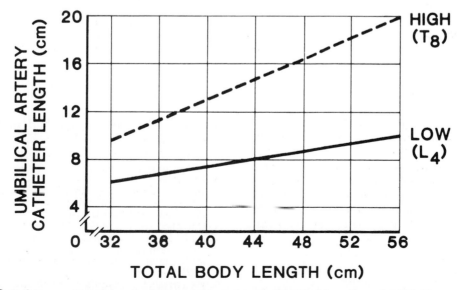

Figure I–2. Catheter position determined from total body length. (Modified from Rosenfield W, Biagtan J, Schaeffer H, et al: A new graph for insertion of umbilical artery catheters. J Pediatr 96:735, 1980.)

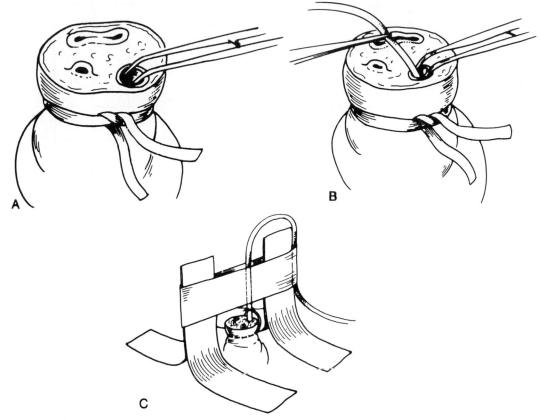

Figure I–3. *A*, Cross section of umbilical cord. Tie in place. Dilatation of artery with iris forceps. *B*, Insertion of catheter into umbilical artery. *C*, Bridge technique used to secure catheter after suturing. Use purse string suture incorporating all three vessels. Tie square knot at the base of the catheter and a second knot 1 cm above the base. The tape bridge further ensures against the line becoming dislodged.

tied in place with a silk suture around the vessel and catheter and sutured to the umbilical stump or taped to the abdominal wall. Disastrous hemorrhage can occur if the catheter is inadvertently pulled out or the stopcocks are disconnected by the activity of the infant. The position of the catheter must be identified by x-ray immediately after insertion.

If the x-ray film obtained following umbilical vessel catheterization indicates that the catheter has been inserted too far, it may be gently withdrawn an estimated amount for appropriate placement. If the catheter is not in far enough, it must be completely withdrawn and a new sterile one inserted after appropriately preparing the area again.

REFERENCES

1. Adams J, Rudolph A: The use of indwelling radial artery catheters in neonates. Pediatrics 55:261, 1975.
2. Dunn P: Localization of the umbilical catheter by post-mortem measurements. Arch Dis Child 41:69, 1966.
3. Goetzman B, Stadalnik R, Bogren H, et al: Thrombotic complications of umbilical artery catheters: a clinical and radiographic study. Pediatrics 56:374, 1975.
4. Oppenheimer D, Carroll B, Garth K: Ultrasonic detection of complications following umbilical arterial catheterization in the neonate. Radiology 145:667, 1982.
5. Rosenfeld W, Biagtan J, Schaeffer H, et al: A new graph for insertion of umbilical artery catheters. J Pediatr 96:735, 1980.
6. Stork E, Carlo W, Kliegman R, et al: Neonatal hypertension appears unrelated to aortic catheter position. Pediatr Res 18:321A, 1984.
7. Todres I, Rogers M, Shannon C, et al: Percutaneous catheterization of the radial artery in the critically ill neonate. J Pediatr 87:273, 1975.
8. Umbilical Artery Catheter Trial Study Group: Relationship of intraventricular hemorrhage or death with the level of umbilical artery placement: A multicenter randomized trial. Pediatrics 90:881, 1992.
9. Wesstrom G, Finnstrom O, Stenport G: Umbilical artery catheterization in newborns. I. Thrombosis in relation to catheter type and position. Acta Paediatr Scand 68:575, 1979.

Conversion of Pounds and Ounces to Grams

Pounds								Ounces								
	0	1	2	3	4	5	6	7	8	9	10	11	12	13	14	15
0	—	28	57	85	113	142	170	198	227	255	283	312	340	369	397	425
1	454	482	510	539	567	595	624	652	680	709	737	765	794	822	850	879
2	907	936	964	992	1021	1049	1077	1106	1134	1162	1191	1219	1247	1276	1304	1332
3	1361	1389	1417	1446	1474	1503	1531	1559	1588	1616	1644	1673	1701	1729	1758	1786
4	1814	1843	1871	1899	1928	1956	1984	2013	2041	2070	2098	2126	2155	2183	2211	2240
5	2268	2296	2325	2353	2381	2410	2438	2466	2495	2523	2551	2580	2608	2637	2665	2693
6	2722	2750	2778	2807	2835	2863	2892	2920	2948	2977	3005	3033	3062	3090	3118	3147
7	3175	3203	3232	3260	3289	3317	3345	3374	3402	3430	3459	3487	3515	3544	3572	3600
8	3629	3657	3685	3714	3742	3770	3799	3827	3856	3884	3912	3941	3969	3997	4026	4054
9	4082	4111	4139	4167	4196	4224	4252	4281	4309	4337	4366	4394	4423	4451	4479	4508
10	4536	4564	4593	4621	4649	4678	4706	4734	4763	4791	4819	4848	4876	4904	4933	4961
11	4990	5018	5046	5075	5103	5131	5160	5188	5216	5245	5273	5301	5330	5358	5386	5415
12	5443	5471	5500	5528	5557	5585	5613	5642	5670	5698	5727	5755	5783	5812	5840	5868
13	5897	5925	5953	5982	6010	6038	6067	6095	6123	6152	6180	6209	6237	6265	6294	6322
14	6350	6379	6407	6435	6464	6492	6520	6549	6577	6605	6634	6662	6690	6719	6747	6776
15	6804	6832	6860	6889	6917	6945	6973	7002	7030	7059	7087	7115	7144	7172	7201	7228
16	7257	7286	7313	7342	7371	7399	7427	7456	7484	7512	7541	7569	7597	7626	7654	7682
17	7711	7739	7768	7796	7824	7853	7881	7909	7938	7966	7994	8023	8051	8079	8108	8136
18	8165	8192	8221	8249	8278	8306	8335	8363	8391	8420	8448	8476	8504	8533	8561	8590
19	8618	8646	8675	8703	8731	8760	8788	8816	8845	8873	8902	8930	8958	8987	9015	9043
20	9072	9100	9128	9157	9185	9213	9242	9270	9298	9327	9355	9383	9412	9440	9469	9497
21	9525	9554	9582	9610	9639	9667	9695	9724	9752	9780	9809	9837	9865	9894	9922	9950
22	9979	10007	10036	10064	10092	10120	10149	10177	10206	10234	10262	10291	10319	10347	10376	10404

Conversion Table to Standard International (SI) Units

Component	Present Unit	×	Conversion Factor	=	SI Unit
Clinical Hematology					
Erythrocytes	per mm³		1		10^6/L
Hematocrit	%		0.01		(1)vol RBC/vol whole blood
Hemoglobin	g/dL		10		g/L
Leukocytes	per mm³		1		10^6/L
Mean corpuscular hemoglobin concentration (MCHC)	g/dL		10		g/L
Mean corpuscular volume (MCV)	μm³		1		fL
Platelet count	10^3/mm³		1		10^9/L
Reticulocyte count	%		10		10^{-3}
Clinical Chemistry					
Acetone	mg/dL		0.1722		mmol/L
Albumin	g/dL		10		g/L
Aldosterone	ng/dL		27.74		pmol/L
Ammonia (as nitrogen)	μg/dL		0.7139		μmol/L
Bicarbonate	mEq/L		1		mmol/L
Bilirubin	mg/dL		17.1		μmol/L
Calcium	mg/dL		0.2495		mmol/L
Calcium ion	mEq/L		0.50		mmol/L
Carotenes	μg/dL		0.01836		μmol/L
Ceruloplasmin	mg/dL		10.0		mg/L
Chloride	mEq/L		1		mmol/L
Cholesterol	mg/dL		0.02586		mmol/L
Complement, C_3 or C_4	mg/dL		0.01		g/L
Copper	μg/dL		0.1574		μmol/L
Cortisol	μg/dL		27.59		nmol/L
Creatine	mg/dL		76.25		μmol/L
Creatinine	mg/dL		88.40		μmol/L
Digoxin	ng/mL		1.281		nmol/L
Epinephrine	pg/mL		5.458		pmol/L
Fatty acids	mg/dL		10.0		mg/L
Ferritin	ng/mL		1		μg/L
α-Fetoprotein	ng/mL		1		μg/L
Fibrinogen	mg/dL		0.01		g/L
Folate	ng/mL		2.266		nmol/L
Fructose	mg/dL		0.05551		mmol/L
Galactose	mg/dL		0.05551		mmol/L
Gases					
P_{O_2}	mm Hg (= torr)		0.1333		kPa
P_{CO_2}	mm Hg (= torr)		0.1333		kPa
Glucagon	pg/ml		1		ng/L
Glucose	mg/dL		0.05551		mmol/L
Glycerol	mg/dL		0.1086		mmol/L
Growth hormone	ng/mL		1		μg/L
Haptoglobin	mg/dL		0.01		g/L
Hemoglobin	g/dL		10		g/L
Insulin	μg/L		172.2		pmol/L
	mU/L		7.175		pmol/L
Iron	μg/dL		0.1791		μmol/L
Iron-binding capacity	μg/dL		0.1791		μmol/L

Component	Present Unit	×	Conversion Factor	=	SI Unit
Lactate	mEq/L		1		mmol/L
Lead	μg/dL		0.04826		μmol/L
Lipoproteins	mg/dL		0.02586		mmol/L
Magnesium	mg/dL		0.4114		mmol/L
	mEq/L		0.50		mmol/L
Osmolality	mOsm/kg H_2O		1		mmol/kg H_2O
Phenobarbital	mg/dL		43.06		μmol/L
Phenytoin	mg/L		3.964		μmol/L
Phosphate	mg/dL		0.3229		mmol/L
Potassium	mEq/L		1		mmol/L
	mg/dL		0.2558		mmol/L
Protein	g/dL		10.0		g/L
Pyruvate	mg/dL		113.6		μmol/L
Sodium ion	mEq/L		1		mmol/L
Steroids					
17-hydroxycorticosteroids	mg/24 h		2.759		μmol/d
17-ketosteroids	mg/24 h		3.467		μmol/d
Testosterone	ng/mL		3.467		nmol/L
Theophylline	mg/L		5.550		μmol/L
Thyroid tests					
Thyroid-stimulating hormone	μU/mL		1		mU/L
Thyroxine (T_4)	μg/dL		12.87		nmol/L
Thyroxine free	ng/dL		12.87		pmol/L
Triiodothyronine (T_3)	ng/dL		0.01536		nmol/L
Transferrin	mg/dL		0.01		g/L
Triglycerides	mg/dL		0.01129		mmol/L
Urea nitrogen	mg/dL		0.3570		mmol/L
Uric acid (urate)	mg/dL		59.48		μmol/L
Vitamin A (retinol)	μg/dL		0.03491		μmol/L
Vitamin B_{12}	pg/mL		0.7378		pmol/L
Vitamin C (ascorbic acid)	mg/dL		56.78		μmol/L
Vitamin D					
Cholecalciferol	μg/mL		2.599		nmol/L
25 OH-cholecalciferol	ng/mL		2.496		nmol/L
Vitamin E (alpha-tocopherol)	mg/dL		23.22		μmol/L
D-xylose	mg/dL		0.06661		mmol/L
Zinc	μg/dL		0.1530		μmol/L
Energy	kcal		4.1868		kj (kilojoule)
Blood pressure	mm Hg (= torr)		1.333		mbar

Modified from Young DS: Implementation of SI units for clinical laboratory data. Style specifications and conversion tables. Ann Intern Med 106:114, 1987.

Conversion Tables

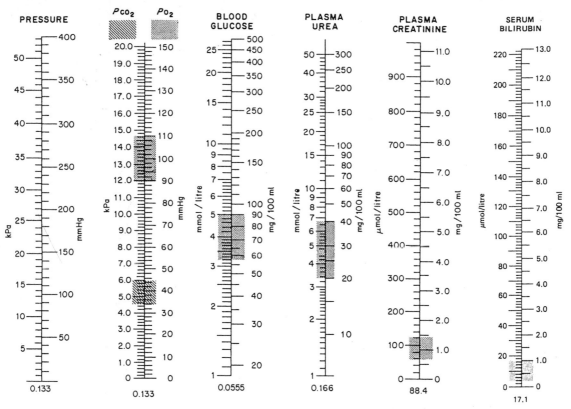

Shading indicates the normal range where appropriate. To convert "old" to "new" units, multiply by the conversion factor at the foot of each column. (Modified from Halliday HL, McClure G, Reid M: Handbook of Neonatal Intensive Care. 2nd ed. Philadelphia: WB Saunders, 1985.)

INDEX

Note: Pages in *italic* indicate illustrations; those followed by t refer to tables.

R

Radiant heaters, 136, 138–139
Radiography, frequency of, 37–38
  safety of, 36–37
Ranitidine, dosage of, 564t
Reactivity, first period of, 74, 116
  second period of, 117
Recommended Dietary Allowances, 163t
Red blood cells, 464–467, 465t, *466*, 574t
  in bilirubin production, 325
  in small for gestational age infant, 113
  transfusion of, 473
Reflexes, primitive, 498
Relative humidity, of incubator, 130
Renal. See also *Kidney(s)*.
Renal artery, blood flow in, 426–427, 426t
  thrombosis of, hypertension from, 439–440
Renal failure, acute, 433–436
  causes of, 433, 434t
  continuous renal replacement therapy for, 435–436
  evaluation of, 434–435
  hemodialysis for, 436
  intrinsic, 434
  medical management of, 435
  peritoneal dialysis for, 435, 435t, *436*
  postrenal, 434
  prerenal, 434
  prognosis of, 436
  renal replacement therapy in, 435–436, 435t, *436*
Renal solute load, calculation of, *149*
Renal vein, thrombosis of, hematuria in, 433
Resistance, 280–281, 288
Resistance units, 399
Respiration, assessment of, after delivery, 77
  chemical control of, 243
  depression of, hypoxia and, 243
  functional residual capacity and, 243–244
  in cold injury, 140
  in newborn, 74
  physical examination of, 117
  pulmonary stretch receptor and, 243–244
Respiratory acidosis, 429
  bicarbonate in, 244
  temperature and, 131
Respiratory distress, congenital heart disease-related, 409–412
  causes of, 410, 410t
  differential diagnosis of, 411
  echocardiography of, 412
  evaluation of, 411–412
  shunts in, 410
  venous admixture in, 410–411
  examination of, 81
Respiratory distress syndrome, 96, 252–255
  air pressure volume curve in, *252*, 253
  arterial oxygen tension in, 269
  cardiac complications of, 257
  communication about, 216
  complications of, 257
  continuous positive airway pressure for, 282, *282*
  diuresis in, 257
  etiology of, 253
  fetal pulmonary maturity and, 14–15
  high-frequency mechanical ventilation in, 294
  hypocalcemia in, 317
  in growth-restricted premature infant, 111, *112*
  lung compliance in, 252, *252*
  mechanical ventilation in, 256

Respiratory distress syndrome *(Continued)*
  monitoring effects on, 269
  neutral thermal environment in, 144
  oxygen monitoring in, 271
  patent ductus arteriosus in, 404
  pathology of, *252*, 252–253
  pathophysiology of, 253, *254*
  phototherapy of, 356
  physiologic abnormalities of, 252, *252*
  premature rupture of membranes and, 31–32
  prevention of, 14–15, 253–254
    corticosteroids in, 32
  radiographic findings in, 320, *320*
  recovery phase of, 257
  signs/symptoms of, 252
  sodium bicarbonate in, 256
  supportive care for, 257, 258t
  surfactant deficiency in, 253, *254*
  surfactant therapy for, 254–255, 255t, 271
    survival in, 528
  treatment of, 255–257
  vs. hypothermia, 145
Respiratory failure, 277
  cardiac vs. pulmonary disease in, 278
  causes of, 277, 278t
  clinical manifestations of, 277–278
  inhaled nitric oxide in, 296
  mechanical ventilation for, 277, 278t
Respiratory frequency, in minute ventilation, 285–286
Respiratory insufficiency of prematurity, 252
Respiratory rate, neonatal, 77
Respiratory syncytial virus infection, 385
  palivizumab for, 385–386
Respiratory system, 243–272
  disorders of, blood pressure in, 251, *251*
    blood volume expansion in, 251
    classification of, 250, 251t
    diagnosis of, 250–252
    differential diagnosis of, 250, 251t
    oxygen therapy for, 246–250
  during transition, 73–74
  in infection, 367
  neonatal examination of, 81–82, 81t
  physical examination of, 121
  transitional evaluation of, 88
Resuscitation, 20, 45–63
  ABCs in, 47, 48
  after rapid delivery, 57–58
  air leaks in, 56
  airway obstruction in, 57
  airway opening in, 49, *49*
  algorithm for, *45*
  anticipation of, 46–47, 46t
  Apgar score in, 47–48, 57, 57t
  apnea in, 57
  approach to, 46–55
  bag-and-mask ventilation in, *51*, 51–52, 57–58, 59
  "best interests of child" in, 542–543
  bradycardia in, 61, 62
  chest compression in, 53–54, *54*
  circulatory support in, 53–55, *54*
  cyanosis in, 61, 62
  drugs in, 54–55
  endotracheal intubation in, *52*, 52–53, *53*, 62
  equipment for, 46, 47, 48t
  estimated fetal weight in, 62
  ethical/legal issues in, 536–540
  evaluation in, 47
  heart rate in, 49–50, 55
  heat control in, 143